D0202313

4TH
EDITION

EMT
Prehospital Care

Mark C. Henry, MD

Professor and Chairman
Department of Emergency Medicine
School of Medicine
Stony Brook University
Stony Brook, New York

Edward R. Stapleton, EMT-P

Associate Professor of Emergency Medicine
Director of Prehospital Education
Department of Emergency Medicine
School of Medicine
Stony Brook University
Stony Brook, New York

EDITED BY *Dennis Edgerly, AAS, EMT-P*

Paramedic Education Coordinator
HealthONE EMS
Englewood, Colorado

With 770 illustrations

MOSBY JEMS

ELSEVIER

MOSBY JEMS
ELSEVIER

11830 Westline Industrial Drive
St. Louis, Missouri 63146

EMT Prehospital Care   978-0-323-05547-5
Copyright © 2010, 2007, 2004 by Mosby, Inc., an affiliate of Elsevier Inc.

All rights reserved. No part of this publication may be reproduced or transmitted in any form or by any means, electronic or mechanical, including photocopying, recording, or any information storage and retrieval system, without permission in writing from the publisher. Permissions may be sought directly from Elsevier's Rights Department: phone: (+1) 215 239 3804 (US) or (+44) 1865 843830 (UK); fax: (+44) 1865 853333; e-mail: healthpermissions@elsevier.com. You may also complete your request on-line via the Elsevier website at http://www.elsevier.com/permissions.

Notice

Knowledge and best practice in this field are constantly changing. As new research and experience broaden our knowledge, changes in practice, treatment, and drug therapy may become necessary or appropriate. Readers are advised to check the most current information provided (i) on procedures featured or (ii) by the manufacturer of each product to be administered, to verify the recommended dose or formula, the method and duration of administration, and contraindications. It is the responsibility of the practitioner, relying on their own experience and knowledge of the patient, to make diagnoses, to determine dosages and the best treatment for each individual patient, and to take all appropriate safety precautions. To the fullest extent of the law, neither the Publisher nor the Authors assume any liability for any injury and/or damage to persons or property arising out of or related to any use of the material contained in this book.

The Publisher

Library of Congress Cataloging-in-Publication Data
Henry, Mark C.
  EMT prehospital care/Mark C. Henry, Edward R. Stapleton; edited by Dennis Edgerly. – 4th ed.
     p. ; cm.
  EMT prehospital care
  Includes bibliographical references and index.
  ISBN 978-0-323-05547-5 (pbk.: alk. paper)
  1. Emergency medicine. 2. Emergency medical technicians.
  I. Stapleton, Edward R. II. Edgerly, Dennis. III. Title. IV. Title: EMT prehospital care.
  [DNLM: 1. Emergency Treatment–methods. 2. Emergency Medical Services–methods. 3. Emergency Medical Technicians. WX 215 H523e 2010]
  RC86.7.H47 2010
  616.02'5-dc22

                                                                                                         2008046550

ISBN: 978-0-323-05547-5

Vice President and Publisher: Andrew Allen
Executive Editor: Linda Honeycutt
Developmental Editor: Kathleen Sartori
Publishing Services Manager: Patricia Tannian
Senior Project Manager: Sarah Wunderly
Design Direction: Amy Buxton

Printed in Canada

Last digit is the print number: 9 8 7 6 5 4 3 2

Working together to grow
libraries in developing countries

www.elsevier.com | www.bookaid.org | www.sabre.org

ELSEVIER   BOOK AID International   Sabre Foundation

To our patients and our communities, who depend on our skills and
our willingness to respond in times of need.
MCH, ERS

To my family for their continued support and love.
MH

To my children, Tara and Edward, who are a source of great pride.
ERS

Author Acknowledgments

We wish to extend our gratitude to the wide variety of friends, coworkers, and Elsevier staff who have contributed their time and expertise in the development of this text.

A special thanks to Kathleen Sartori, who has been a positive force and the "backbone" for the fourth edition. Her diligence and dedication has assured a quality product for all students and instructors who use this book and the related peripherals.

We thank our editor, Linda Honeycutt for her perseverance and support during this project. Her character and integrity has made this project the success that it has become.

We also thank our past editors, Baxter Venable, Margaret Biblis, Selma Kaszczuk, Shirley Kuhn, and Claire Merrick, who provided inspiration and outstanding developmental skills to secure the vital manpower and resources needed to make this project a success.

Our sincere gratitude is extended to Sarah Wunderly, our Senior Project Manager; Amy Buxton, our Senior Book Designer, and Rick Brady, our photographer, for their creative contributions.

We would also like to thank Eric Niegelberg for his dedication and attention to detail in the development of the Student Workbook and other peripherals for this edition.

Finally, we would like to thank Dennis Edgerly who did much of the heavy lifting for this edition. His talents are evident throughout this work.

Publisher
Acknowledgments

Contributors

Dario Gonzalez, MD
Medical Director
New York City Fire Department
New York, New York

Scott Johnson, MD, FACEP
Associate Professor
Department of Emergency Medicine
Stony Brook University
Stony Brook, New York

Robert Levy, MD
Clinical Assistant Professor
Department of Emergency Medicine
Stony Brook University
Medical Director
Setauket Fire Department
Setauket, New York

Victor Tarsia, MD
Department of Emergency Medicine
Stony Brook University
Stony Brook, New York

Reviewers

Dave Aber, NREMT-P, I/C
President
Shore Emergency Educators/DEMS Educators, LLC
Newark, Delaware

Terry L. Bowen, EMT, SEI
Skagit County Medic One
Mount Vernon, Washington

Robert Carter, NREMT-P
Flight Paramedic/Instructor
STAT MedEvac
The Center for Emergency Medicine of Western Pennsylvania
Pittsburgh, Pennsylvania

Peter Connick, EMT-P, EMT I/C
Captain
Chatham Fire-Rescue
Chatham, Massachusetts
Cape Cod Community College EMS Program
Emergency Medical Teaching Services Inc
Dennis, Massachusetts

Jon Steven Cooper, NREMT-P, Instructor III
Baltimore City Fire and EMS Academy
Baltimore, Maryland

Tom Czerniak, MS, EMT-B
Chief
Union Grove-Yorkville Fire Department
Union Grove, Wisconsin

Douglas A. deBest, BS, MPA, EMT-I/C, Fire Officer III
Baroda Fire Department
Baroda, Michigan

Jerry L. Domaschk, NREMT-P
Certified Instructor, EMS Education Coordinator
West Jefferson Medical Center
Marrero, Louisiana

Steven Dralle, BA, LP, EMSC
Vidacare
San Antonio, Texas

Nancy W. ("Cindy") Edwards, AAS, NREMT-P, LP
Coordinator
Bulverde-Spring Branch EMS Training Institute
Spring Branch, Texas

Michael Fisher, AHS, NREMT-P, CCP
Professor
Program Director, Emergency Medical Technology
Director of Human Patient Simulation
Greenville Technical College
Greenville, South Carolina

Jeffery S. Force, BA, NREMT-P
Pikes Peak Community College, Penrose-St. Francis Health
   Services
Colorado Springs, Colorado

Rudy Garrett, AS, NREMT-P, CCEMT-P
Training Coordinator
Somerset Fire/EMS
Somerset, Kentucky

Melissa R. Gladieux, EMT-P
EMS Program and Emergency Preparedness Coordinator
Henry Ford Macomb Hospitals
Clinton, Michigan

William David Hagen, EMT-P
EMT Instructor
American Medical Response
Lawrenceburg, Kentucky

Ricci Hall, NREMT-I, EMT-I/C, BA, MA, MEd, RN
Anna Maria College
Paxton, Massachusetts

Steve Hazelton, NREMT-P
Rutland Regional Medical Center
Rutland, Vermont

Steve Huisman, NREMT-P, EMT-P I/C
Great Lakes EMS Academy
Grand Rapids, Michigan

Mark Johnson, AEMT
AEMT Instructor, AHA Instructor, Medic First Instructor
    and Trainer
State of Idaho EMS Evaluator for State Testing
Ammon, Idaho

Earl W. Klinefelter, EMT-B
Senior EMS Instructor
Skagit County Medic One
Mount Vernon, Washington

Greg Lambert
EMT-I Mass, PHTLS I/C, Sgt. US Army91w Combat Medic,
    AHA BLS Instructor, PEPP I/C, TBI I/C
Quality EMS Educators, Inc.
Worcester, Massachusetts

Joanne McCall, RN, BAS, MA, CEN, CFN, SANE-A
Providence Park Hospital
Novi, Michigan

Mark Milliron, BS, MPA, MS, EMT-Instructor, WEMT
Pennsylvania State University, Department of Health Policy
    and Administration
University Park, Pennsylvania

Eric Niegelberg, MS, NREMTP
Department of Emergency Medicine
School of Medicine
Stony Brook University
Stony Brook, New York

Theresa O'Neil, NREMT-I, N.H. I/C
Androscoggin Valley Hospital, Gorham EMS
Gorham, New Hampshire

Warren J. Porter, MS, BA, LP, PNCCT
EMS Programs Manager
Garland Fire Department
Garland, Texas

Becky A. Ridenhour, PharmD
Progress West Healthcare Center
St. Louis College of Pharmacy
O'Fallon, Missouri

Scott Schaffer, NREMT–P, I/C
EMS Education Coordinator
MidMichigan Medical Center
Midland, Michigan

John J. Scotch II, EMT-P, CIC
FDNY—EMS Academy
Bayside, New York

Maureen Shanahan, RN, BSN, MN
City College of San Francisco
San Francisco, California

Laurie A. Sheldon, MPA, BA, NREMT-NJ
EMT Program Director
Union County College, Cranford, New Jersey
Training Center Manager
Trinitas Hospital Institute of Healthcare & Community
    Education
Elizabeth, New Jersey

Andrew E. Spain, MA, EMT-P
University of Missouri Health Care
Columbia, Missouri

Michael C. Touchstone, BS, EMT-P
Fire Paramedic Services Chief
EMS Training
Philadelphia Fire Department
Philadelphia, Pennsylvania

Margaret E. West, BSN, RN, CEN
Kishwaukee Community Hospital, Kishwaukee College
DeKalb, Illinois

Jon A. Whitmar, NREMT-P, PI
EMS Coordinator
Goshen General Hospital
Goshen, Indiana

Acknowledgment of Previous Edition Contributors

Jonathan Best, EMT-P
CEO
Disaster by Design
Stratford, Connecticut

John Czajkowski
Company Officer
Orange County Fire/Rescue Division
Orange County, Florida

Robert Delagi, EMT-P
Chief, Prehospital Medical Operation
EMS Division
Suffolk County Department of Health
Hauppague, New York

Bob Elling, MPA, REMT-P
Institute of Prehospital Emergency Medicine
Hudson Valley Community College
Albany, New York

Neal Flomenbaum, MD
Chief of Emergency Medicine
Professor of Clinical Medicine
Weil-Cornell Medical College
New York, New York

James M. Floyd, Jr., AS, EMT-B, PI, CTC
St. Vincent Hospitals and Health Services
Indianapolis, Indiana

George Foltin, MD, FACEP, FAAP
Director, Pediatric Emergency Services
Bellevue Hospital Center
Associate Professor of Clinical Pediatrics
New York University School of Medicine
New York, New York

Dario Gonzalez, MD, FACEP
Medical Director
New York City Fire Department
New York, New York

Richard Guerin, EMT-P
New York State Department of Health
Albany, New York

Steve Kidd
Company Officer
Orange County Fire/Rescue Division
Orange County, Florida

James P. Martin, EMT-P
Chief of EMS Training
City of New York Fire Department
Fort Totten, New York

Jonathan Politis, EMT-P
Chief, Town of Colonie, Department of EMS
Colonie, New York

Ray Shelton, PhD, EMT-CC
Nassau County Police Academy
EMS Stress Management Consultant
Hicksville, New York

Donna Stapleton, RNC
Obstetric Nurse
Good Samaritan Hospital Medical Center
West Islip, New York

Andrew Stern, NREMT-P
Health Program Administrator
New York State Department of Health
Albany, New York

Peter Viccellio, MD
Professor and Vice Chairperson
Department of Emergency Medicine, School of Medicine
Stony Brook University
Stony Brook, New York

Preface

Prehospital emergency care is an exciting and challenging endeavor. The steps taken in the first minutes after an incident occurs may make the difference between life and death. Emergency medical technicians (EMTs) make themselves available on the front line every day. They often encounter dangerous and difficult situations as they administer valuable prehospital care. These brave men and women are the foundation of the emergency medical response system in a community. EMTs are recognized by the emergency medical community as a key link in the "chain of survival." Whether a patient experiences a heart attack or sustains a severe injury, the actions of EMTs contribute to patient outcome.

The profession, as well as the duty to prepare and educate EMTs, has evolved greatly since this textbook was first published in 1992. More changes are on the way in light of the *EMS Education Agenda for the Future* and the new *National EMS Education Standards*. Regardless of past changes and changes yet to come, the fourth edition of *EMT Prehospital Care* is keeping step with the profession *and* the education of students just beginning their emergency medical services careers.

At the heart of the EMT's knowledge is the ability to conduct an efficient and organized patient assessment, design a plan of action, institute emergency medical treatment, and make appropriate triage and transport decisions necessary for the patient's survival. The EMT encounters patients of all ages, with multiple conditions, in various and unpredictable environments.

The author team of Dr. Mark Henry and Ed Stapleton has more than 35 combined years of emergency medical experience. We add even more years of experience in this edition by introducing Dennis Edgerly, EMT-P, to this dynamic team. His valuable experience as both a practicing paramedic and an EMS instructor make him a welcome addition.

One of the major strengths of this textbook continues to be the understanding that EMTs are most effective when they can comprehend the "why" and "how" of the actions that they undertake in the field. *EMT Prehospital Care* continues its hallmark expanded coverage of anatomy, physiology, and pathophysiology, its clinically-rich photography throughout the book, and its innovative enrichment tools that are invaluable for learning, reinforcement, and retention. In addition, in response to the evolving education curriculum and standards of the EMT, this edition covers not only the *National Standard Curriculum for the EMT-Basic*, but also addresses the *National EMS Education Standards*. This textbook is also referenced to the *National Registry of Emergency Medical Technicians (NREMT) National EMS Practice Analysis*, which is the basis for NREMT examinations.

Because much of the information in this textbook is likely to be new to the reader, an organizational format that ensures learning and retaining essential knowledge is important. Students must learn new terms, recognize anatomy, grasp concepts of physiology and pathophysiology, become familiar with the signs and symptoms of various injuries and medical conditions, and provide emergency medical care.

A practical study strategy would be use of the "whole-part-whole" approach as follows:

1. *Review the chapter objectives.* The chapter objectives are integrated throughout the text. Review the objectives and keep them in mind as you read the material. The objectives for each lesson are also listed at the end of the chapter so that you can test your knowledge of the *National Standard Curriculum* objectives and the *National EMS Education Standards* after completing the chapter.

2. *Skim the chapter.* Read the outline at the beginning of each chapter to familiarize yourself with the material that is covered in the chapter.

3. *Read The Bottom Line.* Look at the summary and the learning checklist to familiarize yourself with the key terms and focus of the chapter. Reflect on the review questions. Think about how you might answer them now, having just an overview. Note your answers so that after you have read the material, you can retest yourself to compare your understanding of chapter material.

4. *Read section by section.* Begin to read the chapter carefully, stopping to research information or vocabulary that is unclear. Write down words that you do not understand, and return to the text or refer to the glossary for clarification. At the end of each section, attempt to answer the relevant review questions at the end of the chapter. If you have difficulty with a question, review the related material.

5. *Use the tables, boxes, and illustrations.* Tables and illustrations are powerful ways of presenting information. Tables are used to summarize and organize key points. Illustrations include photographs, line drawings, and anatomical drawings to help you visualize relevant anatomic and physiologic facts, key clinical signs, and treatment steps.

6. *Explore the special content.* Read the highlighted features such as the chapter-opening *Scenario* and the *Scenario Follow-up* at the end of each chapter, *Real World, Case-in-Point,* and *Extended Transport* boxes located throughout the chapters. These special features give the student a glimpse of real-life incidents or practical information that impacts patient care in the field.

7. *Review the skills and protocols.* Skills are step-by-step descriptions of how to perform necessary techniques to assess and treat patients, and are specially highlighted for clarity and emphasis. Protocols summarize actions taken when you encounter patients with specific signs and/or symptoms.

They also provide a method for summarizing and condensing key information. *EMT Prehospital Care* recognizes that changes and variations from region to region occur constantly. Therefore we recommend that, whenever possible, you become familiar with your local protocols early in the study of this text.

8. *Perform a self-test.* After reading each chapter, conduct a self-test using the review questions and learning checklist in *The Bottom Line* section. You can also use the workbook or have another student ask you questions based on information taken directly from the book.

9. *Watch the visually-rich DVD.* Included with the text, this DVD features video skills and medical animations that clearly demonstrate anatomy and physiology.

10. *Use the Evolve® Student Resources for* EMT Prehospital Care.
    - **New** *Student Challenge* section tests understanding of presented material.
    - *Anatomy Challenges* reinforce the anatomy and physiology information provided in the text.
    - *Body Spectrum Electronic Anatomy Coloring Book* allows you to color and label anatomy online or on printouts.
    - *Lecture Notes* for PowerPoint slides are an efficient notetaking tool.
    - *English-Spanish Audio Glossary* offers both the definition and pronunciation of common medical terms and conditions.
    - *Heart and Lung Sounds* provides actual audio clips for better understanding of normal and abnormal sounds.

11. *Supplement your studying with the* Workbook for EMT Prehospital Care. This workbook revision reflects all new material. Additional exercises have been added to further increase comprehension. Used in tandem with the textbook, this aid will ensure basic skill knowledge and assist you in passing the EMT certification examination.

12. *Experience Virtual Patient Encounters. Virtual Patient Encounters* is a breakthrough in EMS education! Students can get real-world prehospital experience without leaving the classroom! The *Virtual Patient Encounters* learning triad—your *EMT Prehospital Care* textbook, interactive patient simulation software, and a study guide that ties everything together—offers a state-of-the-art tool for developing critical-thinking skills. You can apply what you are learning in *EMT Prehospital Care* on 15 virtual patients in a variety of prehospital environments. It's an incredible opportunity to make real patient care decisions in a safe environment!

Whenever possible, *EMT Prehospital Care* bases its presentation of material on the standards and guidelines of nationally recognized organizations, such as the American Heart Association, the National Association of EMS Physicians, and the American College of Surgeons.

New to this edition are the Abuse and Assault chapter and the completely revised Patient Assessment chapter. Domestic violence is an ever-increasing problem in our society. The dangers it presents to both the patients and EMTs are real and serious. This chapter allows you to understand basic safety issues and how to approach, treat, and transport the injured. Past editions have featured separate chapters devoted to assessment, from scene size-up to ongoing assessment. Although this edition covers all the assessment topics included in earlier editions, the content has been updated to introduce the new *National Education Standards terminology,* while keeping the language native to the *National Standard Curriculum.* This comprehensive, one-chapter formula has complete coverage all in one place.

The instructor resources to accompany *EMT Prehospital Care* have been completely revised for this edition.

The Instructor's Electronic Resource on CD-ROM provides a variety of tools to help enhance course instruction. The Instructor's Manual provides the following for each chapter in the textbook: *Chapter Objectives,* a *Teaching Focus* statement, a list of desirable *Materials and Resources* for presenting the chapter, *Lesson Checklists, Key Terms* with page references, a *Pretest, Critical-Thinking* questions, detailed *Lesson Plans, Classroom Activities,* and *Discussion Points,* and a *PowerPoint presentation* with speaker notes, illustrations, and imbedded skills video clips. The instructor resources for *EMT Prehospital Care* also feature a comprehensive *Test Bank.* These resources can be accessed via CD and online at the *Evolve® Instructor Resources* website.

EMT Prehospital Care, fourth edition, represents the continued commitment to bringing you the best in all things a textbook can offer: the best and brightest authors; the latest trends and standards in emergency medical care in the prehospital environment; a logical, organized format, consistent, state-of-the-art learning aids, online resources, and electronic assets, and outstanding artwork and illustrations to enhance student learning.

If you have any questions about the components of this learning system, if you would like to place an order, or if you have suggestions about *EMT Prehospital Care,* please contact MOSBYJEMS/Elsevier at 1-800-545-2522 or visit http://www.mosbyjems.com.

Author Biographies

Mark C. Henry, MD

In 1978, Dr. Henry was one of the first physicians trained in emergency medicine to work in New York City. He chaired the first department of emergency medicine in New York City, chaired the New York City EMS Medical Advisory Committee, and was medical director of the first 24-hour paramedic service in Queens, New York.

For more than 27 years, EMTs and paramedics have had the benefit of Dr. Henry's educational expertise. As an educator, speaker, and industry leader, Dr. Henry is well respected by students and peers worldwide.

Dr. Henry has authored or coauthored more than 100 educational and research works, including journal articles and abstracts, textbooks, and book chapters over the course of his career.

Dr. Henry is the current Medical Director of the EMS Program, New York State Department of Health; Chair of the New York State EMS Medical Advisory Committee; and Chair of the New York State EMS BioChem Terrorism Task Force. He is also Professor and Chairman of the Department of Emergency Medicine at Stony Brook University. In 2003, he received the Outstanding Contributor to EMS Award from the American College of Emergency Physicians.

Edward R. Stapleton, EMT-P

With more than 41 years of EMS experience, including 1 year as a combat medic in Vietnam, Ed Stapleton has experienced emergency medical care from a variety of perspectives. In 1974, Ed became one of the first paramedics in the New York City EMS system based in lower Manhattan.

Ed Stapleton has been teaching EMS providers for more than 37 years at both the EMT and paramedic levels. Currently, he is Associate Professor and Director of Prehospital Education at Stony Brook University.

Ed Stapleton has authored or coauthored more than 100 educational and research works, including journal articles, textbooks, films, and videos on EMS, ACLS, and CPR. Included among his accomplishments is his codevelopment of five paramedic training programs in the New York City and Long Island EMS systems, including the first associate degree program in New York state. Today Ed is an acclaimed EMS educator and routinely speaks at EMS and ECC conferences around the world.

Dennis Edgerly, AAS, EMT-P

Dennis Edgerly began his EMS career in 1989 as a volunteer firefighter EMT. He obtained his paramedic certification 1 year later and worked in a high-call volume system in the Denver metropolitan area. Dennis functioned as a field preceptor for new paramedics, as well as a shift supervisor. In 1992 he began working part time for a community hospital, teaching in their EMT-Basic program. He is currently the Education Coordinator for the Paramedic Education Program at HealthONE EMS and Arapahoe Community College in Englewood, Colorado.

Dennis also serves as regional faculty for the American Heart Association, has participated in curriculum revision for the State of Colorado at the EMT-Intermediate level, and was an expert writer for the *National EMS Education Standards*. He is a recognized presenter around the country, has reviewer and contributing author credits for several EMS textbooks, has authored several EMS-related articles, and is a regular contributor to JEMS.com. In 1999, Dennis was named the Colorado EMS Instructor of the Year.

Get the MOST from EMT Prehospital Care, Fourth Edition!

Companion DVD

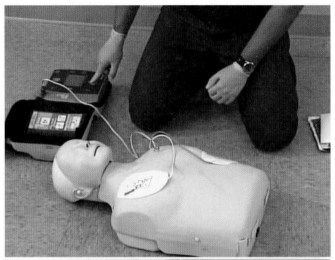

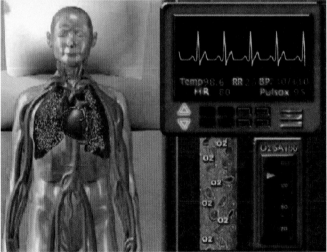

For unmatched visual learning and skills mastery, the Companion DVD complements the text with actual video footage of content from the textbook. You will see concepts come to life with up-close demonstrations of 28 skills, as well as 23 detailed medical animations.

Workbook

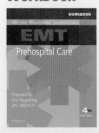

The Workbook to Accompany EMT Prehospital Care, fourth edition, includes approximately 1900 questions in a variety of formats, including multiple choice, matching, fill-in-the-blank, true/false, labeling, case scenarios, and crossword puzzles.

Virtual Patient Encounters

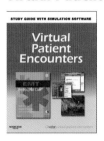

Virtual Patient Encounters will help you develop the critical-thinking and decision-making skills you will need on the job in an engaging and interactive way. Its unique learning triad offers hands-on learning like nothing you have ever experienced. . .

- **EMT Prehospital Care** textbook provides the foundation.
- The **Study Guide** helps you take the information from the textbook and apply it to 15 complex patient care scenarios.
- The **Interactive Patient Care Simulation Software** features scenario-setting videos, virtual assessment tools, treatment protocols, emergency drug information, and intervention wizards that result in realistic emerging conditions!

For the Instructor

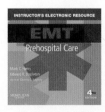

An **Instructor's Electronic Resource** is available on CD-ROM. This resource includes an Instructor's Manual, Computerized Test Bank, and PowerPoint presentations. The Instructor's Manual includes:

- Chapter Objectives
- Teaching Focus
- Instructional Materials
- Lesson Checklist
- Key Terms
- Additional Resources
- Pretest
- Critical-Thinking Questions
- Detailed Lesson Plans
- Discussion Questions
- Classroom Activities

evolve The **Evolve Course Management System** is an interactive learning environment that works in coordination with *EMT Prehospital Care.* It provides Internet-based course content, including the Instructor's Manual, Computerized Test Bank, and PowerPoint presentations. Evolve can also be used to publish your class syllabus, outlines, and lecture notes; set up "virtual office hours" and e-mail communications; share important dates and information through the online class Calendar; and encourage student participation through Chat Rooms and Discussion Boards. Contact your Elsevier sales representative for more information about integrating Evolve into your curriculum.

Contents

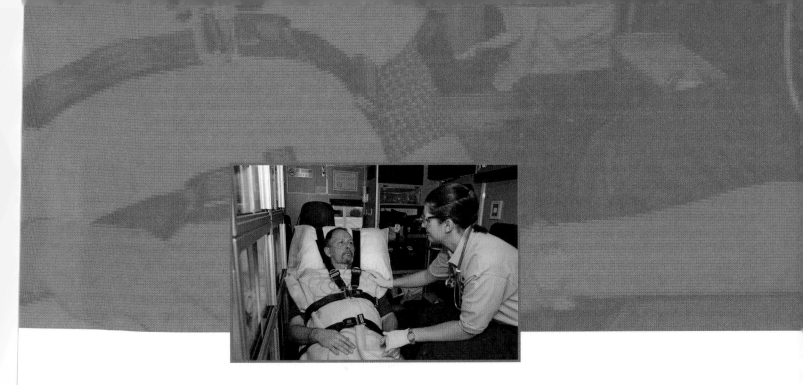

Introduction to Emergency Medical Care

1

CHAPTER OUTLINE

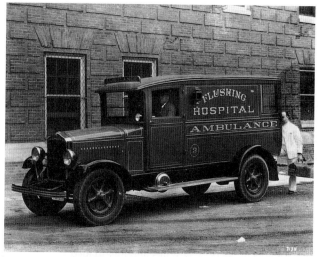

Figure 1-2 An early motorized ambulance. The early models lacked the space and head clearance of modern ambulances. *Courtesy Flushing Hospital, Flushing, New York.*

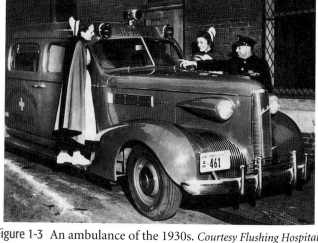

Figure 1-3 An ambulance of the 1930s. *Courtesy Flushing Hospital, Flushing, New York.*

care, they helped focus national attention on the need for the rapid prehospital intervention that had been successfully demonstrated on battlefields. Simple steps were recognized, including bleeding control at the scene, safe patient handling, spinal immobilization, and rapid transportation to organized trauma centers.

In 1966 the U.S. National Academy of Sciences published the landmark paper *Accidental Death and Disability: the Neglected Disease of Modern Society,* documenting that more Americans died from accidental injuries in 1965 than died on the battlefields in Vietnam. Further, if seriously wounded, a person would have a better chance of survival in a combat zone than on an average city street. The newly created Department of Transportation (DOT) and National Highway Traffic Safety Administration (NHTSA), a division of the DOT, were empowered with regulating EMSS, offering $48 million in grants between 1966 and 1973.

In 1973, federal legislation provided funding for the development of EMS systems throughout the United States. After demonstrations of effective trauma systems in Illinois and Maryland, these grants accounted for the rapid growth of EMS systems across the country. Money was allocated for the development of training programs, communication systems, hospital designations, and other essential system components. Many EMS systems developed as a direct result of this legislation and funding.

Medical knowledge and related technology were incorporated into EMS care as new advances became available. For example, in the 1960s, cardiopulmonary resuscitation (CPR) using chest compression and positive-pressure ventilation was introduced, and portable defibrillators to resuscitate victims of cardiac arrest became available. Physicians brought resuscitation equipment into the field to reach their patients earlier, when they had a better chance of survival.

The first advanced life support unit was introduced in Belfast, Ireland, under the direction of Dr. Frank Pantridge. Advanced life support included electrocardiographic

(ECG) monitoring, defibrillation, intravenous (IV) therapy, administration of medications, insertion of endotracheal (ET) tubes, and other invasive medical skills. Dr. William Grace at St. Vincent's Hospital in New York City quickly adopted this innovation so that physicians, nurses, and ambulance personnel could respond to cardiac emergencies in lower Manhattan.

Until this point, only physicians were providing advanced care in the prehospital setting. The introduction of **biotelemetry** (transmission of electrocardiogram [ECG] by radio) extended prehospital care by allowing EMS providers to deliver advanced life support under the direction of a physician at a base hospital. As part of its role in studying cardiovascular emergencies and treatment, every 5 years the American Heart Association (AHA) offers the *Emergency Cardiovascular Care* (ECC) guidelines, adopted by most agencies as the standard of care.

The Physician and Emergency Medical Services

The physician's role in the development of EMS systems has been extremely important. Medical societies such as the American Academy of Orthopedic Surgeons and the American College of Surgeons played a significant part in early EMSS development. The DOT Bureau of Traffic Safety asked these physician groups to develop a standardized curriculum for ambulance personnel. Physicians still work closely with the EMS Division of NHTSA under DOT to ensure the continued development of national training curricula at all levels.

Physician groups such as the American College of Emergency Physicians and the National Association of EMS Physicians have joined their surgical colleagues and have an active leadership role in national EMSS development. Physicians are the "medical conscience" of EMS. All levels of EMS provider function under the direction of a physician advisor or medical director. Medical directors work locally with services to establish protocols, monitor patient care, and provide continuing education.

Although physicians have functioned as prehospital providers in some areas in the United States, their role as field providers has been limited since the 1940s. For many reasons, including resource allocation and costs, nonphysicians currently staff almost all ambulances in North America. In some countries, such as Russia, Norway, France, Brazil, and Germany, physicians still routinely respond in ambulances or helicopters.

The Future of EMS

The *EMS Agenda for the Future*, developed in cooperation with several national organizations, provides recommendations to refine and continue development of EMS systems over the coming years, as follows:

> Emergency medical services (EMS) of the future will be community-based health management that is fully integrated with the overall health care system. It will have the ability to identify and modify illness and injury risks, provide acute illness and injury care and follow-up, and contribute to treatment of chronic conditions and community health monitoring. This new entity will be developed from redistribution of existing health care resources and will be integrated with other health care providers and public health and public safety agencies. It will improve community health and result in more appropriate use of acute health care resources. EMS will remain the public's emergency medical safety net.

The agenda lists 14 essential components: integration of health services, EMS research, legislation and regulation, system finance, human resources, medical direction, education systems, public education, prevention, public access, communication systems, clinical care, information systems, and evaluation.

A partner document to the agenda is the *EMS Education Agenda for the Future*. Focusing on the educational structure for EMS, this document identifies a specific scope of practice for each level, then replaces the "DOT objectives" with "education standards" for each level **(Figure 1-4)**.

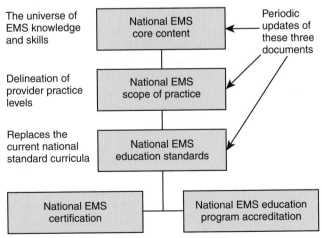

Figure 1-4 The EMS education agenda for the future: a systems approach. A single agency for each function. *Redrawn from National Highway Traffic Safety Administration:* National EMS agenda for the future, *Washington, DC, 2005, US Department of Transportation.*

Overview of the Emergency Medical Services System

As described in the *EMS Agenda for the Future*, EMS systems require many components to function effectively. Each component must be carefully designed and based on the needs of the individual EMSS.

Public Access

Because an EMSS involves a large number of resources, some method of coordination and communication is essential. In many areas, simple and convenient access has been accomplished through the 9-1-1 emergency telephone system. This system allows rapid access to all elements of emergency care and support services, including EMS, fire department, and police. In the 9-1-1 system a central dispatch center coordinates resources and personnel within the system.

Some EMS systems have "enhanced 9-1-1" (E-911) communication systems. E-911 allows the dispatcher to track the caller's exact location. This knowledge becomes important when the caller disconnects, becomes unconscious during the call, or when a bystander unfamiliar with an area calls for help. In the case of some natural disasters a "reverse 9-1-1" system has been used to notify residents of a community to evacuate. With the wide use of cell phones, new technologies are being introduced to track the caller's location and aid response. Some vehicles are now equipped with tracking and monitoring equipment such as Onstar. With this equipment a vehicle can notify the central dispatch center if the vehicle has been involved in a collision and can alert authorities of the vehicle's location.

Other areas still rely on different seven-digit telephone numbers to access emergency assistance.

Elements of a Communication System

A modern EMSS may contain several communication components. A dispatch system receives the call for help and sends the appropriate response vehicles to the scene. An ambulance communication system allows the prehospital provider in the field to communicate with dispatch, with receiving hospitals, and with medical control.

The Dispatch System

The dispatch center receives calls, categorizes them according to priority, provides first-aid instructions to callers, and dispatches the closest appropriate emergency service vehicle (e.g., police, fire), rescue personnel, and equipment. Many emergency service vehicles have vehicle locators so that the dispatcher can see the vehicle's exact location in respect to the call. Dispatch serves as a communication point through which an EMT can call for additional resources. The dispatch center may also relay information from the scene of an incident to the receiving facility and advise the EMT on facility selection and availability of other rescue personnel **(Figure 1-5)**. The dispatcher may also advise the caller or bystanders on initial treatment steps to help the patient until the ambulance arrives.

A formal national training program has been developed to train dispatch personnel to deal with the complexities of their

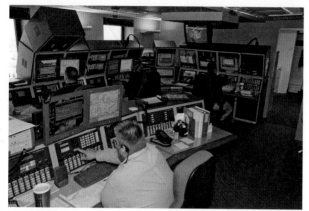

Figure 1-5 A computerized dispatch workstation in a communication center.

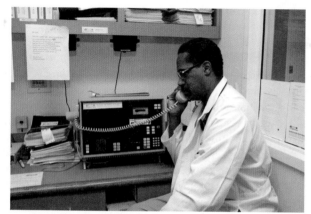

Figure 1-6 Online medical direction. A physician at a hospital communication base station can speak directly with the EMT about a patient's status and give orders regarding treatment and transport.

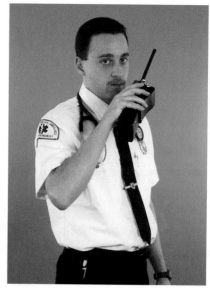

Figure 1-7 An EMT in the field communicates by a portable voice radio. Cellular phones and landline phones are also used to communicate with dispatch or medical direction.

as alerting the trauma team or preparing an isolation room for a patient with a possible infectious disease.

LEARNING OBJECTIVE
- Differentiate the role and responsibilities of the EMT from those of other prehospital care providers.

Levels of Training

A wide range of illnesses and injuries require emergency care. Every year approximately 16 million patients in the United States are transported by ambulance to emergency departments, usually because of chest pain, shortness of breath, abdominal pain, injury from a motor vehicle crash or other accident, convulsions, or general weakness. Persons presenting with imminent childbirth, poisoning, or uncontrolled bleeding are examples of the types of emergencies for which immediate attention is required. For each patient category, distinct interventions can improve the patient's chances for survival.

Patients themselves should know the signs and symptoms of illnesses that require immediate intervention and how to access the EMSS. They also should know some basic self-help measures in the event that immediate help from bystanders is not available.

Lay Rescuers

Often the first person to recognize an emergency condition is another member of the community. For certain conditions that render someone helpless, actions by bystanders and those first to respond can make the critical difference. Simple knowledge, such as how to open an airway or control bleeding, may be all that is necessary to save a life.

When performed in a timely fashion, CPR and use of an *automated external defibrillator* (AED) may save thousands of lives each year (**Figure 1-8**). Training in CPR and other basic first-aid skills may result in certification that permits laypeople to serve as responders in the workplace or other environments.

job. *Emergency Medical Dispatch* (EMD) is now a recognized program. EMD professionals are skilled coordinators of emergency care communication and play a vital role in EMS systems.

Ambulance-to-Hospital Communication Systems

Many EMS systems provide communication from the field personnel to the physician at a base hospital or medical direction center, often referred to as **online medical direction** (**Figure 1-6**; see later discussion). These communication systems may include both voice and biotelemetric components. Field providers may consult medical direction for advice about treatment and transportation decisions or to speak directly with patients who are refusing care or transport to the hospital (**Figure 1-7**).

Biotelemetry allows transmission of ECG data from the patient in the field to the physician at the base hospital or medical control facility. Cellular phones and radio transmission are used for both voice communication and biotelemetry.

Most hospitals have dedicated phones or radio equipment for communication with EMTs in the field. In some cases the hospital makes special preparations for the EMT's arrival, such

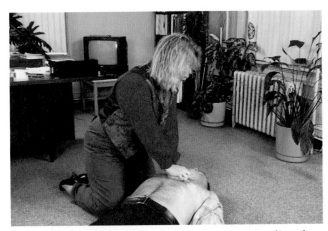

Figure 1-8 A lay responder performs one-person cardiopulmonary resuscitation (CPR).

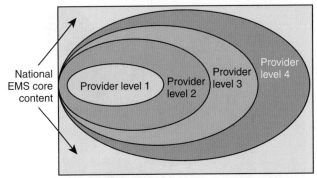

Figure 1-9 Four levels of EMS providers. Provider level 1: Emergency Medical Responder (EMR); level 2: Emergency Medical Technician (EMT); level 3: Advanced EMT; level 4: Paramedic. *Redrawn from National Highway Traffic Safety Administration:* National EMS scope of practice model, *Washington, DC, 2005, US Department of Transportation.*

REAL*World*

In recognition of the importance of bystander care, NHTSA has developed a bystander care program entitled First There, First Care. This campaign identifies target audiences, develops outreach strategies for the general public, and provides tools for conducting local training to teach bystander care.

The program is designed to educate the public on five life-sustaining skills that can be used at a motor vehicle crash: (1) stop to help, (2) call for help, (3) assess the victim, (4) start the breathing, and (5) stop the bleeding. The purpose is to teach the public that bystander involvement can sustain a life until EMS arrives.

The AHA's bystander program is structured around the "chain of survival" concept that defines four critical links for bystanders treating persons with heart attack, stroke, choking, and respiratory and cardiac arrest. The four links include early access to 9-1-1, early CPR, early defibrillation, and early advanced care. Bystanders are encouraged to deliver the first three links in the chain, including CPR and early defibrillation using an AED (see Chapter 12).

This type of program recognizes that the time from collapse to provision of care plays an essential role in victim survival. For example, the chances of survival for victims of cardiac arrest resulting from ventricular fibrillation decrease by 7% to 10% for each minute that passes from the time of collapse until defibrillation is provided. Performance of CPR can extend that critical period by delivering oxygen to the heart and brain until defibrillation is used to restore a normal heart rhythm.

Community education programs that provide the public with basic first-aid skills may be taught by several different community groups. Programs taught in school systems, scuba diving training, Boy Scouts and Girl Scouts, and other organizations educate a significant cross section of the community. Other even more basic actions, such as recognizing the signs of a heart attack and stroke, and calling 9-1-1 for help, are often taught in the mass media to reach even more people in the community.

As an EMT, you should value the contribution made by bystanders since they serve as the "bridge of life support" from collapse to your arrival. You can also play an educational role by becoming a CPR, AED, and first-aid instructor.

Education and Scope of Practice

The NHTSA provides a widely used national curriculum for various levels of EMT. A paradigm shift in EMS education, however, is now underway. The concept is simple: a *core content* of knowledge and skills for EMS providers. The *National EMS Core Content* serves as the total domain of knowledge from which the *National EMS Scope of Practice Model* derives national EMS provider levels. The *National EMS Education Standards* will derive educational objectives to guide EMS training in the future. EMTs at various levels provide the foundation of EMS education for the future. Currently, there are four national levels of EMT described in the scope of practice document (**Figure 1-9**).

Emergency Medical Responders (First Responders). Sometimes a community will plan for a formal response to the call for help by training certain people to administer emergency care before EMTs in an ambulance arrive. For example, EMTs, Advanced EMTs, or paramedics may respond in first-responder vehicles and arrive at a patient's side before the ambulance, shortening the time from the emergency event to patient care. Other trained first responders may include police officers, firefighters, industrial workers, teachers, coaches, and other volunteers.

First responders, or **emergency medical responders (EMRs)**, have a wider range of skills than most bystanders, including management of medical emergencies, childbirth, and specific pediatric emergencies. First responders are often equipped with oxygen, AEDs, and airway equipment and may respond in police cars, fire apparatus, or special first responder vehicles.

First responders may take a course following a national standard. The first responder is trained to recognize emergencies, initiate care, and have the necessary skills to save a life with the use of a minimum of equipment.

Emergency Medical Technician. There are hundreds of thousands of registered EMTs nationwide and the numbers continue to grow. They provide the foundation for prehospital care (**Figure 1-10**). DOT defines an *emergency medical technician* (also called *EMT-Basic*) as someone who has successfully completed a training program according to the NHTSA Emergency Medical Technician National Standard Curriculum or is trained

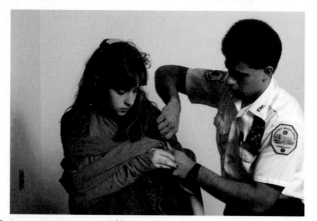

Figure 1-10 An EMT administers treatment to an injured patient.

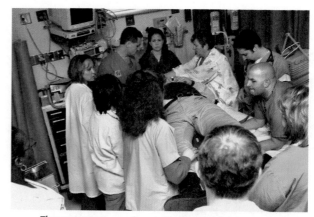

Figure 1-11 A modern emergency department.

within the new educational paradigm meeting the scope of practice proposed by NHTSA and having the requisite knowledge of the EMS core content. This is the course that you are taking now for initial or refresher training.

The EMT curriculum involves attending lectures and receiving practical and clinical instruction in the assessment and management of the acutely ill or injured patient. The EMT provides basic emergency medical care and transportation for critical and emergent patients who access the EMS system. EMTs function as part of a system under medical oversight and perform interventions with basic equipment on an ambulance. EMTs may assist patients with their medications and, under medical direction, may give medication such as aspirin to patients with chest pain and oral glucose to patients with low blood glucose.

In many communities, it is the EMT providing the large portion of out-of-hospital care. In rural areas, they may represent the highest level of EMS care. The EMT's care is based on assessment findings. Their scope of practice is limited to basic skills that are effective and can be performed in an out-of-hospital setting with medical oversight and limited training.

Advanced Emergency Medical Technician. The **advanced emergency medical technician (AEMT)** is also called the *EMT-Intermediate* (EMT-I).

With additional training, EMTs may function at a more advanced level. Various designations are used for advanced EMTs, but the trend is toward standardizing certification to three levels: the EMT, the advanced EMT, and the paramedic.

Advanced training includes skills such as ECG interpretation, advanced or alternative airway management (i.e., ET intubation, dual-lumen airway device), IV fluid therapy, and administration of certain IV medications.

Advanced EMT training is shorter and more focused than the paramedic level. Advanced EMT programs are more often used in rural volunteer EMS systems, where attending longer training programs may not be feasible and call volumes are lower.

Paramedic. The highest level of training for advanced EMTs is usually referred to as **paramedic.** A paramedic has completed a course that followed the standardized national curriculum as prescribed by NHTSA or meets the standards of the new educational paradigm. A paramedic performs advanced techniques, such as ECG interpretation, drug therapy, invasive airway techniques, and manual defibrillation. Paramedic

training is available through programs sponsored by hospitals, community colleges, and other agencies.

Paramedics also may be used for critical care transport operations. In these types of services, EMS providers are involved primarily in the transfer of acutely ill and injured patients from one care center to another. Often EMS providers who function in this role have additional training in specialized devices, such as intravenous pumps (devices that deliver IV fluids more precisely) and balloon pumps (devices that enhance circulation in patients with cardiovascular failure). Paramedics or critical care nurses also are used in medical evacuation (medevac) helicopter programs. These programs often are designed to transport critically ill patients from the scene of the emergency or a local community hospital to specialized care facilities.

The Healthcare System

Emergency Departments

Modern emergency departments (EDs) are vital centers of acute medical and trauma care that serve as the intersection between the prehospital and hospital phases of care (**Figure 1-11**). In the ED the patient is evaluated and treated, and decisions are made about the need for further care, including admission to the hospital, transfer to an operating room, or discharge home. Hospitals may have specialty teams that respond quickly to patients with time-critical illness and injury, such as stroke, trauma, and cardiac conditions.

The standards for EDs also have advanced over the past 25 years. Many communities have developed minimum standards for staff, space, equipment, and availability of specialists (e.g., neurosurgeons, orthopedists). The National EMSS Act of 1973 stimulated much of this progress, citing hospital facilities as a key component of EMS systems. Currently, these standards are set by various organizations, including state departments of health, The Joint Commission (TJC; formerly Joint Commission on Accreditation of Healthcare Organizations [JCAHO]), and other professional organizations.

The acutely ill or injured patient may be admitted to the hospital. Some patients may go directly from the ED to the operating room, cardiac catheterization laboratory, or a critical care unit for additional treatments, monitoring, or both (**Figure 1-12**). Various

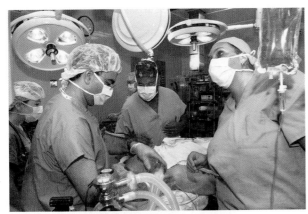

Figure 1-12 Surgery in an operating room may be part of additional emergency treatment.

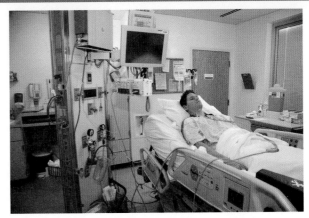

Figure 1-13 Patients may be admitted to a critical care unit.

types of critical care or intensive care units exist for patients with different problems, such as cardiac, respiratory, surgical, pediatric, and high-risk obstetric and neonatal (**Figure 1-13**).

REAL_World_

Of all patients transported to emergency departments, 14% arrive by ambulance. For patients under 15 years of age, 3.8% arrive by ambulance. For patients over 75 years, 40.9% are transported by ambulance.

Can you think of reasons for such a difference at these extremes of age?

Data from Institute of Medicine: *EMS at the crossroads,* Washington, DC, 2006.

Specialty Referral Centers

Some patients have unique needs that require the care of specially trained individuals, using highly specialized equipment. Specialty referral services include trauma centers, burn centers, pediatric intensive care, neonatal (newborn) centers, cardiac centers, and hyperbaric centers for victims of diving injuries or poisoning with carbon monoxide. EMTs may transport certain patients directly to a specialty referral center, at times bypassing other hospitals.

Hospital Personnel

The EMT is part of a larger team of personnel who care for the patient at each phase of the EMSS. These individuals also can serve as a resource for information, feedback about a patient's condition, and continuing education. Mutual respect and appreciation of each team member's contribution are essential to promote effective communication and continuity of care. The hospital team members include the following:

- The physician, who is responsible for the overall management of the patient in the prehospital and hospital phases of care.
- The nurse, who coordinates care in the ED, operating room, critical care units, and other general medical-surgical units in addition to directing patient care duties.
- Other health professionals, such as physician assistants, nurse practitioners, respiratory therapists, radiology technicians, and a host of personnel who tend to the various needs of the patient in the hospital.

Liaison with Other Public Safety Workers

The EMT interacts with various public safety personnel at the scene of a call. Police, fire service, public utility workers, and state and federal law enforcement officers are key resources at general medical or trauma emergencies, crime or motor vehicle crash scenes, mass casualty incidents, and behavioral emergencies. Become familiar with the resources in your region and how to contact them when needed. Understand and respect the roles, responsibilities, and authority of various resources at emergency scenes.

Many systems provide a *tiered* response to certain calls. For example, police or fire service personnel may be dispatched as first responders to provide immediate care (e.g., AED use, bleeding control) before arrival of the ambulance. Police officers often assume responsibility for notification of family, securing valuables or property, and assisting with violent patients or other behavioral emergencies.

When multiple agencies are needed at an emergency incident, the roles and command function are assigned by the nature of the incident. In general, police take charge at any crime scene or where crowd or traffic control may be needed. Fire personnel would take charge at a fire scene. An EMT's primary concern is patient care. The EMT must know the roles of the various agencies in the region so that all can work in a coordinated and a safe, effective manner. An *incident management system,* also known as an "incident command system," has been established to allow for clear lines of authority and responsibilities at the scene of an emergency when many agencies respond and must work together to resolve the emergency situation (see Chapter 28).

Local Emergency Medical Services System

To perform optimally for the patient, EMTs should become familiar with the components of their local EMSS. All the components just described are part of everyday EMT practice. Familiarity with the access and communication system is an essential first step. Knowing the levels of training allows the EMT to interact appropriately with first responders and advanced-level EMTs who may also arrive at the scene. Treatment, triage (sorting according to medical need), and transport protocols should be learned and carried in the vehicle, because they describe the key patient care decisions and interaction with medical direction. Familiarity with the designations of specialty

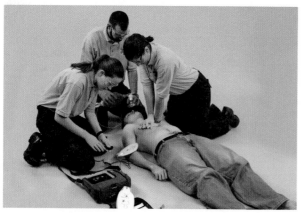

Figure 1-14 EMTs using personal protective equipment during CPR.

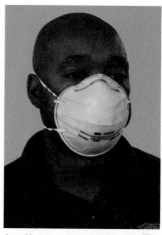

Figure 1-15 A high-efficiency particulate air (HEPA) respirator is an important defense against diseases spread by airborne transmission, such as tuberculosis, chickenpox, measles, and smallpox. *From Chapleau W, Pons P:* Emergency medical technician, *St Louis, 2007, Mosby-Elsevier.*

receiving hospitals is necessary when critical patients with special needs, such as for burn or trauma center care, are identified in the field. EMTs must know the initial steps to take when assisting at a disaster.

Orientation sessions and review of policies and protocols assist the EMT in gathering this important information. Continuing education and studying current local and state EMS updates allow the EMT to retain essential information and stay abreast of change.

> **LEARNING OBJECTIVES**
> * Describe the roles and responsibilities of the EMT related to personal safety.
> * Discuss the roles and responsibilities of the EMT toward the safety of the crew, the patient, and bystanders.

Roles and Responsibilities of the EMT

The work of an EMT is diversified and provides challenge and gratification. As an EMT, you will function in several roles that call for medical, technical, clerical, and social interaction skills. Many of these skills will be acquired during classroom training sessions. Other skills will develop during clinical field experience under the supervision of senior EMTs or instructors.

Primary Responsibilities

Personal Safety and Safety of Others

Primary concern for safety is the first and most important step on every call. Scene safety is the first part of patient assessment. The use of cones and flares, proper positioning of emergency vehicles, and wearing reflective clothing at the scene are all basic defenses against personal injury. Other conditions that may be considered include hazardous materials or toxic gases, aggressive animals, violent patients or bystanders, and electrical hazards.

The risk of exposure to communicable disease is real and should be taken seriously. The primary defenses against disease transmission are **personal protective equipment** (PPE) and handwashing (**Figure 1-14**). Gloves, eye protection, gowns, and high-efficiency particulate air (HEPA) respirator masks are examples of basic PPE carried by an EMT (**Figure 1-15**).

The choice of a particular piece of equipment depends on the circumstances of a given call. For example, gloves are used routinely when exposure to blood or body fluids may occur, such as when bandaging a minor wound. Goggles are used when there is a potential for an eye splash of blood or body fluid. This can happen during suctioning or administration of positive-pressure ventilation. A special mask is used if tuberculosis or another airborne pathogen is suspected (see Chapter 2).

Prevention is the key in matters of safety. Developing good habits early in your clinical experience ensures the safest possible approach. You will learn more about the specifics of safety later in this chapter and in Chapter 2.

Patient Assessment

Assessment is one of your primary responsibilities as an EMT. It involves the systematic collection and analysis of information received through a patient history, vital signs, and a physical examination (**Figure 1-16**). Become a skilled observer who can recognize problems quickly and respond accordingly.

Patient assessment is probably the most difficult skill to master as an EMT because it involves many different areas of knowledge. You will learn to obtain a concise history from a patient who may be in severe pain, confused, or hysterical. This will require patience and much practice. You will learn which facts are relevant to each type of chief complaint and how to avoid unnecessary questioning that wastes time.

Patient Care Based on Assessment Findings

Your training will prepare you to respond to a variety of critical problems, ranging from immobilization of a fractured leg to resuscitation of a cardiac arrest victim (**Figure 1-17**). In some cases, time may not allow a prolonged analysis because many true emergencies require treatment while assessment continues. Significant loss of blood or complete airway blockage requires a reflex reaction that you can develop only with intensive classroom and clinical practice. Other treatments you will learn include CPR, oxygen therapy, assisting at childbirth, management of poisoning and

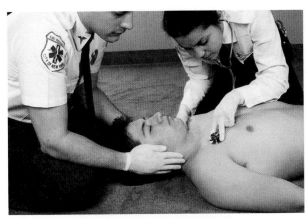

Figure 1-16 An EMT performs patient assessment.

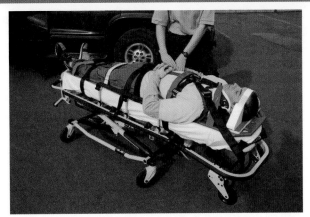

Figure 1-18 The patient is secured to an immobilization device.

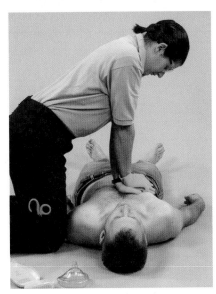

Figure 1-17 An EMT performs cardiopulmonary resuscitation.

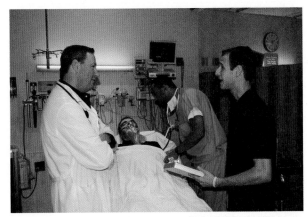

Figure 1-19 An EMT presents a patient history to the emergency physician, providing details gathered from the time of first contact, which can play a major role in diagnosis and treatment.

overdose, treatment of shock states, and psychological first aid. Knowing when to transport a patient and when to choose a special institution (e.g., burn center) is also important.

Lifting and Moving

Many patients you encounter will be injured and require careful handling. A victim with a suspected spinal injury should be immobilized to prevent further injury during transport (**Figure 1-18**). As an EMT, you will become familiar with a variety of spinal immobilization methods, splinting, different types of stretchers, and rapid removal techniques.

The needs of patients vary widely, from an elderly patient who needs a stair chair to be helped to the ambulance, to a seriously injured patient who must be rapidly extricated from a burning automobile. As an EMT, you become an expert in movement, matching a particular strategy with the needs of a patient. You should carefully learn and practice these techniques during and after your EMT course.

Transport and Transfer of Care

If your rapid response to a call results in a preventable injury to yourself, your partner, or a patient, you have defeated your purpose. When you get behind the wheel of an emergency vehicle,

you take on a great responsibility. Although the law allows certain exemptions while you are operating an emergency vehicle, you are still responsible for maintaining control of the vehicle at all times.

You must be familiar with the best possible routes in your area. You should know the traffic patterns at all times of the day and the alternate routes in the event that your original route is obstructed.

The safe and appropriate transport of your patient is another aspect of emergency vehicle operation. Contrary to popular belief, most patients do not benefit from a frantic ride to the hospital with lights flashing and siren blaring.

When you arrive at the ED with your patient, you should be ready to transfer care of the patient to the ED staff. You may need to continue certain aspects of care, such as resuscitation, until the nurse, physician, or other healthcare professional assumes responsibility. You should present a brief report that highlights key aspects of the assessment and treatment performed in the field (**Figure 1-19**).

Record Keeping

Accurate records play an important role in the management of the patient because they become the reference point for information after your departure from the hospital (**Figure 1-20**). Prehospital assessment findings and the chronology of prehospital events and treatments are very important because they

Prehospital Care Report

Agency		Unit #		Trip #		Type of incident ☐ Medical ☐ Trauma ☐ No patient ☐ Refusal		# ___ of ___ Patients		Date of service / /

Incident location				Pt. destination		Transport by	

Attendant	Certification level	Attendant	Certification level	Driver	Certification level

Patient's age	Sex ☐ F ☐ M	Chief complaint	Mechanism of injury

Narrative

Previous medical history

Medications

Allergies   Charted by

Patient Vital Signs

Time	Blood pressure	Pulse rate	Rhythm	Respirations rate	Rhythm/quality	Pupils L	R	Movement of extremities R - arm - L	R - leg - L	Glasgow Eyes	Verbal	Motor	Pulse oximeter SaO2	O2LPM	Cardiac rhythm
	/														
	/														
	/														

IV Therapy / Medications

Time	Solution	Site	Size	Rate	Initials	S/U	Medication	Dose	Route	Time	Time	Time	Time	Order from	Response to treatment

Total infused	cc	Response	

Times

Tone	Responding	On scene	ALS on	Departed	Arr hosp	In service

Patient Information

Name	DOB / /	SS#	Telephone ( )
Address		Next of kin	
City, State, Zip		Relationship	

Hospital notification / Assistance / Call outcome

Med channel #_____	Base physician	☐ Police	☐ Fire	Response code ☐ 2 ☐ 3	☐ Transported to facility
☐ Cellular	☐ Amb dispatch	☐ Sheriff	☐ Other	Transport code ☐ 2 ☐ 3	☐ Care transferred in field
☐ Landline	☐ Other	☐ State Patrol	☐ Air Life ☐ Flight for Life	☐ Helicopter transport	☐ Cancelled

Figure 1-20 A prehospital care report. *Modified from HealthONE EMS Patient Care Report, courtesy HealthONE EMS, Englewood, Colo.*

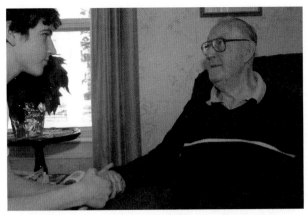

Figure 1-21 An EMT should show compassion.

are the only source of documentation from the scene. When you leave the hospital, physicians and nurses will refer to the prehospital care report to retrieve essential information. You should develop good habits and record pertinent data from the time of the initial patient encounter until arrival at the hospital. Many EMS systems are using electronic prehospital care reports whereas others are still using handwritten forms. Regardless of the type of program your system uses, your documentation must be thorough, chronological, and clear. Accuracy is another necessary ingredient in effective documentation. Times, vital sign values, and other diagnostic findings should be recorded carefully to aid in further assessment of the patient. Your reporting of vital signs provides a baseline that can help track the progress or deterioration of the patient's condition.

Patient Advocacy

At the moment of encounter, you become the primary healthcare representative for the patient during the prehospital phase of care. Patients may not be familiar with the EMSS and depend on you, the EMT, for advice about the best course of action for their problem. Often your actions or advice may be guided by protocols or directives regarding patient care, hospital selection, decisions regarding who can ride with the patient in the ambulance, and many other issues.

It is important to treat patients as a whole and to consider all aspects of their condition, their ability to care for themselves, notification of family members, and other social and psychological issues. A good rule for the EMT is to treat the patient as you would want a family member to be treated under similar conditions. Sometimes such treatment means "going that extra mile" by contacting a family member or advising the nurse at the hospital of the need for social service intervention. As a *patient advocate,* your attitude and actions shift from a purely clinical point of view to a more humanistic approach to patient care (**Figure 1-21**).

At times, patients may present with seemingly minor complaints. Although these may not be emergent problems, stay aware and do not jump to conclusions. Adopting a "help-based" approach rather than a "thrill-seeking" focus will help prevent burnout and poor patient care. What initially may seem minor may easily become serious. Back pain and headaches can be caused by serious vascular problems, such as dissection of the aorta or a hemorrhage (bleeding) in the brain. Flulike

symptoms can be caused by serious conditions such as carbon monoxide poisoning or serious infections (e.g., meningitis, anthrax). Intoxication can often mask a serious underlying injury. Once again, you should focus on the patient.

Other Responsibilities

Public Education

An important responsibility of the EMT is to educate the public and help prevent injuries. Programs such as community CPR classes can go a long way in increasing the chance of survival of a heart attack victim. Bicycle helmet and safety programs help prevent injuries.

Extrication

Although extrication is not a primary EMT responsibility, sometimes you may be called on to gain access to and free people trapped in automobiles. This activity is usually the function of specialized rescue personnel within EMS, police department, or fire department. However, when these units are not immediately available, or when regional systems incorporate these functions into the EMT's protocols, you must be prepared to bring about a safe and efficient rescue. In most situations, you will perform "light extrication," or extrication with the use of basic tools, such as screwdrivers, crowbars, and hacksaws.

If "heavy extrication" is assigned through regional protocols, specialized programs are usually conducted to teach the proper use of the larger and more powerful devices typically used by rescue personnel.

Before extrication can occur, you may need to gain control of the scene. This may mean setting up visual warning devices on a highway or choosing someone to direct traffic or crowd control.

Communications

The proper use of the radio or other communication device is part of your training. Radio communications should be short and clear. The radio is a useful tool for mobilizing essential resources, notifying hospital personnel of the arrival of an acutely ill patient, and documenting unusual circumstances that may have medicolegal implications later. For example, a patient who leaves the scene against your advice and without a proper signature on a release form can be documented by relaying the information to the dispatcher or medical control. Many systems record all conversations to provide another form of documentation.

Importantly, you also must learn to be an effective communicator with patients, family members, and hospital personnel.

Vehicle and Equipment Maintenance

Vehicles and equipment that are well maintained last longer and perform better for you and the patient. It is frustrating and dangerous to attempt resuscitation or another task, only to discover that essential equipment is not serviceable or is missing. Proper inspection and maintenance of the vehicle and restocking equipment are roles of every EMT (**Figure 1-22**). Cleaning the ambulance and equipment is part of a planned program of infection control and respect for EMT and patient safety.

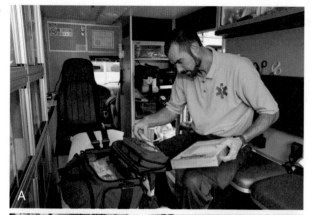

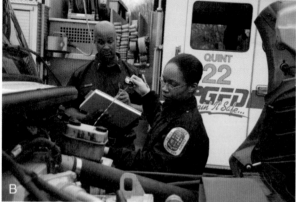

Figure 1-22 **A,** Restocking of the vehicle. **B,** Inspecting the engine.

Professional Attributes of the EMT

As a medical professional, you have a unique and special body of knowledge that is to be used for the benefit of society. You are expected to demonstrate skill and knowledge for the good of the patient. You also are expected to promote high standards of behavior and medical practice within the profession. Also, as a professional, you are expected to add to the body of knowledge to continue to advance progress in emergency medicine.

The term that probably best embodies these basic values is *professionalism.* The dictionary describes professionalism as "acting requisite to the body of knowledge which defines the service and abilities of the professional...according to the oath of the profession." Although the term *professional* is used more loosely now, the expectations of behavior can easily be understood by reading a traditional medical oath. **Box 1-1** provides the EMT's oath.

Appearance and Attitude

A professional appearance and attitude help evoke a sense of confidence in the patient and family members **(Figure 1-23).** Because emergency care providers have little time to establish rapport with their patients, the sight of an EMT in a clean and appropriate uniform helps establish a sense of respect and trust. Of course, wearing a uniform may not always be possible (e.g., a volunteer EMT responding from home or work). Because you often need to gain a stranger's cooperation and trust quickly in EMS, however, you should take advantage of the

---

| **Box 1-1** | Emergency Medical Technician's Oath |

Be it pledged as an Emergency Medical Technician, I will honor the physical and judicial laws of God and man. I will follow that regimen which, according to my ability and judgment, I consider for the benefit of patients and abstain from whatever is deleterious and mischievous, nor shall I suggest any such counsel. Into whatever homes I enter, I will go into them for the benefit of only the sick and injured, never revealing what I see or hear in the lives of men unless required by law.

I shall also share my medical knowledge with those who may benefit from what I have learned. I will serve unselfishly and continuously in order to help make a better world for all mankind.

While I continue to keep this oath unviolated, may it be granted to me to enjoy life, and the practice of the art, respected by all men, in all times. Should I trespass or violate the oath, may the reverse be my lot. So help me God.

© 1994, National Association of Emergency Medical Technicians (NAEMT). Written by Charles Gillespie, MD.

---

fact that you often are judged by your appearance, and dress appropriately.

The attitude of the EMT is even more important than the outer appearance. You should show an interest in your job and possess a sensitive awareness of your environment and the needs of others around you. The provision of medical care is a giving profession and should not be taken lightly. The attributes of *quality* we seek to deliver are well articulated in a report by the Institute of Medicine on quality in America's health care **(Box 1-2).**

You should put the patient's needs first while protecting and preserving the safety of bystanders, other rescuers, and yourself. You are not useful to others if you become a victim yourself. A first step in arrival at the scene of every emergency is to ensure scene safety. EMTs must maintain awareness of the safety of the environment throughout the call, from arrival to transport to the hospital. Evolving or escalating hazards can range from street traffic, violence, fire scenes, and emotionally disturbed patients and family members to communicable diseases.

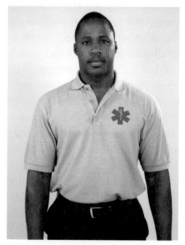

Figure 1-23 A properly attired EMT inspires confidence.
From Aehlert B: Paramedic today: above and beyond, *St Louis, 2010, Mosby-Elsevier.*

Box 1-2	Six Quality Aims of Institute of Medicine (IOM) "Quality Chasm" Report

- Health care should be:
- **Safe**—Avoiding injuries to patients from the care that is intended to help them.
- **Effective**—Providing services based on scientific knowledge to all who could benefit, and refraining from providing services to those not likely to benefit.
- **Patient centered**—Providing patient care that is respectful to and responsive of individual patient preferences, needs, and values, and ensuring that patient values guide all clinical decisions.
- **Timely**—Reducing waits and sometimes harmful delays for both those who receive and those who give care.
- **Efficient**—Avoiding waste, including waste of equipment, supplies, ideas, and energy.
- **Equitable**—Providing care that does not vary in quality because of personal characteristics such as gender, ethnicity, geographic location, and socioeconomic status.

From IOM Committee on Quality of Health Care in America: *Crossing the quality chasm: a new health system for the 21st century,* Washington, DC, 2001, National Academies Press, pp 5-6.

LEARNING OBJECTIVE
- State the specific statutes and regulations in your state regarding the EMS system.

Maintenance of Up-to-Date Knowledge and Skills

Your EMT training is the foundation of your EMS education. Each state establishes license or certification requirements for the practicing EMT that may include written, practical, and clinical requirements. Although there are variations, the NHTSA curricula and the scope of practice documents usually provide the framework for programs throughout the United States. Different states or other countries may also add various training modules that enhance the local or regional provision of prehospital care, such as specialized trauma programs, emergency vehicle operation, extrication training, hazardous materials training, domestic preparedness, and other programs.

Recertification is usually required every 2 to 3 years (although the interval may be longer) and may involve ongoing continuing education (CE) requirements, challenge testing, or attendance at a formalized refresher program. Continuing education takes many forms: attendance at local, state, and national conferences; reading EMS journals; and attending call review. Several national organizations contribute to EMS education. As an EMT, you should also be familiar with the specific statutes and regulations related to EMS in your state.

National Registry of Emergency Medical Technicians

The National Registry of EMTs was developed to establish a high-quality and standardized competency level for all levels of EMTs. The National Registry provides written and practical testing and a continuing education program at the basic and advanced levels. This registry is used by many states to provide reciprocity to EMTs and paramedics. *Reciprocity* is recognition by one state of the validity of the EMT certification granted by another. The National Registry of EMTs also maintains CE requirements that encourage the professional development of EMTs nationwide. EMTs can be registered at either the basic or the advanced level.

National Association of Emergency Medical Technicians

The NAEMT is an organization that represents EMTs throughout the United States. It was founded in 1975 with the support of the National Registry and other national organizations and leaders to serve as a national voice for prehospital providers. The NAEMT maintains three societies that serve other subdivisions of prehospital care: the National Society of EMS Administrators, the National Society of Instructor Coordinators, and the National Society of EMT-Paramedics.

The NAEMT works for legislative change in EMS, provides continuing education, represents EMTs in other national organizations, provides job placement for EMTs, and in general, works for the development and recognition of EMTs nationwide. Among the CE efforts offered by NAEMT are an annual national educational conference and Prehospital Trauma Life Support (PHTLS), a CE trauma program.

American Heart Association

In cooperation with other healthcare organizations, the AHA establishes CPR and emergency cardiovascular care guidelines for both hospital and prehospital providers. Approximately every 5 years, the AHA publishes the *International Guidelines for CPR and Emergency Cardiovascular Care,* which provides recommendations for CPR performance and cardiac protocols used in prehospital care.

LEARNING OBJECTIVE
- Define quality improvement, and discuss the EMT's role in the process.

Quality Improvement

The effectiveness of any organization depends on a continuing process of evaluation and change called **quality improvement (QI).** EMS quality improvement is defined in the National Standard Curriculum for Emergency Medical Technicians as "a system of internal and external reviews and audits of all aspects of an EMS system so as to identify those aspects needing improvement to assure that the public receives the highest quality of prehospital care."

Quality improvement takes many forms and may include the following:
- Reviewing prehospital documentation to ensure appropriate record keeping.
- Reviewing ambulance runs to determine the type of care provided and the quality of care.
- Gathering feedback from patients and hospital personnel on the quality of care.
- Providing continuing education.
- Ensuring preventive maintenance of the emergency vehicle and equipment.
- Maintaining personal skills.

As an EMT, you should be an active participant in the QI process by helping with audits and maintaining a positive attitude about feedback. Viewing QI feedback as a mechanism for personal growth rather than criticism provides the best atmosphere for ongoing individual and system development.

LEARNING OBJECTIVE
• Define medical direction, and discuss the EMT's role in the process.

Medical Direction

Medical direction is defined as the accountability for the medical conduct of EMS personnel by a physician knowledgeable in prehospital emergency care. The type of care provided in the field should be carefully considered and judged to be medically prudent by physicians who are expert in emergency medicine. Depending on the size of the service, more than one physician may share in accepting this responsibility.

Every ambulance service or rescue squad must have physician medical direction. State laws address the practice of medicine and delegate responsibility to *physician extenders,* such as EMTs, paramedics, and physician assistants. The relationship of the EMT to medical direction is best understood by reference to the medical practice act in your state. In general, however, the EMT might be considered to be a designated agent of the medical director and the care rendered an extension of the medical director's authority.

The type of medical direction can vary. The term *medical oversight* has been offered by the National Association of EMS Physicians in reference to system-wide responsibility. Within an EMSS, there may be many individuals who assume responsibilities for medical direction. From the ground up, it would start with the ambulance service medical director, who takes responsibility for the medical conduct of that service's EMTs. Within a region, medical directors from the hospitals and ambulance services may join together to promote uniform treatment protocols. Other physicians may provide online medical direction for particular patients from a medical control console, often located in a regional hospital where physicians familiar with the EMS system offer 24-hour direct contact with the EMTs regarding patient care issues. Some systems only provide this service for advanced EMS providers.

An EMS system medical director may assume responsibility for the medical conduct of the system as a whole. Medical directors of training programs assume responsibility for the clinical accuracy of the educational offerings, provide critical input regarding practical skills, and help to oversee and arrange for clinical rotations.

Online Medical Direction

Online medical direction involves the direct, real-time contact by telephone or radio with a physician who guides treatment, transport, and triage decisions at the scene. The EMT might contact medical direction for a treatment order, such as whether to assist a patient in administration of the patient's nitroglycerin for chest pain. The EMT might contact medical direction for assistance in triage of multiple casualties at the scene. Other uses of online medical direction include a physician resource for patients who are refusing medical assistance but who are believed to have critical illnesses that warrant emergency care.

Offline Medical Direction

Offline medical direction is medical guidance from the physician to the EMT in the form of written protocols, policies, or procedures to guide patient triage, transportation, and transport decisions. Offline medical direction is accomplished without direct voice-to-voice contact. Rather, it is determined in advance by the medical director of the EMSS or a regional or state medical advisory committee. A protocol may consist of standing orders, a requirement to contact medical direction via radio or telephone, or both. *Standing orders* are the aspects of the protocol that the EMT initiates without a requirement to contact medical direction. Some protocols, such as administration of a certain medication, may require contact with medical direction before treatment. Another aspect of medical direction is the responsibility for review of the QI program.

Scenario Follow-up

The motor vehicle crash victim had ultrasound at the bedside, which identified free blood near the spleen. Emergency computed tomography (CT) scan of the head and neck revealed no head injury or neck fracture. The patient was brought emergently to the operating room, where the bleeding from the spleen was stopped, an otherwise fatal injury.

Many people in diverse roles responded to this individual. A fellow motorist, who had read a "First There, First Care" poster, saw the car off the road, called the dispatch center for help, went to the patient's side, and remained there until help arrived. Police and rescue personnel arrived to secure the scene and help extricate the victim. Both an emergency medical responder (EMR) and an emergency medical technician (EMT) cared for the patient. The EMT identified that the patient met criteria for direct transport to a trauma center. This community had organized in advance to identify hospitals willing and able to deliver emergency, lifesaving care to injured patients.

Who saved this life? Without all the partners and prior planning, it may have been lost. The credit goes to all who developed and participated in this emergency medical service system (EMSS).

Summary

EMTs work in cooperation with many people in providing timely and effective medical care. Other workers include lay rescuers, dispatchers, first responders, fire and police personnel, and physicians and nurses in receiving hospitals. As an EMT, you must be familiar with your primary responsibilities, which include personal safety and the safety of others, patient assessment, prompt patient care, safe transportation and transfer, appropriate documentation, and record keeping, and communication of findings with medical directors and hospital personnel. Most important is your responsibility as a patient advocate. You may be the first medical professional the patient encounters in an EMSS. A caring and empathetic attitude is an essential characteristic of an effective EMT. You should review the following learning checklist to reinforce and help retain the information you learned in this chapter. Good luck in your EMS work!

The Bottom Line

Learning Checklist

✓ An emergency medical services system (EMSS) is the planned configuration of community resources and personnel necessary to provide immediate medical care to patients with sudden or unexpected illness or injury.

✓ Although most growth and development of EMS systems occurred over the past 40 years, several key historical events helped to shape EMS over the last century:
- ✓ During the Napoleonic Wars, army surgeon Baron Dominique-Jean Larrey introduced his ambulance volantes.
- ✓ Horse-drawn ambulances were introduced during the Civil War, under the direction of Dr. Jonathan Letterman.
- ✓ During the Korean War in the 1950s, helicopters were used to rapidly evacuate the wounded to mobile army surgical hospitals (MASH units).
- ✓ One of the first hospital-based ambulance services was initiated by Cincinnati General Hospital in the mid-1860s. The first motorized ambulance is said to have been provided by Michael Reese Hospital of Chicago and St. Vincent's Hospital in 1899.
- ✓ CPR and portable defibrillators were introduced in the 1960s.
- ✓ Introduction of biotelemetry in the late 1960s allowed for advanced life support.

✓ Medical societies played a significant part in the development of EMSS, including the National EMT Training Curriculum currently used. The curriculum was an outgrowth of work by these physician groups in the 1960s.

✓ In 1966 the National Academy of Sciences published the landmark paper *Accidental Death and Disability: the Neglected Disease of Modern Society.*

✓ In 1973, federal legislation provided funding for the development of EMSS throughout the United States.

✓ The *EMS Agenda for the Future* is a modern document that defines 14 elements of an effective EMS system.

✓ The *EMS Education Agenda for the Future*, the *National EMS Core Content*, the *National EMS Scope of Practice Model*, and the *National EMS Education Standards* encompass multiple steps intended to enhance effective EMS education and practice.

✓ The National Highway Traffic Safety Administration (NHTSA) provides leadership for EMS on a federal level.

✓ Emergency medical responders (EMRs, or first responders), such as police and firefighters, are often equipped with oxygen, automated defibrillators, and airway equipment and may respond in first-responder cars or police or fire vehicles. They possess knowledge and skills to provide lifesaving interventions while awaiting additional EMS response and can assist higher level personnel on the scene.

✓ Emergency medical technicians (EMTs) provide basic emergency medical care and transportation for critical and emergent patietns who access the EMS system. They perform interventions with basic equipment typically found on an ambulance, under medical oversight, linking the patient from the scene to the emergency healthcare system.

✓ An advanced emergency medical technician (AEMT) provides basic and limited advanced care, including administration of certain drugs.

✓ A paramedic is an allied health professional whose primary focus is to provide advanced emergency medical care for critical and emergent patients. Paramedics possess complex knowledge and skills necessary to perform basic and advanced interventions with equipment found on an ambulance, under medical oversight.

✓ Primary responsibilities of the EMT include personal safety and safety of others, patient assessment, lifting and moving, transport and transfer of care, record keeping, and patient advocacy.

✓ Other responsibilities of the EMT include extrication, communications, and vehicle and equipment maintenance.

✓ EMTs should dress appropriately to instill confidence, show interest in their job, and possess a sensitive awareness of their environment and the needs of others around them.

✓ EMTs should maintain up-to-date knowledge and skills through continuing education and refresher training.

✓ EMTs play several important roles in quality assurance, including reviewing prehospital documentation to ensure accuracy, reviewing ambulance runs to ensure that the prehospital care was appropriate, gathering feedback from patients and hospital personnel on the quality of care, preventive maintenance of the vehicle and equipment, and maintaining personal skills.

✓ Medical direction is the oversight of clinical patient care by a physician.

✓ Online medical direction involves the direct, real-time contact by telephone or radio with a physician who directs treatment, transport, and triage decisions at the scene or while en route to the hospital.

✓ Offline medical direction is medical guidance from the physician to the EMT in the form of written protocols, policies, or procedures that guide patient triage, transportation, and transport decisions.

Key Terms

Advanced emergency medical technician (AEMT) An AEMT provides basic and limited advanced care, including administration of certain drugs under medical oversight to critical and emergent patients who access the EMS system. Also called EMT-Intermediate (EMT-I).

Biotelemetry Method by which biological data are transferred from one location to another by radio or telephone.

Emergency medical responder (EMR) Often arriving before the ambulance, EMRs such as police and firefighters are equipped with oxygen, automated defibrillators, and airway equipment and may respond in first-responder cars or police or fire vehicles. They possess knowledge and skills to provide lifesaving interventions while awaiting additional EMS response and can assist higher-level personnel on the scene.

Emergency medical technician (EMT) EMTs provide basic emergency medical care and transportation for critical and emergent patients who access the EMS system. They perform interventions with basic equipment typically found on an ambulance under medical oversight, linking the patient from the scene to the emergency healthcare system.

Medical direction The active participation of physicians overseeing medical care in an EMS system; includes protocol development, needs assessment of the system, education, quality improvement, and outcome studies, as well as online medical direction. Also called "medical control."

Offline medical direction The accountability by a physician for EMS providers through the use of protocols, quality improvement activities, educational endeavors, and other measures to ensure effective field care.

Online medical direction The accountability of field care by a physician though the use of radio or telephone communications.

Paramedic Allied health professional whose primary focus is to provide advanced emergency medical care for critical and emergent patients. Paramedics possess complex knowledge and skills necessary to perform basic and advanced interventions with equipment found on an ambulance, under medical oversight.

Personal protective equipment (PPE) Variety of safety equipment ranging from gloves, goggles, clothing, and masks to self-contained breathing apparatus (SCBA) designed to protect the EMT at the scene.

Quality improvement (QI) Methods of ensuring a high level of patient care.

Review Questions

1. Which of the following is a system of resources and personnel necessary to provide immediate care to ill and injured patients?
    a. Emergency medical services system
    b. Ambulance service
    c. "Enhanced 9-1-1" dispatching system
    d. Hospital emergency service

2. Which of the following *most* affected the early growth and development of prehospital emergency care?
    a. Disaster drills
    b. Outpatient clinics
    c. War
    d. Laboratory animal research

3. Of the following, which is the leading cause of trauma deaths?
    a. Electrocution
    b. Motor vehicle crashes
    c. Falls
    d. Burn injuries

4. An EMT is caring for a patient with cardiac chest pain and wants to administer aspirin to the patient. The EMT must call and consult with a physician before the aspirin can be administered. This is best described by which of the following?
    a. Offline medical direction
    b. Quality assurance
    c. Online medical direction
    d. Telemetry

Match the following descriptions with the EMS system role *(a-e)*.

Column A	Column B
5. The intersection of hospital and prehospital care.	a. Emergency medical responder
6. Trained individual who provides initial life-sustaining care (AED, CPR) with minimal equipment.	b. Emergency department
7. Responsible for prioritizing calls, communicating with EMS providers, and giving phone instructions to bystanders.	c. Critical care unit
8. Usually the first medical person to see the patient.	d. Emergency medical dispatcher
	e. EMT

9. Which of the following best defines the physician's involvement and participation in all phases of the EMS system to ensure quality care?
    a. Categorization
    b. Standardization
    c. Systemization
    d. Medical direction

For Further Review

In the Student Workbook

- Multiple-choice questions
- Matching questions
- Fill in the blank questions
- Short answer questions
- True/false questions
- Case scenario questions
- Crossword puzzle

On Evolve

- Weblinks
- Lecture notes
- Exercises

Learning Objectives

Cognitive Objectives

- Define emergency medical services (EMS) system.
- Differentiate the roles and responsibilities of the EMT from those of other prehospital care providers.
- Describe the roles and responsibilities of the EMT related to personal safety.
- Discuss the roles and responsibilities of the EMT toward the safety of the crew, patient, and bystanders.
- State the specific statutes and regulations in your state regarding the EMS system.
- Define quality improvement, and discuss the EMT's role in the process.
- Define medical direction, and discuss the EMT's role in the process.

Affective Objectives

- Assess areas of personal attitude and conduct of the EMT.
- Characterize the various methods used to access the EMS system in your community.

References

George Washington Medical Faculty Associates: AED program: AED FAQ's, Washington, DC, 2007.

Gillespie C: Emergency Medical Technician's Oath, 1994, National Association of Emergency Medical Technicians (NAEMT).

Institute of Medicine: Committee on the Future of Emergency Care in the United States Health System: *EMS at the crossroads*, Washington, DC, 2006, National Academies Press.

Institute of Medicine: Committee on Quality of Health Care in America: *Crossing the quality chasm: a new health system for the 21st century*, Washington, DC, 2001, National Academies Press.

McCaig LF, Burt CW: National Hospital Ambulatory Medical Care Survey: 2003 emergency department summary—advance data from *Vital and Health Statistics* 358, Hyattsville, Md, 2005, National Center for Health Statistics.

Miniño AM, et al: *National Vital Statistics Report* 55(19):8, 2007.

National Academy of Sciences–National Research Council: *Accidental death and disability: the neglected disease of modern society*, Washington, DC, 1966, National Academy Press.

National Highway Traffic Safety Administration: *National EMS Core Content*, Washington, DC, 2005 US Department of Transportation.

National Highway Traffic Safety Administration: *National EMS scope of practice model*, DOT HS 810 657, Washington, DC, February 2007, US Department of Transportation.

National Highway Traffic Safety Administration: US Department of Health and Human Services, Public Health Services, Health Resources and Services Administration, Maternal and Child Health Bureau: *EMS agenda for the future*, Washington, DC, 1996, US Department of Transportation.

National Highway Traffic Safety Administration: US Department of Health and Human Services, Public Health Services, Health Resources and Services Administration, Maternal and Child Health Bureau: *Emergency medical services education agenda for the future: a systems approach*, Washington, DC, 2000, US Department of Transportation.

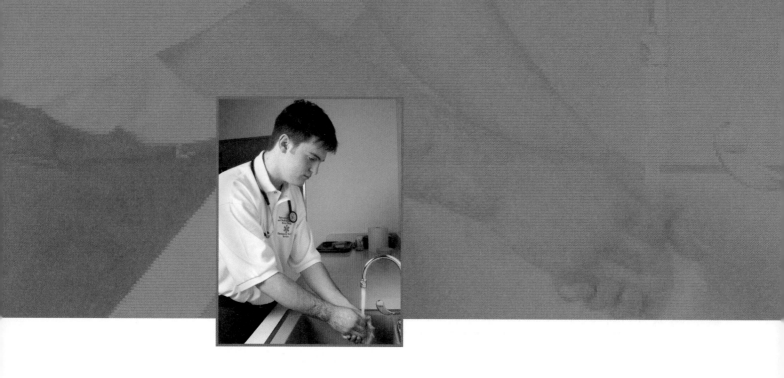

2 Well-Being of the EMT

CHAPTER OUTLINE

Wellness
Scene Safety
Understanding Communicable Diseases
Hazardous Situations
Stress Management
Comprehensive Critical Incident Stress Management
Terminal Illness and Death

Scenario

You arrive at the scene of a two-vehicle collision. One of the four teenage victims is dead, and the others have severe injuries. One young man has a traumatic amputation of the leg with blood spurting from the stump. You are wearing personal protective equipment, including eye protection, mask, gown, and gloves, and apply direct pressure to stop the bleeding. You note the patient has low blood pressure. The other two young men are severely injured; one is unconscious, and the second is pale, weak, and sweating; and they are being attended to by another responding unit.

You exchange your bloody gloves and gown for clean protective equipment and initiate transport of the patient to the trauma center, ensuring that the pressure dressing and bandage control bleeding. As you think about the blood splattered on your protective clothing and the blood at the scene, you know your actions to stop bleeding have helped to save a life. However, your satisfaction from assisting the patient is tempered by the images of the young man dead at the scene.

Emergency medical services (EMS) offer great personal rewards to those who serve as an emergency medical technician (EMT). However, working as an EMT requires both physical and psychological energy. To operate at your best, it is important to maintain personal wellness.

For example, the EMT may encounter stresses and hazards that can be emotionally and physically disabling. Emotional stress is encountered in many situations, such as caring for dying patients and in multiple-casualty incidents (MCIs). Recognizing that you will encounter stress and learning to deal with stress will help you on the job as well as in your personal life.

Physical hazards you will face include communicable disease, hazardous materials, and personal threats of violence. In addition, lifting and moving patients is a physical task. Being physically fit and exercising the appropriate precautions, such as personal protective equipment and using restraints in the moving ambulance, minimizes your chance of personal injury.

One of the greatest rewards in being an EMT is knowing that your actions can contribute to another person's survival. Without your help, the person may have died. There are other patients you will not save. Some patients will die unexpectedly from such events as major trauma or a heart attack. Others will have terminal illness and know they may not survive their next hospital stay.

Not every patient is in critical condition. In fact, most are not critical. However, as an EMT, you must be prepared to encounter dying patients and their families and friends. How you interact with patients and their loved ones when they die or face death will challenge you professionally and personally. What you say and how you act will be remembered long after the incident. Learning about death and dying and how to communicate will help you in this task.

Dealing with stressful encounters can jeopardize your personal well-being and emotional health. We all have limits and need to recognize that stressful events occur in our professional life and learn how best to deal with them. With the right perspective, these stressful events are recognized as part of our duties, handled in a professional and compassionate manner, and present an opportunity for personal and professional growth.

An EMT also faces physical risks. The patients you care for may have infectious diseases. Knowledge of communicable disease transmission and taking actions to limit the risk of acquiring such illness from another is called **infection control** and should be part of your daily practice. Your duty is to provide medical care, to identify and respect potential hazards, and to work with police, fire, and special hazardous materials (**HAZMAT**) teams to conduct your job safely, without jeopardizing your personal safety or that of your patient, fellow rescuers, and bystanders. Paying attention to the personal risks within the EMS profession and taking steps to work within acceptable risks are part of maintaining your well-being.

LEARNING OBJECTIVE
• Explain the need to maintain personal wellness.

Wellness

Wellness is the recognition of a state of positive being, health, and enjoyment of life. It is a state of mental, physical, and spiritual health that leads to positive interactions with family, friends, your community, your environment, and your profession. **Box 2-1** defines major areas of wellness for incorporating in daily life.

Seeking, maintaining, and enjoying personal wellness are key to proper preparation for work and life. You bring your "mental and physical best" to your patients and colleagues. You maintain a balanced life perspective as you deal with illness and injury. You are well fit for the physical tasks of caring for patients unable to walk or move on their own. You bring your keenest sense of purpose to the task at hand. Your attitude reflects your choice of living each day to the fullest.

Box 2-1	Wellness Principles

Environmental wellness: Protecting yourself from environmental hazards and minimizing the negative impact of your behavior on the environment.

Emotional wellness: Maintaining a positive self-concept, dealing constructively with feelings, and developing qualities of optimism and self-confidence.

Intellectual wellness: Keeping an active, curious, and open mind with the ability to think critically about issues, pose questions, identify problems, and find solutions.

Physical wellness: Achieving body health by eating well, exercising, avoiding unhealthy habits, making responsible decisions about sex, being aware of the symptoms of disease, having regular checkups, and taking steps to prevent injuries.

Social wellness: Developing meaningful relationships, cultivating a network of supportive friends and family members, and contributing to the community.

Spiritual wellness: Developing faith in something beyond yourself as well as the capacity for compassion, joy, and forgiveness; finding the meaning and purpose in life, whether through religion, meditation, art, nature, or some other involvement that prioritizes the concern for others.

From http://www.cazenovia.edu/Default.aspx?tabid=465. June 2007.

LEARNING OBJECTIVES
• Explain the need to determine scene safety.
• Discuss how to reduce your chance of occupational injury.

Scene Safety

Scene safety must be your first concern when responding to a call. As an EMT, you encounter many hazards. Some are obvious, such as oncoming traffic. Others may be invisible, such as carbon monoxide from an improperly vented heating system or microorganisms transmitted by coughing or in a patient's blood.

Types of incidents that require assistance from other agencies and use of personal protective gear include hazardous material incidents, rescue operations, violent scenes, and possible exposure to contagious diseases. The EMT who anticipates the need for personal protective equipment, body substance isolation, and assistance from other agencies to make the scene secure will be best able to assist the patient and provide emergency care with the least risk of personal harm to the EMTs, the patient, other agencies, and bystanders.

Ambulance Safety

The most common occupational cause of death for an EMT is motor vehicle related. According to the National Association of Emergency Medical Technicians (NAEMT), each year more than 4000 reportable ambulance crashes result in an average of one death per week. Safe driving and use of restraints are necessary on every call. Most ambulance-related deaths among EMTs and ambulance occupants occur in the patient compartment, often when the EMT is unrestrained (**Table 2-1 and Figure 2-1**).

Case in Point

In May 2001 an EMT, age 26 years, died when her ambulance was struck head-on by a pickup truck at 6:30 AM. The EMT had been riding unrestrained in the patient compartment while attending to a patient during a nonemergency transport. During the collision, the EMT struck the front bulkhead of the patient compartment; she died en route to the hospital from blunt force trauma to the head and chest. The patient and pickup driver also sustained fatal injuries. The ambulance driver had also been driving unrestrained and had multiple serious injuries, including a fractured leg.

The NAEMT Statement on Safety Restraint Use in Emergency Medical Services notes the following:

[There is] limited study of automotive safety engineering testing, but what has been conducted has demonstrated clearly that the use of human restraint systems reduces the [likelihood] of serious injury or death to all occupants. These studies have also demonstrated a need to insure use of over-the-shoulder restraint systems for all patients as well as the securing of all equipment to prevent injury by projectile if an accident occurs.

An occupational study showed the most common injury to EMS workers, although not fatal, was "sprains, strains, and tears." The back was the body part most often injured. Learning to lift and move patients properly and maintaining physical

Table 2-1	Number of Persons Injured in Ambulance Crashes by Injury Severity and Seating Position—United States, 1991-2000		
Injury Severity/ Seating Position	**No.**	**Percent within Injury Severity Group**	**Percent of all Ambulance Occupants**
Possible			
Front left	70	41.7%	
Front right	50	29.8%	
Other enclosed*	34	20.2%	
Other/unknown	14	8.3%	
Total	**168**		**20.6%**
Nonincapacitating			
Front left	81	36.5%	
Front right	54	24.3%	
Other enclosed*	63	28.4%	
Other/unknown	24	10.8%	
Total	**222**		**27.2%**
Incapacitating			
Front left	43	32.8%	
Front right	20	15.3%	
Other enclosed*	50	38.2%	
Other/unknown	18	13.7%	
Total	**131**		**16.0%**
Fatal			
Front left	14	17.1%	
Front right	10	12.2%	
Other enclosed*	48	58.5%	
Other/unknown	10	12.2%	
Total	**82**		**10.0%**
None†	201		24.6%
Unknown†	12		1.5%

From Ambulance crash–related injuries among emergency medical services workers–United States, 1991-2002, *MMWR* 52(8):154-156, 2003.
*Inside the patient compartment.
†Sitting positions irrelevant or unavailable.

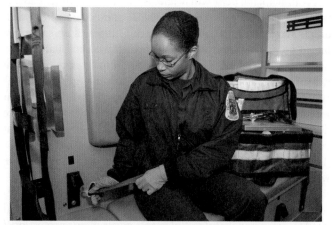

Figure 2-1 The highest risk activity for an EMT is to ride unbelted in the passenger compartment. In a crash the unbelted EMT can be projected onto the patient, putting her at risk as well.

fitness are key to preventing injuries and their accompanying disability. A regular exercise routine of aerobics, resistance training, and "stretching" can help ensure the EMT stays physically healthy. The EMT should eat a well-balanced diet of fruits, vegetables, and grains, as outlined by the US Department of Health and Human Services (HHS) (**Table 2-2**).

Other physical threats by nature of the EMT profession include exposure to communicable disease, hazardous materials, and violent situations. Knowledge about proper precautions and safe practice are key to your well-being.

LEARNING OBJECTIVES

- Discuss the importance of body substance isolation.
- Describe the steps the EMT should take for personal protection from airborne and blood-borne pathogens.
- List the personal protective equipment necessary for each of the following situations:
  - Exposure to airborne pathogens.
  - Exposure to blood-borne pathogens.

Understanding Communicable Diseases

Communicable or contagious diseases are capable of being spread from one person to another. Three elements are necessary for an infectious disease to be spread: a source, a host, and a method of spread or transmission. The common cold is a communicable disease that is well known to everyone. The **source** of the cold is a person who is infected with the cold virus. The **host** is a susceptible person who, if exposed to the source, might become ill with a cold. **Transmission** is the method by which an infectious agent or germ travels from the source to the host. With a cold, transmission might occur when the source sneezes, coughs, or talks, and droplets travel a short distance and contact the nasal mucosa (inner lining of the nose), mouth, or conjunctiva (lining of the eye) of the host. Not all infectious diseases are as benign as the cold. Some are life threatening. As an EMT, you must take precautions to prevent the spread of communicable diseases to and from your patients and others.

At times, a patient clearly has signs of infection; at other times, this may not be so clear. This explains why you should have a basic understanding of infectious diseases and take appropriate precautions for all patient contacts. You should learn how infections are spread, the body's responses when exposed to infectious agents, and actions to take before, during, and after care of an infected patient to block transmission. Armed with this knowledge and after following the guidelines in this text, you can confidently provide the necessary care to sick patients while limiting your own risk.

The precautions taken to prevent the spread of infectious disease are called *infection control*. Once learned, infection control practices become part of everyday behavior.

Infection control practices are routinely followed in hospitals and all other healthcare settings. The Centers for Disease Control and Prevention (CDC) and its associated advisory committees publish and update guidelines that help standardize infection control practices. The CDC has specifically addressed infection control guidelines for emergency workers in response

Table 2-2	Dietary Guidelines	
Food Groups	**Daily Servings**	**Serving Size**
Grains	6-11	3 or more 1-ounce equivalents, at least half from whole grains
Vegetables	3-5	About 2½ cups
Fruits	2-4	About 2 cups
Milk	2-3	About 3 cups per day of fat-free or low-fat or equivalent milk products
Meat and beans	2-3	6 ounces or less: meats, poultry, and fish 4 to 5 servings per week; nuts, seeds, and legumes

Data from US Department of Health and Human Services: *Dietary Guidelines for Americans,* Washington, DC, 2005, DHHS.

to federal law. In addition, the Occupational Safety and Health Administration (OSHA) issues guidelines regarding exposure of emergency personnel to communicable diseases in the course of their work.

Infectious Agents

Infections are caused by **microorganisms** (not visible to the naked eye) that are toxic to the body. These microorganisms include agents classified as bacteria, viruses, fungi, and parasites. Infectious agents multiply and can cause direct and indirect damage to the body. Microorganisms that can be harmful are also called *pathogens*. Not all microorganisms are harmful. For example, certain bacteria inhabit the intestine, where they aid in digestion. Other bacteria are normally found in the upper respiratory tract and on the skin surface. These same bacteria, however, can be harmful if they enter a part of the body where they are not normally found.

Some infections can be treated with medications that inhibit or kill the microorganisms. For example, many antibiotics are used to treat bacterial infections. Penicillin may be taken for a particular type of sore throat (pharyngitis) caused by streptococcal bacteria, commonly called "strep throat." Some antiviral drugs are available, but for many viral infections there is no "cure." Fortunately, many infections are successfully eliminated by the body's own immune system, even if no medication is available.

With many infections, no effective treatment exists once the infection begins. Some infections, such as polio, rubella (German measles), measles, diphtheria, tetanus (lockjaw), pertussis (whooping cough), chickenpox, and hepatitis B, can be prevented through vaccination or immunization. If no immunization or cure is available, as is currently true for acquired immunodeficiency syndrome (AIDS) and hepatitis C, preventing exposure to the microorganism is of the greatest importance.

Spread of Communicable Diseases

Infectious agents spread from a source to a host. A source of infection may be a person, an insect, an object, or another substance that carries or is contaminated by an infectious agent. A *reservoir* is a source in which infectious agents can live and multiply, such as a sewer.

After a microorganism infects a susceptible person or host, it can multiply until symptoms of the disease appear. The time between contact with an infectious agent and the onset of signs and symptoms of the disease is called the **incubation period.** During the incubation period the host may or may not be infectious to others, depending on the particular infection. The period during which a person can transmit an infectious disease to others is called the **communicable period.** The communicable period may be before, during, and even after the occurrence of symptoms of a particular disease. A **carrier** is a person who shows no signs of the disease yet harbors an infectious organism and may be a source of infection to others.

Exposure is a term used to signify coming in contact with, but not necessarily being infected by, a disease-causing agent. The *type* of exposure (how you were exposed) and the *degree* of exposure (how much you were exposed to the agent) can vary greatly, and these factors help determine whether a person is more likely to become ill. For example, the type of exposure necessary to transmit disease varies for each infectious agent. Some diseases, such as measles, can be transmitted through the air (airborne). Other diseases, such as human immunodeficiency virus (HIV), the virus that causes AIDS, are not spread through airborne contact or casual contact but require close contact, such as blood to blood or sexual intercourse for transmission.

Case in Point

Mary, 4 years old, had a cold and coughed and sneezed repeatedly during a car trip with her parents. Both John and Mira were *exposed* to the cold virus when droplets from their daughter's sneezing and coughing contacted the mucous membranes of their eyes and nose. John was not sick until 2 days later, the common *incubation* period for a cold. Then he began to sneeze and cough as well. When he did, he could spread it to others, his *communicable* period. Although exposed, Mira did not become clinically ill.

In terms of degree of exposure, a critical mass of infectious agent usually is required to cause infection. This critical number varies among agents, but in simple terms, the greater the number of microorganisms transmitted to the host, the more significant the exposure. For example, a person who receives a transfusion of contaminated blood has a greater exposure than a person who experiences a "needlestick" with a contaminated needle from the same source.

Some organisms have a greater infective potential than others. For example, hepatitis B virus is much more likely than HIV to cause infection if a healthcare worker is stuck by a needle contaminated with the virus.

Healthcare workers are exposed to patients with infectious conditions as part of their work. Infectious diseases that are spread by healthcare workers or within a healthcare setting are called *nosocomial infections* (**Box 2-2**).

Not everyone who is exposed to a source of infection becomes sick. Understanding which factors and conditions of an exposure can lead to actual infection is part of infection control. These factors include the following:
- Mode of transmission
- Type and duration of contact
- Host susceptibility
- Whether appropriate precautions were used

Box 2-2   Nosocomial Infections

Nosocomial infections (Latin *nosocomium,* "hospital," or Greek *nosokomos,* "one who tends the sick") occur or originate in a hospital or healthcare setting (e.g., ambulance). Nosocomial infections occur between the patient and EMT during a direct patient encounter or indirectly with another EMT or patient by contact with droplets (coughing in an ED hallway) or touching contaminated objects or by airborne transmission. Because people with severe infections are likely to seek medical attention, health care is a high-risk setting for spreading disease, and infection control practices must be closely followed to prevent transmission to others. For example, almost 200 relatives and health workers became ill with the Ebola virus in an African hospital from contact with patients' body secretions, but spread stopped when infection control practices were closely followed and the hospital was resupplied with adequate stock of protective equipment and disinfectants.

Mode of Transmission

The CDC and the Hospital Infection Control Practices Advisory Committee regularly update strategies (e.g., Recommendations for Isolation Precautions in Hospitals) to prevent transmission of infections in health settings. The following description is adapted from these sources for EMTs. The modes of transmission include contact, droplet, airborne, vector, and vehicle (**Figure 2-2**).

Contact Transmission. Contact transmission is the most important and most frequent means of transmission of nosocomial infection and can be divided into two groups: direct and indirect.

Direct Contact. Direct contact involves direct physical transfer between a susceptible host and an infected person. Examples include situations where EMTs move or lift patients, apply dressings, or perform other procedures requiring direct personal contact. Caring for patients generally involves some direct contact.

Indirect Contact. Indirect contact involves personal contact of the susceptible host with a contaminated intermediate object (e.g., instruments, dressings, other infected material) or with contaminated hands that are not washed or gloves that are not changed between patients. If proper care is not taken, personnel can contaminate objects when assembling or handling equipment used for patient care.

A common example of indirect contact is a person with a cold sneezing into his hands and then opening a door. When another person touches the doorknob and then brings the hand to her eye or nostril, exposure to the cold virus occurs by indirect contact.

Several steps may be involved in contact transmission. For example, someone with an active eye infection (conjunctivitis) touches his hand to the infected eye and sometime later shakes another person's hand. This second person now rubs her own eye, thus placing the infectious agent in the eye. This scenario actually occurred in a hospital where conjunctivitis developed in almost 200 people. Many colds also are transmitted in this way (from mouth or nose of an infected person to another's hand, and from this person's hand to mouth or nose). Obviously, handwashing between patient contacts is an essential step in infection control.

Droplet Transmission. Infectious agents may come in contact with the conjunctivae, nose, or mouth of a susceptible person as a result of droplets expelled in coughing, sneezing, or talking by an infected person. This is considered "contact" transmission because droplets usually travel no more than about 3 feet (0.9 meter). Because of this limitation, "close contact" is used to refer to a distance within 3 feet of an infected person. Influenza ("the flu") can be spread by droplet transmission.

Special barrier precautions such as masks are used to prevent droplet transmission. For example, you should wear a mask when working within 3 feet of the patient. A mask should be placed on the patient if he or she will be moved, to limit spread of infection by droplets (e.g., after arrival at emergency department when patient is taken from ambulance and transferred to examination room).

Airborne Transmission. Airborne transmission occurs by the dissemination (to spread or disperse widely) of either droplet nuclei (small-particle residue [≤5 μm in size] of evaporated droplets containing microorganisms that may remain suspended in the air for long periods) or dust particles in the air that contain the infectious agent. Microorganisms carried in this manner can be spread by air currents and inhaled by a susceptible host in the same room or over a longer distance. *Because airborne particles are so small, a special mask is worn for protection by healthcare providers.* Special air handling and ventilation also are required to prevent airborne transmission. The agent is initially spread by talking, sneezing, and coughing. Surgical masks or even oxygen masks worn by a patient reduce transmission by blocking the droplets generated by the patient from entering the air.

Vehicle Transmission. The vehicle route applies to diseases transmitted through contaminated items, such as food, water, medications, devices, or equipment used by hospital workers.

Vector Transmission. **Vectors** carry agents that transmit disease. Vectors can be insects, animals, or inanimate objects. Lyme disease, spread by the deer tick, is an example of a vector-borne disease that is endemic to many areas of the United States. Tularemia is transmitted by contact with blood or body parts of infected animals or insects and is sometimes called "rabbit fever" and "deerfly fever." Malaria is a disease transmitted by mosquitoes. The control of this type of disease is sometimes related to elimination of the vector (e.g., use of insecticides to eliminate mosquitoes).

Type and Duration of Contact

The type and duration of contact are factors that influence the chance of illness after exposure. For example, injecting an infectious agent into the blood represents a more serious exposure than spilling the same agent on the intact skin. A cough directly into your face creates more risk for significant exposure from droplet transmission than if you are 5 feet away. Wearing clothing soaked with blood for an hour during patient care and transport represents a more significant exposure than a splash of blood on intact skin that is washed off minutes later.

Transmission and Infection Control

Major objectives of infection control practices include (1) recognizing the importance of all body fluids, secretions, and excretions in the transmission of infectious diseases in the healthcare setting and (2) having adequate precautions to prevent

MODES OF TRANSMISSION

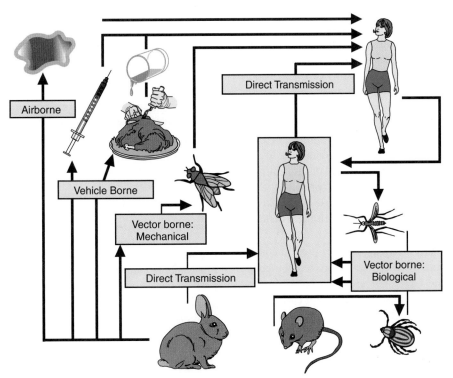

Figure 2-2 Common modes of transmission.

infections transmitted by the airborne, droplet, and contact routes of transmission.

Standard Precautions

Standard precautions should be taken as the first step in infection control, and these measures should be used with every patient. Standard precautions incorporate both *universal* (blood and body fluid) *precautions* (designed to reduce the risk of transmission of blood-borne pathogens) and *body substance isolation* (designed to reduce the risk of transmission of pathogens from moist body substances). Standard precautions apply to blood; all body fluids, secretions, and excretions (except sweat), regardless of whether they contain visible blood; nonintact skin; and mucous membranes. Standard precautions are used in all situations to avoid transmission from both recognized and unrecognized sources of infection in prehospital care.

Transmission-Based Precautions

Transmission-based precautions are used for patients with documented or suspected infection with highly transmissible or important pathogens for which additional precautions beyond standard precautions are warranted. The strategies are specific to different modes of transmission and include airborne precautions, droplet precautions, and contact precautions.

Factors Affecting Infection

Again, not everyone who comes in contact with an infectious agent contracts an infectious disease. In fact, most people do not. Factors that lessen the chance of infection are resistance and immunity. One's ability to fight off infection after exposure to infectious agents is called *resistance.*

Immunity

Immunity is the body's ability to resist infection after exposure to an infectious agent. The body may counteract infectious agents with antibodies or special cells. Beyond the ability of an individual's natural defense system, immunity can be gained by several means. For example, infants have antibodies from the mother that protect them against many common diseases for several months after birth.

Vaccination is a means of acquiring immunity. Vaccines contain microorganisms that are killed or weakened so that exposure to the vaccine is enough to stimulate the immune system but not enough to cause disease. This "primes" the immune system to produce antibodies and defense factors so that the body can respond later to an infection with that particular microorganism.

Vaccination is a standard method currently used to control disease in the world. Standard vaccinations are recommended for all individuals by the CDC. For example, recommended schedules for active immunization of infants and children include vaccinations for polio, diphtheria, tetanus, pertussis, measles, mumps, rubella, varicella (chickenpox), *Haemophilus influenzae,* and hepatitis B. Other vaccinations exist and are recommended on a case-by-case basis. EMTs are among those healthcare workers advised to receive immunization against hepatitis B, influenza (flu), measles, mumps, rubella, and

varicella because they are vaccine preventable and are known to be transmitted in the healthcare setting (**Figure 2-3**).

A person can also acquire immunity to a particular infection from actually having that infection. For example, a person who has had rubella, or German measles, usually is immune and does not contract this disease again if reexposed. Thus, you can become immune to rubella, either through actually having the disease itself or through vaccination against the disease. If you have had the infection, you do not need the vaccine. A person's immune status to diseases such as rubella can be checked with a blood test.

Passive immunity to certain diseases can be conveyed to an exposed individual by injection of antibodies (called immune globulin). So called because it is not produced by the body but injected into it, passive immunity is offered if there has been a high-risk exposure of an unprotected individual. For example, tetanus or hepatitis B antibodies can be given to exposed and susceptible individuals. These persons are considered to be susceptible if their tetanus shots (vaccine) are not up-to-date or if they have not received the hepatitis B vaccine series.

High-Risk Individuals

Some individuals are at high risk for infection because their general health status is poor, their immune system is compromised, natural barriers have been damaged (as in a patient who has sustained burns), or they have had significant exposure.

As an EMT, you are at risk for multiple and more significant exposures than the average person because you care for patients every day. You must also take precautions not to spread disease to your patients. For example, although young, healthy EMTs may not be at high risk for complications of influenza, an elderly or debilitated patient for whom they care can contract it from the EMT and develop fatal complications. Therefore, healthcare workers are advised to obtain the influenza vaccine because of concern for their patients and are advised not to work when they have the flu. General knowledge about how infectious diseases are spread will allow you to practice in a manner that minimizes risk of transmission while a patient is under your care.

REAL*World*

Children and elderly persons both have an increased susceptibility to illness. Children have immature, developing immune systems that are not yet strong enough to fight common infections. For example, the respiratory syncytial virus (RSV) in a healthy adult may cause a runny nose and cough, whereas in a young child, RSV can be lethal, causing severe respiratory distress. Geriatric patients have immune systems that are beginning to slow down. They have a more difficult time recovering from an exposure, resulting in longer illnesses and additional complications. Illnesses such as pneumonia and the flu can cause a geriatric patient to be hospitalized and may result in death.

Specific Communicable Diseases

As an EMT, you do not need to be able to diagnose a specific disease to provide high-quality prehospital care. However, you should understand some of the most frequently encountered conditions and appreciate the range of possible diseases, the

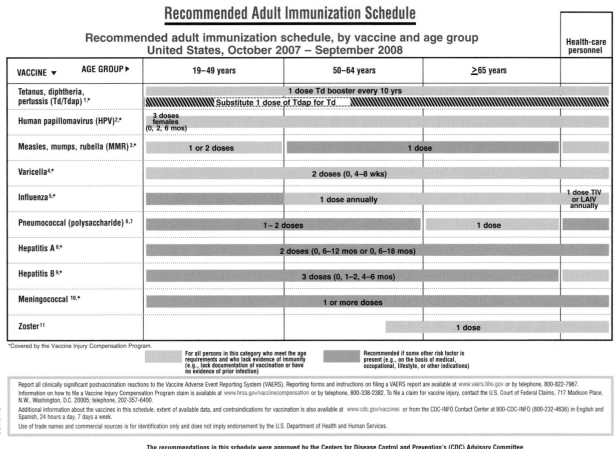

Recommended Adult Immunization Schedule

Recommended adult immunization schedule, by vaccine and age group
United States, October 2007 – September 2008

VACCINE ▼ AGE GROUP ▶	19–49 years	50–64 years	≥65 years	Health-care personnel
Tetanus, diphtheria, pertussis (Td/Tdap) [1,*]	1 dose Td booster every 10 yrs / Substitute 1 dose of Tdap for Td			
Human papillomavirus (HPV) [2,*]	3 doses females (0, 2, 6 mos)			
Measles, mumps, rubella (MMR) [3,*]	1 or 2 doses	1 dose		
Varicella [4,*]	2 doses (0, 4–8 wks)			
Influenza [5,*]		1 dose annually		1 dose TIV or LAIV annually
Pneumococcal (polysaccharide) [6,7]	1–2 doses		1 dose	
Hepatitis A [8,*]	2 doses (0, 6–12 mos or 0, 6–18 mos)			
Hepatitis B [9,*]	3 doses (0, 1–2, 4–6 mos)			
Meningococcal [10,*]	1 or more doses			
Zoster [11]			1 dose	

*Covered by the Vaccine Injury Compensation Program.

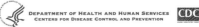 For all persons in this category who meet the age requirements and who lack evidence of immunity (e.g., lack documentation of vaccination or have no evidence of prior infection)

Recommended if some other risk factor is present (e.g., on the basis of medical, occupational, lifestyle, or other indications)

Report all clinically significant postvaccination reactions to the Vaccine Adverse Event Reporting System (VAERS). Reporting forms and instructions on filing a VAERS report are available at www.vaers.hhs.gov or by telephone, 800-822-7967.

Information on how to file a Vaccine Injury Compensation Program claim is available at www.hrsa.gov/vaccinecompensation or by telephone, 800-338-2382. To file a claim for vaccine injury, contact the U.S. Court of Federal Claims, 717 Madison Place, N.W., Washington, D.C. 20005; telephone, 202-357-6400.

Additional information about the vaccines in this schedule, extent of available data, and contraindications for vaccination is also available at www.cdc.gov/vaccines or from the CDC-INFO Contact Center at 800-CDC-INFO (800-232-4636) in English and Spanish, 24 hours a day, 7 days a week.

Use of trade names and commercial sources is for identification only and does not imply endorsement by the U.S. Department of Health and Human Services.

CS115143

The recommendations in this schedule were approved by the Centers for Disease Control and Prevention's (CDC) Advisory Committee on Immunization Practices (ACIP), the American Academy of Family Physicians (AAFP), the American College of Obstetricians and Gynecologists (ACOG), and the American College of Physicians (ACP).

DEPARTMENT OF HEALTH AND HUMAN SERVICES   CDC
CENTERS FOR DISEASE CONTROL AND PREVENTION

These schedules indicate the recommended age groups and medical indications for which administration of currently licensed vaccines is commonly indicated for adults ages 19 years and older, as of October 1, 2007. Licensed combination vaccines may be used whenever any components of the combination are indicated and when the vaccine's other components are not contraindicated. For detailed recommendations on all vaccines, including those used primarily for travelers or that are issued during the year, consult the manufacturers' package inserts and the complete statements from the Advisory Committee on Immunization Practices (www.cdc.gov/vaccines/pubs/acip-list.htm).

Figure 2-3 Vaccination card. *Data from Centers for Disease Control and Prevention:* Recommended adult immunization schedule by vaccine and medical and other indications, United States, October 2006-September 2007, *US Department of Health and Human Services.*

---

importance of infection control, and the relatively low risk of exposure if safe practice patterns are followed.

Fever and chills are common responses to infections. Rashes are seen with many infectious diseases. Some rashes, such as those seen in chickenpox, may be filled with infectious particles and can spread the disease by direct contact.

Cough and sputum can be present with bacterial pneumonia, an upper respiratory tract infection, or tuberculosis. Fever and flank pain are typical of a kidney infection. Fever with a severe headache or a stiff neck, with or without an altered mental status, suggests meningitis. **Table 2-3** provides infection control guidelines for several diseases of concern.

Blood-Borne Diseases

Diseases transmitted by contact with blood carrying an infectious agent are referred to as *blood-borne diseases.* As an EMT, you will come into contact with the blood or blood-tinged body fluids of others when you care for bleeding patients. Therefore, blood-borne infections are of special concern to the EMT.

Acquired Immunodeficiency Syndrome. AIDS was first described in 1982 as a disease of unknown cause that resulted in a defect of cell-mediated immunity. Immunity to many bacterial infections is linked to the production of antibodies (molecules that render the agent harmless). Immunity to fungi, parasites, and other, more unusual infections is mediated or linked primarily through a process called *cell-mediated immunity.* Because of this particular type of impaired immunity, patients with AIDS are susceptible to unusual infections not seen in healthy individuals.

After an extensive search, a virus (HIV) found to be the cause of AIDS was isolated. This virus lives in blood, lymph tissue, and certain other body fluids, and over time it causes the body to lose its natural defenses against disease. When this happens, the body is open to attack by a wide range of illnesses, from mild to life-threatening infections, and an increased occurrence of certain types of tumors.

A common type of pneumonia seen in patients with AIDS that is rarely seen in healthy individuals is *Pneumocystis carinii* pneumonia (PCP).

The most common tumor seen in patients with AIDS is Kaposi's sarcoma, a cancer that affects the skin and the lining of blood vessels. This tumor typically spreads throughout the

Table 2-3   New York State Department of Health Infection Control Guidelines for Prehospital Care Services

Infection	Mode of Transmission	Recommended Precautions	Exposure Follow-up	Relative Risk in EMT Setting
AIDS/HIV (human immunodeficiency virus)	Needlestick, blood splash into mucous membranes (e.g., eyes, mouth), or blood contact of open wound Close contact	Standard precautions for prevention of blood-borne diseases	Scrub exposed area with soap and water. Contact infection control or infectious disease personnel at local hospital if exposure involved blood contact with broken skin, mucous membrane, or needlestick	Low
Chickenpox	Respiratory secretions and contact with moist vesicles Contact, droplet, and airborne	Not a problem for persons who are immune Varicella vaccine for those who are not immune Careful handwashing after contact with moist lesions Persons who are susceptible should avoid contact	Persons who are not immune (i.e., have not had chickenpox) should avoid contact with other susceptible persons who would be at risk for complications (e.g., cancer patients) from days 10-21 after exposure. There is no risk of spread to others (e.g., children at home) until the exposed, susceptible person develops chickenpox	None if immune; significant if not immune
Common cold	Contact with respiratory secretions Contact and droplet	Handwashing Avoid contact of infectious materials with eyes, nose, or mouth	None	Unknown; probably significant if in early stages
Diarrhea *Campylobacter* *Cryptosporidium* *Giardia* *Salmonella* *Shigella* Viral *Yersinia*	Fecal/oral contact	Gloves for direct contact with stool (feces) Handwashing	Contact personal physician if symptoms develop	Unknown; probably low, providing hands are washed after contact with stool
Epiglottitis caused by *Haemophilus influenzae* (usually seen in very young children)	Contact with respiratory secretions Contact, droplet	Masks on crew where possible Do not try to put a mask on a child	Contact infection control or infectious disease personnel at local hospital Rifampin prophylaxis may be recommended if there has been intimate (e.g., mouth-to-mouth) contact with respiratory secretions	Unknown; probably low
German measles (rubella)	Respiratory droplets and contact with respiratory secretions Contact, droplet	Rubella vaccine for nonimmune persons to eliminate risk from potential exposure Masks for susceptible persons	Susceptible persons should avoid contact with other susceptible persons from days 7-21 after exposure Pregnant women who are not immune to rubella should contact their obstetrician	Unknown; susceptible persons are at increased risk
Hepatitis A	Fecal/oral contact	Gloves for direct contact with stool (feces) Handwashing	Contact infection control or infectious disease personnel at local hospital regarding immune (gamma globulin) prophylaxis	Minimal

Disease	Transmission	Prevention	Management	Risk
Hepatitis B	Needlestick, blood splash into mucous membranes (e.g., eye or mouth), or blood contact of open wound. Possible exposure during mouth-to-mouth resuscitation contact	Universal Precautions or prevention of blood-borne disease. Hepatitis B immunization	Hepatitis B immune globulin and hepatitis B vaccine for persons who have not previously received the vaccine or are otherwise immune	Significant (6%-30% chance) if exposed to blood of a hepatitis B carrier and no preexposure or postexposure prophylaxis is provided
Hepatitis C	As with hepatitis B	As with hepatitis B	Role of immune globulin not clear. Contact infection control	Unknown; probably low
Herpes simplex (cold sores)	Contact of mucous membrane with moist lesions; fingers are at particular risk for becoming infected. Contact	Gloves for contact with moist lesions. Handwashing	None	Unknown; probably significant if lesions are present (most people have antibodies)
Herpes zoster (shingles) localized, disseminated (see chickenpox)	Contact with moist lesions. Contact	Not a problem for persons who have had chickenpox. Handwashing after contact with moist lesions	Observe for symptoms if susceptible to chickenpox	Localized; very low and only if a person has not had chickenpox
Influenza	Droplet, airborne	Masks may help reduce exposure. Influenza vaccine	None	Unknown; probably significant during flu epidemics
Legionnaires' disease	No person-to-person transmission	None	None	None
Lice: head, body, pubic	Close head-to-head contact; both body and pubic lice require intimate contact (usually sexual) or sharing of intimate clothing. Contact	Handwashing. Avoid head-to-head contact if head lice present. Body and pubic lice not a problem in this setting	*Head lice:* Observe for nits on hair shafts. Contact physician if significant exposure occurred for consideration of prophylactic shampoo. *Body or pubic lice:* None	Unknown; head may be significant. Body and pubic lice probably not a risk
Measles	Respiratory droplets and contact with nasal or throat secretions; highly communicable. Contact, droplet, airborne	Measles vaccine if no prior history of disease. Masks are not likely to be of significant benefit. Persons susceptible to measles should avoid contact, if possible	Measles immunity should be checked. If susceptible, measles vaccine should be administered and contact with other susceptible persons from the 5th through the 21st day after exposure and/or 7 days after the rash appears should be avoided. Notify the health department	Unknown; probably significant if lesions are present (most people have antibodies)

Continued

Table 2-3 New York State Department of Health Infection Control Guidelines for Prehospital Care Services—Cont'd

Infection	Mode of Transmission	Recommended Precautions	Exposure Follow-up	Relative Risk in EMT Setting
Meningitis *Meningococcus* *Haemophilus influenzae* (usually seen in very young children)	Contact with respiratory secretions Contact, droplet Contact with respiratory secretions Contact, droplet	Masks on crew for close contact Masks on crew where possible Do not try to put a mask on a child	An antibiotic prophylaxis for persons who have given mouth-to-mouth ventilation to a confirmed case Contact infection control or infectious disease personnel at local hospital. An antibiotic prophylaxis may be recommended if there has been intimate (e.g., mouth-to-mouth) contact with respiratory secretions	Unknown; probably low unless mouth-to-mouth ventilation is done Unknown; probably low
Viral	Fecal/oral contact	Thorough handwashing after contact with feces	Contact personal physician if symptoms develop	Unknown; probably low
Mumps (infectious parotitis)	Repiratory droplets and contact with saliva Contact, droplet	Mumps vaccine if no prior history of having disease	If susceptible to mumps, e.g., never had the disease or vaccine, avoid contact with other susceptible persons from the 12th to 26th day after exposure or until 9 days after development of mumps	Unknown; most adults are immune
Scabies	Close body contact Contact	Wash hands and arms carefully after contact	Observe for symptoms (itching, tiny linear burrows or "tracks," vesicles, particularly around fingers, wrists, elbows, and skin folds) and contact physician	Unknown; probably low
Tuberculosis, pulmonary	Airborne	Mask on patient if diagnosis of pulmonary tuberculosis is suspected*	Baseline PPD for previously negative reactors with second PPD in 3 months. Converters to a positive reaction should be seen for medical follow-up	Unknown; depends on level of patient's infectivity and contact time. Most transmission occurs in household setting where duration of exposure is extended
Wounds, infected and draining	Contact—more of a concern for cross-contamination	Wear gloves for contact with infected areas Handwashing	None	Probably none

Modified from *A prehospital care provider's guide to AIDS*, Albany, 1990, New York State Department of Health. Updated with Standard Precautions and Transmission-Based Precautions. *HIV*, Human immunodeficiency virus; *AIDS*, acquired immunodeficiency syndrome; *PPD*, purified protein derivative (tuberculin); *EMT*, emergency medical technician.
*EMTs should use a high-efficiency particulate air (HEPA) mask.

body. HIV also can infect the central nervous system (CNS), causing many different neurologic problems.

Of critical importance to the EMT is that individuals who appear healthy may be infected with the AIDS virus (HIV) for many years with no clinical symptoms. Because no clues point to the presence of infection during this phase, and because anyone may become infected with the virus, it is safest to use standard precautions for all patients.

Human immunodeficiency virus is transmitted by direct contact with body fluids. Common high-risk modes of transmission include the following:

- Needle sharing among intravenous (IV) drug abusers.
- Needlesticks or transfusion of HIV-infected blood or blood products.
- Sexual contact—anal, vaginal, or oral.
- During pregnancy and childbirth, when the mother may transmit HIV infection to the newborn (maternal-to-fetal route).

Human immunodeficiency virus is not transmitted by air or casual contact. The sharing of food, utensils, and water; social contact; contact with nasal or oral secretions through kissing, coughing, or sneezing; sweat; and contact with tears, urine, vomitus, or feces have not been shown to transmit HIV. In addition, toilet seats, bathtubs, showers, handshakes, clothing, linens, and other inanimate objects (other than contaminated needles) are not sources of transmission.

Hepatitis. Hepatitis is an infection of the liver caused by different types of viruses. Hepatitis A virus is spread by oral-fecal routes and is sometimes called "infectious hepatitis." Hepatitis B is contracted in the same manner as described for AIDS. In addition, hepatitis B virus (HBV) can be transmitted by the saliva of an infected person through a bite. Hepatitis C, the most common chronic blood-borne viral infection in the United States, is usually transmitted by blood-borne exposure and less often through sexual contact.

Hepatitis B is of concern to healthcare workers. The CDC estimates that approximately 200,000 new HBV infections occur in the United States each year, and that an estimated 1.25 million Americans are chronically infected with the virus. Patients with chronic infection are at increased risk for chronic liver disease, cirrhosis, and liver cancer.

Precautionary measures taken by EMTs to avoid HBV infection are the same as those taken to avoid HIV. In addition, a vaccination against HBV (90% effective) is available and is recommended for all EMTs. After a possible exposure, passive and active immunity is available that offers some protection against infection. Hepatitis C is also of growing concern to healthcare workers. Currently no vaccine is available to protect against hepatitis C.

Following standard precautions and taking care regarding needlestick injuries are important steps to avoid transmission of these blood-borne pathogens.

Respiratory Secretions and Airborne Exposures

Several diseases of concern to the EMT are spread by respiratory secretions or airborne contact.

Meningitis. Meningitis, or infection of the meninges (the covering of the CNS), can be caused by a virus, a bacterium,

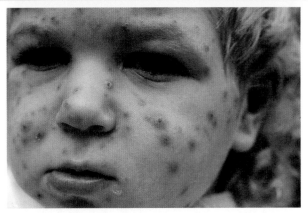

Figure 2-4 Chickenpox is a common communicable disease that is highly contagious. Distinguishing features include the presence of raised, fluid-filled, and crusted regions, all in the same area of the body.

or other organisms. Meningitis can occur with or after a respiratory infection. Meningitis is common in communal environments such as college dormitories. There is a vaccine that can help prevent some forms of the disease. If contracted, the bacterial form can be treated with antibiotics. The viral form is usually allowed to run its course. Symptoms include fever, headache, stiff neck, and altered mental status.

The meningococcus *Neisseria meningitidis* and, to a lesser degree, *H. influenzae* can cause meningitis and are of some concern in cases of close contact with a patient's respiratory secretions and droplets. Follow-up is recommended, and postexposure antibiotics are given in the event of intensive, unprotected contact (not wearing a mask) with infected patients. Close-contact situations that may increase the chance of droplet transmission can occur with mouth-to-mouth resuscitation, close examination of the mouth and nose, endotracheal intubation, or opening or suctioning of the airway. Certain types of viral meningitis can also be spread by fecal-oral routes. Personnel caring for patients with meningitis can decrease their risk by following droplet precautions.

Chickenpox. Chickenpox is a very contagious disease caused by the *varicella* virus. It is spread by respiratory secretions, by contact with the moist vesicles (raised, fluid-filled lesions; **Figure 2-4**), and through the air. Because the disease is so contagious, most adults have had chickenpox during childhood. As an EMT, you should take appropriate precautions with a known or suspected case. If two EMTs are present on the call and one does not know his or her immune status but the other has known immunity, it is safer for the EMT with known immunity to conduct direct patient care.

The same virus, varicella, causes zoster, or "shingles," which usually occurs in patients who have had chickenpox in the past. *Zoster* is a varicella infection along one sensory nerve route, causing pain followed by eruption of the flat, red lesions that quickly become fluid filled (vesicles) and then scab over as in chickenpox. The striking feature of zoster infection is that the distribution of the pain and the rash is along a solitary nerve route.

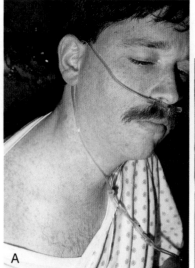
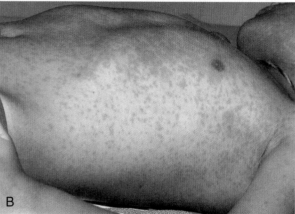

Figure 2-5 **A,** Patient with measles and complications of shortness of breath who required supplemental oxygen and hospitalization. **B,** Child with typical rash of measles on the trunk and face. Discrete lesions are seen on the trunk. These lesions became so multiple on the face that they merged and appeared as one continuous lesion. *Courtesy Dr. Mark Henry.*

Varicella and *variola,* the virus that causes smallpox, are related. A resurgence of interest in smallpox has occurred because of bioterrorism threats (see Chapter 30).

REALWorld

In March 1995 the U.S. Food and Drug Administration (FDA) approved a vaccine to prevent chickenpox (varicella), and in 2005 it was added to the mumps, measles, and rubella (MMR) vaccine, creating the MMRV. Almost all states require the MMRV before a child can begin school, artificially exposing children to the varicella virus early. In immunized areas there has been a dramatic decrease in the number of cases of chickenpox. The vaccine can prevent chickenpox, but patients can still develop shingles.

Measles. Measles, another highly contagious disease, is spread by respiratory droplets and contact with nasal secretions, as well as through the air (**Figure 2-5**). Because "childhood" viruses are generally much worse in adulthood, EMTs should be adequately immunized against them and avoid contact when possible if they have no immunity. Strategies to prevent spread of measles include documentation of immunity in healthcare workers, isolation of patients with fever and rash, and airborne precautions for suspected and proven cases of measles and for patients with fever and rash when the diagnosis is unclear.

Rubella (German Measles). Respiratory droplets and contact with secretions also spread rubella. Women who are pregnant or who are not sure whether they are pregnant should avoid patients with rubella. Healthcare workers are urged to know whether they are immunized against rubella.

Tuberculosis. Tuberculosis is once again a disease of great concern, in part because of AIDS. As an EMT, you should be aware of its existence. The disease is spread by droplet and airborne transmission. Patients with active tuberculosis can be given a mask to wear to block its spread. To prevent airborne exposure, you should wear a special **high-efficiency particulate air (HEPA) respirator** mask if tuberculosis is suspected or has

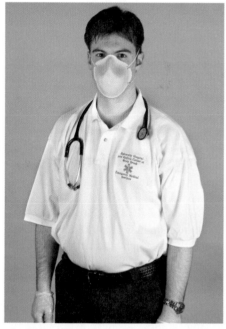

Figure 2-6 The high-efficiency particulate air (HEPA) respirator provides protection against airborne diseases such as tuberculosis, measles, and chickenpox.

been diagnosed (**Figure 2-6**). The HEPA respirator requires a fit test to ensure proper fit and use. Checking for exposure to tuberculosis is part of a physical examination for healthcare workers. This often involves the purified protein derivative (PPD, tuberculin) skin test.

Close Contact

Lice and Scabies. Lice can infect the head, body, or pubic area (**Figure 2-7**). Close contact is required for transmission. Scabies, usually first noted about the fingers, is also spread by close

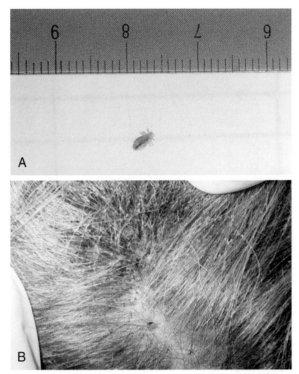

Figure 2-7 **A,** *Pediculus humanus,* or head louse, seen against a millimeter ruler. **B,** Lice, visible in scalp of patient. Eggs, or nits, are also seen along the hair follicles. Nits are seen as small, oval, white objects along the shaft of the hair. *P. humanus* is extremely contagious through direct contact with hair, clothing, or combs of an affected person.

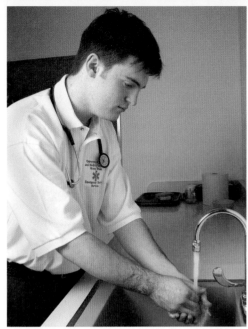

Figure 2-8 Handwashing is the most important measure for blocking the spread of infection. Vigorous scrubbing for 10 to 15 seconds with regular soap, followed by a rinse and drying with paper towels, is recommended.

contact. Although these two conditions are caused by separate agents, they both cause itching and are cured with the same treatment.

Multidrug-Resistant Infections

Patients who have been hospitalized or who recently stayed in a facility (e.g., nursing home) and who have pathogens resistant to multiple antibiotics, especially patients with wound, skin, or urinary infections, should have contact precautions. You may obtain this history from nurses or physicians when called to transport a patient. Contact transmission precautions should be used in addition to standard precautions in these situations. You should wear gloves plus gown, mask, and goggles if the patient is coughing or you are in close contact with possible droplet spread before you enter the environment, and you should change when you leave the facility, before you enter the ambulance, and again in the emergency department (ED) to limit the chance of spreading the bacteria. Knowing how infectious diseases are spread allows EMTs to better understand the need for practicing infection control.

Infection Control

Personal Health Status

The first step in infection control is to determine your personal health status through physical examination and review of your immunization history and status. You should be immunized

in accord with current recommendations to minimize your chances of contracting and spreading infectious diseases.

Your health status should be evaluated periodically. Good health and up-to-date immunizations minimize risks for yourself and your patients. Records of immunizations and personal health status should be available to your medical director for protection of yourself and patients. These records, which should be confidential, are important sources of information should questions regarding exposure arise.

You should not work if you have an illness that may be contagious to patients. Check with your physician or medical director if you have questions about the risk you may present to patients.

Personal Health and Safety Education

An ongoing personal health and safety education program is an essential component of infection control. Knowing about medical practices and updates keeps you aware of hazards and opportunities to reduce risk and improve care. Ongoing continuing medical education programs involve instruction from infection control experts from local hospitals and updates from the CDC and OSHA.

Blocking Spread of Infection

Handwashing. Handwashing remains the most important measure for blocking the spread of infection (**Figure 2-8**). Hands and exposed skin should be washed immediately (as soon as possible) if they are contaminated with blood, body fluids, or potentially contaminated articles and after gloves are removed. You should always wash your hands using ordinary soaps after patient contact and before caring for another patient. A 10- to

15-second scrub reduces the greatest source of transmission of germs. Hands should not be washed in food preparation areas. Paper towels or hand blowers should be used to dry your hands. Lever-operated towel dispensers should be activated before beginning handwashing. If you need to turn off the running water with your hands, you should use the paper towel to avoid secondary contamination.

When handwashing facilities are not available, alcohol-based handrubs and detergent-containing towelettes can be used to clean your hands. When hands are not soiled with dirt or heavily contaminated with blood or other organic material, alcohol-based agents should be used. If your hands are soiled, you should use detergent-based towelettes to cleanse your hands and then use the alcohol-based handrubs for antisepsis, following the manufacturer's instructions.

Aseptic Technique. EMTs should practice *aseptic* (free from germs) technique, especially when caring for open wounds or handling sterile materials that enter the skin or touch normally sterile parts of the body. For example, caution is needed to avoid contaminating a sterile dressing before applying it to an open wound or a needle used to inject epinephrine.

The EMT should ensure that equipment and the ambulance are properly cleaned, disinfected, or sterilized. The level of cleaning required is dictated by the intended use of the equipment. For example, HIV is destroyed by many chemical disinfectants, such as 70% alcohol, hydrogen peroxide, glutaraldehyde, quaternary ammonium chlorides, formalin, germ-killing spray (e.g., Lysol), iodine, and chlorhexidine gluconate–ethanol mix. In addition, fresh solutions, prepared daily, of household bleach (5.25% sodium hypochlorite) in dilutions between 1:10 and 1:100, are effective depending on the amount of organic material (e.g., blood, mucus) present on the surface to be cleaned and disinfected. These agents are capable of viral inactivation within 1 to 10 minutes. Soap and water also readily inactivate the virus, as does exposure to drying. When you use chemical disinfectants, you should understand any special precautions required for any agent you use, including safety precautions, because some disinfectants require special handling (e.g., use of fume hoods).

Universal Precautions. Now part of standard precautions, **universal precautions** refer to the approach to body substances and fluids that may carry a blood-borne pathogen. *Because the EMT cannot tell from outward appearance who is a carrier, the wisest approach is to apply precautions to every (universal) situation.* Blood, semen, vaginal secretions, and body fluids that surround the lungs, heart, brain, joints, abdominal organs, and fetus are included. Breast milk has been linked to cases in infants, acquired through breastfeeding. Other substances, such as urine, feces, nasal secretions, sputum, sweat, tears, and vomitus, are unlikely to contribute to blood-borne infection unless they are mixed with blood. However, because other diseases can be spread through these fluids, use of barrier precautions and handling of all body fluids as potentially infectious is wise.

Personal Protective Equipment. **Personal protective equipment (PPE)** consists of barriers to prevent direct contact with blood or other fluids. Such gear should be routinely available for EMTs to provide **body substance isolation (Figure 2-9).**

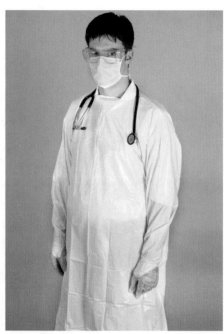

Figure 2-9 Personal protective equipment, including eyewear, masks, gowns, and gloves, should be available to EMTs at all times to provide adequate body substance isolation.

Gloves. Gloves must be standard equipment. Different gloves are required for different purposes, as follows:
- Heavy gloves that meet OSHA requirements should be used for situations involving sharp edges or broken glass.
- Regular disposable medical gloves can be used in most situations.
- Sterile disposable medical gloves should be used for labor and delivery or caring for patients with burn wounds.
- Utility gloves should be used for cleaning vehicles and equipment.

Gloves should be worn in patient care settings for the following reasons.
1. Gloves provide a protective barrier and prevent gross contamination of the hands when touching blood, body fluids, secretions, excretions, mucous membranes, and nonintact skin. The wearing of gloves in specific situations to reduce risk of exposure to blood-borne pathogens is mandated by the OSHA blood-borne pathogens rule.
2. Gloves reduce the likelihood of transmitting microorganisms on the hands to patients during patient care procedures or when touching a patient's mucous membranes or nonintact skin.
3. Gloves reduce the likelihood that the hands of the EMT will transfer microorganisms from one patient to another patient. Gloves are changed between patients and the hands washed after gloves are removed. Failure to change gloves between patient contacts is an infection control hazard.

Wearing gloves does not replace the need for handwashing because gloves may have small defects or be torn during use, and hands can become contaminated during removal of the gloves. Hands should be washed with soap and water or alcohol-based agents after gloves are removed. The EMT should avoid touching personal items (e.g., combs) when wearing gloves.

Table 2-4 Recommended Personal Protective Equipment for Worker Protection against Infectious Disease Transmission in Prehospital Settings

Task or Activity	Disposable Gloves	Gown	Mask	Protective Eyewear
Bleeding control with spurting blood	Yes	Yes	Yes	Yes
Bleeding control with minimal bleeding	Yes	No	No	No
Emergency childbirth	Yes	Yes	Yes, if splashing is likely	Yes, if splashing is likely
Blood drawing	Yes	No	No	No
Starting an intravenous (IV) line	Yes	No	No	No
Endotracheal intubation/dual-lumen airway use	Yes	No	No, unless splashing is likely	No, unless splashing is likely
Oral/nasal suctioning, manually cleaning airway	Yes	No	No, unless splashing is likely	No, unless splashing is likely
Handling and cleaning instruments with microbial contamination	Yes	No, unless soiling is likely	No	No
Measuring blood pressure	Yes	No	No	No
Measuring temperature	Yes	No	No	No
Giving an injection	Yes	No	No	No

Data from *MMWR* 38(S6):3-37, 1989 (supplements).

If you have reusable gloves that have become contaminated with body fluids, you should wash them with soap and water, wipe them with disinfectant, and hang them in an inverted position to air-dry.

REAL*World*

Many patients have an allergy to latex. Latex is a common material used to make disposable gloves. If an EMT wearing latex gloves were to touch a patient with a latex allergy, the patient could experience a severe allergic reaction and could go into anaphylactic shock. If a latex allergy is suspected, the EMT should wear a glove made from vinyl or plastic.

Masks, Eye Protection, and Gowns. When you anticipate that blood will be splashed (e.g., in childbirth or trauma with heavy bleeding), additional barriers should be used to protect your eyes, mucous membranes, and clothing. You should use a face shield or mask that covers the mouth and nose and protective eyewear plus gowns or jumpsuits to protect clothes. An extra change of clothing should be available.

Use of these protective devices can be guided by the situation. **Table 2-4** indicates the appropriate situations in which to use different types of PPE. *Gloves are routinely worn for all patient contacts because it is best to be prepared rather than to be exposed or have to stop and put on gloves before continuing with an assessment.*

These additional barriers also may be used when a risk of contact transmission of pathogens exists, such as exposure to patients soiled with diarrhea or draining abscesses that cannot be covered. The goal in these situations is to prevent spread from the patient and patient's environment to other healthcare settings. This requires changing PPE and washing your hands after patient contact and before entering a new environment such as the ED.

The surgical mask and eye protection also provide a barrier to droplet transmission to the nostrils, mouth, and conjunctivae.

For airborne pathogens, special masks are necessary to block the minute particles that carry the microorganisms. The standard for such masks is an *N95* (N category at 95% efficiency) respirator. One respirator that meets this criterion is a HEPA respirator for patients with suspected tuberculosis and other airborne-transmitted diseases (see Figure 2-6).

Needles and Sharps. Because being stuck by a contaminated needle or other sharp object may represent the highest risk of contracting a blood-borne disease, proper handling of needles and other "sharps" is of the utmost importance. Used needles should never be recapped, bent or broken by hand, removed from disposable syringes, or otherwise manipulated. You should not allow the tip of a needle to touch any part of your body. Instead, you should place the used needle (and any attached disposable syringe) in a puncture-resistant **sharps container** for disposal later (**Figure 2-10**). These containers should be as close as possible to the site where a needle is used. Easy access to a sharps container in the ambulance's patient care area is important, and the sharps container should be brought to the patient's side whenever a needle is used in the course of care.

Taking care to avoid inadvertent needlesticks should be one of your highest priorities. You should pay particular attention if you are handling a needle in a highly charged and active situation, such as a resuscitation or treatment of a patient in critical condition (e.g., when using epinephrine autoinjector [EpiPen] to treat a patient with anaphylaxis).

Isolation and Patient Placement. If you know or suspect that a patient has a contagious disease, you should prevent unnecessary

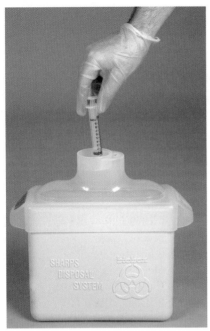

Figure 2-10 All needles and other sharp objects should be properly discarded in a sharps container after use.

exposure to others by isolating the patient or contaminated equipment. Knowledge of the mechanism of transmission guides practice. For example, if you know or suspect that a patient has measles, you should advise the triage nurse of the condition so that you can bring the patient to the appropriate area within the ED where patients with highly contagious infections with airborne transmission are evaluated. Unnecessary contact with contaminated objects by others should be avoided until the objects are cleaned.

Decontamination and Cleaning. Blood spills should be cleaned as soon as possible. Protective precautions should be taken to prevent unnecessary contact by using gloves, boots over shoes, or face and eye PPE as the situation dictates. After wiping up visible material with disposable towels, the soiled toweling should be placed in a plastic bag to prevent contamination with other surfaces. You may use a red plastic bag (common in hospital systems for handling "infectious waste") to mark the contents. Once the visible material is removed, the surface should be cleaned with a diluted 1:100 to 1:10 solution of household bleach or other appropriate germicide. The area should be allowed to air-dry. After cleaning, you should first remove contaminated coverings and then your gloves and place them in the plastic bag. Hands should be washed after you remove the gloves.

The risk of transmission from contaminated linen and clothing is negligible if the material is handled, transported, and laundered in a manner avoiding transfer to others. Soiled linen should be folded or rolled and placed in a plastic or cloth bag for laundering. You should wash your hands after handling. Gloves should be used if the linen is heavily contaminated. If blood soaks through clothing, you can avoid prolonged contact with your skin by changing clothes and washing as soon as practically possible.

Linen can be washed with detergent and bleach in accordance with laundering product recommendations. Clothing can be handled similarly. Detergent washing and drying render materials safe. Dry cleaning is also an effective decontamination method if clothing cannot be laundered.

Waste material should be disposed of in accordance with local or state regulations.

Standard Precautions. Standard precautions incorporate both universal precautions and body substance isolation measures and should be applied to all patients, regardless of their diagnosis or presumed infectious status. Standard precautions apply to blood; all body fluids, secretions, and excretions except sweat, regardless of whether they contain visible blood; nonintact skin; and mucous membranes. They incorporate all measures mentioned earlier. Gloves are used routinely for care of all patients, and other barrier protection is selected based on the possibility of exposure according to the individual patient's condition and type of call (e.g., multiple trauma, spurting blood, childbirth).

Transmission-Based Precautions. Transmission-based precautions should be used in addition to standard precautions when patients have or are suspected of having a highly transmissible disease.

Contact Precautions. In addition to standard precautions, you should use contact precautions for specific patients with known or suspected infection or those who are carrying microorganisms transmitted by direct contact with the patient or indirect contact with patient care items or the patient's environmental surfaces. Gloves should be worn before entering the patient's environment if possible. Gloves should be changed if they are grossly infected with infective material, such as fecal material or wound drainage, followed by handwashing. You should wear a gown if you anticipate that your clothing may contact the patient or infected environment. The gown and gloves should be replaced before leaving the patient's environment to avoid transfer of microorganisms to the ambulance; fresh PPE should then be replaced, with the process repeated if necessary to minimize transporting contamination into the hospital. When possible, you should use single-use equipment and isolate patient care equipment in a plastic bag after use to prevent spread of microorganisms. If multiple-use equipment is required, you should ensure that it is adequately cleaned and disinfected before use with another patient.

Droplet Precautions. Droplet precautions should be used in addition to standard precautions when a patient is known or suspected to be infected with microorganisms transmitted by droplets from sneezing, coughing, or talking or during suctioning or care of the airway. In addition to any standard precautions, a mask and protective eyewear should be worn when working within 3 feet of the patient. If transport or movement is necessary, dispersal of droplets can be minimized by placing a surgical mask on the patient if possible.

Airborne Precautions. Airborne precautions should be used when agents such as tuberculosis, varicella (chickenpox), and rubeola (measles) are suspected. You should wear respiratory protection (HEPA respirator) when entering the room of the patient and during transport and care of patients with known or suspected tuberculosis and other airborne-transmitted diseases.

EMTs without immunity should not enter the room of patients with suspected measles or chickenpox if other EMTs are present who are immune. If susceptible persons must enter the room, they should wear a HEPA respirator. Even persons who are immune to measles or varicella should wear respiratory protection. Many infectious disease experts recommend that everyone use the airborne precautions because, although it is unlikely, some people do contract chickenpox or other diseases a second time, despite prior vaccination.

The EMT should take precautions to limit exposure to others during transport and movement of patients with airborne-spread diseases. During transport, dispersal of droplet nuclei can be minimized by placing a surgical mask on the patient, if possible. The ED should be informed of the suspected need for airborne precautions before patient arrival so movement through the ED can be directed to a negative-pressure room, which is ventilated to minimize airborne spread within the hospital. For example, you might inform ED personnel that a patient with "fever and rash" is en route so they can prepare for the route of entry and destination within the hospital and meet you on arrival.

Postexposure Follow-up

If you are exposed to an infectious disease, you should file a report with your agency and inform the designated infection control officer, medical director, physician, or other designated individual according to policy. You should remember that no one will know you have a blood or body fluid exposure unless you tell them. This is your responsibility. You should know the policy of your agency for your own protection.

For some conditions, prompt follow-up is important. For example, antiviral therapy should be started within hours after a needlestick with possible HIV infection. In most cases, follow-up with the hospital is necessary to confirm the existence of an infectious condition. An assessment is made of the extent of the exposure and the risk to yourself. This information aids your physician in recommending any necessary postexposure care.

Hospitals have infection control programs that follow up on possible contacts of patients who have certain infectious conditions. The federal Ryan White Act requires notification systems to ensure that emergency response employees, including EMTs, are informed when they have been exposed to an emergency medical patient with an infectious, potentially fatal disease (e.g., AIDS) or meningococcemia, a bacterial disease that can be spread by respiratory droplets. Often the diagnosis is made after the EMT has left the patient at the hospital. Hospitals use the prehospital care record as one means of reaching others who might have been exposed to infectious diseases and may need follow-up and evaluation.

Infection control practices are designed to block the spread of infectious disease among patients, healthcare workers, and the general public. Infection control must be practiced until it becomes a habit. The EMT who understands methods of disease transmission and the facts about HBV, HIV, and other contagious diseases incorporates principles and techniques of infection control into his or her daily practice. Such practice lowers the risk to acceptable levels and makes the EMT a sophisticated partner in the care of patients who have infectious conditions. Continued updates in infection control are recommended.

> ### REAL*World*
>
> Failing to report an infectious exposure can have serious consequences for the EMT. As time passes, it may be difficult to locate the patient who was the source of the exposure, and many prophylactic medications must be started within 48 to 72 hours of exposure. If a report is made after this time frame, there may be nothing that can be done other than monitoring the EMT to see if they develop the infectious disease.

The prudent EMT takes actions to prevent significant exposure by following infection control guidelines. These include maintaining personal health status and immunizations, being aware of health and safety, and using actions to block the spread of infection. EMTs and other healthcare professionals must use standard precautions and transmission-based precautions to minimize or prevent transmission of disease. Blocking the spread of infection includes handwashing, using sterile technique, cleaning, disinfecting, and sterilizing equipment after use, wearing PPE, practicing standard and transmission-based precautions, and using simple isolation procedures. **Table 2-5** outlines a protocol that summarizes the approach to a patient with a communicable disease.

Pandemic Flu

Understanding communicable diseases and infection control becomes even more important in the face of a widespread epidemic.

At present the world prepares for **pandemic flu,** which could threaten millions of lives and cause widespread disruption of society. A pandemic flu would involve a highly virulent virus against which the human population has little or no preexisting immunity. The virus would cause illness in humans and have the potential for sustained transmission from person to person.

In such an eventuality, significant challenges would face every sector of society. Health workers might be faced with triage decisions as the hospital sector becomes overloaded. Alternate destinations may need to be used, quarantine of patients and exposed individuals imposed, and judgments made about protection from spread and treatment. The EMT will have a key role in the response. Learning about communicable diseases and model plans as well the plan in your region will be key to a successful response. Web access to state plans and information about the disease are available from www.pandemicflu.gov/. History from 90 years ago provides a lesson to the wise to prepare.

> **LEARNING OBJECTIVE**
> - List the personal protective equipment necessary for each of the following situations:
>   - Hazardous materials
>   - Rescue operations
>   - Violent scenes
>   - Crime scenes

Case in Point

Colorado State Summit

Opening Remarks Prepared for Delivery
By the Honorable Mike Leavitt
Secretary of Health and Human Services
March 24, 2006

The Great Pandemic also touched Colorado.

It first appeared in late September 1918, when some 33 suspected cases were reported at the University of Colorado. It raged across the state through the month of October, sickening those in the valleys, and bringing down residents of high mountain towns.

More than 150 people died in a single week here in Denver. Thousands were afflicted (though actual numbers are unknown).

One of those was Katherine Porter, who would later earn fame and acclaim (including a Pulitzer Prize) for her short stories. One of her best-known works was Pale Horse, Pale Rider, a fictionalized account of her experience in the pandemic.

Porter contracted influenza while working as a journalist for the Rocky Mountain News. She could not be admitted to the hospital at first, because there was no room. Instead, she was threatened with eviction by her landlady and then cared for by an unknown boarder who nursed her until a bed was open at the hospital.

From www.pandemicflu.gov/, June 2007.

Porter was so sick that her newspaper colleagues prepared an obituary and her father chose a burial plot. Her near-death experience changed Porter in a profound way. She said afterward, "It just simply divided my life, cut across it like that. So that everything before that was just getting ready, and after that I was in some strange way altered."

The lives of countless other Coloradoans were also altered.

Residents of Boulder experienced a quarantine. So did all of those living in the entire San Juan Basin (in the southwest corner of the state). All gatherings were cancelled, including schools, sporting events, and social outings. Voters and judges alike were required to wear surgical masks during the November election. People were even prohibited to gather for funerals.

The city of Silverton (located just north of Durango) lost nearly 10 percent of its population, including morticians. Coffins had to be sent from Durango to accommodate the large numbers of the dead.

The pandemic finally faded, leaving echoes of terror and suffering and loss all across the state.

When it comes to pandemics, there is no rational basis to believe that the early years of the 21st century will be different than the past. If a pandemic strikes, it will come to Colorado.

Table 2-5	Protocol for Infection Control

Always
- Wash hands thoroughly after patient contact
- Use Standard Precautions
- Use Transmission-Based Precautions

Category Precautions

Apply to	Gloves	Mask	Gown	Eye Protection
Category 1: Standard Precautions				
Blood Body fluids Body secretions Nonintact skin Mucous membranes	✓ Whenever in contact with blood or body fluids Change gloves before examining mucous membranes or open wounds	✓ Must be worn if spurting blood or splashing is likely, as in childbirth and endotracheal intubation	✓ Should be worn if spurting blood, childbirth, or gross contamination	✓ Must be worn if spurting blood or splashing is likely, as in childbirth and endotracheal intubation
Category 2: Airborne Precautions				
Tuberculosis	✓	✓ Place mask on patient with cough lasting more than 48 hours EMTs must wear HEPA respirator; know your immunity to chickenpox and measles		
Category 3: Droplet Precautions				
Tuberculosis Varicella Rubella Rubeola Meningococcal meningitis	✓	✓ Must be worn when working with patient suspected to be infected with microorganisms transmitted via droplet		
Category 4: Contact Precautions				
Gross contamination	✓ Worn before entering patient's environment; changed if grossly infective material (e.g., fecal matter)	✓ Especially if blood splatter is likely	✓ Especially if blood splatter is likely	

Hazardous Situations

As an EMT, you may be called to a scene where your personal safety is threatened. Examples include situations in which heavy rescue is necessary, hazardous materials are present, or an active fire, threat of explosion, electrical hazard, or threat of violence exists. The EMT's role is to provide emergency medical care after the scene is safe and the patient is removed from the hazardous environment. You do not benefit the patient if you become injured and a patient yourself. EMTs should allow those who are appropriately trained and have the necessary equipment to make the scene safe. You should understand how to approach potentially dangerous scenes and know your role as an EMT with respect to other agencies, such as police, fire, and HAZMAT teams, to make each encounter as safe as possible.

Often you will be alerted by the dispatcher of potential threats at the scene. In other situations, you may be the first to realize that the scene is unsafe. Stay alert on all calls, and anticipate possible dangers. Be familiar with the PPE that can reduce your risk for personal injury.

Rescue (from Latin and Old French, to "shake out" or "wrest away") means to free from confinement, violence, or danger. Patients who require emergency medical care often also require rescue. Many dangers can be encountered in rescue situations and range from environmental to man-made. The specialized techniques available and used in rescue operations are beyond the scope of training in a standard EMT course. In some systems, EMTs are also trained in rescues. In other systems, rescue personnel and EMS personnel work side by side. Common sense and basic principles can be used to identify potentially life-threatening situations. As an EMT, you should know your limitations and be aware of how to call for help.

Rescue and medical skills are guided by the needs of the patient and often are intermingled. For example, as soon as patient access is safe, assessment of the patient's medical needs and initial care may begin before extrication is complete. The medical assessment of the patient may influence the techniques used to rescue a patient.

The primary role of EMT training is to know when and how to use available PPE to allow safe access and treatment to the patient. This requires that you understand the hazards associated with various environments and know when it is safe to gain access or attempt rescue. As an EMT, you will learn some skills to conduct a rescue when safe and necessary and if you are first on the scene. In addition, you will learn patient "packaging" techniques that allow safe extrication and medical care.

The basic safety rule in all circumstances is ensuring the safety of yourself, other rescue personnel, bystanders, and then the patient. The patient is not helped if the EMT and other rescuers become victims. Likewise, exposing bystanders to unnecessary risk may also create more victims.

Identification of Potentially Life-Threatening Situations

The rescue scene may contain possible risks from falling debris, unstable structures, vehicles likely to roll over, and sharp objects. Potential threats also may exist from electricity, fire, explosion, or hazardous materials. Different agencies may be called to help, depending on the hazard, such as the fire department if ongoing fire threatens or victims are trapped in a burning building. Threats from electrical power lines, such as a line on an automobile with victims inside, might require both fire and power company workers to make the scene safe. Threats of explosion might involve experts from the bomb squad before a scene is judged safe.

Electricity

Downed power lines at the scene must be respected and avoided. The electrical company should be notified so that power can be turned off. Electricity seeks the path of least resistance on its path to the ground. You should be especially careful if there is water at the scene, since water is a good conductor of electricity.

Fire

Fire scenes pose risks of burns, smoke inhalation, and structural collapse. The fire department should declare the scene safe before you enter the area.

Explosion

You should beware of risk of explosion—at a fire scene, HAZMAT incident, or in the case of bomb threats. Depending on the circumstance, you may need the assistance of the fire department, HAZMAT crews, or bomb squad.

Rescue Scenes

Protective Clothing

The EMT may need to use protective clothing when entering some rescue scenes to prevent personal injury. Depending on the situation, such protective clothing might include turnout gear, puncture-proof gloves, helmets, protective eyewear, or a combination of these.

Turnout gear is heavy clothing that is puncture resistant and provides some protection from hazardous materials and contact with materials at extremes of temperature, giving protection against cuts, toxic or burning chemicals, cold injury, and burns. Turnout gear also has reflective material to help identify the rescuer at night or in dark environments **(Figure 2-11)**.

Puncture-proof gloves give protection against sharp objects, such as broken glass and other debris at a motor vehicle crash or rescue scene.

Helmets, secured by a chin strap, should be worn when the risk of falling debris exists. Protective eyewear is necessary in situations to protect against falling debris or where shards of glass are present. It is also necessary when fragments may become propelled toward the rescuer.

When heavy or extensive rescue is required, dispatch of heavy rescue units with special skills and equipment should be requested, because they have the experience and equipment to conduct such rescues more safely.

Hazardous Materials

On arrival at any scene where hazardous materials may be present, medical personnel should follow several rules.

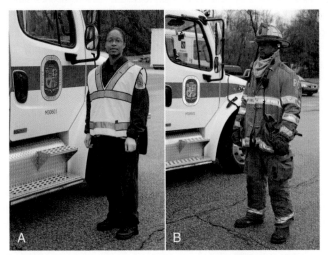

Figure 2-11 **A,** EMT wearing reflective vest. **B,** EMT wearing turnout gear (puncture-resistant heavy clothing).

Safety is the first concern on suspicion of a HAZMAT incident. As an EMT, you should position yourself upwind and uphill from the incident and stay a safe distance away. The type of hazard should be identified from a safe distance, followed by marking off the area, to prevent bystanders and other responders from inadvertently approaching a danger zone, and calling for help. EMTs responding to a potential HAZMAT incident should wear full turnout gear, including a coat, eyewear, helmet, and puncture-proof gloves. However, this gear is modest or minimal protection against vapors and some chemicals. Therefore, if you have taken extra training, you may have and use, when appropriate, a **self-contained breathing apparatus (SCBA)** (mask connected to separate source of fresh air). Chemical protective clothing may be required just to enter the area and provide emergency medical care. Emergency personnel should not use SCBA or any other rescue equipment unless they have received appropriate training and have been assigned these roles within their EMS system. The purpose of wearing this gear is to protect the EMT while he or she provides emergency medical care.

Federal, state, and local agencies have experts who deal with HAZMAT emergencies and whose duty it is to control a hazardous materials scene. The telephone numbers for these agencies, listing a contact person for each, should be available for either the dispatcher or the incident commander whenever a HAZMAT situation is handled. This list should be reviewed and updated on a regular basis. Medical direction may be helpful in assisting with the identification of hazardous materials (see Chapter 28).

The EMT needs to know potential hazards for many reasons. Special equipment and precautions may be required for a safe and efficient rescue. Different materials have different effects on the body. The health hazard of a particular material and whether it needs special treatment are fundamental data needed for patient care.

Scene Safety. On arrival at a HAZMAT incident, your senses can provide extremely valuable information about the safety of the scene. The scene should be observed from a distance whenever possible; binoculars should be used if necessary. You should note if there is a cloud of smoke, indicating that the material was ignited. You should listen for noises that might indicate a leak. If there is a strange odor, you should try to relocate upwind from the source and uphill if possible.

A **placard** is a sign that identifies hazardous materials by color, symbols, category names, and numbers (see Figure 28-6) A vehicle transporting hazardous materials should have a bill of lading or shipping paper containing similar information (see Figure 28-8). The *North American Emergency Response Guidebook for Initial Response to Hazardous Materials Incidents,* published by the U.S. Department of Transportation, should be available in every ambulance or through the dispatcher. This book, organized in outline format for quick reference, lists the health risks and actions for various classes of hazardous materials. The Chemical Transport Emergency Center (CHEMTREC) is a 24-hour, 7-day-a-week telephone resource (1-800-424-9300) providing advice on how to handle chemical emergencies.

Violent Scenes

When approaching a potentially violent scene, you must first be concerned with your own personal safety. The scene should always be controlled by law enforcement personnel before you provide patient care. Entering a potentially violent scene without the necessary support may put you and others at greater risk and may compound the problem.

Threats of personal violence can occur in different scenarios. A crime scene involving the perpetrator of the crime or a mob scene is an obvious threat. At other times, bystanders may become agitated and pose a threat to rescuers. Family members may become distraught and act out with violent threats or actions. If you feel threatened, you should retreat from the situation and call for assistance.

If you are faced with a violent patient, a calm, nonthreatening, and reassuring approach may help defuse the situation. EMTs are not expected to endanger themselves when faced with personal violence.

At times, restraint of violent patients who are a threat to themselves or others may be necessary (see Chapter 17).

Crime Scenes

When involved in patient care at a crime scene, you should not disturb potential evidence any more than necessary to provide emergency medical care. In the course of your duties, if you encounter something with potential importance to a crime scene, you should maintain a **chain of evidence,** or handle the material in such a manner that it can be accounted for from the time it came into your possession until you turned it over to authorities. This chain of evidence should also be documented. For example, a bullet found while transporting a gunshot victim might be inserted in a container and then placed in the pocket of an EMT until it is turned directly over to police or hospital personnel. The EMT would note on the patient's prehospital care record the object found (bullet), the time it was found, and where it was from discovery until transfer to police or hospital personnel, and then ask the receiving agent to sign the record and indicate the time the bullet was transferred. Later, a full accounting of the time this bullet was in the EMT's possession would be clear from the documentation.

LEARNING OBJECTIVES
- Recognize the signs and symptoms of critical incident stress.
- List possible emotional reactions that the EMT may experience when faced with trauma, illness, death, and dying.

Stress Management

Stressful Situations

Many situations are overwhelming. Examples include the death of an infant or child or a patient with whom you have identified because of a similarity in background, age, or profession (e.g., co-worker). Disasters associated with multiple deaths can be traumatic for anyone caring for the victims. The panic, chaos, sights of mutilation, and feelings of being overwhelmed leave their emotional imprint (**Figure 2-12**).

These types of incidents are called **critical stress incidents.** It has been recommended that all personnel participating in disaster rescues and relief undergo a "debriefing," in which feelings can be discussed and, it is hoped, resolved. Cases involving amputations or disfigurement of the body also can be stressful, with lingering images and feelings (see later discussion).

Caring for victims of violent crimes (e.g., rape, assault, attempted murder) and victims of abuse (e.g., child abuse, spouse abuse, parent abuse, family abuse) can provoke feelings of sympathy, disgust, or anger. Maintaining a calm, supportive manner and acting nonjudgmentally toward the patient and his or her family and friends are important.

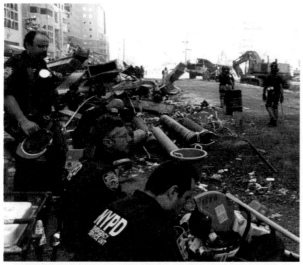

Figure 2-12 Disasters can cause stress to the responders. Be aware of signs of stress, and use critical incident stress debriefing and counseling opportunities.

You may work with law enforcement officials to preserve potential evidence. As always, however, the first priority is patient care.

Although many victims of violence or abuse display rage, anger, despair, violence, disbelief, hysteria, or extreme agitation in response to the event, others may be quiet and withdrawn, feel severely depressed, and experience shame and a profound sense of guilt (e.g., "I brought this on myself").

Particularly in cases of rape, but also in other cases of abuse, the patient has had control taken away. Allowing the patient to regain control is important. You should allow the patient to express his or her feelings, but do not push the patient to reveal specific details not necessary to render prehospital treatment. Although you will need to determine whether any significant injuries are present, more specific questioning is best done by personnel in the hospital.

As an EMT, you should remember that you as an individual are not immune to experiencing personal stress as you render care to patients in the course of your profession.

Recognition of Warning Signs

Dealing with death is difficult for anyone in the healthcare field. Death represents the ultimate inability to care for a patient. EMTs, physicians, nurses, and rescuers cannot save everyone, however, and it is unrealistic to believe that you can; there is no reason to have feelings of guilt when you have done your best. Despite this reality, feelings of helplessness and inadequacy or even embarrassment at being unable to save a patient are common. In some cases, EMTs avoid interacting with the patient's family because of a sense of failure or guilt. Other serious emergency situations, as noted previously, also can be extremely stressful.

Some EMTs may become overly clinical, make inappropriate remarks, or try to relieve tension with humor. At times, EMTs may deny any significant emotional reaction to their work and bury their feelings inside themselves. Some key symptoms, however, often indicate the need to seek help (**Box 2-3**).

The EMT must have an outlet for dealing with his or her inner feelings. This can be accomplished by talking about them with colleagues, a close friend or spouse, a member of the clergy, or a professional counselor. These feelings should not be expressed in front of patients and their families. Each EMT's reaction depends on his or her personality, sense of stability, sense of duty, understanding of personal limitations, and philosophical and religious beliefs.

Box 2-3	Warning Signs of Stress
Sleep difficulty and nightmares	Loss of interest in sexual activity
Irritability with co-workers, friends, or family	Isolation
	Loss of interest in work
Feelings of sadness	Physical symptoms
Anxiety	Hopelessness
Guilt	Alcohol or drug misuse
Indecisiveness	Inability to concentrate
Loss of appetite	

It is vital that every EMT learn to recognize and admit his or her reactions to stress and accompanying feelings and be willing to discuss them.

LEARNING OBJECTIVES
- State the possible reactions that the family of the EMT may exhibit as a result of their outside involvement in EMS.
- State possible steps that the EMT may take to help reduce or alleviate stress.

Balancing Work with Personal Life

Working as an EMT can provide great satisfaction, so much so that the associated feelings of self-worth, excitement, sacrifice for others, and the 24-hour nature of the job can lead to imbalance in your life. As an EMT, you may find that your profession is the main source of satisfaction and that your work takes precedence over personal interests, family, and friends. We all need to pay attention to our mental, physical, and spiritual needs. When pressures of the job distract you from keeping your life in balance, you should take note and make the necessary lifestyle changes.

When you recognize the warning signs of stress or "job burnout," it is important to acknowledge the problem and take action. You should pay attention to your physical needs. Many EMTs change their diets because of the job and work schedules. Foods that consist of simple sugars, such as candy, soft drinks, and desserts, can be replaced by healthy options, such as fruits, fruit drinks, and high-fiber snacks. A diet low in fat and high in complex carbohydrates can increase energy and reduce body weight. These dietary changes, regular exercise, and avoidance of excess caffeine and alcohol decrease tension and irritability while providing the energy for a healthy lifestyle.

Maintaining other interests and hobbies will help you not to become preoccupied with your job and lose touch with other activities that stimulate your mind. You should take time to continue spiritual or religious interests.

Relaxation techniques are also helpful in reducing stress. There are numerous approaches to meditation, breathing, relaxation, and visual imagery. Budgeting a brief period during your day to relax in a quiet environment can significantly reduce stress and restore energy. A variety of books and programs on meditation and relaxation are available, or you can ask for a referral from your physician.

Family and friend commitments and responses also can be factors in stress. The haphazard schedules that affect EMS personnel often become the basis for stress in the family setting. Family members, particularly spouses, may lack a full understanding of the commitments necessary for EMS providers. The spouse or partner may experience fear of separation and resentment at being ignored. On-call schedules can be stressful, since they tend to disturb scheduled events or basic family relaxation time. Families thrive and flourish on shared experiences and can be frustrated with the competition of work commitments.

You should make every attempt to organize a work schedule that allows sufficient attention to your family commitments, relaxation, and exercise. If necessary, you may find it helpful to request assignment to the less busy sectors of your EMS response area to reduce stress.

At times, an EMT may benefit from professional help. Professional counselors can help identify the causes of stress and provide a plan for reducing stress at work and at home. They can also provide support during particularly difficult periods of stress.

Comprehensive Critical Incident Stress Management

Critical Incident Stress

As an emergency responder, you regularly undergo experiences that an ordinary person might never encounter. You are trained to respond to these events in a calm, controlled manner—to make a difference in someone's life through your knowledge and actions.

As an EMT, you handle critical or major incidents as a professional, doing the things that need to be done. However, it is also important to take a professional attitude toward yourself. The stress generated by a critical incident can be a danger to your well-being. You must acknowledge this danger as seriously as any other hazard you face in the field. Denial of your own needs may cause unintended consequences that can affect your health, family, and career.

A program in comprehensive critical incident stress management involves several components, all designed to lessen the powerful stress a critical incident can create. You should take advantage of these opportunities in your region.

Preincident Stress Education

Preincident stress education sessions are designed to familiarize emergency responders with the nature of emergency service stress. In these sessions, responders learn the signs and symptoms of cumulative stress and critical incident stress. The stress of providing emergency service and the stress encountered in home and family life are discussed. Particular attention is directed to the potentially powerful effect of critical incident stress on the responder. The educational sessions create an awareness of the physical, emotional, and cognitive symptoms that can occur either immediately after a critical incident or in the following days, weeks, or months.

Emergency responders are taught the importance of recognizing symptoms, talking about their feelings, and taking specific action steps to lessen symptoms. The critical incident stress debriefing process is also explained.

A program of preincident stress education teaches emergency responders the following measures to reduce stress:
- Develop an awareness of the effect emergency stress creates.
- Develop a positive attitude toward managing stress symptoms.
- Learn the action steps to take for immediate and long-term stress management.

On-Scene Support

Many signs and symptoms of stress can occur immediately at the scene of a critical incident. The purpose of on-scene support is to identify and assist distressed emergency workers with the stress reactions they may be experiencing (**Figure 2-13**).

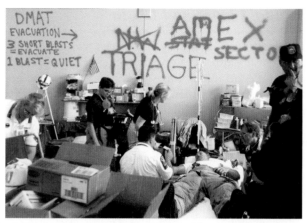

Figure 2-13 At the scene of a critical incident, professionals who recognize signs and symptoms of stress among co-workers can often refer them to on-scene personnel who have been trained in critical incident stress management. Disaster management assistance teams often stage their operation at the perimeter of a disaster scene for treatment of victims and responders, such as this team staged at the American Express building near the World Trade Center.

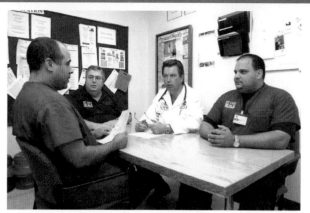

Figure 2-14 Critical incident stress debriefing sessions should be conducted 24 to 72 hours after the incident with a qualified counselor.

Mental health professionals who have received specialized training in critical incident stress can provide support during critical incident rescue activity. On-scene support may also be provided by peer support personnel who function not as mental health professionals but as experienced peers who have been trained in critical incident stress management. Inner-perimeter peer support and mental health personnel should have training in disaster scene operation to prepare them for the powerful stress this type of incident can create.

One-on-One Support

Although critical incident stress debriefings involve a group of emergency responders, group debriefing is not always necessary. In some cases, single responders may benefit from one-on-one support from a qualified peer or mental health professional. This support may be provided at the scene or may occur in the days following the incident. One-on-one support is designed to provide assistance to a single responder experiencing distress and needing short-term support to sort through the emotions the incident has created. One-on-one support does not take the place of professional counseling. If, in the opinion of the peer counselor, the individual needs professional assistance, a referral should be made to an appropriate mental health professional.

Defusing

Defusing is an early intervention that occurs either at the scene or shortly after responders have returned to quarters. The goal of defusing is to stop the negative stress process that may occur in the hours immediately after a critical incident, thus minimizing its influence. A defusing session is led by a trained mental health professional or peer counselor who provides information about the stress response and allows for brief discussion. The defusing process usually lasts approximately 30 minutes.

Critical Incident Stress Debriefing

In times of severe stress, such as a disaster, death of a child, or mutilation, **critical incident stress debriefing** (CISD) is used to deal immediately with feelings that may cause long-term emotional harm **(Figure 2-14).** Many EMS systems have a formal CISD team consisting of mental health professionals and peer counselors.

After a disaster or other stressful event, the CISD team meets with the EMS providers, usually within 24 to 72 hours. The session consists of sharing common experiences and expressing feelings, fears, and reactions surrounding the event. The CISD session is not designed to be an investigation or interrogation of the event, but rather an opportunity to diffuse feelings that otherwise might be internalized and provide the basis for a future source of stress and emotional illness. All information expressed during the CISD session is confidential and should not be discussed with friends, family, and co-workers not involved in the process.

At the conclusion of the session, the CISD professionals evaluate the information and offer suggestions to the group on overcoming stress. CISD is a valuable process because the intervention is immediate. Feelings are expressed quickly and not internalized for long periods, which helps avoid ongoing stress and related emotional problems. You should familiarize yourself with the local CISD resources available through your EMS system.

Follow-up Services

After a critical incident, it is necessary to keep a close watch on all concerned personnel. In the days following the incident, including the days after a debriefing has been conducted, referral of some responders for additional counseling may be necessary. Supervisors and line officers should pay close attention to their staff, watching for additional signs of physical and emotional stress reactions.

Follow-up service with medical and mental health agencies should be preplanned, thus allowing them to be prepared and ready to provide the required assistance.

Disaster Support Services

Disaster support services provide the resources needed to maintain disaster scene activity and long-term recovery. These services include federal and local agencies that provide immediate support through specialized equipment, additional personnel, housing and food services, and medical supplies.

Spouse and Family Support

Emergency service strains families and taxes relationships. Critical incidents not only take a toll on the emergency responder, but also can be devastating to the family.

After a critical incident, provision should be made for spouse and family support of responders involved. This assistance may consist of debriefing, stress education, support groups, or referral to family counseling.

Community Outreach Programs

Long-term recovery from a critical incident may require the use of various community outreach programs. For example, support groups can provide continued assistance to the responder and family members who have identified issues that need resolution. A list of outreach services should be made available through the CISD program.

Other Health and Welfare Programs

Programs that promote the health and wellness of emergency responders are essential to long-term success in the emergency services field.

Emergency service units should develop training programs to educate their staff to the need for good health. These programs should include stress management training, exercise, diet, and nutrition information. An excellent approach to responder wellness includes significant life partners in these training programs.

Additional health and welfare programs may include couples and parenting workshops that are designed to lessen the stress encountered within the family. The intent of such workshops is that a healthy family promotes a healthy emergency responder.

LEARNING OBJECTIVE
- Describe the steps in the EMT's approach to the family confronted with death and dying.

Terminal Illness and Death

When treating a terminally ill patient, you should allow the patient to express his or her feelings (**Figure 2-15**). You should not contradict if the patient indicates that he or she is dying. Often the patient is seeking human warmth and communication and wants the final moments of life to be honest and direct. Such a desire should be met with compassion and acknowledgment. Offering false assurances is inappropriate. You should listen empathetically with respect and provide the patient privacy, dignity, and some sense of control.

A patient with a chronic terminal illness may experience a variety of emotional responses. Five stages of grief characterize a patient's potential reaction to dying: denial, anger, bargaining, depression, and acceptance (**Table 2-6**). These stages need not occur in any particular sequence but are typically encountered. With knowledge of these responses to dying, you will be better prepared to react appropriately and empathetically to patients with terminal illness. For example, a patient may direct anger toward you as the EMT. You should recognize this as a reaction

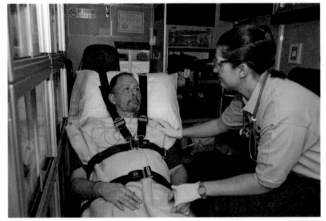

Figure 2-15 Compassion, understanding, and effective listening are crucial to caring for patients who have a terminal illness.

Table 2-6	Stages of Grief	

Stage	Emotional Response	EMT Response
Denial	Patient denies seriousness of situation to buffer the pain of the event. This may occur with acute emergencies or chronic terminal illness.	If denial impairs patient's judgment to seek medical attention, make an effort to convince patient to go to the hospital.
Anger	Patient may project feelings of anger at family or staff and create a situation that leads to isolation.	Don't take anger or insults personally. Be patient, tolerant, and empathetic. Use effective listening skills. Don't be judgmental.
Bargaining	Patient may attempt to negotiate to extend life.	Be attentive but not judgmental.
Depression	Patient may experience profound sadness, despair, grief, and depression. Patient is usually silent and retreats to his or her own world.	Allow patients to express self and experience the natural feelings of loss associated with death.
Acceptance	Patient ultimately accepts the situation but is not necessarily happy.	Use effective listening skills. The family may require support during this phase.

to dying and not take it personally. Acting in a calm, supportive manner usually benefits such patients. If the illness has been known for some time, the patient and family have had time to adapt to the approaching death, and emotions tend to be less charged.

When arriving on the scene, you should assess the patient's and family's knowledge of the patient's condition. For example, the family may know that the patient has terminal lung cancer, but the patient may not have been told. In this circumstance it is not wise for you to be the first to inform the patient of the diagnosis. However, if the patient knows the diagnosis and wants to discuss it, do not hesitate to use words that the patient uses, such as "cancer" or "death." If death appears imminent, (e.g., you cannot obtain a blood pressure measurement), it is appropriate to alert the family. You could say, "The patient has very weak vital signs," or, "The signs of life are very weak."

The patient or family may want the patient transported to the hospital, which they hope might provide comfort, pain relief, and support. Treatment of secondary complications, such as infection, may substantially prolong life or may help make the patient more comfortable. At other times, such as when patients are struggling for breath, the patient and/or family may seek emergency care, and appropriate medical protocols should be followed.

In general, the family should be allowed to be with the patient and travel with the patient to the hospital. If the patient or patient's family refuses treatment, it is best to contact medical direction for guidance. The medical direction physician can advise on the appropriateness of withholding treatment according to local and state guidelines and laws regarding "do not resuscitate" (DNR) orders or *living wills* (in which the patient has determined that particular types of treatment should not be initiated). A patient can revoke a previously executed DNR order or change a living will when faced with death. If there is any doubt about withholding treatment, you should err on the side of treating the patient (see Chapter 3).

When approaching the family of a person who has died, you should be prepared for a variety of emotional responses, including denial, guilt, grief, anger, hysteria, withdrawal, and physical reactions. Of course, on arrival at the scene, treatment of the patient is the first priority, and cardiopulmonary resuscitation (CPR) should be initiated unless it is specifically contraindicated by local or state guidelines. Be honest and straightforward, and keep the family informed. You should encourage emotional responses of grief and loss such as crying.

You should respect a family's wishes to be alone or to see the body of the deceased. If the body is mutilated, the mutilated parts should be covered and good judgment used about the potential impact on loved ones. Suggest that the family members seek follow-up counseling with their family physician, a member of the clergy, or other resources to help them through the grieving process. You might ask if there is anyone you can call for them as a way to extend help.

Particularly with unexpected deaths, as in cases of suicide or the death of younger patients who have been in good health, the family's emotional reaction can be very strong. The family is often in a state of disbelief or may show signs of feelings of guilt. It is essential that you be supportive and make no judgmental comments, such as, "You should have brought him to the hospital," or, "If only you had called earlier." If the family expresses guilt, you should be supportive and avoid any comments that imply they were responsible for wrongdoing. In other circumstances, a family may want to blame others for the death, including those who provided emergency care. Such comments should not be taken personally but recognized as part of the grief and loss reaction of certain individuals.

In many cases, a family may call for an ambulance long after the patient has died. The patient might be found dead in bed or might have been left alone for some time before discovery. Signs of **rigor mortis** (rigidity of muscles after death) or **dependent lividity** (black-and-blue discoloration of most gravity-dependent body portions) indicate death, and in these circumstances, you should confirm to the family what they no doubt suspect, that their loved one has died.

Scenario Follow-up

The patient has been transferred to the trauma team. Although your patient has lost a limb, his life has been saved. You have protected yourself from possible blood-borne infection through practice of standard precautions and use of protective equipment. You have not had an exposure that put you at risk. You stopped the patient's bleeding at the scene by securing a pressure bandage over the dressing. You cared for the patient en route to the hospital, secured by protective restraints in the back of the ambulance. You cleaned yourself, your equipment, and the vehicle after the call, using appropriate germicides. You carefully separated "infectious waste," placing contaminated linen and bandages in a biohazard bag. You are prepared for the next patient.

You talk with your partner about the victims after the call. Your agency has a critical incident stress debriefing program, and you and your partner are invited to speak about the event the next day. You notice that your supervisor is paying careful attention to you in the days that follow, to be sure that you are well.

Summary

Ensuring your well-being is best accomplished by recognizing that you have personal, emotional, and physical limitations. Stressful and hazardous situations are often encountered when you are asked to provide emergency medical care. When you encounter signs of stress in your own life, you should take advantage of counseling and critical incident stress debriefing. Choosing a lifestyle that prepares you physically and emotionally for your job helps to prevent burnout.

To protect yourself physically, you should anticipate situations in which you might be exposed to communicable disease, violence, and other potentially life-threatening situations, such as electricity, explosion, fire, or hazardous materials. Motor vehicle fatalities are the greatest occupational risk for EMTs, reminding one to drive safely and use proper restraints. Scene safety, including standard precautions for infection control, should be integrated as part of your routine approach to all patients. You should work with appropriate agencies, such as fire, police, and HAZMAT teams, and remember that your primary role is to render emergency medical care without risking undue harm to yourself or others.

The Bottom Line

Learning Checklist

✓ EMTs make scene safety their first concern when responding to a call for help. Anticipate the need for assistance from other agencies and for personal protective equipment (PPE) should you encounter hazardous materials (HAZMAT) incidents, rescue situations, violent or crime scenes, or possible exposure to airborne or blood-borne infectious microorganisms.

✓ Most fatalities in ambulance crashes occur in the patient compartment. Securing the patient and the EMTs and equipment in the compartment is an essential safety step.

✓ Body substance isolation is the use of PPE to protect the EMT from exposure to airborne or blood-borne or body fluid pathogens and includes use of gloves, masks, gowns, and eyewear. The type of body substance exposure anticipated guides indications for use of specific gear.

✓ To protect yourself from airborne-transmitted pathogens, you should wear a high-efficiency particulate air (HEPA) respirator.

✓ To protect from droplet spread, a face mask and face shield or protective eyewear should be worn.

✓ Protection from contact spread (e.g., blood-borne pathogens) requires gloves for contact with blood or bloody body fluids, eye protection and masks for possible blood splatter, and gowns if childbirth, spurting blood, or major trauma is anticipated.

✓ Contact transmission precautions also are used for other non–blood-borne infections, including chickenpox, draining abscesses, patients with uncontrolled diarrhea or urination, and patients with multidrug-resistant infections.

✓ Standard precautions should be used for every patient, with transmission-based precautions added as indicated by the patient's condition.

✓ To protect yourself at the scene if heavy rescue is needed, you should use PPE, including turnout gear with puncture-proof gloves, helmets, and protective eyewear. If hazardous materials are present at the scene, you may also need to use HAZMAT suits and self-contained breathing apparatus, if you have been trained in their use.

✓ Warning signs of stress include irritability with others, difficulty sleeping, anxiety, guilt, indecisiveness, loss of appetite, disinterest in sex, isolation, misuse of alcohol and drugs, and loss of interest in work.

✓ Because of their outside involvement in EMS, an EMT's family might exhibit lack of understanding, fear of separation and being ignored, frustration with scheduling, and inability to plan or share activities.

✓ The EMT can help manage stress by recognizing signs of stress; making lifestyle changes to promote physical, mental, and spiritual well-being; balancing work with recreation, family, and personal interests; planning a schedule that allows for time with family and friends; and seeking peer support and professional help when necessary.

✓ After cases of trauma, illness, death, and dying, an EMT might experience guilt, helplessness, feelings of inadequacy, and being a target of the patient's or family's anger or blame.

✓ When confronted with death or dying, a family member may exhibit disbelief, guilt, grief, blame, anger, denial, withdrawal, and physical reactions.

✓ The EMT must respect the need for dignity, communication, and privacy of the family confronted with death or dying. Listen empathetically, use a gentle tone of voice, be careful not to give false assurances, and allow them as much as possible to be with the patient.

Key Terms

Body substance isolation Procedures used to protect the EMT from contact with communicable diseases, including the use of gloves, goggles, masks, and gowns.

Carrier A person who shows no signs of disease yet harbors an infectious organism and may be a source of infection to others.

Chain of evidence An accountability of evidence at a crime scene. Any evidence should be accounted for from the time it came into your possession until it is turned over to the authorities.

Communicable Classification of disease in which the causative agent may pass or be carried from one person to another directly or indirectly.

Communicable period The time period during which a person can transmit an infectious disease to others.

Critical incident stress debriefing Psychological, emotional, and educational group process to lessen the impact of a critical incident.

Critical stress incident A particularly overwhelming incident that results in emotional stress.

Dependent lividity Black-and-blue discoloration of most gravity-dependent body portions, seen after death.

Exposure Process of coming in contact with, but not necessarily being infected by, a disease-causing agent.

HAZMAT Term referring to a hazardous materials incident or the special team to handle it.

High-efficiency particulate air (HEPA) respirator Specialized filtering mask designed to protect the EMT from airborne pathogens.

Host A susceptible person who, if exposed to a source of infectious disease, may become ill.

Immunity The body's ability to resist infection after exposure to an infectious agent. The state of being protected from (immune) from disease.

Incubation period The time period between contact with an infectious agent and occurrence of signs and symptoms of infection.

Infection control The practice of specific actions to block the spread of infectious agents.

Microorganisms Organisms not visible to the naked eye.

Pandemic flu virulent virus against which humans have little or no preexisting immunity; casues illness in humans and has the potential for sustained transmission from person to person.

Passive immunity Immunity that is injected into a body (not produced by it), such as injection of an antibody against tetanus.

Personal protective equipment (PPE) A variety of safety equipment used to prevent direct contact with blood and other body fluids, including gloves, eye protection, masks, and gowns, or used to prevent contact with hazardous materials, including turnout gear, chemical-resistant clothing, and self-contained breathing apparatus.

Placard Specialized signage used to identify various hazardous materials.

Rigor mortis Rigidity of muscles after death.

Self-contained breathing apparatus (SCBA) Specialized mask and regulator used by rescue personnel in environments that may be dangerous, such as those containing smoke, carbon monoxide, or other hazardous materials.

Sharps container Special container designed for the disposal of needles and other sharp instruments used in conjunction with the care of a patient.

Source A person, insect, object, or other substance that carries or is contaminated by an infectious agent.

Standard precautions Incorporate the older universal precautions and body substance isolation. Precautions used in all situations to avoid transmission from both recognized and unrecognized sources of infection. Standard precautions apply to the blood, body fluids, secretions, excretions (except sweat), nonintact skin, and mucous membranes.

Transmission Method by which an infectious agent travels from the source to its host.

Transmission-based precautions Special precautions beyond standard precautions that are used for patients documented or suspected to be infected with highly transmissible disease.

Turnout gear Heavy clothing that is puncture resistant and gives some protection from hazardous materials and materials at extremes of temperature.

Universal precautions The approach to protect oneself in every patient contact against exposure to body substances and fluids that may carry blood-borne pathogens such as HIV, hepatitis B virus, or hepatitis C virus.

Vaccination Inoculation with a vaccine to establish immunity to a particular disease.

Vector Insects, animals, or inanimate objects that carry and transmit disease. For example, malaria is transmitted by mosquitoes.

Review Questions

1. How should you respond when the family wants to view the body of a deceased loved one?
   a. Encourage them to avoid it, to prevent hysterical reactions
   b. Tell them that they can view it at a later time
   c. Allow them to view the body
   d. Make them wait until the physician arrives

Case History for Questions 2 and 3
You are dispatched to a call for a patient with difficulty breathing and terminal lung cancer. At the scene, you encounter a 45-year-old man in moderate distress, conscious, and aware of his condition. He responds angrily to almost every request or comment made to him.

2. Which of the following is most correct in regard to this patient's reaction?
   a. Is common with dying patients
   b. Suggests insensitivity on your part
   c. Must be dealt with firmly
   d. Should be actively converted by cheerfulness

3. What is the most effective method for dealing with this patient?
   a. Empathetic listening
   b. Firm interaction and directions
   c. A detached clinical approach
   d. Distracting him from his problems

4. Which approach can an EMT take after the death of a patient when the EMT has associated feelings of helplessness, guilt, and isolation?
   a. Share feelings with a peer counselor
   b. Take additional clinical training
   c. Reason it out through positive thinking
   d. Relate to it as a natural part of life and "go on"

5. A major disaster, such as the death of children in a fire, may require a more organized response by EMTs to resolve negative feelings. What is this process called?
   a. Critical incident stress debriefing
   b. Encounter group
   c. Catharsis
   d. Psychotherapy

6. When should standard precautions be used?
   a. Patients with AIDS
   b. All patients
   c. Contagious patients
   d. Infected patients

7. Which of the following best describes diseases capable of being spread from one person to another?
   a. Pathogens
   b. Communicable
   c. Infectious
   d. Bacterial

8. An EMT is transporting an ill geriatric patient with a weakened immune system. Which of the following would be the best method of protecting the patient?
   - a. Mask on the patient and on the EMT
   - b. Mask on the patient
   - c. Mask on the EMT
   - d. No additional precautions are necessary.

9. Which of the following can be defined as coming in contact with, but not necessarily being infected by, a disease-causing agent?
   - a. Indirect contact
   - b. Interface
   - c. Exposure
   - d. Casual contact

10. Which of the following defines the transfer of a microorganism from the spray produced during coughing, sneezing, or talking by an infected person?
   - a. Vapor transmission
   - b. Spray transmission
   - c. Droplet transmission
   - d. Mist transmission

11. For which of the following diseases is a vaccination available for prevention?
   - a. HIV
   - b. Hepatitis B
   - c. Hepatitis C
   - d. Common cold

12. With suspected tuberculosis, what precautions should be taken?
   - a. Standard
   - b. Airborne
   - c. Droplet
   - d. Standard, droplet, and airborne

13. What is the simplest and most effective measure for blocking the spread of infection?
   - a. Avoiding physical contact with patients
   - b. Using alcohol on infection sites
   - c. Handwashing after every patient contact
   - d. Wearing a gown with every patient contact

14. When splash from a bleeding artery is possible, in addition to wearing gloves, what are the recommended precautions?
   - a. Mask, protective eyewear, and gowns
   - b. Mask only
   - c. Protective eyewear only
   - d. Gown and protective eyewear only

15. Which of the following would be *least* helpful when trying to obtain information at the site of a potential hazardous materials incident?
   - a. Shipping papers
   - b. Color of the vehicle
   - c. Placards on the vehicle
   - d. Driver of the vehicle

16. What is the EMT's first priority when dealing with a potentially violent patient?
   - a. Self-protection
   - b. The patient's protection
   - c. The legal implications
   - d. Restraining the patient

17. After running a call in which an infant died, you find your EMT partner crying in the break room. You try to talk to him, but he continues to cry. Which of the following could you request to help your partner now?
   - a. Critical incident stress debriefing
   - b. Priest
   - c. Emergency physician
   - d. Defusing

For Further Review

In the Student Workbook

- Multiple-choice questions
- Matching questions
- Fill-in-the-blank questions
- Short answer questions
- Crossword puzzle

On Evolve

- Weblinks
- Lecture notes
- Exercises

Learning Objectives

Cognitive Objectives

- Explain the need to maintain personal wellness.
- Explain the need to determine scene safety.
- Discuss how to reduce your chance of occupational injury.
- Discuss the importance of body substance isolation.
- Describe the steps the EMT should take for personal protection from airborne and blood-borne pathogens.
- List the personal protective equipment necessary for each of the following situations:
  - Exposure to airborne pathogens
  - Exposure to blood-borne pathogens
  - Hazardous materials
  - Rescue operations

- Violent scenes
- Crime scenes
- Recognize the signs and symptoms of critical incident stress.
- List possible emotional reactions that the EMT may experience when faced with trauma, illness, death, and dying.

- State the possible reactions that the family of the EMT may exhibit as a result of their outside involvement in EMS.
- State possible steps that the EMT may take to help reduce or alleviate stress.
- Describe the steps in the EMT's approach to the family confronted with death and dying.

References

Ambulance crash–related injuries among emergency medical services workers—United States, 1991–2002, *MMWR* 52(8):154-156 2003.

Centers for Disease Control and Prevention: Guidelines for prevention of transmission of human immunodeficiency virus and hepatitis B virus to health-care and public-safety workers: a response to PL 100-607, The Health Omnibus Programs Extension Act of 1988, *MMWR Suppl* 38(S6):3-37 1989.

Centers for Disease Control and Prevention: Nutrition resources for health professions. http://www.cdc.gov/nccdphp/dnpa/nutrition/health_professionals/. November 2007.

Maguire BJ, Hunting KL, Guidotti TL, Smith GS: Occupational injuries among emergency medical services personnel, *Prehosp Emerg Care* 9(4):405-411 2005.

National Association of Emergency Medical Technicians: Statement on safety restraint use in emergency medical services. http://www.naemt.org/aboutNAEMT/restraint+position.htm. June 2007.

www.pandemicflu.gov/.

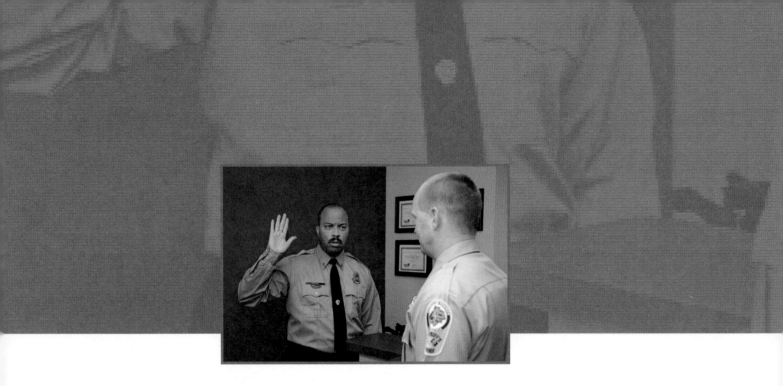

Medicolegal
3 and Ethical Issues

CHAPTER OUTLINE

Ethical Responsibilities

Scope of Practice

Equipment

Negligence

Consent

Refusal of Treatment and Transport

Abandonment

Intoxicated, Irrational, and Emotionally Disturbed Patients

Resuscitation Issues

Donor and Organ Harvesting

Medical Identification Insignia

Crime Scenes

Risk Management

Scenario

You respond to a call from the family of a 45-year-old man with lung cancer who is turning blue and gasping for breath. The patient is not responsive. You learn from the family that the patient has incurable cancer and only weeks to live. He has a "do not resuscitate" order that directs medical personnel not to perform positive-pressure ventilations or chest compressions if his breathing or heart stops. In light of this information, you seek to understand more clearly exactly why the family called for help.

Laws pertaining to emergency medical services (EMS) and healthcare providers provide the basis for the conduct of emergency medical technicians (EMTs) in regard to patients, the medical directors, and society. The services that an EMT is expected to provide are outlined in the Scope of Practice section in this chapter. EMTs provide care only with a patient's consent. Sometimes the consent must be implied because patients may not be mentally competent (e.g., they are unconscious) or of legal age to formally give their consent (expressed consent).

At times, patients may refuse care or transportation to a hospital. Knowing the rules governing consent and patients' rights allows EMTs to provide the best care to patients while respecting their legal rights.

For example, information obtained during patient care is held confidential. At times, however, laws require certain information, such as suspected child abuse or highly communicable diseases, to be released to officials. Knowing the medicolegal aspects of EMS allows EMTs to conduct themselves in the manner expected of them by society.

Ethical Responsibilities

The "Golden Rule"

"Do unto others as you would have them do unto you." This time-tested philosophy provides a sound basis for defining ethical practices within all aspects of medical care. It implies that the individual is acting in a manner that he or she believes to be in the best interest of the patient. As an EMT, you must make the patient's emotional and physical needs your first priority. In many cases, personal convenience, comfort, and self-interest may interfere with providing the best possible care for the patient.

For example, it may be easier to walk a patient from the scene than to provide the appropriate stretcher or chair transport, or it may be tempting to deliver a patient to a nearby but less suitable emergency department (ED) at the end of your shift. These are examples of clearly unethical practices. Such practices, which place the convenience of the EMT over the needs of the patient, destroy the essence and intent of quality prehospital care. Remember, patients are vulnerable because they are ill or injured, and they rely on the health profession to act in their interest.

Ethics and Competence

The Golden Rule implies that you will provide care to others the same way you would want care given to you or your family. Quality care is caring and competent. The EMT needs to have the knowledge and skills to recognize and treat critical conditions properly. The EMT has a professional and ethical responsibility to maintain competence in the practice of prehospital care. This includes a serious effort to acquire the skills taught in an initial training program as well as a continued effort to polish those skills to a level of "mastery" and to reinforce knowledge.

Remaining skillful in prehospital care requires diligence and careful self-evaluation. After passing the initial certification examination, many states require attendance at refresher courses every few years to qualify for recertification. You probably will see some conditions, such as tension pneumothorax, once a year or less. To keep knowledge and skills current, you can read journals, attend lectures, participate in call review sessions, and practice clinical skills so that you are prepared to recognize a patient's problem even if you rarely see it. EMS educators offer "refresher" courses with this in mind.

An EMS agency's quality improvement (QI) program may review both individual cases and the agency's overall performance. Goals can include improvement in many different activities, such as response times, patient care, and communication. You should become involved with local QI efforts. For example, EMTs might meet with their medical directors at call review sessions to review the assessment and care given in the field. Call review sessions provide an opportunity to compare the prehospital impression with the ED diagnosis and to critique the care, all in an effort to find ways to improve patient care.

An EMS program designed to promote ethical practice is ICARE. ICARE is a pneumonic identifying the traits to be held by those in EMS. ICARE stands for:

- I–ntegrity
- C–ompassion
- A–ccountability
- R–espect
- E–mpathy

Schools and EMSS adopting the ICARE philosophy award fellow students and co-workers with ICARE pins when they witness acts reflecting the ICARE philosophy. You can learn more about ICARE at http://www.icarevalues.org/.

> **REAL**World
>
> Remaining current in knowledge and skills requires a combination of refresher training and continuing education. Refresher training reviews information and skills previously learned but most likely not frequently used. Continuing education is keeping up-to-date on changes in medicine and healthcare or learning new information. It is important for the EMT to appreciate that the knowledge and skills learned today will be different 10 years from now. There is continual research in health care, resulting in changes in medical practice. An effective, competent EMT must remain current.

> **LEARNING OBJECTIVE**
> - Explain the importance, necessity, and legality of patient confidentiality.

Confidentiality

By the nature of the work, the EMT enters into some very private situations and circumstances. All patients have the right to know that the information they give in order to be treated will be kept confidential. Indeed, without a truthful and honest history, it is difficult to make an accurate assessment of the patient's problem. In turn, as an EMT you have a responsibility to regard information provided in a patient's history, physical assessment, and treatment as confidential. The patient-EMT relationship, as with the patient-physician relationship, is based on the mutual trust that what is revealed will be kept confidential and used for the benefit of helping the patient. It is a very special relationship.

Release of confidential patient information requires a written release from the patient. For patients not capable of giving expressed consent, such as minors or mentally incompetent individuals, confidential information is not given unless legal guardianship has been established and has authorized such release.

Exceptions to the requirement for a written release of information from the patient are limited but include the following:
1. Other healthcare providers who need the information to continue the patient's care (e.g., hospital personnel)
2. The need for EMTs to report incidents such as child abuse or gunshot wounds, as required by state law
3. Third-party payment billing forms
4. Response to legal subpoena

These exceptions specify not only *what* information is required to be reported but also *to whom*. Although information such as alleged child abuse is required to be reported to authorities and hospital personnel, this does not mean it is no longer confidential and now public information. Rather, the rules of release specifically address *who* may receive the report as an exception to the rule that patient information is only released with the patient's consent.

You may be thrust into a situation in which you must deal with reporters. The press and TV cameras usually appear at the scene of major incidents. Events involving EMS often make the "news." While pursuing a story, the media may try to get the EMT to reveal confidential information. An EMT's first obligation is to the patient, and you must respect this relationship above all else. Sometimes the EMT may provide the media with general facts regarding an incident, consistent with the local policy established in your service. However, it is a better practice, whenever possible, to consult with your supervisor, administrator, or medical control physician before releasing any information to the press. Your agency may have a spokesperson to handle such requests. Your obligation to the patient should be honored.

Case in Point

You encounter a well-known businessman who collapsed in a section of town known for drug activity. When he was found, drug paraphernalia was in his pocket, and he had track marks over the veins of his left arm. You suspect a drug overdose. A reporter who recognizes the man approaches you and asks why he collapsed. What do you do?

Recognizing the patient's right to confidentiality, you do not divulge information you gather in the course of patient care to anyone not involved in the care of the patient.

Requests for information may come from family members, co-workers, or friends. In general, let the patient or the ED physician divulge personal information regarding the diagnosis or care of the patient.

REAL*World*

In most cases when a child has been injured, parents can and should be notified and informed of the child's injury and current status. In the case of sexual assault, sexually transmitted disease, and pregnancy, however, many states not only allow a minor to seek medical care without consent from a parent or guardian, but also often consider that this information is privileged and cannot be shared with the parents or guardian unless requested by the child. It is the responsibility of the EMT to be familiar with the laws regarding confidentiality in his or her area.

HIPAA

A federal law protecting patient privacy, the Health Insurance Portability and Accountability Act of 1996 (**HIPAA**), took effect in 2003. Because of the widespread use of electronic records and communication and the potential to have patient information transmitted without the patient's knowledge or consent, rules were established for many parties who would have access to patient information, including insurance companies, health maintenance organizations (HMOs), and providers of medical care, including EMTs.

Specifically outlined in HIPAA rules are provisions for patients' access to their medical records and more control over how their private, personal health information is used and disclosed (disseminated), regardless of *how* it is communicated. Agencies and their health providers are required to develop and follow written privacy procedures, provide training for their employees, and have a designated privacy officer. HIPAA provides for limited disclosures of health information for specific public responsibilities, including emergency circumstances; identification of the body of a deceased person, or the cause of death; public health needs; research that involves limited data or has been independently approved by an institutional review board (IRB) or privacy board; oversight of the healthcare system; judicial and administrative proceedings; limited law enforcement activities; and activities related to national defense and security.

Become aware of the HIPPA provisions within the agency from which you provide emergency medical care. The website http://www.hhs.gov/ocr/hipaa/ provides detailed information and answers to frequently asked questions.

LEARNING OBJECTIVE
• State the conditions that require an EMT to notify local law enforcement officials.

Reporting Requirements

Local laws may require EMTs and other emergency personnel to report certain conditions to the police, health department, and other authorities. Circumstances that may be reportable include the following:
- Child abuse
- Geriatric abuse
- Family violence and abuse
- Violent crimes

- Certain infectious diseases
- Patients transported against their will
- Patients who are mentally incompetent (e.g., intoxicated with injuries)
- Animal bites
- Wounds from guns and knives
- Deaths

You should familiarize yourself with local laws and protocols to determine your responsibility in these areas, because local and state reporting requirements differ. Often the hospital rather than the EMT may be legally required to report a condition, but information provided by EMS may be part of this report.

REAL*World*

When dealing with a suspected reportable event, the EMT must be sure to report but not accuse. For example, if called by a father to provide care for his child, who appears to have been abused, an EMT is required to report these suspicions. However, just because the father was the person caring for the child at the time of the call does not mean he was the abuser. Making false accusations are slanderous and can result in legal actions against the EMT. Report; don't accuse.

LEARNING OBJECTIVE
- Define the EMT scope of practice.

Scope of Practice

The **scope of practice** refers to the range of activities and limitations of a given medical provider. State EMS laws define the practice of prehospital care. These laws address such issues as minimum training standards, medical control, vehicle and equipment specifications, and licensure or certification requirements. They may also specify formation and duties of EMS councils and EMS medical advisory committees.

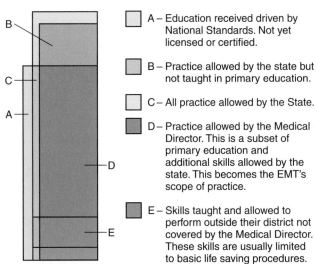

A – Education received driven by National Standards. Not yet licensed or certified.

B – Practice allowed by the state but not taught in primary education.

C – All practice allowed by the State.

D – Practice allowed by the Medical Director. This is a subset of primary education and additional skills allowed by the state. This becomes the EMT's scope of practice.

E – Skills taught and allowed to perform outside their district not covered by the Medical Director. These skills are usually limited to basic life saving procedures.

Figure 3-1 The relationship among education, certification, scope of practice, and medical oversight. *Modified from National Highway Traffic Safety Administration:* National EMS Scope of Practice Model, *Washington, DC, 2005, US Department of Transportation.*

The scope of practice establishes what an EMT legally can and cannot do in the course of emergency medical evaluation and treatment. For example, the EMT might use an oropharyngeal airway and a bag-mask resuscitator to ventilate the lungs of a patient who is not breathing, but the EMT would not perform needle cricothyroidotomy (insertion of needle through neck into windpipe). The scope of practice essentially describes what you can and cannot do during a patient encounter. The scope of practice is further defined by state and regional treatment protocols (**Figure 3-1**).

The *National EMS Scope of Practice Model* outlines a useful framework for understanding an individual EMT's scope of practice based on the notion that education, certification, licensure, and credentialing represent four separate but related activities (**Box 3-1**).

Standard of Care

The guiding standard of effective medical practice is referred to as the **standard of care.** Standard of care deals with the questions, "Did you do the right thing, and did you do it properly?"

Box 3-1   EMS Scope of Practice

Education includes all of the cognitive, psychomotor, and affective learning that a provider has undergone throughout his or her life. This includes entry-level and continuing professional education, as well as other formal and informal learning. Clearly, many individuals have extensive education that, in some cases, exceeds their EMS skills or roles.

Certification is an external verification of the competencies that an individual has achieved and typically involves an examination process. While certification exams can be set to any level of proficiency, in health care they are typically designed to verify that an individual has achieved minimum competency to assure safe and effective patient care.

Licensure represents permission granted to an individual by the State to perform certain restricted activities. Scope of practice represents the legal limits of the licensed individual's performance. States have a variety of mechanisms to define the margins of what an individual is legally permitted to perform.

Credentialing is a local process by which an individual is permitted by a specific entity (Medical Director) to practice in a specific setting (EMS agency). Credentialing processes vary in sophistication and formality.

For every individual, these four domains are of slightly different relative sizes. However, one concept remains constant: an individual may only perform a skill or role for which that person is:

- Educated (has been trained to perform the skill of role), AND
- Certified (has demonstrated competence in the skill or role), AND
- Licensed (has legal authority issued by the State to perform the skill or role), AND
- Credentialed (has medical oversight to perform the skill or role).

From National Highway Traffic Safety Administration: *National EMS Scope of Practice Model,* Washington, DC, 2005, US Department of Transportation.

The term *standard of care* is used to describe the body of knowledge, laws, policies, common practices, standards, and guidelines that provide the basis of prehospital and other medical care.

Laws, rules, and regulations govern your practice as an EMT. The extent of regulation varies from region to region. State or local statutes may specifically define the practice of prehospital care. In addition, the standard of care can be defined by **protocols,** which may incorporate or refer to authoritative medical sources, such as international guidelines for performance of CPR. Protocols may be developed or modified by state and local medical directors and allow EMTs to operate under *standing orders* (prewritten treatment directives) or by online telephone or radio communications.

The standard of care may address both limitations on your role as well as requirements to perform specific skills in a specific situation. For example, EMTs may be legally required to attempt resuscitation of every cardiac arrest victim, with only a few specified exceptions.

An EMT's evaluation under the standard of care also involves comparison with others functioning at a similar level. In a lawsuit, EMTs are often brought in as expert witnesses to establish how they would have acted in similar circumstances.

Equipment

When responding to an emergency call, you are expected to provide care with equipment, medications, and medical devices appropriate for your level of training and certification. This includes having available the equipment essential to the treatment of common emergencies. It is important to check all equipment, including the vehicle, at the beginning of each shift and to replace or repair missing or malfunctioning items before responding to your first call. You should carefully document equipment failure that occurs during the treatment of a patient and report it to administrative personnel.

LEARNING OBJECTIVES
- State the conditions necessary for the EMT to have a duty to act.
- Discuss the issues of abandonment, negligence, and battery and their implications to the EMT.

Negligence

In general, **negligence** is a deviation from the accepted standard of care that results in injury to the patient. To establish negligence (at other times called "medical malpractice"), however, four elements must be present:
1. Duty to act
2. Breach of duty
3. Damage
4. Causal connection

Duty to Act

For litigation to be successful, the complainant's attorney must first establish that the EMT had a duty to the patient. An EMT, whether volunteer or paid, has a **duty to act** when responding to a patient while working in EMS. Other situations that might establish a duty to act for an EMS service or individual EMT include the following:
- A patient calls for an ambulance, and the dispatcher confirms that an ambulance will be sent.
- An ambulance service has a written contract with a municipality or community.
- An ambulance passes the scene of an emergency, whether inside or outside their primary areas of response.
- As per specific state regulations regarding duty to act.

On the other hand, an off-duty EMT usually has no initial duty to act when encountering an emergency situation. The EMT may have ethical or moral reasons to intervene, but there is usually no legal mandate. An off-duty EMT can establish a duty to act by becoming involved with the patient, but the standard of care to which the EMT is held may differ from what is required of the same EMT in the course of work. In some states, an EMT not on duty and acting as a "Good Samaritan" is held liable only for "gross negligence," a tougher legal standard meant to encourage citizens to act to help one another.

Breach of Duty

A **breach of duty** refers to a negligent action or omission that has violated the standards of care expected from an EMT under the circumstances. Every medical provider is expected to act with reasonable care to prevent injury to the patient. EMTs may breach their duty by *commission,* such as performing a procedure incorrectly or performing acts outside their scope or deemed otherwise negligent, or by *omission,* such as failing to act in the circumstances required.

Damage

To initiate a complaint of negligence, or medical **malpractice,** the plaintiff must also demonstrate damage, either physical or psychological. If the patient was not injured after an omission of treatment or the alleged use of improper methods by an EMT, no basis for a lawsuit exists.

Causal Connection

The final element necessary to initiate a successful lawsuit is a clear connection between the patient's injury and actions taken or omitted by the EMT. Demonstrating injury is not enough; the complainant must prove that the injury was caused by the actions or omissions of the EMT who had a duty to act. For example, if a patient was paralyzed after an injury and sued the EMT, the patient would be required to prove that the paralysis was related to an action or inaction on the part of the EMT and was not a result of the traumatic event. A **causal connection** must exist.

A successful lawsuit requires the presence of all four elements: duty to act, breach of duty, damage, and causal connection (**Table 3-1**).

Case in Point

A Land's End ambulance responds to a man reported to be exhibiting bizarre behavior in the park. On arrival, a 20-year-old man is speaking gibberish. You notice he is sweaty and has a rapid pulse but otherwise appears normal. You notice a Medic Alert tag on his wrist that lists diabetes. Your partner rushes to the ambulance for the oral glucose gel. He returns and says he cannot find any gel, so you initiate transport to the hospital.

At the hospital the patient is treated immediately. The nurse says his glucose level is very low, based on the bedside test. He receives intravenous glucose, which results in a gradual recovery. His brother arrives at the hospital a short time later; when he hears that there was no glucose at the scene, he threatens to sue.

Failure to stock the ambulance with a medication necessary for emergency treatment would be a breach of duty by omission and could support a charge of negligence. A delay in correcting the patient's low blood sugar level could result in brain damage, and the minutes lost because the ambulance did not administer glucose may have contributed to such an injury and may be a causal connection. However, this patient recovered fully, so there were no damages. Although duty to act and breach of duty could be established in this case, without damages a claim of medical malpractice would not be supported.

Table 3-1	Elements Necessary to Establish Negligence
Element	**Explanation**
Duty to act	Patient-provider relationship must be established
Breach of duty	Improper act or failure to act
Damage	Patient must have sustained physical or psychological damage
Causal connection	Injury resulted from improper action or failure to act

"Good Samaritan" Legislation

Federal and state laws often provide institutions, medical professionals, government agencies (e.g., military services), and individuals an extra degree of protection from lawsuits in certain situations. In some cases, such as with the military and certain governmental agencies, you may not be allowed to sue by law. Other laws are designed to protect people who come to the aid of an ill or injured person in a "volunteer" capacity. These laws might raise the bar for negligence to a "gross negligence" standard. Negligence is the failure to meet the standard of care a reasonable EMT in the community would meet. *Gross negligence* is willful and wanton recklessness that would be so careless as to be dangerous.

Specific laws designed to protect the private citizen who is functioning in a nonprofessional capacity and without an expectation of remuneration are often referred to as "Good Samaritan" laws. These laws were developed to encourage medical professionals and laypersons to provide aid without undue fear of litigation.

Good Samaritan laws help protect the EMT from civil charges, such as claims of malpractice and negligence. However, gross negligence may result in criminal charges that are not covered under a Good Samaritan law.

Some laws are specific about what is and is not covered. For example, the responsibility to drive an ambulance safely might be clearly separate from any Good Samaritan protection offered for the medical encounter. In New York state, for example, Public Health Law: Article 30—Emergency Medical Services, states the following:

3013: Immunity from Liability

3. Nothing in this section shall be deemed to relieve or alter the liability of any such voluntary ambulance service or members for damages or injuries or death arising out of the operation of motor vehicles.

LEARNING OBJECTIVES
- Define consent, and discuss the methods of obtaining consent.
- Differentiate between expressed (informed) and implied consent.
- Explain the role of consent by minors in issues of care.

Consent

Before treating a patient, you must obtain the consent of the patient, parent, or guardian. This reflects the principle of *autonomy,* or self-determination, that a person has the right to be self-directing, especially regarding decisions to enter into a medical relationship with health professionals.

The EMT provides care to individuals only with their consent. In a hospital, patients are usually asked to sign a statement of consent. In emergency prehospital care, this is not usually done. Because of the emergency situation, a verbal approval or other indication of agreement, such as a nod, may be the form of consent. An unconscious patient may receive emergency treatment by implied consent, as discussed later.

The EMT should understand basic concepts of consent and seek to obtain consent for care in all cases. However, consent is not always possible. For example, you may encounter patients who are disoriented, minors with no parent or guardian immediately available, and individuals who are mentally handicapped and incapable of providing consent. Consent may take several forms, as described next.

Expressed (Informed) Consent

Expressed consent, or **informed consent,** must be obtained from every conscious, mentally competent adult. A mentally competent patient is older than the legal adult age and able to make an informed decision. For consent to be *informed,* the patient must be made aware of the risks, benefits, and consequences of the care provided and alternatives to the care. In prehospital care the EMT needs to inform patients of the steps of procedures and related risks. A patient must then *express* his or her consent verbally or with affirming gestures, such as a nod or holding out an arm for examination or treatment.

Documenting that you fully informed the patient is especially important when a patient wants to withhold consent. If a patient or patient's family refuses medical treatment, you must inform them of the potential consequences of delayed treatment before the patient or patient's relative signs a release form. Signing a "release against medical advice" form should meet expressed consent standards. This means that the patient should have a reasonable understanding of the potential consequences of his or her actions.

Prehospital Research

A special area of consent that may arise in the practice of EMS is related to research. Research studies may be conducted in your EMS system to evaluate the effectiveness of certain treatments or procedures. Research studies are approved by *institutional review boards* (IRBs), which may be based at hospitals or universities within state departments of health. As part of their responsibilities, IRBs may prescribe steps for acquiring patient consent. This may involve reading and signing a consent agreement or giving verbal consent. In the case of cardiac arrest research or research related to unconscious patients who cannot give consent, public awareness and input required before IRB approval may be achieved on a community-wide basis through local media or meetings with community groups. The purpose of this process is to respect the autonomy of individuals. You must become familiar with the consent procedures of research studies to ensure compliance with research protocols and respect of patient autonomy. National courses sponsored by the National Institutes of Health (NIH) and others that deal with research and human subjects are well worth your time and will deepen your respect for the patient's (and human) rights and the ethical obligations of research involving people.

Implied Consent

Implied consent refers to circumstances in which verbal or written consent is not possible but a reasonable person would want and expect emergency treatment to be rendered. For example, when you encounter an unconscious person, you should provide treatment because a reasonable person would want such actions to be taken under these circumstances. This concept also applies to persons unable legally to give consent, such as children with no parent or guardian immediately available or mentally incompetent individuals. As previously mentioned, a parent or guardian should provide consent in these circumstances; however, if the delay caused by seeking such consent would adversely affect the health or life of the patient, the EMT should pursue treatment.

Other Types of Consent

Children and mentally incompetent individuals are not legally able to give expressed consent. Rather, EMTs must obtain consent from the parent or legal guardian, unless implied consent is more appropriate for the patient's condition. An individual is capable of consenting when he or she is a mentally competent adult or an emancipated minor. An **emancipated minor** is an individual who is younger than the legal adult age but who is living independently of his or her parents, is financially self-supporting, is or was married, is or was a parent, or actively enlisted in the armed forces. You should check the specific definitions of an emancipated minor in your state.

LEARNING OBJECTIVE
- Discuss the implications for the EMT in patient refusal of transport.

Refusal of Treatment and Transport

As an EMT, you will encounter patients who refuse medical treatment. A person has the right to refuse care if he or she is mentally competent and therefore capable of making a clear judgment. Also, a patient has the right to withdraw from treatment at any time, even after some treatment has been rendered. You run the risk of a charge of "false imprisonment" if you forcibly transport a patient against his or her expressed wishes. You may also leave yourself open to charges of **assault** and **battery** if you touch and provide emergency care to a patient without his or her consent.

When a patient who refuses care appears in need of medical assistance, you should make every attempt to convince the patient to go to the hospital. Family members, friends, and physicians at medical control provide an excellent resource in these difficult situations.

Ensure that the patient understands the consequences of not seeking medical attention. One test is to have the patient repeat, in his or her own words, your assessment of the possible condition and possible consequences of refusing care, so that you are more assured that he or she has understanding when making this decision. For example, a patient might be asked to state and sign, "I understand that my chest pain might be a serious cardiac condition and I might sustain sudden death," as an addition to the standard "refusal of medical attention" release.

If the patient still refuses medical care, he or she should sign a "refusal of treatment" release form. You should carefully document your assessment and treatment, attempts to encourage further care, and names of witnesses or police officers. These forms generally require the signature of a witness. Signatures of family members, friends, and police are preferred over other EMS personnel on the scene to ensure objectivity. Again, to be an "informed" refusal of services, the patient must understand the potential consequences of refusing medical care before signing the release form (**Figure 3-2**).

Patients whose mental competence may be altered by drugs, alcohol, illness, or injury present special problems. In these circumstances, you should seek assistance from law enforcement, family members, and medical control. Use your best judgment, and err on the side of transport.

Abandonment

As an EMT who is part of an EMS system, you assume the responsibility of providing care to an ill or injured patient from the time you arrive on the scene until you transfer the patient to the care of hospital personnel. **Abandonment** is a legal term that describes a situation in which an EMT or other health professional discontinues a patient-provider relationship without giving the patient time or opportunity to obtain continuation of care at the same level or higher. This includes circumstances in which an EMT on the scene leaves a patient who is in need of emergency care and transportation to a hospital or when an EMT prematurely discontinues care.

For a case of abandonment to hold up in court, complainants must first establish that they were owed a duty and that the duty was breached.

Charges of abandonment are also possible if a patient who refused care was incompetent, such as a child or an adult with altered mental status, yet was left at the scene. If the EMT suspects that a patient who refuses care is not capable of making a reasonable judgment, he or she should make every attempt to transport that patient to the hospital. If the patient adamantly refuses, you should secure the aid of family, medical control, and police officers. In some cases, transporting the patient against his or her will may be appropriate and necessary. If available in such circumstances, you should seek administrative or legal advice.

REFUSAL OF TRANSPORT AND TREATMENT
PLEASE READ THIS DOCUMENT

This form has been given to you because you have refused treatment or transportation to the hospital by Emergency Medical Service personnel. Your health and safety are our primary concerns. Even though you have decided not to accept our offer of treatment or transport to the hospital, please remember the following:

1. We recommend that you be evaluated and treated by a physician.

2. Your decision to refuse treatment and transport may result in delay, which may result in worsening of your condition.

3. Medical evaluation or treatment may be obtained by calling your personal physician or by going to any hospital's Emergency Department.

4. You may change your mind about transport. Please do not hesitate to contact us. We will not hesitate to return to assist you.

5. **Do not wait!** When medical treatment is needed, it is usually better to get it sooner than later.

DIAL 911
IF YOU NEED
EMERGENCY MEDICAL SERVICES

_____   _____
Attending EMS Personnel   Date/Time

_____
Patient Signature

Figure 3-2 "Refusal of care" form. *Courtesy HealthONE EMS, Englewood, Colo.*

Intoxicated, Irrational, and Emotionally Disturbed Patients

The management of emotionally or mentally disturbed patients represents an area of high legal risk for both hospital and prehospital personnel. Because these patients are often held against their expressed wishes, charges of false imprisonment and battery are sometimes brought in relation to an injury sustained during the restraining process.

The EMT should always exercise caution when removing patients against their will. Generally, such actions are taken to prevent patients from injuring themselves or others. In such circumstances, many state and local governments permit the police to help remove the patient under the concept of "protective custody." If conditions permit, you should contact the patient's family or physician to encourage the patient to submit to care. With violent or suicidal patients, however, this is sometimes not possible.

When forcible removal is necessary, care should be taken not to harm the patient. "Soft" restraints should be available and used in these circumstances. Handcuffs are discouraged because of the injury likely to occur during the patient's struggle. Precise documentation is essential to record the circumstances that warranted the use of force. Extreme care should be exercised not to use subjective words or phrases to describe the patient's behavior. Instead, specifically document the patient's behavior; for example, "The patient attempted to strike the EMTs and police during the patient interview," or "The patient stated that he was going to kill himself." In most states, patients may also be forcibly removed under a court order or multiple-physician order. You should consult with your administrative staff about the policy within your organization.

Case in Point

It is well past midnight. A man in his 40s who is well known in the community for his alcoholic binges is lying on the street. People looking out the window from an apartment building down the block called 9-1-1. You note that he has a bruise on his forehead and abrasions on his hand, consistent with a fall to the sidewalk. He is breathing adequately, and his breath smells of alcohol. His pupils are equal and reactive, and he has a pulse, but he will not let you take a blood pressure reading because he keeps pulling his arm away. He does not converse with you, but between four-letter words he periodically slurs phrases you understand such as "get off me" and "leave me alone." You ask him if he wants to come to the hospital, but all you get in reply is more cursing and refusals. You tell him if he wants to stay, he will have to sign a release. You know that will not happen.

Continued

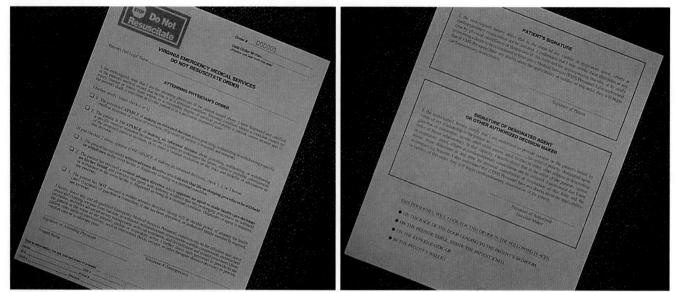

Figure 3-3 "Do not resuscitate" (DNR) request (DNR order). *Courtesy Virginia Office of Emergency Medical Services. In Shade B et al:* Mosby's EMT-Intermediate textbook for the 1999 National Standard Curriculum, *ed 3, St Louis, 2007, Mosby-Elsevier.*

You and your partner have seen the man in this condition before. He is obviously intoxicated. His bruises and abrasions do not appear to be severe injuries. You wonder whether you should call a patrol car to help you transport or witness the fact that the patient is refusing care. You are uncertain about whether you should force him to come along to the hospital. You are tempted to leave him according to his wishes and trust he will sleep it off by morning.

Your partner overhears a call for a motor vehicle crash four blocks away, and you look at each other and decide to go to that call. You tell the patient that you will be back and to think over his decision. You then tell the dispatcher the last case refused care and you are on your way to the car crash.

You become very involved caring for the crash victims. When you return 2 hours later to check on your first patient, he is no longer there.

The next day as you report for duty, your supervisor asks you to explain what happened with your first call. You find out that another ambulance was called an hour later and transported the same man, now unarousable, to the trauma center, where he was taken to the operating room for evacuation of an epidural hematoma (blood clot) compressing the brain.

Discussion

There are many questions to ponder in this case. Although fictional, this case is based on other cases that have filled the incident files of many EMS systems. Patients with chronic substance abuse problems and behavior problems are difficult for EMS and public agencies called to their aid, often by strangers. Was this patient abandoned? Could this patient have made an informed refusal of medical attention? Did this patient's condition obviously require transport to the hospital? If so, should he have been restrained if necessary and brought against his will? Should the police have been called to the scene? If so, what might they have done to help? Should medical control have been called for advice while EMS was at the scene? Were the EMTs correct to leave for a call that sounded more like an emergency? Although not always easy to answer, these questions need to be posed in every EMS region so that you can plan in advance for difficult situations in which your judgment and knowledge of consent, refusal, abandonment, restraint, and medical care will be tested.

> **LEARNING OBJECTIVE**
> * Discuss the importance of DNR orders, advance directives, and local or state provisions regarding EMS application.

Resuscitation Issues

Proxies

Patients, especially those with terminal or chronic illness, may express consent for, or refusal of, future medical care while they can still make decisions for themselves. Although it is customary to initiate cardiopulmonary resuscitation (CPR) for individuals through the doctrine of implied consent, some individuals may not wish to have resuscitative efforts initiated on their behalf. Because expressed consent is not possible once patients are incapacitated, laws allow for ways to make decisions in advance. Examples include a "do not resuscitate" order or an advance directive, or a patient may designate a healthcare proxy who will make decisions in his or her place. By these means, healthcare providers are able to honor the wishes of patients even after they have lost the capacity to communicate directly.

Do not resuscitate (DNR) orders (or DNR requests) direct healthcare providers not to perform resuscitation if breathing or circulation stops (**Figure 3-3**). In general, these are written orders from a physician. They may be communicated to EMTs in different ways, whether a patient is at home, in a nursing home, or at another healthcare facility. DNR orders are quite specific in that they deal with respiratory and cardiac arrest. They do not direct stopping treatment for other conditions, such as administration of oxygen for shortness of breath and administration of glucose for hypoglycemia.

Advance directives are more specific statements regarding a wider range of patient consents and refusals. For example,

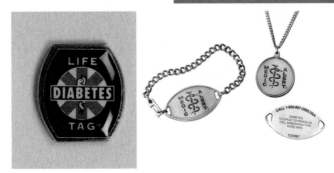

Figure 3-4 Medical identification jewelry. *Courtesy MedicAlert™ Foundation, Turlock, Calif. From Chapleau W:* Emergency first responder: making the difference, *St Louis, 2004, Mosby-JEMS.*

patients may leave instructions about their consent for such treatments as artificial nutrition and hydration, dialysis, transplantation, and blood transfusions if they become mentally incapacitated or otherwise unable to communicate.

A **healthcare proxy** is an individual named to make decisions for a person about health care if that person becomes incapacitated.

Case in Point

A patient has metastatic cancer and is undergoing chemotherapy and other treatment to prolong her life. She called 9-1-1 when she fell and has pain in her hip. She is aware that her time is limited. She does not want to have CPR if her breathing or heart stops. She has spoken to her physician and has DNR forms completed so that her wishes may be known when her time to die arrives. If her family calls an ambulance and she has a cardiac arrest, the EMTs will become aware of her directive and act accordingly. In the current situation, however, where the fall may have resulted in a broken hip, she needs and desires emergency care.

Because options for advance directives, DNR decisions, and their applicability to EMS can vary from state to state, you should become knowledgeable about your laws in your own region so that you can carry out your patients' wishes.

Extended Transport

Extended transport of patients who have valid DNR orders may place the EMT in a precarious situation, especially if the transport crosses county (or borough) lines. First, the EMTs must make sure they have an original copy of the DNR order. For DNR orders to be considered valid by EMS or receiving facilities, typically the paperwork must be intact and not otherwise torn or mutilated, and it must be the original document. Photocopies are not accepted in some states. Second, if the patient dies during transport, the ambulance must stop within the county in which the patient died, and the coroner for that jurisdiction must be notified. In many states it is illegal to transport a dead body across county lines. Third, the EMTs must remain with the body, and the body must remain in the ambulance, until the coroner or their proxy arrives to take custody of the body. It is also illegal in some states to move a dead body or leave it unattended. Before the transport the EMTs may consider notifying the coroner's office of the regions through which they will be transporting the body, and they must be familiar with local laws.

LEARNING OBJECTIVE
- Discuss the considerations of the EMT regarding issues of organ retrieval.

Donor and Organ Harvesting

Individuals may decide in advance to donate organs. These wishes can be indicated on a driver's license or separate donor card. In general, you should treat a potential organ donor the same as any other patient. If you become aware of a patient's organ donor status, communicate this information to the hospital or medical direction when appropriate so that steps are taken to attempt to carry out the patient's wishes.

Medical Identification Insignia

At times, a patient may indicate an advance directive to you by medical identification insignia. For example, DNR bracelets might be used to indicate DNR status. Other patients may wear bracelets or necklaces (jewelry) that indicate a preexisting medical condition such as diabetes, allergies, heart disease, or epilepsy (**Figure 3-4**).

LEARNING OBJECTIVE
- Delineate the actions that an EMT should take to assist in preserving a crime scene.

Crime Scenes

If you need to render emergency care at the scene of a crime, the following additional considerations apply:
- Ensure safety of yourself and fellow responders. Do not enter a crime scene where you may be in danger. Wait for police to make the scene safe.
- Notify police personnel through dispatch if you are first on the scene.
- Try not to disturb any item at the scene unless emergency care requires it.
- If possible, do not cut through holes in clothing made by knife or gunshot wounds.

You should keep other items that might be important as evidence and transport them with the patient in such a manner as to preserve their evidentiary value if the items were to be introduced in court. This is called a **chain of evidence,** or custody. Evidence collected should be under the direct observation or control of the EMT or police or otherwise placed in a secure, locked compartment. When turned over to the hospital or legal authorities, the item should be signed for on the prehospital care record as documentation that it was transferred. Later, if the materials are introduced as evidence in a court of law, the documentation can help identify who had control of the material at all times.

Risk Management

Risk management refers to practices by healthcare providers that reduce the possibility of a lawsuit or other legal or professional actions taken against you, your medical director, or your agency. In general, the best prevention of legal problems is providing quality emergency care. This includes acting according to the standard of care, carefully documenting your actions, and acting in the best interest of the patient.

Act According to Standard of Care

First and foremost, you should act according to the current standard of care, within your scope of practice and the local protocols established for your agency and EMS system. You may seek online consultation with your medical control physician. When in doubt, you should use your best judgment and act in the best interest of the patient.

Document Actions Carefully

The prehospital care record is the backbone of a defense in any lawsuit against an EMT. Most lawsuits come to the attention of the EMT months or sometimes years after an incident. Your individual recollection of circumstances and actions is likely to be extremely vague and blurry. The prehospital care record is the primary reference point in these cases. Effective documentation ensures continuity of patient care and protection to all healthcare providers. Assessment steps, treatments, times, and other significant events should be documented.

Act in the Patient's Best Interest

Although interaction with the patient and family members is usually brief, the nature of the circumstances is likely to generate strong and sometimes turbulent emotions. The patient and family view you as the individual charged with lifesaving responsibilities. Your attitude and demeanor should reflect an appropriate sense of the significance of the circumstances. Patients and families may often manifest anger or impatience during their care or the care of their loved one. An understanding and tolerant attitude is essential to avoid destructive and often unnecessary confrontation. It helps to imagine how you might behave under similar circumstances.

Scenario Follow-up

The patient's family explains that they were not sure if the patient was suffering and sought help in case he was experiencing undue pain or anguish. They noted he has had fever and chills for the past 2 day as his breathing became more labored. As you continue assessing the patient, your partner calls medical control for advice and direction.

You are advised to transport the patient to the hospital and give supplemental oxygen. While you will respect the patient's directive not to resuscitate him if his heart stops beating or if he stops breathing, you respect the patient's wish to have other emergency medical care, such as treatment for pneumonia.

Summary

The educational curriculum, medical protocols, ethics, and laws that guide EMTs help define the scope of practice and the interactions expected between EMTs and society. Ethical considerations of the EMT include maintaining competence, obeying community laws and professional guidelines, working in harmony with other members of the healthcare team for the good of the patient, and generally upholding the dignity of the profession. Specific laws address other important issues, such as consent, confidentiality, and special reporting situations. Patient autonomy is an essential right of individuals, and mechanisms to respect the wishes of people once they have lost their capacity—such as advance directives, DNR orders, healthcare proxies, and organ donation authorizations—should be understood as they pertain to patients where you practice. Although lawsuits in EMS are rare, the legal definitions of duty to act, breach of duty, injury to a patient, and a causal connection are important to understand as expectations of society from the health profession. Laws, codes, or ethics and medical protocols cannot address every foreseeable situation, and EMTs must rely on good judgment and act in the best interest of the patient. Take a moment to review the EMT Code of Ethics issued by the National Association of EMTs (**Box 3-2**).

| Box 3-2 | The EMT Code of Ethics |

Professional status as an Emergency Medical Technician and Emergency Medical Technician-Paramedic is maintained and enriched by the willingness of the individual practitioner to accept and fulfill obligations to society, other medical professionals, and the profession of Emergency Medical Technician. As an Emergency Medical Technician at the basic level or an Emergency Medical Technician-Paramedic, I solemnly pledge myself to the following code of professional ethics:

A fundamental responsibility of the Emergency Medical Technician is to conserve life, to alleviate suffering, to promote health, to do no harm, and to encourage the quality and equal availability of emergency medical care.

The Emergency Medical Technician provides services based on human need, with respect for human dignity, unrestricted by consideration of nationality, race, creed, color, or status.

The Emergency Medical Technician does not use professional knowledge and skills in any enterprise detrimental to the public well-being.

The Emergency Medical Technician respects and holds in confidence all information of a confidential nature obtained in the course of professional work unless required by law to divulge such information.

The Emergency Medical Technician, as a citizen, understands and upholds the law and performs the duties of citizenship; as a professional, the Emergency Medical Technician has the never-ending responsibility to work with concerned citizens and other healthcare professionals in promoting a high standard of emergency medical care to all people.

The Emergency Medical Technician shall maintain professional competence and demonstrate concern for the competence of other members of the Emergency Medical Services healthcare team.

An Emergency Medical Technician assumes responsibility in defining and upholding standards of professional practice and education.

The Emergency Medical Technician assumes responsibility for individual professional actions and judgment, both in dependent and independent emergency functions, and knows and upholds the laws which affect the practice of the Emergency Medical Technician.

An Emergency Medical Technician has the responsibility to be aware of and participate in matters of legislation affecting the Emergency Medical Technician and the Emergency Medical Services System.

The Emergency Medical Technician adheres to standards of personal ethics which reflect credit upon the profession.

Emergency Medical Technicians, or groups of Emergency Medical Technicians, who advertise professional services, do so in conformity with the dignity of the profession.

The Emergency Medical Technician has the obligation to protect the public by not delegating to a person less qualified any service which requires the professional competence of an Emergency Medical Technician.

The Emergency Medical Technician will work harmoniously with, and sustain confidence in, Emergency Medical Technician associates, the nurse, the physician, and other members of the emergency medical services healthcare team.

The Emergency Medical Technician refuses to participate in unethical procedures and assumes the responsibility to expose incompetence or unethical conduct of others to the appropriate authority in a proper and professional manner.

Gillespie C: *EMT Code of Ethics,* 2007, National Association of Emergency Medical Technicians (NAEMT).

The Bottom Line

Learning Checklist

✓ Practice the Golden Rule when treating patients: "Do unto others as you would have them do unto you."

✓ EMTs have an ethical and professional duty to remain competent through continuing education, call review, and other activities that ensure maintenance of knowledge and skills.

✓ EMTs have a responsibility to regard information provided in a patient's history, physical assessment, and treatment as confidential, except during the transfer of information to other healthcare providers, for third-party billing forms, in response to a legal subpoena, or when required by state law.

✓ EMTs and other emergency personnel may be required by law to report certain conditions to the police, health department, and other authorities, including infectious disease exposure, child or elder abuse, family violence, assaults, wounds from guns and knives, animal bites, and deaths.

✓ EMTs must function within a scope of practice defined broadly by their education, certification, licensure (in some states), and credentialing. More specifically defined by state and local laws, regulations, policies, guidelines, and protocols, the scope of practice is the duties and services that an individual with specific credentials may legally perform.

✓ The standard of care refers to the body of knowledge, laws, policies, protocols, standards, and guidelines that provide the basis of prehospital and other medical care. The standard of care means the EMT does the right thing and does it properly. The standard of care is used to judge the actions and omissions of prehospital personnel.

✓ Negligence is a deviation from the accepted standard of care resulting in injury to the patient. For medical malpractice to be established, four elements must be present: a duty to act, breach of duty, damage, and causal connection.

✓ Federal, state, and Good Samaritan laws often provide an extra degree of protection from lawsuits. Some laws are designed to protect government employees, whereas the Good Samaritan laws generally are for laypersons and EMTs who come to the aid of an ill or injured person in a voluntary (off-duty) capacity.

✓ Before treating a patient, you must obtain the consent of the patient or a parent or guardian for children or incompetent individuals. This may include expressed consent, in which a competent adult makes an informed decision about care, or implied consent, when a clear need for emergency care exists and the patient is unconscious, a minor, or an incompetent individual.

✓ A person may refuse care if he or she is a mentally competent adult and therefore capable of making a clear judgment. Make every attempt to convince the patient to receive needed care and be transported to the hospital. Patients who refuse care should sign a release documented by a witness.

✓ An EMT who prematurely discontinues care or fails to treat a patient in need may be guilty of abandonment.

✓ Patients with terminal or severe illnesses may express consent or refusal for medical care before it becomes necessary through DNR orders, advance directives, or healthcare proxies.

✓ Individuals can express their desire to donate organs on a driver's license or on a separate donor card. When appropriate, communicate this fact along with the patient presentation to the hospital or medical control so that appropriate steps are taken to carry out the patient's wishes.

✓ When caring for a patient at a crime scene, do not disturb the crime scene unless required for the care of the patient. Maintain any potential evidence under your control until transferred to police or hospital personnel, to maintain the chain of evidence.

✓ The best way for EMTs to prevent lawsuits is to act according to the standard of care and in the best interest of the patient and to document those actions on the appropriate prehospital care report.

Key Terms

Abandonment Discontinuation of a professional provider-patient relationship without providing the patient the time or opportunity to obtain continuation of care at the same level or higher.

Advance directive Specific statement or documentation made by an individual to withhold care, such as blood transfusions or CPR, if that person becomes mentally incapacitated or otherwise unable to communicate.

Assault Creating the fear of injury (e.g., lifting a fist in a threatening manner).

Battery The act of physically touching someone without that person's expressed consent.

Breach of duty A negligent act or omission that has violated the standards of care expected from an EMT under the circumstances.

Causal connection A clear connection between the patient's injuries and actions taken or omitted by a healthcare provider.

Chain of evidence An accountability of evidence at a crime scene. (Account for any evidence from the time it comes into your possession until you turn it over to the authorities.)

Do not resuscitate (DNR) Legal order signed by a physician that allows withholding of lifesaving measures in the event of a respiratory or cardiac arrest.

Duty to act Legal requirement to evaluate and treat a patient.

Emancipated minor Individual who is younger than the legal adult age but who is living independently, is (or was) married, or is (or was) a parent.

Expressed consent Consent given by a patient for treatment to be performed. This consent may be given verbally or through an affirming gesture such as a nod of the head.

Healthcare proxy Legal empowerment of a third party to make decisions regarding the health care of an individual.

HIPAA Health Insurance Portablitiy and Accountability Act; federal law protecting the privacy and dissemination of patients' medical and health information.

Implied consent Type of consent in which verbal or written consent is not possible but circumstances warrant that a reasonable person would want and expect emergency treatment to be rendered.

Informed consent Consent made when the patient has been made fully aware of the risks, benefits, and consequences of the care being provided and any alternatives to that care.

Malpractice Legal finding that negligence has occurred.

Negligence Deviation from the accepted standard of care that results in injury to the patient. For negligence to occur, there must be a duty to act, a breach of duty, injury to the patient, and a causal connection.

Protocol Written procedure for a clinical treatment.

Scope of practice Range of duties and services that may be performed by a given medical provider.

Standard of care The body of knowledge, laws, policies, common practices, standards, protocols, and guidelines that provide the basis for care; doing the "right thing" properly.

Review Questions

1. The activities and limitations that define the practice of a given medical provider are known as what?
   a. Scope of practice
   b. Standard of practice
   c. Emergency doctrine
   d. Legislative guidelines

2. Which of the following would best meet the definition of "doing the right thing properly" within the EMT's scope of practice?
   a. Protocol compliance
   b. Risk management
   c. Duty to act
   d. Standard of care

3. A duty to act, a breach of duty, an injury to the patient, and a causal connection between the injury and the EMT's actions are all elements of which of the following?
   a. Abandonment
   b. Negligence
   c. Malfeasance
   d. An EMS system

4. Your ambulance is on the scene. A 72-year-old woman has tripped on the curb and injured her hip. She is awake and alert, actively conversing with you. You explain the splinting procedure you intend to perform, and she nods her head. Which type of consent is being used to treat this patient?
   a. Implied
   b. Applied
   c. Expressed
   d. Presumed

5. Your ambulance is on the scene. A 54-year-old woman is having a heart attack. During treatment of this patient, you hear another call for a child who is choking approximately 1 mile away. You may be guilty of which of the following if you leave your patient and respond to the child who is choking without assuring continuation of care?
   a. Malpractice
   b. Abandonment
   c. Negligence
   d. Breach of duty

6. Your ambulance is dispatched to the scene of a "man down." On arrival, you find a 52-year-old unconscious patient. Which type of consent may be used to treat this patient?
   a. Informed
   b. Presumed
   c. Implied
   d. Surrogate

7. Who is an emancipated minor?
   a. Individual who is younger than the legal adult age but who is living independently of his or her parents
   b. Child who is injured at school and the parent is at work
   c. Patient who has been judged mentally incompetent by the court
   d. Individual who is younger than the legal adult age but who is injured while at work

8. The Good Samaritan laws are designed to protect whom against what?
   a. EMTs, against legal action resulting from abandonment of the patient
   b. EMTs, against legal action resulting from gross negligence in the driving of the ambulance
   c. EMTs, against legal action if CPR is not started for a patient in witnessed cardiac arrest and who is pronounced dead at the scene
   d. Volunteers, functioning in a nonprofessional capacity and without an expectation of remuneration

9. Which of the following documents is created specifically to avoid the application of CPR in the field or the hospital, usually signed by the patient and a physician?
   a. Refusal of aid
   b. Advance directive
   c. Terminal illness
   d. "Do not resuscitate" order

10. Which of the following persons is authorized to make broad medical decisions on behalf of a patient who may be incapacitated or unconscious?
    a. Executor
    b. "Living will" administrator
    c. Healthcare proxy
    d. Trustee

11. When documenting a patient's refusal of care, in addition to having the refusal form signed by the patient and a bystander and ensuring that the pateint does not have altered mental status, which of the following should the EMT do?
    a. Exaggerate the consequences to emphasize the need for care to the patient
    b. Make the patient call his doctor while on scene
    c. Prepare to restrain the patient
    d. Have the patient verbalize the possible consequences of refusing care

12. Responding to a report of shortness of breath, you discover a patient in cardiac arrest. You see on the nightstand a valid DNR order for the patient. The wife comes into the room crying and begs you to do all you can. How should you respond?
    a. Do not resuscitate the patient, and offer support for the wife
    b. Follow the wife's wishes, and attempt resuscitation
    c. Begin resuscitation in the house for the wife's benefit, but stop in the ambulance
    d. Pretend to do CPR, and ventilate the patient for a short time to make the wife feel better

For Further Review

In the Student Workbook

- Multiple-choice questions
- Fill-in-the-blank questions
- Short answer
- Case scenario
- Crossword puzzle

On Evolve

- Weblink
- Lecture notes
- Exercises

Learning Objectives

Cognitive Objectives

- Explain the importance, necessity, and legality of patient confidentiality.
- State the conditions that require an EMT (EMT-Basic) to notify local law enforcement officials.
- Define the EMT scope of practice.
- State the conditions necessary for the EMT to have a duty to act.
- Discuss the issues of abandonment, negligence, and battery and their implications to the EMT.
- Define consent, and discuss the methods of obtaining consent.
- Differentiate between expressed (informed) and implied consent.
- Explain the role of consent by minors in issues of care.
- Discuss the implications for the EMT in patient refusal of transport.
- Discuss the importance of DNR orders, advance directives, and local or state provisions regarding EMS application.
- Discuss the considerations of the EMT in issues of organ retrieval.
- Delineate the actions that an EMT should take to assist in preserving a crime scene.

Affective Objectives

- Explain the role of EMS and the EMT regarding patients with DNR orders.
- Explain the rationale for the needs, benefits, and use of advance directives.
- Explain the rationale for the concept of varying degrees of DNR orders.

References

Gillespie C: *EMT Code of Ethics*, 2007, National Association of Emergency Medical Technicians (NAEMT).

Human Participant Protection Education for Research Teams, http://cme.cancer.gov/clinicaltrials/learning/humanparticipant-protections.asp. May 2007.

National Highway Traffic Safety Administration: *EMS agenda for the future*, Washington, DC, 1996, US Department of Transportation.

National Highway Traffic Safety Administration: *National EMS Scope of Practice Model*, DOT HS 810 657, Washington, DC, February 2007, US Department of Transportation.

State of New York Public Health Law Article 30, Emergency Medical Services, updated Sept. 29, 2006, New York.

US Department of Health and Human Services: Protecting the privacy of patients' health information. http://www.hhs.gov/news/facts/privacy.html. May 2007.

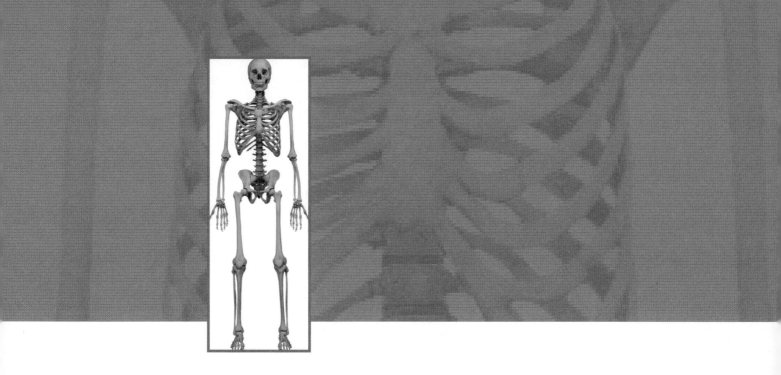

4 The Human Body

Scenario

Called to the scene of a stabbing, you find a 25-year-old man with blood spurting from his left arm and stab wounds to the left chest in the midclavicular line and to the left upper quadrant of the abdomen. The patient is awake and breathing. You apply direct pressure to the arm to control bleeding. You take vital signs and note a rapid and weak pulse and a blood pressure of 80 over 60. The skin is pale and moist. You ready the patient for transport to the trauma center and call ahead during transport, describing the patient's condition and physical findings.

Knowledge of anatomy and physiology is essential for you to function as an EMT. The opening scenario illustrates how you will often use anatomic landmarks to assess the patient, perform a variety of procedures, and communicate with other healthcare professionals. Understanding how the body works will also help you to recognize abnormal conditions and decide on the appropriate treatment.

The study of anatomy and physiology is the study of the body's structure and function. Anatomy is the study of the structure of body parts, and physiology is the study of processes and activities of living organisms. As in other chapters, **bold** terms and others in *italics* are used. This will help you learn important and essential terminology. Bold terms are those you will routinely use as an EMT and are called "key terms." These are also listed at the end of the chapter so that you can test your knowledge and review the terms that you do not remember. Terms in *italics* are important words that will help you learn many concepts discussed in this text and will be important as you read other medical textbooks.

LEARNING OBJECTIVE
- Identify and define the following topographic terms: medial, lateral, proximal, distal, superior, inferior, anterior, posterior, midline, right and left, midclavicular, bilateral, and midaxillary.

Anatomic Terms

Normal Anatomic Position

To describe the relation between body parts, you use anatomic terms and imagine the body in the *anatomic position*. The anatomic position refers to a body standing erect with the feet together, the arms at the sides, and the palms and the head facing forward (**Figure 4-1**). Anatomic terms are always applied to the body in the anatomic position, regardless of the actual position of the body.

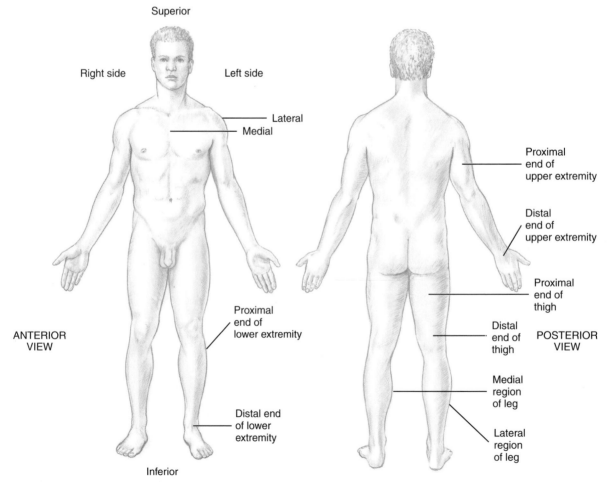

Figure 4-1 The standard anatomic position: body erect, palms forward. This allows for a standard reference for communicating anatomic relationships. *Modified from Applegate EJ: The anatomy and physiology learning system, ed 3, Philadelphia, 1995, Saunders.*

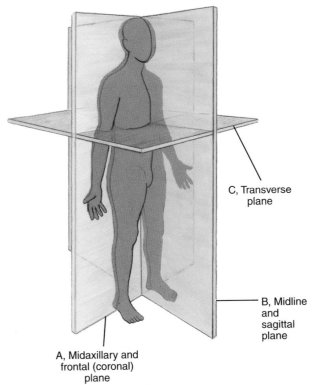

Figure 4-2 Body planes. **A,** An imaginary plane that divides the body into anterior and posterior portions runs along the midaxillary line. **B,** The midline plane separates the body into right and left halves. **C,** A transverse plane separates the body into superior and inferior portions. *Modified from Applegate EJ: The anatomy and physiology learning system, ed 3, Philadelphia, 1995, Saunders.*

C, Transverse plane

B, Midline and sagittal plane

A, Midaxillary and frontal (coronal) plane

In the anatomic position, any part farther from the ground or closer to the head is referred to as **superior**. Any part closer to the ground or the feet is referred to as **inferior**. For example, the knee is superior to the ankle. The heart is inferior to the head.

Structures toward the front of the body are said to be **anterior** or **ventral**. Structures toward the rear of the body are **posterior** or **dorsal**. In the anatomic position, the *sternum* (breastbone) is anterior to the heart; the spine is posterior.

Reference to the **midline** of the body is easy if you imagine a line running through the nose, sternum, and *umbilicus*, or navel, separating the body into right and left halves (**Figure 4-2**). If a structure is farther away from the midline, it is said to be **lateral**. Many organs or parts of the body are **bilateral** and are right and left of the midline. For example, breath sounds heard equally on both sides might be described as "clear and equal bilaterally." Conversely, if a structure is closer to the midline, it is said to be **medial**. For example, the arm is lateral to the torso; the nose is medial to the eyes. A **midclavicular** line passes through the middle of the *clavicle(s)* (collarbones) parallel to the midline. This anatomic reference is useful when placing a stethoscope to check the patient's breath sounds over the lungs.

A **midaxillary** line is an imaginary line passing vertically through the *axilla* (armpit). This line divides the body into

anterior and posterior halves. This landmark is also used to check a patient's breath sounds on the lateral aspect of the chest.

On the extremities, additional terms are sometimes used to describe location. **Proximal** means closer to the trunk, and **distal** means farther away from the trunk. For example, the elbow is proximal to the hand, and the foot is distal to the knee. The palm of the hand is termed the *palmar* surface, and the sole of the foot is termed the *plantar* surface.

Other useful terms include *superficial* and *deep,* which are used to describe distance from the surface of the body. For example, a wound might be described as "superficial" if it scrapes the outermost layer of skin and "deep" if it punctures through the skin and underlying tissues.

Central and **peripheral** refer to the distance from the center of the body. For example, arteries and veins in the extremities are referred to as "peripheral vessels." The major arteries and veins that leave and enter the heart would be appropriately referred to as "central vessels."

For some students, the relationships of the arms and hands can be confusing. To avoid confusion, you should always refer to the picture of the anatomic position, where the arms are at the sides and the palms are facing *forward* (see Figure 4-1). In this position, the thumb is lateral and the little finger is medial. When dealing with the extremities, the anatomic meanings of the words "arm" and "leg" may also be confusing. In anatomy, the *arm* refers to the upper arm only, from the shoulder to the elbow. The *leg* refers to the lower leg, from the knee to the ankle.

Terms Relating to Position and Movement

Special terms are used to describe body position and movement. The body standing upright is called *erect,* and lying on its back, **supine.** If the body is lying facedown, it is **prone.** A body lying on its side is in the *lateral recumbent* (or *recovery*) position. The lateral recumbent position is further described by which part of the body is positioned on the ground or stretcher. For example, a patient lying on the left side would be in the *left lateral recumbent position.*

Movement away from the midline is referred to as **abduction** (*ab,* "away"). Movement toward the midline is called **adduction** (*ad,* "toward"). For example, raising the arm from the side upward would be abduction; returning the arm to the side would be adduction. In the hand, abduction and adduction refer to movement with respect to an arbitrary line drawn through the third finger. When the fingers are spread apart, they are abducted; when the fingers are held together, they are adducted (**Figure 4-3**).

Flexion and **extension** describe motion around a joint. When a joint is bent and the two parts are brought closer together, they are in flexion, or flexed. When the joint is straightened, the two parts are said to be in extension, or extended (**Figure 4-4**). The head is flexed when it is bent forward toward the chest and extended when it is brought back to anatomic position or slightly beyond. When the head is further extended toward the back, it is said to be *hyperextended.*

Medial rotation is used to describe motion of a limb when the anterior surface of the limb is rotated to face medially. *Lateral rotation* is used when the anterior surface rotates to face laterally

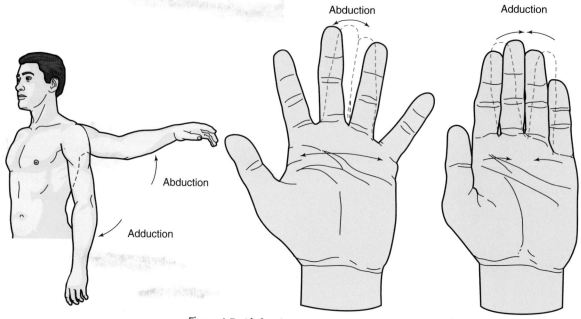

Figure 4-3 Abduction versus adduction.

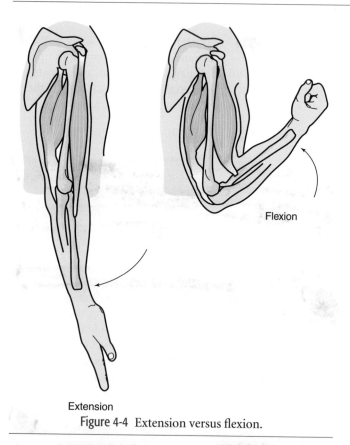

Extension

Figure 4-4 Extension versus flexion.

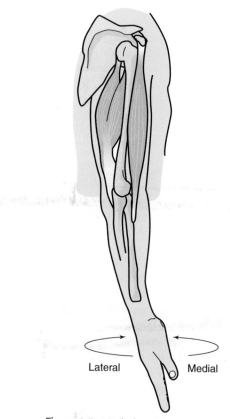

Figure 4-5 Medial and lateral rotation.

(Figure 4-5). For example, medial rotation describes rotation of the arm from the anatomic position to a position where the anterior surface faces the trunk instead of forward.

LEARNING OBJECTIVE
- Describe the anatomy and function of the following major body systems: respiratory, circulatory, musculoskeletal, nervous, and endocrine.

Body Systems

The organization of the human body has six levels, starting with the smallest particles, *atoms* and *molecules*, and concluding with the body as a whole **(Figure 4-6).**

The *cell* is the fundamental unit of all living things. There are one-celled animals and large animals such as humans made up

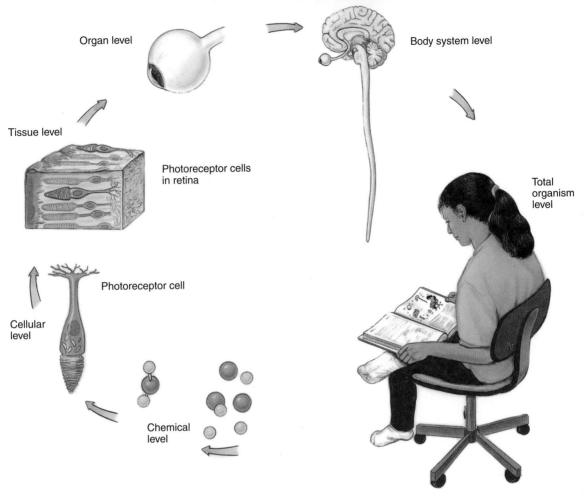

Figure 4-6 Organizational scheme of the body. *From Applegate EJ:* The anatomy and physiology learning system, *ed 3, Philadelphia, 2006, Saunders.*

of trillions of cells. Cells have common characteristics, such as a cell membrane and nucleus, but cells also can specialize and serve a specific function.

When many specialized cells are grouped together to serve a common function, they compose a *tissue*. There are four basic types of tissue, as follows:

- *Muscle tissue* is composed of cells that can contract to allow motion.
- *Nerve tissue* conducts impulses used to direct body functions and for communication.
- *Epithelial tissue* is a protective covering that can allow certain substances to pass through while prohibiting the passage of others.
- *Connective tissue* provides structure, attachment, and protection.

An *organ* is a structure composed of several types of tissues that work together to serve a particular function. The *stomach* is an organ that contains several tissues. For example, epithelial tissue lines the inside and outside of the stomach, muscular tissue mechanically churns the food, and nerve tissue regulates the activities. Collectively, these tissues work together to give the stomach its specialized ability and role in the digestion and transport of food.

A body system or *organ system* is a group of organs that work together to perform a complex function. For example, the stomach and several other organs, including the mouth, esophagus, gallbladder, liver, pancreas, intestines, and rectum, form the digestive system. Other major organ systems include the skeletal, muscular, respiratory, circulatory, nervous, endocrine, urinary, reproductive, and integumentary (or skin).

Each body system has a specific role in the body's activities and functions. Understanding the contributions of each body system will help you appreciate the body as a whole.

Skeletal System

The *skeletal system* gives structure and support to the body and serves to protect vital organs. In conjunction with the muscles, the skeleton allows for movement.

The body contains 206 bones (**Figure 4-7**). Bones are a form of connective tissue that is hardened by the deposition of calcium. Bone is a living substance and capable of growth and repair. Other forms of connective tissue in the skeletal system include cartilage, ligaments, and tendons. *Cartilage* is a softer form of connective tissue that allows for flexible support. For example, the sections of the ribs that connect to the sternum

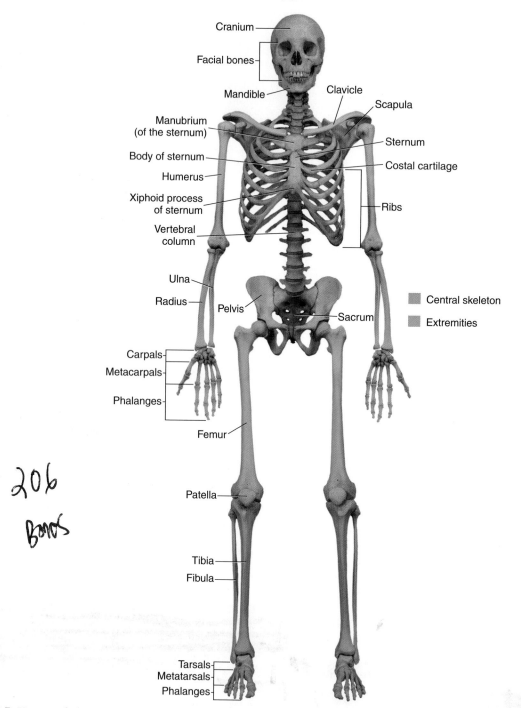

Cranium
Facial bones
Mandible
Manubrium (of the sternum)
Body of sternum
Humerus
Xiphoid process of sternum
Vertebral column
Ulna
Radius
Pelvis
Carpals
Metacarpals
Phalanges
Femur
Patella
Tibia
Fibula
Tarsals
Metatarsals
Phalanges

Clavicle
Scapula
Sternum
Costal cartilage
Ribs
Sacrum

■ Central skeleton
■ Extremities

206 Bones

Figure 4-7 Human skeleton, with major bones identified. *From Aehlert B: Paramedic practice today: above and beyond, St Louis, 2010, Mosby-Elsevier.*

are made of cartilage to allow movement of the chest during breathing. This also allows you to perform chest compressions during CPR on the lower half of the sternum where the cartilage is more extensive. *Ligaments* attach bone to bone and provide structure to joints. When a ligament is torn, a joint may become unstable and dislocate from its normal anatomic position. *Tendons* attach muscle to bone. For example, when the biceps muscle of the arm contracts, the tendon pulls the bone of the forearm to cause flexion. If the tendon completely tears, mobility will be weak or lost.

Skull

The *skull* is made up of the bones of the cranium and the face **(Figure 4-8)**. The *cranium* encases the brain and, in the adult, has about a 1-liter(L) internal capacity that is fully occupied by the brain, *cerebrospinal fluid* (CSF), and blood vessels. The cranium serves mainly to protect the delicate brain tissue within. Sometimes, however, the sharp edges of broken skull bones can tear into brain tissue underneath. The cranial and spinal (vertebral) cavities surround the brain and spinal cord, or *central nervous system* (CNS) **(Figure 4-9)**.

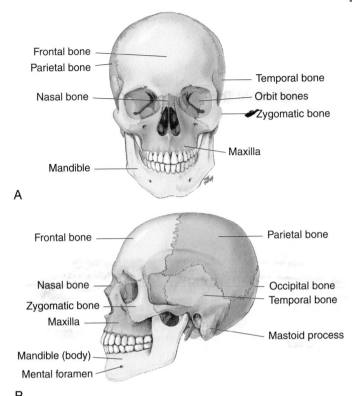

A

B

Figure 4-8 Human skull. **A,** Frontal view. **B,** Lateral view. *Modified from Applegate EJ: The anatomy and physiology learning system, ed 3, Philadelphia, 2006, Saunders.*

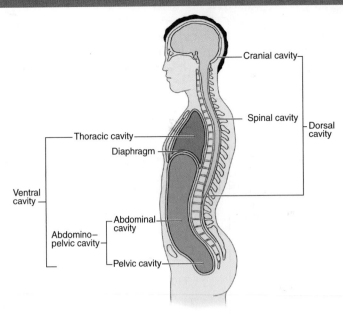

Figure 4-9 Major cavities in the body. *Modified from Applegate EJ: The anatomy and physiology learning system, Philadelphia, 1995, Saunders.*

hollow opening called the *spinal canal*. The *spinal cord* extends downward from the brain through a hole in the base of the skull and is protected within the spinal canal.

REAL*World*

Geriatric patients may develop a spinal condition known as *kyphosis*. Kyphosis is the abnormal curvature of the spine resulting in a rounded appearance of the back, or humpback. Severe cases can make airway management and immobilization difficult for the EMT.

Thoracic Cavity

The *thoracic cavity* begins just below the neck and extends down to the *diaphragm*, a respiratory muscle that separates the thorax (chest) and abdomen. The rib cage surrounds the thoracic cavity on both sides and provides structure for ventilation and protection of the organs within. The upper 10 pairs of ribs are attached to the sternum on the anterior side and to the thoracic spine on the posterior side. These ribs are attached to the sternum by *costal cartilage*. The eleventh and twelfth pairs of ribs are not attached to the sternum. They are attached only to the eleventh and twelfth thoracic vertebrae and are referred to as "floating" ribs.

The sternum is composed of three separate bones: the upper manubrium, the middle body, and the lower *xiphoid process*. When performing chest compressions, the heel of your hand is positioned on the lower half of the sternum, where the costal cartilage allows the most mobility or movement. The upper part of the sternum has less costal cartilage attached and is therefore less mobile. If you compress the upper sternum during CPR, a fracture is more likely to occur.

The *clavicles*, or collarbones, lie over the anterior upper ribs and extend from the sternum to the shoulders. The *scapulas*

Facial Bones

The *orbit bones* that surround the eyes, the nasal bones, and the *maxilla* make up the front of the skull. The *zygomas* (or *zygomata*) connect the *temporal bones* with the maxilla and are easily palpated where the cheek meets the temple just anterior to the ear. The *mandible*, or lower jaw, is connected to the rest of the skull at the *temporomandibular joints*.

Spinal Column

The spinal column consists of 33 bones called **vertebrae** that give support to the neck, thorax, abdomen, and pelvis. The spinal column can be divided into the following five sections **(Figure 4-10):**
- *Cervical*—the 7 vertebrae that form the neck.
- *Thoracic*—the 12 vertebrae to which the ribs are attached.
- *Lumbar*—the 5 vertebrae forming the lower back.
- *Sacral*—the 5 fused vertebrae that form the sacrum, or back of the pelvis.
- *Coccygeal*—the 4 fused vertebrae that form the coccyx, or tailbone.

The fifth cervical vertebra may be referred to as C5, the fourth lumbar vertebra as L4, and so on. Other initials used to designate vertebrae are T for thoracic and S for sacral.

The cervical, thoracic, and lumbar vertebrae are separated by cartilaginous (composed of cartilage) disks that allow for varying degrees of mobility in addition to support and cushioning between bones. The fused sacral vertebrae offer support and protection to the pelvis. In the center of the spinal column is a

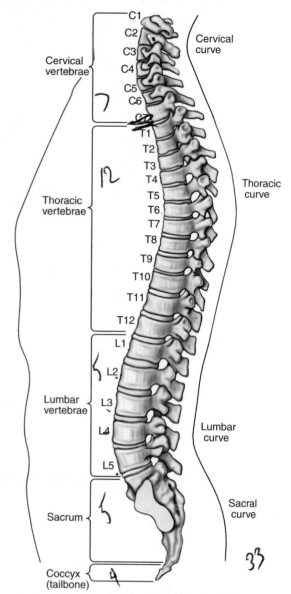

Figure 4-10 Vertebral column. *From Herlihy B, Maebius N: The human body in health and illness, Philadelphia, 2000, Saunders.*

Contained within the thoracic cavity are the heart, lungs, and great vessels. The esophagus travels through the middle of the thoracic cavity posterior to the airway.

The thoracic cavity is subdivided into two smaller spaces, the *mediastinum* (in the center) and the *pleural spaces* on either side. The mediastinum is occupied by the heart, great vessels, esophagus, *trachea* (windpipe), and main stem *bronchi*. The *lungs* occupy the pleural spaces.

Abdominopelvic Cavity

The *abdominal cavity* is bounded by the diaphragm superiorly and the bony *pelvic cavity* inferiorly (see Figure 4-9). Posteriorly, it is protected by the spine. The sides and anterior portions are protected by layers of muscle. Additional protection over the superior portion is provided by the lower ribs.

The abdominal cavity contains several organs of digestion, including the stomach, small and large intestines, liver, gallbladder, and pancreas, as well as the kidneys and the *ureters*, which are organs of excretion. The *spleen* is also contained within the abdominal cavity.

The pelvic cavity is the lowermost portion of the abdominal cavity. The pelvic girdle is a ring of bones formed by the sacral section of the spinal column posteriorly and three additional bones: the *ilium* (two, left and right), the *ischium* (two), and the *pubis* (two). They provide protection to the pelvic organs within, including parts of the lower intestine, the rectum, and the *urinary bladder* as well as the reproductive organs in females. The top of the ilium bone is called the *iliac crest*. The point where the pubic bones meet anteriorly is called the *symphysis pubis* (**Figure 4-11**).

Abdominal Quadrants. The abdominopelvic cavity can be divided in various ways to describe the location of pain, tenderness, or other physical findings. A common system is to divide the abdomen into quadrants by two imaginary lines that intersect at the umbilicus, or navel. Horizontal and vertical lines through the umbilicus form right and left upper quadrants and right and left lower quadrants. Some organs are contained within a single quadrant and others lie in more than one (**Figure 4-12**). Knowledge of the location of organs within different quadrants of the abdomen is used when assessing patients. For example, bleeding from the liver would be suspected after a stab wound to the right upper quadrant.

Upper Extremities

The upper extremities (arm and forearm) consist of the shoulder, the arm, the elbow, the forearm, the wrist, and the hand (**Figure 4-13**). The only bone in the arm is the *humerus*. The shoulder is formed by the *articulation* (joining) of the humerus with the scapula. The head of the humerus fits against the *glenoid process* of the scapula to form a *ball-and-socket joint*. The shoulder receives support from attachments between the scapula and the clavicle at the acromion (the lateral tip of the scapula). The muscles of the shoulder give this joint added stability.

Bones in the forearm are the *radius and ulna*. The radius is on the lateral side (thumb side) of the forearm in the anatomic position. The ulna is on the medial side. The elbow is the joint formed by the articulation of the humerus, radius, and ulna. The tip of the elbow can be palpated posteriorly. This process is called

(scapulae), or shoulder blades, lie over the upper posterior ribs and attach to the clavicles and *humerus* to form the shoulder. The bony tip of the shoulder is the *acromion*.

The diaphragm is a dome-shaped muscle that forms the base of the thoracic cavity. It contracts and pushes downward into the abdomen to allow air to enter the lungs during *inspiration* (breathing in). The diaphragm relaxes and rises within the thoracic cavity during *expiration* (breathing out). As mentioned, the diaphragm forms the division between the thoracic and abdominal cavities. Because it moves with breathing, the boundary between these two cavities may move as well, which should be considered when evaluating penetrating injuries.

The attachments of the diaphragm are the xiphoid process of the sternum, the lower six ribs, and the upper lumbar vertebrae. There are openings in the diaphragm for the *aorta* (major artery), *vena cava* (major vein), and esophagus (food pipe).

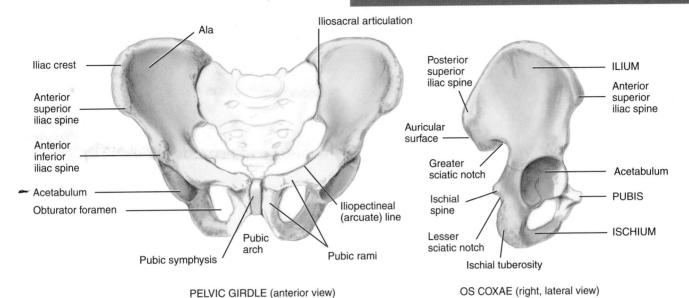

Figure 4-11　Pelvic cavity. *From Applegate EJ: The anatomy and physiology learning system, ed 3, Philadelphia, 2006, Saunders.*

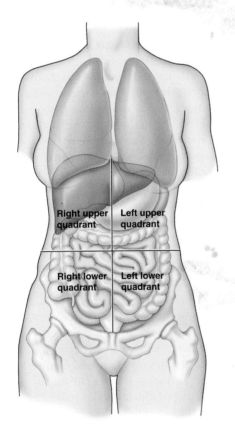

Figure 4-12　Abdominal quadrants. *From Herlihy B, Maebius N: The human body in health and illness, Philadelphia, 2000, Saunders.*

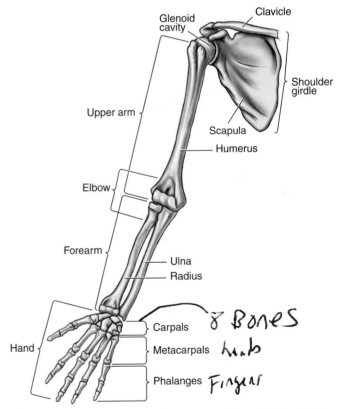

Figure 4-13　The upper extremity. *From Herlihy B, Maebius N: The human body in health and illness, Philadelphia, 2000, Saunders.*

the *olecranon.* The wrist is made up of eight bones called *carpal* bones. The hand is made up of *metacarpal* bones and *phalanges.*

Lower Extremities

The **femur** is the bone of the thigh and is the largest bone in the body. The head of the femur and the acetabulum, or socket, of the pelvis form the hip joint. The *greater trochanter*

is the prominent lateral portion of the proximal femur (**Figure 4-14**).

The bones of the lower leg are the *tibia* and the *fibula.* The tibia, the major weight-bearing bone, is larger and located medially. It is covered by a thin layer of skin and soft tissue anteriorly and is easily palpable. The fibula is a thinner bone that lies lateral to the tibia.

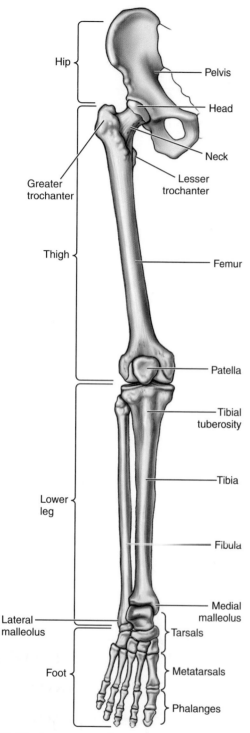

Figure 4-14 The lower extremity. *From Herlihy B, Maebius N: The human body in health and illness, Philadelphia, 2000, Saunders.*

The femur, the tibia, and the *patella* (kneecap) form the knee joint. The patella is a triangular bone that is situated in the tendon of the *quadriceps muscle* (which extends the knee) at the anterior aspect of the knee. The patella is felt below the skin on its anterior surface. Its posterior surface articulates with the femur. The patella aids in extension of the knee.

The ankle is made up of seven bones called *tarsal* bones. The foot is composed of metatarsal bones and phalanges (see Figure 4-14).

Joints

Joints are sites where bones are joined to bones, allowing for connection and movement. Two examples of joints are ball-and-socket and hinged. Ball-and-socket joints (e.g., hip, shoulder) allow for a wide range of motion. Hinge joints, such as the elbow and knee, permit motion in one plane and flexion and extension only. Other types of joints include pivot joints, gliding joints, saddle joints, and condyloid joints. **Figure 4-15** shows the different types of joints and their related motion. Take a moment to move the related joints on your body to better appreciate the normal range of motion.

Muscular System

The muscles are tissue capable of contraction, or shortening. They are attached and designed so that the power of their contraction results in movement. Muscles also give the body shape and provide protection for some internal organs. There are three types of muscles, as follows:

- Voluntary, or *skeletal* (striated)
- Involuntary, or *smooth*
- Cardiac

Skeletal *(voluntary)* muscles are any muscles that are normally controlled by a person's will. They are attached to bones and comprise the major muscle mass of the body (**Figure 4-16**). Contraction of the smooth *(involuntary)* muscles results in automatic functions such as *peristalsis,* or waves of contraction causing movement of food through the digestive tract. Smooth muscle is found in walls of many tubular structures within the body. They may respond to such stimuli as stretching or changes in temperature. *Cardiac* muscle, found only in the heart, has its own blood supply, which cannot be interrupted for long without injury or cell death. Cardiac muscle has the ability to contract on its own, a property called *automaticity.*

Respiratory System

The respiratory system brings oxygen into the body and rids the body of *carbon dioxide,* the waste product. It is composed of the nose and mouth, the *nasopharynx* and *oropharynx,* the *larynx,* the trachea, the bronchi, and the lungs (**Figure 4-17**).

The respiratory system allows an exchange of gases with the outside environment. The nose, nasopharynx, and oropharynx are designed to filter, moisten, and warm or cool the air, as needed, before it reaches the delicate *alveoli,* or air sacs, in the lungs. The larynx (which also contains the vocal cords), the trachea, and the bronchi conduct air to the lungs. The diaphragm and the muscles of the chest cause the thoracic cavity to expand and contract like a bellows to create airflow during ventilations.

Upper Airway

The upper airway is composed of the nose, mouth, pharynx, larynx, and the upper part of the trachea (**Figure 4-18**).

Nose and Mouth. The first portion of the airway is the nasal passage. The nasal passage consists of external and internal sections. The external section includes the nose, which is formed by cartilage and skin and opens at the nares, or nostrils. The upper portion contains the nasal bone, and the entire nose is

(Text continued on p. 80)

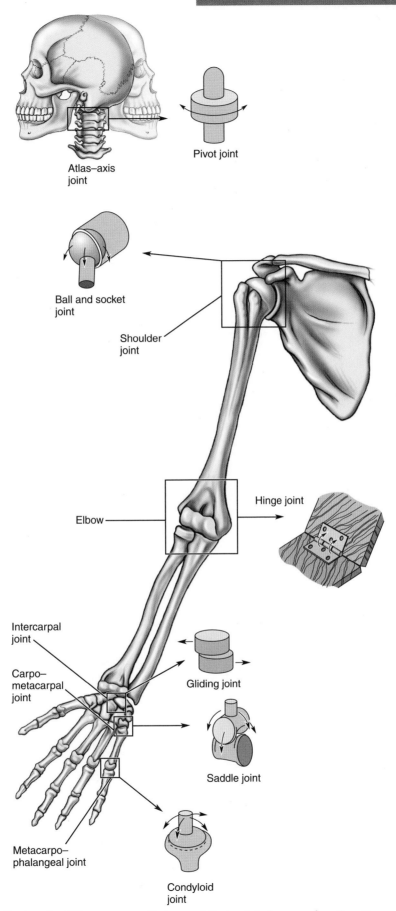

Pivot joint

Atlas–axis
joint

Ball and socket
joint

Shoulder
joint

Hinge joint

Elbow

Intercarpal
joint

Carpo–
metacarpal
joint

Gliding joint

Saddle joint

Metacarpo–
phalangeal
joint

Condyloid
joint

Figure 4-15 Types of joints. Review the different types of joints and their related range of motion. *From Herlihy B, Maebius N: The human body in health and illness, Philadelphia, 2000, Saunders.*

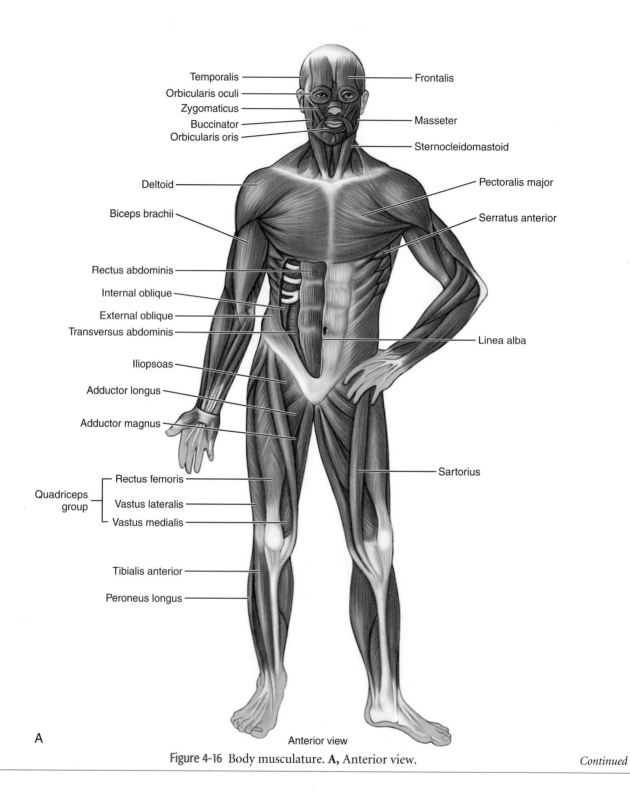

Temporalis

Orbicularis oculi

Zygomaticus

Buccinator

Orbicularis oris

Frontalis

Masseter

Sternocleidomastoid

Deltoid

Biceps brachii

Pectoralis major

Serratus anterior

Rectus abdominis

Internal oblique

External oblique

Transversus abdominis

Iliopsoas

Adductor longus

Adductor magnus

Linea alba

Sartorius

Quadriceps group
Rectus femoris
Vastus lateralis
Vastus medialis

Tibialis anterior

Peroneus longus

A

Anterior view

Figure 4-16 Body musculature. **A,** Anterior view.

Continued

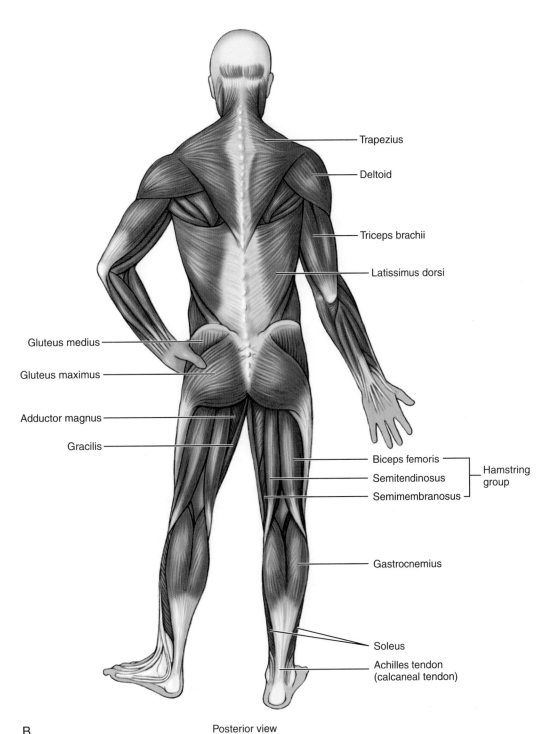

Trapezius

Deltoid

Triceps brachii

Latissimus dorsi

Gluteus medius

Gluteus maximus

Adductor magnus

Gracilis

Biceps femoris
Semitendinosus — Hamstring group
Semimembranosus

Gastrocnemius

Soleus

Achilles tendon (calcaneal tendon)

B

Posterior view

Figure 4-16—cont'd B, Posterior view. *From Herlihy B, Maebius N:* The human body in health and illness, *Philadelphia, 2000, Saunders.*

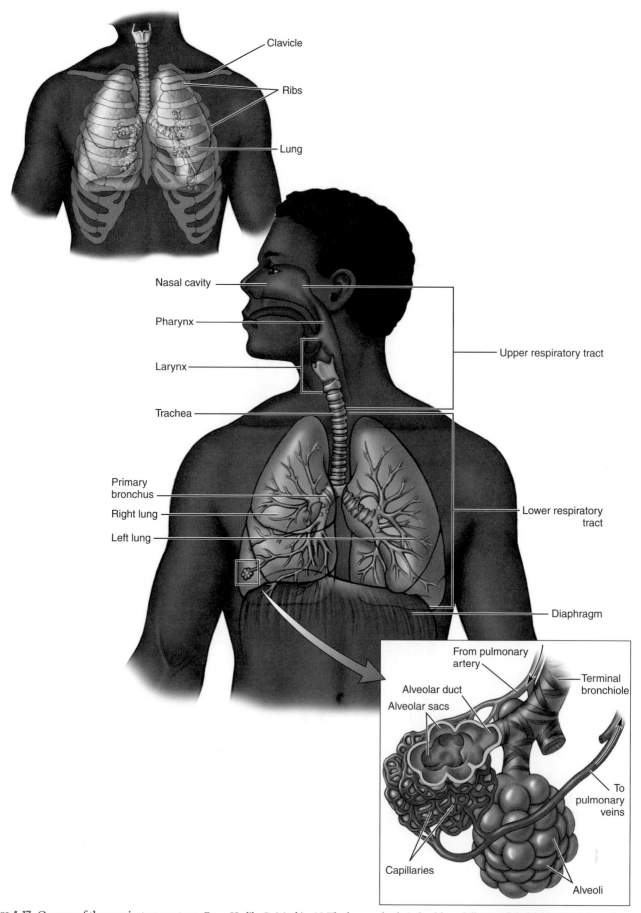

Figure 4-17 Organs of the respiratory system. *From Herlihy B, Maebius N:* The human body in health and illness, *Philadelphia, 2000, Saunders.*

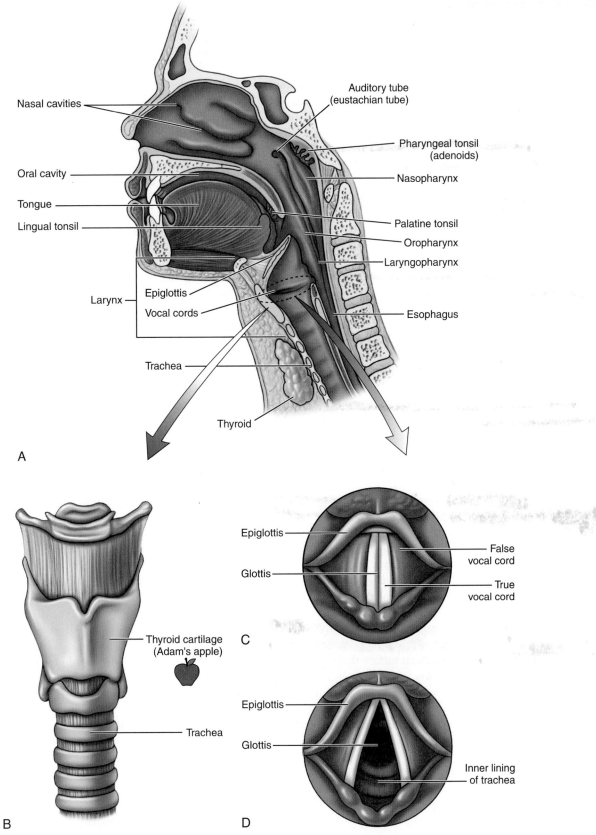

Figure 4-18 **A,** Features of the upper respiratory tract. **B,** Larynx showing thyroid cartilage. **C,** Vocal cords and glottis (closed). **D,** Vocal cords and glottis (open). *From Herlihy B, Maebius N:* The human body in health and illness, *Philadelphia, 2000, Saunders.*

divided into two compartments by the *nasal septum,* which is made of cartilage and bone. Three functions of the airway that begin at the nose are filtering, moistening, and warming the air that is breathed in. The nose also provides the function of smell.

Injuries to the nose are of concern to the EMT because fractures of nasal bones can compromise the *patency* (openness) of the airway, and bleeding from the nose in unconscious patients may lead to aspiration of blood into the lungs.

Pharynx. The passage extending from the back of the nasal cavity down to the esophagus and larynx is called the *pharynx.* Each part of the pharynx is further classified according to its relation to other structures: the *nasopharynx,* the *oropharynx,* and the *laryngopharynx.* This portion of the airway anatomy may become obstructed when the tongue falls back against it in an unconscious patient or when swelling of pharyngeal tissue develops as a result of allergic reactions or trauma.

Larynx. Most anterior in the laryngopharynx is the larynx, or "voice box." This structure is formed by cartilage, bone, and ligaments and contains the vocal cords. The vocal cords serve two primary functions: creating voice and preventing foreign objects that have slipped past the epiglottis from entering the lungs. When foreign material attempts to enter the airway, the vocal cords, which are muscular bands within the larynx, spasm and close shut (laryngospasm).

The two main cartilages forming the larynx are the thyroid and cricoid cartilages. The *thyroid cartilage* is superior and is commonly referred to as the "Adam's apple." The *cricoid cartilage* is inferior and forms a circle just above the trachea. A membrane lies just between these two structures and is called the *cricothyroid membrane.*

Epiglottis. The **epiglottis** is a flap of cartilage that covers the larynx during swallowing to prevent food from entering the lungs. However, a disease of the epiglottis that can cause rapid swelling of this structure can result in progressive obstruction of the airway. This is called *epiglottitis* and most often affects young children. This is a problem that you may encounter as an EMT because swelling can progress rapidly and cause respiratory distress.

Trachea. Extending down from the larynx is the **trachea** (windpipe). It is a hollow tube with several horseshoe-shaped rings of cartilage on the anterolateral surface that support and provide structure for this portion of the airway. Posteriorly, the trachea is composed of a muscular wall that permits food to move freely down the esophagus, which is located directly behind the trachea. In infants, the trachea is so pliable that great care must be taken not to hyperextend the neck to open the airway. Much like a hose when bent, an infant's trachea may kink and cause an obstruction. Take a moment to feel the tracheal rings just above your sternum in the anterior portion of your neck.

Lower Airway

Bronchi. At approximately the second *intercostal* space (e.g., between the first and second ribs), the trachea subdivides into two tubes made of cartilage called bronchi (**Figure 4-19**). Each main stem bronchus (singular term) extends into the left lung and the right lung, respectively.

Bronchioles. Much like a tree, the bronchi in turn subdivide to form smaller and smaller bronchi. As they become smaller, they contain less cartilage and more muscle. At about the 15th generation of division, these tubes lose cartilage and become totally muscular and are referred to as *bronchioles.* Bronchioles are the smallest type of airway tube and can change in diameter because of their muscular quality.

A major factor in the disease of asthma is bronchial constriction, which increases the work of breathing by narrowing the airways and increasing the resistance to airflow. Drugs called bronchodilators that dilate the smooth muscle of the bronchioles are used to treat asthmatic patients. You may assist patients with asthma by administering inhaled bronchodilator medications.

Alveoli. The final results of all the subdivisions of the tracheobronchial tree are the alveoli. These microscopic air sacs are the portion of the lungs where gas exchange takes place. Alveoli arise in grapelike clusters at the end of the bronchioles. The wall of an alveolus (singular term) is one cell thick. The walls must be thin to permit the exchange of gas with blood in the adjoining capillaries (smallest units of a blood vessel). The ability of the lung to exchange oxygen with the blood also depends on the total number of functional alveoli in contact with capillaries. The alveoli in a normal adult would cover an area greater than 50 m^2, or the approximate surface area of a tennis court, if spread out. This massive surface area permits the delivery of oxygen during rest and when oxygen demands increase, such as during exercise. In diseases such as *emphysema,* in which the alveoli are damaged or destroyed, patients have less ability to take up oxygen from the lungs. Often, the only way for these patients to achieve adequate oxygen delivery to tissues is to inhale enriched concentrations of oxygen through oxygen delivery devices (see Chapter 6).

Lungs. The bronchi, bronchioles, and alveoli together form two cone-shaped organs called *lungs.* Each lung is divided into lobes, which are separate sections of lung tissue. The left lung has two lobes, and the right lung has three lobes. In patients with lung cancer, lobes or even an entire lung may need to be removed to prevent the spread of the disease. The vast surface area of the alveoli permits survival with a relatively small portion of lung tissue intact.

Both lungs are suspended within the chest cavity. The lungs lie on either side of the mediastinum, a space occupied by the heart, great vessels, trachea, main stem bronchi, esophagus, and nerves.

The lungs of an adult can hold approximately 6 L. With each breath, we breathe in about 500 mL (0.5 L) of air, which is referred to as the tidal volume (V_T). About 3000 mL (3 L) is available for deep inhalation and is known as the *inspiratory reserve volume* (IRV). About 1400 mL is available for deep exhalation and is known as the *expiratory reserve volume* (ERV). The remaining 1100 mL is known as the *residual volume* (RV) and always remains within the lungs.

Muscles of Respiration

The chest movement that results in air exchange between the atmosphere and the alveoli occurs by actions of the muscles of respiration. These muscles change the diameter of the chest

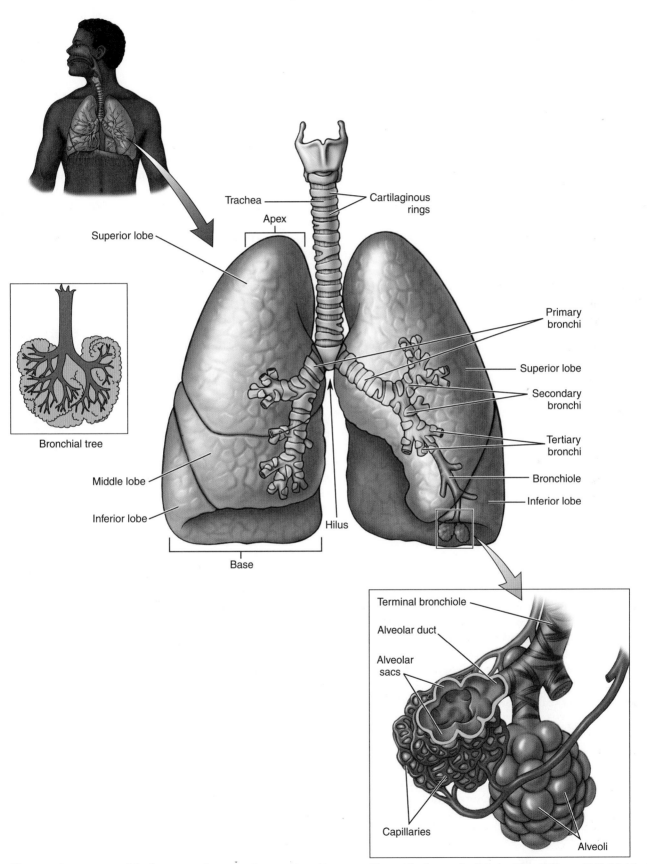

Figure 4-19 Features of the lower respiratory tract. *From Herlihy B, Maebius N: The human body in health and illness, Philadelphia, 2000, Saunders.*

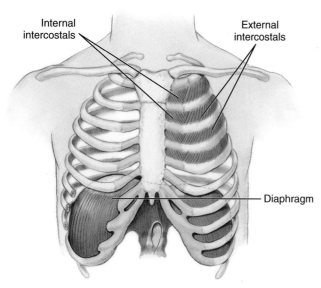

Figure 4-20 Muscles of respiration. *Modified from Applegate EJ: The anatomy and physiology learning system, ed 3, Philadelphia, 2006, Saunders.*

cavity by contracting and relaxing and therefore create a "bellows effect," resembling the device used by blacksmiths to fan a fire. In normal, quiet breathing, the principal muscle of respiration is the diaphragm, aided by the external intercostals (**Figure 4-20**). The diaphragm, which is a dome-shaped muscle at rest, separates the chest and abdomen in the inferior portion of the thoracic cavity.

Inhalation is an active process that occurs when the diaphragm contracts downward and "flattens" out while the external intercostals pull the ribs upward and outward, thereby increasing the anterior-posterior, superior-inferior, and lateral-lateral dimensions of the chest cavity. When the chest cavity increases in size, the pressure within the chest cavity becomes lower than the pressure in the atmosphere, and air rushes into the tracheobronchial tree (**Figure 4-21**). Air continues to rush in until the pressure within the lungs becomes equal to the atmospheric pressure. This is the end of inhalation.

Exhalation occurs as a result of relaxation of the muscles of respiration and the elastic recoil of lung tissue. As the chest cavity becomes smaller, the pressure inside the lungs increases, causing air to be pushed out. Exhalation is essentially a passive process. The end of exhalation occurs when the pressure inside the lungs is once again equal to atmospheric pressure.

Accessory Muscles of Respiration

During quiet breathing, the diaphragm and external intercostals are more than capable of providing the appropriate volumes of air needed to sustain effective oxygen levels. However, during strenuous exercise or in cases of respiratory disease or trauma, the **accessory muscles** of breathing come into play. There are two types of accessory muscles: muscles of inspiration and muscles of expiration.

The accessory muscles of inspiration primarily increase the size of the thoracic cavity by pulling the ribs further in the upward direction and increasing intrathoracic diameters. These

muscles include the *scalene* muscles in the neck, which elevate the upper ribs; the *sternocleidomastoids,* which pull and elevate the sternum; and the *parasternals,* which pull up on the cartilaginous portion of the ribs adjacent to the sternum. These accessory muscles add to the efforts of the external intercostals and diaphragm to increase the volume of air entering the lungs. This can occur during exercise, with respiratory compromise from disease or injury, or when destruction of the airway creates greater resistance to airflow.

Accessory muscles of expiration are used when more rapid forceful breathing is needed and when obstructive processes exist. The muscles are the *internal intercostals,* which pull the ribs down and inward, and the abdominal muscles, which pull the lower ribs downward and compress the abdominal contents, pushing the diaphragm upward to decrease the size of the thorax.

During patient assessment, active accessory muscle use provides a key warning signal of respiratory distress. Bulging of the neck muscles, retraction of the spaces between the ribs, and active abdominal muscle use collectively comprise this warning signal.

> ### Case in Point
>
> You arrive at a camp where a child has sudden onset of shortness of breath. The patient has a history of asthma and allergies to dust. After the first night at camp, this 8-year-old girl is sitting upright in a chair in the nurse's office, with prominent use of neck muscles during breathing. While you listen to her breath sounds, which are high-pitched during expiration, you notice retractions between the ribs as well.
>
> The narrowing of the bronchioles in asthma results in resistance to airflow, typically heard as wheezing. The accessory muscle use is a sign of increased work of breathing. Children, with their softer, growing bones, may have obvious retractions of the muscle between the ribs, with intercostal muscle contraction.

Physiology of Respiration

The adequacy of breathing is determined by evaluating two parameters: the **tidal volume** (the amount of air per breath) and the *respiratory rate*. The tidal volume multiplied by the respiratory rate is called the *minute volume*, or volume of air breathed in 1 minute. The normal respiratory rate is between 12 and 20 breaths/min, and the normal tidal volume (at rest) is approximately 500 mL, or about a pint of air. As an EMT, you will not be able to record a specific tidal volume; however, well-defined visible chest expansion usually indicates an adequate tidal volume. This is used as a guide during positive-pressure ventilation (forcing air into the body by using mouth-to-mouth, mouth-to-mask, or bag-valve-mask ventilation) that an adequate volume has been delivered.

Nervous System Regulation

Similar to a home heating system, the body has a "thermostat" that monitors respiratory function. As certain changes take place, it turns breathing "on" or "off." Messages from this system are sent to the muscles of breathing and cause them to contract and relax. This regulation or control is the function of the brain and peripheral nerves that stimulate these muscles.

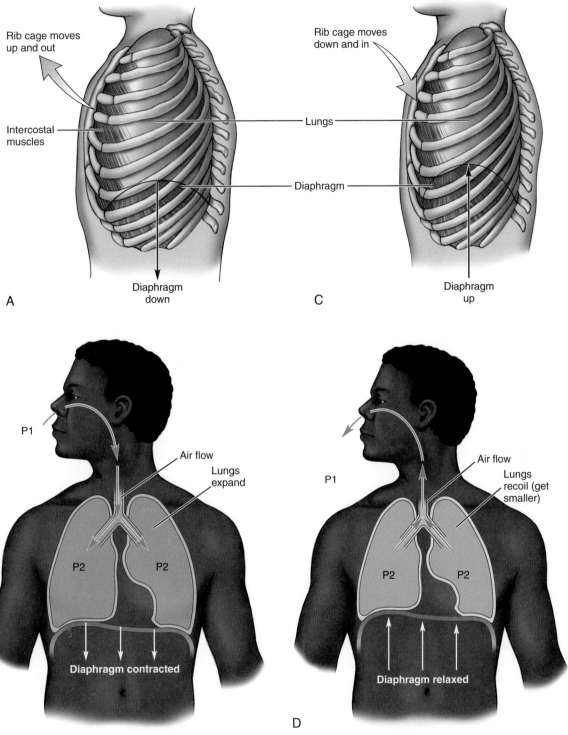

Figure 4-21 Respiration. **A** and **B,** Inspiration. When the muscles of inspiration contract, the chest cavity enlarges. The pressure of the air within the airway and alveoli *(P2)* falls below atmospheric pressure *(P1)*. Air rushes into the lungs. **C** and **D,** Expiration. When the muscles of inspiration relax, the elastic recoil of the lungs and the chest wall decreases the size of the chest cavity. This increases the pressure within the airway and alveoli *(P2)* in relation to the atmosphere *(P1)*. Air then rushes out through the airway until the pressure within the lungs and that of the atmosphere equalize (P1 = P2). *From Herlihy B, Maebius N: The human body in health and illness, Philadelphia, 2000, Saunders.*

There are essentially two methods of nervous control: unconscious (or automatic) and conscious (or voluntary). Our breathing is automatically controlled most of the time. However, we can voluntarily slow down, speed up, increase, and decrease our volume of breathing. As you sit reading this text, your unconscious controls dominate, unless you "override" these mechanisms and consciously alter your pattern of respiration.

Automatic control consists of the following:

- Sensors or receptors that monitor blood levels of carbon dioxide (CO_2), oxygen (O_2), and acidity (pH) to determine the body's respiratory and cardiovascular needs. These sensors are located in the carotid arteries in the neck and in the aorta, the main artery leading out of the heart. Other sensors are located within the brain itself.
- Nerves that provide feedback to the respiratory centers in the brain.
- Nerves that travel from the brain to the muscles of respiration to control the rate and depth of breathing.

The voluntary control of breathing comes from the higher brain centers, which communicate through the automatic control centers by nerve pathways extending into the brainstem.

As we take each breath, we change the levels of oxygen and carbon dioxide and blood acidity. When we increase the rate and depth of breathing, blood O_2 levels tend to increase, whereas CO_2 levels decrease as we "blow off" carbon dioxide. Conversely, as we decrease our respiratory rate and depth, blood O_2 levels decrease, whereas CO_2 levels increase as we "retain" carbon dioxide.

The blood acidity will change because some carbon dioxide in the blood takes the form of acid. Thus, more CO_2 equals more acid; less CO_2 equals less acid.

Metabolism also changes the levels of oxygen, carbon dioxide, and acid. Metabolism represents the sum of cellular activity. As cells become more active, they consume more oxygen and produce more carbon dioxide or waste.

The respiratory centers are constantly monitoring these parameters. When O_2 levels decrease or CO_2 levels increase, messages are sent from the brain to increase the respiratory rate and depth.

To review the functions just described, monitor your own respiratory patterns during exercise, or hold your breath and notice the drive that forces you to take your next breath. As we discuss the various respiratory emergencies, this concept of *neuroregulation* will be constantly useful.

Alveolocapillary Cellular Exchange

Diffusion is the tendency of molecules (e.g., O_2) to move from an area of higher concentration to an area of lower concentration. The movement of oxygen and carbon dioxide across the *alveolocapillary membranes* occurs as a result of this principle. Capillary blood moving past the alveolar surface is lower in O_2 content and higher in CO_2 than the gas within the alveoli. Oxygen moves into circulating blood through the mechanism of diffusion and attaches to the *hemoglobin* molecule. The hemoglobin molecule is a pigment found in the red blood cell that is responsible for carrying oxygen. It gives oxygen-rich blood its red color. Carbon dioxide, which is in a higher concentration in the blood than in the alveoli, in turn leaves the blood and

enters the alveoli and is exhaled. Take a moment to review this principle by examining **Figure 4-22.**

Blood is then pumped through the rest of the body, where it gives oxygen to the body's cells and picks up carbon dioxide, the waste product of metabolism in the cells.

Adequate versus Inadequate Breathing

During patient assessment, you will assess the rate, rhythm, quality, and depth of a patient's breathing to determine whether it is adequate or if assistance is needed. The normal rate of breathing varies with age (**Table 4-1**). The rhythm of breathing is usually regular, with slight variation and occasional sighs. The quality of breathing is assessed with breath sounds, chest expansion, and effort. Chest rise is an indication of tidal volume. Additional signs of inadequate breathing include changes in skin color; signs of increased muscular effort such as *retractions, nasal flaring,* and *"seesaw breathing"*; or irregular and inadequate terminal *(agonal)* respiratory efforts.

Understanding the difference between adequate and inadequate respirations is critical in your decision making as an EMT. You will use this information to decide if you need to administer supplemental oxygen or provide positive-pressure ventilation (see Chapter 6).

Infants and Children

The anatomy of the infant and child has many important differences from that of the adult. In general, the child's airway is smaller and therefore more easily occluded by secretions or foreign bodies. The tongue takes up proportionally more room in the mouth of a child and can obstruct the airway in an unconscious patient. Because the trachea is softer in infants and children, it may kink; therefore it is important not to hyperextend the neck when opening the airway (**Table 4-2**). The narrowest section of the airway in an infant or small child occurs at the cricoid cartilage and is often the point of obstruction in a medical condition called *croup.*

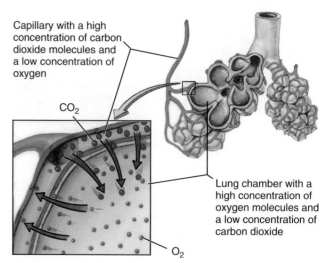

Capillary with a high concentration of carbon dioxide molecules and a low concentration of oxygen

CO_2

Lung chamber with a high concentration of oxygen molecules and a low concentration of carbon dioxide

O_2

Figure 4-22 Diffusion of oxygen (O_2) and carbon dioxide (CO_2) in the lungs. *Modified from Applegate EJ: The anatomy and physiology learning system, Philadelphia, 1995, Saunders.*

REAL*World*

As the body ages, the ability of the lungs to relax during exhalation decreases, resulting in an increased residual volume (RV). An increased RV results in a decreased inspiratory reserve volume (IRV). Because of this, geriatric patients may have difficulty increasing their respiratory function when necessary.

Circulatory System

The circulatory system is the transport system of the body. It has many functions. It delivers oxygen and nutrients to the tissues and returns the waste products of metabolism (carbon dioxide and cellular wastes) to the lungs for elimination and the kidneys for excretion from the body. It also transports specialized cells to areas of the body where they are needed to repair injured tissues, combat foreign bacteria, and control bleeding. By reducing or increasing the amount of blood in contact with the skin, the circulatory system helps regulate body temperature as well.

Because the tissues are most dependent on an adequate supply of oxygen for survival, any compromise in circulatory function can lead to tissue damage or death. Because the most oxygen-dependent tissues are the brain and heart, EMTs look for the signs of inadequate oxygenation when examining these organ systems. Although all organ systems are affected by lack of oxygen, rapid assessment of brain and circulatory function must be given priority in the early part of every examination. You must be able to recognize the indicators of cardiovascular failure quickly and administer prompt emergency treatment.

Table 4-1	Adequate versus Inadequate Breathing	
	Adequate	**Inadequate**
Rates		
Adult	12-20 breaths/min	Outside normal ranges
Child	15-30 breaths/min	Outside normal ranges
Infant	25-50 breaths/min	Outside normal ranges
Rhythm	Regular	Irregular
Quality		
Breath sounds	Present and equal	Diminished or absent
Chest expansion	Adequate and equal	Inadequate or unequal
Effort		Accessory muscle use; noisy
Depth	Normal chest rise	Inadequate/shallow
Skin	Normal	Pale or cyanotic (blue); cool and clammy
Retractions	None	Present, especially in infants and children
Nasal flaring	Not present	Present, especially in infants and children
Seesaw breathing	Not present	Alternate use of chest and abdominal muscles during breathing
Agonal (gasping) breaths	Not present	May be seen just before death

Proper functioning of the circulatory system depends on three interdependent components:
- Heart
- Blood vessels
- Blood

The *blood* is the fluid in which oxygen and nutrients are transported. The *blood vessels* are the pathways that direct blood to the various cells of the body. The *heart* is the pump that provides the driving force necessary to keep the blood circulating.

Heart

The heart is a muscular pump that generates the driving force for blood to flow to all parts of the body. The force must be sufficient to open the vessels so that blood can pass through and *perfuse* the body's organs and tissues.

The heart is located in the chest cavity between the sternum and the thoracic spine, just left of center (**Figure 4-23**). It is positioned between the two lungs in a space known as the *mediastinum* and occupies an area about the size of a fist. The *apex* of the heart is located to the left and rests on the left diaphragm. Its impulse can be felt anteriorly at the level of the fifth or sixth rib.

The heart is surrounded by a two-layered sac called the *pericardium*. The pericardium is a protective covering that separates the heart from the other organs in the mediastinum. The inner layer lines the heart wall and is separated from the outer layer by a small amount of fluid. This fluid serves as a lubricant between the pericardial layers as the heart beats.

Layers of the Heart. The heart muscle itself is made up of three layers (**Figure 4-24**):
- *Epicardium*—an outer layer, actually the inner or visceral layer of the pericardium.
- *Myocardium*—a middle layer, the muscular portion that performs the work of contraction.
- *Endocardium*—a smooth inner layer, lining the chambers of the heart.

The endocardium continues into the blood vessels that enter and leave the heart. Its function is to provide a surface lining within the heart and vessels that prevents the clotting of blood. When this layer is disrupted or diseased, clotting is likely to occur.

Heart Chambers. The inner portion of the heart is divided into four chambers. The upper chambers, the *right atrium* and *left*

Table 4-2	Anatomic Airway Differences between Children and Adults
Structure	**Pediatric Characteristic Compared with Adult**
Mouth and nose	Structures are smaller and more easily obstructed
Pharynx	Tongue takes up more space in mouth and may obstruct airway
Trachea	Narrower, obstructed more easily; softer, more pliable
Cricoid cartilage	Less developed and less rigid
Diaphragm and chest wall	Diaphragm relied on more for breathing, softer chest wall

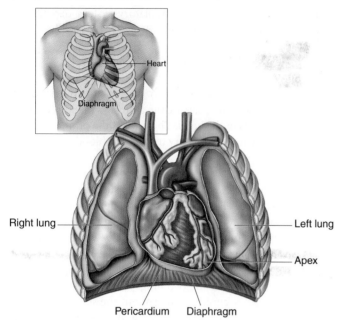

Figure 4-23 The heart within the chest cavity. *From Herlihy B, Maebius N: The human body in health and illness, Philadelphia, 2000, Saunders.*

atrium, are the receiving chambers for blood returning to the heart from the lungs and the rest of the body (**Figure 4-25**). Because these chambers serve primarily as collecting areas for blood, they have relatively thin walls.

The two lower chambers, the *right ventricle* and *left ventricle,* are the pumping chambers and have thicker walls. The left atrium is located above the left ventricle, and the right atrium is located above the right ventricle. The two atria beat simultaneously pumping blood into the ventricles, followed by simultaneous contraction of the two ventricles. The right and left sides of the heart are separated by the *septum.* The septum, or wall, divides the heart into two separate circulatory systems. These systems are considered two distinct systems, as follows:

- Pulmonary circulation
- Systemic circulation

Pulmonary Circulation—Right Ventricle. The pulmonary circulation pumps blood through the lungs, where it picks up oxygen and releases carbon dioxide for exhalation from the body. The pump for the pulmonary circulation is the right ventricle. Blood returning to the heart from the pulmonary circulation is saturated with oxygen and collects in the left atrium.

Systemic Circulation—Left Ventricle. The systemic circulation transports and delivers oxygen-rich blood (and other nutrients) to the rest of the body, where it is needed for energy. At the same time, it picks up carbon dioxide and other waste products of metabolism. The pump for the systemic circulation is the left ventricle. Blood returning to the heart from the systemic circulation collects in the right atrium. Thus, blood is returned to the pulmonary circulation to begin the cycle once again.

Follow the blood flow in **Figure 4-26** to understand how blood flows through both the pulmonary and the systemic circulation.

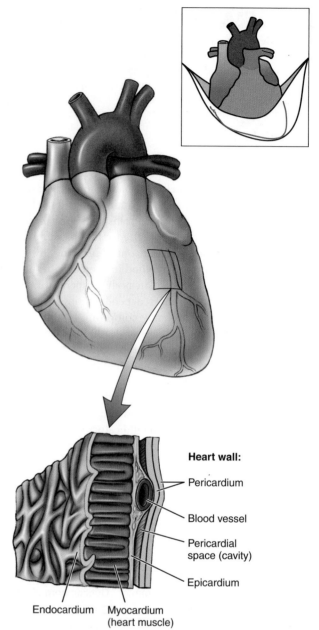

Figure 4-24 The pericardium has two layers. The visceral pericardium, or inner layer, closely adheres to the surface of the heart. The parietal pericardium, or outer layer, consists of a more loosely attached, thin membranous covering. Layers of the heart: endocardium (smooth inner lining), myocardium (thick muscular layer), and epicardium (thin outer covering). *From Herlihy B, Maebius N: The human body in health and illness, Philadelphia, 2000, Saunders.*

Valves—One-Way Flow. Although the atria and ventricles are contracting, a one-way flow of blood is maintained by the presence of *valves.* During *systole* (ventricular contraction), the blood in the ventricles is pumped out of the heart through the arteries. During *diastole* (ventricular relaxation), blood flows into the empty ventricles from the atria, where it has been collecting. There is a valve at both the inlet and outlet of each ventricle to maintain the direction of blood flow from the atrium to the ventricle to the artery.

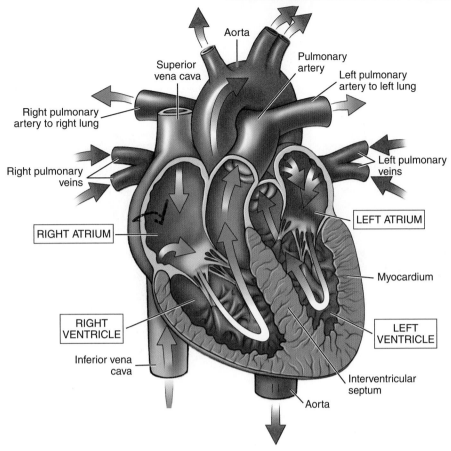

Figure 4-25 Chambers of the heart. *From Herlihy B, Maebius N: The human body in health and illness, Philadelphia, 2000, Saunders.*

The valves are composed of flaps of tissue that are cupped in one direction. If pressure is exerted on one side of the valve, it opens. If pressure is exerted on the other side, it closes (**Figure 4-27**). Closure of the valves signals the beginning and end of ventricular contraction. The main heart sounds heard through a stethoscope are caused by the closing of these two sets of valves.

Conduction System. The *conduction system* is composed of a series of specialized tissues that order the rhythmic relaxation and contraction of the myocardial cells. The heart must have an orderly relaxation and contraction of its atria and ventricles to function as a pump. The conduction system is organized to ensure that the atria contract first, followed by the ventricles. So while the ventricles relax, the atria contract and help fill the ventricles with blood. Then the ventricles contract and pump blood out of the heart through the arteries.

The conduction system starts with the *sinoatrial node,* the *pacemaker* of the heart located in the right atrium. The sinoatrial node discharges, or fires, about 60 to 100 times a minute in an adult and begins an electrical impulse that ultimately spreads through the atria and then through the ventricles.

Disturbances in the conduction system result in various abnormalities. These include too slow a heartbeat, too fast a heartbeat, an irregular heartbeat, or in the most extreme case, no heartbeat at all (**cardiac arrest**).

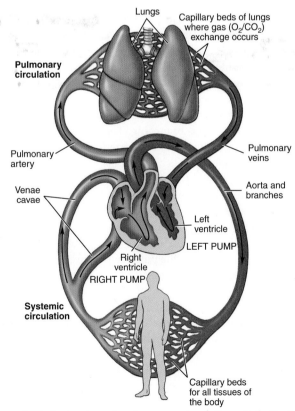

Figure 4-26 Systemic and pulmonary circulation. *From Herlihy B, Maebius N: The human body in health and illness, Philadelphia, 2000, Saunders.*

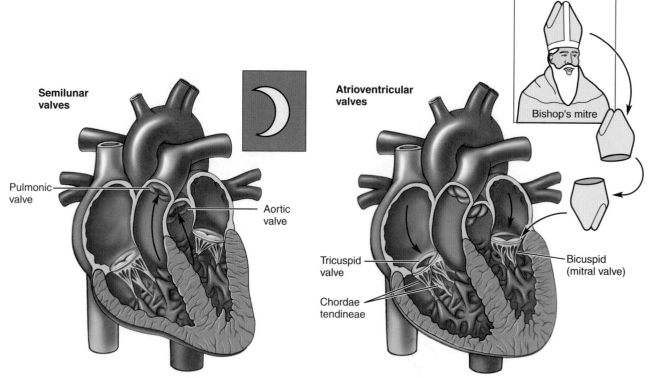

Figure 4-27 Valves of the heart. *From Herlihy B, Maebius N: The human body in health and illness, Philadelphia, 2000, Saunders.*

Blood Vessels

There are three major types of blood vessels: arteries, veins, and capillaries. Together they form a branching network that directs the blood through every part of the body. **Arteries** direct blood flowing away from the heart. **Veins** direct blood returning to the heart. **Capillaries** are located between the arteries and veins; they are thin-walled vessels that come in close contact with the cells so that the exchange of oxygen, nutrients, and waste products between the blood and cells can occur.

The vascular system has often been compared to a tree because of the continuous branching. The arterial system subdivides until it reaches the size of the arteriole, whose diameter is approximately that of a hair. The capillary network begins beyond the arterioles and further subdivides to ensure close contact with the cells. The capillaries then start to reconnect, thereby forming the smallest veins, called the *venules.* The venules begin to unite and form larger and still larger tubes called veins, which ultimately connect with the inferior or superior vena cava on one side of the circuit and the pulmonary veins on the other.

There is not sufficient blood to completely fill the body's vascular tree. Blood is directed to those tissues that have the greatest need at a given time. This is primarily accomplished by the constriction and relaxation of the arterioles, which are regulated by the *autonomic nervous system.*

The vessels have the ability to vary their diameter by dilation (opening) or constriction (narrowing). If all vessels were in a state of dilation, the normal blood volume could not fill the vascular space. Therefore, at any given time, some vessels are dilated while others are constricted, depending on the relative needs throughout the body.

For example, when a person is running, the blood vessels in the skeletal muscles are dilated while the vessels within the gastrointestinal tract are constricted. When performing heavy physical exercise, blood is directed toward the muscles doing the greatest work. The weightlifter, after curling weights, speaks of the "pump" felt in the biceps, which become engorged with additional oxygen-bearing blood. Likewise, after a heavy meal you might feel a bit sluggish or tired because the blood is directed to the digestive system to pick up nutrients from the food. People are warned not to swim after eating because there may not be sufficient blood to perfuse both the digestive system and the skeletal muscles at the same time. Also, the warning that a cramp might develop in a muscle is based on the fact that insufficient oxygen is being delivered to meet the demands of the muscles used for swimming.

Major Arteries. The arteries are composed of three layers (**Figure 4-28**). There is a smooth inner lining called the *endothelium,* a tough protective outer layer of connective tissue, and a middle layer that is quite elastic in the aorta but becomes more and more muscular as the arteries decrease in size. The elastic middle layer in the aorta and larger arteries allows them to withstand the high pressure of blood pumped from the left ventricle. They can initially expand as blood enters during systole and then contract during diastole. This contraction also serves to propel the blood forward.

Blood leaves the heart through either the *pulmonary artery* or the *aorta* (**Figure 4-29**).

Pulmonary Artery. The pulmonary artery leaves the right ventricle and branches into the right and left pulmonary arteries, which carry blood to the two lungs. These pulmonary arteries in turn subdivide until they become the capillaries that surround the alveoli in the lungs. At this site, diffusion of oxygen and carbon dioxide takes place. In contrast to all other arteries in the body, the pulmonary artery carries blood that is low in oxygen.

Aorta. The left ventricle pumps out oxygenated blood through the aorta. The aorta is a very elastic vessel approximately 1 inch

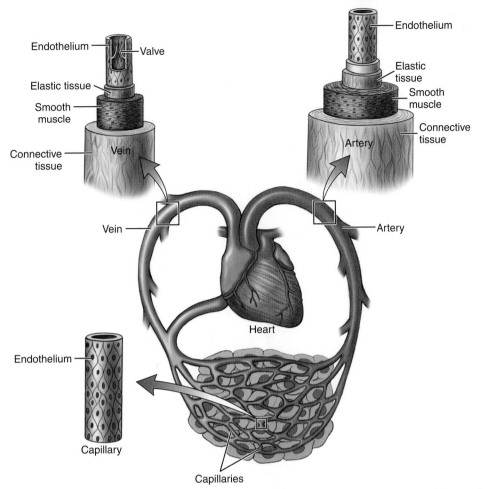

Figure 4-28 Layers of arteries, capillaries, and veins. *From Herlihy B, Maebius N: The human body in health and illness, Philadelphia, 2000, Saunders.*

(2.5 cm) in diameter where it leaves the heart. It is initially directed upward and called the *ascending aorta*. It then curves backward and to the left at the aortic arch. At the level of the fourth thoracic vertebra, the aorta begins to descend downward along the spine, where it is named the *thoracic aorta*. It is then called the *abdominal aorta* as it crosses the thorax and abdomen. It continues in the abdomen to the level of the fourth lumbar vertebra, where it divides into the right and left *common iliac arteries.*

Coronary Arteries. The first arteries to branch off the aorta are the *coronary arteries,* which exit just above the aortic valve and form a network around the heart. The heart is the first organ to receive oxygenated blood. The pressure in the aorta is the driving force for the blood that flows through the coronary arteries.

The coronary arteries enter the myocardium and branch into capillaries, which give nutrients and oxygen to the heart and pick up waste products. It is estimated that 5% of the blood in the systemic circulation is devoted to the coronary circulation to ensure that the constantly pumping heart has adequate energy to do its work.

Arteries to the Head and Upper Extremities. The next group of arteries to branch off the aorta is directed to the head and upper extremities. The *common carotids* bring blood to the head and neck. They divide to form the internal and external carotids.

The *internal carotids* provide the main source of blood supply to the brain. The *carotid pulse* is checked in an unresponsive patient. To palpate the carotid pulse, first find the Adam's apple (the thyroid cartilage), then slide the tips of your fingers laterally toward the sternocleidomastoid muscles of the neck. You should never compress both carotid arteries at once because this may obstruct most of the blood flow to the brain.

The *subclavian* and *brachiocephalic* arteries give rise to branches feeding the thorax, brain, and spinal cord and then continue to the upper limbs. The name changes as each artery continues, from *axillary* in the axillary region to *brachial* in the upper arm, and then divides into the *radial* and *ulnar* arteries in the forearm that extend down into the hand. The brachial and radial arteries are used to check blood pressure and pulse rate and quality. The brachial artery can be palpated medially, just proximal to the crease of the elbow. The brachial artery is used to determine blood pressure with a blood pressure cuff (sphygmomanometer) and a stethoscope. The radial artery is palpated on the anterior and radial (thumb) side of the wrist and is the major artery of the lower arm. The ulnar artery can also be palpated on the anterior but ulnar (little finger) side of the wrist.

Arteries to the Thorax, Abdomen, and Lower Extremities. The *thoracic* and *abdominal* aortas divide into multiple branches along their course to the tissues and organs in the thorax and

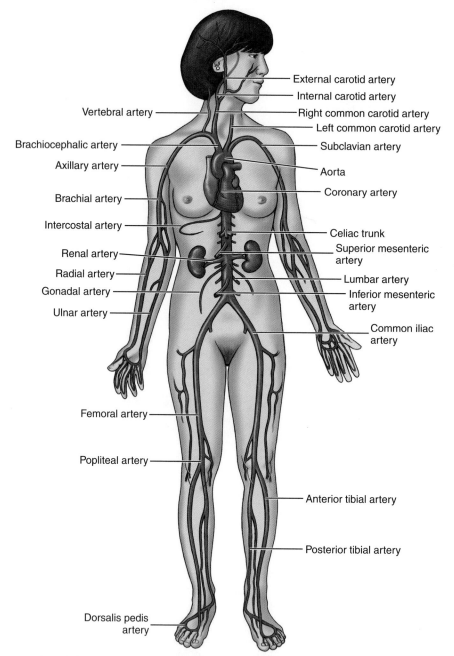

Figure 4-29 Major systemic arteries. *From Herlihy B, Maebius N:* The human body in health and illness, *Philadelphia, 2000, Saunders.*

abdomen. The common iliac arteries are formed by the division of the abdominal aorta. The external iliac arteries extend to the *inguinal ligament* (crease where thigh joins pelvis at groin), where they enter the thighs and are named the femoral arteries. The *femoral artery* is easily palpable at the level of the inguinal ligament, halfway between the superior iliac crest and the symphysis pubis.

The femoral artery gives rise to the *popliteal artery,* beginning in the lower thigh. The popliteal artery passes behind the knee, where it may be palpated, and then divides to form the anterior and posterior tibial arteries. The *anterior tibial artery* passes between the tibia and fibula and is palpable on the anterior surface of the tarsal bones in the foot, where it is called the *dorsalis pedis.* The *posterior tibial artery* passes down the calf and

is palpable just posterior to the bony prominence of the distal tibia (medial malleolus of ankle).

Arterioles. The terminal branches of the arteries, the arterioles, are the smallest tubes in the arterial network. Their middle wall primarily consists of circular smooth muscle, which constricts or relaxes at the direction of the autonomic nervous system. The tone of the muscles in the arterioles (constricted or relaxed) regulates the amount of blood permitted to flow into the capillaries beyond.

Vasoconstriction occurs when the muscular wall of the vessel contracts, decreasing its inner diameter. *Vasodilation* occurs when the muscular wall relaxes, thereby increasing its inner diameter. These changes in the arterioles' diameter are important in controlling the body's blood pressure.

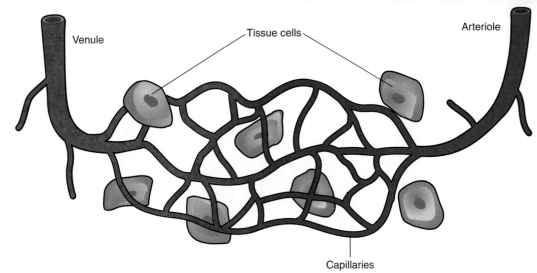

Figure 4-30 The capillaries are microscopic vessels that consist of walls that are one cell thick and permit the movement of gases, fluid, and small particles to alveoli and tissue cells as blood flows through (perfuses) an organ. *From Herlihy B, Maebius N: The human body in health and illness, Philadelphia, 2000, Saunders.*

Capillaries. The capillaries extend out from the finer branches of the arterioles. The capillary walls are only one cell thick and therefore permit the passage of water, gases, small molecules, and other substances carried in the blood. The diffusion of oxygen and nutrients and the exchange of waste products between the blood and the body cells can occur only at the capillary level. The capillaries are in close contact with all the body's tissues. The capillary network is so extensive that if placed end to end, it would extend for 60,000 miles (**Figure 4-30**).

Because the capillary walls are so thin, they cannot withstand much pressure. The arterioles reduce the pressure of blood before it enters the capillaries. The extensive size of the capillary network provides a greater space for the blood to fill, which also helps to reduce pressure.

Veins. The basic structure of the walls of the veins is similar to that of the arteries. Veins consist of a smooth internal lining, a tougher protective outer lining, and a middle layer that is elastic and muscular in nature. This middle layer is not as thick as that found in the arteries because pressure in the veins is much less. However, the veins can expand and contract to accommodate changes in blood volume and normally contain greater than half the circulating blood volume.

Venous Reservoir. Of the total blood volume, approximately 25% is in the heart and pulmonary circulation, 15% in the arterial circulation, and 4% in the capillary bed. The remaining approximately 56% lies within the veins.

Because the veins contain more than half the blood volume, they serve as a reservoir of blood within the vascular tree. The muscular and elastic middle wall allows the veins to contract or expand to accommodate changes in blood volume. For example, if a sudden loss of blood volume occurs, the nervous system can tell the muscles in the veins to constrict. Blood from the venous reservoir is then redistributed to help maintain blood pressure.

Major Veins. The major veins tend to run beside the major arteries. Many of the veins share the names of the arteries that lie parallel to them (**Figure 4-31**). The *pulmonary vein* brings oxygen-rich blood back from the lungs to the left atrium so that the left ventricle can pump it to the body. The *superior vena cava* is the major vein that returns blood from the upper body to the heart. The *inferior vena cava* receives branches from the organs in the abdomen and the lower body and empties into the right atrium.

Blood

The average adult's body contains 5 to 6 L of blood. The amount of blood volume is proportionate to the size of the patient. For the adult, an estimate of 70 mL of blood per kilogram of body weight is used. Infants and small children have about 80 mL of blood per kilogram. Blood consists of both liquid and cellular components. The liquid portion of blood is called the *plasma;* it constitutes 55% to 65% of the blood volume. The plasma consists mostly of water in which other elements and particles are dissolved. The cellular component of blood consists of *red blood cells* (RBCs), *white blood cells* (WBCs), and *platelets.* The cellular component makes up 35% to 45% of the total blood volume (**Figure 4-32**).

Red Blood Cells. The RBCs (also called *erythrocytes*) constitute the largest portion of the cellular component. They carry oxygen and carbon dioxide. RBCs contain a large protein called *hemoglobin,* which binds oxygen at the alveoli to form *oxyhemoglobin.* Oxyhemoglobin is bright red in color and accounts for the pink appearance of the lips and nail beds. Hemoglobin binds oxygen in the lungs and then releases it to the tissues of the body that are oxygen depleted. Hemoglobin that is not bound to oxygen is more blue or purple in appearance. This explains why patients who are oxygen deprived may appear *cyanotic,* especially in the nail beds or the lips, where many small vessels are visible at the skin's surface.

Hemoglobin and Oxygen Transport. Normally, 98% of the oxygen carried in the blood is bound to hemoglobin. The other 2% is dissolved in the plasma. Without hemoglobin, the blood

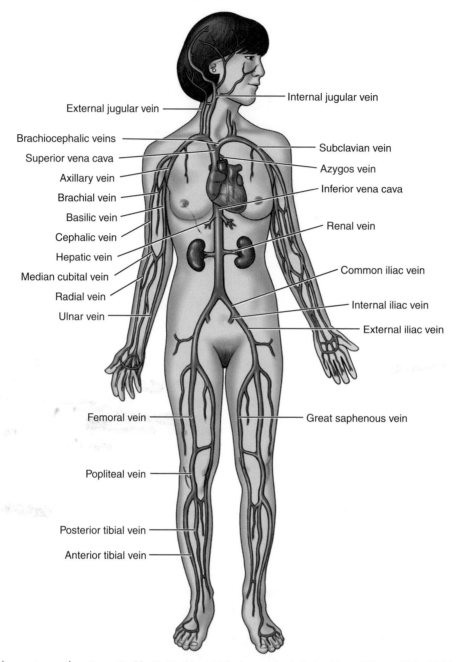

Figure 4-31 Major system veins. *From Herlihy B, Maebius N:* The human body in health and illness, *Philadelphia, 2000, Saunders.*

could not carry enough oxygen to meet the body's needs. When patients have a normal number of RBCs, the body usually extracts only one fourth of the total supply of oxygen bound to hemoglobin during circulation. There is more than enough to meet the body's needs. However, patients who have a low number of RBCs may not be able to carry enough oxygen to meet the body's needs. In cases of severe blood loss, transfusion of RBCs may be required to restore the blood's oxygen-carrying ability.

The amount of oxygen dissolved in the plasma alone is not adequate to support the body's needs. If supplemental oxygen is breathed, more oxygen is dissolved in the plasma. However, even with 100% oxygen the dissolved oxygen cannot meet the body's needs by itself; rather, it supplements the oxygen carried

by the hemoglobin. The main role of oxygen therapy is to ensure full saturation of the hemoglobin with oxygen.

Red blood cells have an average life expectancy of 120 days. As individual RBCs reach the end of their life span, they are replaced by new cells that are produced in the bone marrow.

White Blood Cells. The principal role of WBCs (also called *leukocytes*) is to combat and eliminate infecting organisms and foreign materials. They are fewer in number than RBCs and have a much shorter life span. WBCs pass through the walls of microscopic vessels and accumulate at the site of an infection. Once there, they break down and attack the offending organism or foreign substance, consume some of the breakdown products, and help direct the remaining pus (wastes) out of the body. A splinter left embedded in a finger shows this process. Initially,

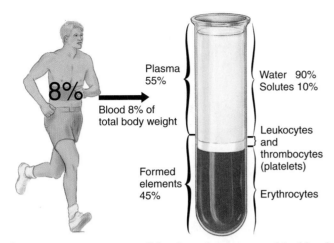

8%

Plasma 55%

Water 90%
Solutes 10%

Blood 8% of
total body weight

Leukocytes
and
thrombocytes
(platelets)

Formed
elements
45%

Erythrocytes

Figure 4-32 Composition of blood. Leukocytes are white blood cells (WBCs); erythrocytes are red blood cells (RBCs). *Modified from Applegate EJ: The anatomy and physiology learning system, ed 3, Philadelphia, 2006, Saunders.*

erythema (redness) and warmth are noted around the puncture site as the white cells begin to assemble at the wound. Later, a pus formation may be observed around the splinter. The pus consists of fluid, dead bacteria, dead tissue cells, and WBCs.

In other infections such as pneumonia, the number of WBCs in the blood increases as the body combats the infecting organisms. An increase in WBC count is one indication of an infection.

Platelets. Platelets are fragments of cells that circulate in the blood and are necessary for clotting to begin. Together with proteins in the plasma, the platelets form a *thrombus* (blood clot) when exposed to any surface other than the normal lining of a blood vessel. The clotting process is called *thrombosis* and usually takes 5 to 6 minutes. Without healthy platelets, an individual will bleed excessively after sustaining even a small cut and will have a tendency to bruise easily. Platelet function may be altered by many drugs, including common agents such as aspirin.

The plasma proteins involved in clotting are equally important for bleeding control. Some patients, such as those with hemophilia, have a deficiency of the proteins used for clotting and can bleed excessively. Patients with severe liver disease may also have a deficiency of clotting proteins and can have prolonged or excessive bleeding.

Blood Pressure

Blood pressure is the force exerted by the blood volume on the walls of the vessels. Pressure inside the blood vessels exerts a force in all directions. The one-way valves and the containing walls of the vessels enable the pressure to force blood forward through the circulatory system.

When blood is pumped into the arteries during ventricular contraction (systole), the amount of blood in the arteries increases and the pressure rises. The pressure measured during systole is the **systolic blood pressure.** As the heart relaxes (diastole), blood continues to move forward through vessels of lower pressure. The contraction of the elastic walls of the arteries aids blood flow during diastole. The amount of blood

volume remaining in the arteries decreases, and thus the blood pressure falls. The pressure measured during diastole is called the **diastolic blood pressure.**

Normal systolic blood pressure is estimated by calculating 100 millimeters of mercury (mm Hg) plus the patient's age (up to 140 mm Hg). Normal diastolic blood pressure is 65 to 90 mm Hg. In general, blood pressure is 8 to 10 mm Hg lower in women than in men.

Perfusion

Normally, blood flow is matched to meet the body's energy requirements on an organ-by-organ basis. Blood perfuses the tissues in sufficient quantity to meet each organ's oxygen needs. Each tissue and organ has some independent control over its own blood flow by its ability to regulate the flow through the capillaries in direct response to its oxygen needs. The arterioles, the smallest arteries that adjoin the capillaries, open or close in response to the level of oxygen in the tissues.

When the tissues need more oxygen, the arterioles open. This permits blood to flow through the area. When the tissues have sufficient oxygen, the arterioles close.

Shock. Shock, or **hypoperfusion,** is the failure of the circulatory system to adequately perfuse and oxygenate the tissues of the body. There are many causes of shock, but ultimately all result in inadequate tissue **perfusion** and oxygenation. Shock is caused by a disruption of any of the components of the circulatory system and may be present in varying degrees. In some cases it may be slight and self-correcting; in others it may be severe enough to result in death. The onset of shock may be immediate or delayed. Because the early recognition of shock is important in ensuring prompt treatment and correction of the underlying cause, the EMT must be familiar with the signs and symptoms of this life-threatening condition.

The ability to assess shock is aided by knowledge of the "compensatory mechanisms" that the body uses to survive. These compensatory mechanisms work to keep the mind alert and the blood pressure normal until the last moments. Thus the EMT who is aware of the signs of shock and the ways the body tries to compensate is able to recognize and treat patients in the early stages of shock, when they have the greatest chance of survival.

When a person is in shock, some organs are not perfused even though they have immediate oxygen needs. Less important organs are sacrificed first to allow perfusion of the more vital systems (brain and heart). Eventually, even the vital organs are underperfused in shock, and death follows if the condition is left uncorrected.

When shock is present, there is not enough blood flow through the organs and tissues to meet the body's needs at rest. Patients are weak and unable to sustain muscular activity.

Several signs and symptoms indicate shock. Some or all of the following may be present in a patient who is in shock **(Table 4-3):**
- Weakness
- Change in skin color, such as cyanosis (a blue-gray color), or a pale color
- Rapid and weak pulse
- Clammy and cool skin

| Table 4-3 | Signs and Symptoms of Shock |

Sign or Symptom	Cause
Pale, cool, clammy skin	Redistribution of blood from skin to more vital organs
Cyanotic skin	Poor perfusion and oxygenation
Rapid, weak pulse	Pulse increases to compensate for decreased perfusion
	Pulse weak from decreased blood pressure
Rapid, shallow breathing	Rapid breathing to compensate for decreased perfusion and oxygenation
Restlessness, anxiety, mental dullness	Poor circulation to the brain
Low blood pressure	Heart failure, low circulating blood volume, dilation of blood vessels
Nausea and vomiting	Central nervous system response

- Rapid and shallow breathing
- Restlessness and anxiety
- Altered mental state (as shock progresses)
- Low or decreasing blood pressure (in late shock)

Nervous System

One of the major goals of emergency care is to ensure brain viability. Therefore the EMT needs to be familiar with the functions of the nervous system. Most deaths from trauma result from direct injury to the nervous system. In addition, because the brain is the controlling center for other vital organ systems, such as respiration and circulation, brain dysfunction may result in cardiopulmonary failure and death. Because of the interdependence of the heart, lungs, and brain, signs of brain function are used to assess the status of other vital organs.

The nervous system is the controlling organ of the body. It is the center of consciousness and the intellectual, emotional, and behavioral functions that make up many of the characteristics of personality and human behavior. It receives and interprets stimuli from the internal and external environment, and it directs and regulates other organs and tissues. Some of its activity is conscious or willful, but much brain activity is unconscious or involuntary in response to the environment.

The nervous system is composed of two main divisions:
- Central nervous system—the computer
- Peripheral nervous system—the communicator

The *central nervous system* (CNS) receives information about the outside environment and about functions within the body itself. In turn, it organizes and analyzes this information and formulates a response that directs the activities of the organs, muscles, and other tissues.

The CNS receives and transmits information by nerves or special tracts of nerve tissue that extend through the CNS and extend out into the *peripheral nervous system* (PNS). The PNS is composed of the nerves outside the CNS, extending from both the brainstem and spinal cord. The PNS carries messages to the spinal cord and the brain by sensory nerves. The PNS also

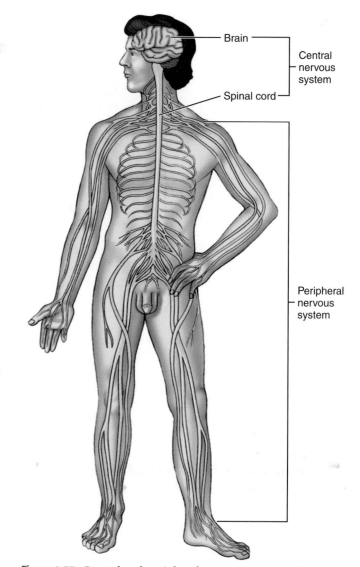

Figure 4-33 Central and peripheral nervous systems. *From Herlihy B, Maebius N: The human body in health and illness, Philadelphia, 2000, Saunders.*

carries messages back to the muscles and to the various organs by the motor nerves (**Figure 4-33**).

Central Nervous System

The CNS is composed of the *brain, brainstem,* and *spinal cord* (**Figure 4-34**). The brain and spinal cord are covered by layers of tissue, bathed in spinal fluid, and encased in the cranium and spinal column.

The brain is the central computer. It processes sensory input from sensory nerves and organizes responses that are then transmitted back to the body by outgoing motor nerves. Sensory input includes sight, hearing, smell, taste, and touch. Temperature, pain, vibration, pressure, and tickle are all variations of feeling. Special receptors in the ear and special nerve pathways relay input concerning balance and equilibrium. In addition, the brain receives input about the oxygen and carbon dioxide content of the blood as well as about the body's circulatory and nutritional status. All this information is processed at incredible speeds, as evidenced by a person's reaction to

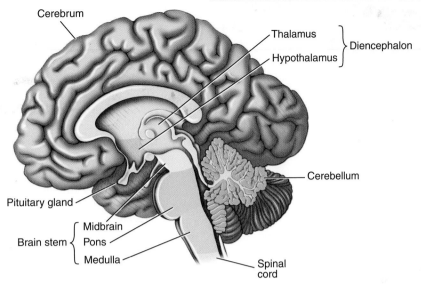

Figure 4-34 Midline section of the brain. *From Herlihy B, Maebius N: The human body in health and illness, Philadelphia, 2000, Saunders.*

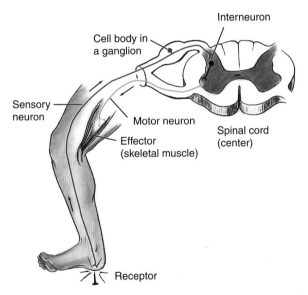

Figure 4-35 The reflex arc. *From Applegate EJ: The anatomy and physiology learning system, ed 3, Philadelphia, 2006, Saunders.*

a startling noise or noxious taste or odor. So much information is received by the brain at any one time that usually we are conscious of only about 1% of the sensory input.

Cerebrum. The largest and most superior portion of the brain is called the *cerebrum*. The cerebrum is divided down the middle into right and left halves called *hemispheres*. Generally, the right hemisphere controls the left side of the body, and vice versa. The hemispheres are further subdivided into different lobes or sections that have specific and distinct functions. They are named by their location with respect to the overlying skull bones; for example, the *frontal* lobe is the area responsible for intellectual functions and motor control of skeletal muscles. The *occipital* area is the center for receiving and processing visual stimuli, and the *temporal* area receives smell and hearing signals.

Brainstem. The brainstem is the lower part of the brain. Some nerve centers in the brainstem monitor and direct respiratory and circulatory function. Damage to certain parts of the brainstem can result in abnormal breathing patterns or cessation of breathing.

Cerebellum. The *cerebellum* is an outpocketing of the brain located behind or posterior to the brainstem. It is primarily concerned with coordination of movement and balance.

Spinal Cord. The spinal cord emerges from the brainstem and is a continuation of nerve tracts from all parts of the brain. It has its own processing centers as well. One example is reflex action. For example, stepping on a nail will cause an immediate reaction to remove your foot before the brain receives the message that damage has occurred (**Figure 4-35**). This type of action can occur through the reflex arcs along each segment of the spinal cord.

Voluntary and Involuntary Divisions

The nervous system can be divided into voluntary and involuntary functions. Voluntary functions are willful actions, such as running to catch a train. The *autonomic nervous system* is concerned with control of involuntary body functions, including control of the heart, the smooth muscles within organs such as the digestive tract, and the glands.

Voluntary Nervous System. The voluntary nervous system connects the CNS with sensory nerves that receive information from the skin and special sense organs (sight, hearing, smell, taste, pain). We are aware of these sensations. The motor nerves of the voluntary nervous system then carry information back to the body, directing conscious actions such as the control of our skeletal muscles. As the name implies, the voluntary nervous system controls activities that require willful or conscious action. For example, when you lift the lid off a hot pot of soup on the stove, the voluntary nervous system gauges how long your hand can tolerate the heat from the handle while you stir the soup before you must put the lid back down.

Involuntary Nervous System. The involuntary *(autonomic)* nervous system is composed of the special tracts of nerves and nerve centers that control vital body functions, such as heart rate, constriction/dilation of blood vessels, digestion, and heat regulation. Sensory nerves carry such information as the oxygen content in the blood, blood pressure, and body temperature to special centers in the brain, where this information is analyzed. In response, the brain sends messages by the motor nerves back to the various organs and tissues, directing or modifying their activity. Such activities may result in a change in heart rate, respiratory rate, or the amount of sweating from the skin; release of hormones; and constriction or dilation of the muscle in the walls of the blood vessels. The autonomic nervous system functions automatically, without our conscious control.

The autonomic nervous system has the following two main divisions:
- Parasympathetic nervous system
- Sympathetic nervous system

In general, these two divisions have opposite effects on a given organ or tissue. For example, the parasympathetic division slows the heart's rate, whereas the sympathetic division speeds it up. These two divisions, with their opposite effects, tend to counterbalance each other.

Parasympathetic Nervous System. The parasympathetic nervous system is most active during quiet or nonstressful conditions. For example, the parasympathetic nervous system plays an important role in digestion. Immediately after eating, the parasympathetic nervous system directs blood to the digestive tract to permit absorption of nutrients into blood.

Sympathetic Nervous System. The sympathetic nervous system, on the other hand, prepares the body for stressful situations. This is commonly called the "fight or flight" response. Imagine someone is chasing and trying to hurt you. You might prepare for fight or flight. Your pupils dilate to increase the amount of light and improve vision. Blood flows to your skeletal muscles so that you can fight or run. Your heart pumps faster, and your breathing is deeper and more rapid. All these responses are mediated through the sympathetic nervous system. In general, when one division of the involuntary (autonomic) nervous system is active, the other is at rest. This explains why after eating a large meal, you should not immediately exercise, because your blood supply will be directed to your digestive tract, and circulation to your muscles will be low, causing cramps to occur.

REAL*World*

Many geriatric patients take medications that work by altering the effects of the sympathetic nervous system. If a patient taking one of these medications were to experience a medical emergency requiring the response of the sympathetic nervous system, the patient would not be able to compensate appropriately. This medication would not allow the heart rate to increase, and the patient might not be able to maintain the blood pressure.

Integumentary System (Skin)

The skin is the largest organ of the body, providing a protective covering and insulation. It separates the internal from the external environment. It is a barrier to infection and loss of body fluids and is important for regulation of body temperature (**Figure 4-36**).

Epidermis

The surface or outermost layer of the skin is called the *epidermis*. The epidermis is nonvascular (does not contain blood vessels) and is made up of four separate sublayers. The epidermis is "impermeable," which means it cannot be penetrated by microorganisms, and it is responsible for preventing water loss from the cells underneath. The most superficial layer of the epidermis is dead tissue that is constantly rubbed or flaked away and replaced by the living cells underneath, which migrate upward. The layers of the epidermis become filled with a protein called *keratin* as they move upward toward the skin surface. This protein is partly responsible for the skin's impermeable barrier.

The epidermis is also responsible for the color of the skin. It contains a special pigment called *melanin* that helps protect the body from the sun's radiation. This pigment contributes to the color of the skin and is produced deep within the layers of the epidermis.

Skin color is also influenced by blood flow in the skin capillaries within the dermis. Increased flow, as occurs in a hot environment, causes the skin to appear pink or flushed. When blood flow to the skin is reduced, as in shock or cold temperatures, the skin may appear pale.

Dermis

The *dermis* is composed of dense connective tissue that contains the nerves, blood vessels, sweat and sebaceous glands, and hair follicles. The connective tissue gives strength to the skin and serves to anchor and support the other structures. The nerves in the dermis have various specialized endings that can perceive different sensations, such as pressure, vibration, pain, and warmth/cold. If this layer of skin is completely damaged, as occurs in third-degree burns, there will be no sensory perception. The blood vessels within the dermis play an important role in temperature regulation. They can constrict to prevent heat loss to the environment and dilate when the body needs to give off heat.

The *sweat glands* play an important role in the regulation of body temperature as well. *Evaporation* is an important means of cooling, particularly in extremely hot environments or when internal heat production builds up rapidly (as in exercise). The *sebaceous glands* secrete an oily substance called *sebum,* which helps moisturize the skin. Injuries that spare part of the dermis may allow for regrowth of new skin from cells that make up the hair follicles and sweat glands. Injuries such as burns that destroy all structures within the dermis require skin grafting.

Case in Point

An elderly man was burned when he overturned a pan of boiling water. You note that the anterior area of both legs and the dorsum of his feet are red, and that he has multiple blisters, some as large as 3 cm.

Blisters, a sign of a second-degree burn, are an accumulation of fluid between the epidermis and the dermis.

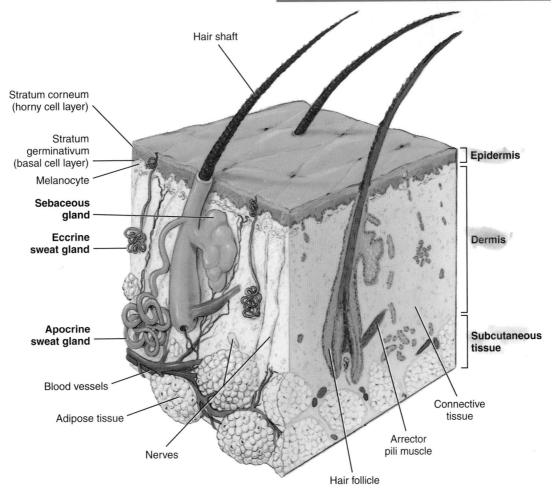

Figure 4-36 Structure of the skin. *Modified from Jarvis, C: Physical examination and health assessment, ed 3, Philadelphia, 2000, Saunders.*

Mucous Membranes

As skin continues into a body orifice, it changes its character. The tough layer of the epidermis is replaced by *mucous membranes*. Mucous membranes line the internal surface of the body organs, such as the oropharynx, nasopharynx, ureters, bladder, lungs, intestines, and vagina. This membrane is rich in mucous glands, which secrete a lubricating fluid (mucus) to protect the body from invading organisms.

Subcutaneous Tissue

Beneath the skin is a layer of fat and connective tissue called the *subcutaneous tissue*. It serves as a body insulator, and the fat can be used for energy as needed. Beneath the subcutaneous tissue is the *fascia*, a fibrous membrane covering that separates the subcutaneous tissue from the skeletal muscles.

Endocrine System

The endocrine system is also a regulatory system (**Figure 4-37**). Endocrine tissue is gland tissue that secretes special chemicals within the body or into the blood. These special chemicals, called *hormones*, can influence body functions distant from the site where they are produced. The hormones help regulate metabolism as well as influence reproduction, growth, and response to stress.

The major hormones that are helpful for the EMT to understand are epinephrine (or **adrenaline**) and insulin. **Epinephrine** is secreted by the adrenal glands, located above the kidneys. This hormone is released in times of stress and is part of a survival mechanism that enhances the activity of the sympathetic nervous system. **Insulin** is secreted by the pancreas and regulates metabolism of glucose.

Other hormones include *growth hormone* (from pituitary gland), *thyroxine* (from thyroid gland), *testosterone* (from testes), and *estrogen* (from ovaries).

Digestive System

The digestive system is the source of all nutritional intake except for oxygen. Throughout the digestive system, food is processed both mechanically and chemically to allow its absorption into the blood. Water is absorbed by the digestive tract as well. Foodstuffs that cannot be used by the body are eliminated through the rectum and anus as feces.

Food first enters through the mouth, where it is broken down mechanically by the teeth and tongue and is mixed with saliva to begin chemical processing (**Figure 4-38**). As food is swallowed, it is moved from the oropharynx into the esophagus. The epiglottis closes to protect the trachea during swallowing. Food moves along the esophagus by *peristaltic contractions* of

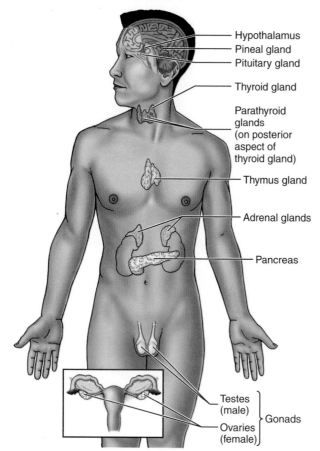

Figure 4-37 Major endocrine glands. *From Herlihy B, Maebius N: The human body in health and illness, Philadelphia, 2000, Saunders.*

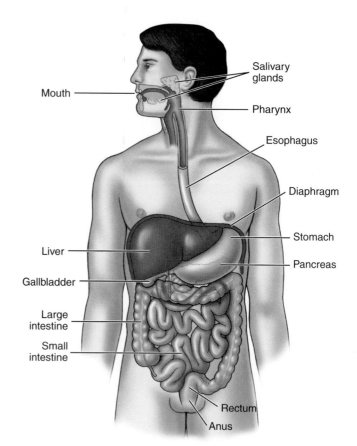

Figure 4-38 Organs of the digestive system. *From Herlihy B, Maebius N: The human body in health and illness, Philadelphia, 2000, Saunders.*

the smooth muscle that lines the esophageal walls. This wavelike contraction of smooth muscle that propels substances forward, called *peristalsis,* is found throughout the digestive tract from the esophagus to the anus. Food passes from the esophagus into the stomach, where it is churned and mixed with stomach acid and other secretions to continue chemical processing. Food leaves the stomach as *chyme* (partially digested food) through the *pylorus,* a sphincter-type muscle at the end of the stomach. It enters the *duodenum,* or the first part of the small intestine, where pancreatic secretions neutralize the stomach acids and break down the chyme into smaller units. The liver secretes *bile* to aid in fat absorption. The gallbladder stores bile until it is needed.

Small Intestine

The small intestine is the main site for absorption. The small intestine begins with the *duodenum* at the outlet of the stomach, then continues as a long tube that is initially called the *jejunum* and later, as the nature of the intestinal walls changes, the *ileum.* After the chemical and mechanical processing has broken the chyme into sufficiently small components, these fragments can enter the blood vessels within the intestinal walls. The blood from the intestines passes through a capillary bed within the liver on its return to the general circulation. The liver serves to filter blood and is concerned with the storage, breakdown, and synthesis of the proteins, carbohydrates, and fats that are the basic constituents

of food. "Interconversion" of proteins, fats, and carbohydrates, or the changing of one form of food constituent to another (e.g., from fat to carbohydrate), also takes place in the liver.

Large Intestine

The large intestine absorbs excess water as the unused foods are converted to feces, which are excreted through the anus. The large intestine begins in the right lower quadrant at the *cecum.* Off the cecum is the *appendix.* The large intestine continues as the *ascending colon* as it passes upward to the right upper quadrant, travels across the abdomen as the *transverse colon,* then descends along the left side as the *descending colon,* where it changes to the *sigmoid colon* in the left lower quadrant. Feces are stored in the descending and sigmoid colon before passing into the rectum and through the anus during defecation. The sigmoid colon and rectum lie within the pelvis.

Whereas the digestive system functions automatically, contractions and sensations within the intestines and stomach stimulate us to eat food and to eliminate feces. Although involuntary muscle is found from the esophagus to the rectum, there is voluntary muscle in the mouth and pharynx for chewing and swallowing and at the anal canal for control of defecation.

Urinary System

The urinary system, which is composed of the *kidneys,* the *ureters,* the *urinary bladder,* and the *urethra,* filters the blood and excretes excess water and waste products (**Figure 4-39**). For example, if

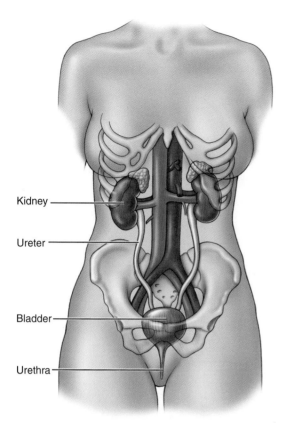

Figure 4-39 Components of the urinary system. *From Herlihy B, Maebius N: The human body in health and illness, Philadelphia, 2000, Saunders.*

you drink more water than you need, you must eliminate the excess, or it will dilute the concentration of the blood and body fluids.

The kidneys filter the blood and reabsorb essential ingredients while selectively excreting excesses and waste products. The urine that is formed is transferred by peristalsis through the ureters to the bladder, where it is stored. The bladder is emptied during urination, when urine is released through the urethra.

Lymphatic System

Lymphatic vessels transport fluid *(lymph)* from the tissues of the body back to the blood vessels. There are *lymph nodes* throughout the body that filter the fluid during its passage and remove foreign particles along the way. Other organs of the lymphatic system include the *tonsils,* the *spleen,* and the *thymus* gland.

Reproductive System

The female reproductive organs, located within the pelvis, are the *ovaries,* the *fallopian tubes,* the *uterus,* and the *vagina* **(Figure 4-40, A)**. The eggs travel from the ovaries through the fallopian tubes to the uterus. If fertilized by sperm, the egg will implant on the wall of the uterus. If the egg is not fertilized, it will be discharged during menstruation.

In the male the testes are located in the scrotum. Spermatozoa manufactured by each testis travel through the *vas deferens* and then the *prostate,* where sperm are mixed with secretions to form *semen* and ejaculated through the urethra in the penis **(Figure 4-40, B)**.

Understanding the Relevance of Anatomy and Physiology

The vital organ systems are the nervous, respiratory, and circulatory systems. These three systems are intimately interrelated. Failure of any one system may rapidly lead to collapse of the other two. For this reason, primary emphasis in emergency assessment and treatment in the prehospital phase of care is directed to these three organ systems. Failure of any one of these three vital organ systems can lead to clinical death in seconds or minutes **(Table 4-4)**.

Tracing the need for oxygen demonstrates this interdependence. When breathing stops, the level of oxygen in the blood begins to fall. After a few minutes, the brain no longer has enough oxygen delivered to maintain consciousness. The heart and other tissues keep extracting the oxygen that remains in the lungs and the blood, causing the oxygen content to drop lower and lower. Eventually, there is inadequate oxygen to power heart contractions, and circulation stops.

The brain can function for only 10 seconds (or less) if deprived of oxygen. Lack of oxygen flow to the brain, as evidenced by no pulse and respirations, causes the condition known as *clinical death.* If the brain is deprived of oxygen for 4 to 6 minutes, biological death begins. *Biological death* defines a state of sustained oxygen deprivation after which recovery without brain damage is unlikely.

The time to biological death is modified by certain factors or conditions. For example, children are more tolerant of periods of cardiac arrest than are adults. A cool body temperature lowers the body's metabolism and improves the chances of recovery. Drowning often arouses reflexes that improve the chances of recovery as well (e.g., the mammalian diving reflex is a reaction to cold water that shuts off major blood flow throughout the body, except to the brain, heart, and lungs).

Case in Point

A 68-year-old man is experiencing a myocardial infarction, or heart attack. The injured and dying heart muscle is causing his blood pressure to drop (hypotension) and fluid to back up into his lungs, resulting in shortness of breath and hypoxia. The hypotension and hypoxia result in the patient becoming unconscpious.

Sudden and Unexpected Death

The common causes of sudden and unexpected death are cardiovascular disease, cerebrovascular disease, and accidental injuries. Understanding how these conditions lead to clinical death and the time intervals involved in the dying process helps the EMT accomplish the following:

- Focus on the conditions the EMT will be facing in the community.
- Understand the priorities built into standardized approaches to assessment and treatment.
- Recognize the importance of rapid delivery of definitive medical care for critical patients.

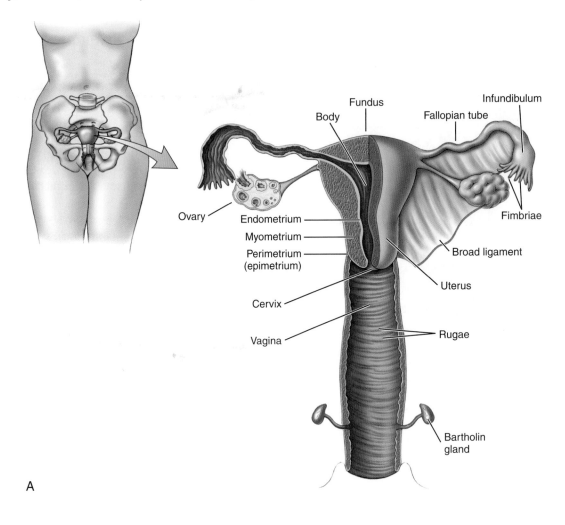

A

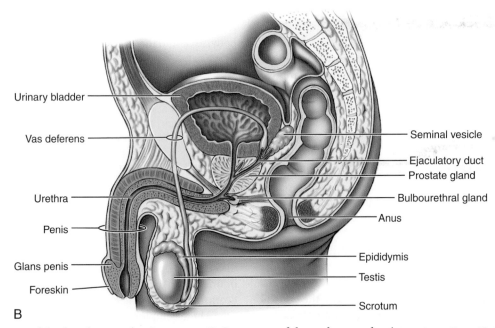

B

Figure 4-40 **A,** Organs of the female reproductive system. **B,** Structures of the male reproductive system. *From Herlihy B, Maebius N: The human body in health and illness, Philadelphia, 2000, Saunders.*

| | Table 4-4 | Interrelationships of Vital Organs | | | |

Organ	Function	Some Causes of Organ Failure	Signs of Failure	Response of Rescuer
Brain	Maintains consciousness Controls breathing	Stroke Injury Electric shock Drug overdose	Unresponsive to stimuli	Check for breathing
Lungs	Oxygenate blood Remove carbon dioxide	Drowning Airway obstruction Chest injury Suffocation Asphyxiation	No breathing or inadequate breathing	Provide positive-pressure ventilation
Heart	Circulates blood	Myocardial infarction Electric shock	No pulse	Provide circulation by external chest compression and/or defibrillation

Scenario Follow-up

The victim of the stabbing shows signs of significant blood loss, with a low blood pressure and rapid, weak pulse. The spurting blood from the arm is consistent with an arterial injury. Direct pressure is often enough to prevent further blood loss. The wound to the upper chest can cause both collapse of the lung and bleeding within the chest cavity. The wound to the left upper quadrant may have injured the spleen, a blood-rich organ. Surgery may be required to stop internal bleeding. When less blood returns to the heart, the amount of blood pumped from the ventricles decreases, making the pulse feel "weak." To compensate for the decreased blood flow, the heart rate is increased in an attempt to maintain cardiac output sufficient to perfuse the vital organs.

Summary

Anatomy and physiology constitute the basis for understanding in all aspects of medical education. By understanding the structure and function of the human body, you will improve your understanding of patient assessment and treatment. Anatomy will help you appreciate the causes of pain and the severity of blunt and penetrating trauma by body region and location. Physiology will help you appreciate the changes in vital signs and other physical findings that you may encounter as an EMT. Take a moment to review the learning checklist to reinforce the key concepts in this chapter.

The Bottom Line

Learning Checklist

✓ Define the following anatomic terms: torso, anterior (ventral), posterior (dorsal), medial, lateral, bilateral, proximal, plantar, palmar, distal, superficial, deep, midline, midaxillary, and midclavicular.

✓ Define the following terms related to position: supine, prone, and lateral recumbent (recovery position).

✓ Define the following terms related to movement: abduction, adduction, flexion, extension, medial rotation, and lateral rotation.

✓ The skeletal system gives structure and support to the body and serves to protect vital organs. In conjunction with the muscles, it allows for body movement.

✓ Bones, cartilage, and ligaments are forms of connective tissue.

✓ There are 206 bones in the body. The major bones of the body are:
  ✓ Skull
  ✓ Spinal column: 7 cervical, 12 thoracic, 5 lumbar, 5 sacral, 4 coccygeal
  ✓ Thorax: 12 ribs, sternum
  ✓ Pelvis: iliac crest (wings), pubis (anterior), ischium (inferior)
  ✓ Upper extremities: scapula, clavicle, acromion, humerus, olecranon, radius and ulna, metacarpals, phalanges
  ✓ Lower extremities: greater trochanter, acetabulum, femur, patella, tibia and fibula, medial and lateral malleoli, metatarsals, phalanges

✓ There are several types of joints, including ball-and-socket joints, which allow for a wide range of motion, and hinge joints, which allow for flexion and extension.

✓ There are three types of muscle: voluntary or skeletal muscle (provides motion), involuntary or smooth muscle (lines body structures such as blood vessels and the digestive tract), and cardiac muscle (the heart).

✓ The respiratory system brings oxygen into the body and rids the body of carbon dioxide, the waste product.

✓ The respiratory system is composed of the nose and mouth, nasopharynx and oropharynx, larynx and epiglottis, trachea, bronchi, bronchioles, alveoli, and lungs.

✓ The diaphragm and the muscles of the chest cause the thoracic cavity to expand and contract like a bellows to create airflow during ventilation. Inhalation occurs when the diaphragm and intercostal muscles contract and enlarge the thoracic cavity. Exhalation occurs when the diaphragm and intercostals relax, decreasing the size of the thoracic cavity.

✓ Oxygen and carbon dioxide exchange occurs at the level of the alveoli and capillaries through the process of diffusion.

✓ During strenuous exercise or in respiratory disease or trauma, the accessory muscles of breathing help increase the respiratory volumes.

✓ Adequate breathing is characterized by a normal respiratory rate (adult, 12-20 breaths/min; child, 15-30; infant, 25-50), regular rhythm, and normal quality of breathing (breath sounds present and equal, chest expansion adequate and equal).

✓ Inadequate breathing is characterized by a respiratory rate outside the normal range, irregular rhythm, and abnormal quality of breathing (breath sounds diminished or absent, chest expansion inadequate or shallow, or use of accessory muscles). Other signs of inadequate breathing include pallor, cool or cyanotic skin, retractions, nasal flaring, seesaw breathing, and agonal respirations.

✓ The circulatory system is the transport system of the body. It delivers oxygen and nutrients to the tissues and returns the waste products of metabolism (carbon dioxide and cellular wastes) to the lungs and kidneys for excretion. It also transports specialized cells to areas of the body where they are needed to repair injured tissues, combat foreign bacteria, and control bleeding.

✓ The circulatory system consists of the heart, blood, and blood vessels. The blood consists of plasma and cells: white blood cells (combat infection), red blood cells (transport oxygen and carbon dioxide attached to hemoglobin), and platelets (clotting).

✓ The major arteries of the body are the aorta, pulmonary, carotid, coronary, femoral, radial, brachial, posterior tibial, and dorsalis pedis.

✓ The major veins of the body are the pulmonary (brings oxygen-rich blood to left atrium) and vena cava (brings oxygen-poor blood to right atrium).

✓ The major pulse points of the body are the carotid, femoral, radial, brachial, posterior tibial, and dorsalis pedis.

✓ Blood pressure consists of two components: systolic pressure is that exerted on the walls of the artery when the ventricle contracts; diastolic pressure is that exerted on the walls of the artery when the ventricle relaxes.

✓ Inadequate circulation (shock or hypoperfusion) is characterized by pallor, cyanosis, cool and clammy skin, rapid and weak pulse, rapid and shallow breathing, restlessness, anxiety or mental dullness, nausea or vomiting, and low blood pressure.

✓ The nervous system controls the voluntary (e.g., muscular movement) and involuntary functions (e.g., heart rate) of the body.

✓ The nervous system consists of the central nervous system (brain and spinal cord) and the peripheral nervous system (sensory nerves carry information to the brain, and motor nerves carry information away from the brain).

✓ Reflexes are automatic muscular movements mediated through a reflex arch in the spinal cord.

✓ The skin consists of three layers: epidermis (outermost layer), dermis (deeper layer containing major structures such as sweat glands and hair follicles), and subcutaneous or fatty tissue layer.

Key Terms

Abduction Movement away from the midline.

Accessory muscles Muscles found in the neck, chest, and abdomen that can increase the forces of inhalation and exhalation in patients in respiratory distress.

Adduction Movement toward the midline.

Adrenaline See *Epinephrine*.

Anterior Toward the front of the body.

Artery Muscular blood vessel that carries blood away from the heart.

Bilateral Occurring or appearing on two sides.

Capillary Thin-walled blood vessel where exchange of nutrients and waste products occurs between blood and tissue fluid through diffusion.

Cardiac arrest Cessation of a functional heartbeat.

Central Situated at, in, or near the center.

Diastolic blood pressure Blood pressure measured during the relaxation phase (diastole) of the heart. The pressure at which the sounds heard through a stethoscope disappear or significantly diminish.

Distal Farther away from the trunk.

Dorsal Toward the back (or ventral) surface.

Epiglottis Flap of cartilage that covers the larynx during swallowing to prevent food from entering the lungs.

Epinephrine Hormone secreted by the adrenal glands that increases sympathetic activity throughout the body. Effects include increased heart rate, force of contraction, bronchodilation, and rate of breathing; increased blood flow to skeletal muscles with decreased flow to other organs (digestive and skin); and increased blood glucose. Also called *adrenaline*.

Extension Straightening of a joint.

Femur The thighbone, the largest bone in the body.

Flexion Bending of a joint.

Hypoperfusion Decreased blood flow through an organ, as in shock. Prolonged hypoperfusion can result in permanent cellular dysfunction and death.

Inferior Toward the feet.

Insulin Hormone produced by the pancreas; necessary for glucose metabolism.

Lateral Toward the side of the body.

Medial Toward the midline of the body.

Midaxillary An imaginary line on the body that extends from the armpit down through the lower chest wall.

Midclavicular An imaginary line on the body that extends from the middle section of the clavicle down through the lower chest wall.

Midline An imaginary line that divides the body into right and left halves.

Perfusion Fluid passing through an organ or part of the body. The surrounding and bathing of a tissue or cell with blood or the fluid part of blood.

Peripheral Away from the center of the body.

Posterior Structures toward the rear of the body.

Prone Lying facedown or on the ventral or anterior surface of the body.

Proximal Closer to the trunk.

Shock State resulting from failure of the circulatory system to perfuse and oxygenate the vital organs of the body adequately.

Superior Toward the head.

Supine Position of the body when a person is lying on his or her back.

Systolic blood pressure Blood pressure measured during the contraction phase (systole) of the heart, noted by the first sound heard through a stethoscope when blood pressure is obtained.

Tidal volume Volume of air inspired and expired during one breath. Normal tidal volume at rest for an adult is approximately 500 mL.

Trachea Hollow tube with several horseshoe-shaped rings of cartilage on the anterolateral surface that support and provide structure for this portion of the airway; the "windpipe."

Vein Blood vessel that returns blood to the heart.

Ventral Toward the abdomen, or anterior.

Vertebrae The irregular bones that form the spinal column.

Review Questions

Questions 1-6. Match the definition in column B to the correct term in column A.

Column A	Column B
1. Lateral	a. Toward the rear of the body
2. Proximal	b. Away from the midline
3. Superior	c. Lying faceup
4. Posterior	d. Movement toward the body
5. Supine	e. Toward the point of origin
6. Adduction	f. Toward the head

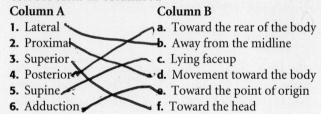

7. In the normal anatomic position, the body is erect with feet together and parallel, arms extended, and palms and head facing which direction?
   a. Medially
   b. Posteriorly
   c. Anteriorly
   d. Laterally

Questions 8-10. Match the function in column B to the type of muscle in column A.

Column A	Column B
8. Voluntary or skeletal muscle	a. Walking
9. Involuntary or smooth muscle	b. Pumping of blood
10. Cardiac muscle	c. Constriction of blood vessels

11. When eating or drinking, what is the respiratory structure responsible for preventing aspiration of food and other materials into the airway?
    a. Bronchiole
    b. Carina
    c. Pharynx
    d. Epiglottis

12. Which of the following are the chambers of the heart that receive blood from the lungs and body tissues?
    a. Septa
    b. Sinuses
    c. Atria
    d. Ventricles

13. What is the major vein that delivers blood back to the heart from the body or systemic circulation?
    a. Aorta
    b. Pulmonary
    c. Coronary
    d. Vena cava

14. Which of the following is the protein responsible for the transport of oxygen and carbon dioxide?
    a. Plasma
    b. Thrombin
    c. Hemoglobin
    d. Fibrinogen

15. Which of the following is part of the central nervous system?
    a. Cranial nerves
    b. Autonomic nervous system
    c. Spinal cord
    d. Optic nerve

16. The heart, lung, and brain depend on each another to maintain vital functions. Which of the following reasons best explains why a patient stops breathing after cardiac arrest?
    a. Lack of oxygen to the brainstem
    b. Loss of voluntary breathing control
    c. Damage to the cerebrum
    d. Toxicity of blood

17. A patient has a gunshot wound to midabdomen, just above the umbilicus, and signs of shock. Which structure in this area can cause rapid loss of blood?
    a. Stomach
    b. Descending aorta
    c. Gallbladder
    d. Spleen

For Further Review

In the Student Workbook
- Multiple-choice questions
- Matching questions
- Fill-in-the-blank questions
- Case scenario questions
- Labeling questions
- Crossword puzzles

On Evolve
- Weblinks
- Lecture notes
- Exercises

Learning Objectives

Cognitive Objectives
- Identify the following topographic terms: medial, lateral, proximal, distal, superior, inferior, anterior, posterior, midline, right and left, midclavicular, bilateral, and midaxillary.
- Define the following topographic terms: medial, lateral, proximal, distal, superior, inferior, anterior, posterior, midline, right and left, midclavicular, bilateral, and midaxillary.
- Describe the anatomy and function of the following major body systems: respiratory, circulatory, musculoskeletal, nervous, and endocrine.

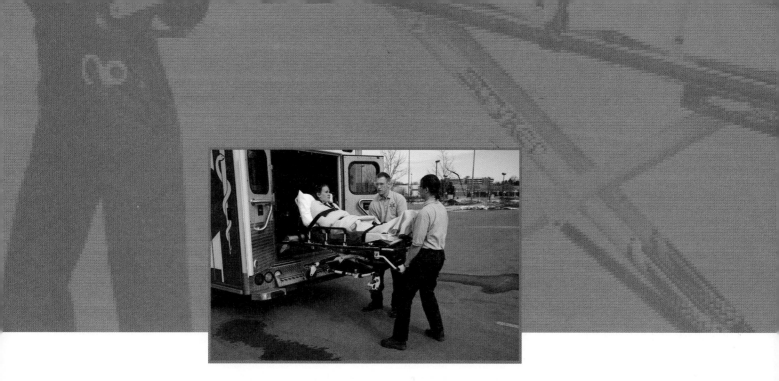

5 Lifting and Moving Patients

CHAPTER OUTLINE

Body Mechanics
Principles of Moving Patients
Equipment
Patient Positioning
Skills

Scenario

You respond to a call for a "multiple-vehicle collision" with two other emergency medical services (EMS) units. The police are on the scene controlling traffic. After safely positioning your ambulance, you attend to a 25-year-old woman who was thrown from her car and is lying supine in a pool of gasoline. Her car's engine is engulfed in fire 15 feet away. You quickly grasp the patient's shirt at the shoulder region and drag her away from danger and begin your assessment.

An emergency medical technician (EMT) from a second unit evaluates the driver of another car and finds that she is experiencing severe airway difficulty. He coordinates with two other EMTs to extricate her rapidly from the car by using a long spine board.

A paramedic from a third unit finds a victim who was thrown from a car into a nearby ditch that is 10 feet deep. The patient weighs more than 300 pounds. The paramedic recruits two other EMS providers and a police officer to lift the victim from the ditch with spinal immobilization and place him in a basket stretcher for removal over the rough terrain. The lift requires careful coordination and a balanced lifting team with an even number of persons. They are strategically positioned so that the two larger and stronger persons are at the head of the patient. On clear command from the team leader, the victim is lifted. All team members position themselves close to the device and lift with their thigh muscles while keeping their backs in the locked-in position. They are careful not to twist their bodies during the lift.

The selection of the appropriate lift-and-carry technique is as much a part of your patient's care as bandaging, splinting, or administering oxygen therapy. In the case of a suspected spinal injury victim, choosing the appropriate lift and carry is frequently the most important aspect of care.

As an EMT, you will need to be an expert in lifting and carrying techniques. Each situation requires its own unique strategy and equipment for lifting and moving the patient. This may include the use of cot stretchers, scoop stretchers, spine boards, basket stretchers, and a variety of other lifting and moving devices. Factors such as available personnel, terrain, hazards, and, most important, the condition of the patient influence the manner by which you remove and transport the patient from the scene. Optimally, a trauma patient should not be moved until he or she has been fully immobilized and prepared for transport. There are, of course, exceptions to this rule. If remaining on the scene to attach a spine board or other specialized device will endanger the patient (e.g., fire), you must remove the patient from the area first and deal with specific injuries later.

Improper lifting and carrying of the patient may be hazardous to your patient and to yourself. A back injury can last a lifetime and can be career ending. Protecting yourself from this possibility should be a major concern. Learning and practicing the proper scientific techniques for lifting and carrying patients, as described in this chapter, can help minimize the chance that you will sustain an injury.

LEARNING OBJECTIVES
- Define body mechanics.
- Discuss the guidelines and safety precautions to follow when lifting a patient.
- Explain the rationale for properly lifting and moving patients.

Body Mechanics

Lifting Techniques

The scientific use of specific methods of efficiently lifting large weights to avoid injury is known as **body mechanics.** The human body is composed of a system of levers and support structures that, if used correctly, can support a great deal of weight. However, if they are used incorrectly, severe and permanent injury can result. General guidelines for lifting include the following:
- Know your physical capabilities and limitations.
- Seek help when needed.
- Do not attempt to move a patient if you believe you cannot lift the person.

Safety Precautions

The long bones are the strongest bones of the body. The largest of these is the femur, which also is surrounded by the largest and strongest muscle group in the body. You should use these support units when attempting to lift heavy objects. You should never lift with your back because the back muscles that support the spinal column are relatively small and weak and more prone to injury. Use your legs by bending them before lifting while keeping your back as straight as possible (do not twist while lifting).

When lifting a patient from the ground, you should communicate clearly and frequently to your team members. You need to position your feet properly for balance by placing one foot in front of the other. Always get as close as possible to the person and device you are lifting, and keep your arms close to your body as you lift (**Figure 5-1**). This technique places your center of gravity closer to the patient, giving you more leverage and, in effect, making the patient lighter. This position also helps you

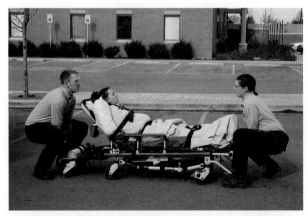

Figure 5-1 Proper body mechanics when lifting.

Box 5-1	Guidelines for Lifting

1. When holding or moving a stretcher, keep your back straight and tighten the muscles of your abdomen and buttocks. These muscles provide the main support for your back.
2. Maintain a firm grip on the device or the patient, and lift and move it or the patient slowly and smoothly and in unison with your partner.
3. Avoid twisting or using sharp, jerky movements, which can result in injury to you or discomfort to the patient.
4. Always maintain firm footing. Try not to keep your muscles contracted for a long time because this induces fatigue and increases the possibility of muscle strain or injury.
5. Communicate clearly and frequently with your partner.
6. Practice basic fitness to prevent back injuries; weak back and abdominal muscles are conducive to back injury.
7. Use good posture and proper lifting techniques while moving patients.
8. Know your own physical limitations, and use other resources available at the scene, including prehospital providers, police, and occasionally bystanders.

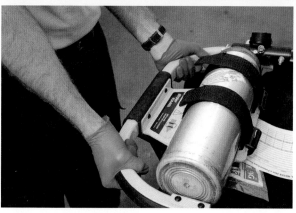

Figure 5-2 Power grip.

Box 5-2	Guidelines for Carrying

1. Determine the weight to be lifted.
2. Become familiar with your own abilities and the abilities of your partner.
3. Communicate with the lifting team, and coordinate the lift.
4. Keep the weight as close to your body as possible.
5. Lock your back, and do not twist during the lifting process.
6. Flex at the hips, not the waist, and bend at knees.
7. Do not hyperextend the back by leaning back from the waist.
8. Use correct lifting techniques to lift the stretcher.
9. Partners should be similar in strength and height.

maintain your balance. A seesaw demonstrates the value of this technique. When you sit toward the center of the seesaw, your partner raises you more easily. As you move toward the end, lifting you becomes much more difficult.

Box 5-1 reviews the key methods for effective lifting and avoiding injuries.

> **LEARNING OBJECTIVE**
> • Describe the safe lifting of cots and stretchers.

Safe Lifting of Cots and Stretchers

When lifting cots and stretchers, you support the combined weight of the device and the patient. Stretchers and cots can be more difficult to handle because the patient is positioned higher off the ground, making the device less stable. Become familiar with the weight of the patient, and use two or more people to execute a lift. You should consider the overall mechanics of the lift and ensure that enough help is available to provide a smooth and appropriate lift of the device. The team should be balanced, with an even number of people on each side of the device. The size and strength of available personnel should be considered when placing helpers around the device.

An effective method for lifting an extremely heavy device is called a **power lift** or **squat lift** (**Skill 5-1**). The power lift is a technique used by body builders to maximize lifting power and avoid injury.

When lifting, use the **power grip** to maintain control over the device. Your palms and fingers should be in complete contact with the device during the lifting process. Fold your fingers at the same angles, and your hands should be at least 10 inches (25 cm) apart (**Figure 5-2**).

When lowering the device, use the power lift in reverse. You should always avoid bending at the waist. Bending at the waist distributes the weight to your back muscles and increases the probability of back injury.

> **LEARNING OBJECTIVES**
> • Describe the guidelines and safety precautions for carrying patients and equipment.
> • Discuss one-handed carrying techniques.
> • Describe correct and safe carrying procedures on stairs.

Carrying

General Guidelines

Patients may have to be carried a significant distance from the scene to the vehicle. As with lifting, you should adhere to effective guidelines during transport of the patient up or down stairs, up or down hills, and along flat or rough terrain. When possible, a device that can be rolled should be used (**Box 5-2**). These guidelines are similar to those discussed for lifting because the same body mechanics are needed to avoid injury.

Specific Techniques

The **one-handed carrying technique** is used when multiple personnel are available for the carry and team members are placed strategically around the device. As with any device, lift and carry with the back in straight alignment or the **locked-in position.** With one-handed techniques, it is particularly important not to lean to either side to compensate for any imbalance.

This will strain the muscles of your back or side and increase the potential for injury. As with carrying a heavy suitcase, you should maintain a straight posture while you are carrying a stretcher.

Carrying a patient up and down stairs can be particularly challenging because of the effect of the incline on the distribution of weight. In general, the personnel at the bottom of the device are expected to carry a heavier load and may have to elevate it to keep the device level. Team members at the upper position of the device may have to bend their knees to maintain the device at a safe angle during ascent or descent. In general, a stair chair is a more effective and safer method for transport on stairs, but it is not suitable for patients who are unconscious or who have suspected spinal injury. As with all lifting and carrying, the following measures should be followed:

- Keep your back in locked-in position.
- Flex at the hips (not the waist).
- Bend at the knees, not with the back.
- Keep your weight and arms as close to the device as possible.
- Have stronger personnel positioned at the bottom.
- Use a stair chair whenever possible.

> **LEARNING OBJECTIVES**
> - State the guidelines for reaching and their applications.
> - Describe correct reaching for log rolls.

Reaching

Many back injuries occur when reaching or stretching during the lifting and carrying process. If you have ever worked in a close space and stretched in the same position for an extended period, you can understand the potential for injury. This is why prehospital providers should be in excellent physical condition, maintaining both strength and flexibility. You should pay particular attention to good body mechanics, as follows:

- Keep your back in the locked-in position.
- Avoid the hyperextended position when reaching overhead.
- Avoid twisting while reaching or stretching over an obstacle or patient.
- Avoid reaching more than 15 to 20 inches (38-50 cm) in front of your body.
- Avoid situations in which prolonged (>1 minute) strenuous effort is needed.
- Keep the weight close to the body.
- Push from the area between your waist and shoulder.
- If the weight is below waist level, use the kneeling position.
- If possible, avoid pushing or pulling from an overhead position.
- Keep your elbows bent, with your arms close to your sides.

A common procedure that requires reaching is the **log roll.** Correct log rolls involve the following principles:

- Keep your back straight while leaning over the patient.
- Lean from your hips.
- Use your shoulder muscles to execute the procedure.

The technique of log rolling a patient onto a long spine board is illustrated in Skill 24-1.

> **LEARNING OBJECTIVE**
> - State the guidelines for pushing and pulling.

Pushing and Pulling

Most movement to and from the ambulance involves pushing and pulling. Although this seems like a simple process, keep in mind the following important considerations:

- In general, pushing is safer and more effective than pulling because you are less likely to use your back muscles.
- Keep your back in the locked-in position.
- Keep the line of pull through the center of your body by bending at the knees. For example, when pulling a cot stretcher, the mattress should be on a straight line with your waist.
- Keep weight close to the body.
- Push from the area between the waist and the shoulder.
- If weight is below the level of your waist, use the kneeling position if possible.
- Avoid pushing or pulling from an overhead position.
- Keep your elbows bent with your arms close to your side.

> **LEARNING OBJECTIVES**
> - Discuss the general considerations of moving patients.
> - Describe three situations that may require an emergency move.

Principles of Moving Patients

General Considerations

The technique you select to move a patient depends on several factors, including the position in which the patient is found, the patient's condition, presence or absence of suspected spinal injury, urgency of the clinical situation, and presence of immediate danger at the scene. Whenever possible, select a move that is designed to provide maximum benefit to the patient's condition. This may require thoughtful planning before execution.

In general, the patient should be moved immediately and with careful planning only when he or she is in immediate danger (see Emergency Moves), such as in the following circumstances:

- When fire, explosion, or hazardous materials threaten the patient or personnel.
- You must access a severely injured patient who is trapped behind a stable patient.
- Lifesaving care requires placing the patient in the supine position.

In other situations the patient should be moved quickly, not immediately (see Urgent Moves), because of a life-threatening condition. In these cases, some methods are faster but still minimize the chances of aggravating existing injuries. Weigh the potential risks to the patient and others against the need for specific interventions in each situation.

A person who is bleeding internally from a severe chest injury may lose the entire blood volume if rapid surgical

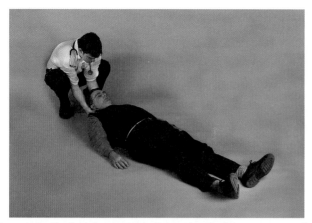

Figure 5-3 Clothes drag. Grasp the patient's shirt or coat at the shoulder region, and support the patient's head against your forearms while dragging the person to a safe location.

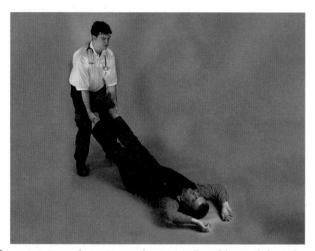

Figure 5-4 Foot drag. Grasp the patient's ankles and drag the patient to a safe location.

intervention is not obtained in a timely manner. In this case, you cannot take the time to apply a short spine board but must rapidly extricate the patient and transport the person to a trauma center while performing essential life support measures en route.

A patient with a complete airway obstruction that cannot be relieved by basic life support procedures also requires rapid transport.

You may be unable to secure the scene safely at highway automobile crashes; caring for a patient in such a setting places you and the patient in jeopardy.

As an EMT, you must integrate "time to transport" into your overall strategy for selecting the appropriate move for the patient.

Emergency Moves

When an immediate threat of death to the patient or the rescuer exists, an **emergency move** is necessary. An emergency move is one in which the patient is moved before any assessment. As previously stated, certain situations require the use of an emergency move.

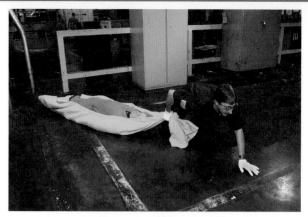

Figure 5-5 Blanket drag.

The greatest consequence to an emergency move is the possibility of harming a patient with a suspected spinal injury. Moving the patient along the long axis of the body can minimize this risk. The patient can be dragged from the feet or from the shoulders with minimal flexion, extension, or twisting to the spine. When the patient is being moved from a vehicle that is on fire, effectively considering inline immobilization may not be possible, but the rationale for such a move is obvious—life over limb.

The move chosen for each situation depends on the number of personnel available, the terrain over which you must move the patient, and the size of the patient. You should never attempt to lift a patient whom you cannot fully support.

Drag Techniques

The simplest technique, which is also practical for quickly moving a patient in almost all situations, is the **clothes drag** technique. In this technique, you grasp the patient's shirt, sweater, or jacket and drag the patient, always along the long axis of the body (**Figure 5-3**). When you cannot access the head of the patient, the **foot drag** is an alternate technique for quickly moving the patient from a dangerous situation (**Figure 5-4**).

If a blanket is available, the **blanket drag** is preferable to the clothes or foot drag. It permits a long-axis pull without dragging the patient's clothes or skin on the ground and is therefore gentler on the patient (**Figure 5-5**).

The patient may also be moved by lifting and supporting the upper torso and dragging the patient to safety (**Figure 5-6**).

Urgent Moves

For patients who are critically ill or injured, such as those in shock, respiratory arrest, or an altered mental state, an "urgent" move may be necessary. Patients who are thought to have internal bleeding in the chest, abdomen, or brain require surgical intervention. Excessive time in the field is likely to result in fatal blood loss. Transport of these patients should begin after applying immediate lifesaving skills. At ground level, injured patients can be rapidly transported on a long spine board, and noninjured patients can be transported on a stretcher in the appropriate position. When patients are critically injured in a vehicle, they can be removed by the **rapid extrication procedure (Skill 5-2).**

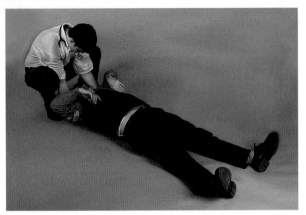

Figure 5-6 Drag using the patient's torso.

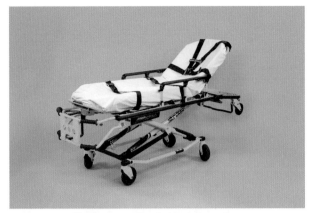

Figure 5-7 Wheeled cot stretcher.

Nonurgent Moves

When deciding to transport, select the device best suited to provide a safe and comfortable ride for the patient. Medical patients most often require a **wheeled cot stretcher,** which can be adjusted for sitting or lying in the supine or lateral recumbent positions. Trauma patients may require several other devices. These devices are primarily designed to ensure proper immobilization of the spine to prevent spinal cord injury that might result from the twisting or bending of the spinal column. The major danger connected with moving a patient quickly in an emergency is the possibility of worsening an existing spinal injury. Splinting before transport protects extremities, but if time does not permit, the patient may be splinted to the long spine board.

A wheeled cot stretcher is the most common transport device for patients without suspected spinal injuries. Although many techniques are available for transferring a patient from a bed to a wheeled cot stretcher, the following methods are used most often:

• Direct ground lift (**Skill 5-3**)
• Extremity lift (**Skill 5-4**)
• Direct carry (**Skill 5-5**)
• Draw sheet method (**Skill 5-6**)

LEARNING OBJECTIVE
• Identify the following patient carrying devices: wheeled ambulance stretcher, portable ambulance stretcher, stair chair, scoop stretcher, long spine board, short spine board (vest-type device), basket stretcher, and flexible stretcher.

Equipment

Stretchers are the most frequently used devices in prehospital care and include the wheeled stretcher, the portable stretcher, the scoop stretcher, the basket stretcher, and the flexible stretcher. Other types of equipment used for moving prehospital patients include the stair chair and the long and short spine boards.

Wheeled Stretcher

The wheeled stretcher is the preferred device for transporting patients along smooth terrain (**Figure 5-7**). It permits the movement of the patient along level ground without unduly tiring the EMTs. Because the stretcher becomes top-heavy in the upright position, care should be taken in rougher terrain to avoid tipping it. Because of its weight and bulkiness, the wheeled cot stretcher is the least effective device for moving a patient over rough terrain or down stairs. In these circumstances the folding stretcher, scoop stretcher, or basket stretcher is preferred.

There are two types of wheeled cot stretchers: the multilevel stretcher and the two-level stretcher.

The multilevel cot permits height adjustment at a few levels to allow for certain activities such as cardiopulmonary resuscitation (CPR), ventilation techniques, and movement of the stretcher along level ground. Both multilevel and two-level stretchers permit easy transfer of the patient from a bed to the stretcher and back to another bed again. Some two-level stretchers permit loading and removal of the stretcher without lifting. This device has large wheels that coincide with the height of the ambulance floor. Once these wheels are planted on the floor, a lever can release the base of the stretcher, allowing it to roll freely into the ambulance.

Most wheeled cot stretchers have other features. Most permit adjustment of the head of the stretcher at several angles, ranging from completely supine to sitting upright at 90 degrees. Some stretchers allow for the patient to be in full Trendelenburg position or to have the legs or knees elevated. Adjunctive equipment, such as intravenous (IV) poles, oxygen-carrying devices, and devices that carry monitor defibrillators, may be attached to the wheeled stretcher. Some stretchers have motors that raise and lower the device. The motor helps providers avoid injury by decreasing the need to manually raise and lower the stretcher, but it also adds weight.

Moving the Stretcher

Standard procedures in the movement of stretchers help to ensure a smooth and safe transfer of the patient. The foot end of the stretcher should always go first, except when you are loading the patient into the ambulance. This procedure is particularly important when going down stairs because the stretcher is heavier at the head end; the EMT who is at the bottom already carries a greater load because that end of the stretcher must be elevated to prevent the patient from sliding off the device.

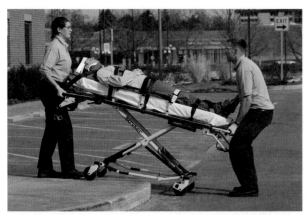

Figure 5-8 EMTs should be positioned at each end of the stretcher, facing each other and moving the stretcher toward the patient's feet.

The stretcher should be rolled along the ground with one EMT at each end of the stretcher (**Figure 5-8**). This facilitates negotiation of narrow or crowded passages and allows smooth, natural movement. While rolling the stretcher along level ground, each EMT should maintain a firm grip because a top-heavy stretcher may tilt and fall if it hits a crack, crevice, or bump. On moderately rough terrain, you may have to carry the stretcher end to end, facing the other EMT. This approach, known as the *end carry,* provides less protection from the stretcher tipping on its side but is preferable in narrow spaces. If the terrain is extremely rough, the *side carry,* in which one EMT is positioned on each of the four sides of the stretcher, is the most stable method of carrying the stretcher. The disadvantage of this technique is that more personnel are needed.

A wide variety of wheeled stretchers are available. You should be familiar with the device you are using and follow the manufacturer's recommendations. When loading a patient or a wheeled stretcher in and out of the ambulance, you must have sufficient lifting power. For extremely obese patients, as many as four to six rescuers may be needed. The techniques of loading and unloading a stretcher in and out of the ambulance are illustrated in **Skills 5-7** and **5-8**.

REAL*World*

The incidence of obesity in America has reached epidemic proportions. To adjust for the increase in patient size, transport equipment has been modified and reinforced. Newer stretchers can routinely support weights of 500 to 800 pounds (225-360 kg) and can be purchased with side extension panels to accommodate larger patients. Some ambulances are fitted with ramps and winches to help load heavy patients. Ambulances modified with equipment to make the transport of obese patients easier and safer are known as *bariatric ambulances.*

Portable Stretchers

Portable stretchers are lightweight devices that can be folded and stored (**Figure 5-9**). Unlike the bulky wheeled cot stretcher, portable stretchers permit easy transfer of a patient down stairs and over rough terrain. As with wheeled cot stretchers, portable

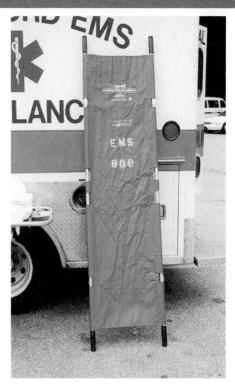

Figure 5-9 Portable stretcher.

stretchers should be carried end to end. Unlike the wheeled cot, they can also be loaded from that position.

Stair Chair

The **stair chair** is a device designed to move patients who are able to assume the sitting position to the ambulance. It is a primary lifting and carrying device in urban EMS systems, where narrow stairways make the use of a cot stretcher difficult and sometimes dangerous. The stair chair should never be used for patients with a suspected spinal injury or for patients who are or may become unconscious. The patient should be transferred to a wheeled cot stretcher when you reach the ambulance because the stair chair is not intended for transport purposes within the ambulance environment.

The extremity lift method is preferred for loading a patient into the stair chair. Before being moved, the patient should be instructed not to grasp for the handrails because this action may cause the EMT to lose balance. To avoid falls, it may be appropriate to secure the patient's hands if the patient is disoriented or is a child.

The chair can be tilted back and rolled along smooth, level terrain. When using a stair chair, the head of the patient must always be at the top when traveling down stairs because the weight will be too great if you go head-first; the chair may also have a tendency to fold. You should move the patient one step at a time. Rushing the patient down the stairs using one foot after the other significantly increases the chance of injury. When descending stairs, the EMT at the patient's head should support the chair firmly, with the hands at the outermost portion of the bar, and should always be at the top position of the carry. The EMT at the foot may have to elevate the lower portion of the chair to prevent the wheel from hitting the stairs. Whenever possible, a "spotter," such as a police officer, should be positioned below the EMT at the foot for extra support in the event that one of the EMTs trips (**Skill 5-9**).

Scoop or Orthopedic Stretcher

The **scoop stretcher** is a specialized device that facilitates easy lifting of supine patients. The aluminum frame consists of a rectangular tube with shovel-type flaps for sliding under the patient. The stretcher splits lengthwise into two equal halves so that the patient can be "scooped" off the ground with minimal patient movement. Before sliding the halves of the stretcher under the patient, you should adjust the scoop stretcher to a length just longer than the patient. Each half should then be positioned under the patient while the edges of the stretcher are carefully guided one side at a time. The head end of the stretcher is connected first, and then the hips are lifted slightly to allow connection of the bottom half and avoid pinching the patient. For spinal injury patients, cervical immobilization should be maintained throughout this procedure. The patient then should be placed on a long spine board or a wheeled cot stretcher and secured by straps before moving (**Skill 5-10**).

Long Spine Board

There are several varieties of **long spine boards** (LSBs) (**Figure 5-10**), but all provide essentially the same function: rigid support for the spinal column to prevent further injury. The long spine board is the *primary* device (used alone without a short spine board) for removing patients who are lying supine or laterally recumbent. It is also used with the rapid extrication of motor vehicle crash victims. Additionally, the long spine board is used as a *secondary* support device for patients removed with a short spine board.

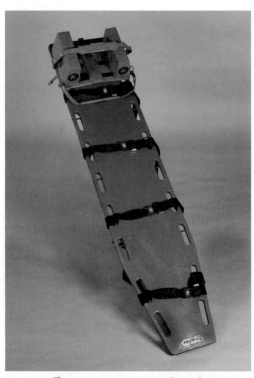

Figure 5-10   Long spine board.

REALWorld

Because of anatomic differences, pediatric and geriatric patients need to be handled differently when being placed on a long spine board. In pediatric patients, the head is proportionally larger than the body. This requires extra padding under the child's shoulders to maintain the neck in an inline position. Pediatric boards are designed to allow for this variant. Geriatric patients can develop spinal changes such as kyphosis (increased curvature of spine) and require extra padding around the neck and lower back to support the spine properly.

EXTENDEDTransport

When transporting a patient who is immobilized on a long spine board for long distances, the patient can become uncomfortable and develop back pain. Consider placing a pad or blanket between the patient and the board. Place adequate padding in the voids, and consider placing pillows under the patient's knees, allowing for a slight bend to help flatten the back and make the patient more comfortable.

Short Spine Board and Vest-Type Device

The **short spine board** is used to immobilize and extricate victims of motor vehicle crashes who are found in the sitting position. The short spine board is designed to extend from the base of the buttocks to just above the head. It is attached to the patient by straps or cravat bandages while maintaining cervical immobilization.

The *vest-type device* is an evolution of the short spine board. Its semirigid form permits easy and fast application and provides effective immobilization of the spine (**Figure 5-11**).

Basket Stretcher

The **basket stretcher** (Stokes basket or litter) is an extrication device ideal for removing patients on rough terrain or during high-angle rescues, during which a patient must either be lowered from a height or lifted, as from a ditch or well. The basket stretcher is constructed of hard plastic or wire mesh

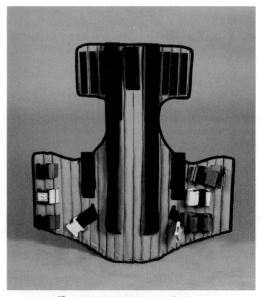

Figure 5-11   Vest-type device.

with a metal frame. Before the patient is placed in a basket stretcher, it must be well padded to prevent further injury to the patient.

Flexible Stretcher

The **flexible stretcher,** or **rescue stretcher** (Reeves stretcher), is useful for carrying a patient through narrow corridors or over difficult terrain (**Figure 5-12**).

Case in Point

Two EMTs responded to a 57-year-old woman with severe difficulty breathing. They administered high-concentration oxygen and placed the patient in the sitting position on a cot stretcher. During transport the patient became lethargic and sleepy and exhibited slow, shallow breathing. One EMT quickly placed a cardiac board behind the patient, lowered the head of the stretcher, and began assisted positive-pressure ventilation.

Patient Positioning

Special terms are used to describe the body position and movement. The body standing upright is called *erect,* and lying on the back is *supine* (**Figure 5-13, A**). If the body is lying facedown, it is *prone.* A body lying on its side is in the **lateral recumbent position,** or **recovery position** (**Figure 5-13, B**). The lateral recumbent position is further described by which part of the body is positioned on the ground or stretcher. For example, a patient lying on the left side would be said to be in the *left lateral recumbent position.*

Patients are transported in various ways, including the **Trendelenburg position** (body supine with feet elevated 8-12 inches and head down), the **Fowler's position** (sitting position; **Figure 5-13, C**), or the **shock position** (**Figure 5-13, D**).

The patient's condition is the main consideration when positioning the patient on the scene and during movement. The

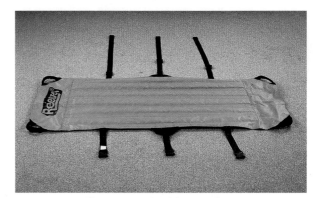

Figure 5-12 Flexible stretcher.

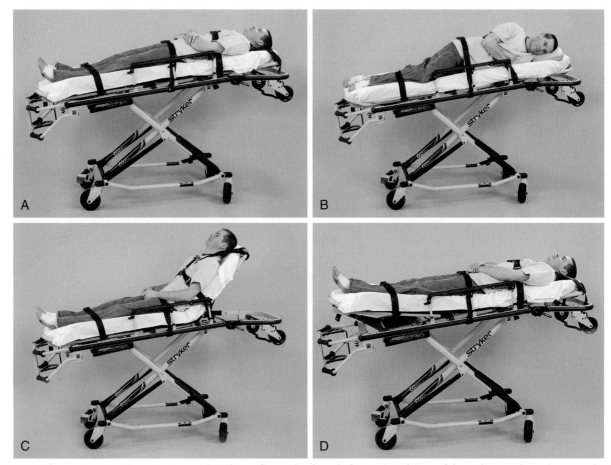

Figure 5-13 Body positioning. **A,** Supine position: lying flat on back with face upward. **B,** Left lateral recumbent (recovery) position. **C,** Fowler's (sitting) position. **D,** Shock position: lying supine with legs elevated 10 to 12 inches.

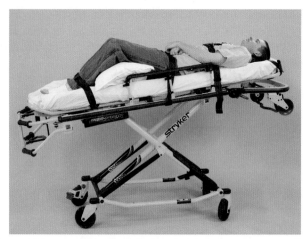

Figure 5-14 Patients with abdominal pain may gain some relief by flexing the knees because it relaxes the abdominal muscles.

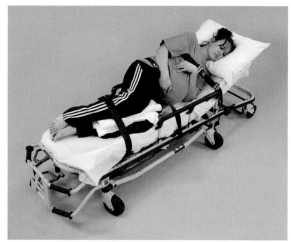

Figure 5-15 Position of choice for transporting a pregnant patient.

moving device should be comfortable and support the appropriate position. Factors such as airway maintenance, patient comfort, suspected spinal injury, and shock dictate the device chosen and the position of the patient.

Patients with Dyspnea or Chest Pain

Patients with dyspnea (difficulty breathing) or chest pain are generally transported in a semireclining or fully upright position on a wheeled cot stretcher. You should be guided by the patient, who is able to express a preferred position of comfort. Patients with shortness of breath usually prefer the full upright position because it allows maximum use of the diaphragm and chest muscles. However, patients with difficulty breathing who become sleepy or lethargic should be placed in the supine position to facilitate airway management and positive-pressure ventilation.

Unresponsive Patient without Suspected Spinal Injury

The primary concern for unconscious patients is airway management. If breathing is adequate, the patient should be placed in the recovery or left lateral recumbent position on a wheeled cot stretcher without twisting the body (see Figure 5-13, *B*). This position helps prevent aspiration if the patient vomits. Patients in need of positive-pressure ventilation or CPR must be placed in the supine position on a long spine board or on a cardiac resuscitation board.

Patients with Abdominal Pain

Patients with acute abdominal distress usually are most comfortable in the supine or lateral recumbent position with their knees bent. Some wheeled cot stretchers can be adjusted to support the knees in this position, or a pillow can be used to prop up the knees (**Figure 5-14**).

Patients in Shock

A patient in shock (hypoperfusion) should be placed in the supine position with the legs elevated 8 to 12 inches to facilitate increased venous blood flow to the heart (see Figure 5-13, *D*).

Patients with Suspected Spinal Injury

Patients who have multiple injuries and suspected spinal injuries should be transferred on a long spine board (LSB) to provide full body immobilization. As previously mentioned, the initial method of immobilization may vary. Patients found in the sitting position are usually removed on a short spine board or with a vest-type device and then transferred to an LSB. Remove patients who are found supine or who are in need of rapid extrication with an LSB. The LSB is then placed directly on the wheeled cot stretcher.

Pregnant Patients

If possible, women in the late stages of pregnancy (6-9 months) who are injured or in shock should not be placed flat on their backs. This position causes the bulk of the fetus to compress the vena cava, thereby seriously affecting blood return through the veins. Most pregnant women are uncomfortable in this position even if they are uninjured. The left lateral recumbent position is the position of choice, but a semireclining position is appropriate if the patient is uncomfortable in that position. Pregnant patients who have suspected spinal injury can be placed on a long spine board with the board then tilted to the left to relieve pressure on the vena cava (**Figure 5-15**).

Nausea and Vomiting

Patients with nausea and vomiting should be transported in a position of comfort with the EMT positioned to manage the airway effectively.

Scenario Follow-up

This case illustrates three distinct circumstances requiring different lifting strategies for safe removal of patients. The first patient was in imminent danger from fire and needed to be relocated to a safe location, with potential spinal injuries still a consideration. A drag technique was used to preserve reasonable allignment of the spine while quickly moving the patient.

The second patient was not in danger from the environment but showed signs of airway compromise. Care and transport could not be delayed by applying a short spine board. The rapid extrication technique was used to ensure effective spinal immobilization while not delaying transport.

The final patient was removed from a ditch. A cot strecher could not be used because it would be difficult to negotiate over rough terrain. The EMS providers also made sure they had sufficient personnel to execute the lift safely. They were also careful to use their legs and not their backs during the lifting process.

Summary

Lifting and moving will be an essential part of your daily activities as an EMT. Back injuries are "the plague" of prehospital care. Injuries to the spine from poor lifting technique can cause severe lifelong pain, lost working days, and even the end of an EMS career. However, simple preventive measures can be taken that significantly reduce the chance of back injury and make you a more effective prehospital provider. You should learn proper techniques to prevent injuries to you, your partners, and the patient. Simple techniques, including staying close to the lifting device, maintaining a straight posture, and lifting with your strong leg muscles rather than your back muscles, can greatly reduce the chances of injury.

The prevention of back injuries starts with basic fitness. Weak back and abdominal muscles are a perfect setup for back injury. You should try to stay in shape and should pay particular attention to good posture and proper lifting techniques during patient movement.

Lifts with team members should be coordinated to ensure a smooth and unhurried lift, with all team members lifting in unison. Frantic and hurried approaches to lifting are likely to result in injury to you and possibly the patient. Lifting techniques should be practiced in the classroom, or your clinical preceptor can be requested to review basic techniques before your first run.

Again, prevention is the key to a healthy back and to being a useful prehospital provider. Take a moment to review the learning checklist to test and reinforce essential knowledge of lifting and moving and review those areas that are unclear.

Skills

| Skill | 5-1 | *Power Lift* |

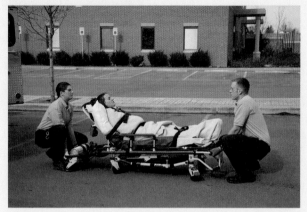 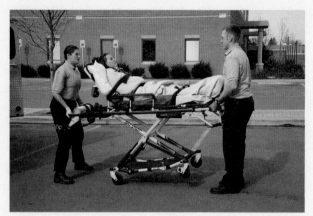

1. Keep your back locked, place your feet a comfortable distance apart, tighten your abdominal muscles. Bring the center of your body over the object so that the lift will be as vertical as possible.

2. Allow the upper body to rise before the hips as you rise. Straighten your legs as you lift, keeping your back in the locked-in position.

| Skill | 5-2 | *Rapid Extrication* |

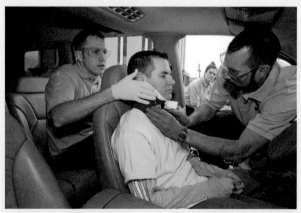 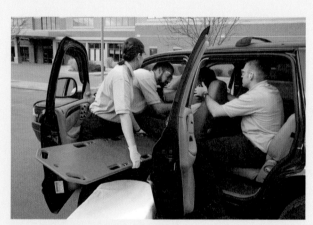

1. The first EMT immobilizes the patient's head from the back. The second EMT sizes and places a neck collar.

2. A third EMT prepares the stretcher and places the backboard under the patient's leg.

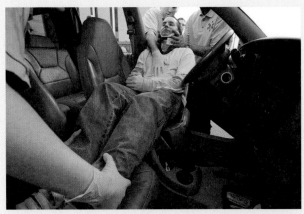

3. In unison, the second EMT takes control of the patient's neck as the first EMT moves to rotate the patient onto the backboard. A fourth EMT, positioned next to the patient in the vehicle, moves the patient's legs across the seat.

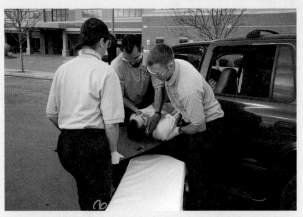

4. The patient is placed flat on the backboard. Maintaining control of the patient's head and neck, the EMTs slide the patient onto the backboard.

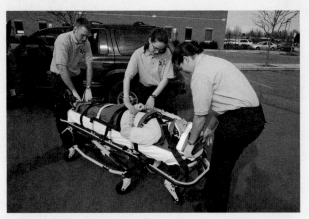

5. After being moved out of the vehicle and onto the stretcher, the patient is strapped to the backboard and secured to the stretcher.

Skill | 5-3   *Direct Ground Lift*

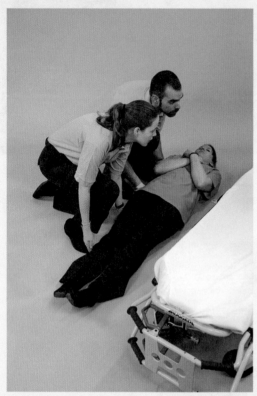

1. Two (or three) EMTs line up on the side of the patient and drop to one knee. To maintain balance, both EMTs should be kneeling on the same knee.

2. Fold the victim's arms across the chest. The EMT at the patient's head places one arm under the patient's neck and shoulder and cradles the head while placing the other arm under the patient's lower back. The second EMT places one arm under the buttock region and the other arm just below the patient's knees.

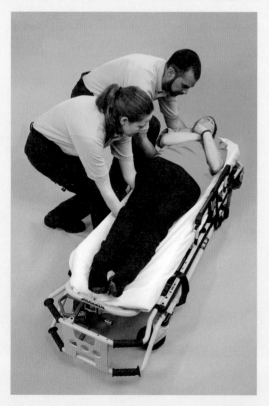

3. On command, both EMTs smoothly lift the patient onto their elevated thighs. The EMTs then carefully load the patient onto the stretcher in unison.

Skill | 5-4   *Extremity Lift*

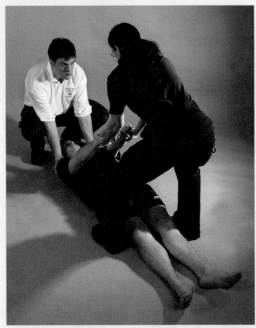

1. One EMT is positioned at the patient's head and a second EMT at the patient's knees. The EMT at the patient's head lifts the shoulders while the second EMT straddles the patient's knees and grasps the patient's wrists. In unison, the two EMTs pull the patient to a sitting position.

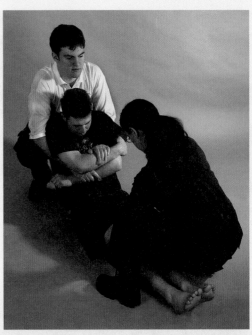

2. The first EMT then grasps the patient under the armpits and supports the patient's wrists. The second EMT supports the patient with one hand behind each knee.

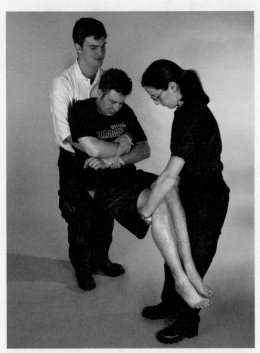

3. Both EMTs rise smoothly to an upright position.

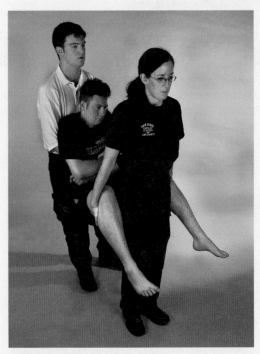

4. The EMT holding the legs can then turn 180 degrees to facilitate forward movement of the patient to the stretcher.

| *Skill* | 5-5 | | *Direct Carry* |

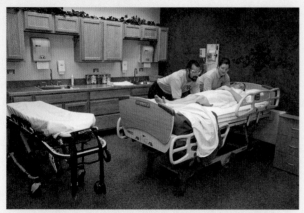

1. Place the stretcher at a 90-degree angle to the patient's bed. Prepare the stretcher by releasing the belts. The two EMTs then prepare the patient for movement and take their place alongside the patient.

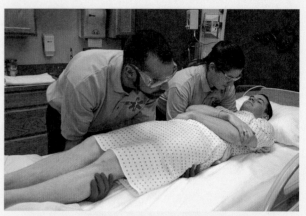

2. The EMTs slide their hands under the patient's back, providing support to the shoulders and head, pelvis, and legs.

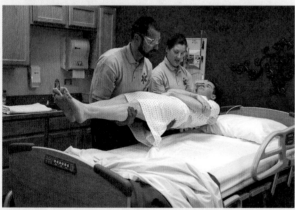

3. At the same time, both EMTs pull the patient toward them and lift the patient from the bed. The patient is carried to the stretcher.

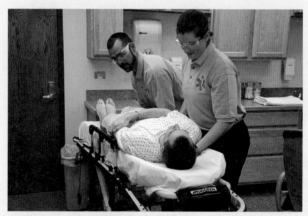

4. The patient is gently placed onto the stretcher, covered, and secured appropriately.

Skill | 5-6   **Draw Sheet Method**

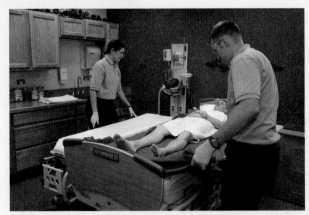

1. The EMTs move to each side of the patient. The stretcher is prepared by releasing the belts and lowering it to the height of the patient's bed. The patient's bedding is untucked and then gathered toward the patient.

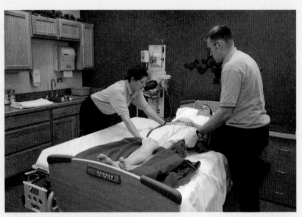

2. Each EMT grabs the sheet or blanket under the patient, with one hand at the shoulders and one hand below the hips.

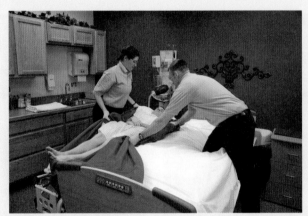

3. At the same time, the EMTs slide the patient onto the stretcher. The patient is then covered and secured as appropriate.

Skill | 5-7   *Loading the Ambulance*

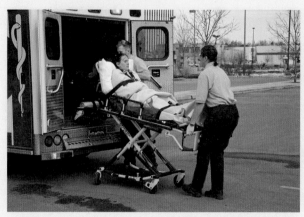

1. The two EMTs wheel the stretcher in the raised position to the back of the ambulance. The EMT at the head of the stretcher guides the front wheels into the back of the ambulance.

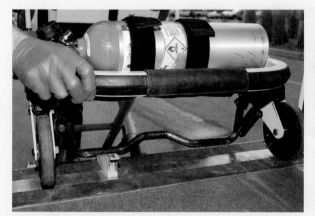 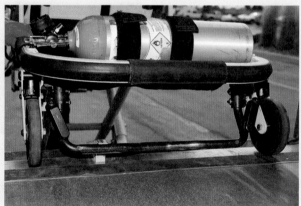

2. The EMT at the head of the stretcher makes sure the locking bar slides over the locking bracket mounted on the floor of the ambulance.

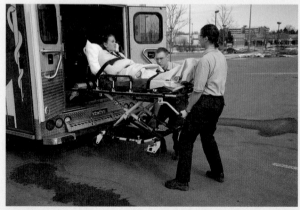 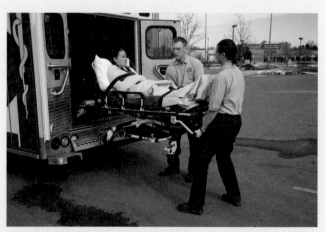

3. The EMT at the foot of the stretcher lifts the stretcher and squeezes the release mechanism for the wheels, allowing them to be raised.

4. The second EMT raises the wheels.

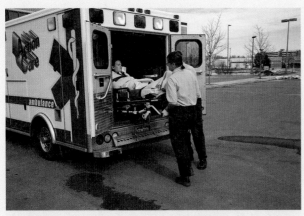

5. The EMT at the foot of the stretcher walks forward, pushing the stretcher into the ambulance.

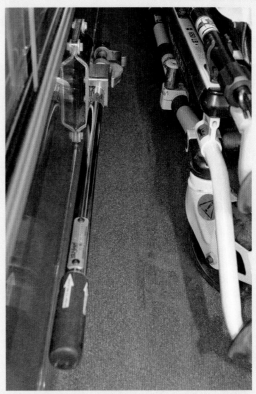

6. After it is in the ambulance, the stretcher should be slid into the locking mechanism, ensuring the mechanism locks in place.

Skill | 5-8   *Unloading the Ambulance*

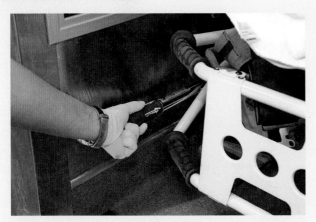

1. Push the red release handle on the locking mechanism to release the stretcher. Slide the stretcher out of the locks.

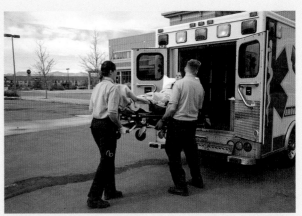

2. The EMT at the foot of the stretcher walks backward, lifting the stretcher to keep it in a level position.

Continued

Skill | 5-8   *Unloading the Ambulance—cont'd*

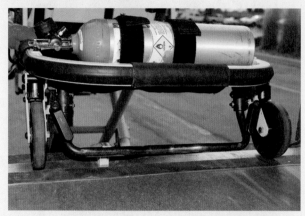

3. The second EMT makes sure the locking bar catches on the locking bracket to keep the stretcher from falling to the ground.

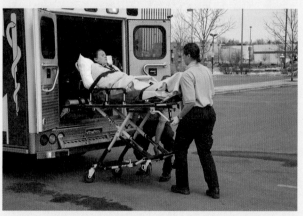

4. The EMT at the foot of the stretcher releases the wheels, and the second EMT slowly lowers the wheels to the ground. Both EMTs must verify the wheels have been locked into place.

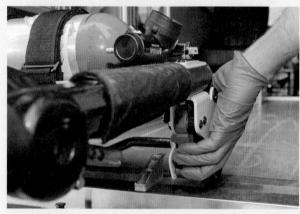

5. The second EMT pushes the release lever for the locking bar, allowing the stretcher to roll freely.

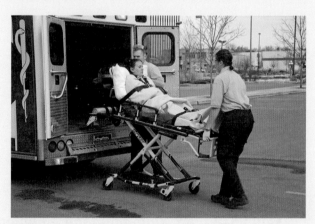

6. The second EMT takes control of the head of the stretcher while the EMT at the foot maintains control of that end.

Skill | 5-9 *Using a Stair Chair*

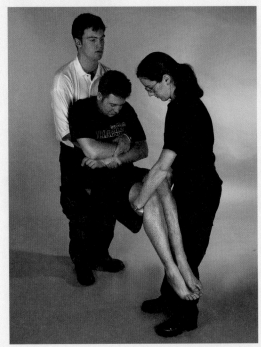

1. Move the patient into the chair by using the extremity lift.

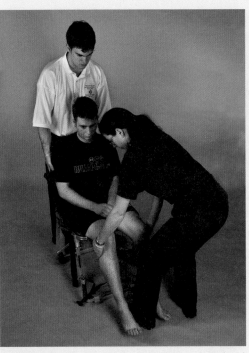

2. Secure the patient's hands (if necessary) and tilt the device.

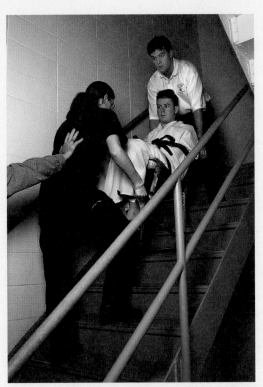

3. Tilt the chair back to move to ground level. Use a spotter to move down the stairs.

Skill | 5-10   *Using a Scoop Stretcher*

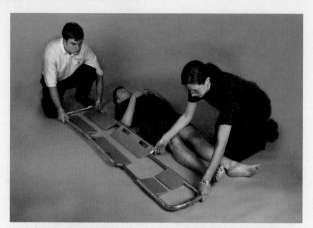

1. Measure and adjust the length of the device next to the patient.

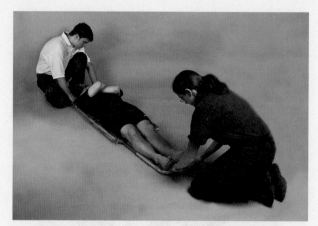

2. Carefully slide the stretcher under both sides of the patient. Lock the head and the feet sections of the scoop stretcher, and strap the patient in place. Place the patient on the secondary device, and secure in place.

The Bottom Line

Learning Checklist

✓ Safe lifting involves the use of the legs, not the back, and lifting as close to the device as possible.

✓ Guidelines for lifting include considering the weight to be lifted and need for additional help, knowing your own limitations, positioning your feet properly, lifting without twisting, and communicating frequently and clearly with other team members.

✓ When lifting cots and stretchers, use an even number of people—at least two—to ensure balance.

✓ The power lift, or power squat, is ideal for individuals with weak knees or thighs and should be performed in the locked-in back position using abdominal muscles for support.

✓ The power grip is used with hands at least 10 inches apart to hold the device securely and with the fingers bent at the same angle.

✓ Ideally, when carrying on level ground, use devices that can be rolled; when on stairs, use stair chairs.

✓ When carrying, consider the weight to be lifted and need for additional help; know your own and your crew's limitations and work in a coordinated manner; keep your weight as close to the device as possible and your back in the locked-in position (do not hyperextend back).

✓ When reaching, keep your back in the locked-in position (avoid twisting), and never reach more than 15 to 20 inches from the body.

✓ When pushing or pulling, push rather than pull, keep the line of pull through the center of the body by bending the knees, and push from the area from the waist to the shoulder. If the weight is below the waist, use a kneeling position.

✓ Move patients immediately (before assessment) using emergency moves only when they are in danger (explosions, fire, hazardous materials), when they block access to a severely ill or injured patient, or when lifesaving care requires placing them in the supine position.

✓ Move patients quickly using the rapid extrication procedure (urgent move) when they have an immediate life-threatening condition such as airway obstruction, shock, or altered mental state.

✓ When emergency moves are used, move the patient along the long axis of the body using the clothes drag, blanket drag, or other appropriate procedure.

✓ Urgent moves out of vehicles can be done with the rapid extrication procedure.

✓ Nonurgent movement of a patient to a stretcher can be done with the direct ground lift, extremity lift, direct carry, or draw sheet lift.

✓ Stretchers and other devices for transporting patients include cot stretchers, folding stretchers, spine boards (long and short), stair chairs, scoop stretchers, and flexible stretchers.

✓ Transport patients in a position appropriate to their condition:

   ✓ Recovery position for an unresponsive patient without spinal injury.

   ✓ Position of comfort for patients with chest pain or dyspnea.

   ✓ Immobilized position for patients with suspected spinal injuries.

   ✓ Legs elevated 8 to 12 inches for patients in shock.

   ✓ On the left side or tilted on a long spine board for pregnant patients.

   ✓ Position of comfort for patients who are experiencing nausea or vomiting while being closely monitored by EMT.

Key Terms

Basket stretcher Type of stretcher useful for removing patients on rough terrain or during high-angle rescues, in which a patient must be lowered from a height or lifted, as from a ditch or well.

Blanket drag Rescue evacuation technique in which a blanket is used to drag the patient from the hazardous situation.

Body mechanics The scientific use of specific methods of efficiently lifting large weights so as not to injure oneself.

Clothes drag Rescue evacuation technique that uses the patient's clothing to drag the patient along the long axis of the body from a hazardous situation.

Emergency move Various lifting and moving techniques used to remove someone rapidly from a hazardous situation.

Extremity lift Rescue evacuation technique in which one person supports the patient's legs and the other person supports the torso to remove the patient from a hazardous situation.

Flexible stretcher (rescue stretcher) Type of stretcher that can be used to carry a patient through narrow corridors or over difficult terrain.

Foot drag Rescue evacuation technique that uses the patient's feet to drag the patient along the long axis of the body from a hazardous situation.

Fowler's position Posture assumed by the patient when the head of the bed is elevated; sitting position.

Lateral recumbent position Position of the body when the person is lying on his or her side.

Locked-in position Technique in which the back is maintained in straight alignment during a lift so as not to cause strain or injury.

Log roll Rotation technique used to slide an immobilization device under a patient, with minimal flexion, extension, or rotation of the spinal column.

Long spine board Long, flat, rigid device, usually made of plastic, used to maintain spinal immobilization.

One-handed carrying technique Carrying technique used when multiple personnel are available for the carry and persons are placed strategically around the device.

Portable stretcher Type of stretcher that can be easily carried to and from the scene of an emergency.

Power grip Technique for holding a stretcher with your palms and fingers in complete contact with the device to ensure a safe transport.

Power lift (squat lift) Effective lifting method that maximizes lifting power while avoiding injury.

Rapid extrication procedure Specialized rescue removal technique used to extricate a patient quickly with minimal flexion, extension, or rotation of the spinal column.

Recovery position Position of the person lying on his or her side, to help maintain a clear airway.

Scoop stretcher Specialized device consisting of an aluminum frame and a rectangular tube with shovel-type lateral flaps for sliding under the patient.

Shock position Placement of a patient supine with the legs elevated 8 to 12 inches to facilitate venous return.

Short spine board Device used to immobilize and extricate patients who are found in a sitting position; evolved into *vest-type device*.

Stair chair Folding chair used to carry patients who can assume the sitting position.

Trendelenburg position Position in which patient is supine on a surface inclined 45 degrees, with patient's head at the lower end and legs at the upper end.

Wheeled cot stretcher Primary transport stretcher used by prehospital providers. The stretcher has a wheeled base and comes in a variety of types.

Review Questions

1. Which of the following predetermined methods of efficiently lifting large weights should be used to avoid injury?
   a. Body mechanics
   b. Lift science
   c. Lifting physics
   d. Physiology of lifts

2. While observing two EMTs lifting a stretcher, the supervisor noted they were using their backs to generate power. After the call, he advised the EMTs to use a different muscle group as the primary means for generating power. Which muscle group did he suggest?
   a. Lower back
   b. Upper back
   c. Legs
   d. Pelvis

3. When lifting a stretcher, your back should be maintained in which of the following positions?
   a. Curved outward
   b. Locked in
   c. Very loose
   d. Slightly bent

4. What should be the state of your abdominal muscles when lifting a stretcher?
   a. Tightened
   b. Relaxed
   c. Alternating between relaxed and tightened
   d. Pushed outward

5. When carrying a device, how should the weight be maintained in relationship to the body?
   a. About 10 inches from the body
   b. As close to the body as possible
   c. Above waist level
   d. Above shoulder level

6. How should the EMT be positioned when carrying with one hand?
   a. Leaning slightly toward the object
   b. Leaning slightly away from the object
   c. Bending at the waist.
   d. Avoiding leaning to either side

7. You respond to a patient with difficulty breathing who lives in a fourth-floor walk-up. What transport device is most appropriate for removing the patient to the ambulance?
   a. Wheeled cot stretcher
   b. Scoop stretcher
   c. Stair chair
   d. Portable stretcher

8. Which of the following should be avoided when reaching overhead?
   a. Using the hyperextended position
   b. Locking the back
   c. Bending at the knees
   d. Leaning from the hips

9. You are log rolling a patient onto a spine board with three other EMTs. The EMT at which patient location should deliver the commands to ensure coordination of the move?
   a. Head
   b. Shoulder
   c. Hip
   d. Lower legs

10. When pushing a device, you should push from the area between the waist and which location?
   a. Knees
   b. Shoulders
   c. Midthigh region
   d. Ankles

11. You respond to a call and find the patient in a kitchen with an active fire that has engulfed the walls, ceiling, and floor. You suspect the patient may have spinal injuries. Your partner has not yet arrived with the stretcher. What lift would be most apprpriate for removal of the victim?
    a. Clothes drag
    b. Arm carry
    c. Chair carry
    d. Firefighter's carry

12. You respond to a climber who has fallen in an area with rough terrain. You park the ambulance approximately 200 yards (180 m) from the patient. Which of the following devices is best suited for moving the patient back to the ambulance?
    a. Wheeled cot stretcher
    b. Stair chair
    c. Basket stretcher
    d. Long spine board

For Further Review

In the Student Workbook

- Multiple-choice questions
- Matching questions
- Fill-in-the-blank questions
- Case scenario questions
- Skill check questions

On Evolve

- Weblinks
- Lecture notes
- Exercises

Learning Objectives

Cognitive Objectives

- Define body mechanics.
- Discuss the guidelines and safety precautions to follow when lifting a patient.
- Describe the safe lifting of cots and stretchers.
- Describe the guidelines and safety precautions for carrying patients and equipment.
- Discuss one-handed carrying techniques.
- Describe correct and safe carrying procedures on stairs.
- State the guidelines for reaching and their application.
- Describe correct reaching for log rolls.
- State the guidelines for pushing and pulling.
- Discuss the general considerations of moving patients.
- Describe three situations that may require the use of an emergency move.
- Identify the following patient-carrying devices:
  - Wheeled ambulance stretcher
  - Portable ambulance stretcher
  - Stair chair
  - Scoop stretcher
  - Long spine board
  - Short spine board (vest-type device)
  - Basket stretcher
  - Flexible stretcher

Affective Objective

- Explain the rationale for properly lifting and moving patients.

Psychomotor Objectives

- Working with a partner, demonstrate techniques for the transfer of a patient from an ambulance stretcher to a hospital stretcher.
- Working with a partner, (1) prepare each of the following devices for use, (2) transfer a patient to the device, (3) properly position the patient on the device, (4) move the device to the ambulance, and (5) load the patient into the ambulance:
  - Wheeled ambulance stretcher
  - Portable ambulance stretcher
  - Stair chair
  - Scoop stretcher
  - Long spine board
  - Short spine board (vest-type device)
  - Basket stretcher
  - Flexible stretcher

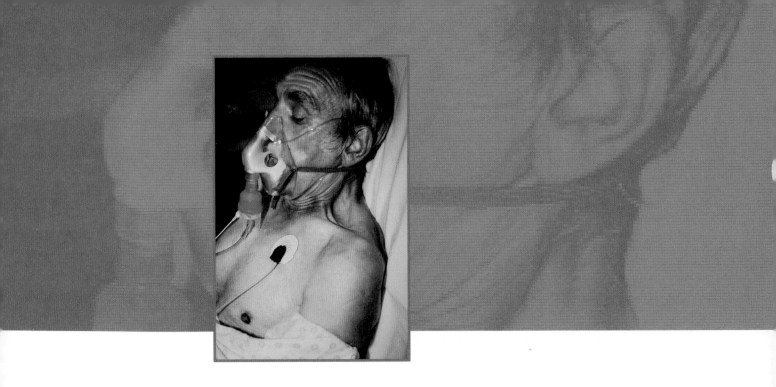

6 Airway

CHAPTER OUTLINE

Scenario

You are called to the home of an elderly man with a complaint of shortness of breath. You enter to find the patient sitting upright in a chair with his arms folded over the dining room table. He speaks a few words but cannot speak a full sentence. He has clammy skin and bluish discoloration of the lips. His breathing is rapid, and gurgling sounds are audible. There is obvious accessory neck muscle use. Frothy sputum is noted at the lips. The patient has a blood pressure of 120/78 mm Hg, pulse rate of 120 beats/min, respiratory rate of 32 breaths/min, and a pulse oximetry reading of 85%. He has a history of congestive heart failure and has had two previous episodes of severe shortness of breath requiring emergency care. You provide supplemental oxygen with a nonrebreather mask and remove some of the oral secretions with suction.

Management of airway, ventilation, and oxygenation represents the first and most critical step in the care of any ill or injured patient. Humans are oxygen-dependent organisms. You can exist for 30 days without food, 3 days without water, but only minutes without air. As an emergency medical technician (EMT), you will assess the patient's airway, breathing, and circulation (ABCs) on every call. You should be an expert in managing an airway, providing positive-pressure ventilation, and administering supplemental oxygen.

Understanding the anatomy and physiology of the respiratory system will aid your understanding of both assessment and treatment of respiratory emergencies. You will assess the airway and breathing of every patient and look for signs of adequate versus inadequate breathing. You must recognize when the airway is clear and breathing is adequate. Likewise, you must be able to identify when the airway is not clear and breathing is inadequate. You will be able to clear and maintain an airway by using the following methods:

- *Manual techniques* include the head-tilt/chin-lift, jaw thrust, and obstructed-airway maneuvers.
- *Suctioning*
- *Mechanical techniques* include adjuncts such as the oropharyngeal or nasopharyngeal airway.

When a patient has inadequate breathing (inadequate ventilation), you must assist with positive-pressure ventilation (artificial ventilation) by using a mouth-to-mask device, bag-mask device, or flow-restricted, oxygen-powered ventilator. You will learn how to give supplemental oxygen by nasal cannula, nonrebreathing masks, or positive-pressure ventilation devices. You will also learn about how to care for special patient populations, including infants and children and patients with stomas or facial injuries.

Respiratory emergencies call for rapid evaluation and treatment. A patient with slow and inadequate breaths who is unresponsive and cyanotic is on the brink of cardiopulmonary arrest. By maintaining an airway, providing positive-pressure ventilations, and giving supplemental oxygen, you can save a patient's life.

With all patients, you should use your general impression and a quick assessment to judge whether problems with the airway and breathing are present. You will learn to quickly distinguish patients with adequate breathing from those who have respiratory distress and respiratory failure. For patients with respiratory distress, you will intervene with supplemental oxygen, possible medication, patient positioning, and rapid transport, with ongoing assessment for signs of respiratory failure. For patients with respiratory failure, you must ensure an open airway and provide positive-pressure ventilations with supplemental oxygen to support respiration and life.

Looking for signs of respiratory distress and distinguishing between respiratory distress and respiratory failure will become second nature to you as a professional EMT. As you continue with your training, you will encounter many conditions that can cause respiratory emergencies for which treatment centers on airway, breathing, and oxygenation.

> **LEARNING OBJECTIVE**
> - Identify and label the major structures of the respiratory system on a diagram.

Anatomy and Physiology

The respiratory system serves three main functions (**Figure 6-1**):

1. Delivery of oxygen from the atmosphere to the blood
2. Removal of carbon dioxide (the waste product of the body's metabolism) from the blood to the atmosphere
3. Creation of voice by the movement of air past the vocal cords

Airway and Alveoli

The airway is a series of tubes that extend from the mouth and nose down into the lungs. The air passage must be clear of obstructions for easy air passage and normal breathing.

Nose

The first portion of the airway is the nasal passage. The nasal passage consists of external and internal sections. The external section includes the nose, which is formed by cartilage and skin and opens at the nares, or nostrils. The upper portion contains the nasal bone, and the entire nose is divided into two compartments by the *nasal septum*, which is made of cartilage and bone. The following three functions of the airway begin at the nose:

1. Filtering
2. Moistening
3. Warming the air before it enters the lungs

Pharynx

The passage extending from the back of the *nasal cavity* down to the esophagus and larynx is called the pharynx (**Figure 6-2**). Each part of the pharynx is further classified according to its relation to other structures, as follows:

- Nasopharynx
- Oropharynx
- Laryngopharynx (or hypopharynx)

The pharynx may become obstructed when the tongue falls back against it in an unconscious patient or when swelling of pharyngeal tissue results from allergic reactions or trauma.

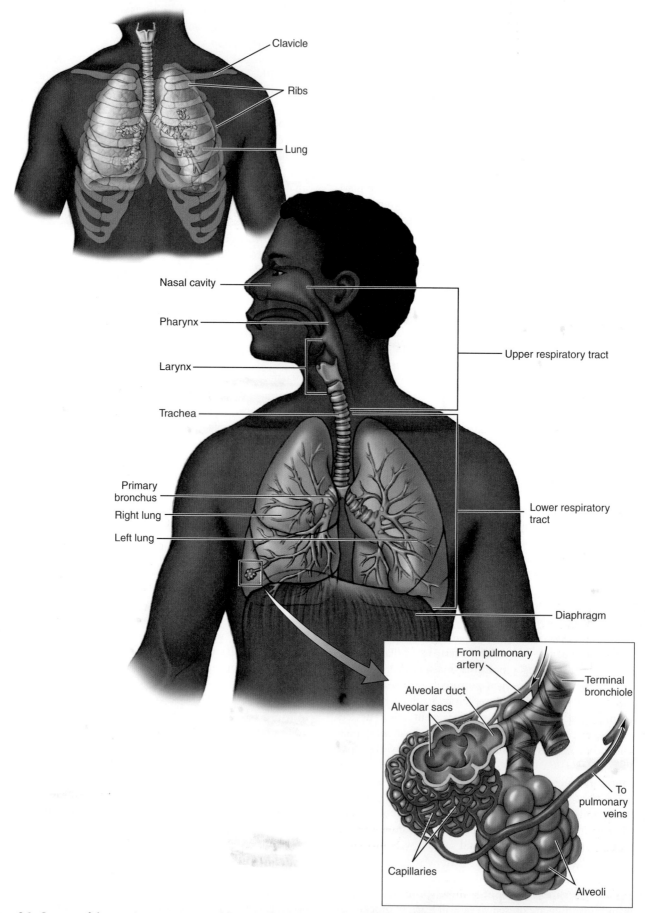

Figure 6-1 Organs of the respiratory system. *From Herlihy B, Maebius N: The human body in health and illness, ed 3, St Louis, 2007, Saunders.*

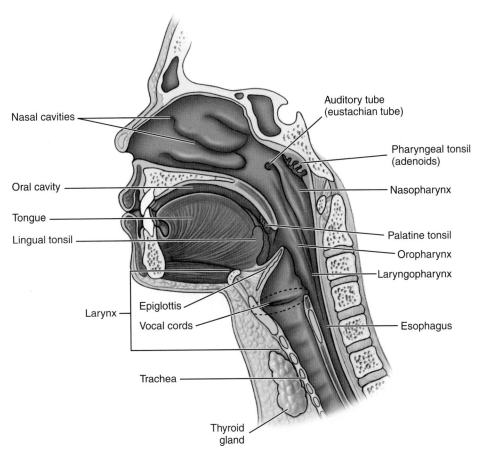

Figure 6-2 Features of the upper respiratory tract. *From Herlihy B, Maebius N: The human body in health and illness, ed 3, St Louis, 2007, Saunders.*

Epiglottis and Larynx

The epiglottis is a flap of cartilage that covers the larynx during swallowing to prevent food from entering the lungs. **Epiglottitis,** an infection of the epiglottis that causes swelling, can obstruct the upper airway. Patients with epiglottitis may require rapid transport for surgical intervention at the hospital to clear the airway.

The larynx is easily palpated in the anterior neck and is formed by cartilage, bone, and ligaments. It contains the *vocal cords,* which serve two primary functions:

1. Creating the voice.
2. Preventing foreign objects that have slipped past the epiglottis from entering the lungs. When foreign material enters the airway, the vocal cords, which are muscular bands within the larynx, go into spasm and close shut.

The two main cartilages forming the larynx are the thyroid cartilage and cricoid cartilage. The *thyroid cartilage* is superior and is commonly referred to as the "Adam's apple." The *cricoid cartilage* is inferior and forms a circle just above the trachea. Compressing the cricoid cartilage downward will collapse the esophagus, which lies behind it, reducing the chance for gastric distention during positive-pressure ventilation and gastric regurgitation or vomitus passing into the larynx.

The cricothyroid membrane separates the cricoid and thyroid cartilage. At times, physicians or paramedics may pass a needle through or surgically open the cricothyroid membrane to create an airway when an obstruction exists above the larynx. This procedure is called a *cricothyroidotomy.*

Trachea

Extending down from the larynx is the trachea. It is a hollow tube with several horseshoe-shaped rings of cartilage anteriorly that give support (**Figure 6-3**). The posterior surface of the trachea is a muscular wall. As with the cricothyroid membrane, the trachea can be used to gain access to the airway. The process of surgically making an entrance into the trachea to provide an airway is called a **tracheostomy.** You may encounter some patients who have a permanent tracheostomy. Take a moment to feel the tracheal rings just above your sternum in the anterior portion of your neck.

Bronchi and Bronchioles

The trachea subdivides into two tubes (left and right) made of cartilage called *bronchi* that direct air into the left and right lungs.

Much like a tree, the bronchi in turn subdivide to form smaller and smaller bronchi. As the bronchi subdivide, they

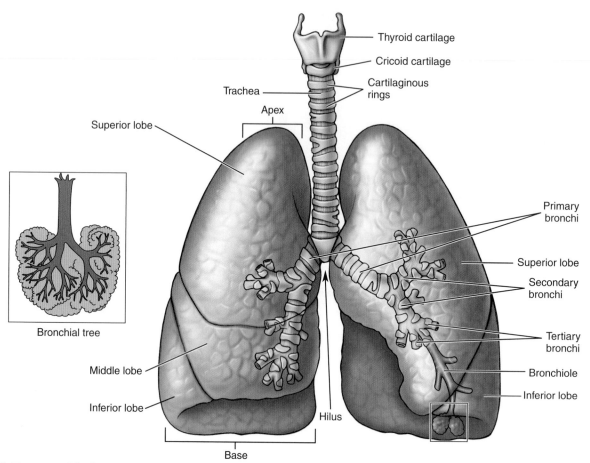

Figure 6-3 Features of the lower respiratory tract. *From Herlihy B, Maebius N: The human body in health and illness, ed 3, St Louis, 2007, Saunders.*

become smaller and smaller and have less cartilage and more muscle. Bronchioles are the smallest type of airway tube and have a muscular quality that allows the tubes to change in diameter as the muscles constrict or dilate. **Asthma** is a disease that results in bronchiole constriction and secretions. The narrowed airways increase the work of breathing. Drugs that dilate the smooth muscle of the bronchioles (e.g., albuterol) are used to treat asthma and are called *bronchodilator* medications.

Alveoli

The tracheobronchial tree continues to subdivide until it ends at the alveoli. Alveoli are the microscopic air sacs within the lung where gas exchange takes place. Alveoli arise in grapelike clusters at the end of the bronchioles. The wall of an alveolus is one cell thick. The walls must be thin to permit the exchange of gas with blood in the adjoining capillaries. The ability of the lung to exchange oxygen effectively with the blood depends on the total number of functional alveoli in contact with capillaries. The alveoli in a normal adult would cover an area greater than 50 square meters when spread out (about the size of a tennis court). When the alveoli are damaged or destroyed (as in **emphysema**) or filled with fluid (as in congestive heart failure or

pneumonia), patients have less ability to diffuse oxygen from the lungs into the capillaries.

Lungs and the Muscles of Breathing

Lungs

The bronchi, bronchioles, and alveoli together form two cone-shaped organs called lungs. The lungs are suspended within the thoracic cavity and are separated by the *mediastinum*, a space occupied by the heart, great vessels, trachea, main stem bronchi, esophagus, and nerves. The ribs, thoracic spine, scapula, and muscles surround the lungs and provide protection and function. The clavicle and neck are superior, and the diaphragm, the primary muscle of respiration, is inferior.

The outer surface of the lungs and the inner surface of the chest wall are lined with thin, membranous sheaths called *pleurae*. The pleura of the lung and the pleura of the chest wall are in direct contact with each other. A lubricating film between the two surfaces permits smooth movement of the lung within the chest during breathing. When inflammation (swelling) occurs between the pleurae or when scarring results from a disease or injury, the normal smooth process is interrupted, and pain occurs during breathing. Pain made worse by breathing is called **pleuritic chest pain.**

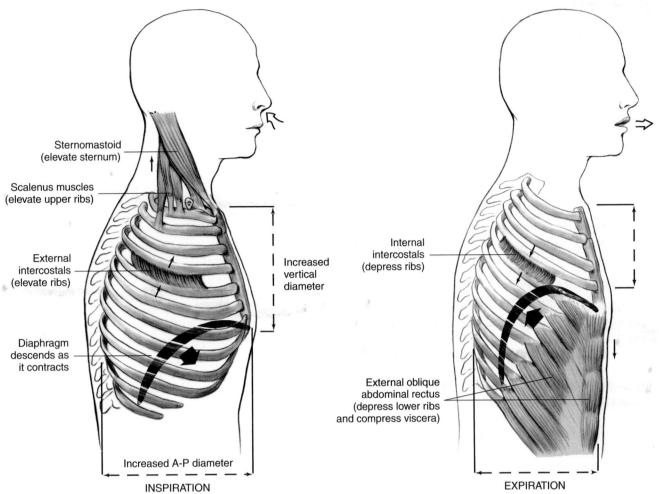

Figure 6-4 Muscles of inspiration and expiration. *From Jarvis C: Physical examination and health assessment, ed 4, Philadelphia, 2004, Saunders.*

Muscles of Respiration

The muscles of respiration change the diameter of the chest cavity as they contract and relax and cause air to move in and out of the lungs, which is known as *breathing*. In normal, quiet breathing, the principal muscle of respiration is the diaphragm, aided by the external intercostal (between the ribs) muscles (**Figure 6-4**). The diaphragm, a dome-shaped muscle at rest, contracts downward and "flattens" out while intercostals pull the ribs upward and outward, thereby increasing the size of the chest cavity.

As the chest cavity increases in size, the pressure within the chest cavity becomes lower than atmospheric pressure. Some describe this as a "negative pressure" (compared with atmospheric pressure). As a result of unequal pressures, air moves through the nose and mouth, down the trachea, and into the lungs. Air continues to move in until the pressure within the lungs equals the atmospheric pressure. This is the end of inspiration.

Normal exhalation begins when the muscles relax and the chest cavity returns to normal size. As the chest cavity becomes smaller, the pressure increases within the chest and air moves back through the bronchioles and bronchi and out the nose and mouth. Exhalation stops when the pressure of air inside the chest cavity is equal to atmospheric pressure.

The flow of air in and out of the lungs is called *ventilation* and is a direct result of the rhythmic contraction and relaxation of the muscles of respiration. Inhalation is an active process with work done by muscles. If the respiratory muscles stop contracting, breathing stops. When breathing stops, you will need to force air into the lungs by providing positive pressure with a mouth-to-mask device, a bag-mask device, or an oxygen-powered resuscitator. When the muscles of respiration fail, positive pressure is needed to expand the lungs and deliver oxygen to the alveoli and remove carbon dioxide.

Accessory Muscles of Respiration

During normal breathing, contraction and relaxation of the diaphragm and external intercostals are more than capable of providing the volume of air needed to deliver oxygen. When more air exchange is needed, the **accessory muscles of respiration** are also used to give added volume with each breath. The two types of accessory muscles are the muscles of inspiration and the muscles of expiration.

The accessory muscles of inspiration increase the size of the thoracic cavity by pulling the ribs farther upward. These muscles include certain neck muscles, which elevate the upper ribs, and the sternocleidomastoid muscles, which pull and elevate the sternum. Accessory muscle use is seen in normal people during exercise and also in patients with respiratory problems who are working harder to breathe at rest.

Accessory muscles of expiration include the internal intercostals, which pull the ribs down and inward, and the abdominal muscles, which pull the lower ribs downward and compress the abdominal contents, which pushes the diaphragm upward. Both actions decrease the size of the thorax and force out more air.

Active accessory muscle use provides a key warning signal of respiratory distress. During patient assessment, you should watch for bulging of the neck muscles, retraction of the spaces between the ribs, and active abdominal muscle use.

Physiology of Respiration

An adequate amount of air must be inhaled and exhaled each minute to meet the body's needs. This is called the **minute volume.** The minute volume is determined by the volume of air in each breath (tidal volume) multiplied by the respiratory rate.

The normal respiratory rate of an adult is 12 to 20 breaths per minute (breaths/min). The normal tidal volume (at rest) for an adult is approximately 500 milliliters (mL). Thus the normal minute volume for an adult is 6000 to 10,000 mL of air per minute, or 6 to 10 L/min.

As an EMT, you can assess minute volume. Visible chest rise indicates adequate tidal volume. Respiratory rate is a vital sign measurable by observation. Visible chest rise at a normal rate of 12 to 20 breaths/min would be a good indicator of adequate minute volume and thus adequate ventilation. Contrast this to a patient with a slow respiratory rate, such as 6 or 8 breaths/min, or a patient with a normal rate but no noticeable chest rise and barely audible breath sounds. In either case, the respiratory rate or tidal volume is decreased, which can indicate a low minute volume and inadequate ventilation. When a decreased minute volume is recognized, the EMT must intervene and help the patient breathe faster or deeper, or both.

Alveolar, Capillary, and Cellular Exchange

Diffusion is the movement of molecules, such as oxygen (O_2) and carbon dioxide (CO_2), from an area of higher concentration to an area of lower concentration. For example, if perfume is sprayed in one corner of a room, the perfume molecules will diffuse throughout the room until they are in equal concentration in all four corners. This is a physical law. Because O_2 is in higher concentration in the alveoli, it moves into the capillaries (where O_2 concentration is lower) across the alveolocapillary membrane, by diffusion. Similarly, CO_2, in higher concentration in the capillaries, moves into the alveoli by diffusion. O_2 is carried in the blood by the hemoglobin molecule, which is found in red blood cells. O_2 attached to hemoglobin gives blood its red color. When the blood reaches the tissues, O_2 leaves the hemoglobin and moves from the capillaries to the cells, which have a lower O_2 concentration than the blood. At the same time, CO_2 (in higher concentration in the cells) moves into the blood.

> **LEARNING OBJECTIVES**
> - List the signs of adequate breathing.
> - List the signs of inadequate breathing.

Adequate versus Inadequate Breathing

Look for signs of adequate or inadequate breathing when approaching all patients (**Table 6-1**). Patients who have inadequate breathing may complain of **dyspnea,** a subjective feeling of difficulty in breathing or shortness of breath. Dyspnea is the most common symptom associated with respiratory emergencies. When the respiratory system begins to fail and breathing cannot support organ and body system function (including the brain), patients may exhibit an altered mental state or become sleepy or unresponsive. Remember, the brain is the most oxygen-dependent organ. In patients with respiratory problems change in mental status is of great concern and usually indicates the need for positive-pressure ventilation with a high concentration of oxygen.

Respiratory emergencies can range from respiratory distress to respiratory failure to respiratory arrest. As an EMT, you are expected to distinguish between respiratory distress and respiratory failure because the treatments are different. All patients with respiratory emergencies require administration of oxygen. Patients in respiratory failure and respiratory arrest also require positive-pressure ventilation because their own breathing is inadequate to support life.

Respiratory Distress

Respiratory distress is a condition in which the patient has to work harder to breathe. Signs of respiratory distress include increased respiratory rate, increased accessory muscle use, and nasal flaring; the patient may also assume a position to aid the breathing muscles (tripod or bolt upright) (**Figure 6-5, A**). Patients with respiratory distress may have difficulty speaking in complete sentences. They may appear agitated or restless. *However, the patient in respiratory distress is able to compensate for the underlying problem and get enough oxygen to maintain mental responsiveness and muscle tone, and to move air.* You will usually note signs of respiratory distress as you approach the patient and form a general impression. Respiratory distress is treated by maintaining a clear airway, administering supplemental oxygen, placing the patient in a position of comfort, and if indicated, assisting in administration of bronchodilator medication.

Increased effort to breathe can be exhausting, and a patient in respiratory distress may progress to respiratory failure. As an EMT, your goal is to recognize respiratory distress early and respond quickly to help support adequate oxygenation and breathing.

Respiratory Failure

Respiratory failure is inadequate ventilation to support life. The patient in respiratory failure is not able to maintain mental status, display muscle tone, or move adequate amounts of

Table 6-1	Adequate versus Inadequate Breathing	
	Adequate	**Inadequate**
Rates		
Adult	12-20 breaths/min	Outside normal ranges
Child	15-30 breaths/min	Outside normal ranges
Infant	25-50 breaths/min	Outside normal ranges
Rhythm	Regular	Irregular
Quality		
Breath sounds	Present and equal	Diminished or absent
Chest expansion	Adequate and equal	Inadequate or unequal
Effort	No visible effort	Accessory muscle use, noisy
Depth	Normal chest rise	Inadequate/shallow
Skin	Normal	Pale or cyanotic (blue), cool and clammy
Retractions	None	Present, especially in infants and children
Nasal flaring	Not present	Present, especially in infants and children
Seesaw breathing	Not present	Alternate use of chest and abdominal muscles during breathing
Agonal or gasping breaths	Not present	May be seen just before death

air to the lungs (**Figure 6-5, B**). Respiratory failure can occur by several mechanisms. Examples include problems with brain function (e.g., stroke, head injury, drug overdose) in which the respiratory center is depressed and ventilations are slow and infrequent. Muscle fatigue after prolonged respiratory distress can also lead to inadequate tidal volumes. Injuries to the chest wall can compromise chest movement and result in inadequate volume. Obstruction of the upper or lower airway can also limit ventilation and oxygen exchange. Any of these conditions can lead to respiratory failure and severe hypoxia. Key signs of respiratory failure are related to low blood oxygen level and include altered responsiveness and sleepiness, generalized weakness, and cyanosis. In addition, the patient may have a decreased respiratory rate, little or no chest rise, and decreased

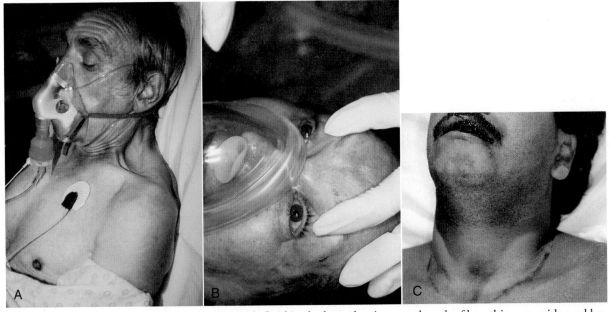

Figure 6-5 **A,** Respiratory distress. This elderly man with fluid in the lungs has increased work of breathing, as evidenced by bulging neck muscles, retractions above the clavicles, and sitting in a bolt-upright position. He is able to maintain his position, is mentally aware, and is moving air in and out of his lungs. **B,** Respiratory failure. This patient with opioid overdose has inadequate ventilations, evidenced by a slow respiratory rate, depressed mental status, and weak muscle tone. The patient is not moving sufficient air to support life and requires positive-pressure ventilation. **C,** Respiratory arrest. This patient was struck by lightning, collapsed immediately, and was found in respiratory arrest. The patient's life was saved by the immediate administration of positive-pressure ventilation. Note the burn mark about the neck from a necklace heated by the lightning.

breath sounds. *Patients with respiratory failure require positive-pressure ventilation.*

The distinction between respiratory distress and respiratory failure is not always clear. The distinction is really whether the patient is able to maintain enough air movement into the lungs to support life without assisted ventilation. When in doubt, you should attempt positive-pressure ventilations and evaluate the patient's response. Ventilations should be continued if the patient accepts your help with little or no resistance or discomfort. A patient who accepts ventilation is showing you that assistance is needed. On the other hand, if a patient actively resists your efforts and is moving air with his or her own efforts, you should stop ventilations and reevaluate the patient. Ongoing assessment of the patient is very important because a patient may later tire and be unable to continue the effort to breathe and will require (and not resist) positive-pressure assistance (**Box 6-1**).

Respiratory Arrest

Respiratory arrest is the complete cessation of breathing. Respiratory failure can progress to respiratory arrest. If untreated, respiratory arrest can progress to cardiac arrest. With cardiac arrest, the patient's chance of survival is greatly diminished. Respiratory arrest can occur suddenly from conditions such as electrocution, lightning strikes, or spinal cord injury (**Figure 6-5, C**).

Box 6-1	Technique to Provide Assisted Ventilation

Use with Patient Who Is Breathing

Assess the need to provide ventilatory support.

1. Any patient with a reduced minute volume (breathing rate and depth) must receive ventilatory support and supplemental oxygen.
2. Some patients will be in respiratory arrest and will require 10-12 ventilations per minute (1 breath every 5-6 seconds).
3. Some patients will have reduced tidal volume and a rapid rate and may need volume support through assisted ventilations.
4. Some patients will have reduced minute volume (hypoventilation) and will require their respiratory rate and volume to be assisted by ventilation.

Use with Patient Who Has Rapid Breathing

1. Explain the procedure to responsive patients.
2. Place the mask over the patient's nose and mouth.
3. Initially assist ventilation at the rate at which the patient has been breathing. Squeeze the bag each time the patient begins to inhale.
4. Over the next 5 to 10 seconds, slowly adjust the rate and the delivered tidal volume until an adequate minute volume is achieved.

Use with Patient Who Is Hypoventilating

1. Place the mask over the patient's nose and mouth.
2. Squeeze the bag at the time the patient begins to inhale.
3. Over the next 5 to 10 breaths, slowly adjust the rate and the delivered tidal volume until an adequate minute volume is achieved (10-12 breaths/min with chest rise).

Signs of Adequate and Inadequate Breathing

You should look for signs of adequate versus inadequate breathing in every patient. If signs of increased work of breathing or inadequate breathing are present, determine whether the patient is in respiratory distress or respiratory failure because treatment differs. All patients with respiratory problems need supplemental oxygen. Patients in respiratory failure and respiratory arrest need positive-pressure ventilation.

Rate of Breathing

The normal respiratory rate varies with age; again, the normal adult rate is 12 to 20 breaths/min. The normal rate for children is 15 to 30 breaths/min, and for infants, 25 to 50 breaths/min. Slow respiratory rates alone may indicate the need for positive-pressure ventilation and supplemental oxygen, especially if other signs of inadequate breathing are present. Rates higher than the normal range can be a sign of respiratory distress. However, many conditions can result in increased respiratory rates with no airway or lung problem. For example, a patient may be trying to rid the body of excess acid from metabolic problems (e.g., diabetic ketoacidosis), or a patient may have increased drive to breathe because of a drug overdose (e.g., salicylates/aspirin). In these conditions, **tachypnea** (increased respiratory rate) does not indicate inadequate breathing. However, because the cause for rapid breathing is not always clear to an EMT, supplemental oxygen is routinely provided.

The respiratory rate can change for many reasons. For example, a patient may have a sudden attack of asthma and may initially have an increased respiratory rate. Over time, if the asthma is severe and the patient becomes fatigued from the increased work of breathing, the rate may gradually slow and pass through a "normal" range as the patient tires. Depending on when you encounter this patient, you may note an increased rate, a normal rate, or a decreased rate of respirations. The respiratory rate should be evaluated within the overall assessment of the patient and should be repeated during the ongoing assessment.

When dealing with patients in respiratory distress, the respiratory rate and other vital signs should be evaluated at least every 5 minutes.

Rhythm of Breathing

To evaluate breathing you should also look at the rhythm of the breaths. Is it regular, with a consistent rise and fall of the chest wall over time, or irregular? An irregular pattern may be found with certain illnesses and brain injuries. A patient may have patterns of increasing and decreasing rates and tidal volumes interspersed with periods of no breathing. **Agonal breathing**, or slow, irregular gasping breaths, can be seen during the early onset of cardiac arrest (**Figure 6-6**).

Quality of Breathing

The quality of breathing can be assessed by looking at chest and abdominal movements, observing use of accessory muscles of breathing, listening for breath sounds, and feeling air movement through the mouth and nose. You can also inspect the

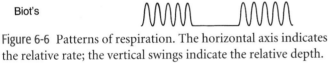

Normal

Cheyne-Stokes

Ataxic

Central neurogenic
hyperventilation

Terminal respiratory
depression

Apneustic

Biot's

Figure 6-6 Patterns of respiration. The horizontal axis indicates the relative rate; the vertical swings indicate the relative depth. *From Sanders MJ: Mosby's paramedic textbook, ed 3, St Louis, 2005, Mosby.*

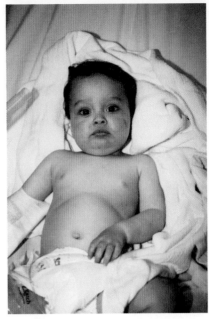

Figure 6-7 Seesaw breathing.

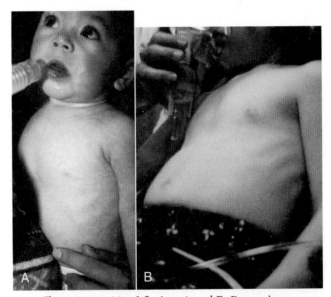

Figure 6-8 **A,** Nasal flaring. **A** and **B,** Retractions.

skin and evaluate the patient's mental state. Identifying abnormal findings may give clues to the underlying problem.

Chest and Abdominal Movement. Visible chest and abdominal movements at a rate normal for the patient's age characterize normal breathing. Equal chest expansion should be present on both sides of the chest. In contrast, a patient who has multiple rib fractures may have normal expansion on only one side of the chest.

Effort of Breathing. Use of accessory muscles is usually obvious with inspection, particularly in children because they have softer rib cages. Look for prominent neck muscles bulging and **retractions (Figure 6-8, B),** which are exaggerated indentations between the ribs or above and under the sternum. Retractions may indicate inspiration through narrowed or obstructed airways or an increased work of breathing because lungs are "stiff" from the accumulation of fluid. The abdominal muscles may be prominent during breathing, indicating forced exhalation.

An infant may have movement of the abdominal and chest wall muscles in opposite directions, with chest retraction and abdominal distention, called **seesaw breathing.** This type of breathing is often seen with upper airway obstruction (**Figure 6-7**). Other infants and small children struggling to breathe may have noticeable **nasal flaring,** or widely dilated nostrils (**Figure 6-8, A**). For a complete discussion on the assessment of breathing in children, see Chapter 25.

Breath Sounds. Sounds of breathing may be heard with or without a stethoscope. To assess breath sounds, listen with the stethoscope to both sides of the chest. Are breath sounds

REAL*World*

All patients, but especially children, can tire easily if they are forced to use accessory muscles for a prolonged period. As they tire, they may appear to be relaxing and want to sleep; this is not the case. These patients are progressing into respiratory failure and need assistance from the EMT.

present and equal, diminished, absent, or unequal on both sides? Diminished or absent breath sounds in both lungs may indicate respiratory failure and very low tidal volumes. When absent or diminished breath sounds are noted on one side, a collapsed lung or massive bleeding in the chest cavity may be present. You may hear wheezing or a high whistling sound during exhalation, as in asthma or bronchitis. Alternately, you may hear crackles created by fluid in the alveoli. You will learn more about the technique of auscultation and specific breath sounds in later chapters.

You may also hear audible breath sounds without a stethoscope. Because breathing is normally quiet, these sounds are usually abnormal and may indicate respiratory distress or obstruction. Audible breath sounds include snoring, gurgling, stridor, wheezing, grunting, and gasping (**Box 6-2**).

Skin

Cyanosis, or a blue-gray skin color, is a sign of oxygen-depleted hemoglobin in the blood. You should inspect the patient's lips and tongue, which are your best indicators of *central* cyanosis. Cyanosis of the extremities may be caused by circulatory problems to the limbs, particularly in small infants; therefore you should always check the lips. Remember that the absence of cyanosis does not mean that there is good oxygenation. Pale, cool, or clammy skin might also be seen in patients with respiratory distress.

Mental Status

Alterations in mental status that may be observed as a result of hypoxia range from agitation and restlessness to lethargy (sleepy appearance) to coma. Patients with respiratory emergencies who have mental status changes require supplemental oxygen treatment and, if indicated, positive-pressure ventilation.

Case in Point

You are called to a college dormitory for an unconscious patient. Two young men meet you at the door and tell you that their friend took an overdose and they cannot wake him. You put on gloves as you enter the dorm room and find a 20-year-old man lying on his bed, which has a small amount of vomited material. You hear infrequent gurgling sounds but see no visible chest rise. His lips are blue, and he is unresponsive. You put on a mask and protective eyewear. You immediately open the airway with the head-tilt/chin-lift maneuver and suction secretions from the airway; then you look, listen, and feel for breathing. The gurgling ceases, and you feel breaths with minimal chest rise at a rate of 8 breaths/min. A pulse is present.

You insert an oropharyngeal airway and begin positive-pressure ventilations at a rate of 12 breaths/min with a bag-mask device. Your partner attaches the bag-mask to oxygen at a flow rate of 15 L/min. The man's lips become pink, but he remains unresponsive. Vital signs show a pulse rate of 100 beats/min and regular, blood pressure 100/70 mm Hg, and respiratory rate 12 breaths/min and assisted; the patient is unresponsive to pain. The pupils are small and equal and minimally responsive to light. There is equal chest rise bilaterally and clear breath sounds with positive-pressure ventilation. As you continue positive-pressure ventilation, you prepare the patient for transport and attach a pulse oximeter that shows oxygen saturation of 97%.

This scenario is consistent with an opioid overdose, which classically causes loss of consciousness, small pupils, and death from inadequate breathing.

LEARNING OBJECTIVES
- Describe the steps in performing the head-tilt/chin-lift.
- Relate mechanism of injury to opening the airway.
- Describe the steps in performing the jaw thrust.

Box 6-2   Audible Breath Sounds

- A *snoring* sound indicates obstruction of the upper airway caused by collapse of soft tissues in the oropharynx or the tongue.
- *Gurgling* is a sound created by air moving through fluid. It sounds similar to blowing through a straw beneath water. This usually indicates the presence of fluid in the upper airway.
- **Stridor,** also called *crowing,* is a high-pitched sound usually heard on inspiration and suggests upper airway obstruction.
- **Wheezing** is a high-pitched, "whistling" noise usually occurring on exhalation. It is generally associated with a lengthening of the expiratory phase of breathing. Narrowing of the lower airways, as in asthma, often causes wheezing.
- **Grunting** is a sound heard at the end of exhalation. This sound is caused by contraction of the diaphragm against partially closed vocal cords in an effort to keep the small airways open during exhalation.
- *Gasping* is characterized by short, irregular breaths with a rapid inspiratory phase associated with severe respiratory distress and fatigue.

Opening the Airway

There are three goals in airway management:
1. Establish and maintain a patent airway
2. Ensure adequate ventilation
3. Ensure adequate oxygenation

The first step in any emergency is to ensure a *patent* (open) airway. Once the airway is established, it must be maintained. Methods of airway control include the following:
- Manual techniques
- Suctioning
- Mechanical techniques

Manual Techniques

Manual airway techniques are used as the first step in opening the airway. They are also used in conjunction with mechanical techniques to maintain an open airway.

Immediate opening of the airway is the first and most basic skill of emergency care. The most common cause of airway obstruction occurs when the tongue falls to the back of the throat as the muscles of an unconscious patient relax (**Figure 6-9**). Because the tongue is attached to the lower jaw, bringing the jaw forward lifts the tongue away from the back of the throat, and the airway opens. Two techniques are routinely used to open the airway: the head-tilt/chin-lift and the jaw thrust.

Head-Tilt/Chin-Lift

To perform the head-tilt/chin-lift, place the index and middle fingers of one hand under the bony part of the lower jaw. Then place the other hand on the patient's forehead and lift the patient's lower jaw upward with one hand while tilting the forehead back with the other (**Figure 6-10**). Lift the lower

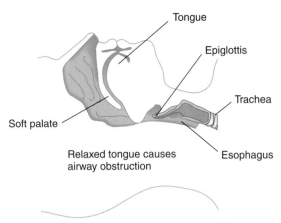

Figure 6-9 In the relaxed or unconscious state, the tongue may fall against the back wall of the pharynx and block the upper airway. *From McSwain N, Paturas J: The basic EMT: comprehensive prehospital patient care, St Louis, 2003, Mosby.*

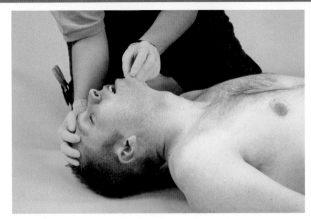

Figure 6-10 Head-tilt/chin-lift.

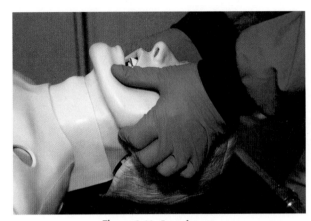

Figure 6-11 Jaw thrust.

jaw upward until the teeth are almost touching but the mouth is not closed.

Jaw Thrust

The jaw thrust, or modified jaw thrust, should be used for unresponsive patients with suspected cervical spine injury (or unknown mechanism of injury) because this maneuver opens the airway without extension of the neck. If ventilations are ineffective in the neutral position, it may be necessary to slightly extend the neck.

Place one hand on either side of the patient's head, with your elbows on the surface on which the patient is lying. Place your index and middle fingers beneath the angle of the jaw just below the ears, and lift the jaw upward while opening the mouth with your thumbs on the lower lip (**Figure 6-11**).

LEARNING OBJECTIVES
- State the importance of having a suction unit ready for immediate use when providing emergency care.
- Describe the techniques of suctioning.

Suctioning

General Considerations

Suctioning is the act of introducing a soft or rigid catheter into the airway to vacuum out liquid and small, solid secretions. With some suction units, removing solid particles from the airway is difficult. In these cases, particles may have to be removed manually with a gloved hand by turning the head to the side to aid drainage. Vomiting, drowning, bleeding, and lung secretions are all sources of airway obstruction in unconscious or lethargic patients. A gurgling sound in an unconscious patient is a sign of fluid in the airway. Timely removal of these substances ensures a patent airway and more adequate ventilation and oxygenation. To perform procedures related to management

of the airway, you should use standard precautions, including wearing goggles, gloves, and a face mask as indicated.

Suction equipment consists of a suction machine, which may be a portable, battery-operated model or a hand-operated device. There are also wall-mounted, in-board suction units located in the ambulance (**Figure 6-12**).

Suction devices should be checked regularly and should be capable of removing thick secretions and providing negative pressures of at least 300 mm Hg (80-120 mm Hg for children; 100 mm Hg for infants). A soft catheter or rigid device is connected to the machine by tubing and placed in the patient's mouth before suction is initiated. Some catheters have an opening at the base that activates suctioning; in some cases, suctioning is initiated by pushing a button on the machine. The catheter or rigid device should be placed into the oropharynx with the suction not activated. Once the device is in place, suction should be applied while rotating the tip of the catheter to avoid plugging by pharyngeal tissue. To avoid hypoxia, suctioning should not be performed for more than 15 seconds (**Skill 6-1**). A shorter suctioning time is used in infants and children.

If the patient has copious secretions or particles that cannot be removed quickly and easily by suctioning, log-roll the patient, or if on a long spine board, turn the board on its side and clear the patient's oropharynx. If the patient produces frothy secretions as rapidly as suctioning can remove them, suction for

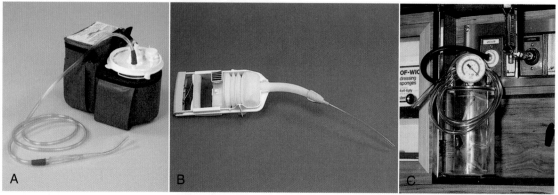

Figure 6-12 **A,** Battery-operated suction device. **B,** Hand-operated suction unit. **C,** Inboard suction device with large collection chamber.

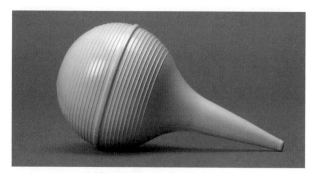

Figure 6-13 Bulb suction.

15 seconds, provide positive-pressure ventilation for 2 minutes, and then suction again for 15 seconds. Seek medical direction in this type of situation.

Infants and Children

A rigid catheter should be used to suction the upper airway of infants and children. Care should be taken not to touch the back of the airway. In general, less suction time is used for infants and children than adults because pediatric patients may become hypoxic with prolonged suctioning. Nasal suctioning is performed with a bulb suction device (**Figure 6-13**) or with a small, soft catheter with low to medium vacuum.

> **LEARNING OBJECTIVES**
> * Describe how to measure and insert an oropharyngeal airway.
> * Describe how to measure and insert a nasopharyngeal airway.

Mechanical Techniques

Mechanical airway devices maintain a clear route to the lungs by keeping the tongue away from the pharyngeal wall. The principal airway adjuncts are the oropharyngeal and nasopharyngeal airways.

Oropharyngeal Airway

The **oropharyngeal airway (OPA)** is a basic airway device designed to elevate the tongue away from the oropharynx *in unconscious patients without a gag reflex*. Although airway devices

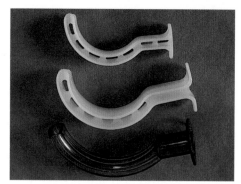

Figure 6-14 Oropharyngeal airways. *From McSwain N, Paturas J: The basic EMT: comprehensive prehospital patient care, St Louis, 2003, Mosby.*

are available in a variety of sizes, the basic design is essentially the same (**Figure 6-14**). The OPA consists of a curved plastic device that extends from just anterior to the lips down to the base of the tongue in the oropharynx. The outer portion has a flange that extends over the opening of the mouth to help prevent the device from slipping into the airway. **Skill 6-2** illustrates the insertion of an OPA.

Nasopharyngeal Airway

The **nasopharyngeal airway (NPA)** has the same purpose as the OPA: keep the tongue away from the pharynx. It is used when an OPA cannot be tolerated, such as when a patient has a gag reflex. It is also useful when the mouth cannot be opened because of trauma or clenching of the teeth. The NPA should not be used in patients with severe, direct facial injury or possible skull fracture. The NPA consists of a soft rubber tube that, when properly positioned, extends from the nares down into the oropharynx (**Figure 6-15**). It also has a lip that extends around the outside of the nose to prevent slippage into the airway. **Skill 6-3** illustrates the insertion of an NPA.

> **LEARNING OBJECTIVES**
> * Describe how to ventilate a patient artificially with a pocket mask.
> * List the steps in performing mouth-to-mouth artificial ventilation.

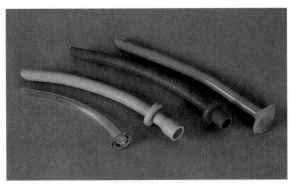

Figure 6-15 Nasopharyngeal airways. *From McSwain N, Paturas J: The basic EMT: comprehensive prehospital patient care, ed 2, St Louis, 2003, Mosby.*

Table 6-2 Methods for Ventilating a Patient*		
Method	**Advantages**	**Disadvantages**
Mouth-to-mask device	Reliable volume delivery Two-hand seal Ability to feel lung expansion	Fatigue of rescuer
Two-person bag-mask device	Two-hand seal Higher oxygen delivery Ability to feel lung expansion	
Flow-restricted, oxygen-powered ventilation device	Highest oxygen delivery Two-hand seal Good volume delivery	Use in adults only High pressure can further injure patients with chest trauma. Inability to feel lung expansion
One-person bag-mask device	Higher oxygen delivery Ability to feel lung expansion	One EMT may have difficulty maintaining seal, so less volume may be delivered than with mouth-to-mask method.

*In order of preference.

Positive-Pressure Ventilation

Once an airway has been established, the need for ventilation must be determined. If a patient has inadequate breathing, respiratory failure, or respiratory arrest, the EMT must "breathe" for the patient. This is called **rescue breathing** or **positive-pressure ventilation.** Several techniques are available to force air positively into the lungs (**Table 6-2**). Methods for artificially ventilating a patient include the following:

- Mouth-to-mouth or mouth-to-nose
- Mouth-to-mask or mouth-to-barrier device
- Bag-mask ventilation
- Flow-restricted, oxygen-powered ventilation device

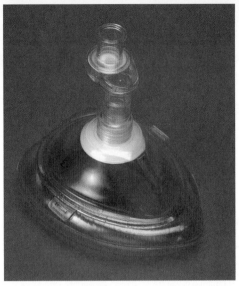

Figure 6-16 A mouth-to-mask device consists of a mask, a one-way valve, and on some units an oxygen inlet to provide enriched concentration of oxygen.

You must use a conscientious approach with each technique to ensure adequate ventilation. "Adequate ventilation" is assessed on the basis of chest rise and other indicators of oxygenation, such as skin color. When providing care for the airway, you should always wear gloves and mask and protective eyewear if splashing or spraying of blood, secretions, or vomitus is likely.

When functioning as an EMT you should always use a barrier device or some other means to provide positive-pressure ventilation. However, in a lay rescuer situation you may not have a barrier device available and choose to provide rescue breathing using mouth-to-mouth resuscitation. We will not review this technique since it was covered in your Basic Life Support training. Although not commonly done, this procedure may help to save a life.

Mouth-to-Mask or Mouth-to-Barrier Device

As an alternative to mouth-to-mouth or mouth-to-nose rescue breathing, barrier devices such as masks or face shields are available to protect the EMT from direct contact with the patient's bodily fluids. The mouth-to-mask device or pocket mask is a transparent, semirigid mask that, when properly placed, seals around the patient's mouth and nose with an air-filled bladder. A one-way valve is either incorporated into the mask or can be attached to the device to prevent the patient's exhaled air from reaching the EMT. The advantages of mouth-to-mask ventilation include the ability to provide supplemental oxygen and the elimination of direct contact with the patient's mouth or nose (**Figure 6-16**). The mouth-to-mask device is an extremely reliable form of ventilation because you can use two hands to create a mask seal, and you experience a "sense of lung compliance" while delivering a rescue breath. When providing mouth-to-mask breathing, breathe until you achieve chest rise over a 1-second period.

Supplemental oxygen can be delivered to some mouth-to-mask devices through a port on top of the mask. Flow rates of 15 L/min of oxygen will result in delivery of O_2 concentrations of approximately 50% (**Skill 6-4**).

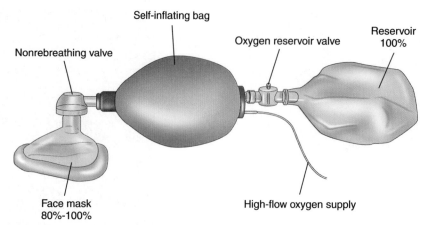

Figure 6-17 A bag-mask with an oxygen reservoir can deliver approximately 90% oxygen. The reservoir can consist of long tubes or plastic bags that collect oxygen between breaths. *From McSwain N, Paturas J:* The basic EMT: comprehensive prehospital patient care, *St Louis, 2003, Mosby.*

Mouth-to-face shield devices are composed of a plastic sheet that separates the patient from the provider. When delivering a rescue breath, you must pinch the patient's nose and deliver a slow breath over a 2-second period through the valve or filter in the center of the shield. For EMTs, a pocket mask is preferred over a face shield for rescue breathing.

> **LEARNING OBJECTIVES**
> - Describe the steps in artificially ventilating a patient with a bag-mask device while using the jaw thrust.
> - List the parts of a bag-mask system.
> - Describe the steps in artificially ventilating a patient with a bag-mask device.
> - Describe the signs of adequate artificial ventilation using the bag-mask device.
> - Describe the signs of inadequate artificial ventilation using the bag-mask device.

Bag-Mask

The **bag-mask device** is the most common mechanical aid used in emergency care to initially administer positive-pressure ventilation. It also can be the most unreliable unless it is used properly. The typical bag-mask consists of a bag that has a capacity of approximately 1600 mL of air and a one-way valve that ensures flow of air to the patient. Exhaled air escapes into the environment through an exit port on the valve. A mask is attached to a universal opening next to the valve. The mask should be transparent (so that you can observe for possible vomiting) and capable of achieving an adequate seal.

The bag-mask has an oxygen inlet that provides increased oxygen concentrations to the patient. A bag-mask with an oxygen-collecting reservoir is capable of delivering 90% to 100% oxygen (**Figure 6-17**). You should familiarize yourself with the type of bag-mask used in your region.

Other features of a bag-mask device include the following:
- A self-refilling bag that is disposable or is easily cleaned or sterilized

- A non-jamming valve that allows a maximum oxygen inlet flow of 15 L/min
- Standardized fittings of 15 and 22 mm
- A true nonrebreather valve
- Ability to perform at all environmental extremes
- Availability of infant, child, and adult sizes

You should closely monitor chest rise when using the bag-mask device because delivery of low tidal volumes is a common complication when the seal between the patient's face and the mask is inadequate (**Skill 6-5**). If the chest does not rise, you will need to reevaluate. You should first try repositioning the patient's head. If air is escaping from under the mask, or if the abdomen is rising, you should reposition your fingers and the mask. If the chest still does not rise, you should check for an airway obstruction. If the airway is obstructed, follow the appropriate steps to relieve the obstruction. If the chest still does not rise, you may need to use an alternative method of positive-pressure ventilation (e.g., pocket mask, manually triggered device). You should always consider the use of airway adjuncts such as the OPA or NPA to help keep the airway open.

Cricoid Pressure

During positive-pressure ventilation, air can enter the esophagus and cause gastric inflation and increase the chance of vomiting and aspiration. To prevent this from occurring, **cricoid pressure,** or the *Sellick maneuver,* can be used when sufficient personnel are available to compress the esophagus between the cricoid cartilage and the thoracic spine. This maneuver closes the esophagus and reduces the chances of air entering the esophagus during positive-pressure ventilation and helps prevent regurgitation. **Figure 6-18** illustrates the location and technique of applying cricoid pressure.

> **LEARNING OBJECTIVE**
> - Describe the steps in artificially ventilating a patient with a flow-restricted, oxygen-powered ventilation device.

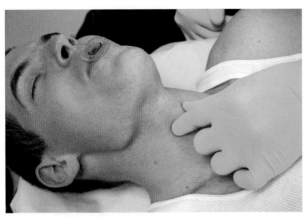

Figure 6-18 Cricoid pressure. Locate the thyroid cartilage (Adam's apple) and slide down the groove just below (cricothyroid membrane); the prominence just below that point is the cricoid cartilage. Provide firm pressure downward to compress the esophagus during ventilation with a mask device.

Flow-Restricted, Oxygen-Powered Ventilation Devices

A **flow-restricted, oxygen-powered ventilation device** can achieve the highest delivered oxygen concentrations of any positive-pressure apparatus (**Figure 6-19**). This oxygen-powered device delivers 100% O_2 to the patient's airway. It is activated by a lever or button located on the valve or by the negative pressure (demand) created by a breathing patient's inspiratory effort. The valve and regulator reduce the delivered pressure to about 60 cm of water (H_2O) and flow rates of 40 L/min, which is a safe level for the adult patient. When the airway pressure exceeds 60 cm H_2O, the oxygen is vented into the atmosphere, and an audible alarm sounds. An inspiratory relief valve serves as a backup to avoid overexpansion of the lungs. Do not use this device in infants and small children (**Box 6-3**).

LEARNING OBJECTIVES
- Define the components of an oxygen delivery system.
- Identify a nonrebreather face mask, and state the oxygen flow requirements for its use.
- Describe the indications for using a nasal cannula versus a nonrebreather face mask.
- Identify a nasal cannula, and state the flow requirements for its use.

💿 Oxygen Therapy

Oxygen is a colorless, odorless gas that is plentiful in our environment. Normal atmospheric air contains approximately 21% O_2. Anyone in respiratory distress or failure should receive supplemental oxygen. Other patients with no breathing difficulty may also benefit, including patients with chest pain, stroke, trauma, or poisoning (e.g., carbon monoxide).

Emergency medical technicians carry supplemental oxygen in tanks or cylinders for delivery through various devices to the

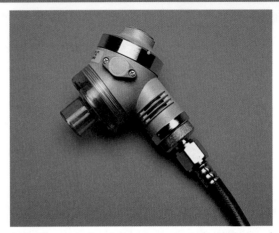

Figure 6-19 Flow-restricted, oxygen-powered ventilation device. *From McSwain N, Paturas J: The basic EMT: comprehensive prehospital patient care, St Louis, 2003, Mosby.*

Box 6-3	Flow-Restricted, Oxygen-Powered Ventilation Device

Method 1: No Suspected Spinal Injury

1. After opening airway, insert correct size of oral or nasal airway and attach adult mask.
2. Position thumbs over top half of mask, index and middle fingers over bottom half. Place apex of mask over bridge of nose, then lower mask over mouth and upper chin. Use ring and little fingers to bring jaw up to mask. Connect flow-restricted, oxygen-powered ventilation device to mask if not already done. Trigger the flow-restricted, oxygen-powered ventilation device until chest rises.
3. Repeat one breath every 5-6 seconds. If chest does not rise, reevaluate.

Method 2: Suspected Spinal Injury

1. After opening airway, insert correct size of oral or nasal airway and attach adult mask. Immobilize head and neck; have assistant hold head manually, or use your knees to prevent movement. Position thumbs over top half of mask, index and middle fingers over bottom half. Place apex of mask over bridge of nose, then lower mask over mouth and upper chin. Use ring and little fingers to bring jaw up to mask without tilting head or neck.
2. Connect flow-restricted, oxygen-powered ventilation device to mask, if not already done.
3. Trigger the flow-restricted oxygen-powered ventilation device until chest rises. Repeat every 5-6 seconds. If chest does not rise, reevaluate.

---

patient. Oxygen from the tank flows through a regulator, which reduces pressure to safe levels for the lungs. An O_2 administration device (nonrebreather mask, nasal cannula) is connected to the regulator by oxygen tubing.

Oxygen Cylinders

Oxygen cylinders are extremely strong and contain a proportionately large quantity of gas that is stored at very high pressure, usually 2000 pounds per square inch (psi). These cylinders are

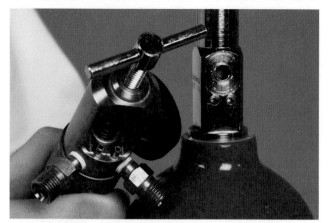

Figure 6-20 An oxygen pin index system consists of two small holes below an opening on the cylinder valve (where gas exits the cylinder). These holes interface with the pins on a regulator that prevents the misplacement of an oxygen regulator on a cylinder containing a different gas (e.g., nitrous oxide).

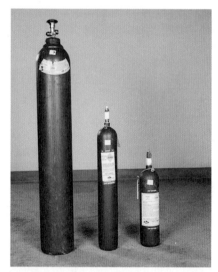

Figure 6-21 Oxygen cylinders sizes D, E, and M.

color-coded green, which identifies them as containing oxygen. Cylinders containing other gases are identified by different colors. This reduces the chance of inadvertently administering the wrong gas. Another safeguard for portable oxygen cylinders is called the **pin index safety system.** This method varies the openings at the top of the cylinder valve so that the tank accepts a special regulator designed only for oxygen (**Figure 6-20**). The holes include one opening through which air flows out of the cylinder and two other openings that receive stabilizing pins that extend from the regulators.

Cylinder Sizes

Oxygen cylinders are available in several sizes (**Figure 6-21**). The smaller sizes are referred to as D or E cylinders. These tanks are portable and designed to bring oxygen to the patient's side. Larger cylinders are identified as M, G, or H and are used to store large quantities of gas in the emergency vehicle. As the

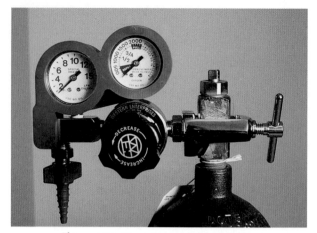

Figure 6-22 Bourdon gauge regulator.

Box 6-4	Volumes of Oxygen Cylinders				
D cylinder	350 L	M cylinder	3000 L	H cylinder	6900 L
E cylinder	625 L	G cylinder	5300 L		

size of the cylinder increases, so does the volume of gas it can contain (**Box 6-4**).

Regulators

The regulator is a device that reduces the very high pressure of gas within the cylinder to a level that will not injure the patient. Regulators can be classified as either single or double staged. *Single-staged regulators* have only one phase of pressure reduction and usually result in an exiting pressure of 40 to 70 psi. This is the most common type of regulator used in EMS. *Double-staged regulators* reduce gas pressure in a two-step process. First, the pressure is reduced as the gas enters the regulator to approximately 700 psi and is then further reduced at the interface with the liter flow gauge to 40 to 70 psi. This two-staged reduction has the advantage of saving wear and tear on the reducing valve and serves as an additional safety measure.

All regulators have a pressure gauge that measures tank pressure. A full tank should measure approximately 2000 psi. Some regulators also have a flowmeter that records the flow rate of gas leaving the cylinder. These flowmeters usually range from 0 to 25 L/min. Three types of flowmeters are used in EMS. A *Bourdon gauge flowmeter* uses a pressure gauge to measure flow rates to the delivery device (**Figure 6-22**).

A *pressure-compensated flowmeter* (Thorpe tube flowmeter) uses a gravity-regulated ball on a vertical meter to record flow (**Figure 6-23**). The liter flow is read at the center of the ball as it rises. The pressure-compensated flowmeter has the advantage of being more accurate because it measures actual flow. If the tubing on a device is clogged or kinked, the flow rate will not accurately reflect the actual amount of gas delivered to the patient. The pressure-compensated flowmeter is the type usually found on oxygen systems inside the ambulance.

The *constant-flow selector valve flowmeter* uses a flow marking at the adjustment dial to indicate flow rates.

Cylinder Calculations

Knowing the cylinder size, the pressure in the tank, and the rate of oxygen delivery to the patient *(flow rate),* you can calculate the approximate time a tank will last during O_2 administration. For example, an E cylinder containing 1200 psi and opened to deliver 8 L/min O_2 will last approximately 35 minutes. This conclusion is reached by applying the following formula:

$$\text{Time (min)} = \frac{(\text{Tank pressure[psi]} - 200\,\text{psi}) \times \text{Constant}}{\text{Flow rate (L/min)}}$$

The pressure gauge notes the tank pressure. The figure 200 is subtracted from this pressure to ensure the cylinder does not run empty before it is changed. This value is then multiplied by a constant, which is a figure that controls for the variance in cylinder size (**Box 6-5**). The product of this multiplication is then divided by the liter flow.

In theory, this formula predicts the point at which the cylinder must be changed. However, if you are using large quantities of oxygen, such as positive-pressure ventilation with a demand valve, closely monitoring the pressure gauge is the safest and most convenient method. **Skills 6-6** and **6-7** demonstrate the assembly and disassembly of an oxygen system.

Case in Point

You are transporting a patient who is receiving 15 L/min of oxygen by a nonrebreather mask. The estimated transport time is 20 minutes. On your E cylinder, the pressure gauge reads 1200 psi. Do you have enough oxygen for this patient, or should you prepare to change tanks en route?

$$\text{Time (min)} = \frac{(1200\,\text{psi} - 200\,\text{psi}) \times 0.28}{15\,\text{L/min}} = 18\tfrac{2}{3}\ \text{minutes}$$

At a rate of 15 L/min, you have between 18 and 19 minutes of oxygen left in the tank. You should be ready to change tanks before you arrive at the hospital.

Oxygen Administration Devices

When patients are ventilating adequately but are in need of supplemental oxygen, free-flow oxygen devices are used. The two devices used most often in EMS are the nasal cannula and the nonrebreather mask. Each device has advantages and disadvantages and should be selected accordingly.

Nasal Cannulas

Nasal cannulas, or nasal prongs, are low-flow, low-concentration O_2 delivery devices. The cannulas do not deliver the total quantity of gas consumed by the patient; the patient breathes O_2 delivered from the nasal cannula along with room air. The nasal cannula delivers a low-to-medium O_2 concentration (24%-40% O_2 at flow rates of 2-6 L/min). As a rule, you should not administer more than 6 L/min O_2 through a nasal cannula because this amount will dry the nasal mucosa and will not increase delivery concentrations.

Nasal cannulas are useful in treating any condition in which low-to-medium O_2 concentrations are needed, such as chronic obstructive pulmonary disease, asthma, and uncomplicated

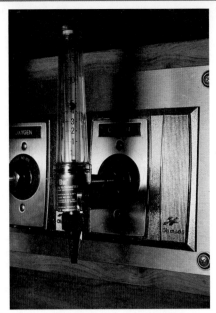

Figure 6-23 Pressure-compensated flowmeter.

Box 6-5	Constants by Tank Size				
D Cylinder	0.16	M Cylinder	1.56	H Cylinder	3.14
E Cylinder	0.28				

chest pain. In EMS, however, patients who require supplemental oxygen generally receive it by a nonrebreather mask. Nasal cannulas are also valuable when patients cannot tolerate the restrictive feeling of a mask, a common finding among dyspneic and hypoxic patients (**Skill 6-8**).

Nonrebreather Mask

A **nonrebreather mask** is a high-flow, high-concentration O_2 delivery device. It is the best device to use when a patient requires high O_2 concentrations. The nonrebreather mask can achieve concentrations up to 90% O_2 at flow rates of 10 to 15 L/min, the rate adequate to keep the O_2 reservoir bag inflated at the end of inspiration. A nonrebreather mask consists of a reservoir bag beneath a one-way valve that prevents the patient from exhaling into the bag ("nonrebreather") (**Figure 6-24**).

Oxygen is administered by first attaching the oxygen tubing and providing a flow rate of at least 8 L/min while keeping your finger over the valve to fill the bag. You should then place the mask around the patient's face and pull the elastic straps to secure the mask. Leakage around the mask decreases O_2 delivery. When the patient inhales, the bag should not fully collapse. If this occurs, the delivered O_2 should be increased by 2 liters/min increments until the bag remains partially inflated at the end of each breath (**Skill 6-9**).

The nonrebreather mask is excellent for patients who require supplemental oxygen and have adequate ventilatory volumes. It is used for the treatment of respiratory distress, shock, and any other cause of poor tissue oxygenation.

Table 6-3 lists O_2 delivery capabilities of the nasal cannula and nonrebreather mask.

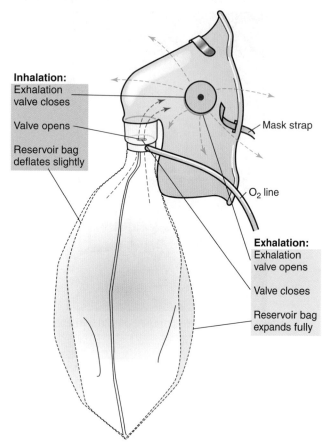

Inhalation:
Exhalation valve closes

Valve opens

Reservoir bag deflates slightly

Mask strap

O₂ line

Exhalation:
Exhalation valve opens

Valve closes

Reservoir bag expands fully

Figure 6-24 A nonrebreather mask works by using an oxygen collection device below the mask, where oxygen collects before inhalation. A one-way valve separates the reservoir from the mask and directs exhalation out through the sides of the mask. With a tight-fitting mask, this device results in approximately 90% oxygen delivery to the patient.

Table 6-3	Oxygen Delivery by Device	
	Approximate Concentration of Oxygen Delivered	**Flow Rate Device**
Nasal cannula	24%-40%	2-6 L/min
Nonrebreather mask	90%	10-15 L/min

Every oxygen device on the ambulance should be checked so that it is always available on an emergency basis (**Box 6-6**).

Pulse Oximetry

A pulse oximeter is a device that monitors oxygen saturation through measurements of light transfer through capillary beds and hemoglobin. It is attached to the tip of the patient's finger over a nail bed or to an earlobe and reads the transmission of red and infrared (IR) light through the capillary bed below (**Figure 6-25**). Pulse oximeters use a *colorimeter* to measure red and IR light waves to determine the *percent of oxygen saturation* of hemoglobin. When fully saturated with O_2, hemoglobin assumes a bright-red color. Hemoglobin that is well saturated with O_2 absorbs more IR light waves and fewer red light waves

Box 6-6   Safety Issues Related to Oxygen Use

- Monitor the tank pressure frequently.
- Do not smoke or use an open flame within 10 feet (3 m) of oxygen equipment.
- Do not use near electrical equipment that gives off sparks.
- Do not use oils or other flammable substances around oxygen equipment.
- Store cylinders in a cool, well-ventilated area, and secure them in place at all times.
- Close all valves when oxygen is not in use.
- Never attempt repair of cylinders or regulators.
- Never position yourself or the patient above the valve of the cylinder.

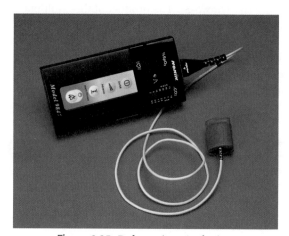

Figure 6-25 Pulse oximeter device.

than unsaturated hemoglobin. On the other hand, unsaturated hemoglobin absorbs more red light waves and fewer IR light waves. The difference in the rate of absorption of these light waves is used to generate a numeric value of percent O_2 saturation. Normal hemoglobin saturation is 93% to 100%. A reading of 95% or higher is a good indication that oxygenation is adequate in most patients. A lower value suggests the presence of hypoxia and should be managed through adjustments in O_2 administration and positive-pressure ventilation, if needed. A reading below 90% when a patient is receiving high-concentration O_2 is an indication for positive-pressure ventilation.

The EMT should use care when interpreting information from a pulse oximeter. The accuracy of a pulse oximeter can be affected by several variables. Excessive ambient light can alter the reading of a pulse oximeter. Any condition that reduces circulation to the peripheral arteries may generate a falsely low reading. These conditions include cardiac arrest, hypotension, hypothermia, and the use of drugs that cause vasoconstriction. Patients who have carbon monoxide (CO) poisoning may generate a falsely high reading because of the bright-red color of CO-saturated hemoglobin. Because of these limitations, **pulse oximetry** should be considered an adjunct to patient assessment, but never as the sole indicator of the effectiveness (or ineffectiveness) of oxygen therapy.

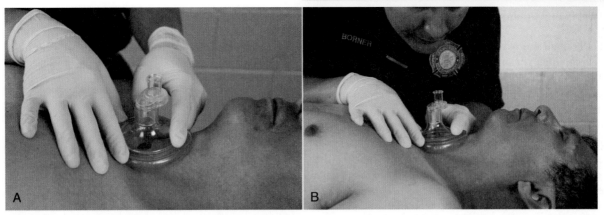

Figure 6-26 Mask-to-stoma ventilation. *From Chapleau W, Pons P:* Emergency medical technician: making the difference, *St Louis, 2007, Mosby-Elsevier.*

Pulse oximeters should not be the only tool for confirming placement of an endotracheal tube. Data from the device are too slow and unreliable as a source of feedback and decision making. Additionally, most patients intubated by EMTs will be in cardiac arrest, limiting the value of pulse oximetry. In patients who have effective perfusion, however, the pulse oximeter is an important continuous-monitoring device that is used with other signs of hypoxia to guide you in the care of the patient.

Humidification

A humidifier is a water-filled bottle that moisturizes the inspired oxygen. It is useful for loosening secretions and preventing drying of the airway. In some system protocols, humidified oxygen is preferred for the treatment of children (to help loosen secretions), when available, and for conditions such as smoke inhalation. However, short periods of O_2 administration without humidification are not harmful.

When humidification is used, you should take care to prevent contamination of the humidification device. The device should be changed after each use.

> **LEARNING OBJECTIVES**
> - List the steps in performing mouth-to-stoma artificial ventilation.
> - Demonstrate bag-mask artificial ventilations for the infant and child.
> - Demonstrate oxygen delivery for the infant and child.

Special Patient Populations

Patients with Stomas

You may encounter patients who have a permanent or temporary breathing tube or opening in their trachea or larynx. These artificial permanent openings, called **stomas,** are also named for their location: **tracheostomy,** when the opening is in the trachea, and **laryngectomy,** when part of the larynx has been removed. The stoma or the tube protruding through it may become obstructed with secretions and require suctioning. If these patients require positive-pressure ventilation, you can breathe directly through the opening or through the tube. To ventilate the stoma, an infant or child mask should be used

and placed directly over the stoma (**Figure 6-26**). Extension of the head and neck is not necessary during stoma ventilation. Squeeze the bag as usual and observe chest rise. If you are unable to breathe through the stoma, attempt to breathe through the upper airway. Some patients still have communication with the upper airway and may be effectively ventilated with the techniques previously described. With these patients, you may need to cover the opening of the stoma during ventilation through the mouth and nose.

If the patient has a tube coming out of the stoma (tracheostomy tube), you can attach a bag-mask device directly to the tube and ventilate (**Figure 6-27**).

Infants and Children

The airway in infants and children differs in important ways from that of an adult:
- The internal diameter of a child's airway is smaller at all levels: from the nose and mouth and pharynx, through the larynx and trachea, and extending through the bronchi and bronchioles.
- The tongue is also larger in relation to the airway and thus has greater potential to cause obstruction.
- The narrowest part of a child's airway is at the ring formed by the cricoid cartilage. In the adult airway the vocal cords are the narrowest part of the airway.
- The cartilage that forms the larynx and trachea in the child is softer than the firm cartilage in the adult, an important fact to consider during opening of the pediatric airway.
- Because the chest wall is softer, infants and children tend to depend more on the action of the diaphragm muscle for breathing.

These differences in the infant and child airway have practical implications in airway management. For example, the head position for opening the airway varies with age. For infants (<1 year) the head is placed in the sniffing or neutral position to avoid bending and kinking the soft trachea. For toddlers and small children (1-8 years) the neck is extended slightly but not hyperextended. The relatively large tongue in the child makes maneuvers to keep the tongue from obstructing the airway especially important. For example, when inserting an OPA, a tongue blade is used to displace the tongue. Rotating the OPA in the usual manner may damage the soft tissues of the child's palate.

Given the small size of an infant's airway, small obstructions (e.g., swelling, mucus) can result in significant blockage of airflow. Although 1 to 2 mm of airway edema in an adult may be inconsequential, it becomes a significant obstruction in an infant.

Infants prefer to breathe through the nose. In fact, infants are considered obligate nose breathers. Blockage of the nasal passages from mucus or swelling can significantly narrow the airway and increase a baby's work of breathing. If an infant with an upper respiratory infection (e.g., common cold) also has a disease of the lower airway, this blockage in the nasal pharynx may be sufficient to worsen the baby's condition. Suctioning the baby's nasal passages with a bulb suction or soft catheter with low to medium suction may significantly improve the condition. Humidification of supplemental oxygen that the child breathes can also help by loosening any encrusted mucus or secretions.

When providing bag-mask ventilation to an infant or child, you must adjust your technique to account for the decreased size and differences in the airway. For the infant, place the head in the neutral position; for a child, place the head with slight extension. You should never hyperextend the neck of an infant or a child. As with the adult, squeeze the bag only enough to initiate chest rise. This is particularly important with infants and children because they are prone to gastric distention. If the bag-mask has a pop-off valve, you may need to disable this valve to achieve effective ventilation. Most authorities recommend that a bag-mask device used for resuscitation should have either an override feature for the pop-off (pressure release) valve, to use high pressures when necessary to ventilate the patient adequately, or no pop-off valve at all. For example, a child with an incomplete upper airway obstruction, such as croup, may require higher pressures to overcome the higher resistance from the narrowed airway. If a pop-off valve was not disabled in such a case, air would be released through the valve rather than into the patient.

Case in Point

You are called to a health clinic where a 2-year-old girl has shortness of breath. She was awake most of the night with a barking cough, and the mother took her by bus to the clinic at 9 AM. You hear stridor and note nasal flaring and suprasternal and intercostal retractions. She is lethargic, and the clinic states her respirations are slowing to 12 per minute. You begin to administer supplemental ventilation with a bag-mask, timing the positive-pressure ventilation with the patient's own effort. The air seems to escape from the pressure release valve. You turn off the valve and see the chest rise with subsequent breaths.

Patients with Facial Injuries

Because of the rich blood supply to the face, blunt injuries can cause severe bleeding. This can make airway management very difficult. Suctioning should be readily available for patients with facial injuries, and bleeding in the cheek and mouth area can be controlled with direct pressure. You may need to turn the head of the patient to aid drainage.

Patients with Dental Appliances

As a rule, dentures should remain in place during standard airway management. Dentures give form to the face and help create a better seal with a mask device (e.g., bag-mask). If a patient has dentures or other dental appliance, watch that the appliance does not become loose or obstruct the airway. If the dental appliance becomes dislodged during care, you should remove it and continue ventilating the patient.

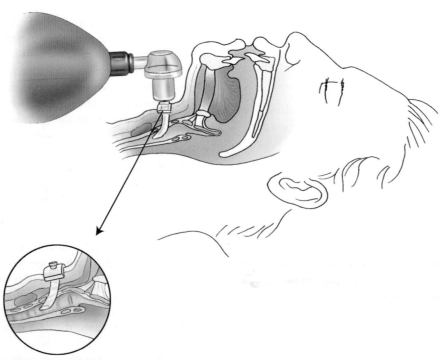

Figure 6-27 Ventilating through a stoma with a bag-mask device and tracheostomy tube. *From McSwain N, Paturas J: The basic EMT: comprehensive prehospital patient care, St Louis, 2003, Mosby.*

Patients with Chronic Obstructive Pulmonary Disease

Control of breathing is both conscious and unconscious. Although we do not ordinarily think about breathing, we have the ability to take a deep breath or hold our breath at will. Most of the time, however, breathing is controlled by centers in the brain and brainstem that react to messages from the body's receptors in the brain about the amount of oxygen, carbon dioxide, and acid in the blood. If the blood O_2 level is too low or if CO_2 levels are too high, the brain will direct an increase in rate and depth of ventilation.

The unconscious control is so strong that it can override our conscious input over breathing. For example, hold your breath and notice the drive that eventually forces you to take your next breath. The ordinary control of ventilatory drive is the CO_2 level in the blood. When CO_2 level rises, the brainstem directs an increase in respiratory rate to eliminate the "excess" CO_2 and return the level to normal. When there is a chronic CO_2 buildup caused by severe and long-standing lung disease, the brain may become desensitized to carbon dioxide. In this circumstance, low oxygen content in the blood is the main stimulus to breathe.

Knowledge of the respiratory drive control can be helpful during oxygen therapy. Some patients with **chronic obstructive pulmonary disease (COPD)** may have very high CO_2 levels, and their drive to breathe is based on low O_2 levels in the blood. These patients are likely to have respiratory emergencies and require supplemental oxygen. Administering high concentrations of oxygen can increase the blood O_2 level to a point where the drive to take a breath is turned off, possibly resulting in hypoventilation or even respiratory arrest. Thus, when treating patients with COPD, oxygen should be administered with close monitoring of the patients' ventilations.

When patients with COPD are severely hypoxic, in shock, or in respiratory distress, high-concentration oxygen should be administered with monitoring of the patient for possible respiratory depression or arrest. If the patient starts to hypoventilate, give positive-pressure ventilation.

LEARNING OBJECTIVE
- Describe the signs of foreign body airway obstruction.

Airway Obstruction

When you encounter a patient with complete airway obstruction or partial airway obstruction with poor air exchange, you should perform basic life support airway obstruction procedures in an attempt to clear the obstruction. If basic life support maneuvers are unsuccessful after three cycles, you should rapidly transport the patient to the hospital, continuing your efforts en route.

Choking

Severe obstruction of the airway can cause death within minutes. Obstructions of the airway can occur from several mechanisms. The tongue may obstruct the pharynx because of relaxation of the muscles of the lower jaw. This is the most common cause of airway obstruction. The epiglottis can block entrance of the airway in unconscious victims. Bleeding from head and facial injuries or regurgitation of stomach contents may also obstruct the upper airway, particularly if the patient is unconscious. The airway may also obstruct when there is swelling of the tissues of the face, neck, or internal airway associated with an anaphylactic reaction, epiglottitis, or croup.

Choking in adults caused by foreign bodies usually occurs during eating when food becomes lodged in the pharynx, glottis (opening of the vocal cords), or trachea. However, a variety of other foreign bodies can cause choking in children and adults.

Recognition of Airway Obstruction

Encounters with conscious victims of severe airway obstruction by a foreign body are rare for EMTs because the obstruction is usually cleared before their arrival, or the patient becomes unconscious from hypoxia. However, you may occasionally witness an episode of choking.

Foreign bodies may cause either mild or severe airway obstruction. With *mild* airway obstruction, the victim is responsive and can cough forcefully and may be able to talk, although frequently there is wheezing between coughs. As long as signs of mild airway obstruction continue, the victim should be encouraged to continue coughing and breathing efforts. At this point, you should not interfere with the victim's own attempts to expel the foreign body but should stay with the victim and monitor these attempts.

The victim with choking may immediately demonstrate mild airway obstruction that progresses to severe. Signs of *severe* (or complete) airway obstruction include a weak, ineffective cough, high-pitched noises while inhaling, increased respiratory difficulty, an inability to talk, and possibly cyanosis.

With severe (or complete) airway obstruction, the victim is unable to speak, breathe, or cough and may clutch the neck with the thumb and fingers. Movement of air is absent. Ask the victim, "Are you choking?" If the victim cannot speak, provide abdominal thrusts. If the airway obstruction is not relieved, the victim's blood oxygen saturation will fall rapidly because the obstructed airway prevents entry of air into the lungs. The victim will become unresponsive, and death will follow rapidly if prompt action is not taken.

Relief of Choking

The abdominal thrust is recommended for relief of choking. By elevating the diaphragm, an abdominal thrust can force air from the lungs. Each individual thrust should be administered with the intent of relieving the obstruction. It may be necessary to repeat the thrust multiple times to clear the airway. Care should be taken during performance of abdominal thrusts because it is possible to damage internal organs, such as a rupture or laceration of the abdominal or thoracic viscera, during the maneuver.

Abdominal Thrusts with Victim Standing or Sitting

Stand behind the victim, wrap your arms around the victim's waist, and proceed as follows. Make a fist with one hand. Place the thumb side of your fist against the victim's abdomen, in the midline slightly above the navel and well below the tip of the xiphoid process. Grasp the fist with your other hand, and press the fist into the victim's abdomen with a quick upward thrust. Repeat the thrusts until the object is expelled from the airway or the victim becomes unresponsive. Each new thrust should be a separate and distinct movement, administered with the intent of relieving the obstruction (**Skill 6-10**).

If a person is too short to reach around the waist of a responsive victim, abdominal thrusts may be performed with the victim sitting or lying down.

Abdominal Thrusts with Responsive Victim Lying Down

Place the victim in the supine position (face up). Kneel astride the victim's thighs, and place the heel of one hand against the victim's abdomen, in the midline slightly above the navel and well below the tip of the xiphoid. Place your second hand directly on top of the first. Press both hands into the abdomen with quick upward thrusts. If you are in the correct position, your arms will be positioned over the midabdomen, unlikely to direct the thrust to the right or left. You can use your body weight to perform the maneuver (see Skill 6-10).

Chest Thrusts with Victim Standing or Sitting

Chest thrusts may be used as an alternative to the abdominal thrust when the victim is in the late stages of pregnancy or is extremely obese. Stand behind the victim, with your arms directly under the victim's armpits, and encircle the chest. Place the thumb side of one fist on the lower half of the victim's sternum (in the same location as a chest compression), taking care to avoid the xiphoid process and the margins of the rib cage. Grab the fist with your other hand and perform backward thrusts until the foreign body is expelled or the victim becomes unresponsive (see Skill 6-10).

Chest Thrusts with Responsive Victim Lying Down

This maneuver may be used when the victim is in the late stages of pregnancy or when the person cannot apply abdominal thrusts effectively to an unconscious, extremely obese victim. The person should place the victim on his or her back and kneel close to the victim's side. The hand position and technique for the application of chest thrusts are the same as for chest compressions during cardiopulmonary resuscitation (CPR). In the adult, for example, the heel of the hand is on the lower half of the sternum. Each thrust should be delivered with the intent of relieving the obstruction.

Finger Sweep and Tongue-Jaw Lift

The *finger sweep* should be used only in the unresponsive victim with a foreign body airway obstruction. This sweep should not be performed if the victim is having seizures.

With the victim face up, open the mouth by grasping both the tongue and the lower jaw between the thumb and fingers and lifting the mandible *(tongue-jaw lift)*. This action draws the tongue away from the back of the throat and from a foreign body that may be lodged there. This maneuver alone may be sufficient to relieve an obstruction. If you see an object, insert the index finger of your other hand down along the inside of the cheek and deeply into the victim's throat, to the base of the tongue. Then use a hooking action to dislodge the foreign body and maneuver it into the mouth so that it can be removed. It

is sometimes necessary to use the index finger to push the foreign body against the opposite side of the throat to dislodge and remove it. If the foreign body comes within reach, grasp and remove it. Be careful to avoid forcing the object deeper into the airway.

Relief of Foreign Body Airway Obstruction in Unresponsive Victim

Victims of foreign body airway obstruction may initially be responsive and then may become unresponsive. In this circumstance, you will know that a foreign body airway obstruction is the cause of the victim's symptoms. Victims of foreign body airway obstruction may be unresponsive when initially encountered by the EMT. In this circumstance, the EMT will probably not know that the victim has a foreign body airway obstruction until repeated attempts at rescue breathing are unsuccessful.

If a victim of choking collapses and becomes unresponsive, perform CPR. When opening the airway, perform a tongue-jaw lift and look for the object. If you see it, remove using a finger sweep. If you cannot see it, continue attempts at rescue breathing and chest compressions.

If you encounter a victim of choking who is unresponsive, you may not know it until you ventilate. At that point, you will feel resistance to airflow, and there will be no chest rise. If this occurs, reopen the airway and try again. If air does not go in (no chest rise), start CPR. Each time you open the airway, look for the foreign body. If you see it, remove it using a finger sweep (see Skill 6-10).

Foreign body airway obstruction in infants and children is discussed in Chapter 25.

Scenario Follow-up

The elderly patient with a history of congestive heart failure is having another episode of pulmonary edema. His lung sounds reveal crackles throughout both lung fields. The frothy sputum is another finding consistent with excess fluid in the lungs. Administration of high-concentration oxygen increased the amount of O_2 crossing the wet alveoli, improving O_2 saturation of hemoglobin, as noted by the increased pulse oximetry reading and the patient no longer being cyanotic.

Summary

Airway and breathing are evaluated in every patient as part of the initial assessment. Signs of adequate versus inadequate breathing are actively sought. Assessment of mental status, muscle tone, and air movement, as well as central cyanosis, helps distinguish patients with respiratory distress from those with respiratory failure. Patients with respiratory failure require positive-pressure ventilation.

For all patients, knowing when and how to maintain the airway and administer positive-pressure ventilation and supplemental oxygen are keys to management. Initial airway management is performed by using manual maneuvers such as the head-tilt/chin-lift and jaw thrust, and suctioning if necessary. When continuous airway control is needed, the insertion of an oropharyngeal or nasopharyngeal airway may be necessary. Positive-pressure ventilation with supplemental oxygen is provided by methods such as mouth-to-mask or two-person bag-mask, when possible, while observing chest rise. Supplemental oxygen should be administered as soon as possible in the care of patients according to the needs of the given patient. Patients who are in respiratory distress or in shock usually require a high concentration of oxygen delivered by the nonrebreather mask. During ongoing assessment, you should evaluate the patient to ensure adequate oxygenation and ventilation.

Skills

Skill | 6-1   *Suctioning*

RIGID CATHETER

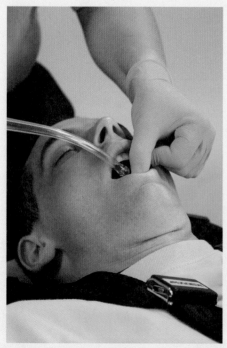

1. Connect the rigid catheter to the suction line. Turn on the suction unit, and ensure the presence of negative pressure.

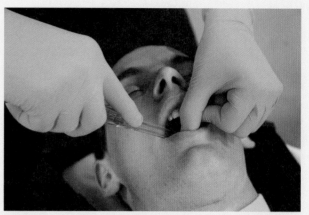

3. Initiate suctioning by closing off the hole on the rigid catheter or turning on the suction device. Suction from side to side for no more than 15 seconds.

SOFT CATHETER

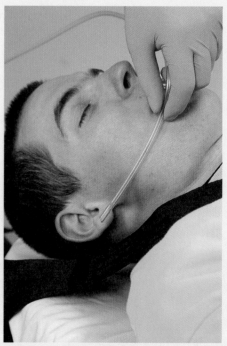

1. Use personal precautions. Attach the soft catheter, and measure it from the corner of the mouth to the earlobe.

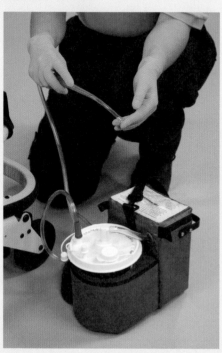

2. Using personal precautions, open the patient's mouth by the cross-finger technique. Place the tip of the catheter into the posterior pharynx.

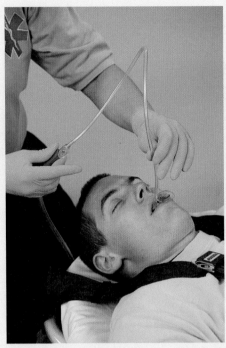

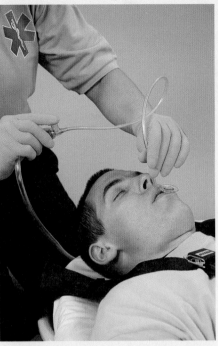

2. Insert the catheter into the oral cavity without suction. Insert only to the base of the tongue.

3. Apply suction. Move the catheter tip from side to side in a twisting motion. Suction for no more than 15 seconds at a time. If necessary, rinse the catheter and tubing with water to prevent obstruction from dried material.

Skill | 6-2   ***Inserting an Oropharyngeal Airway (OPA)***

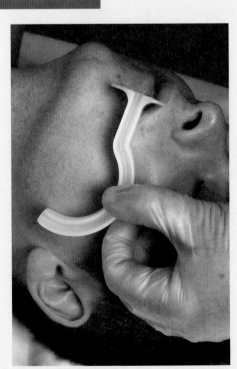

1. Use personal precautions. Measure the airway from the corner of the mouth to the angle of the jaw to ensure proper sizing.

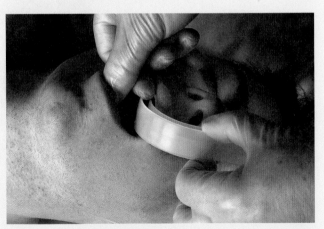

2. Place the index finger of one hand on the top teeth and the thumb on the lower teeth; apply pressure in opposite directions. Insert the device into the mouth with the tip pointing toward the roof of the mouth.

Continued

Skill | 6-2   *Inserting an Oropharyngeal Airway (OPA)—cont'd*

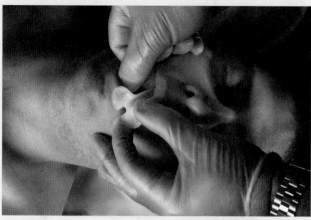

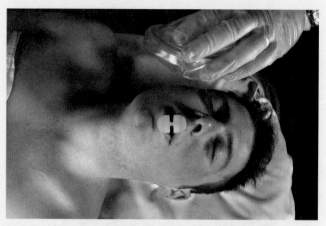

3. Advance the OPA along the hard palate until you reach the soft palate, then rotate into position. If the patient begins to gag, remove the airway immediately, and do not attempt reinsertion; this could result in vomiting and aspiration. Insert the OPA without undue interruption of ventilation. Generally, ventilations should not be interrupted for more than 10 seconds.

4. Once the airway is in place, test the patency by ventilating the patient, or look, listen, and feel for breathing. If you cannot ventilate the patient, remove the airway, maintain manual maneuvers, and reinsert the device when possible.

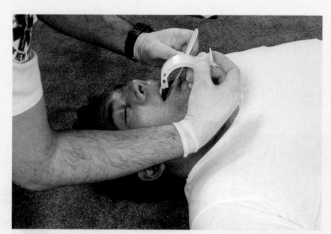

5. The OPA can also be inserted by restraining the tongue with a tongue blade and inserting the device while following the normal curvature of the mouth and pharynx.

Skill | 6-3 *Inserting a Nasopharyngeal Airway (NPA)*

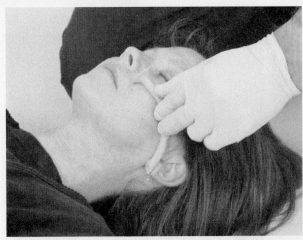

1. Use personal precautions. Measure the airway from the nose to the angle of the jaw to ensure proper sizing.

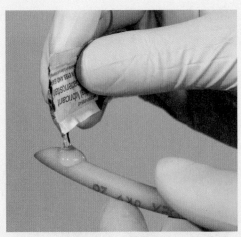

2. Lubricate the outside of the tube with a water-soluble gel to decrease irritation to the nasal passage and to ease insertion.

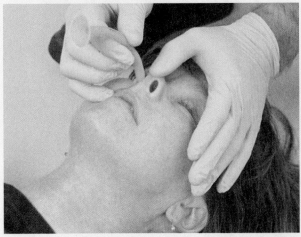

3. Slowly insert the NPA into the nasal passage with the bevel facing toward the septum. Do not force it in or nasal bleeding may occur, resulting in potential aspiration. Gentle, firm pressure sometimes results in dilation of one nasal passage and facilitates insertion. If you cannot successfully insert the tube in one nostril, try the opposite nostril.

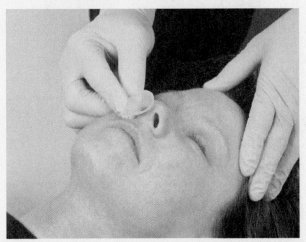

4. Once the airway is in place, test the patency by ventilating the patient, or look, listen, and feel for breathing. If you cannot ventilate the patient, remove the airway, maintain manual maneuvers, and reinsert the device when possible.

Skill | 6-4   *Mouth-to-Mask Device*

METHOD 1: NO SUSPECTED SPINAL INJURY

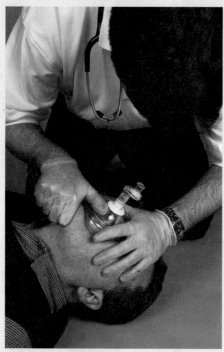

1. Position yourself adjacent to the patient's head. Apply the mask to the patient's face using the bridge of the patient's nose as a guide for correct position. The mask should be connected to high-flow oxygen at 15 L/min.

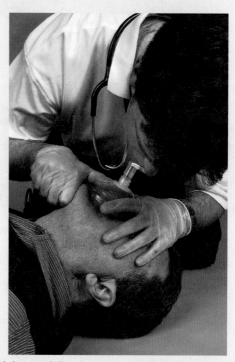

2. Seal the mask by placing your index finger and thumb of the hand closer to the top of the patient's head along the border of the mask and placing the thumb of your other hand along the lower margin of the mask. Place the remaining fingers of your other hand along the bony margin of the patient's jaw.

Lift the jaw while performing the head-tilt/chin-lift maneuver. Compress firmly and completely around the outside margin of the mask to provide a tight seal. Give slow breaths by blowing your exhaled air into the one-way valve attached to the mask. Breaths should be given over 2 seconds. The patient's chest should rise with each breath.

METHOD 2: SUSPECTED SPINAL INJURY

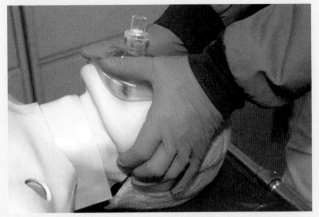

1. Position yourself directly above the patient's head. Apply the mask to the patient's face using the bridge of the patient's nose as a guide for correct position. Use the thumb and heel of each of your hands to make a complete seal around the edge of the mask. Use your remaining fingers to lift the angle of the jaw.

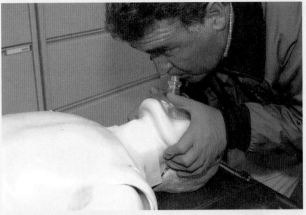

2. While lifting the jaw, squeeze the mask with your thumbs and heels of your hands to achieve an airtight seal between the mask and the patient's face. Give slow breaths by blowing your exhaled air into the one-way valve attached to the mask. Breaths should be given over 1 second. The patient's chest should rise with each breath.

Skill | 6-5   *Bag-Mask Ventilation*

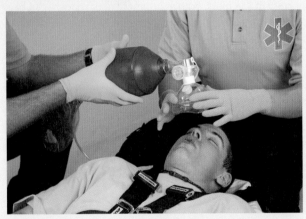

1. After opening the patient's airway, insert the correct size of oral or nasal airway device, and attach the correct mask size (adult, infant, or child). The EMT at the patient's head places a hand on each side of the mask.

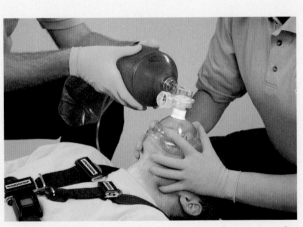

2. Maintaining a head-tilt/chin-lift position, the EMT at the patient's head places the mask on the patient's face, creating a seal around the patient's nose and mouth.

Continued

Skill | 6-5   *Bag-Mask Ventilation—cont'd*

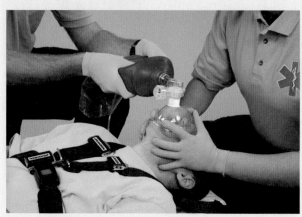

3. Connect the bag-mask to high-flow oxygen if not already done. A second EMT squeezes the bag, watching for chest rise.

4. If a neck injury is suspected, use the jaw thrust; the thumbs seal the mask to the patient's face, and the fingers lift the jaw forward.

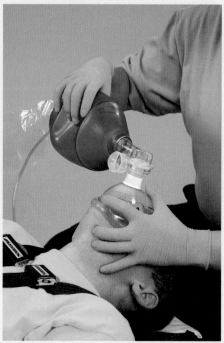

5. If you are the only EMT present, use one hand to grasp the mask with your thumb and index finger, placing the mask on the patient's face, and using your other fingers to bring the jaw up to the mask. With your other hand, squeeze the bag, watching for chest rise. You may need to use your leg to be able to deflate the bag-mask completely.

Skill | 6-6   *Setting Up an Oxygen System*

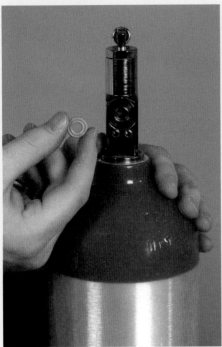

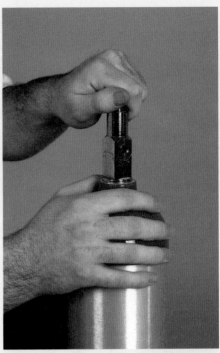

1. Confirm that the cylinder contains oxygen by identifying the color and pin index grouping. Check to ensure a rubber washer (the O-ring) is in place at either the cylinder opening or the regulator opening.

2. To clear dust from the opening, open the main valve at the top of the cylinder slowly until gas starts to come out, then immediately close the valve.

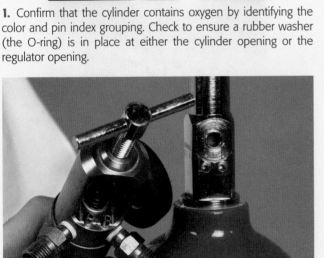

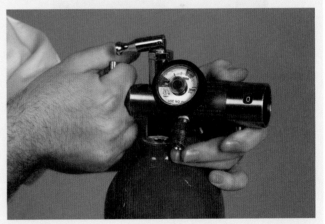

3. Attach the regulator by carefully aligning the pin index from the regulator into the cylinder holes.

4. Tighten the clamp with firm hand pressure to ensure an adequate seal.

Continued

Skill | 6-6 *Setting Up an Oxygen System—cont'd*

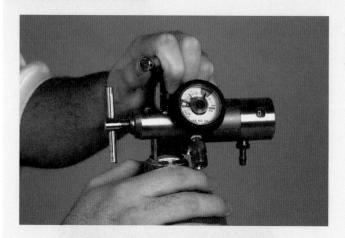

5. Open the valve two full turns. Check the pressure gauge, which should record approximately 2000 psi. If the cylinder leaks, turn off the main valve, and check the connection and firmness of the attachment.

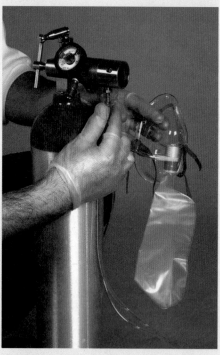

6. Attach the tubing or delivery device to the regulator and adjust liter flow.

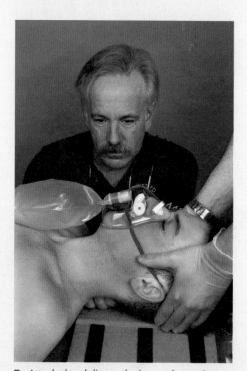

7. Attach the delivery device to the patient.

Skill | 6-7   *Discontinuing an Oxygen System*

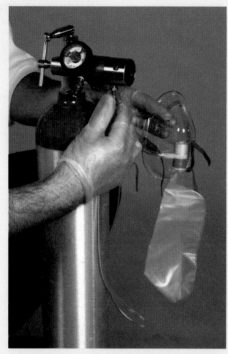

1. Remove the oxygen delivery device from the patient. Turn off the flow of oxygen.

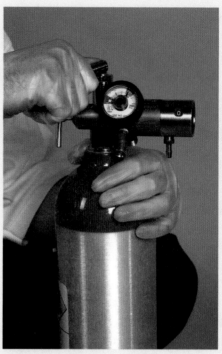

2. Turn off the main valve at the top of the cylinder.

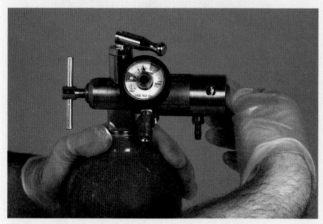

3. Open the flowmeter valve to bleed oxygen out of the system.

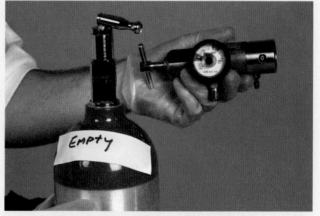

4. Detach the regulator by loosening the clamp; mark the cylinder as empty, and store in the appropriate area.

Skill | 6-8 *Applying a Nasal Cannula*

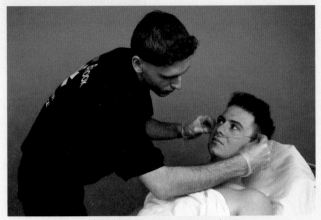

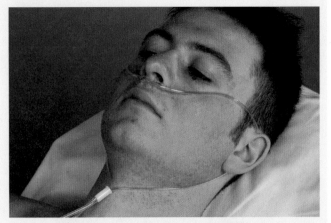

1. Use personal precautions. Place the nasal cannula prongs into the nares.

2. Guide the tubing around the patient's ears and under the chin. Adjust the fit of the device under the chin.

Skill | 6-9 *Applying a Nonrebreather Mask*

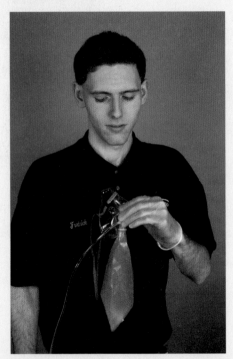

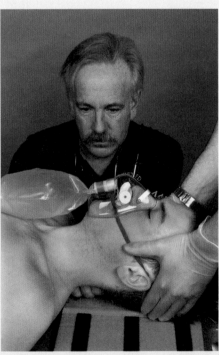

1. Use personal precautions. Prefill the reservoir bag with oxygen by placing two fingers inside the mask and closing off the valve.

2. Extend the elastic strap, and place the mask over the patient's head. Cinch the metal band on the patient's nose, and adjust the elastic strap to fit the patient.

Skill | 6-10   *Adult Choking*

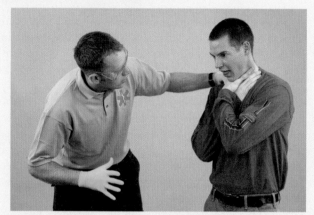

1. Ask, "Are you choking?"

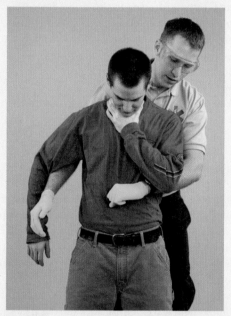

2. Move behind the choking victim, and place one hand on the person's abdomen above the umbilicus and below the ribs. Reach around the victim with your other hand and grab the first hand, holding firmly.

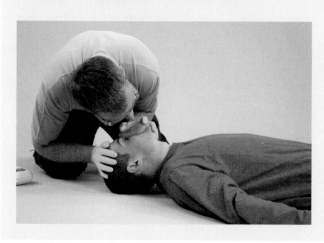

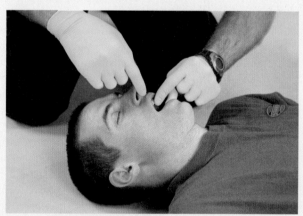

3. Give abdominal thrusts. (Use chest thrusts for pregnant or obese victims.) Repeat thrusts until object is expelled or the victim becomes unresponsive.

4. If the victim becomes unresponsive, help the person safely to the ground. Perform a tongue-jaw lift, followed by a finger sweep to remove the object if you see it.

5. Attempt to ventilate the patient.

6. If unable to ventilate, begin CPR (see Skill 12-2). Every time you attempt a breath, look for the object and remove it if you see it.

7. Repeat steps 4, 5, and 6 until effective.

The Bottom Line

Learning Checklist

✓ The respiratory system brings oxygen into the body and rids the body of carbon dioxide, the waste product.

✓ The respiratory system is composed of the nose and mouth, nasopharynx and oropharynx, larynx and epiglottis, trachea, bronchi, bronchioles, alveoli, and lungs.

✓ The diaphragm and the muscles of the chest cause the thoracic cavity to expand and contract like a bellows to create airflow during ventilation. Inhalation occurs when the diaphragm and intercostal muscles contract and enlarge the thoracic cavity. Exhalation occurs when the diaphragm and intercostals relax, decreasing the size of the thoracic cavity.

✓ Oxygen and carbon dioxide exchange occurs at the level of the alveoli and capillaries through the process of diffusion.

✓ During strenuous exercise or with respiratory disease or trauma, the accessory muscles of breathing help to increase the respiratory volumes.

✓ Adequate breathing is characterized by a normal respiratory rate (adult, 12-20; child, 15-30; infant, 25-50 breaths/min), regular rhythm, and normal quality of breathing (breath sounds present and equal, chest expansion adequate and equal).

✓ Inadequate breathing is characterized by a respiratory rate outside the normal range, irregular rhythm, and abnormal quality of breathing (breath sounds diminished or absent, chest expansion inadequate or shallow, or use of accessory muscles). Other signs of inadequate breathing include pale, cool, or cyanotic skin; retractions; nasal flaring; seesaw breathing; and agonal respirations.

✓ Respiratory distress involves a breathing problem requiring increased work of breathing to ensure adequate oxygenation and ventilation. Signs of respiratory distress include increased respiratory rate, accessory muscle use, nasal flaring, and assumption of a position to aid the muscles of breathing (tripod position or sitting bolt upright). A patient with respiratory distress may have difficulty speaking in complete sentences but is able to maintain mental status and muscle tone and to move air.

✓ Respiratory failure is inadequate ventilation to support life. The patient in respiratory failure is not able to maintain mental status or muscle tone and is unable to move adequate amounts of air to the lungs. Patients with respiratory failure require positive-pressure ventilation.

✓ Respiratory arrest is the complete cessation of breathing. Respiratory failure can progress to respiratory arrest and, if untreated, to cardiac arrest. Respiratory arrest can occur suddenly from conditions such as electrocution, lightning strikes, or spinal cord injury.

✓ The airway is opened by using the head-tilt/chin-lift or the jaw thrust for patients with suspected spinal injury or when the mechanism of injury is unknown.

✓ Suctioning can be used to clear liquid or small solid secretions with a soft or rigid catheter. You should never suction for more than 15 seconds. You may need to turn the patient's head to aid drainage. Log-roll the body as a unit if spinal injury is suspected.

✓ An oropharyngeal airway can be used for a patient who is unconscious or has no gag reflex to keep the tongue away from the back of the pharynx when ventilation devices are used.

✓ A nasopharyngeal airway can be used to maintain the tongue away from the back of the pharynx when the patient cannot tolerate an oropharyngeal airway.

✓ Positive-pressure ventilation can be provided by using a mouth-to-mask device, bag-mask device, or a flow-restricted, oxygen-powered ventilation device.

✓ Mouth-to-mask ventilation is a reliable method of positive-pressure ventilation because it allows the EMT to create a mask seal with two hands, feel the compliance of the chest wall during rescue breaths, and administer supplemental oxygen.

✓ Bag-mask ventilation is the most common method of positive-pressure ventilation used in emergency care. Adequate tidal volumes must be ensured because a mask seal leak may reduce the volume of air delivered to the patient. The two-person approach to bag-mask ventilation helps reduce the chance for mask seal leak and ensure adequate tidal volumes.

✓ Cricoid pressure can be used to compress the esophagus and prevent gastric inflation during positive-pressure ventilation.

✓ Oxygen is stored in green steel or aluminum cylinders (size D, E, or M) and used with regulators to deliver gas to administration devices.

✓ The two most common free-flow oxygen devices used to deliver supplemental oxygen include the nasal cannula (24%-40% oxygen) and nonrebreather mask (up to 90% oxygen).

✓ Pulse oximetry is a useful adjunct to assess oxygen saturation of the blood. In general, oxygen saturation is 95% or greater; if it is below 90% when the patient is receiving high-concentration oxygen, positive-pressure ventilation may be indicated.

✓ When delivering supplemental oxygen to patients with chronic obstructive pulmonary disease (COPD), be prepared to assist with positive-pressure ventilations because some patients may have hypoventilation from high-concentration oxygen.

✓ Patients with a laryngectomy or stoma can be ventilated directly through the opening in the neck to provide positive-pressure ventilation.

✓ Basic life support airway obstruction procedures are performed to clear a foreign object.

✓ Choking in adults caused by foreign bodies usually occurs during eating.

✓ Signs of severe (or complete) airway obstruction include a weak ineffective cough, high-pitched noises while inhaling, increased respiratory difficulty, and inability to talk and possibly cyanosis.

✓ Abdominal thrusts are recommended for relief of choking.

✓ When treating patients with COPD, oxygen should be administered with close monitoring of the patient's ventilations.

Key Terms

Accessory muscles of respiration Group of muscles found in the neck and abdomen that facilitate forced inhalation and exhalation in patients in respiratory distress.

Agonal breathing Irregular gasping breaths that can be seen during the early onset of cardiac arrest.

Asthma Acute obstructive respiratory disease with narrowing of the lower airways; often precipitated by infection or an allergic response.

Bag-mask device Mechanical aid used to administer positive-pressure ventilation; usually consists of a bag with oxygen inlet, unidirectional valve, mask, and oxygen reservoir.

Chronic obstructive pulmonary disease (COPD) Long-term lung disease in which air becomes trapped in the alveoli as a result of bronchospasm, mucus plugs, or collapse of the bronchioles. Greater force is needed for these patients to exhale.

Cricoid pressure Compression of the esophagus between the cricoid cartilage and the thoracic spine to reduce the chances of air entering the esophagus during positive-pressure ventilation and help prevent gastric distention and regurgitation.

Cyanosis Bluish discoloration of the mucous membranes or skin caused by oxygen-depleted hemoglobin.

Dyspnea Difficulty breathing.

Emphysema Disease caused by a destruction of alveoli and the loss of elastic recoil within the lung; a type of COPD.

Epiglottitis Inflammation of the epiglottis, usually caused by a bacterial infection; usually affects children but can be seen in adults. Severe cases can cause obstruction of the trachea.

Flow-restricted, oxygen-powered ventilation device Manually triggered positive-pressure ventilator administered by using oxygen under pressure.

Grunting Rhythmic sound heard at the end of exhalation; a key sign of respiratory distress in infants.

Laryngectomy Surgical removal of part of the larynx.

Minute volume Total volume of air inhaled in a minute; tidal volume multiplied by respiratory rate.

Nasal cannula Low-flow oxygen delivery system consisting of a thin tube with prongs at the end that slip into the nares, capable of delivering 24% to 40% oxygen.

Nasal flaring Characteristic flaring of the nostrils in infants and small children that suggests the presence of respiratory distress.

Nasopharyngeal airway (NPA) Soft rubber tube that extends from the nares down into the oropharynx, used to elevate the tongue away from the oropharynx.

Nonrebreather mask Low-flow, high-concentration oxygen (O_2) delivery device consisting of a reservoir bag (of O_2) beneath a one-way valve that prevents the patient from exhaling into the bag; used when high O_2 concentrations are needed, up to 90%.

Oropharyngeal airway (OPA) Mechanical airway device designed to elevate the tongue away from the oropharynx when the patient is unconscious.

Pin index safety system Safety system of gas cylinders that allows tanks of different types of gas to accept special regulators designed specifically for that gas.

Pleuritic chest pain Pain made worse by breathing.

Positive-pressure ventilation The act of forcing air into the lungs.

Pulse oximetry Measurement of hemoglobin oxygenation by a pulse oximeter; read as percentage oxygen saturation.

Rescue breathing Providing artificial ventilation for patients who cannot breathe on their own.

Respiratory arrest Cessation of breathing.

Respiratory distress Condition in which there is an increased work of breathing.

Respiratory failure State that results when the respiratory system becomes so ineffective that it can no longer support life.

Retractions The drawing in of soft tissues between the ribs, above the clavicle, and below the sternum; retractions reflect increased work of breathing.

Seesaw breathing Physical finding in small children and infants characterized by alternate use of abdominal and chest wall muscles and indicating respiratory distress.

Stoma Permanent opening in the trachea or larynx.

Stridor Harsh, high-pitched sound created by air flowing through a narrowed upper airway, usually heard on inspiration.

Tachypnea Rapid breathing.

Tracheostomy Surgical opening of the trachea to provide an airway.

Wheezing High-pitched whistling sounds created by narrowed bronchioles.

Review Questions

1. To prevent aspiration, which of the following structures covers the trachea during swallowing?
   a. Pharynx
   b. Epiglottis
   c. Thyroid cartilage
   d. Cricoid cartilage

2. Which respiratory structure can be palpated just superior to the sternum?
   a. Bronchus
   b. Trachea
   c. Epiglottis
   d. Larynx

3. Which of the following terms refers to the amount of air inhaled and exhaled during one breath?
   a. Residual volume
   b. Minute volume
   c. Total volume
   d. Tidal volume

4. Which term refers to a bluish discoloration of the skin caused by oxygen-depleted hemoglobin?
   a. Jaundice
   b. Pallor
   c. Cyanosis
   d. Anoxic erythema

5. Which terms refers to a high-pitched sound emitted from a narrowed upper airway that usually occurs on inspiration?
   a. Wheezing
   b. Stridor
   c. Grunting
   d. Crackles

6. When performing positive-pressure ventilation, you can check for effective ventilation based on which of the following?
   a. Chest rise
   b. Skin color
   c. Pupil response
   d. None of the above

7. Which of the following is the most common problem with excessive ventilation?
   a. Pneumothorax
   b. Gastric distention
   c. Oxygen toxicity
   d. Air embolism

8. Which oxygen administration device provides the highest oxygen delivery to the patient?
   a. Nasal cannula
   b. Pocket mask
   c. Nonrebreather mask
   d. Simple face mask

9. Patients with respiratory distress would most likely receive all the following treatments *except:*
   a. Supplemental oxygen
   b. Transport in the position of comfort
   c. Positive-pressure ventilation
   d. Suctioning of the airway

10. Which of the following criteria best distinguish respiratory failure from respiratory distress?
    a. Gurgling, shortness of breath, accessory muscle use
    b. Increased respiratory rate, pale clammy skin, wheezing
    c. Depressed mental status, poor muscle tone, cyanosis
    d. Nasal flaring, seesaw breathing, gurgling

11. The treatment for respiratory failure includes which of the following?
    a. Positive-pressure ventilation
    b. Supplemental oxygen
    c. Maintaining an open airway
    d. All of the above

12. After inserting an oropharyngeal airway (OPA), what should you do if the patient begins to gag and choke?
    a. Remove the airway
    b. Use a smaller airway
    c. Lubricate the airway
    d. Tape the airway in place

13. When sizing an OPA, measure from the corner of the patient's mouth to the:
    a. Angle of the jaw
    b. Top of the ear
    c. Cheekbone
    d. Trachea

14. The major complication of one EMT using a bag-mask device is:
    a. Overventilation and pneumothorax
    b. Low tidal volumes caused by leakage from mask seal
    c. Rupture of the bag during exhalation
    d. Valve failure caused by clogging

15. A bag-mask used with an oxygen reservoir is capable of achieving a maximum of approximately _____ oxygen delivery to the patient's airway.
    a. 40% to 60%
    b. 50% to 60%
    c. 70% to 90%
    d. 90% to 100%

16. When suctioning the upper airway, activate the negative pressure:
    a. When the tip is in the oropharynx
    b. Before insertion
    c. At the entrance of the mouth
    d. Halfway between the teeth and the pharynx

17. A patient with a respiratory emergency who is extremely cyanotic and lethargic would be best treated with which of the following devices?
    a. Nasal cannula
    b. Bag-mask device
    c. Simple face mask
    d. Nonrebreather mask

18. All the following are signs of inadequate breathing *except:*
    a. No visible chest rise
    b. Retractions of the chest wall
    c. Nasal flaring
    d. Respiratory rate of 16 breaths/min

19. You have a patient with shortness of breath who is lethargic, is wheezing bilaterally, and has respirations of 12 per minute and a pulse oximetry reading of 80%. You administer high-concentration oxygen via a nonrebreather mask. The pulse oximetry increases to 84%. What further treatments are indicated for this patient?
    a. Positive-pressure ventilation
    b. Cricoid maneuver, CPR
    c. Oropharyngeal intubation, cricothyrotomy
    d. FBAO, suction

20. What should the paramedic do for a 45-year-old man choking on a piece of steak during dinner and coughing forcefully?
    a. Perform back blows
    b. Attempt a finger sweep
    c. Monitor the patient
    d. Give abdominal thrusts

For Further Review

In the Student Workbook

- Multiple-choice questions
- Matching questions
- Fill-in-the-blank questions
- Case scenario questions
- Skill check questions

On Evolve

- Anatomy challenge
- Weblinks
- Lecture notes
- Exercises

Learning Objectives

Cognitive Objectives

- Identify and label the major structures of the respiratory system on a diagram.
- List the signs of adequate breathing.
- List the signs of inadequate breathing.
- Describe the steps in performing the head-tilt/chin-lift.
- Relate mechanism of injury to opening the airway.
- Describe the steps in performing the jaw thrust.
- State the importance of having a suction unit ready for immediate use when providing emergency care.
- Describe the techniques of suctioning.
- Describe how to ventilate a patient artificially with a pocket mask.
- Describe the steps in artificially ventilating a patient with a bag-mask device while using the jaw thrust.
- List the parts of a bag-mask ventilation system.
- Describe the steps in artificially ventilating a patient with a bag-mask device.
- Describe the signs of adequate artificial ventilation using the bag-mask device.
- Describe the signs of inadequate artificial ventilation using the bag-mask device.
- Describe the steps in artificially ventilating a patient with a flow-restricted, oxygen-powered ventilation device.
- List the steps in performing mouth-to-mouth and mouth-to-stoma artificial ventilation.
- Describe how to measure and insert an oropharyngeal airway.
- Describe how to measure and insert a nasopharyngeal airway.
- Define the components of an oxygen delivery system.
- Identify a nonrebreather face mask, and state the oxygen flow requirements for its use.
- Describe the indications for using a nasal cannula versus a nonrebreather face mask.
- Identify a nasal cannula, and state the flow requirements for its use.
- Describe the signs of foreign body airway obstruction.

Affective Objectives

- Explain the rationale for basic life support artificial ventilation and airway protective skills taking priority over most other basic life support skills.
- Explain the rationale for providing adequate oxygenation through high inspired oxygen concentrations to patients who previously may have received low concentrations.

Psychomotor Objectives

- Demonstrate the steps in performing the head-tilt/chin-lift.
- Demonstrate the steps in performing the jaw thrust.
- Demonstrate the techniques of suctioning.
- Demonstrate the steps in providing mouth-to-mouth artificial ventilation with body substance isolation (barrier shields).
- Demonstrate how to use a pocket mask to ventilate a patient artificially.
- Demonstrate the assembly of a bag-mask unit.
- Demonstrate the steps in artificially ventilating a patient with a bag-mask device.
- Demonstrate the steps in artificially ventilating a patient with a bag-mask while using the jaw thrust.
- Demonstrate artificial ventilation of a patient with a flow-restricted, oxygen-powered ventilation device.
- Demonstrate how to ventilate a patient artificially with a stoma.
- Demonstrate how to insert an oropharyngeal airway.
- Demonstrate how to insert a nasopharyngeal airway.
- Demonstrate the correct operation of oxygen tanks and regulators.
- Demonstrate the use of a nonrebreather face mask and state the oxygen flow requirements for its use.

- Demonstrate the use of a nasal cannula and state the flow requirements for its use.
- Demonstrate bag-mask artificial ventilations for the infant and child.
- Demonstrate oxygen delivery for the infant and child.
- Demonstrate artificial ventilation of a patient with a stoma.
- Demonstrate the techniques of foreign body airway obstruction removal.

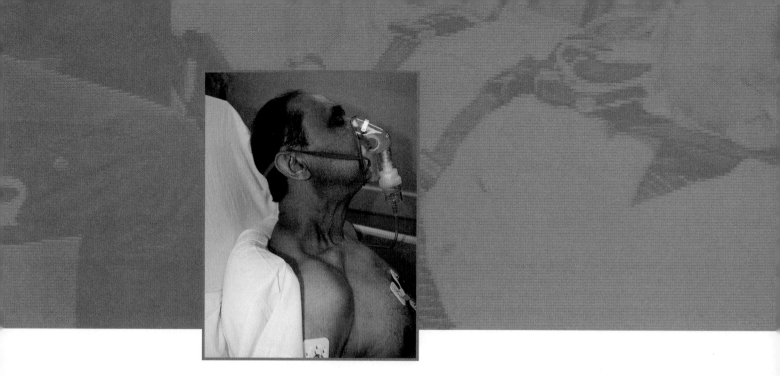

7 Patient Assessment

CHAPTER OUTLINE

Overview
Scene Size-up
Initial (Primary) Assessment
Patient History
Focused (Secondary) Assessment
Ongoing Assessment or Reassessment
Skills

Scenario

You are dispatched to a motor vehicle crash at a busy intersection. On arrival, you note that two vehicles are involved. One car is struck on its side and has significant deformity. The other car has overturned on its roof. You see two people lying on the street. Four people are trapped in two of the cars. You and your partner put on protective gear, including helmets, eyewear, heavy-duty gloves, and turnout coats, in anticipation of the rescue and the possibility of contact with blood or body fluids.

As you continue your scene size-up, your partner positions the ambulance and traffic cones to divert cars safely away from the crash scene. You notify the dispatcher on the portable radio that police, rescue, and additional emergency medical services (EMS) units are needed at the scene for continuing scene safety, gaining access and extrication, and managing and transporting at least four patients.

After making the scene safe, you quickly begin triage of the patients and, with your partner, assessment and treatment of the most severely injured patient, a 23-year-old man who is alert and complaining of difficulty breathing and pain in his chest. His skin is pale, cool, and sweaty, and he has a rapid and weak radial pulse. You administer high-concentration oxygen using a nonrebreather mask. While maintaining inline immobilization of the spine, you coordinate a rapid extrication using a long spine board.

With the patient out of the vehicle, you perform a focused (secondary) examination that reveals active accessory muscle use, absent breath sounds on the left side of the chest, and tenderness in the upper-right quadrant of the abdomen. His vital signs are pulse, 110 breaths/min; respirations, 26 breaths/min and labored; and blood pressure 100/70 mm Hg. You complete packaging of the patient, and during transport, you notify the trauma center of the impending arrival and provide a brief history.

LEARNING OBJECTIVES
- Identify the components of an initial (primary) assessment.
- Explain the importance of an initial (primary) assessment.

Overview

Comprehensive and systematic patient assessment is the foundation of emergency medical care. Patient assessment includes the scene size-up, initial (primary) assessment, and focused (secondary) assessment, including patient history and in some cases a detailed physical examination. Each phase of assessment has an important and distinct purpose.

In the **scene size-up,** the emergency medical technician (EMT) ensures the safety of the providers, patients, and bystanders. This includes using personal protective equipment and identifying any hazards, such as traffic, fire, or violence. During the scene size-up, the EMT also determines the number of patients, the mechanism of injury, and if additional resources may be needed, by performing triage of the scene, if required.

In the **initial (primary) assessment** the EMT provides the essential lifesaving treatment, including identifying the need for

rapid transport. The **focused (secondary) assessment,** which includes the focused history and physical examination, provides additional information to initiate decision making and treatment. Collectively, the approach to patient assessment needs to be sequential and systematic to ensure safety and to provide treatments in the appropriate order.

LEARNING OBJECTIVES
- Explain the rationale for crew members to evaluate scene safety before entering.
- Recognize hazards and potential hazards.
- Describe common hazards found at the scene of a trauma and a medical patient.
- Determine whether the scene is safe to enter.

Scene Size-up

To professional EMS personnel, the observations and actions taken in the opening scenario speak volumes about the importance of an effective scene size-up. In a well-organized scene size-up, the following critical actions occur:

- Police respond and secure the scene on the open roadway, keep bystanders at a safe distance, and ensure that roads approaching and leaving the scene are clear for emergency responders.
- When approaching a scene that involves potential hazardous materials, you should remain uphill and upwind until the scene has been evaluated and cleared by hazardous materials (HAZMAT) personnel.
- Rescue personnel assist in gaining access to the patients, including *disentanglement* (movement of wreckage that is trapping victims) and *extrication* (process by which people are removed from vehicles and other situations).
- Consider weather and other environmental threats that may be a hazard to the patient or personnel.
- Additional units respond to manage the multiple victims who have sustained significant *mechanisms of injury* (the forces that cause the injuries).
- As additional EMS units arrive, you direct them to the most severely injured patient s determined during triage.
- The most life-threatening conditions are managed first. Patients are transported to the hospital in priority order.

By taking a few moments to size up the scene and communicate their findings, EMTs address safety issues for themselves, their co-workers, the patients, and the public. Once **scene safety** has been addressed, EMTs begin patient **triage** (sorting patients according to priority) and the initial (primary) assessment of patients.

The choices you make and the actions you take may make the difference between life and death for the patients, bystanders, and, most importantly, you. Many EMS providers have died exercising the best intentions but poor judgment. The irony of these situations is that they were ultimately not able to help the patient, but instead became patients themselves.

This section addresses general principles of sizing up a scene and, most importantly, ensuring safety at the scene. **Table 7-1** provides examples of key scenarios and actions related to scene safety.

Table 7-1	Scene Safety Scenarios and Action

Scenario	Action
You respond to a call for an "attempted suicide." On arrival, you enter the patient's kitchen and smell gas and note that the oven door is open.	Quickly extricate patient to a safe area outside the house, and contact dispatcher to have the appropriate resource personnel respond.
While responding to a motor vehicle crash, you observe from a distance an overturned tanker truck and a large smoke cloud above the scene. Several victims are lying around the truck.	Remain upwind, and contact dispatcher to have personnel respond who have the appropriate personal protective equipment and resources needed to evaluate safety at the scene.
You respond to a home for an "unconscious female." When you knock on the door, a large, aggressive dog barks and growls from the other side.	Retreat to a safe location, and contact dispatcher so that animal control experts can respond to secure the scene.
You respond to a call for a shooting in a large apartment building. When you arrive in front of the building, you note the police have not yet responded.	Retreat to a safe location, and wait for the police to arrive. If needed, notify dispatcher to expedite police response.
You respond to a pedestrian struck during a severe snowstorm. The patient is lying on the ground, exposed to the elements.	Make sure that the scene is safe through the use of traffic cones or other devices, and quickly remove the patient to a warm, safe location.

Scene Size-up and Patient Assessment

Scene size-up is an assessment of the scene and its surroundings. The scene size-up provides valuable information to the EMT and includes information necessary to ensure protection of the EMT, the patients, and bystanders. You will evaluate information in a short time as you approach a patient. The scene size-up includes information about the following:

1. Need for personal protection
2. Safety of the scene
3. Nature of illness for medical patients
4. Mechanism of injury for trauma patients
5. Number of patients
6. Need for additional help
7. Need for stabilization of patient's spine

Figure 7-1 provides an overview of the steps in the scene size-up.

You will be able to anticipate some factors through information from the dispatcher, which you then confirm or reassess after arrival at the scene. Scene size-up is an ongoing process. You constantly reassess scene information throughout the call.

Scene size-up is actually the beginning of *patient assessment,* an orderly approach to medical and trauma patients that uses the following sequence: scene size-up, initial (primary) assessment, focused (secondary) assessment, ongoing assessment or reassessment, and communication and documentation (**Table 7-2**). Maintaining a consistent order during scene size-up and patient assessment helps ensure that you gather essential information and take appropriate actions in a timely manner. This approach provides the greatest benefit to the patient while maintaining the safety of all involved.

Standard Precautions: a Review

Standard precautions should be used as the first step to protect you and others from the spread of contagious disease. Standard precautions apply to exposure or contact to (1) blood; (2) all body fluids, secretions, and excretions

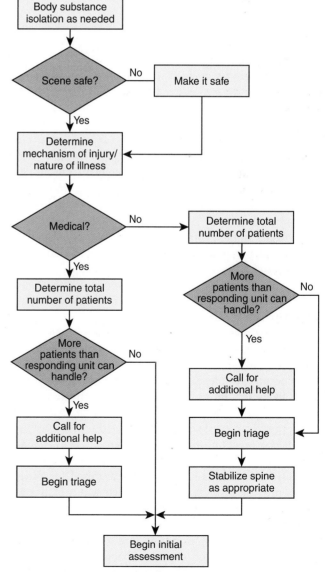

Figure 7-1 Algorithm for scene size-up.

Table 7-2	Overview of Patient Assessment	

Assessment Component	Specific Observations	Actions
Scene size-up	Mechanism of injury/nature of illness	Take appropriate body substance isolation precautions
	Is scene safe?	Make scene safe
	Are more resources needed?	Call for additional help
		Consider stabilization of the spine
Initial (primary) assessment	Establish and maintain the airway	CPR and AED
	Check for responsiveness	Positive-pressure ventilations
	Check for life-threatening conditions	Administer oxygen
	Check airway, breathing, and circulation	Stop any bleeding
		Make transport decision
Focused (secondary) assessment	Reconsider mechanism of injury or history	Treat patient based on assessment findings
Chief complaint, history, and physical examination	Perform history and physical examination	Contact medical direction as needed
	If indicated, perform rapid assessment	Reevaluate transportation decision
	Monitor vital signs	
	Complete SAMPLE history	
Head-to-toe survey	Perform on trauma patient, as indicated	Reevaluate rapid assessment
	Consider for medical patients	Look for additional findings
		Manage secondary injuries and wounds appropriately
Ongoing assessment or reassessment	Repeat initial (primary) assessment	Look for trends in the vital signs and response to treatment
	Repeat vital signs	Provide additional treatments as needed
	Repeat focused (secondary) assessment regarding patient complaint or injuries	

CPR, Cardiopulmonary resuscitation; *AED,* automated external defibrillator.

(except sweat), regardless of whether they contain visible blood; (3) nonintact skin; and (4) mucous membranes. Use standard precautions in all situations to avoid transmission from both recognized and unrecognized sources of infection from patients.

The degree of protection required will vary. For example, as you approach a trauma scene where exposure to blood is likely, it makes good sense to have gloves on as you approach the patient. If you see blood spurting from a wound or know you are about to be involved in an emergency childbirth, wear gloves, gown, mask, and protective eyewear.

As you approach patients, you should carry protective gear on your person or in a trauma, airway, or other kit so that the items are readily available if needed.

Once you become involved with patient care, you will be less likely to stop to don personal protective equipment (PPE). Therefore, you should use the scene size-up as your first opportunity to assess the need for the degree of body substance protection. You will supplement your standard precautions with transmission-based precautions as indicated. *Transmission-based precautions* are used for patients documented or suspected to be infected with highly transmissible or important pathogens for which additional precautions beyond standard precautions are warranted. These strategies include airborne precautions, droplet precautions, and contact precautions. (Review Chapter 2 to be sure you are familiar with these recommendations so that you can act accordingly.)

Scene Safety

Personal Protection

One of the basic principles of EMS operations is scene safety. You must assess the scene for potential danger to you, other rescuers, the public, and the patient. Not all patients in need of rescue can be rescued. Certain situations present such significant hazards to both personnel and the public that attempted rescue may be both futile and fatal. A risk-benefit analysis is essential. The EMT who runs into a burning building without assessing the safety of the scene may become an unnecessary additional victim. If the scene is unsafe, you should not enter until it can be made safe or request persons trained in specialized rescue to gain access and retrieve the patient. For example, rescue of a patient who is trapped in a toxic, enclosed space must wait until EMS personnel trained in the use of a self-contained breathing apparatus (SCBA) can gain access and remove the patient. For a patient who is unconscious in an apartment with an aggressive dog, the EMT may have to wait until police or specialized animal control officers can secure the dog before gaining access. In general, ***do not enter a scene until you are absolutely sure that it is safe.***

The first questions to ask when approaching the scene are as follows:
• Will I be safe in the environment?
• Is it safe to approach the patient?

A *life-safety hazard* is any situation in which EMS personnel are risking serious injury or death as the result of entering the

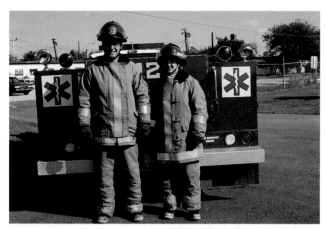

Figure 7-2 The EMT wears protective clothing as indicated by the scene survey.

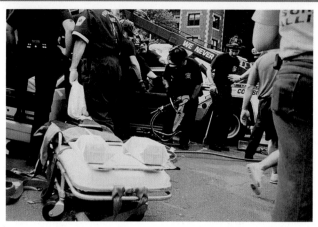

Figure 7-3 During the scene size-up, note whether a motor vehicle crash will require a "heavy" rescue team to extricate the victim.

scene, such as when an EMT stops to assist an injured motorist on a dark, unmarked roadway. Again, your value to the patient is lost if you are injured or killed.

Protective Gear

Your protective "envelope" is the most important factor in reducing injury. A complete protective envelope consists of the following **(Figure 7-2):**

- Head gear
- Eye protection
- Respiratory protection (if required)
- Gloves
- Boots
- Coat

The type of PPE required will vary and may not be available on your ambulance. For example, in dealing with toxic emergencies, personnel must be protected from exposure by inhalation or contact with skin, depending on the type of suspected or known toxin and its properties. The type of PPE carried by EMS personnel varies greatly from service to service. Check with your EMS service to identify the protective equipment available, and ensure that you are properly trained in its use. When you are not given specific PPE that may be necessary to enter a scene (e.g., SCBA), wait for the appropriate rescue personnel to arrive at the scene.

Crash/Rescue Scenes

The greatest and most common hazard encountered by EMTs is the traffic surrounding motor vehicle crashes. Risks to EMTs are reduced by wearing bright clothing and reflective vests and using **traffic delineation devices** appropriately. Traffic cones, flares, and the lights on the ambulance should be used to alert oncoming traffic that there is a hazard ahead and to protect those operating at the scene. Although traffic control is usually a police function, situations occur that require EMTs to be knowledgeable about traffic hazards. Many EMTs have been badly injured and killed in traffic situations. EMTs must be alert to traffic hazards at all times.

Once the hazards are eliminated and you are wearing protective clothing, medical treatment for the patient becomes your priority.

Scene Survey: Approach to the Crash Scene. The decisions you make when approaching a crash scene determine the effectiveness of the patient's rescue. You have the capability of making a rescue safe and efficient or disastrous **(Figure 7-3).**

You should take the following steps when approaching the scene:

1. Stop (ideally, 100 feet [30 m] away, uphill, and upwind).
2. Look and listen. Observe what is happening. How many cars are involved? How many victims?
3. Assess resources. Are the resources you may need currently with you or available to you in a timely manner?
4. Determine whether a rescue attempt will pose an undue risk of injury to you or other personnel. If the risk is greater than the benefit, you should take actions that will reduce the risk. For example, if a vehicle is fully engulfed in flames on your arrival, you would not attempt to rescue the occupants without attempting to extinguish the fire first. Routinely conducting a risk-benefit analysis makes you an effective member of the rescue team.
5. When approaching the vehicle, do a windshield survey **(Figure 7-4).** Are the victims moving? Are they conscious? Are they attempting to exit the vehicle?
6. During your approach to the vehicle, quickly check for downed electrical wires in the immediate vicinity. If wires are down, use the following precautions:
   - Do not touch anything.
   - Retreat to a position of safety.
   - Protect all bystanders by establishing a hazard zone.
   - Advise the occupants of the vehicle not to attempt to exit.
   - Contact the appropriate support service (local utility) to shut the power off and move the wires.
7. Evaluate the stability of the vehicle and determine whether it can be entered safely:
   - Will the vehicle turn over?
   - Is the vehicle on its side? On its wheels?
   - Is the vehicle secure and stable in its position?
   - Does the vehicle rock?
   - Could the movement of the vehicle or a rescue attempt cause injury to the patient because the vehicle still has the capability of moving?

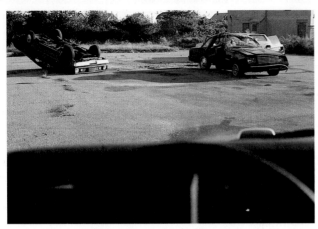

Figure 7-4 Windshield survey.

The potential for severe injury to both personnel and victims from an unstable vehicle is great. A vehicle resting on its side presents a significant hazard and should be stabilized. It may be necessary to place *chocks* (wedges used to stabilize a vehicle) or other structural supports strategically around the vehicle to prevent it from falling during the rescue attempts. People skilled and knowledgeable in crash vehicle rescue should supervise this activity (see Chapter 26).

Knowing your personal limitations in relation to the rescue scene is very important. The place to try new rescue equipment and technique is in a structured training program, not in the field, where the lives of the victims and personnel may be at risk. Specialized training programs are available for EMS providers, including HAZMAT, domestic preparedness (bioterrorism), EMT tactical rescue (Special Weapons and Tactics [SWAT]), ice rescue, swift-water rescue, high-angle rescue, low-angle rescue, confined-space rescue, and other programs. Your decisions to participate in such programs should be made in conjunction with your EMS system manager or medical director to ensure that you will be able to use the related skills. However, you may also participate in these programs to expand your general knowledge and skills even if you are not allowed to use them in your day-to-day activities. Specialized courses are discussed further in Chapters 26 (Ambulance Operations), 27 (Gaining Access), and 28 (Disasters and Hazardous Materials).

Traffic Delineation Devices. Traffic delineation devices are essential to maintain the safety of the scene. Reflectors, flares, traffic cones, and battery-operated lights are recommended. All these devices have merit; the EMT must decide which device best fits the needs of a particular situation. The benefits and hazards of particular devices must be considered when deciding to use them. For example, *flares,* although clearly visible at night, are of less benefit in the daytime. In addition, if gasoline has spilled at the scene, flares represent a fire hazard and add to the risks already present.

A primary hazard to consider is the oncoming, inebriated or sleeping driver. These individuals operate their vehicles on muscle memory; they seem to be driving on "automatic pilot." The use of *traffic cones* is more effective with these hazardous

drivers. When a vehicle hits and runs over a traffic cone, the sound of the cone's impact continues as it is dragged beneath the undercarriage of the vehicle. This noise may return sleepy or drunken drivers to a level of consciousness that enables them to avoid an oncoming collision and keeps them from swerving into the scene.

When positioning traffic delineation devices (cones, flares, reflectors), you should consider the posted speed limit. A good rule is to place these devices at least three times the distance (in feet) of the posted speed limit. For example, if the speed limit is 30 miles per hour, the first delineation device should be placed no closer than approximately 90 feet from the crash site. This allows all individuals approaching the scene to react and stop in time (**Figure 7-5**).

Blind turns represent another problem. Devices must be placed before the turn begins and throughout the entire turn to alert drivers that a hazard exists ahead.

Crime Scenes

You should not enter a crime scene until police officers have secured the scene. Otherwise, you might confront the perpetrator and either subject yourself to personal injury or compound the situation. When responding to a call for a violent situation (e.g., shooting, stabbing), you should wait for police to arrive at the scene and follow their directions before approaching the patient.

Some scenes may pose threats of personal violence that are not obvious from the dispatch information. On arrival at any scene where signs or indications of violence exist, retreat to a safe position and notify the dispatcher to send police to the scene before you enter.

If you inadvertently find yourself in a place with a violent person when you are responding to a call, you should remember the following principles:

1. Do not block escape of a violent person, and do not challenge the individual.
2. Identify yourself as a medical provider so that your role is not confused with that of a police officer.
3. Acknowledge that the person seems upset, and emphasize that you are there to help.
4. Explain exactly what you are doing in a calm and reassuring voice.
5. Maintain a safe distance, and do not make any quick moves.
6. Encourage the person to state what is troubling him or her, and respond honestly to the person's questions.

Review Chapter 17 (Behavioral Emergencies) for more information on dealing with distressed patients.

Environmental Hazards

The environment may pose a danger to you or others. For example, you should not attempt a water rescue unless you are trained to do so and have the proper equipment at hand. Instead, you should call for an appropriate rescue team. Unless you are trained in water rescue, a victim overcome by water may inadvertently pull you under during a rescue attempt.

Winter and icy conditions may pose different hazards. For example, a victim who falls through thin ice requires special

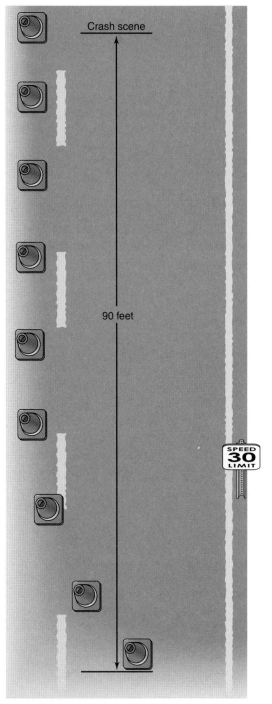

Figure 7-5 Placement of traffic delineation devices. Three times (in feet) the posted speed limit.

considerations for a safe rescue. Steep slopes might make rescue and patient access and extrication difficult. You will need to consider multiple and varied environmental conditions when you ask the question, "Is it safe to approach the patient?"

Protection

Patients. Patients benefit when the EMT takes measures to ensure their personal protection, such as providing traffic diversion at a crash scene or calling for special resources. However, the EMT can take special measures to offer additional protection to the patient. For example, removing the patient from a hazardous environment, such as an active highway, a home with a gas leak, or a vehicle filled with carbon monoxide, is a lifesaving action before formal patient assessment and treatment are begun. Rescue personnel who enter a location that has a suspected gas leak must have the appropriate protection. Providing shelter and maintaining body temperature are important patient care tasks. A pedestrian struck and lying on an icy street is subject to *hypothermia* (general cooling of the body). Extrication from a vehicle might carry the risk of patient exposure to broken glass and sharp pieces of metal. Covering the patient with a rescue blanket or other protective device before extrication will minimize this danger.

Bystanders. Bystanders are drawn to the scene of a motor vehicle crash or emergency. Some bystanders might stop to offer assistance and first aid; others may be drawn by curiosity. In some situations the EMT should take action to help protect bystanders from becoming victims. For example, traffic control at a crash scene helps protect everyone. Isolating a toxic spill and establishing a safe zone will help avoid further injuries.

> **LEARNING OBJECTIVES**
> - Discuss common mechanisms of injury and nature of illness.
> - Discuss the reason for identifying the total number of patients at the scene.
> - Explain the reason for identifying the need for additional help or assistance.

Mechanism of Injury and Nature of Illness

Once an emergency scene has been made safe, direct your attention to the patient. The scene and surroundings, along with dispatch information, provide early clues about the mechanism of injury or nature of illness. **Mechanism of injury** refers to the manner in which an injury occurred during trauma. This can involve the type, strength, and direction of injuring forces. **Nature of illness** refers to the type of medical symptoms that a patient exhibits or other clues, such as empty pill bottles, syringes, or exposure to allergens (e.g., bee sting).

Trauma Patients

You can determine the mechanism of injury from inspection of the scene and from the patient, family, or bystanders. Reconstructing the forces of injury helps to anticipate injury patterns. You may learn from bystanders or observation of the scene that a medical problem occurred and may have contributed to the injury. For example, if a patient working on a roof on a hot day fainted before falling off a ladder, this event may suggest an underlying medical problem.

You should determine the total number of patients and initiate a mass casualty plan as needed. If the responding crew can manage the situation after the appropriate notifications have been initiated, consider spinal precautions, begin initial (primary) assessment, and if necessary, begin triage.

Table 7-3	Mechanisms of Injury and Associated Injuries		
Mechanism	**Common Associated Injuries**	**Mechanism**	**Common Associated Injuries**
Head-on collisions	Head and spinal trauma	Rear-end collision	Head and spinal trauma
	Chest and abdominal trauma		Whiplash
	Flail chest		
	Pneumothorax	Rotational collision	Varies according to vector; person
	Internal hemorrhage		closest to impact point sustains
	Lower extremity trauma		most force of impact
	Knee, femur, hip	Falls	Type of injury depends on impact
	Upper extremity trauma		point
	Protection injury	Feet first	Calcaneus (heel)
			Lower extremity
Side collision	Head and spinal trauma		Spine
	Chest and abdominal trauma		
	Lateral chest wall injury	Outstretched arm	Wrist, elbow, humerus, shoulder
	Flail chest		
	Pneumothorax		
	Internal hemorrhage	Penetrating knife injuries	Type of injury depends on size,
	Upper extremity trauma		direction, and location
	Shoulder, clavicle, humerus	Missile injuries	Type of injury depends on velocity,
	Lower extremity trauma		location, and range
	Hip and acetabulum		

Significant Mechanism of Injury

Significant mechanisms of injury warrant a thorough search for clues on the body. Over time, physicians and prehospital personnel learn to associate certain mechanisms of injury with a significant chance of death or serious disability (**Table 7-3**).

In motor vehicle crashes, knowledge of the speed of impact is an important clue. The higher the speed of the vehicle, the greater is the energy transmitted to the patient, because energy varies directly with the velocity squared (**Figure 7-6**). Sometimes a driver can tell you the speed of impact. Knowing the posted speed limit is another clue.

Knowledge of the mechanism of injury also helps anticipate certain injury patterns. For example, a person who falls from a height and lands on the feet is likely to have the force transmitted up the lower extremities and the spine (**Figure 7-7**). An unrestrained driver who strikes a tree may have injuries from collision of the steering wheel and the chest, the windshield and the head and neck, and the dashboard with the lower extremity (**Figure 7-8**). A vehicle passenger struck by a side collision with intrusion of the vehicle into the passenger compartment might have injuries to the lateral chest wall, the head and neck, and the lower extremity. Incorporate this information in your physical examination of the patient to identify specific injuries. Try to reconstruct the mechanism of injury from your observations of the environment, the patient, and the history gathered from the patient and bystanders who may have witnessed the event. Document this important information, and relay it to the hospital staff.

Hidden Injuries

Seat belts and airbags modify the forces sustained by the body in motor vehicle crashes and have helped prevent death and serious injury. Ascertaining whether safety devices were used by

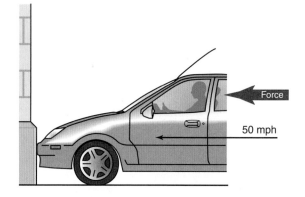

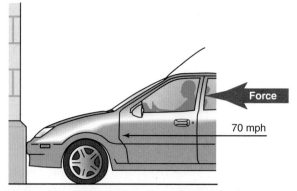

Figure 7-6 Kinetic energy increases with speed (velocity squared) of the vehicle. *Modified from McQuillan KA, Flynn Makic MB, Whalen E:* Trauma nursing: from resuscitation through rehabilitation, *ed 3, Philadelphia, 2002, Saunders.*

victims of crashes is important. This information can be obtained by questioning the patient and others at the scene and inspecting the vehicle and the patient (**Figure 7-9**).

Patients who have used safety devices may still have serious injuries. For example, the force of the accident can be great enough to cause injury even though the safety device was in use. In other situations, shearing forces from deceleration may have damaged internal organs without external signs of injury. Safety devices may also have been improperly used. For example, a motorized shoulder belt worn without manually fastening the

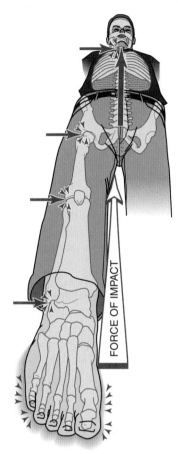

Figure 7-7 Impact forces to the heel with location of related injuries to the extremity and spine. *Modified from McQuillan KA, Flynn Makic MB, Whalen E. Trauma nursing: from resuscitation through rehabilitation, ed 4, Philadelphia, 2009, Saunders.*

lap belt can cause serious neck injury. A loose lap belt can ride up on the abdomen, causing compression of abdominal organs and spinal injury (**Figure 7-10**). At times, wearing only a lap belt can result in spinal injury from hyperflexion of the lower spine.

Airbag deployment itself does not guarantee that a victim is free of injury. For example, airbags may not be effective without simultaneous use of a seat belt. In some circumstances a patient, especially if short and sitting close to the steering wheel, may still have hit the steering wheel even though the airbag deployed. Because of this possibility, it is recommended that the EMT "lift and look" when caring for crash victims. *Lift* the deployed airbag, and *look* at the steering wheel to see whether it has been deformed, an indication of potentially serious internal injury.

Infants and Children

Significant mechanisms of injury for infants and children include bicycle collisions, being struck by vehicles, and falling from smaller heights. Infants and children younger than 5 years are often injured from falls. Children between ages 6 and 12 years are often injured in motor vehicle crashes as passengers, pedestrians, or bicyclists hit by a car.

Children should use age-specific and size-specific safety devices. All states have safety device utilization laws that require use of special seats for infants and toddlers.

Medical Patients

You should determine from the patient, family, or bystanders why EMS was activated and how many patients are at the scene. Someone other than the patient usually makes the initial 9-1-1 call. It may be a family member, someone in the school or workplace, or a bystander. Valuable information can be gained from this person at the scene about the nature of the illness.

The scene may offer clues to the patient's medical condition. Look for oxygen tanks and tubing. Is there a wheelchair or walker present, indicating the patient has difficulty ambulating? Look for medications, and bring any medications to the hospital with the patient.

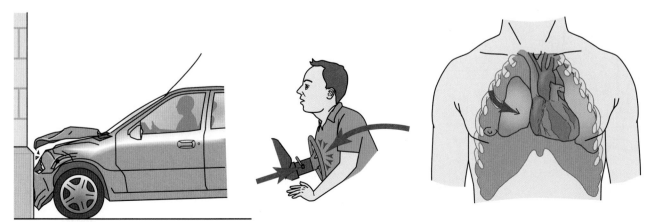

Figure 7-8 Compression forces in a front-end collision caused by the chest striking the steering wheel. Injuries include multiple rib fractures, lung collapse, cardiac damage, and internal hemorrhage. *Modified from McQuillan KA, Flynn Makic MB, Whalen E. Trauma nursing: from resuscitation through rehabilitation, ed 4, Philadelphia, 2009, Saunders.*

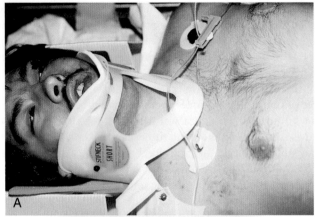

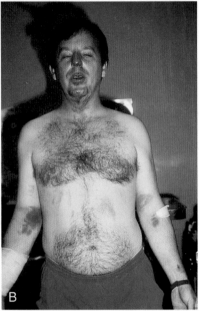

Figure 7-9 **A,** Contusions and abrasions from striking the steering wheel. **B,** Abrasions resulting from deployment of an airbag. The patient survived a high-speed collision.

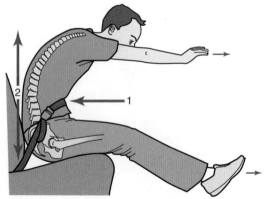

Figure 7-10 An improperly worn lap belt may cause soft tissue injury in the abdomen or fracture to the lower spine. *Modified from Connolly JF:* DePalma's the management of fractures and dislocations: an atlas, *Philadelphia, 1981, Saunders.*

Multiple Patients

If there are more patients than the responding unit can handle, call for additional help. Making this call for additional help before contact with the patient is particularly important because EMTs are less likely to call for help once they become involved in patient care. In addition, some patients may benefit from advanced life support care provided by Paramedics or Advanced EMTs (EMT-Intermediates). For example, when treating a cardiac arrest patient with an automated external defibrillator (AED), the patient may remain in ventricular fibrillation or convert to another cardiac arrest heart rhythm that benefits from the use of advanced airway management or medications to stabilize the patient. An **advanced life support (ALS) intercept** is a valuable tool of the EMT. Other conditions that might benefit from an ALS intercept include airway obstructions not cleared by basic maneuvers, patients in unstable condition resulting from fast or slow heart rhythms, patients whose ventilation cannot be managed effectively with basic airway and ventilation techniques, and numerous other conditions in which ALS interventions may be lifesaving. These interventions are discussed in later chapters. Remember to identify the need for an ALS intercept early to gain the maximum benefit for the patient.

If several patients are at the scene, you should begin triage of the patients so that care can be rendered according to medical priority, pending arrival of additional help. When ongoing hazards or numerous patients are present, you may need to initiate a **multiple-casualty incident** plan, an approach used to manage both large-scale and small-scale multipatient responses (see Chapter 28).

LEARNING OBJECTIVES
- Identify the components of an initial (primary) history.
- Summarize the reasons for forming a general impression of the patient.
- Discuss methods of assessing altered mental status.
- Explain the importance of forming a general impression of the patient.
- Explain the value of performing the initial (primary) assessment.
- State reasons for management of the cervical spine once the patient has been determined to be a trauma patient.

Initial (Primary) Assessment

The initial assessment, or primary assessment, is a rapid means of assessing patient condition, life threats, and priorities of care. It is performed on all patients after ensuring scene safety. The initial (primary) assessment is directed toward identifying and treating the most life-threatening conditions by forming a general impression of the patient and quickly evaluating the three most critical organ systems (nervous, respiratory, and circulatory) in a rapid but systematic manner. If a life-threatening condition is found, initiate treatment or transport immediately as you continue care. **Figure 7-11** provides an overview of the initial (primary) assessment process.

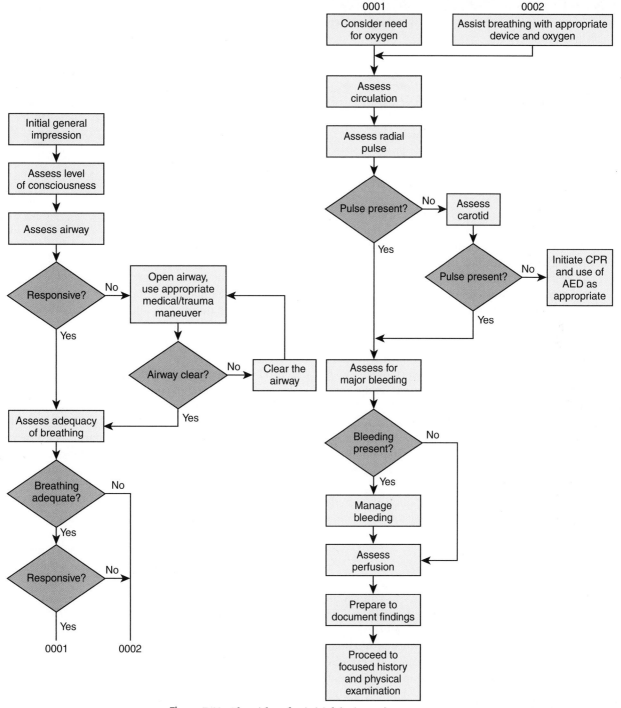

Figure 7-11 Algorithm for initial (primary) assessment.

General Impression

You form a **general impression** of the patient to determine the priority of care. The patient may be stable, potentially unstable, or unstable. The general impression is based on your immediate assessment of the environment and the general appearance of the patient.

You can quickly assess many aspects of the respiratory, circulatory, and nervous systems from observation alone. The patient's mental status may be obvious and may range from the awake, talking individual to the patient who appears unconscious.

Similarly, a patient talking normally with unlabored breathing is showing that the airway is patent and that breathing is adequate. Contrast this to a patient sitting bolt upright with bulging neck muscles, head in the "sniffing position," and rapid and labored breathing.

The general appearance of the skin may give clues to the status of circulation. Pale, sweaty skin may be noticeable as you approach the patient. The patient may have obvious cyanotic lips or extremities or exhibit jaundiced or yellow skin. Contrast this to the patient who has pink and normal, dry skin that is evident as you walk in the room.

The clues regarding neurologic, respiratory, and circulatory status are all designed to help you judge the severity of the patient's condition, even before you perform the "ABCs" (airway, breathing, circulation) during your initial (primary) assessment.

The general impression includes the following elements:
• Whether the patient's condition is unstable or life threatening, such as serious trauma or cardiac or respiratory arrest.
• Whether the condition is medical in nature or the result of trauma.
• Basic information regarding age and gender.

The information from the general impression will influence treatment. For example, a 50-year-old man who clutched his chest and then experienced cardiac arrest is best treated at the scene with an AED. If he received a gunshot wound and then collapsed, this man is best treated in the operating room. The EMT's response to these two circumstances will dramatically differ based on the general impression of the patient. In general, trauma patients with serious injuries require rapid transport to the hospital because surgical intervention often is required to stabilize the patient's condition. This may include surgery to control internal bleeding, evacuation of blood within the brain, or other lifesaving procedures.

Medical patients, such as those with cardiac arrest, may benefit from interventions on the scene before transport. For example, in cases of cardiac arrest, an AED is best applied as quickly as possible to give the patient a greater chance to live. Often, as described earlier, an ALS intercept may be helpful to stabilize patients with life-threatening conditions. For example, a patient who has a complete airway obstruction that cannot be cleared using basic life support techniques may benefit from ALS procedures.

Life-Threatening Conditions

If the patient has a life-threatening condition, you should begin treatment immediately. In an unresponsive patient, the tongue may block the airway. Inadequate breathing or perfusion or severe bleeding are other life-threatening conditions you may encounter. You should treat a life-threatening condition as soon as possible after identifying it. While treatment is under way, you or your partner should continue assessing the patient, looking for other conditions that may need care. The range of lifesaving treatment includes airway management and positive-pressure ventilation, supplemental oxygen, cardiopulmonary resuscitation (CPR), defibrillation with an AED, bleeding control, ALS intercept, and rapid transport. You can make the decision to rapidly transport the patient at any time during the course of the initial (primary) assessment with subsequent treatment and evaluation rendered en route.

Spinal Immobilization

All patients who have suspected spinal injury should be appropriately immobilized. You should establish early manual stabilization of the neck and head and maintain manual stabilization

---

| Box 7-1 | AVPU Mnemonic to Assess Mental Status |

Alert—Patient communicates clearly without any stimuli. Normally, a patient should be able to express his or her name, the location, and the date. This is called **orientation** to person, place, and time (oriented ×3). In some cases, patients can be oriented to one or two but not all three; for example, a patient can be oriented to name and time but not place. Normal responses for infants and children vary with age (see Chapter 25).
Verbal—Patient responds to verbal stimuli.
Painful—Patient does not respond to verbal stimuli but does respond to painful stimuli.
Unresponsive—Patient is unresponsive to both verbal and painful stimuli.

---

until the patient is immobilized on a long spine board. These precautions are important to protect the spinal cord from any further damage during care and transport if a spinal injury is suspected.

Assessment of Mental Status

Central nervous system (CNS) function is evaluated quickly by assessing the level of consciousness. The mental state (status) is the most sensitive indicator of CNS function. Therefore the patient's response to verbal and physical stimuli is determined during the initial (primary) assessment (**Skill 7-1**, Establishing Responsiveness). Most patients will be awake and communicating without any stimuli. If the patient does not communicate normally, you should provide verbal and, if necessary, painful stimuli and evaluate the response according to the mnemonic **AVPU (Box 7-1).** Note the patient's facial expressions. Does he appear to be in pain or look scared? Facial expressions may offer good insight to the emotional state of the patient. Pay attention to the patient's thought process and speech. Are his thoughts logical or is he making statements that don't make sense? Is he using the correct words, and is he able to speak easily, or does he struggle to form words?

LEARNING OBJECTIVES
• Discuss methods of assessing the airway in the adult, child, and infant.
• Demonstrate the techniques for assessing the airway.

Airway Assessment

The next priority is to ensure that the patient has an open airway and adequate ventilation. An open airway in a responsive patient is best noted by observing normal speech, crying, or effortless breathing. If the airway is open, assess the adequacy of breathing. If the patient is unresponsive, you may need to open the airway to check for breathing. Basic methods used to open the airway include the following:
• Head-tilt/chin-lift
• Jaw thrust without head-tilt
• Tongue-jaw lift

The head-tilt/chin-lift procedure involves tilting the patient's forehead back, lifting the chin, and moving the tongue away from the back of the pharynx. The jaw thrust without head tilt is used in patients with suspected cervical spine injuries or when the mechanism of injury is unknown. This maneuver displaces the jaw forward and lifts the tongue away from the pharynx without extending the cervical spine. Patients found in a prone positions (on the stomach) may need to be placed in a supine position (on the back) to maintain the airway (**Skill 7-2**).

An alternative maneuver for patients with a cervical spine injury is the tongue-jaw lift. This may be the method of choice in patients with a fractured mandible (jaw), which might make the jaw thrust maneuver less effective. If the jaw thrust or tongue-jaw lift does not open the airway, use the head-tilt/chin-lift, because opening the airway takes priority over concern for suspected spinal injury.

All three of these maneuvers achieve the same result. They move the lower jaw forward and carry the tongue (which is attached to the lower jaw) away from the back of the throat. This opens the airway and allows passage of air if the patient is breathing.

When performing an initial (primary) assessment, you may note sounds such as snoring, stridor, or gurgling. *Snoring* suggests obstruction by the tongue and is usually controlled by basic airway maneuvers (head-tilt/chin-lift or jaw thrust) or insertion of an oropharyngeal or nasopharyngeal airway. *Stridor* suggests the presence of obstruction in the upper airway caused by swelling, inflammation, or foreign body. *Gurgling* is associated with fluid in the airway. After opening the airway, if secretions are present or if the airway is obstructed, use suctioning or obstructed airway maneuvers as indicated.

Skill 7-3 illustrates the steps in opening the airway.

LEARNING OBJECTIVES

- Describe methods used for assessing whether a patient is breathing.
- State the type of care to provide the adult, child, or infant with adequate breathing.
- State the type of care to provide the adult, child, or infant without adequate breathing.
- Differentiate between a patient with adequate breathing and one with inadequate breathing.

Breathing Assessment

Once the patient's airway is opened, the adequacy of ventilation and oxygenation must be evaluated. For a responsive patient, breathing may be normal, rapid (>24 breaths/min), or slow (<8 breaths/min). Breaths may also be shallow or deep with respiratory distress. Normal respiration, respiratory distress, and respiratory failure are discussed in detail in Chapter 6.

Quiet breathing may be difficult to evaluate, especially in environments that are noisy or distracting, such as in the street or during transport in an ambulance. Three senses (looking, listening, and feeling) maximize the information that can be gathered to establish the presence and help gauge the adequacy of breathing. You should look, listen, and feel for **signs** of adequate versus inadequate breathing (**Skill 7-4**). Infrequent or shallow breaths accompanied by other signs of respiratory ineffectiveness may reveal inadequate breathing. Alterations in

Table 7-4	Assessing Adequate versus Inadequate Breathing	
Parameter	**Normal Range**	**Inadequate**
Rate		
Adult	12-20 breaths/min	Outside normal ranges
Child	15-30 breaths/min	Outside normal ranges
Infant	25-50 breaths/min	Outside normal ranges
Rhythm		
Regular	Consistent rise and fall of the chest	Irregular
Quality		
Breath sounds	Present and equal	Diminished or absent
Chest expansion	Adequate and equal	Inadequate or unequal
Effort		Accessory muscle use; noisy
Depth	Normal chest rise	Inadequate/shallow
Other		
Skin	Normal	Pale or cyanotic (blue), cool and/or clammy
Retractions	None	Present, especially in infants and children
Nasal flaring	Not present	Present, especially in infants and children
Seesaw breathing	Not present	Alternate use of chest and abdominal muscles during breathing
Agonal or gasping breaths	Not present	May be seen just before death

consciousness may also indicate inadequate oxygenation of the brain (**Table 7-4**).

If breathing is not adequate, you should provide supplemental oxygen and determine the need for airway adjuncts and ventilatory assistance. Even if breathing is adequate and the patient is responsive, administration of oxygen may still be indicated, depending on the chief complaint and further assessment findings. An open airway must be maintained in all unresponsive patients. The decision to ventilate the patient's lungs and the specific techniques and indications for airway adjuncts and positive-pressure ventilation are addressed in Chapter 29.

LEARNING OBJECTIVES

- Describe the methods used to assess a pulse.
- Differentiate among obtaining a pulse in an adult, child, and infant.
- Discuss the need for assessing the patient for external bleeding.

Circulation Assessment

Pulse Check

After checking responsiveness, the airway, and breathing, check the patient's pulse. Check the carotid pulse on any patient who is unresponsive. For responsive patients, check the radial pulse for rate and quality (**Figure 7-12**). The pulse rate may be normal (60-100 beats/min), fast (>100 beats/min), or slow

(<60 beats/min). It may also be weak (faint) or strong (bounding). If the radial pulse is faint or absent, check the carotid pulse. If the patient is younger than 1 year, palpate a brachial pulse. You should check for a femoral pulse if the brachial pulse is faint or absent.

If there is no pulse, you should use the following interventions:

- Start CPR and attach an AED. Specially modified AEDs can be used with infants and younger children. Check for the protocol and AED used in your emergency medical services system (EMSS).
- If the patient is in cardiac arrest as a result of trauma, begin CPR and, if appropriate, attach the AED. This will be dictated by local protocol. Most trauma patients in cardiac arrest will not have a cardiac rhythm that requires a shock; however, some trauma patients may be in ventricular fibrillation and

an AED may indicate shock advised. For example, *commotio cordis* is a rare condition in which generally young and otherwise healthy individuals are struck on the chest by a baseball or other object and suddenly collapse from trauma-induced ventricular fibrillation.

Identification of Life-Threatening Bleeding

Identify life-threatening bleeding. Severe bleeding can result in rapid death if it is not treated immediately. The patient may have to be log-rolled to assess for bleeding because there may be wounds on the other side of the body. Rapid external blood loss must be controlled with appropriate techniques, including direct pressure, elevation, pressure points (in an extremity), and, if all else fails, a tourniquet (see Chapter 20).

LEARNING OBJECTIVES

- Describe normal and abnormal findings when assessing skin color.
- Describe normal and abnormal findings when assessing skin temperature.
- Describe normal and abnormal findings when assessing skin condition.
- Describe normal and abnormal findings when assessing skin capillary refill in the infant and child.

Signs of Perfusion

Examination of the skin is an important part of assessing circulation. The skin can provide clues regarding perfusion and oxygenation. Use inspection and palpation to assess the following:

- Skin color
- Skin temperature
- Moisture
- Capillary refilling time

Skin Color

Inspect the nail beds, oral mucosa, and conjunctiva for skin color (**Figure 7-13**). These areas contain many capillaries close to the surface and are the most reliable regardless of pigmentation. In infants and children, color of the palms of the hands and soles of the feet can also be assessed. Normal skin color is pink, indicating perfusion with oxygenated blood.

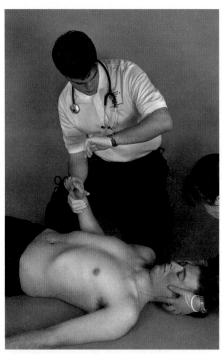

Figure 7-12 Locate the radial pulse at the base of the thumb on the anterolateral aspect of the wrist.

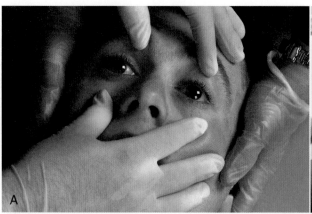
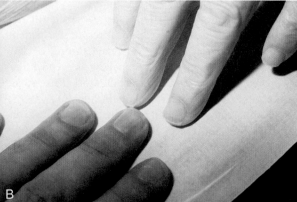

Figure 7-13 **A,** Inspect the sclerae and conjunctivae for appearance. **B,** Note color of skin and nail beds for important clues. Normal skin and nails are contrasted with the pale color seen with severe deficiency of red blood cells.

Abnormal skin colors include the following:

- Pale; may indicate poor perfusion or reduced blood flow or low hemoglobin (**Figure 7-14**).
- Cyanotic (blue-gray); may indicate inadequate oxygen in the blood or poor perfusion (**Figure 7-15**).
- Flushed; may be a sign of exposure to heat or carbon monoxide.
- Jaundiced (yellowish tint); may indicate liver abnormalities (**Figure 7-16**).

Skin Temperature and Condition

You should assess skin temperature and condition (temperature and moisture) by feeling the patient's skin.

Normal temperature is described as "warm." Hot skin temperature can indicate fever. Cool, cold, or clammy (cool and moist) skin can indicate poor perfusion. The condition of skin (e.g., dry, moist, or wet) is a description of the amount of moisture on the skin. Moist, cool, pale skin can be a sign of adrenaline release (epinephrine) to counteract shock or hypoperfusion, a life-threatening condition.

Assess **capillary refilling time** by pressing the nail down against the nail bed until blanching occurs and then releasing and counting the seconds until normal color returns. *Delayed capillary refill* is defined as failure of normal color return within 2 seconds, about the time it takes to say "capillary refill" (**Figure 7-17**). Delayed capillary refilling time may indicate poor perfusion. Be aware that other conditions (e.g., cold temperature, local injuries to extremity) may also cause delayed capillary refill.

When you note signs of circulatory compromise, you should initiate early transport and essential life support. Early transport to the hospital is particularly important when a condition (e.g., internal bleeding) may require surgical intervention.

LEARNING OBJECTIVES

- Differentiate among assessing the altered mental status in the adult, child, and infant.
- Distinguish among methods of assessing breathing in the adult, child, and infant.
- Compare the methods of providing airway care to the adult, child, and infant.

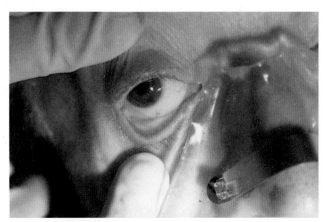

Figure 7-14 Note the pale conjunctivae caused by a deficiency of red blood cells (anemia). Skin pallor is also seen with hypoperfusion.

Infants and Children

Be sure to alter your assessment techniques for infants and children (**Table 7-5**). For further review and discussion, see Chapters 4 and 25 for a complete discussion of airway, breathing, circulation, and neurologic assessment and treatment considerations for infants and children.

LEARNING OBJECTIVE

- Explain the reason for prioritizing a patient for care and transport.

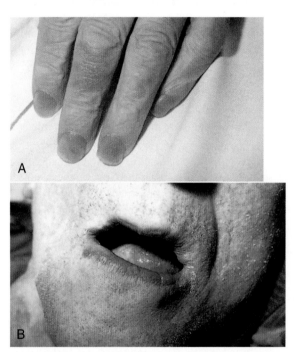

Figure 7-15 **A,** Cyanosis of nail beds is caused by poorly oxygenated red blood cells. The extremities of infants and small children may have a cyanotic appearance when cold. **B,** Cyanosis of the lips from poorly oxygenated red blood cells. Cyanosis is always an indication for supplemental oxygen and often for positive-pressure ventilation.

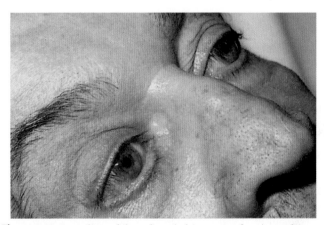

Figure 7-16 Jaundice of the sclera (white part of eye) resulting from liver disease.

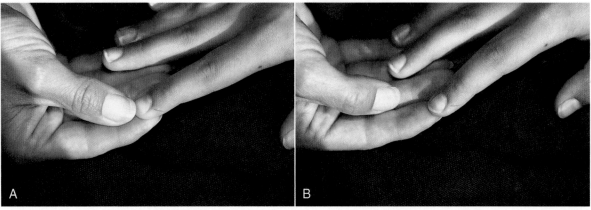

Figure 7-17 Capillary refilling time test. **A,** Press the nail over the nail bed to squeeze blood out of the capillaries under the nail. Pallor or blanching will occur. **B,** Release the nail and observe time to return to normal color. Usually it is immediate. Delayed capillary refilling time is defined as taking more than 2 seconds for return of normal color.

Table 7-5	Differences in Assessment for Infants and Children	
Parameter	**Infants**	**Children**
Mental state/Responsive?	Alertness; can be consoled?	Responses vary by age from infant to adult
	Distracted?	
	Age-specific according to developmental scale in infants and children	Age-specific according to mental state and developmental scale in infants and children
	Muscle tone	
Airway	Place infant's head in sniffing or neutral position when opening airway; do not hyperextend.	Slightly extend head and neck if no trauma is present
	Stridor	Stridor (more common in infants and children from croup, epiglottitis)
Adequacy of breathing	Look for nasal flaring, seesaw breathing, and retractions of chest wall.	Look for nasal flaring and retractions of chest wall
	Grunting	Grunting
Care for inadequate breathing	Suction nasal secretions	Suction nasal secretions
	Smaller volumes of air during positive-pressure ventilation (Look for chest rise.)	Smaller volumes of air (look for chest rise)
	Rate of ventilations: 1 breath every 3 seconds (20 breaths/min)	Rate of ventilations: 1 breath every 3 seconds (20 breaths/min) up to age 8; 15 breaths/min over age 8
Obtaining a pulse	Brachial pulse	Same as for adult: radial and carotid pulses
Assessing perfusion	Capillary refilling time should occur within 2 seconds.	Capillary refilling time should occur within 2 seconds.
	Also assess skin color, temperature, and condition.	Also assess skin color, temperature, and condition.

Identification of Priority Patients

Lifesaving treatments, such as opening the airway, positive-pressure ventilation, oxygen therapy, and immobilization of the spine, are provided as needed during the initial (primary) assessment. You will also make the decision of whether to evaluate further and treat the patient or to transport the patient immediately. Patients in unstable condition with problems that require immediate hospital care should be transported without delay to the appropriate medical facility (**Box 7-2).**

Summary: Initial (Primary) Assessment

During the initial (primary) assessment of the patient, the EMT forms a general impression of the patient from observations of the patient and the environment. Apparent, life-threatening

Box 7-2 **Patients with Priority Conditions Who Require Early Transportation Decision**

Consider rapid transport if the initial (primary) assessment identifies priority patients with conditions such as:

- Poor general impression
- Unresponsiveness (no gag or cough reflex)
- Responsiveness but not following commands (altered mental status)
- Difficulty breathing
- Shock (hypoperfusion)
- Complicated childbirth
- Chest pain with systolic blood pressure <100 mm Hg
- Uncontrolled bleeding
- Severe pain in any location

conditions are noted as the EMT determines the **chief complaint** (the reason EMS was summoned) from the patient, family, or bystanders. The EMT identifies the nature of illness or the mechanism of injury and performs a rapid and orderly assessment for responsiveness, airway, breathing, and circulation to identify any need for immediate intervention to maintain life. The EMT decides if the patient is a priority patient who requires rapid transport to the hospital.

With experience and practice, you will perform the initial (primary) assessment quickly yet thoroughly so that critical problems are identified and treated early. Your general impression and knowledge of the chief complaint, nature of illness, or mechanism of injury will govern your subsequent actions. Review the algorithm in Figure 7-11 and think of the steps, decision points, and therapeutic interventions incorporated in the initial (primary) assessment.

LEARNING OBJECTIVE
- Differentiate between a sign and a symptom.

Patient History

The history of the patient focuses on the patient's chief complaint and signs and symptoms of the present illness. It is a rapid assessment of conditions that may require emergency care or the need for early transport to the hospital. It includes a **history of the present illness,** with special emphasis on the **signs** and **symptoms,** patient complaint, and observable evidence (e.g., OPQRST) and rest of the **SAMPLE** history (allergies, medications, pertinent past medical history, last oral intake, events leading to present illness), rapid assessment of specific body regions, and baseline vital signs. Treatment may be provided based on the findings of this examination. Care may be continued with a more detailed (secondary) history and physical examination, as appropriate, en route to the hospital (**Figure 7-18**).

Sources of a History

A number of potential sources are available for collecting a patient history; the best source is an alert, competent patient who can clearly express the chief complaint and clarify the history of

the present illness. The patient is also most likely to be aware of the nuances of the past history. However, some patients may be unresponsive or disoriented or may have a severe mental illness. The patient may also be an infant or young child who cannot communicate. In these cases the closest family member may be the best source for a history. If necessary, you may also use the patient's friends, bystanders at the scene, public safety workers, or other individuals who may be able to provide information. Bystanders and public safety workers may describe only what they saw and heard before your arrival, but this additional information can be helpful in the assessment and treatment of the patient.

Reliability of a History

A history is only as good as the truth it reveals about the current and past history of the patient. In some circumstances, however, patients, family members, and others may provide false or inaccurate information. For example, patients who have been drinking or taking illegal drugs may deny it because of legal concerns or embarrassment. If you note evidence of alcohol intake (e.g., breath odor) or drug use (e.g., needle marks on patient's arm), you may want to explore the questions further in a private location away from family members and others.

Symptoms such as chest pain that may be associated with serious illness also may result in denial. Normal protective mechanisms lead individuals to deny such symptoms because of the fear of serious complications and death. The patient may also trivialize such symptoms by saying, "It's just indigestion." It is important for you to err on the side of exploring these symptoms further and encourage the patient to seek medical attention. Other reasons for an inaccurate history may include a history of sexually transmitted diseases, pregnancy in younger patients, poor memory in patients with dementia, and general confusion caused by epilepsy, diabetes, or other disorders that may affect brain function. If you are unsure or concerned about the accuracy of data, notify the physician or nurse on arrival at the hospital.

LEARNING OBJECTIVES
- Describe the unique needs for assessing an individual with a specific chief complaint with no known prior history of the problem.
- Differentiate between the history and physical examination performed for responsive patients with no known prior history and for responsive patients with a known prior history of the problem.

Chief Complaint

The history is often the key to assessing and managing the medical patient and points to areas of the body that require physical examination. Patients with a specific chief complaint but no prior known history of the problem will need to have their conditions sufficiently explored to identify the underlying problem. Other patients, such as those with asthma, may know the cause of their chief complaint because they are familiar with their illness. The extent of the history and the scope of the physical examination will vary from patient to patient.

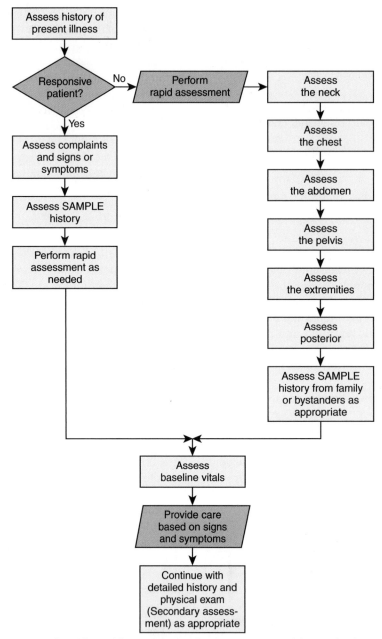

Figure 7-18 Algorithm of focused (secondary) assessment of the medical patient.

Case in Point

Chief Complaint and No Prior History of the Problem

An 11-year-old boy complains of shortness of breath. The scene is safe, and initial (primary) assessment reveals an anxious and alert young man sitting bolt upright and speaking in short phrases with regular respirations, retractions of the neck muscles, and audible wheezing. History reveals his shortness of breath began a half-hour ago after he arrived at his friend's home. He has never had a similar problem. On eliciting further elements of the SAMPLE history, he notes that whenever he has been near cats over the past 2 months, his eyes have teared and his nose became congested. As he relates this history, you notice a long-haired cat enter the room.

Chief Complaint with Prior History of the Problem

An 18-year-old woman complains of shortness of breath. The scene is safe, and initial (primary) assessment reveals an anxious and alert young woman sitting upright, speaking in short sentences, with regular respirations,

retractions of neck muscles, and audible wheezing. She tells you that she has asthma and that this episode is similar to past attacks that were often triggered by a cold or upper respiratory tract infection. She has had a stuffy nose and sore throat for a few days. She has a metered-dose inhaler of albuterol, which she uses when she has an asthma attack, but at present it is empty. She is now having difficulty breathing and finds it difficult to walk.

Discussion

These two examples contrast the scenarios of patients with and without a prior history of a problem. Although both patients appear to have bronchoconstriction or asthma, the second patient understood that her problem was a recurrence of asthma and recognized the signs and symptoms. The first patient had developed shortness of breath for the first time. A more detailed history, gathering information about his "allergies" and other signs, including the presence of the cat, was necessary to point

Continued

toward an impression of possible bronchoconstriction secondary to an allergic reaction.

In general, medical patients are divided into categories of "responsive" and "unresponsive." With responsive patients, you first obtain the SAMPLE history from the patient. This is followed by the physical examination, which is focused on the chief complaint and the signs and symptoms. Third, you obtain baseline vital signs.

With unresponsive patients or patients with altered mental status, you should first complete a rapid assessment of all body regions to ensure that findings are not overlooked. This rapid medical assessment is followed by obtaining baseline vital signs. A SAMPLE history should be sought from family or bystanders at the scene as soon as practically possible.

LEARNING OBJECTIVES
- Identify the components of the SAMPLE history.
- Explain the importance of obtaining a SAMPLE history.

History of Present Illness

The history of the present illness is frequently the most significant part of assessment for the medical patient. It is the patient's story of significant events related to and surrounding the current problem that resulted in the EMS call. The patient usually begins by describing the main problem, the chief complaint, such as, "I have chest pain," "I can't breathe," or "It's the worst headache I've ever had." You should begin a systematic and chronological gathering of relevant information associated with the chief complaint. This history of the present illness includes pertinent past medical history.

Many serious diseases or conditions are often suspected primarily on the basis of the patient history. A heart attack may first be suspected in the prehospital setting because of information in the history (e.g., "This chest pain is just like my heart attack 3 years ago").

The history is obtained by following a set sequence during the interview. All medical professionals perform this to collect relevant data efficiently. Properly taken, a history proceeds in an orderly manner that allows information gathered to be processed with physical signs to achieve a working impression (**Figure 7-19**).

This process includes a SAMPLE history. Remember that the SAMPLE history uses a mnemonic to ensure that you collect key information. Again, the components of SAMPLE are as follows:
- **S**igns and symptoms
- **A**llergies
- **M**edications
- **P**ertinent past medical history
- **L**ast oral intake
- **E**vents leading to the present illness

Signs and Symptoms of the Present Illness

For medical patients, the chief complaint may be associated with a variety of signs and symptoms. For example, a patient with shortness of breath may also complain of leg swelling and chest pain. A patient with chest pain may also complain of nausea, vomiting, sweating, pain in the arm and jaw, and shortness of breath. You should always ask patients whether they have other complaints or abnormal sensations associated with their present illness.

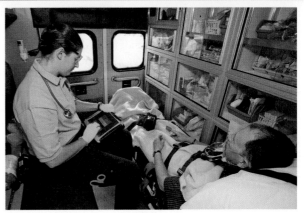

Figure 7-19 Taking a history while evaluating other signs and findings.

Table 7-6	OPQRST: Questions about History of Present Illness

Phase of OPQRST	Explanation
Onset	Determine when the problem occurred and what the patient was doing when it occurred.
Provocation	What, if anything, makes the symptom worse, and what makes it better?
Quality	How does the patient describe the symptom? What does it feel like?
Radiation	Does the pain radiate to other areas of the body?
Severity	How severe is the problem compared with the symptom in past experiences (e.g., "the worst headache in my life")? Rate pain on a scale of 1 to 10, with 1 barely perceptible and 10 the worst pain ever experienced.
Time (duration)	How long has the patient experienced the problem?

One method to help you remember to ask common questions about particular chief complaints is the mnemonic **OPQRST** (**o**nset, **p**rovocation, **q**uality, **r**adiation, **s**everity, **t**ime) (**Table 7-6**). This method is particularly useful for patients with pain and respiratory symptoms.

Onset. Ask the patient to describe when the complaint first occurred (**onset**) and the patient's activity at the onset or immediately before the event (e.g., running, sitting, on awakening, eating). If there are associated complaints, have the patient express the order in which each sign or symptom occurred. For example, "I have been short of breath for 2 days, and an hour ago I had chest pain."

Provocation. Have the patient relate any behavior that makes the symptoms worse or better (**provocation**), for example, "Walking increases the pain," or "When I sit down, it goes away."

Quality. The subjective description of the complaint in the patient's own words is known as the **quality.** For example, if pain is the complaint, ask the patient to describe the pain; typical answers include crushing, viselike, tearing, sharp, dull, and pressure.

Radiation. Pain may spread to another body part or area (**radiation**). Ask the patient whether the pain travels. Chest pain from a blocked coronary artery in the heart may radiate to the arms, neck, or jaw. Back pain can radiate down the leg. If radiation of the pain is noted, relay the information in your patient presentation to the receiving hospital or medical direction.

Severity. Asking patients to use a 10-point (or 5-point) scale to gauge the degree, or **severity,** of their pain is often helpful. For example, ask them to rate the pain from 1 to 10, with 1 barely perceptible and 10 the worst pain they have ever had. Later, during reassessment, ask patients to use the same scale to rate their pain. This might help you monitor whether your treatment has been effective.

Time (Duration). Have the patient tell you the **time,** or duration, of the chief complaint and significant associated complaints.

Allergies and Medications

Be sure to inquire specifically about any history of allergies, including allergic reactions to medications. Ask whether the patient is taking any medications. Bring the medications to the hospital if they are readily available. An older person may not be able to describe the name of a specific disease, but the conditions might be suspected by medical direction because of the medications. In addition, if directed, you can use certain medications, such as nitroglycerin, epinephrine, and metered-dose inhalers (bronchodilators), to assist the patient.

Pertinent Past Medical History

Always ask about pertinent past medical history. Of note are any hospitalizations, surgeries (operations), current medications, and whether the patient is currently under a physician's care. Certain diseases, such as heart problems, diabetes, chronic pulmonary disease, and hypertension, are often progressive and place the patient at risk for emergency conditions. General questions about the patient's overall health status can become important. For example, an older patient who is exhibiting flu symptoms may be asked about a flu immunization. Patients who appear to have respiratory or cardiovascular symptoms should be asked about a smoking history. **Table 7-7** lists questions about current health status that may be important to the patient history.

Last Oral Intake

Inquire about the patient's last oral intake. This information may provide some indication of the patient's underlying condition and is particularly important in diseases such as diabetes. You may also note compliance (or noncompliance) in taking prescribed medications.

Events Leading to the Present Illness

Ascertain the chronology of events leading to the call for help if not already clear from the answers to previous questions. Depending on the circumstance, and particularly with unresponsive patients, determine whether the patient has had any recent trauma. For example, a patient found unresponsive may have a subdural hematoma caused by a head injury months earlier.

Table 7-7	Questions Regarding Current Health Status
Question Area	**When Appropriate**
Current medications	Always appropriate to ask about.
Allergies	Always appropriate to ask about.
Tobacco	Appropriate for most medical problems.
Alcohol, drugs, and related substances	Appropriate for most medical problems.
Diet	Appropriate for most medical problems, especially when you suspect diabetes and allergies.
Screening tests	Important for allergies and when a particular past medical history is suspected (e.g., heart attack, diabetes, infectious disease).
Immunizations	Important for patients with flu symptoms and children with suspected infectious disease.

History According to Type of Patient

The questions you will ask during the history will vary depending on the specific complaint or situation. Although the OPQRST format is well suited to complaints of pain or respiratory distress, other situations (e.g., emergency labor, poisoning) may require additional questions. These questions will become clear as you learn more about various medical conditions that require EMS assistance.

> **LEARNING OBJECTIVES**
> - Differentiate between the assessment performed for a patient who is unresponsive or has an altered mental state and other medical patients requiring assessment.
> - Describe the needs for assessing an individual who is unresponsive.

Responsive Patient

The history and physical examination for responsive medical patients are *focused*. When patients are responsive and can give a clear history, the questioning and physical examination are directed toward the chief complaint rather than the complete head-to-toe approach. For example, for a patient with shortness of breath, a physical examination would be directed toward the head and neck and chest; the legs may be evaluated for swelling. As you learn more about specific conditions, you will understand where to focus your attention during the physical examination.

Unresponsive Patient or the Patient with Altered Mental Status

If the patient is unresponsive or has altered mental status, or if the presenting problem is not clear, perform a **head-to-toe survey (Figure 7-20).** In these patients, you must be sure that trauma is not playing an underlying role or that other findings are not overlooked. Inspect and feel for injury and signs of injury as well as the other signs in different body regions during the head-to-toe survey (see Table 7-11).

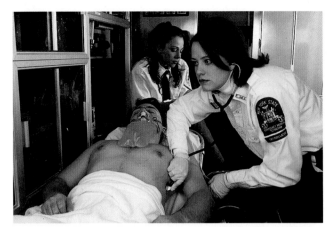

Figure 7-20 Performing a physical examination of a medical patient.

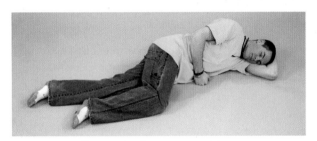

Figure 7-21 Recovery position.

For the unresponsive medical patient, seek the history of the patient's condition from family, friends, or bystanders. A search for a medical identification tag or bracelet may provide helpful clues. Proceed with assessing vital signs, and place the patient in the recovery position to protect the airway during transport (**Figure 7-21**).

Respecting Privacy and Patient Autonomy

Be sensitive to a patient's right to privacy during questioning and the physical examination. You should inform the patient about what you intend to do before beginning your physical examination to gain the patient's cooperation and to ensure that you are acting with the patient's consent.

After you have completed the focused (secondary) history and physical examination of the medical patient, assess the baseline vital signs and provide emergency medical care based on signs and symptoms and your findings.

Challenging Issues Related to Histories

You may encounter many potentially challenging circumstances while collecting a history. **Table 7-8** addresses common patient situations that may present a challenge and suggestions for taking an effective history.

Summary: Patient History

For responsive medical patients, the physical examination is focused on the parts of the body likely to be related to the nature of illness; therefore the history (chief complaint, history of present illness, rest of SAMPLE history) is usually completed before the physical examination. For unresponsive patients and for patients in whom the nature of illness is not clearly defined, you

Table 7-8	Special Patient Challenges when Collecting a History
Patient	**Helpful Suggestions**
Silent	Be sensitive to the patient's silence. Try to observe nonverbal clues. For example, an abused patient may be afraid of abuser in the room.
Overly talkative	Try not to become impatient, and summarize frequently in a focused manner.
Anxious	Anxiety is natural. Be patient, and provide reassurance as needed.
Angry and hostile	Understand that hostility can be natural in stressful situations. Do not react with anger; it will cause the situation to deteriorate.
Intoxicated	Be accepting, not challenging. Treat with dignity.
Crying	Consider cause of crying. Be sympathetic.
Depressed	Be alert for signs of depression, and include them in your history.

will use the more thorough head-to-toe approach and then attempt to gather or complete the history from family and bystanders. Baseline vital signs are assessed, and emergency care is provided. Your partner may obtain the vital signs as you gather more history.

Elicit the nature of the illness by a SAMPLE history format and OPQRST-type questions to describe more fully the present illness. Use questions specific to the chief complaint (**Box 7-3**). For example, a patient with chest pain requires different questions than the patient with altered mental state. You will learn the key questions for each chief complaint as you read about the various conditions in later chapters.

For patients with a prior history of illness similar to the chief complaint, available medications may be valuable in the emergency treatment. As an EMT, you will be prepared to assist the patient with medications for certain medical emergencies according to local medical direction. When life-threatening conditions are determined at any point in the examination, you may intervene with emergency treatment and/or prioritized transportation.

> **LEARNING OBJECTIVES**
> - Identify the components of a focused (secondary) assessment.
> - Explain the importance of a focused (secondary) assessment.
> - Discuss the reason for performing a focused (secondary) assessment.

Focused (Secondary) Assessment

From the scene evaluation, you determine the mechanism of injury and form a general impression of the patient. During the initial (primary) assessment, you evaluate responsiveness, breathing, and perfusion in a search for life-threatening conditions. If such conditions exist, treatment is initiated (e.g., positive-pressure ventilations, bleeding control), and a transport decision is considered. However, many patients will have significant injuries not identified by the initial (primary) assessment alone. Therefore, after the initial (primary) assessment and before you begin further history and physical assessment, *reconsider* the mechanism of injury to determine whether the patient needs (1) a head-to-toe survey or (2) a focused physical examination.

When the mechanism of injury is severe, a head-to-toe-survey is necessary to identify other serious conditions that require emergency care. You should conduct a systematic but quick review of each body area for injuries that may have occurred away from the point of impact or penetration. Because it is rapid, you will only observe for significant signs and symptoms in each body region. When possible, a more comprehensive examination is performed by using the **detailed physical examination.** This is usually performed during transport to the hospital for patients with significant mechanisms of injury.

The mechanism of injury guides the physical examination. If the mechanism is significant, a head-to-toe survey is conducted. If the mechanism is not significant, a **focused physical examination** of the affected part may be sufficient. In critical patients who have problems with their airway, breathing, and circulation, the EMT may never get to the second examination. Treatment remains focused on maintaining breathing and circulation, as with the patient in cardiac arrest.

LEARNING OBJECTIVES
- Identify the components of vital signs.
- Explain the value of performing the baseline vital signs.
- Defend the need for obtaining and recording an accurate set of vital signs.

Baseline Vital Signs

Vital signs are measurements of the functions of vital body systems and are good indicators of abnormal conditions. The vital signs described in the U.S. Department of Transportation (DOT) EMT-Basic Curriculum include the following:
- Respirations
- Pulse
- Blood pressure
- Temperature
- Pupils

The interpretation of vital signs plays a central role in determining prehospital management. Vital signs serve as a basis for initiating specific treatments (e.g., oxygen therapy, ventilation, shock management) and provide a baseline or initial value to measure the effectiveness of therapy. After acquiring a baseline reading, trends in changing vital signs can also be observed. Evaluating the significance of vital signs is done in the context of norms.

Norms are the general ranges of vital signs that are considered normal. For example, the normal pulse rate for adults should be between 60 and 100 beats/min. Norms were established by observing typical ranges among healthy individuals. However, athletes may have pulse rates well below 60 beats/min and still be considered normal.

Vital signs should always be considered in the context of the entire situation. Variables such as stress, anxiety, age, and medications may alter the expected norms. EMTs may ask certain patients, such as athletes or those with a history of **hypertension** (high blood pressure), what is "normal" for them.

Box 7-3	Questions to Ask According to Presenting Problem*

Respiratory
- Onset?
- Provokes?
- Quality?
- Radiates?
- Severity?
- Time?
- Interventions?

Cardiac
- Onset?
- Provokes?
- Quality?
- Radiates?
- Severity?
- Time?
- Interventions?

Altered Mental Status
- Description of the episode
- Onset?
- Duration?
- Associated symptoms?
- Evidence of trauma?
- Interventions?
- Seizures?
- Fever?

Allergic Reaction
- History of allergies?
- "What were you exposed to?"
- "How were you exposed?"
- Effects?
- Progression?
- Interventions?

Poisoning/Overdose
- Substance?
- "When did you ingest/ become exposed"?
- "How much did you ingest?"
- Over what time period?
- Interventions?
- Estimated weight?

Environmental Emergency
- Source?
- Environment?
- Duration?
- Loss of consciousness?
- Effects—general or local?

Obstetrics
- "Are you pregnant?"
- "How long have you been pregnant?"
- Pain or contractions?
- Bleeding or discharge?
- "Do you feel the need to push?"
- Last menstrual period?

Behavioral
- "How do you feel?"
- Determine suicidal tendencies.
- Is the patient a threat to self or others?
- Is there a medical problem?
- Interventions?

Modified from National Registry of Emergency Medical Technicians.
*The questions to ask about the presenting problem will vary according to the circumstances.

Case in Point

You respond to a 28-year-old man who was struck by an automobile. There is no evidence of external bleeding. You record baseline vital signs: respirations, 20 and shallow; pulse 110, weak, and regular; blood pressure, 106/70; skin pale, cool, and sweaty. You suspect that the patient may be bleeding internally. You place him in the shock position with legs elevated 12 inches and administer high-concentration oxygen. Follow-up vital signs taken 5 minutes later are respirations, 20 and shallow; pulse 120, weak, and regular; blood pressure, 100/80; skin pale, cool, and sweaty. These vital signs reflect a slightly increased pulse rate consistent with a trend observed in patients with continued bleeding. You continue to assess the patient's vital signs every 5 minutes to monitor the progress of his condition as you are en route to the hospital.

LEARNING OBJECTIVES
- Describe the methods to obtain a breathing rate.
- Identify the characteristics that should be evaluated during a breathing assessment.
- Differentiate among shallow, labored, and noisy breathing.

Respirations

Normal breathing is characterized as the smooth rise and fall of the abdomen and chest wall. The accessory muscles of breathing are not used. The process of breathing is evaluated according to rate and quality.

Rate. To evaluate breathing, you should be stationed at the side of the patient for a clear view of the chest and abdominal regions. The patient's breathing should be observed without the patient's awareness because the patient may vary breathing with conscious controls. Observing the margin of the chest and abdomen, count the number of breaths occurring in a 30-second period and multiply by two. The normal respiratory rate in adults is 12 to 20 breaths/min. The rate in children tends to be fastest during infancy and gradually decreases to adult rates with age (Table 7-9).

A patient's rate of breathing may be slow, normal, rapid, or stopped completely (respiratory arrest). Identifying abnormal rates will allow you to recognize the need for administering supplemental oxygen and positive-pressure ventilation (see Chapter 6).

Quality. Quality of respiration is categorized as follows:
- Normal
- Shallow
- Labored
- Noisy

Table 7-9	Normal Respiratory Rates
Patient Age	**Normal Rate**
Adult (>10 yr)	12-20 breaths/min
Child (2-10 yr)	15/30 breaths/min
Infant (birth-2 yr)	25-50 breaths/min

Normal breathing occurs quietly with little effort and with bilateral chest movement.

Shallow breathing results in minimal movement of the abdominal and chest wall.

Labored breathing occurs when respiratory effort is increased. This can result from an obstructed airway, fluid in the lungs, or collapse of the lungs.

At times it is evident from across the room that a patient has labored breathing. Patients may be sitting bolt upright or leaning forward; children may have their head and neck thrust forward, seated and perched on both hands in the **tripod position;** and signs of accessory muscle use and abnormal sounds may be evident from a distance. **Nasal flaring** and **retractions** of the chest wall may be especially noticeable in infants and children (**Figure 7-22**). Retractions are inward depressions of muscular areas between the ribs, above the clavicles, and below the sternum.

Noisy respirations refer to sounds emitted during breathing. Sounds heard externally, without the use of a stethoscope, usually indicate an obstructive process in the upper or lower airways. Such sounds include the following:
- **Grunting**—Rhythmic sound that is abnormal, deep, short, and hoarse and heard at the end of exhalation.
- **Gurgling**—Sound created by air moving through fluid, similar to blowing through a straw beneath water. This usually indicates the presence of fluid in the upper airway.
- **Wheezing**—High-pitched, "whistling" sounds created by narrowed bronchioles in the lower airway. This is often noted with asthma, an allergic reaction, or bronchitis.
- **Crowing (stridor)**—Harsh, high-pitched sound usually heard on inspiration. It is indicative of upper airway obstruction involving the vocal cords or epiglottis.
- **Snoring**—Harsh, low-pitched sound usually caused by the tongue partially blocking the upper airway. An unconscious patient may have this type of obstruction.
- **Gasping**—Short breaths with a rapid inspiratory phase associated with respiratory distress and fatigue.

Sounds of breathing may also be auscultated through a stethoscope. The technique of auscultating breath sounds is explained in Chapter 6.

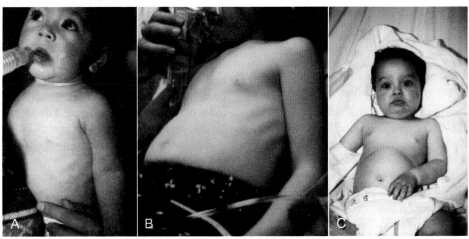

Figure 7-22 Signs of labored breathing in children. **A,** Nasal flaring; **B,** retractions; **C,** abdominal distention.

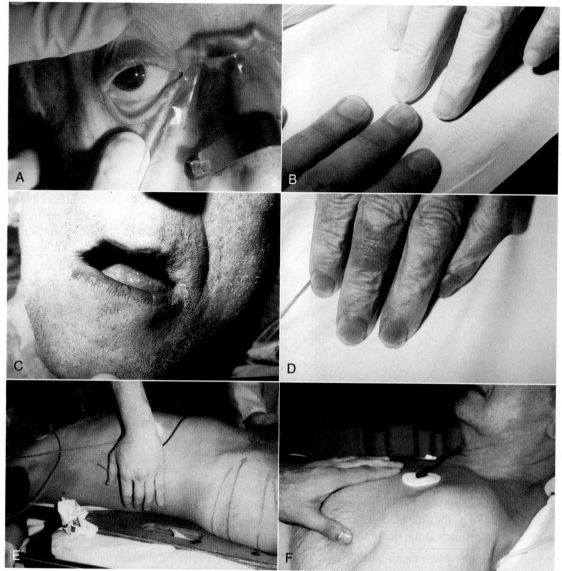

Figure 7-29 Note the color of the skin and nail beds for important clues. **A,** Pale conjunctivae. **B,** Normal skin and nails are contrasted with pale color seen with severe deficiency of red blood cells. **C** and **D,** Cyanotic lips and nail beds. **E,** Flushed skin (contrasted with normal hand). **F,** Jaundice.

occur in extreme heat conditions as the body attempts to bring blood to the surface for heat removal. It also can occur when a person has been poisoned with carbon monoxide, causing the hemoglobin on the red blood cells to assume a bright-red color. Again, flushed color to the skin must be assessed on the basis of the presenting problem.

Jaundiced Skin. Jaundiced, or yellow, skin usually indicates problems related to the liver or gallbladder. The liver produces a substance called *bile* that is stored and excreted from the gallbladder through ducts into the small intestines. When the ducts in the liver or gallbladder become obstructed from inflammation or disease, the bile and a yellow pigment of bile called *bilirubin* build up in the blood and are deposited in the patient's skin, causing **jaundice.**

Skin Temperature. Skin temperature is usually assessed by feeling the patient's forehead with the back of your ungloved hand. Note whether the patient's skin feels normal (warm), cool, or hot.

If the patient's skin feels cool, you can further assess the skin by placing the back of your hand (with the glove retracted so you feel with your skin) on a more central area of the trunk, such as the abdomen. For example, you might place your hand on the abdomen underneath the patient's clothing. The skin feels cool with shock or other conditions that limit perfusion. The skin feels hot with conditions such as fever or other heat-related emergencies.

Moisture. In addition to feeling for skin temperature with the back of your hand, it is important to feel for moisture on the skin. Normal skin is warm and dry to the touch. Skin that feels slightly moist and cool is called "clammy." Excessive sweating is called *diaphoresis.* Cool, clammy skin is found in patients in shock. Hot and dry skin may be found in patients with heat-related emergencies.

Capillary Refill Time. Another method for assessing perfusion in children and infants, capillary refill time is tested by first pressing the nail bed to whiten or "blanch" the nail. The return

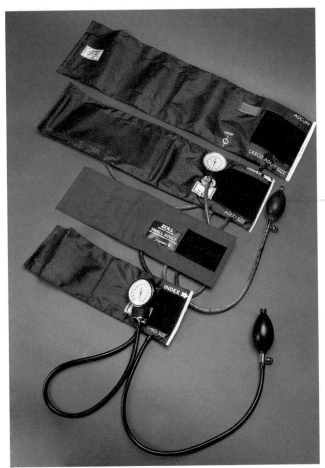

Figure 7-30 Different-sized blood pressure cuffs. Use the correct-sized cuff for the patient to avoid incorrect readings.

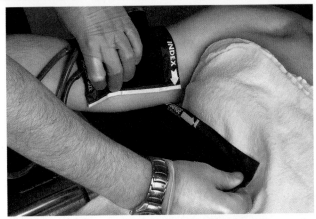

Figure 7-31 Using index and range lines to check cuff size. The cuff is applied so that the inflation bag is centered over the brachial artery using the markings on the cuff. When a cuff fits properly, the index line should fall between the two range lines.

to a pink color is then timed. Normal capillary refilling time is less than 2 seconds. A longer time reflects poor perfusion. Remember always to relate your findings to the patient's overall condition. Note that an increased capillary refilling time could indicate that perfusion is only decreased to an exposed area of the skin, such as occurs in the hands during cold weather.

LEARNING OBJECTIVES
- Describe the methods to assess blood pressure.
- Define systolic pressure.
- Define diastolic pressure.
- Explain the difference between auscultation and palpation for obtaining a blood pressure.

Blood Pressure

Blood pressure is a measure of the force that blood exerts on the walls of the arteries. It is determined by the following two factors:
- The amount of blood ejected from the heart each minute.
- The space within the arteries that the blood occupies.

The measurement of blood pressure reflects two phases of the heart's cycle: systole (contraction) and diastole (relaxation). As the heart contracts during systole, blood is propelled from the left ventricle into the aorta and is distributed to the other arteries, generating an increase in pressure on the walls of the

arteries. At its peak, this pressure reaches approximately 120 mm Hg in a young, healthy person. As the ventricle relaxes in diastole, the pressure in the arteries begins to drop. The pressure drops to approximately 80 mm Hg (young healthy person), and then the next contraction occurs; thus, during the heart's normal cycle, the pressure does not drop to zero. Changes in heart function, blood vessel diameter, and total blood volume may alter blood pressure.

Blood pressure is measured with a **sphygmomanometer.** The cuff is placed around the arm above the elbow; most cuffs have markings that aid in the correct placement. The cuff should be snug enough so as not to move freely, but not so tight as to cause discomfort to the patient.

Sizing the Blood Pressure Cuff. Various sizes of blood pressure cuffs are available, from pediatric through large adult (**Figure 7-30**). Selecting the correct size is important; a cuff that is too small may result in a falsely high reading, and a cuff that is too large may result in a falsely low reading. Several methods are used to measure blood pressure cuff size. The simplest method is to use the standard line markings that are on the cuff to check the proper size. When the cuff is the correct size, the lines of the cuff should fall between the markings (**Figure 7-31**).

In the adult, width of the cuff should be one-third to one-half the circumference of the arm. For children, width of the bladder within the cuff should not exceed two-thirds the length of the child's arm (from armpit to crease in elbow). The length of the bladder should encircle approximately three-quarters the circumference of the child's arm. If the bladder encircles the entire arm, it is too large.

Methods for Measuring Blood Pressure. Blood pressure can be measured using auscultation or palpation. **Auscultation,** the preferred method, involves listening to sounds emitted from an artery while its diameter changes from a collapsed to a fully opened state (**Skill 7-5**).

Palpation is used when you cannot ascertain blood pressure by auscultation, possibly because of environmental noise or very low blood pressure, such as in shock. As you release the pressure in the cuff, feel for the distal pulse, usually the radial

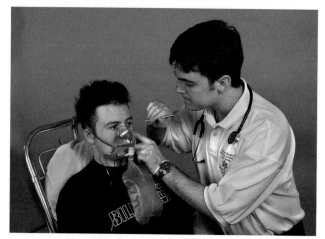

Figure 7-32 Pupil check.

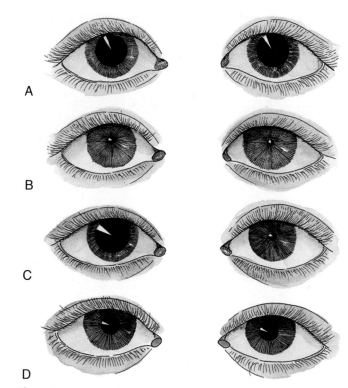

Figure 7-33 **A,** Pupil dilation; **B,** pupil constriction; **C,** unequal pupils; **D,** normal pupils. *From NAEMT:* Prehospital trauma life support, *ed 5, St Louis, 2002, Mosby.*

or brachial, and determine the point at which blood first flows through the artery **(Skill 7-6);** record this number as the systolic pressure. You cannot determine the diastolic pressure by palpation, so you should record the blood pressure as "120/palp" or "120/p."

Normal and Abnormal Blood Pressure Readings. The normal values for adult blood pressure vary with age. A general rule for the systolic pressure is 100 mm Hg plus the patient's age, up to 140 to 150 mm Hg. The diastolic range is 65 to 90 mm Hg. Women tend to have blood pressures 8 to 10 mm Hg lower than men of the same age. Children and young adults normally have lower pressures (see Chapter 25).

Many factors and disease states affect blood pressure. Stress, anxiety, drugs, metabolic disturbances, and CNS diseases and injuries are common causes of increased pressure. Shock states, drugs, heart rhythm disturbances, and simple fainting are associated with decreased pressures. Again, the significance of variations must be evaluated in the framework of the entire clinical situation. Questioning patients about their normal blood pressure is important when you are considering its significance.

Blood pressure should be measured in all adults and children older than 3 years. Because the vital signs of infants and children can vary over a broad range in both sickness and health, the general assessment (e.g., sick appearance, unresponsiveness) is often more valuable than the actual number.

REAL*World*

Measuring blood pressure in a moving ambulance can be a challenge because of ambient sounds and movement over rough terrain. A blood pressure by palpation is a useful adjunct in such conditions. If changes are noted during palpation, it may be appropriate to stop the ambulance briefly to validate any concerns.

LEARNING OBJECTIVES
- Describe the methods used to assess the pupils.
- Identify normal and abnormal pupil size.
- Differentiate between dilated (large) and constricted (small) pupil size.
- Differentiate between reactive and nonreactive pupils and equal and unequal pupils.

Pupils

An important diagnostic sign during examination of the head is the status of the pupils **(Figure 7-32).** Pupillary function is measured according to the following parameters:
1. Diameter
2. Reactivity to light
3. Equality of size

The pupil is the central, round, black portion of the eye that normally changes diameter in relation to light. When exposed to bright light, the pupil should **constrict,** or become smaller. Conversely, in a dark environment pupils should be **dilated,** or become larger. When a pupil changes in response to light, it is said to be *reactive.* When a pupil does not respond to light, it is *nonreactive.* The two pupils should be round, equal in size, and equally reactive to light. *PERRL* is an acronym for remembering the normal response of pupils: *Pupils* are *Equal, Round,* and *Reactive* to *Light.*

Abnormal findings in the examination of pupils may indicate a metabolic problem or brain injury. For example, pupils that are constricted or pinpointed may be associated with an overdose of certain opiate drugs (e.g., heroin) or may be caused by damage to certain areas of the brain. Pupils may be dilated because of a severe lack of oxygen (hypoxia), brain death, or ingestion of toxic substances. Pupils that are unequal may be caused by injury to one side of the brain.

As an EMT, you are not expected to know every cause of variations in pupil findings, but you should be prepared to evaluate, carefully document, and report your findings to hospital personnel **(Figure 7-33).**

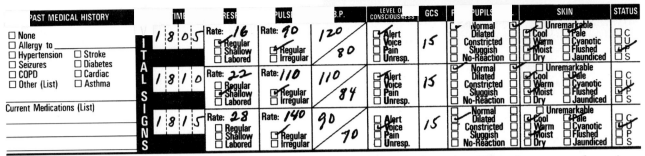

PAST MEDICAL HISTORY	TIME	RESP	PULSE	B.P.	LEVEL OF CONSCIOUSNESS	GCS	PUPILS		SKIN	STATUS

Figure 7-34 Repeat vital signs should be documented completely to track changes in the patient. These changes can play an important role in decision making at the hospital.

> **LEARNING OBJECTIVES**
> - State the importance of accurately reporting and recording baseline vital signs.
> - Explain the rationale of recording additional sets of vital signs.

Vital Signs Assessment

You should continually monitor a patient's vital signs while you are on the scene and during transport. As a rule, vital signs should be reassessed, at a minimum, every 15 minutes for patients in stable condition and every 5 minutes for patients in unstable condition. You should also reassess vital signs after medical interventions, such as repositioning the patient or administrating medications (e.g., nitroglycerin, albuterol). line status of the patient compared with changes that occurred during treatment and transport. This plays an important role in decision making at the hospital (**Figure 7-34**).

> **LEARNING OBJECTIVES**
> - State the reasons for performing a rapid trauma assessment.
> - Determine when the rapid assessment may be altered to provide patient care.

Rapid Assessment

The approach to the trauma patient varies by the relative severity of the mechanism of injury. Obviously, you will evaluate a patient with a minor cut on the hand from a kitchen knife differently than someone who was struck by a vehicle. Your assessment for the patient with a minor cut will focus on the hand, evaluating the nature of bleeding, circulation, and motor and sensory function in the hand. The patient who was struck and thrown by a vehicle will require a rapid (head-to-toe) trauma assessment of the entire body.

Case in Point

Consider the following two scenarios to clarify the use of a focused physical examination versus the head-to-toe survey.

Head-to-Toe Survey: Significant Mechanism of Injury

You respond to a call for "man down" and find a 24-year-old man who has fallen from a two-story window. The scene is safe. You applied gloves, mask, and eyewear while approaching the scene. You estimate the height of the fall at 20 feet. Your general impression reveals a man who is lying supine and appears conscious and complaining of pain in the ankle, where you note obvious deformity. Co-workers advise you that he fell while cleaning windows and landed on his feet. Your partner stabilizes the man's head and cervical spine, and you perform an initial assessment. The patient is responsive, alert, and oriented and is breathing rapidly with normal chest rise. He has a weak and rapid pulse with no evidence of external bleeding. While a third EMT prepares for transport, you administer high-concentration oxygen by a nonrebreather mask and perform a head-to-toe survey.

You cut away the patient's clothing, and using the DCAP/BTLS mnemonic, you rapidly examine the head, neck, chest, abdomen, pelvis, and upper and lower extremities. After examining the neck, you apply a cervical collar. You also check for breath sounds while examining the chest and perform a sensorimotor examination in the upper and lower extremities. While log rolling the patient onto a long spine board, you check his back and buttocks. Your head-to-toe survey reveals tenderness, deformity, and swelling of the left ankle and pain and tenderness of the hip and lower back region. Baseline vital signs are respirations 20 breaths/min and adequate, pulse 110 beats/min and weak, and blood pressure 90/70 mm Hg. You immediately transport the patient and notify the hospital of his impending arrival.

Focused History and Physical Examination: Mechanism of Injury Not Significant

You respond to an office building for an "injured female." You apply gloves while approaching the scene. On arrival at the scene, you find a 72-year-old woman who has twisted her ankle while walking on an uneven surface. She did not fall but has severe pain in the left ankle and cannot stand. Your general impression reveals a patient who is alert, sitting up, and has normal skin color and moisture. While your partner takes baseline vital signs, you examine the ankle. You note that the ankle is swollen and tender on the lateral surface. The patient has a distal pedal pulse and can move her toes. The foot has a normal color and temperature, and normal capillary refilling time is present in the toes. The patient also has normal sensation and movement of the foot and toes. Her vital signs are respirations 12 breaths/min and regular, pulse 84 beats/min and regular, and blood pressure 130/80 mm Hg. You splint the ankle, place the patient on a stretcher, and take a SAMPLE history during transport.

Analysis of the Cases

These two cases illustrate the key difference between a significant and a nonsignificant mechanism of injury. Both patients injured their ankles and had a chief complaint of ankle pain. However, the patient with a significant mechanism of injury clearly had the potential for multiple serious injuries in other locations of the body and required a head-to-toe survey to look for more clues. The other patient essentially "twisted" her ankle and required focused attention to the site of the injury to identify signs of injury and possible complications to nerves and blood supply to the ankle.

Assessing mechanism of injury allows you to quickly plan your overall approach to a patient to ensure identification of life-threatening injuries for patients with significant mechanisms of injury, and to care appropriately and efficiently for patients who do not have a significant mechanism of injury.

Reconsidering the Mechanism of Injury

During the scene size-up, the specific mechanism of injury is one of the first details you should determine when arriving at the scene of an emergency. *Significant mechanisms of injury* warrant a thorough search for signs of their impact on the body. Over time, physicians and prehospital personnel have learned to associate certain mechanisms of injury as capable of causing, or likely resulting in, death or serious disability (see Table 7-3).

The issue of injury severity is so important in emergency medical services decision making that the American College of Surgeons (ACS) developed a triage scheme that incorporates the mechanism of injury in the decision regarding whether a patient should be transported to a trauma center. (See **Figure 7-35** and note the list of significant mechanisms of injury.)

Knowledge of a mechanism of injury also helps you anticipate certain injury patterns. For example, a person who falls from a height and lands on the feet is likely to have the force transmitted up the lower extremities and the spine. Other factors that may help in determining types of injuries include the location of penetrating injuries, velocity of firearms, point of impact during a collision or fall, point of impact in a pedestrian injury, and type of blunt object that strikes a victim in a violent episode.

Hidden Injuries

As discussed earlier, identifying whether victims of motor vehicle crashes were wearing safety devices is important. This information can be obtained by questioning the patients and others at the scene and by inspecting the vehicle and the patient.

You should remember that the force of collision may still cause serious injury despite safety devices. Safety devices may also have been improperly used. A shoulder or lap belt that is worn alone can cause serious injuries. A loose lap belt can ride up the abdomen, causing compression of abdominal organs and spinal injury.

You should remember to "lift and look" when caring for crash victims when an airbag has been activated. Lift the deployed airbag, and look at the steering wheel to see whether it has been deformed, an indicator of potentially serious internal injury to the chest and abdomen.

Infants and Children

Significant mechanisms of injury for infants and children include bicycle collisions, impact from vehicles, and falls from lesser heights. Children should use age-specific and size-specific safety devices. All states have safety device utilization laws that require use of special seats for infants and toddlers (see earlier discussion).

Elderly Patients

Older patients can be seriously injured by lesser mechanisms of injury and should be carefully evaluated for potential bone injury, even with relatively minor mechanisms such as low falls. For example, a slip and fall on the floor is a common cause of hip fracture as people age. The elderly patient may also have a different response to an injury than a younger counterpart. Typically, older patients do not compensate as well for serious injury and tend to decompensate (become worse) more quickly. They may also be taking medications that affect vital signs.

Chapter 31 provides a comprehensive review of older patients.

Detailed Physical Examination

You will perform a head-to-toe survey on all patients with significant mechanism of injury to look for signs and symptoms of injuries. In the responsive patient, symptoms should be sought before and during the trauma assessment. If the patient is unresponsive, a head-to-toe survey is indicated. The detailed examination in a patient with a medical complaint may help determine the underlying disease process. Treatments provided by the EMT will depend on the physical exam. Typically, detailed examination and ongoing assessment or reassessment are completed in the ambulance en route to the hospital.

If the mechanism of injury raises the possibility of spinal injury, or if the patient has head trauma or an altered mental state, you should continue to maintain manual spinal stabilization while you conduct the head-to-toe survey. Consider whether the condition requires rapid transportation to the receiving hospital or if an ALS intercept is warranted.

DCAP/BTLS

As you inspect and palpate, you should look and feel for certain injuries and signs of injury. The mnemonic **DCAP/BTLS** indicates the signs you should seek and record for each body area examined, as follows:

- **D**eformities
- **C**ontusions
- **A**brasions
- **P**unctures/penetrations
- **B**urns
- **T**enderness
- **L**acerations
- **S**welling

These injuries are frequently encountered, and their findings are significant to EMTs and receiving hospitals (**Figure 7-36**).

Deformities. A **deformity** is a structural distortion or bend that alters the normal appearance of the body or a body part. Broken bones (fractures), dislocations, and soft tissue swelling are causes of deformity in trauma patients. Different types of deformities are caused by different underlying conditions. For example, angulation of long bones, protuberance of the bone end against soft tissues, and overriding or separation of bone fragments by opposing muscles can result in visible and palpable deformities. The grating of one bone fragment against another generates a sensation to the examiner's fingers known as **crepitus**, or *crepitation*.

Contusions. A **contusion** can be defined as a *bruise*, an injury to part of the body without a break in the skin. When blunt or compression forces are applied to the skin, the capillaries or larger vessels may leak or rupture. This may be accompanied by slight swelling from leakage of plasma into the injured area. Tenderness or pain may be present at the site of injury.

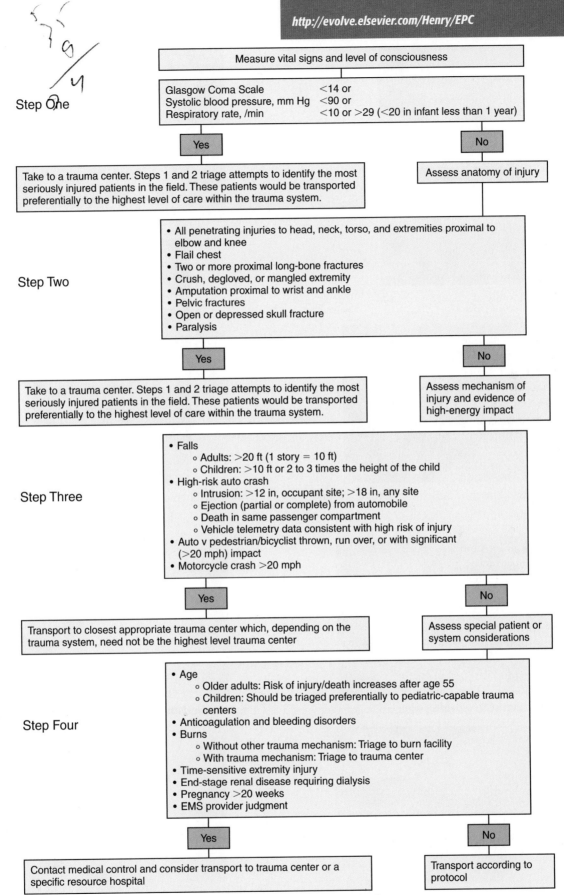

Step One

Measure vital signs and level of consciousness

Glasgow Coma Scale	<14 or
Systolic blood pressure, mm Hg	<90 or
Respiratory rate, /min	<10 or >29 (<20 in infant less than 1 year)

Yes / **No**

Take to a trauma center. Steps 1 and 2 triage attempts to identify the most seriously injured patients in the field. These patients would be transported preferentially to the highest level of care within the trauma system.

Assess anatomy of injury

Step Two

- All penetrating injuries to head, neck, torso, and extremities proximal to elbow and knee
- Flail chest
- Two or more proximal long-bone fractures
- Crush, degloved, or mangled extremity
- Amputation proximal to wrist and ankle
- Pelvic fractures
- Open or depressed skull fracture
- Paralysis

Yes / **No**

Take to a trauma center. Steps 1 and 2 triage attempts to identify the most seriously injured patients in the field. These patients would be transported preferentially to the highest level of care within the trauma system.

Assess mechanism of injury and evidence of high-energy impact

Step Three

- Falls
  - Adults: >20 ft (1 story = 10 ft)
  - Children: >10 ft or 2 to 3 times the height of the child
- High-risk auto crash
  - Intrusion: >12 in, occupant site; >18 in, any site
  - Ejection (partial or complete) from automobile
  - Death in same passenger compartment
  - Vehicle telemetry data consistent with high risk of injury
- Auto v pedestrian/bicyclist thrown, run over, or with significant (>20 mph) impact
- Motorcycle crash >20 mph

Yes / **No**

Transport to closest appropriate trauma center which, depending on the trauma system, need not be the highest level trauma center

Assess special patient or system considerations

Step Four

- Age
  - Older adults: Risk of injury/death increases after age 55
  - Children: Should be triaged preferentially to pediatric-capable trauma centers
- Anticoagulation and bleeding disorders
- Burns
  - Without other trauma mechanism: Triage to burn facility
  - With trauma mechanism: Triage to trauma center
- Time-sensitive extremity injury
- End-stage renal disease requiring dialysis
- Pregnancy >20 weeks
- EMS provider judgment

Yes / **No**

Contact medical control and consider transport to trauma center or a specific resource hospital

Transport according to protocol

When in doubt, transport to a trauma center

Figure 7-35 American College of Surgeons (ACS) triage scheme. Note the mechanisms of injury list to appreciate significant factors. From ACS Committee on Trauma: Resources of optimal care of the injured patient, Chicago, 2006.

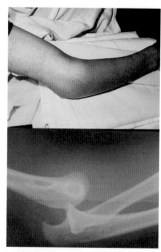

Deformity of elbow dislocation.

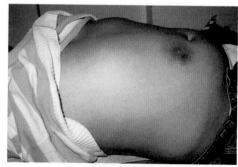

Contusion on abdomen caused by a kick the previous day.

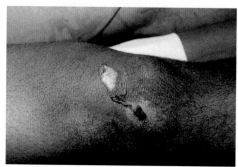

Abrasion wounds to kneecaps caused by fall to the ground.

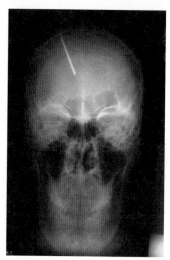

Radiograph of **puncture** from a nail gun.

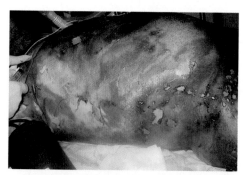

Burn; third-degree burn.

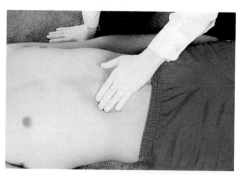

Tenderness during palpation of abdomen.

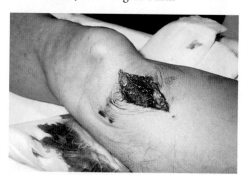

Laceration to thigh caused by circular saw.

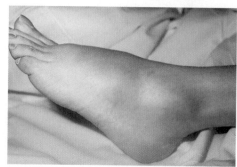

Swelling and dislocation from fracture of foot and distal leg.

Figure 7-36 Atlas of a DCAP/BTLS

Contusions can be accompanied by leakage of blood from injured vessels. This bleeding may be visible just under the skin as a black-and-blue area and is called *ecchymosis*. The color changes to green-brown and then to yellow over time as the blood products break down and are absorbed. When blood collects beneath the skin, it is known as a *hematoma* (literally a tumor or swelling containing blood).

Abrasions. An **abrasion** is a scraping of the surface of the skin or mucous membrane. It may result in the breaking of superficial capillaries, causing an oozing of blood at the skin's surface. Although often very painful, abrasions themselves do not usually result in significant blood loss. As with other open wounds, abrasions are subject to infection.

Puncture or Penetration. A **puncture** occurs when a sharp instrument is driven through the skin's outer layer. Punctures can be very deceiving. A small puncture wound may be caused by an object, such as an ice pick, that has penetrated to a significant depth, causing damage to underlying structures.

Burns. A burn may result from thermal, chemical, or electrical injury. Burns are categorized according to depth, as follows:
- *Superficial* (first-degree) burns involve the upper level of the skin (epidermis) and are characterized by a reddened appearance to the skin, such as a sunburn.
- *Partial-thickness* (second-degree) burns involve the upper and lower layers of the skin (dermis) and are characterized by blistering with or without reddening of the skin.
- *Full-thickness* (third-degree) burns extend through the upper and lower layers of the skin. They may appear black and charred, yellow-brown, dark red, or white and translucent. Often the veins are visible at the skin's surface.

Tenderness. **Tenderness** is pain that is elicited on palpation. *Palpation* should be gentle to minimize the patient's discomfort.

Lacerations. A **laceration** is a tearing of the skin or other soft tissues resulting from a blunt tearing force or from a sharp object. The extent of surrounding tissue damage is a function of the mechanism of injury. Blunt forces that tear the skin also may cause significant damage to the surrounding tissues. In contrast, a sharp object is more likely to cause an incision-type wound and cause little damage to the tissue surrounding the wound.

Swelling. *Swelling* is an abnormal enlargement of a body part or organ caused by an increased volume of fluid in blood vessels or between cells. Swelling may be obvious during palpation, when indentations from your fingers leave an imprint in the tissue.

LEARNING OBJECTIVES
- State the reasons for performing a head-to-toe survey.
- Describe the areas included in the head-to-toe survey, and discuss what to evaluate.
- Give examples and explain why patients should receive a head-to-toe survey.

Head-to-Toe Survey

The head-to-toe order of this examination helps ensure that all body parts are included. In all body regions, you should look for and note the signs of injuries described earlier by the mnemonic

Table 7-11	Head-to-Toe Survey	
Body Region	**DCAP/BTLS**	**Other Signs**
Head	DCAP/BTLS	Crepitation
Neck	DCAP/BTLS	Crepitation Jugular venous distention Tracheal deviation
Chest	DCAP/BTLS	Crepitation Breath sounds at four locations: midclavicular line at the apices and midaxillary line at the bases Paradoxical motion of the chest wall
Abdomen	DCAP/BTLS	Firm, soft Distended
Pelvis	DCAP/BTLS	Crepitation Gentle compression for tenderness and motion
Lower extremities	DCAP/BTLS	Distal pulse Sensation Motor function
Upper extremities	DCAP/BTLS	Distal pulse Sensation Motor function
Roll patient over and examine the back	DCAP/BTLS	

DCAP/BTLS: Look for deformities, contusions, abrasions, punctures or penetrations, burns, tenderness, lacerations, and swelling.

DCAP/BTLS (**Table 7-11**). Remember, you are inspecting and feeling for these types of injuries in all body regions. When assessing patients with medical complaints, body systems are evaluated to help determine the cause of the illness and to establish treatment plans.

You should tell responsive patients that you need to check them briefly to determine whether other injuries are present. For patients who have a significant mechanism of injury but no complaints, explaining the purpose of your head-to-toe survey is especially important. Remember, you treat and evaluate patients with their consent. You should respect a patient's privacy as much as possible during the head-to-toe survey.

During the head-to-toe survey, you may have to alter your approach to provide patient care. For example, if a patient's breathing becomes inadequate during the head-to-toe examination, you would stop to provide supplemental oxygen, positive-pressure ventilation, or both measures. Any life-threatening condition noted during assessment may cause you to alter your sequence to initiate treatment or prioritize transport.

Head

The head should be examined for evidence of injuries. When examining the head of a suspected trauma patient, you should always assume the presence of a neck injury. Observe and palpate the skull and face carefully. Palpation should be gentle to avoid compressing bone fragments into the brain if a skull

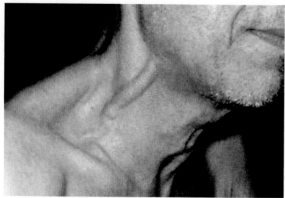

Figure 7-37 Distended neck veins. *From Swartz MH:* Textbook of physical diagnosis, *ed 5, St Louis, 2006, Saunders.*

fracture exists. You might note crepitus or a grating sensation on your fingertips from overriding bone fragments. Note any bruising to the head. Bruising behind the ears (Battle's sign) or bruising around both eyes (raccoon eyes) may be a sign of basilar skull fracture. Using a penlight, look at both eyes, noting the responsiveness of the pupils. Both pupils should respond equally. Nonresponsive or unequal pupils could suggest a head injury, stroke, or drug use. Look at both ears and assess for fluid and blood. Open the mouth and look for swelling, blood, teeth, or other potential sources of obstruction.

Neck

Examination of the neck offers valuable information about the status of the respiratory and cardiovascular systems as well as signs of soft tissue and possible cervical spine injury. You should observe the neck and palpate for signs of injury, especially wounds, contusions, and deformity.

Active neck muscles (accessory muscles) during respiratory efforts suggest impairment or obstruction of respiratory function requiring increased work of breathing. The larynx and trachea, which are located midline just above the suprasternal notch, should be palpated. **Tracheal deviation** to either side of the neck and the development of **subcutaneous emphysema** (air beneath the skin) can occur from injury to the airway or chest. Subcutaneous emphysema is characterized by a crackling sensation (similar to squeezing cellophane wrapping) beneath the skin's surface, also called crepitus. When crepitus is severe, the neck might appear swollen or enlarged (see Chapter 22).

Neck Veins. The external jugular veins, which extend down to the clavicle on both sides of the neck, should be examined for distention (**Figure 7-37**). **Jugular venous distention** (distended neck veins) can indicate backup in the venous system returning to the heart (see Chapter 12). Flat external jugular veins in the supine patient may be a sign of decreased blood pressure.

Cervical Collar. If either the mechanism of injury or the examination findings (e.g., tenderness or deformity in the spine) indicate possible spinal injury, you should apply a cervical collar.

Chest

The thorax should be observed and palpated on the anterior, posterior, and lateral planes. Open wounds should be identified and promptly sealed with an airtight dressing. Areas of suspected fractures should be closely observed for signs of paradoxical motion of breathing (**Figure 7-38**). This is characterized by injured sections of the thorax moving in the opposite direction of the uninjured sections. These types of injuries are detailed in Chapter 22. Subcutaneous emphysema may also be observed or felt (crepitus) and may be associated with an underlying lung injury.

You should observe the chest for symmetrical expansion. Decreased movement on one side of the chest, called *splinting,* suggests underlying chest injury.

Look for the use of accessory muscles, which may indicate a respiratory problem such as asthma or emphysema (see Chapter 11).

Examine the lungs and listen to the lungs with the diaphragm (flat) end of the stethoscope at four locations. At each location, listen to at least one complete respiratory cycle. Listen to the apices (top portion of the chest) of the lungs at the midclavicular line bilaterally just below the clavicles. Also, listen to the bases of the lungs on each side in the midaxillary line at the level of the nipples. The lower border of the lung normally moves from the sixth rib to the eighth rib along the lateral chest wall during inhalation and exhalation. You should note whether breath sounds are present, absent, or equal. Identify sounds such as wheezing, stridor, or crackles.

Abdomen

Examination of the abdomen should begin with inspection for injury and distention. Distention may be characterized by a bloated appearance, which can be caused by air or fluid collecting within the abdomen. Feel to determine whether the abdomen is soft or firm. Gently palpate the four quadrants of the patient's abdomen and note whether they are tender or rigid. If the patient is conscious and complaining of abdominal pain, ask the patient to point to the area of pain, and assess that area last. Assess for abdominal masses, which may indicate bowel obstruction or abdominal aneurysm.

Pelvis

Inspect and palpate the pelvis and hip region. If no pain is noted, gently compress the iliac crests of the pelvis toward each other (medially) and posteriorly, observing for tenderness or movement. If the patient complains of pain, or if there is movement of these normally fixed bones, you must suspect a pelvic fracture exists. Care and gentleness are essential during this examination to avoid complicating underlying fractures. You should not compress the pelvis if the patient has pain. Compression should be stopped if you feel any movement or cause pain.

You should also look for the presence of **priapism,** an abnormal persistent erection of the penis caused by a spinal injury, tumor, or drugs.

Lower Extremities

When examining the lower extremities, you should observe and palpate bilaterally while moving downward to compare one leg with the other. Subtle evidence of swelling and deformity may be noted only when you recognize the relative difference between the two legs. The importance of this finding is reinforced by the fact that when a liter of blood is lost into the tissues of

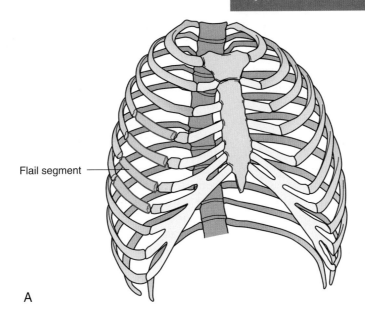

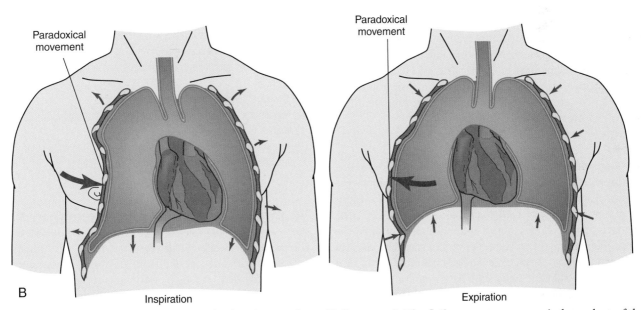

Figure 7-38 Paradoxical motion. A, Ribs are broken in two places (flail segment). The flail segment can move independent of the rest of the chest wall. B, Movement in opposite direction of the rib cage during breathing. When the chest wall expands during inspiration, the flail segment is "sucked inward" from the loss of structural support. During this phase the lung near the flail segment is functionally "exhaling" while the remainder of the lung is inhaling. When the chest wall decreases in size during expiration, the flail segment is "pushed outward" from the loss of structural support. During this phase the lung near the flail segment is functionally "inhaling" while the remainder of the lung is exhaling. This combination results in ineffective ventilation.

the thigh from a femur fracture, the circumference increases by only 1 to 2 cm. In the absence of trauma, swelling of both legs may indicate heart failure and swelling of one leg, a blood clot.

When palpating the lower extremities, you should start at the top and work down the extremity. The entire extremity should be palpated completely around. Certain bones, including the patella, tibia, metatarsals, and phalanges, are palpable on the surface. Feel for deformity and any evidence of crepitus.

Certain types of fractures in the lower extremity may cause the leg to assume a specific posture. For example, a fracture of

the hip (head and neck of femur) can cause the leg to rotate externally and shorten. A posterior hip dislocation results in internal rotation, adduction (upper leg bent toward midline), and flexion at the knee. These are classic findings and are covered in Chapter 23.

The final aspect of the lower extremity examination is the evaluation for circulation and nerve function. An injury may lacerate or put pressure on nerves and blood vessels. Two locations to check for a pulse are the **dorsalis pedis,** located on the dorsal surface of the foot, and the **posterior tibial,** behind the medial malleolus (protruding bone at medial side of ankle). Absence of pulses should always be reported to the emergency department (ED) staff and documented in the patient's record. To evaluate nerve function, ask the patient to flex and extend the foot and, if there is no pain, press the foot against the examiner's hand. Ask if the patient can feel you touching the bottom of the feet.

Upper Extremities

The upper extremities should be inspected and palpated bilaterally starting at the clavicles and shoulders and working down toward the hands. Check for sensation in the arms, hands, and fingers. To evaluate motor function, ask the patient to move the hands, spread the fingers, and squeeze your fingers. Ask the patient to push and pull your hands. Check the radial pulse, located on the anterior, lateral surface of the wrist just proximal to the thumb.

Log-Roll the Patient

Using spinal precautions, roll the patient to inspect and palpate the posterior surface of the body for injuries or signs of injury. Take special note of the thoracic and lumbar spine, palpating along the bone for signs of injury and tenderness. This may be done, if possible, when you are transferring a patient to a long spine board. For patients with unstable pelvic injuries, as evidenced by movement of the pelvic area or DCAP/BTLS in that body region during your physical examination, you might use a scoop stretcher for transfer to the long spine board to avoid further injury to the pelvic girdle.

Summary

Skill 7-7 illustrates the steps in performing a head-to-toe survey.

During the focused (secondary) assessment for trauma patients, reconsider the mechanism of injury you assessed in the scene evaluation and initial (primary) assessment. If the mechanism of injury is significant, perform a rapid head-to-toe physical examination (head-to-toe survey) to search for injuries or signs of injury (DCAP/BTLS) in all body regions. Continue to stabilize the spine as you reassess the ABCs. After assessing the head and neck, apply a cervical collar if you suspect injury to the spine, and then continue to assess the chest, abdomen, pelvis, and extremities. Log-roll the patient to assess the posterior body areas. Assess baseline vital signs and collect a SAMPLE history. For patients who do not have a significant mechanism of injury, focus the physical examination on the injured body part.

Patients with No Significant Injury

You may encounter patients with localized injuries who do not have a significant mechanism of injury. In these situations, you should focus your attention directly on the affected body part. A rapid head-to-toe survey is not necessary for a patient with a cut finger. However, you will have still performed your scene size-up and initial (primary) assessment and reconsidered the mechanism of injury to arrive at this point. After doing so, closely evaluate the injury to decide on appropriate care. For example, a cut finger might have avulsed tissue or partial or complete amputation. This focused (secondary) assessment affects how you treat and where you transport the patient. With all patients, you should assess baseline vital signs and collect a SAMPLE history.

Assessment of Baseline Vital Signs

Early in the initial (primary) assessment, you should note the patient's adequacy of breathing and circulation. Next, formally evaluate the pulse, respirations, blood pressure, and temperature.

Vital signs are an important objective measurement of the patient's vital functions. Low blood pressure, slow pulse rate, and very slow or very rapid ventilatory rates are examples of findings that can affect treatment, transportation decisions, or both aspects of care. In addition, because these are the baseline vital signs, subsequent measures might show improvement, deterioration, or no change. Taking baseline vital signs and periodically reassessing the patient help you observe response to treatment or deterioration from progression of the injury or illness. For example, massive internal bleeding might first be noted by an increase in the pulse and respiratory rate with a normal blood pressure. Over time, the blood pressure might start to fall as the patient loses more and more blood.

LEARNING OBJECTIVES

- Discuss the reasons for repeating the initial (primary) assessment as part of the ongoing assessment.
- Describe the components of the ongoing assessment or reassessment.
- Describe trending of assessment components.
- Explain the value of performing an ongoing assessment or reassessment.
- Explain the value of trending assessment components to other health professionals who assume care of the patient.

Ongoing Assessment or Reassessment

The **ongoing assessment** or **reassessment** is a reevaluation of the patient with a repeat of the initial (primary) assessment, vital signs, focused (secondary) assessment, and a check of the effectiveness of treatment and other interventions. Because a patient's condition may suddenly deteriorate, the ongoing assessment or reassessment is routinely used for every patient to look for changes in condition, monitor effectiveness of therapy, and detect life-threatening conditions. By performing the ongoing assessment at frequent intervals, you can observe dynamic changes in a patient's status. Changes in condition and repeated vital signs are documented and examined for trends that may indicate improvement or deterioration and help the hospital staff arrive at a diagnosis.

EXTENDED*Transport*

Providers with an extended transport time must be extremely diligent about ongoing assessment or reassessment activities. Particular attention should be paid to mental status, vital signs, and the need for positive-pressure ventilation. Whenever possible, you should be positioned in such a way so as to maintain visual and verbal contact. Before transport, you should prepare equipment that may be needed quickly should the patient decompensate en route to the hospital.

Table 7-12	Components of Ongoing Assessment	
Component	**Example**	**Photo Examples**
Repeat initial (primary) assessment.	General impression. Reassess mental state. Maintain open airway. Monitor breathing. Reassess pulse for rate and quality. Monitor skin color and temperature. Reestablish patient priorities.	Looking, listening, and feeling with the oxygen mask on the patient in the ambulance.
Monitor vital signs.	Blood pressure Pulse Respiratory rate Temperature	Taking the patient's blood pressure in the ambulance.
Repeat focused (secondary) assessment.	Patient-specific assessment relative to patient complaint or injuries.	Checking breath sounds in back of the ambulance.
Check interventions.	Check adequacy of interventions: Oxygen delivery Positive-pressure ventilations Management of bleeding Splints	Checking the patient's pedal pulses to evaluate distal circulation.

The condition of an emergency patient can improve, deteriorate, or remain unchanged. Assessment must be ongoing so that the EMT is continuously aware of the patient's status and can respond accordingly. The EMT must have up-to-the-minute information about the patient's status to answer, for example, the following questions:

- Has the patient with chest pain responded to administration of oxygen? Did the pain decrease?
- Is there evidence of internal bleeding in the crash victim with a significant mechanism of injury?
- What does assessment of the extremity show after a traction splint was applied to the patient's painful, swollen, deformed left thigh?
- Is there evidence of adequate ventilation in the patient receiving ventilation with a bag-mask and high-concentration oxygen?

Key components in the ongoing assessment or reassessment include the following (**Table 7-12**):
1. Repeat the initial (primary) assessment.
2. Monitor the patient's vital signs.
3. Repeat the focused (secondary) assessment relative to the patient's complaints or injuries.
4. Check the adequacy of interventions.

Repeat Examinations

Repeating the initial (secondary) assessment ensures that the ABCs are continuously monitored and that the search for life-threatening conditions is continuous and ongoing and thus takes high priority. Vital signs provide objective information about the patient's breathing and circulatory status, which can be compared with prior measurements as well as normal values. Focused parts of the history and physical examination might be assessed on the basis of the patient's chief complaint or injury. The adequacy of continuing emergency treatment is reassessed to ensure proper administration and judge its effectiveness in treating the patient's condition.

The frequency and manner in which an ongoing assessment or reassessment is conducted depend on the condition of the patient and length of time the EMT spends with the patient. In general, patients in unstable condition are checked every 5 minutes, whereas patients in stable condition are checked every 15 minutes.

Findings should be recorded after each assessment so that documentation is accurate. As you repeat your examinations, you might notice a **trend,** or tendency, for improvement or deterioration of the patient's condition. This information is important for you and other health care providers caring for the patient. For example, a patient with chest pain who complains of pain rated as "10" (on a scale of 1 to 10) on your initial (primary) assessment might tell you the pain is a "5" after 5 minutes of oxygen therapy and "0 or 1" just before arrival at the hospital 5 minutes later. This trend of diminishing pain is important to both you and the physicians at the hospital. A patient with a gunshot wound to the trunk might have initial vital signs showing blood pressure of 120/80 mm Hg and a pulse of 100 beats/min, with cool and clammy skin. Five minutes later the ongoing assessment or reassessment reveals blood pressure of "100/palp" and a pulse of 120 beats/min, with pale, cool, and clammy skin. The trend of decreasing blood pressure and increasing pulse over a short period indicates probable internal bleeding, which is of great importance to you and to the trauma surgeon in caring for the patient.

The ongoing assessment or reassessment usually follows the focused (secondary) assessment. However, the condition of the patient may not allow a detailed examination. For example, in a patient with multiple trauma who requires positive-pressure ventilation and control of major bleeding, the critical lifesaving interventions are the focus of the EMT. In this case the ongoing assessment should be repeated every 5 minutes while patient management is in progress.

LEARNING OBJECTIVE
- Recognize, respect, and respond to the feelings that patients might experience during assessment.

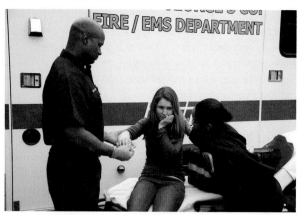

Figure 7-39 Empathy and emotional support are a critical part of good patient care, especially in small children and older adults.

Emotional Needs of the Patient

As in all phases of assessment, you should be sensitive to the feelings a patient might experience (**Figure 7-39**). Early on, identify yourself and state that you are an EMT and are there to assist the patient. As the case proceeds, the patient may look to you for an indication of the seriousness of the injury or illness. Be careful about direct or indirect communication. For example, you might encounter a patient with a devastating injury, such as paralysis of the lower extremities or a lethal wound or illness, who is still responsive. To a patient who has just been paralyzed from a fall, the results of reassessment of motor and sensory function may be overwhelming. Be empathetic and sensitive to the feelings such a patient might experience. You should be honest, but at the same time you should not draw conclusions beyond your scope of practice about the ultimate outcome for the patient.

Components of Ongoing Assessment or Reassessment

Repeat Initial (Primary) Assessment

The ongoing assessment or reassessment should begin by repeating the components of the initial (primary) assessment:
- Assess for life-threatening and priority conditions.
- What is your general impression?
- Does the patient look better, worse, or unchanged?

Reassess Mental Status

The patient's mental status should be quickly evaluated using AVPU:
- Is the patient alert?
- Does the patient respond to verbal or painful stimuli?
- Is the patient totally unresponsive?

Maintain Open Airway

- Is the airway still open? (Can the responsive patient talk or cry?)
- In an unresponsive patient, do you see, hear, or feel air movement or chest expansion?
- Is further intervention needed as a result of a change in a patient's condition, such as suctioning or insertion of an oropharyngeal airway?

Monitor Breathing for Rate and Quality

You should reassess the adequacy of breathing by observing for chest rise, respiratory rate, skin color, and signs of increased work of breathing, such as retractions, accessory muscle use, and nasal flaring or seesaw breathing in infants. If signs of inadequate breathing are present, you should begin positive-pressure ventilation and administer supplemental oxygen as appropriate.

Reassess Pulse for Rate and Quality

- Check the radial pulse in the adult and child older than 1 year and the brachial pulse in the infant younger than 1 year.
- Check the carotid pulse if you cannot detect a radial pulse in adults and children; check the femoral pulse if you cannot detect a brachial pulse in infants.
- For an unconscious patient, check the carotid pulse.
- Note the rate and quality (e.g., normal, thready or weak, bounding).

Monitor Skin Color and Temperature

- Check the skin color and temperature to help assess the patient's perfusion.
- Look at the nail beds, lips, and eyes (conjunctivae) for the normal pink color or an abnormal color, such as pale, cyanotic, or flushed.
- Feel the skin to reassess temperature and moisture.
- Assess capillary refilling time in infants and children younger than 6 years, and note whether it is greater or less than 2 seconds.

Reestablish Priority Patients

Reassess the priority status of the patient for transport. Does your reassessment show a condition that would benefit from expedited transport or air transport, bypass to a specialty receiving hospital, or an ALS intercept?

Reassess and Record Vital Signs

Take the blood pressure, and document the vital signs. Compare follow-up vital signs with the initial and any other previous vital signs, and note any trends.

Repeat Focused (Secondary) Assessment

On the basis of nature of illness and chief complaint or mechanism of injury and your knowledge of the patient at this point, include pertinent aspects of the focused (secondary) assessment in your ongoing assessment or reassessment. For example, ask a patient complaining of shortness of breath and chest pain about these complaints during your reassessment. You might ask, "Mrs. Smith, do you still have chest pain? How would you rate it on that 1 to 10 scale now? How is your breathing?"

Answers to pertinent questions and the results of your repeat focused (secondary) assessment (e.g., breath sounds, inspection of neck for neck veins, accessory muscle use) should be documented and compared with previous findings.

Check Interventions

Ensure Adequacy of Oxygenation and Ventilation. Evaluate the patient's ventilation and oxygenation by observing chest rise and rate. Also, check mental status, skin color, pulse rate, and

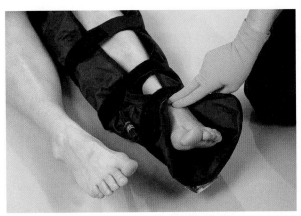

Figure 7-40 Checking a distal pulse after a splint has been applied is part of periodic reassessment of distal circulation and sensorimotor function of an injured extremity.

general condition of the patient to help evaluate the effectiveness of therapy. If the adequacy of positive-pressure ventilation is questionable, you should reevaluate your technique and possibly the delivery system.

Ensure Control of Major Bleeding. Major external bleeding should be controlled in the field by direct pressure, elevation, use of pressure points if necessary, and as a last resort, tourniquets. Reassess the adequacy of control of major external bleeding. If adequacy of control is questionable, the technique may need to be readjusted. For example, you might need to reinforce the dressing or use a blood pressure cuff for increased pressure over the bleeding site. In extreme cases, if a life-threatening condition exists and other measures have failed, a tourniquet might be applied.

Ensure Adequacy of Other Interventions. You should periodically assess any other interventions, such as splinting and spinal immobilization. For example, when applying a splint to an extremity, periodically reassess the distal circulation and sensory and motor function (**Figure 7-40**). If a traction splint has been applied, check that it is still in proper position with sufficient traction.

Scenario Follow-up

The opening scenario illustrates the comprehensive management of an EMS call, from scene size-up through transport. The first priority is always safety of the providers, patients, and bystanders. Taking the appropriate standard precautions and securing the scene of a motor vehicle crash to divert traffic are essential for this type of call. Rather than focusing on a single patient, the providers appropriately reviewed the number of patients and mechanisms of injury and quickly performed triage. Additional units were called through

dispatch, and the most seriously injured patient was selected for treatment. After initial assessment it was determine that the patient was unstable and required rapid extrication. On removal, a focused (secondary) assessment was performed, and additional data suggested significant chest and abdominal injuries requiring definitive care at the hospital. Transport was initiated as soon as possible, and the trauma center was notified during transport. En route to the hospital the patient was continuously reassessed, and care was transferred to the trauma team at the hospital, including a more detailed history.

Summary

This chapter presents the basic structure or foundation for a complete patient assessment at an EMS scene. The scene size-up is the first critical step in patient assessment, and "Is it safe to approach the patient?" the first question asked. You should assess the need for personal protective rescue gear, standard precautions, and transmission-based precautions.

Once you have addressed the safety of the rescuers, patients, and bystanders, form a general impression of the patient from your observations of the patient and the environment. During this initial (primary) assessment, determine the mechanism of injury, nature of illness, and number of patients. Perform a rapid and orderly assessment for responsiveness and airway, breathing, and circulation (ABCs) to identify any need for immediate intervention to maintain life. Decide if the patient is a priority patient who requires rapid transport to the hospital.

During the focused (secondary) assessment, reconsider the mechanism of injury. If significant, perform a rapid head-to-toe physical examination (DCAP/BTLS). Continue to stabilize the spine as you reassess the ABCs.

Assessing vital signs and taking a SAMPLE history are key to the focused (secondary) assessment. Vital signs represent an essential measurement of the patient's condition. They are often the basis for the treatments provided in the field and provide an important measure of any improvement or deterioration in the patient's status during the prehospital phase of care. The SAMPLE history records critical information on the events surrounding the call in addition to important data regarding the patient's medical history. The OPQRST-type questions more fully describe the present illness. Use questions specific to the chief complaint.

The ongoing assessment or reassessment has four key components: initial (primary) assessment, vital signs, pertinent aspects of focused (secondary) assessment, and a check of the interventions. Patients in critical condition are reassessed every 5 minutes. Accurate documentation of the findings is important.

Skills

| *Skill* | 7-1 | *Establishing Responsiveness* |

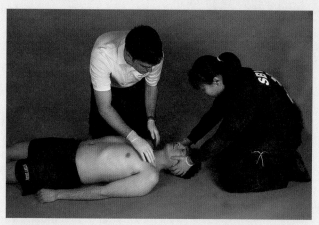

1. If the patient is suspected as having sustained trauma, one EMT should maintain inline manual stabilization of the head and neck while the other EMT performs the initial (primary) assessment. If the patient is not communicative, ask loudly, "Are you OK?"

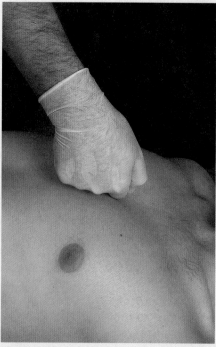

2. If the patient does not respond to verbal stimuli, tap on the patient's chest. Vigorously rub the sternum (breastbone) or firmly pinch the neck muscles.

You can do this with the patient in the same position as when you arrived.

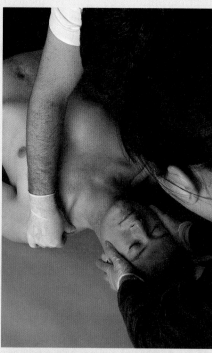

3. An unresponsive patient who is found in a position other than supine should be rolled into the supine position. If spinal injury is suspected, do this while maintaining alignment of the patient's spine.

Skill | 7-2   *Placing a Patient in the Supine Position*

ONE-PERSON PROCEDURE WHEN PATIENT IS FOUND PRONE

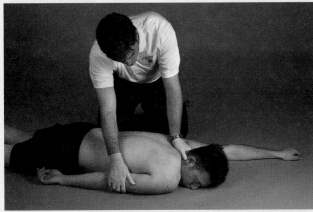

1. Support the patient's cervical spine, and hold the arm next to the chest with the hand.

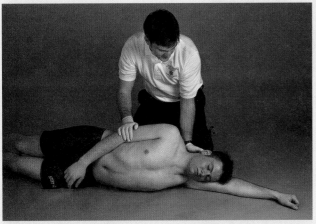

2. Carefully rotate the patient while maintaining alignment of the spine.

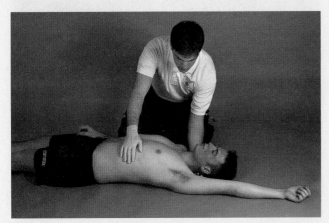

3. Place the patient in the supine position.

TWO-PERSON PROCEDURE WHEN PATIENT IS FOUND PRONE

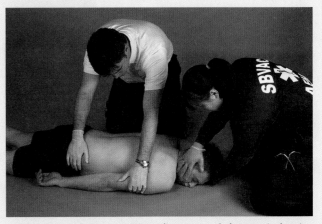

1. The first person maintains alignment of the cervical spine while the second person supports the shoulder and hip region.

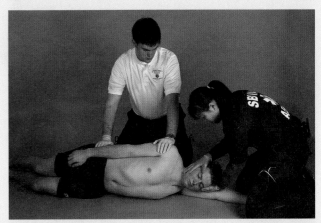

2. Both providers smoothly rotate the patient to the lateral position on command of the first person.

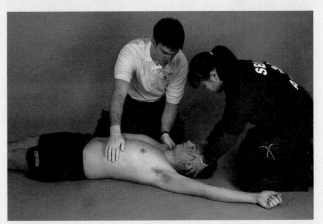

3. Carefully rotate the patient to the supine position.

Skill | 7-3   *Opening the Airway*

HEAD-TILT/CHIN-LIFT

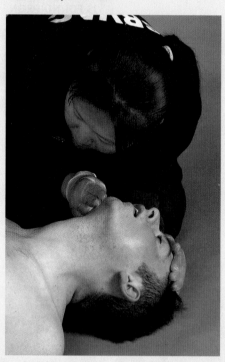

1. Place one hand on the forehead and the fingers of the hand closest to the feet along the patient's jawbone.

2. Apply a gentle, tilting force to the forehead while lifting the chin upward with your fingers, taking care not to close the mouth.

JAW THRUST

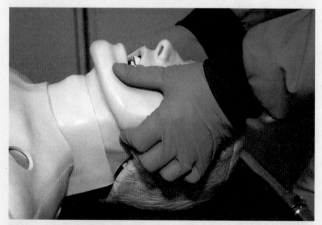

1. Place both thumbs on the patient's maxilla (cheekbone) and your index and middle fingers on both sides of the mandible where it angles toward the ear.

2. Apply upward pressure with your fingers to displace the jaw forward without tilting the head.

TONGUE-JAW LIFT

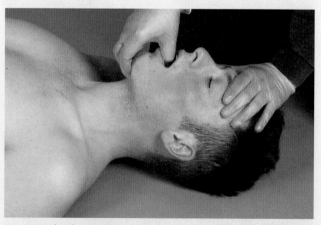

1. Grasp the lower jaw with your thumb and index and middle fingers, placing your thumb inside the lower teeth and your fingers along the margin of the mandible inferiorly.

2. While stabilizing the head with your other hand, pull the jaw forward.

Skill | 7-4   *Assessing Breathing*

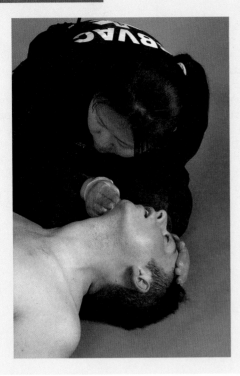

1. Look, listen, and feel for breathing. Look for movement of the chest and abdomen and use of accessory muscles and retractions. Listen for air exchange.

2. If necessary, feel for warm breath against your cheek.

3. For unresponsive patients and responsive patients with signs of respiratory distress, maintain an open airway, administer high-concentration oxygen, and determine the need for assisted ventilations. For patient with respiratory failure or respiratory arrest, provide positive-pressure ventilation. (See Chapter 6 to review signs of respiratory failure.)

Holes in the chest wall must be sealed with a three-sided airtight dressing because they can lead to rapid ventilatory failure (see Chapter 22).

Skill | 7-5   *Measuring Blood Pressure by Auscultation*

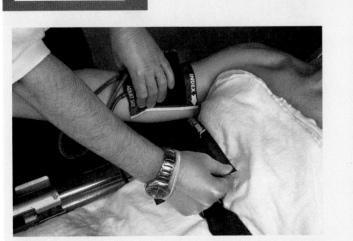

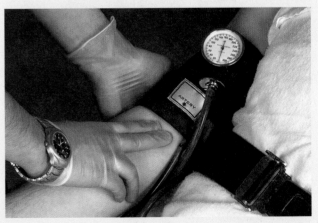

1. The blood pressure cuff is placed on the arm just above the elbow, with the bladder portion of the cuff centered over the brachial artery using the marking on the cuff.

2. Locate the brachial pulse point in the crease of the anterior side of the elbow in a straight line up from the little finger.

Continued

| *Skill* | 7-5 | *Measuring Blood Pressure by Auscultation—cont'd* |

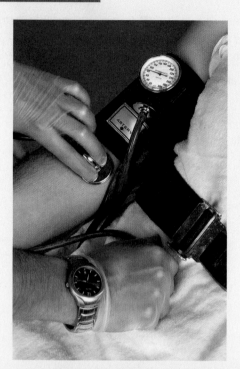

3. Your stethoscope is placed over the pulse point. Close the valve located above the bulb of the sphygmomanometer, and pump air into the cuff until the mercury (Hg) or dial on the gauge stops undulating as it moves upward. In most cases, this occurs between 150 and 200 mm Hg. Listen for pulse sounds with the stethoscope over the brachial artery. If sounds are heard at this point, continue pumping until sounds disappear; then pump 20 mm Hg further. At this point, you will have totally occluded the flow of blood past the site of the cuff. When the pressure in the cuff exceeds the pressure within the artery, no blood can flow through, and you will hear no pulse sounds. Release the valve slowly (about 3 mm/sec) and listen for the soft sounds created by blood beginning to flow as the pressure in the cuff goes below the highest pressure within the blood vessel. Because the artery remains partially occluded, the blood flow that occurs is turbulent. This turbulence creates the sounds heard over the brachial artery distal to the occlusion.

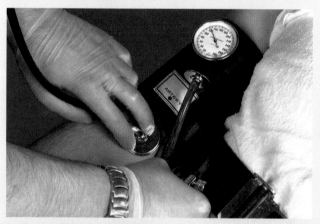

4. The first sound will reflect flow during the systolic phase (contracting phase) of the heart. Therefore the first sound is referred to as the systolic blood pressure.

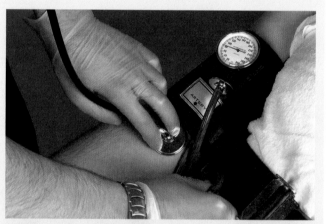

5. Continue to release pressure and listen until the sounds disappear or suddenly diminish in volume. This point will be reached when the pressure in the cuff is less than the blood pressure during the heart's diastole, or relaxation phase, allowing blood to flow without turbulence. The point where the sounds disappear or significantly diminish in volume is recorded as the diastolic blood pressure.

Record the measured values by placing the systolic reading over the diastolic reading by using a diagonal line to divide the two values (e.g., 120/80).

Skill | 7-6 — *Measuring Blood Pressure by Palpation*

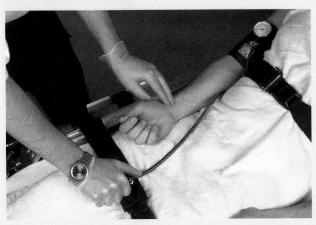

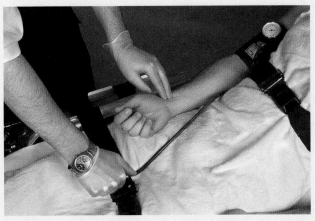

1. After applying the cuff, monitor the radial pulse and pump up the pressure until the pulse disappears.

2. Slowly release the pressure until the pulse first reappears. This point establishes the systolic blood pressure. When taking the pressure by this method, you cannot determine the diastolic measurement because the changes that occurred in auscultation are audible but not detectable by palpation.

Record the measured values by placing the systolic reading over the letter "P" (for palpation) and using a diagonal line to divide the two values (e.g., 120/P).

Skill | 7-7 — *Performing a Head-to-Toe Survey*

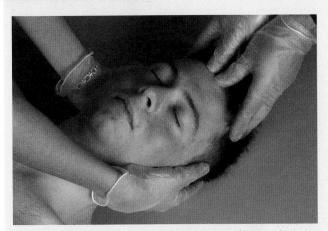

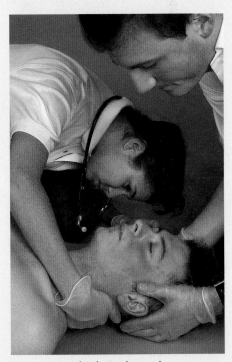

1. Inspect and palpate the head for injuries and signs of injuries (DCAP/BTLS).

2. Inspect and palpate the neck.

Continued

Skill | 7-7   *Performing a Head-to-Toe Survey—cont'd*

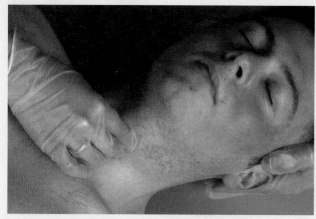

3. In palpation of the trachea, look and feel for crepitation, tracheal deviation, and neck vein distention.

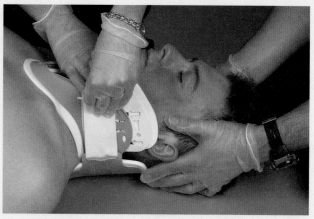

4. Apply a cervical collar.

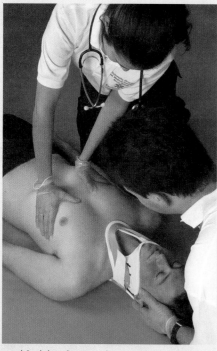

5. Inspect and feel the chest, and note any crepitation or paradoxical motion of the chest wall.

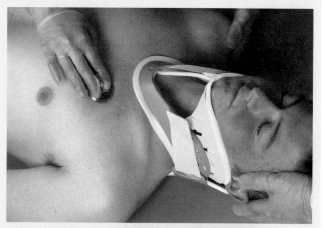

6. Asculate breath sounds on the anterior chest wall.

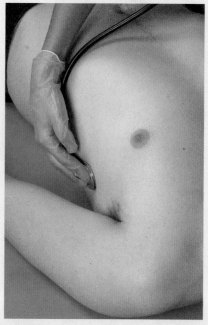

7. Auscultate breath sounds on the lateral chest wall.

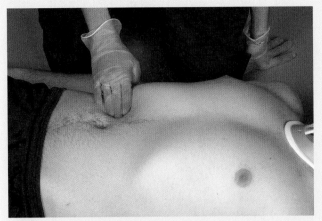

8. Inspect and palpate the abdomen. Note if firm, soft, or distended.

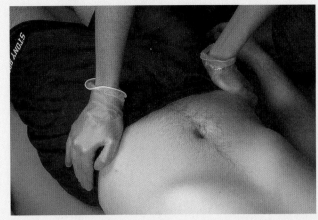

9. Inspect and palpate the pelvis. If no pain, gently compress to detect tenderness or motion.

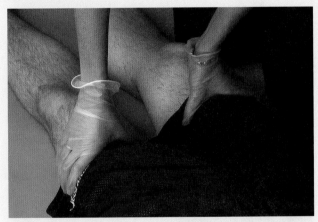

10. Inspect and palpate the lower extremities.

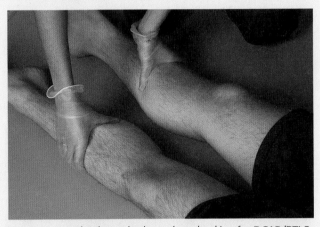

11. Inspect and palpate the lower leg, checking for DCAP/BTLS.

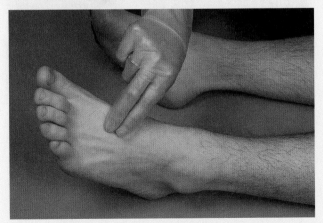

12. Check distal pulse. Palpate the dorsalis pedis.

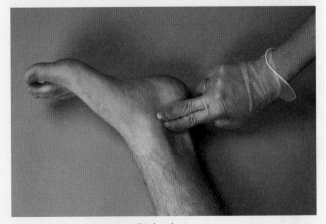

13. Palpate the posterior tibial pulse.

Continued

Skill | 7-7 *Performing a Head-to-Toe Survey—cont'd*

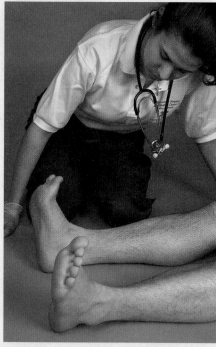

14. Check motor ability. Ask the patient to flex the foot against your hand.

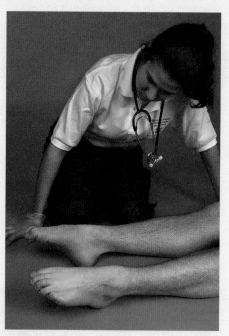

15. Ask the patient to extend the foot.

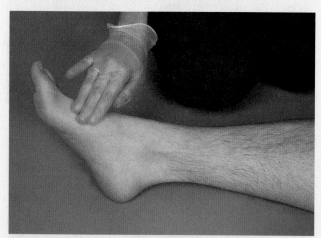

16. Check sensation. Have the patient close the eyes and state when you touch the legs and feet.

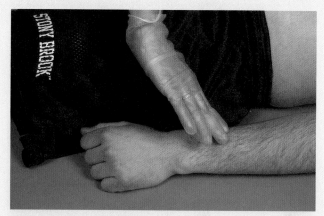

17. Inspect and palpate the upper extremity.

18. Check sensation. Have the patient close the eyes and state when you touch the arms, hands, and fingers.

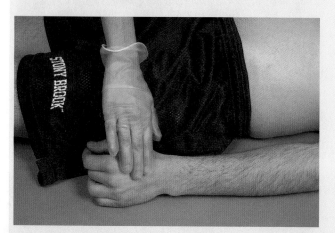

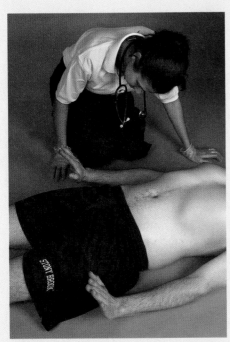

19. Check motor ability. Have the patient move his or her hands.

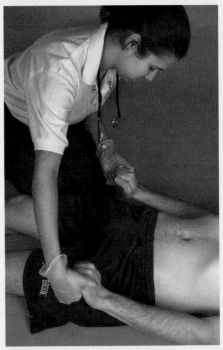

20. Have the patient spread his or her fingers and squeeze your fingers. Ask the patient to pull and push your hands.

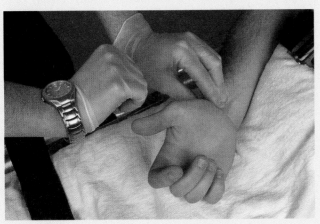

21. Check the radial pulse.

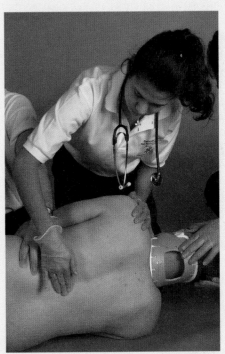

22. Log-roll the patient and check the back.

The Bottom Line

Learning Checklist

✓ During the scene size-up, the EMT determines if the scene/ situation is safe, takes appropriate substance precautions, determines the mechanism of injury or nature of illness, determines the number of patients, requests additional help if necessary, begins triage, and considers stabilization of the spine as appropriate.

✓ Scenes where potential hazards might be encountered include crash and rescue scenes; presence of toxic substances; crime scenes; and environmental conditions such as ice, water, and unstable surfaces.

✓ The scene is evaluated before the EMT enters, to ensure the scene is safe for providers, patients, and bystanders; to call for additional resources; to take appropriate personal protection and precautions; to anticipate the numbers and needs of patients (e.g., medical vs. trauma); and to determine whether triage and spine stabilization are indicated.

✓ Hazards at the scene of a motor vehicle crash include oncoming traffic, gasoline spills, fire, unstable vehicles, glass and sharp metal, slippery or unstable surfaces, and downed power lines.

✓ Resources that may be requested after a scene size-up include law enforcement, fire, rescue, hazardous materials experts, advanced life support (ALS), and utilities.

✓ Determine the nature of illness and why EMS was activated on medical cases by using information gathered from the scene as well as from the patient, family, or bystanders. Remember that someone besides the patient usually makes the call for help.

✓ Determine the mechanism of injury for trauma patients by inspecting the scene and talking to the patient and bystanders to help anticipate associated injuries and whether a medical condition was related to the trauma.

✓ When you determine the number of patients is more than the responding unit can handle, call for additional help and begin triage to determine the medical priority for treatment.

✓ The initial (primary) assessment is a means of assessing patient condition and priorities of care.

✓ The general impression is the first step of initial (primary) assessment, when you note the patient's age and gender, nature of illness or mechanism of injury, and any obvious life-threatening conditions.

✓ Look for life-threatening conditions in your initial (primary) assessment so that treatment can be given immediately.

✓ Lifesaving treatments include controlling bleeding; opening and maintaining the airway; and providing supplemental oxygen, positive-pressure ventilations, automated external defibrillation, and CPR.

✓ Assess mental status quickly during initial (primary) assessment by the AVPU mnemonic: alert, responds to verbal stimuli, responds to pain, or unresponsive.

✓ Assess the airway with the appropriate technique: head-tilt/ chin-lift for medical patients and jaw thrust for trauma patients with suspected cervical spine injury. In unresponsive patients, maintain an open airway. Oropharyngeal or nasopharyngeal airway may be needed for continued airway control.

✓ Assess breathing with the "look, listen, and feel" method: look for chest and abdominal movements, accessory muscle use, and retractions; listen for air movement and abnormal sounds of breathing; and if necessary, feel for warm air from the lips and mouth.

✓ For all patients with inadequate breathing, give high-concentration supplemental oxygen, use airway adjuncts, and assist ventilations if indicated.

✓ Assess circulation with the pulse check by using the radial pulse in children and adults and the brachial pulse in infants. Use the carotid pulse in unresponsive patients or when unable to feel a pulse in the arm. For infants, use the femoral pulse.

✓ Assess circulation and perfusion by assessing the skin, nail bed, conjunctivae, and mucous membranes for color, temperature, and condition (moisture); note cyanosis or pale, cool, clammy skin as signs of hypoperfusion.

✓ Assess capillary refilling time as part of the assessment for perfusion in infants and children, noting a delay of more than 2 seconds for normal color to return as a possible indication of hypoperfusion.

✓ Assess an infant's airway by placing the head in a sniffing, or neutral, position, being careful not to hyperextend the neck; just slightly extend the head and neck of a child (1-8 years old) if no trauma is present.

✓ In infants and children, look carefully for signs of nasal flaring, seesaw breathing (alternate use of chest and abdominal muscles during breathing), and retractions of the chest wall when assessing for inadequate breathing.

✓ Initiate rapid transport, and consider ALS backup for patients with findings such as poor general impression, unresponsiveness with no gag or cough, responsiveness but not following commands, difficulty breathing, shock or hypoperfusion, complicated childbirth, or chest pain with low blood pressure.

✓ At the beginning of the focused (secondary) assessment, you should reconsider the mechanism of injury/illness to guide the scope of the evaluation.

✓ Patients with a specific chief complaint with a prior known history will often recognize their illness and may have medications on hand that can be used in emergency treatment.

✓ The mechanism of injury guides the physical examination. If the mechanism of injury is significant, you should conduct a head-to-toe survey. If the mechanism of injury is limited, a focused physical examination of the affected part may be sufficient.

✓ Remember to look for "hidden injuries" that may result from safety devices such as seat belts and airbags.

✓ Perform the head-to-toe survey on patients with a significant mechanism of injury that may result in life-threatening injuries or injuries to multiple body parts.

✓ The mnemonic DCAP/BTLS can guide you during the head-to-toe survey to check for any deformities, contusions, abrasions, punctures, burns, tenderness, lacerations, and swelling.

✓ In the responsive medical patient, perform a focused (secondary) physical examination based on the chief complaint and history of the present illness and the rest of the SAMPLE history.

✓ In the unresponsive medical patient, perform a head-to-toe survey and then obtain as complete a history as possible from family and bystanders.

✓ The mnemonic OPQRST (onset, provocation, quality, radiation, severity, time) can be used to guide you during the collection of the history of the present illness to clarify complaints and factors surrounding the event.

✓ A SAMPLE history (signs/symptoms, allergies, medications, pertinent past medical history, last oral intake, events leading to present illness) is taken from the patient, family, and bystanders to identify life-threatening conditions and problems that may have caused or will complicate the patient's condition.

✓ Baseline vital signs, including respirations, pulse, blood pressure, and mental state, are evaluated to help identify potential respiratory and circulatory compromise and brain injury.

✓ Check key areas of the body, such as the head, neck, and chest, for crepitus to identify bony injury or injury to the respiratory system.

✓ Look for jugular venous distention in the neck to identify backup of blood in the venous system returning to the heart.

✓ Look for deviation of the trachea to either side of the neck, which can occur from injury to the airway or chest.

✓ Evaluate breath sounds to identify injury to the respiratory system, such as a collapsed lung.

✓ Assess the abdomen for distention, rigidity, and tenderness to identify potential serious organ damage and bleeding.

✓ Check the extremities for distal pulses, sensation, and motor function to identify circulatory compromise and injury to the nerves or nervous system.

✓ Log-roll patients and examine the back to avoid missing serious injuries.

✓ On a patient with no significant mechanism of injury (e.g., cut hand), perform the focused (secondary) assessment on the specific injury site.

Key Terms

Abrasion Scrape on the surface of the skin or mucous membrane.

Advanced life support (ALS) intercept Call for ALS to acquire resources on the scene that can be lifesaving for the patient (e.g., intubation).

Auscultation Method of listening for sounds produced within the body; usually performed with a stethoscope.

AVPU Mnemonic used to remember the responses during assessment of a patient's mental status: *A*, alert; *V*, response to verbal stimuli; *P*, response to painful stimuli; *U*, unresponsive.

Blood pressure The force exerted by the blood volume on the walls of the vessels.

Capillary refilling time Diagnostic test in which the nail bed is compressed to empty the capillaries and determine the time it takes to refill (for color to return); also *capillary refill time.*

Chief complaint The reason, best stated in the patient's own words, for the medical problem that prompted the patient to seek emergency medical assistance.

Conjunctiva Membrane that lines the interior surface of the eyelids and covers the anterior surface of the sclera of the eye.

Constrict To narrow and become smaller.

Contusion Compression or blunt-force injury with no skin break in which blood vessels may leak or rupture; bruise.

Crepitus Grating or crackling sound or sensation caused by air beneath the skin or broken bone ends rubbing together; also called *crepitation.*

Crowing See *stridor.*

Cyanosis Bluish discoloration of the mucous membranes or skin resulting from oxygen-depleted hemoglobin.

DCAP/BTLS Mnemonic used to remember possible physical findings identified during the head-to-toe survey: **d**eformities; **c**ontusions; **a**brasions; **p**unctures or penetrations; **b**urns; **t**enderness; **l**acerations; **s**welling.

Deformity Structural distortion or bend that alters the normal appearance of the body or a body part.

Detailed physical examination Deliberate and comprehensive head-to-toe assessment to identify secondary injuries; part of focused (secondary) assessment.

Dilate To widen or become larger.

Dorsalis pedis Artery in the foot that is palpable on the dorsal (top) surface of the foot.

Focused physical examination Physical examination directed to the specific area of injury for patients with limited injuries or specific medical complaints; part of focused (secondary) assesssment.

Focused (secondary) assessment Part of assessment devoted to identifying history and physical findings needed to treat the patient.

Gasping Short breaths with a rapid inspiratory phase associated with respiratory distress and fatigue.

General impression First part of the initial (primary) assessment during which EMT notes the patient's age and gender, nature of illness or mechanism of injury, and any obvious life-threatening conditions.

Grunting Rhythmic sound heard at the end of exhalation; key sign of respiratory distress in infants.

Gurgling Sound created by air moving through fluid in the airway.

Head-to-toe survey Rapid examination to identify signs and symptoms in unresponsive patients with a significant mechanism of injury.

History Information about the patient, including the chief complaint, history of the present illness, past medical history, medications, and allergies; gathered during an interview with the patient, family, or bystanders.

History of the present illness Portion of the history that clarifies the chief complaint or presenting problem through a series of questions (e.g., OPQRST).

Hypertension Increased blood pressure.

Initial (primary) assessment Early part of assessment devoted to identifying and treating life-threatening conditions related to airway, breathing, circulation, and mental status.

Jaundice Yellowing of the skin or sclera of the eye caused by a buildup of bilirubin in the blood.

Jugular venous distention Enlargement of the neck veins associated with increased venous pressure.

Laceration Tear or cut in the skin or other tissues.

Mechanism of injury Manner in which an injury was incurred; knowing the mechanism helps in recognizing the type and extent of injury.

Multiple-casualty incident Event involving more than one patient that requires more resources than the responding units can provide.

Nasal flaring Characteristic flaring of the nostrils in infants and small children suggesting the presence of respiratory distress.

Nature of illness Type of medical complaint that a patient exhibits.

Ongoing assessment Reevaluation of the patient (repeat initial [primary] assessment, vital signs, focused [secondary] assessment, check of interventions); or **reassessment.**

Onset When and how a patient's complaint first occurred.

OPQRST Mnemonic used to remember the key questions in the history of present illness: **o**nset; **p**rovocation; **q**uality; **r**adiation; **s**everity; **t**ime.

Oral mucosa The lining of the mouth.

Orientation A person's awareness of person, place, and time.

Palpation The act of feeling with the hand; applying light pressure with the fingers to the surface of the body to determine the condition of the parts underneath.

Posterior tibial Artery passing just behind the ankle bone, where it is palpable between the medial malleolus and the Achilles tendon.

Priapism Abnormal sustained penile erection.

Provocation Any factor that causes or worsens a patient's complaint.

Puncture To pierce or penetrate with a pointed object or instrument.

Quality Subjective description of the complaint in the patient's own words.

Radiation In assessment of the patient's chief complaint, the spread of pain from one area of the body to another.

Retractions The drawing in of soft tissues between the ribs, above the clavicle, and below the sternum; reflects increased work of breathing.

SAMPLE Mnemonic used to remember the key questions in a patient history: **s**igns and symptoms, **a**llergies, **m**edications, **p**ertinent past history, **l**ast oral intake, and **e**vents leading up to the present illness.

Scene safety First step in the scene size-up phase of patient assessment; ensures safety of the providers, patients, and bystanders by effectively securing the scene.

Scene size-up First phase of patient assessment that includes scene safety, appropriate use of personal protective equipment, and determination of the mechanism of injury or nature of illness.

Severity Measurement of the degree of pain a patient is experiencing.

Sign Any objective evidence of disease or dysfunction; a clue to the patient's condition that can be observed (seen, smelled, heard, or felt) by the EMT.

Snoring Harsh, low-pitched sound usually caused by the tongue blocking the airway.

Sphygmomanometer Device for measuring blood pressure.

Stridor Harsh, high-pitched sound created by air flowing through a narrowed upper airway, usually heard on inspiration; also called *crowing.*

Subcutaneous emphysema Entrapment of air beneath the skin as a result of trauma to the airways, lungs, esophagus, or skin; characterized by deformity and crepitus of the skin.

Symptom Anything that the patient perceives as part of his or her complaint and communicates to the EMT.

Tenderness Pain that is elicited on palpation.

Time Duration of the chief complaint and significant associated complaints.

Tracheal deviation Position of the trachea to either side of the midline of the neck.

Traffic delineation devices Devices used to alter traffic flow around an emergency scene.

Trend Tendency toward improvement or deterioration in a patient's condition.

Triage To sort or choose; the sorting of patients according to injury priority.

Tripod position Position characterized by sitting upright and leaning forward with the head and neck thrust forward; generally associated with respiratory distress.

Vital signs Measurement of the function of the vital body systems, including respirations, pulse, blood pressure, temperature, and pupils.

Wheezing High-pitched whistling sounds created by narrowed bronchioles.

Review Questions

1. A downed electrical wire is crackling and jumping on the ground within 6 feet of a pedestrian struck by a car. The victim appears to be unconscious. What actions should you take?

   a. Retreat to a safe position and wait until utility personnel and police arrive

   b. Displace the wire with a wooden stick while your partner drags the patient to safety

   c. Drag the patient to safety since the wire is at a safe distance

   d. Approach the victim wearing a rubber jumpsuit

2. You arrive at a scene and observe a pregnant patient crowning. You decide that you must deliver the baby. What protective equipment should you wear? *(Select all that apply.)*
   a. Jumpsuit
   b. Gloves
   c. Protective eyewear
   d. Gown
   e. Mask

3. You arrive at a farm and are informed that a worker entered a silo and passed out. You approach upwind and learn that a second worker went after him and has passed out in the silo as well. Your scene size-up would lead to which of the following actions?
   a. Hold your breath while you enter the silo to pull out the victims.
   b. Ensure rescuers entering the silo have a self-contained breathing apparatus.
   c. Ask for volunteers who can swim long distances underwater.
   d. Wear an oxygen mask to enter the silo.

4. Scene size-up at a multiple-casualty incident reveals an overturned tanker truck with a noxious odor and three victims lying adjacent on the ground. Ideally, where should you park your vehicle with respect to the scene?
   a. Uphill and downwind
   b. Uphill and upwind
   c. Downhill and upwind
   d. Downhill and downwind

5. Which of the following are reasons to identify the number of patients at the scene before initiating patient care? *(Select all that are appropriate.)*
   a. Triage may be necessary
   b. Calling early for additional units saves time
   c. Need to initiate the multiple-casualty incident plan
   d. To determine the mechanism of injury

6. What is the first step of initial (primary) assessment, when you note the patient's age and gender, nature of illness or mechanism of injury, and obvious life-threatening conditions?
   a. General impression
   b. Scene survey
   c. Secondary survey
   d. Neurologic examination

7. In a responsive patient, the best way to evaluate the patency of the airway is by observing if the patient:
   a. Has a normal pulse
   b. Can talk clearly or cry
   c. Has normal skin color
   d. Has normal skin temperature

8. You find a man who has fallen off a 20-foot ladder and is unresponsive. You should first:
   a. Perform a head-tilt/chin-lift
   b. Maintain spinal immobilization
   c. Take a blood pressure reading
   d. Inspect the cervical spine

9. If you encounter a responsive patient with chest pain who is alert and breathing 26 times per minute, which device should you use to administer oxygen?
   a. Nasal cannula
   b. Bag-mask
   c. Nonrebreather mask
   d. Oxygen-powered resuscitator

10. You respond to a patient who was struck by a vehicle. His skin is pale, cool, and sweaty. This may indicate:
    a. Poor perfusion
    b. Liver disease
    c. Low body temperature
    d. High blood pressure

11. Which of the following locations are used for inspecting color when assessing perfusion? *(Select all that apply.)*
    a. Eyes (conjunctivae)
    b. Nail beds
    c. Lips and face
    d. Earlobe

12. Which of the following are signs of respiratory distress in infants and children? *(Select all that are appropriate.)*
    a. Nasal flaring
    b. Flushed skin
    c. Retractions
    d. Stridor or grunting

13. Gathering information from bystanders, identifying hazards, securing the scene, and calling for specialized assistance are all components of which of the following?
    a. Initial (primary) assessment
    b. Scene size-up
    c. Secondary survey
    d. Dispatch review

14. Which maneuver are you performing when you tilt the head back with one hand while lifting the lower margin of the jaw with the index and middle fingers of the other hand?
    a. Jaw thrust with head tilt
    b. Chin pull
    c. Head-tilt/jaw-lift
    d. Head-tilt/chin-lift

15. Which is the best way to evaluate an adequate breath during positive-pressure ventilation?
   a. Observing chest rise
   b. Counting to 3 for each breath
   c. Feeling the chest wall for expansion
   d. Checking the pulse rate

16. To palpate the carotid pulse, place your fingers:
   a. At the groove between the larynx and the muscle in the neck
   b. At the angle of the jaw adjacent to the muscle
   c. Just above the suprasternal notch
   d. Just above the clavicle, adjacent to the trachea

17. Capillary refilling time is considered abnormal when refill takes more than:
   a. 0.5 second
   b. 1.0 second
   c. 1.5 seconds
   d. 2.0 seconds

18. The *P* of the AVPU mnemonic of mental state evaluation refers to a patient's ability to respond to:
   a. Purposeful stimuli
   b. Painful stimuli
   c. Persistent stimuli
   d. Pulsatile stimuli

19. Which artery is routinely used to monitor the rate, regularity, and quality of the pulse?
   a. Radial
   b. Femoral
   c. Carotid
   d. Ulna

20. Which of the following questions reflects the best way to inquire about the quality of chest pain in a medical history?
   a. Was your chest pain "squeezing" in nature?
   b. How would you describe the pain in your own words?
   c. Did the pain feel as if someone was standing on your chest?
   d. Was the pain sharp or dull?

21. The sequence of events, activity at the onset of the problem, location and radiation of pain, and aggravating and relieving factors are examples of which of the following?
   a. History of present illness
   b. Past medical history
   c. Scene size-up
   d. Chief complaint

22. Fill in the term for each of the following components of the OPQRST approach:
   O ___onset___
   P ___provocation___
   Q ___quality___
   R ___radiation___
   S ___severity___
   T ___time___

23. What does the *C* in DCAP/BTLS stand for?
   a. Circulation
   b. Crepitation
   c. Contusion
   d. Conjunctiva

24. Which of the following are examples of significant mechanisms of injury? *(Select all that apply.)*
   a. Fall from a chair
   b. Ejection from a vehicle
   c. Bicycle injuries in children
   d. Vehicle-pedestrian collision

25. Which of the following steps are appropriate in the head-to-toe survey? (Select all that are appropriate.)
   a. Looking and feeling for DCAP/BTLS
   b. Listening for breath sounds with a stethoscope
   c. Checking for abdominal distention
   d. Checking for motor response in feet

26. Which of the following is the method used by EMTs for assessing basic mental status?
   a. Using AVPU mnemonic
   b. Noting pattern of speech
   c. Evaluating retention of information
   d. Observing eye movement

27. The best location for assessing adequate breath sounds on the anterior surface of the body is at the apices (top of lung field) at the
   a. Anterior axillary line
   b. Midsternum
   c. Midclavicular line
   d. Nipple line

28. Which of the following refers to movement of a section of the chest wall in the opposite direction of the remaining chest wall during ventilation?
   a. Paradoxical motion
   b. Thoracic deviation
   c. Mediastinal shift
   d. Thoracic paradoxus

29. The iliac crests of the pelvis are gently compressed posteriorly and:
   a. Anteriorly
   b. Medially
   c. Laterally
   d. Superiorly

30. Which of the following are compared when examining the lower extremities?
   a. One leg to the other
   b. Upper thighs to lower legs
   c. Lower extremities to upper extremities
   d. Anterior-posterior diameter to lateral diameter

31. The posterior tibial pulse is located behind which of the following structures?
  a. Medial ankle bone
  b. Midthigh region
  c. Hip region
  d. Kneecap (patella)

32. Which pulse can be palpated on the anterior portion of the wrist, just proximal to the thumb?
  a. Brachial
  b. Ulnar
  c. Radial
  d. Humeral

33. Which of the following is most directly evaluated by having the patient flex and extend the foot?
  a. Sensory function
  b. Mental state
  c. Motor function
  d. Brainstem function

For Further Review

In the Student Workbook

- Multiple-choice questions
- Matching questions
- Fill-in-the-blank questions
- Short answer questions
- True/false questions
- Case scenario questions
- Crossword puzzle

On Evolve

- Anatomy challenges
- Weblinks
- Lecture notes
- Exercises

Learning Objectives

Cognitive Objectives

- Identify the components of an initial (primary) assessment.
- Recognize hazards and potential hazards.
- Describe common hazards found at the scene of a trauma and a medical patient.
- Determine whether the scene is safe to enter.
- Discuss common mechanisms of injury and nature of illness.
- Discuss the reason for identifying the total number of patients at the scene.
- Explain the reason for identifying the need for additional help.
- Summarize the reasons for forming a general impression of the patient.
- Discuss methods of assessing altered mental status.
- State reasons for management of the cervical spine once the patient has been determined to be a trauma patient.

- Discuss methods of assessing the airway in the adult, child, and infant.
- Describe methods of assessing whether a patient is breathing.
- State the type of care to provide the adult, child, or infant with adequate breathing.
- State the type of care to provide the adult, child, or infant without adequate breathing.
- Differentiate between a patient with adequate breathing and one with inadequate breathing.
- Describe the methods used to obtain a pulse.
- Differentiate among obtaining a pulse in an adult, child, and infant.
- Discuss the need for assessing the patient for external bleeding.
- Describe normal and abnormal findings when assessing skin color.
- Describe normal and abnormal findings when assessing skin temperature.
- Describe normal and abnormal findings when assessing skin condition.
- Describe normal and abnormal findings when assessing skin capillary refilling time in the infant and child.
- Differentiate among assessing for altered mental status in the adult, child, and infant.
- Distinguish among methods of assessing breathing in the adult, child, and infant.
- Compare the methods of providing airway care to the adult, child, and infant.
- Explain the reason for prioritizing a patient for care and transport.
- Differentiate between a sign and a symptom
- Describe the unique needs for assessing an individual with a specific chief complaint with no known prior history of the problem.
- Differentiate between the history and physical examination performed for responsive patients with no known prior history and responsive patients with a known prior history of the problem.
- Identify the components of the SAMPLE history
- Differentiate between the assessment performed for a patient who is unresponsive or has an altered mental state and other medical patients requiring assessment.
- Describe the needs for assessing an individual who is unresponsive.
- Identify the components of a focused (secondary) assessment.
- Discuss the reason for performing a focused (secondary) assessment (history and physical examination).
- Identify the components of vital signs.
- Describe the methods to obtain a breathing rate.
- Identify the characteristics that should be evaluated during a breathing assessment.
- Differentiate among shallow, labored, and noisy breathing.
- Describe the methods to obtain a pulse rate.
- Identify the information obtained in the assessment of the pulse.
- Differentiate among a strong, weak, regular, and irregular pulse.
- Describe the methods to assess skin color, temperature, conditions, and capillary refill in infants and children.

- Identify normal and abnormal skin colors.
- Differentiate among pate, blue, red, and yellow skin color.
- Identify normal and abnormal skin temperatures.
- Differentiate among hot, cool, and cold skin temperatures.
- Identify normal and abnormal skin conditions.
- Identify normal and abnormal capillary refill in infants and children.
- Describe the methods to assess blood pressure.
- Define systolic pressure.
- Define diastolic pressure.
- Explain the difference between auscultation and palpation for obtaining a blood pressure.
- Describe the methods used to assess the pupils.
- Identify normal and abnormal pupil size.
- Differentiate between dilated (large) and constricted (small) pupil size.
- Differentiate between reactive and nonreactive pupils and equal and unequal pupils.
- State the importance of accurately reporting and recording baseline vital signs.
- State the reasons for performing a rapid trauma assessment.
- Determine when the rapid assessment may be altered to provide patient care.
- Discuss the reasons for reconsidering the mechanism of injury.
- State the reasons for performing a head-to-toe survey.
- Describe the areas included in the head-to-toe survey, and discuss what to evaluate.
- Give examples and explain why patients should receive a head-to-toe survey.
- Discuss the reasons for repeating the initial (primary) assessment as part of the ongoing assessment or reassessment.
- Describe the components of the ongoing assessment or reassessment.
- Describe trending of assessment components.

Affective Objectives

- Explain the importance of an initial (primary) assessment.
- Explain the rationale for crew members to evaluate scene safety before entering.
- Serve as a model for others explaining how patient situations affect your evaluation of mechanism of injury or nature of illness.
- Explain the importance of forming a general impression of the patient.
- Explain the value of performing an initial (primary) assessment.

- Explain the value of performing the baseline vital signs.
- Defend the need for obtaining and recording an accurate set of vital signs.
- Explain the rationale of recording additional sets of vital signs.
- Explain the importance of obtaining a SAMPLE history.
- Explain the importance of a focused (secondary) assessment.
- Explain the value of performing an ongoing assessment or reassessment.
- Explain the value of trending assessment components to other health professionals who assume care of the patient.
- Recognize, respect, and respond to the feelings that patients might experience during assessment.

Psychomotor Objectives

- Observe various scenarios and identify potential hazards.
- Demonstrate the skills that should be used to obtain information from the patient, family, or bystanders at the scene.
- Demonstrate the techniques for assessing mental status.
- Demonstrate the techniques for assessing the airway.
- Demonstrate the techniques for assessing if the patient is breathing.
- Demonstrate the techniques for assessing if the patient has a pulse.
- Demonstrate the techniques for assessing the patient for external bleeding.
- Demonstrate the techniques for assessing the patient's skin color, temperature, condition, and capillary refilling time (infants and children only).
- Demonstrate the skills associated with obtaining blood pressure.
- Demonstrate the skills associated with assessing the pupils.
- Demonstrate the ability to prioritize patients.
- Demonstrate the patient assessment skills to use when assisting a patient who is responsive with no known history of the problem.
- Demonstrate the patient assessment skills to use when assisting a patient who is unresponsive or has an altered mental state.
- Demonstrate the head-to-toe survey to use when assessing a patient based on a significant mechanism of injury.
- Demonstrate the skills involved in performing the ongoing assessment or reassessment.
- Attend to the feelings that unresponsive patients or those with altered mental status might be experiencing.

References

Bickley LS, Bates A: *Guide to physical assessment,* ed 9, Philadelphia, 2007, Lippincott–Williams & Wilkins.

Guyton AC, Hall JE: *Textbook of medical physiology,* ed 11, Philadelphia, 2006, Saunders-Elsevier.

Mawlavi A et al: Dorsalis pedis arterial pulse: palpation using a bony landmark, *Postgrad Med J* 78:746-747, 2002. © 2002 Fellowship of Postgraduate Medicine.

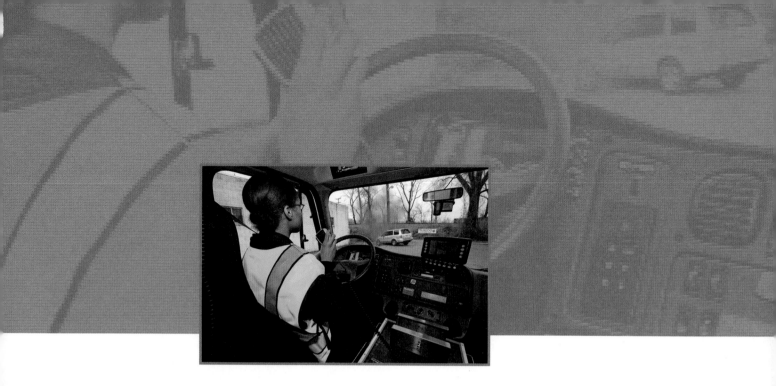

8 Communications

CHAPTER OUTLINE

Scenario

You are en route to the hospital with a patient experiencing respiratory distress. During transport the patient stops breathing. You immediately provide positive-pressure ventilation with a bag-mask device. Your partner calls the receiving hospital and provides essential patient information and your estimated time of arrival. Members of the hospital "code team" meet you at the emergency department door. As you transfer care of the patient to the physicians and nurses, you give your verbal report to the staff, summarizing the information given over the radio and providing updates from your ongoing assessment and treatment en route. The hospital seems fully prepared for this patient. They have the airway and ventilation equipment ready and immediately insert an endotracheal tube and attach the patient to a ventilator. You are impressed by the number of personnel present at the bedside and the level of preparedness for this patient, who stopped breathing just minutes ago.

Prehospital care requires many resources that ultimately affect the survival of the acutely ill or injured patient. Communication systems play an important role by receiving the call for help, dispatching first responders and emergency medical services (EMS) providers, coordinating the emergency response, and relaying information from prehospital to hospital staff. Communication systems serve as the "central nervous system" of EMS by coordinating all essential activities among the scene, ambulance, and hospital. These systems provide a way to communicate the conditions at the scene to the dispatcher, give medical direction for advice on assessment or patient care, and notify the receiving hospital of the impending arrival of a seriously ill or injured patient.

Effective communication in EMS also involves the routine collection and exchange of information with patients, family members, bystanders, first responders, and healthcare providers. Good communication includes several important variables, including accuracy, confidentiality, and use of a systematic approach to collect and communicate essential information. It also includes emotional or affective elements to calm people at the scene and express caring and empathy to the patient and family members.

> **LEARNING OBJECTIVE**
> • Explain the rationale for providing efficient and effective radio communications and patient reports.

Effective communication requires an understanding of the elements of an EMS communication system, adherence to principles of communication, and knowledge of the information that must be conveyed to the dispatcher and hospital team. Communication occurs in many ways, including mobile two-way or portable radios to regional base stations through repeater systems that can boost and strengthen the signal. Most portable radios function on the basis of "line of sight." Radio communication may not be possible in valleys or around mountains. Cellular phones are also frequently used in EMS systems. Emergency medical dispatchers coordinate the communication system and receive the call for help, dispatch the appropriate units, provide updates and clarifications throughout the call, and dispatch additional resources as needed. Dispatchers also may provide prearrival instructions over the phone to the bystander before EMS providers arrive.

Communication includes direct conversations between you and the patient. Some patients, such as hearing- or visually impaired patients, children, and elderly persons, may require special communication principles. Patients who speak a foreign language may require an interpreter, such as a family member, to collect a history.

The final and often most important communication occurs on arrival at the hospital, where the history of the call must be presented clearly and concisely to emergency department (ED) staff. In essence, EMS communications provide the link from the scene through prehospital care and into the hospital. The quality of this communication can play an important role in identifying life-threatening conditions, communicating care that was provided in the field, and establishing the need for ongoing care at the hospital.

Communication Systems

System Components

Communication systems are formed by many components; each component has its own specific function, but all are vital to a good communications network. The **base station** is a radio located at a stationary site, such as a communications center, ambulance headquarters, or hospital, that provides a hub for communications throughout the EMS network (**Figure 8-1**). **Mobile two-way radios,** which are capable of transmitting and receiving information, are located in vehicles (**Figure 8-2**). Typically, vehicular radios transmit with less power than those at the base stations, usually between 20 and 50 watts. The typical transmission range for a vehicular radio is 10 to 15 miles (16-40 km) over average terrain. Hand-held or portable radios transmit with even less power, usually between 1 and 5 watts, and are limited in range (**Figure 8-3**).

Repeater systems are used in many EMS communication systems. These components receive a radio signal from

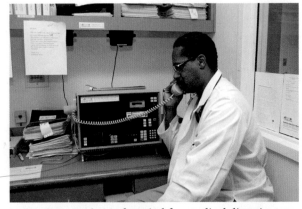

Figure 8-1 Base station at hospital for medical direction. *From Chapleau W, Pons P: Emergency medical technician: making the difference, St Louis, 2007, Mosby-Elsevier.*

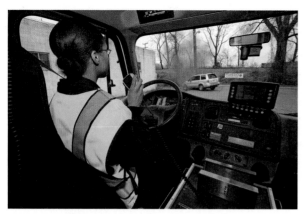

Figure 8-2 Mobile two-way radio.

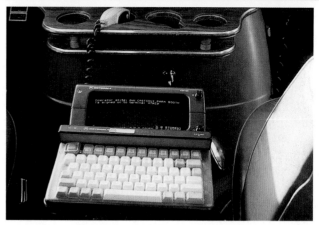

Figure 8-4 Mobile data terminal.

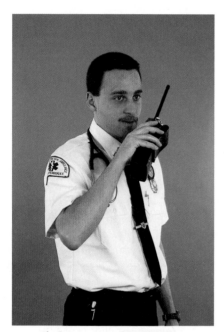

Figure 8-3 Hand-held radio.

a low-power radio (portable or ambulance radio) on one frequency and retransmit the message at a higher power on another frequency. Repeater systems relay signals to the dispatch center or base hospital. Repeaters are receivers and transmitters that are often strategically located on high ground or on tall buildings. They may also be situated in the emergency vehicle specifically to boost and relay the portable radio signal. Modern technological advances now allow use of digital radio equipment and cellular telephones, and the future use of *telemedicine* raises the possibility of communicating with video transmissions from the scene to medical direction or the receiving hospital (see later discussion).

Communications can transmit more than verbal information. For example, **biotelemetry** is a method by which biological data are transferred from one location to another by radio. In EMS systems, telemetry is used to transmit a patient's electrocardiogram to a base hospital. Electrocardiographic information is coded or digitized and then decoded at the base

hospital to its original form. These data are often transmitted by telephone lines, including cell phones.

Some systems have **computerized mobile data terminals** mounted in the ambulance **(Figure 8-4).** These terminals allow the dispatcher to communicate by a computer screen, thereby decreasing the amount of voice transmission over the airwaves. The use of visual data decreases the likelihood of errors in communications that may occur from verbal misunderstandings. The field personnel can also enter data into the system to communicate with the dispatcher. The dispatcher can maintain a visual status display of each unit to aid in strategically selecting units for calls. Another feature of mobile data terminals is the ability to recall the history of a unit during a shift or throughout the response day.

Radio Communications

Communications in EMS systems are one part of a large, complex network of radio communications that must be coordinated to ensure that information moves freely and appropriately through the airwaves. The **Federal Communications Commission (FCC)** is the government agency responsible for regulating all aspects of radio communications in the United States. The FCC establishes technical standards for radio equipment, allocates radio frequencies, and licenses and regulates those who use and repair radio equipment.

Communications Center

The **communications center** does the following **(Figure 8-5):**
- Receives requests for emergency assistance
- Performs triage (determines the priority of the complaint)
- Dispatches appropriate responders
- Provides prearrival instructions to the caller
- Coordinates EMS and other emergency resources (e.g., fire, police, "heavy" rescue, hazardous materials [HAZMAT] personnel, hospitals)
- Notifies the hospital of the impending arrival of the patient

The individual who receives calls for assistance is the **receiving operator,** or call taker. The person who communicates with field personnel is the **dispatcher.** Depending on the size of the

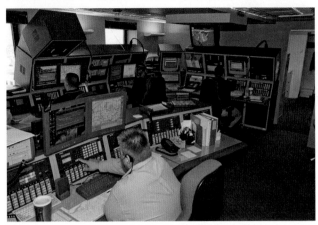

Figure 8-5 Communications center.

system, the receiving operator and dispatcher may be the same person. In very small systems, the emergency medical technician (EMT) may receive the call at the ambulance headquarters and respond directly.

Emergency Medical Dispatch

Dispatchers and receiving operators should possess good communication skills and should be knowledgeable in emergency care because they must perform triage to dispatch either EMTs or advanced life support (ALS) personnel. They may also need to notify other special services such as the police department, HAZMAT teams, or extrication teams. The receiving operator or dispatcher obtains the following information:
1. The call location
2. Nature of the medical problem
3. The resources required
4. Name and location of the caller

In systems that use **emergency medical dispatch** (EMD) the specially trained dispatcher may remain on the line after notifying the appropriate response personnel to give basic first-aid instructions over the phone to the person who placed the call for help. Emergency medical dispatch training is a comprehensive program based on the U.S. Department of Transportation (DOT) EMS Dispatcher National Standard Curriculum.

To ensure optimal coordination, field personnel must communicate at prescribed intervals with the dispatcher. Typically this includes the following time points:
• When the call is received
• When the unit begins its response
• On arrival at the scene
• When leaving the scene
• On arrival at the hospital
• When the unit is available for the next assignment

Communication may also occur in special circumstances, such as calling for additional help and mobilizing special resources (e.g., police, fire, HAZMAT personnel) after scene size-up.

LEARNING OBJECTIVES
• List the proper methods for initiating and terminating a radio call.
• Describe the attributes for increasing the effectiveness and efficiency of verbal communications.
• State legal aspects to consider in verbal communication.

Principles of Radio Communication

Radio communication requires special skills and techniques to ensure the clear and accurate transfer of information. Because many units may be competing for time over the same airwaves, radio communications are more concise than conversations over the telephone.

When making initial radio contact, you should never interrupt another radio transmission unless you have emergency priority radio traffic. Most systems use unit codes or names to identify each caller to the dispatcher. In your initial contact, identify yourself by announcing your code to the dispatcher. After acknowledgment by the dispatcher, you can proceed with your brief transmission. You should speak in a normal (or monotone) voice with the microphone a few inches away from your mouth. The tendency is to speak too loudly or quickly when providing patient care in a serious situation, which may garble your message. Unlike telephone conversations, radio allows only one person to speak at a time. While you speak, you must hold down a button, which prevents you from being interrupted by the person to whom you are speaking. This is another reason to keep your messages brief.

At the end of each exchange between you and the other party, give a signal, such as saying "over," to indicate that you are finished speaking and are ready to receive the other person's response. Likewise, you should wait until you hear the same code ("over") from the other party before you press the button to speak again. Some radios send out an automated "beep" or tone to signal the beginning or ending of a transmission. When speaking on the radio, keep principles of good radio communication in mind (**Box 8-1**).

LEARNING OBJECTIVES
• State the proper sequence for the delivery of patient information.
• Identify the essential components of a verbal report.
• Explain the importance of effective communication of patient information in the verbal report.
• List the correct radio procedures in the phases of a typical call.

Communication with Medical Direction

Many EMS systems provide for direct online communication with a physician medical director located at the receiving hospital or at a centralized medical direction facility. EMTs may consult with EMS physicians for medical orders and other triage, treatment, or transport decisions or assistance with patients who may be refusing medical attention. EMTs should be thoroughly familiar with local communications protocol regarding consultation with an online physician.

| Box 8-1 | Principles for Radio Communication |

Radio Operations

- Turn the radio on and adjust the volume.
- Use EMS frequencies only for EMS communications.
- Listen to frequency and be sure it is clear before beginning a transmission.
- Press the "press to talk" button on the radio and wait for 1 second before speaking.
- Speak with lips 2 to 3 inches from the microphone.

General Communication Principles

- Address the unit being called, then give the name of your unit (and number if appropriate).
- Wait for the signal (e.g., "go ahead") from the receiving unit to indicate that you may start your transmission. A response such as "stand by" may be given instead, which means wait until further notice.
- Speak clearly and slowly in a monotone voice.
- Keep the transmission brief. If a transmission takes longer than 30 seconds, stop at that point, and pause for a few seconds, so that emergency traffic can use the frequency if necessary.
- Avoid meaningless phrases such as "be advised."
- Courtesy is assumed, so there is no need to say "please," "thank you," and "you're welcome."
- Do not give a patient's name or other identifying information such as a Social Security number over the air. The airwaves are public, and scanners are popular. EMS transmissions may be overheard by more listeners than the EMS community.
- Remain objective and impartial when describing patients. An EMT may be sued for slander if someone's reputation is damaged in this way.
- Use "we" instead of "I." An EMT rarely acts alone.
- Do not use profanity on the air. The FCC takes a dim view of such language and may impose substantial fines.
- Say "over" when the transmission is finished. Obtain confirmation that the message was received.
- Reduce background noise as much as possible (e.g., close the ambulance window).

Accuracy

- Use clear text.
- Use the standard format for transmission of information.
- Avoid overuse of codes, especially those that are not standardized.
- When transmitting a number that may be confused (e.g., a number in the teens), give the number and then the individual digits.
- Avoid words that are difficult to hear, such as "yes" and "no." Use "affirmative" and "negative."
- Avoid diagnosing the patient's problem.

| Box 8-2 | Essential Elements of a Patient Report to Medical Direction or a Receiving Facility |

- Unit and level of provider identification
- Estimated time of arrival
- Age and gender of patient
- Patient's chief complaint
- Brief history: brief, pertinent aspects of the history of the present illness and major past illnesses
- Patient's mental status
- Patient's baseline vital signs
- Pertinent findings of the physical examination
- Emergency medical care given
- Patient's response to emergency medical care
- Report update, as needed

| Box 8-3 | Sample Presentation |

"Base, this is EMT Unit 42. We are en route to University Hospital with a 10-minute ETA. We are transporting a 52-year-old male complaining of squeezing chest pain radiating to the jaw and left arm that he rates as 10 on a scale from 1 to 10. The pain started approximately 30 minutes ago at rest and was not relieved by three nitroglycerin. The patient has a history of angina and hypertension and takes nitroglycerin and Acupril. He describes the pain as similar to his previous episodes of chest pain but more severe. He is alert and oriented with respirations of 20 and regular, pulse 84 and regular, and blood pressure of 110/74. His skin is pale, cool, and sweaty. Physical exam is otherwise normal. We have administered oxygen by nonrebreather and placed the patient in the position of comfort. His pain and vital signs remain unchanged."

You should conclude with the prehospital treatments that were administered and how the patient has responded (**Box 8-3**).

Deal in facts as assessed by you and your crew. Because physicians base their treatment on your information, accuracy is essential. You may be asked to provide your prehospital impression of the patient's problem. You should follow this same format when transferring care to ALS personnel who arrive at the scene after you have already begun to give care.

The information you provide guides appropriate prehospital decisions and helps the hospital to prepare for the patient by having the right room, equipment, and personnel available. Depending on the system, the dispatcher or the EMT notifies the hospital of the patient's status and the estimated time of arrival so the hospital can prepare to receive the patient.

Radio communications should be organized, concise, and pertinent.

A standard medical presentation format should be used when presenting a patient (**Box 8-2**). Give the name of the EMS unit, the estimated time of hospital arrival, and the level of prehospital provider. Include the patient's age, gender, chief complaint, history of the present illness and brief pertinent history, the patient's mental status, baseline vital signs, and results of the physical examination (including pertinent negative findings).

REALWorld

Most EMTs can administer medications or assist a patient with their medication only after receiving an order from medical direction. The order can be received only after the EMT has given a clear description of the patient being treated. If the report from the EMT is not clear and accurate, the physician at the hospital may refuse a requested order, not allowing the patient to receive the required medication. In addition to being professional, good radio communication skills benefit patients.

On arrival at the hospital, you will provide the hospital staff with the patient report (**Figure 8-6**). Start by introducing the patient by name, if it is known, and summarize the information presented over the radio, including the following:

- The patient's chief complaint
- Any medical history not previously given
- Additional treatment provided en route
- Any additional vital signs or changes in vital signs obtained during transport

In addition to your verbal report, you will also leave a written prehospital care report (see Chapter 9).

The dispatcher should be notified when you arrive at the hospital, when you leave the hospital, when you return to your station, and when you are available for another call. **Table 8-1** summarizes the communications made by an EMT during the various phases of a typical call.

Telemedicine

The new frontier in EMS communication with medical direction is **telemedicine,** the process of bidirectional communication between a physician and EMS provider in the field using an audio and video system. This allows the physician to view actual physical findings, direct the examination and treatment of the patient, and observe the patient's changing condition (**Figure 8-7**).

System Maintenance

Communication equipment should be checked regularly to ensure that it is operational. In addition, special routine maintenance is required by qualified technicians on a regular basis (e.g., to ensure that a radio is not drifting from its assigned frequency).

Again, as technology changes, new equipment is incorporated into EMS communications. For example, cellular telephones are used in many regions to contact medical direction and are often made available as a backup system if radio communications fail.

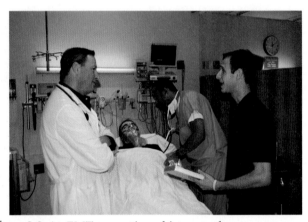

Figure 8-6 An EMT presenting a history to the emergency physician at the hospital.

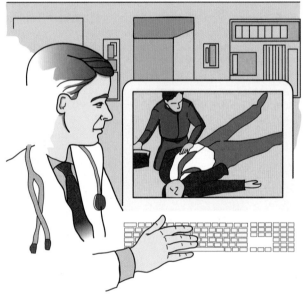

Figure 8-7 Emergency department physicians can monitor and guide care provided by EMTs on scene over the radio and via video monitors.

Table 8-1	Communications at Various Phases of a Typical EMS Call	
Phase	**To Whom**	**What Is Communicated by EMT**
To the scene	Dispatcher (or other agencies as appropriate)	Call received Unit en route Estimated time of arrival
At the scene	Dispatcher	Arrival at the scene: communication of scene size-up and call for additional resources as needed
	Medical direction	Patient's assessment findings
To the facility	Dispatcher	En route to facility
	Receiving hospital	Patient status and estimated time of arrival
At the facility	Hospital staff	Verbal report: brief summary of information given over radio and any history not given previously, in addition to other treatments and vital signs en route and other pertinent information gathered but not transmitted
To the station	Dispatcher	Leaving facility and estimated time back in service
At the station	Dispatcher	Readiness for service

LEARNING OBJECTIVES
- Discuss the communication skills used to interact with the patient.
- Discuss the communication skills used to interact with the family, bystanders, and individuals with other agencies while providing patient care, as well as the different skills used to interact with the patient and with others.

Interpersonal Communication

Communication is an essential component of prehospital care. As an EMT, you work as a key member of a team. Team members must share information on every call. To be effective, you must be familiar with the equipment used to transmit information, the basic principles of radio reporting, and the format of a prehospital care report. Communications should be concise, organized, and accurate. You also should be effective at interpersonal communications. A direct, honest, clear, and respectful approach is the foundation that promotes understanding when dealing with patients, bystanders, and other healthcare providers.

Although individual situations demand different types of interaction and each EMT has a unique style, some general guidelines for communicating with patients, families, and bystanders are listed in **Box 8-4.**

Special Considerations

Elderly Patients and Children

Elderly patients should be treated with respect. You should move the elderly patient with extra care and a gentle touch. You should be sensitive to the spouse's concerns and allow the spouse to travel with the patient if possible. Remember not to address the patient by first name unless you are given specific permission to do so. In communicating with elderly patients, allow them adequate time to answer questions before asking the next one. You should never assume that they are hearing impaired. Even if the patient is hearing impaired, speaking louder is not an effective strategy because sound becomes distorted at higher volumes.

Children and infants also need special attention. Objects such as a doll or special blanket may help the child feel more secure.

Box 8-4	Guidelines for Interpersonal Communication

1. **Focus.** Focus your attention directly on the patient and maintain eye contact. Conversation between EMTs that is directed away from the patient may upset or anger some patients.
2. **Develop contact with the patient.** Introduce yourself, informing the patient that you are an EMT and explaining your function. When practical, position yourself at eye level or lower than the patient. This is especially important for children.
3. **Tell the truth.** Although you may wish to limit what you say, speak truthfully and do not falsely reassure the patient. If you do not know the answer to a question, admit it.
4. **Communicate effectively.** Do not use medical terminology that the patient may not understand. Conversely, do not talk down to the patient.
5. **Use effective body language.** Your body posture and gestures should be calm and nonthreatening. Aggressive body language can be frightening to the patient.
6. **Speak clearly.** Speak slowly, clearly, and distinctly. With the patient who is hearing impaired, this may require a slightly louder voice; however, avoid shouting, which may frighten the patient.
7. **Explain treatments.** Explain what you are going to do before doing it.
8. **Use the patient's name.** Use the patient's proper name. Do not refer to a patient as "Mom" or "Dear" or "Honey." Referring to patients who are your seniors by their first names can be interpreted as being disrespectful. Also, trying to be the patient's "pal" or to "be cool" with the patient is inappropriate and phony. The novice EMT may believe such an approach may be more persuasive or may make it easier to enlist the patient's cooperation. However, professional demeanor will be much more effective and much less likely to create a situation in which the patient refuses to cooperate.
9. **Allow for a response.** Allow the patient ample time to respond to questions and not be rushed. This requires expert judgment by the EMT, who must balance the time allowed for the patient to talk against the urgent need to stabilize the patient.
10. **Be helpful and considerate.** Be aware of the patient's comfort. Is the patient cold? Is he or she in a comfortable position (if it is safe to reposition the patient)? Should a friend or family member accompany the patient?
11. **Look beneath the surface.** Try to sense the concerns and meanings beneath the patient's words. People call for an ambulance for a reason. A patient who states that he just needs his heart medications renewed may have actually had chest pain all night. Patients may deny their symptoms, but be alert when they have a sudden interest in keeping a clinic appointment, in refilling medications, or in wanting a "checkup."
12. **Be professional.** Maintain a professional and calm demeanor at all times. Do not show anger or personalize a patient's negative remarks. Many people deal with stress and illness by becoming angry, making inappropriate remarks, or hurling insults. This is just as much a part of the patient's illness as the chest pain or shortness of breath. During times of stress, patients may not have the emotional strength or maturity to show appreciation for the EMT's efforts. Thus, do not be disappointed by the patient who is hostile toward you while you are putting forth your best efforts. The EMT must always be at his or her professional best, even when the job feels like a thankless one.
13. **Anticipate problems with communication.** Is the patient disoriented, angered, or hearing impaired? What does the patient expect to happen? If there is resistance to your efforts, who is resisting?
14. **Assume understanding.** Always assume that the patient can understand what you are saying, even if it appears that he or she cannot. Avoid inappropriate remarks, and do not talk about the patient as if he or she is not there. For example, stroke patients may be unable to speak yet can understand everything that is being said.

You should interact with both the parent and the child. When caring for a sick or injured child, allow the parent to accompany the child if possible. If the child sees the parent accept the EMT, the child will be less fearful. As with adults, you should be honest with the child; do not make promises that cannot be kept. For example, avoid saying that the child will "not get a shot" at the hospital when this is uncertain.

Hearing-Impaired and Visually Impaired Patients

Hearing-impaired patients should be treated as having normal intelligence. You should always look directly at the patient when speaking and determine whether the patient can read lips. If the patient cannot read lips, communicate with short, written questions. You should not become impatient with the slow pace sometimes necessary for this type of communication. While performing procedures on the patient, you should call attention to what is being done and, if necessary, write an explanation. Learning the alphabet in sign language, as well as simple signs for pain, time, and so on, is simple and worth the small effort involved. When a patient is hearing impaired, the EMT should not attempt to communicate by shouting.

Visually impaired patients have heightened senses of hearing, touch, and smell. You should maintain physical contact with the patient and explain in detail what is being done or where the patient is being moved. If the patient has a service animal such as a dog, bring it with the patient or make arrangements to care for the animal. During transport, periodically inform the patient about what is happening.

Foreign Language

Patients who speak another language or who speak minimal English should be interviewed through a translator. Speaking loudly in a language not understood by the patient is obviously ineffective. Some EMTs carry a manual of simple phrases in other languages to communicate with such patients. When attempting to communicate with a patient who speaks minimal English, both the EMT and the patient can misinterpret or may not understand what the other is saying. The patient may answer a question that is different from the one you asked. If you find that the patient is having difficulty understanding, proceed with the interview in the patient's native language. You can use visual clues to assist in translating questions and answers. Several manuals are also available for EMS providers that contain key phrases that may be helpful. The dispatch center may also have interpreters available to you.

Cultural Considerations

Different cultures may have variations on what are considered acceptable forms of communication. The EMT should be alert to these differences to avoid miscommunication. For example, in the Asian culture it is not acceptable for women to show anger or pain, so they may try to smile to avoid placing their burden on others. This may lead the EMT to judge the severity of the patient's condition incorrectly. Other cultures may not permit a woman to bare her face in the presence of man other than her husband. The EMT must be sensitive to these variations, remaining professional and a patient advocate, and must treat patients while respecting their cultural beliefs.

Altered Mental Status

When approaching the confused or disoriented patient, you should communicate in simple terms and try to determine what is causing the confusion. Detailed explanations should be avoided. If the patient can respond, do not rush the person. Allow ample time for the patient to focus and respond to your questions.

As with confused patients, mentally challenged patients should be assisted by giving simple explanations and reinforcement. You should determine the level of communication appropriate for the patient because some mentally challenged patients are capable of simple communication. Be sure to distinguish mental abnormalities from physical abnormalities. As discussed previously, you should always assume that the patient can understand what you are saying, and you should be careful not to say something that could insult the patient.

Verbal Defusing Strategies

Some patients may be unfriendly and may resist going to the hospital. At times, patients may become verbally and physically combative. In such cases the EMT's first priority is the patient's safety. If necessary, the patient should be positioned with physical restraints, or the EMT may need to leave the scene. In many cases, however, the EMT may be able to take control of the situation using only words. The EMT should not become caught up in the patient's anger or anxiety. For example, if a patient is yelling at you, there is no reason to yell back. Allow the patient to yell, and then calmly ask what you can do to help. The following suggestions may help *defuse* a situation (make it less "charged" or tense):

- Always be polite
- Be firm, but not angry or mean
- Never call the patient names
- Allow the patient to express his concerns by asking the patient such questions as, "Why don't you want to go to the hospital?" or "What is your concern about answering some of our questions?"
- Maintain a relaxed posture, allowing the patient to maintain her own space

REALWorld

Communicating with children and geriatric patients can offer additional challenges. Geriatric patients may have difficulty hearing and seeing and may be slower at gathering their thoughts. It is important to be polite; always address older patients as "Mr." or "Mrs." (as appropriate). Ask one question at a time, and wait for an answer. Face them when you talk with geriatric patients, and speak loud enough for them to hear. If communication is difficult, consider other means (e.g., pen and paper).

When talking with children, remember you may be one of their first encounters with the medical community. Younger children especially are frightened the first time they are sick or injured. Be reassuring in your tone of voice. Do not use medical words such as "abdomen," but rather assess their "tummy," and do not work quietly, because this may heighten their anxiety. Allow mom or dad to remain close.

Case in Point

Two EMTs respond to find an 89-year-old woman at home sitting in a chair complaining of difficulty breathing. One EMT positions himself in front of the patient so that she can see and hear him better. He assesses for a pulse while his partner delivers supplemental oxygen. The first EMT notices that the patient's pulse is irregular, which can be a sign of a new medical problem, but also a normal finding in some geriatric patients. More history is required. As he begins to talk to the patient, the EMT notices that she appears to have difficulty hearing him. He notices a hearing aid lying on the table next to her, and he helps her place it in her ear. The patient does not recall the purpose of all her medications, so the EMTs collect the drugs to take to the hospital. As they load the patient into the ambulance, she requests that the EMTs make sure the stove is turned off and lock the doors. The EMTs do so, returning the patient's keys to her purse, and begin transport.

Scenario Follow-up

As you prepare to leave the hospital, one of the physicians comes over and says, "Thanks for that patient report. In a few words, you painted a clear and accurate picture of the patient's condition. It really helps us work as a team." You radio the emergency medical dispatcher as you depart from the hospital, updating your status and availability for another call. The dispatcher thanks you for your quick return to services and gives you the address and chief complaint of another patient calling 9-1-1 for help.

This case illustrates the importance of effective and timely communication in the EMS environment. Notification via radio during transport to the hospital allows the emergency department team to prepare adequately for the imminent arrival of the patient. This may also involve the mobilization of special team members from the hospital area, including anesthesiologists, respiratory therapists, trauma surgeons, cardiologists, neurologist, pediatricians, and other personnel who may be needed, depending on the nature of the emergency. In emergency care, seconds count and can make the difference between life and death. Communication over the radio must be clear, concise, and include the information needed for hospital and EMS personnel to react appropriately.

Summary

Effective communication is an essential skill for the EMT. Whether communicating by radio or providing a history to ED personnel, a structured and concise approach is critical to the rapid and accurate exchange of information. Radio and telephone systems are important tools to prepare hospitals for the imminent arrival of patients in critical condition. Remember to apply key principles of communication when using the radio or when communicating with the patient, bystanders, and medical personnel. The time saved by proper notification can mean all the difference for the patient.

The Bottom Line

Learning Checklist

✓ EMS communication systems include mobile two-way or portable radios to regional base stations through repeater systems that can boost and strengthen the signal.

✓ Emergency medical dispatchers coordinate the communications system and receive the call for help, dispatch the appropriate units, provide updates and clarifications throughout the call, and dispatch additional resources as needed.

✓ Principles of radio communication include making sure the frequency is clear before transmission, pressing the "press to talk" button and waiting before communicating, and speaking clearly and slowly in a monotone voice with lips 2 to 3 inches away from the microphone.

✓ General radio communication principles include identifying yourself and the unit you are calling, waiting for "go ahead" to speak, keeping transmissions brief, and avoiding codes and meaningless phrases.

✓ General radio communication principles also include not giving the patient's name or other identifying information (e.g., Social Security number) over the airwaves, not using profanity, using "affirmative" and "negative" to convey yes or no answers, and using EMS frequencies.

✓ Emergency medical dispatchers may also provide first-aid directions over the phone to the bystander before EMS providers arrive.

✓ Telecommunications can allow the physician in the emergency department to see what the EMTs see in the field by way of digital video, allowing the physician to better guide their care.

✓ Effective interpersonal communication includes eye contact, honesty, clear language, use of the patient's proper name, and an opportunity for the patient to offer information and respond to questions.

✓ Presentation to medical direction should include the name of the EMS unit; estimated time of arrival; level of prehospital provider; patient's age, gender, and chief complaint; history of the present illness; SAMPLE history; mental status; vital signs and physical examination; prehospital treatments; and how the patient responded.

✓ Communication with children and the elderly and patients who are hearing impaired or visually impaired requires special communication principles.

✓ Some situations can be "defused" by the appropriate use of words and gestures.

Key Terms

Base station Central coordination area of a communication system that is in contact with other components of the system.

Biotelemetry Transmission of biological data by a radio or other form of communication to a distant location such as a hospital.

Communications center Part of the communication system that coordinates receiving calls, triage, dispatch, and other activities of an EMS system.

Computerized mobile data terminal Terminal located in the ambulance that allows the EMTs to communicate with the dispatcher by computer screen; units can also be tracked.

Dispatcher Individual who receives the call for help and dispatches the appropriate resources through the EMS system.

Emergency medical dispatch Nationally recognized method for training dispatchers in the systematic questioning of people calling 9-1-1 and, when necessary, providing phone-directed instructions.

Federal Communications Commission (FCC) Government agency responsible for regulating all aspects of radio communications in the United States.

Mobile two-way radio Radio contained within vehicles that allows transmission through the dispatch or medical direction system.

Receiving operator Individual who receives the call for assistance.

Repeater system Strategically based receiver and transmitter that accept signals from a portable unit or mobile radio and relay them with a more powerful transmitter.

Telemedicine Bidirectional audiovisual communication between EMT at scene and medical direction.

Review Questions

1. Which type of communication is most often used in the patient compartment of an ambulance?
   a. Hand-held portable radios
   b. Mobile radios
   c. Transceivers
   d. Telemetry

2. Approximately how much power does a hand-held or portable radio use to transmit?
   a. 1 to 5 watts
   b. 10 to 20 watts
   c. 20 to 50 watts
   d. 50 to 100 watts

3. Which of the following devices receive a radio signal from a low-power radio (portable or ambulance radio) on one frequency and retransmit the message at a higher power on another frequency?
   a. Receivers
   b. Repeaters
   c. Transmitters
   d. Digitals

4. What is the name of the government agency that is responsible for regulating all aspects of radio communications in the United States?
   a. Radio Communication Center
   b. Dispatch Communications Center
   c. Center for Radio Control
   d. Federal Communications Commission

5. Who is the person who communicates with field personnel?
   a. Dispatcher
   b. Communication technician
   c. Emergency operator
   d. Receiving operator

6. How many inches away from your mouth do you hold a radio while speaking?
   a. 2 to 3
   b. 5 to 6
   c. 8 to 10
   d. 10 to 12

7. What should you do when initiating a radio call?
   a. Wait for the receiving unit to say "go ahead" before you send your initial message.
   b. Use "yes" and "no" to indicate your acceptance or refusal of their response.
   c. Speak in a voice that is louder than usual for clarity of transmission.
   d. Use codes extensively to reduce air time and summarize communications.

8. Which of the following would be least appropriate when speaking to a hearing-impaired patient?
   a. Maintain eye contact
   b. Shout in a loud voice
   c. Use written notes
   d. Allow the patient to see your lips

9. Which of the following is most likely to gain the desired response from a patient or bystander?
   a. Allow sufficient time for a response
   b. Be personal by using terms such as "dear" or "honey"
   c. When possible, use medical terminology to show professionalism
   d. Keep your hands in your pocket to avoid distraction

10. In most cases, which of the following would be the least important piece of information for an EMT's presentation to medical direction or hospital staff?
    a. Patient's age and gender
    b. Mental status
    c. Physical examination findings
    d. Immunization history

For Further Review

In the Student Workbook

- Multiple-choice questions
- Short-answer questions
- Case scenario questions

On Evolve

- Weblinks
- Lecture notes
- Exercises

Learning Objectives

Cognitive Objectives

- List the proper methods of initiating and terminating a radio call.
- Describe the attributes for increasing the effectiveness and efficiency of verbal communications.
- State legal aspects to consider in verbal communication.
- State the proper sequence for the delivery of patient information.
- Identify the essential components of a verbal report.
- Explain the importance of effective communication of patient information in the verbal report.
- List the correct radio procedures in the following phases of a typical call:
  To the scene
  At the scene
  To the facility
  At the facility
  To the station
  At the station
- Discuss the communication skills used to interact with the patient.
- Discuss the communication skills used to interact with the family, bystanders, and individuals from other agencies while providing patient care, as well as the different skills used to interact with the patient and with others.

Affective Objective

- Explain the rationale for providing efficient and effective radio communications and patient reports.

Psychomotor Objectives

- Perform a simulated, organized, and concise radio transmission.
- Perform an organized, concise patient report that would be given to the staff at a receiving facility.
- Perform a brief, organized report that would be given to an ALS provider arriving at a scene where the EMT was already providing care.

References

American Geriatrics Society, National Council of State Emergency Medical Services Training Coordinators: *Geriatric education for emergency medical services (GEMS)*, Sudbury, Mass., 2003, Jones and Bartlett.

LeBaron M: *Bridging cultural conflicts: a new approach for a changing world*, San Francisco, 2003, Jossey Bass.

Novinger T: *Intercultural communication*, Austin, 2001, University of Texas Press.

Thompson GJ: *Verbal judo: the gentle art of persuasion*, New York, 2004, HarperCollins.

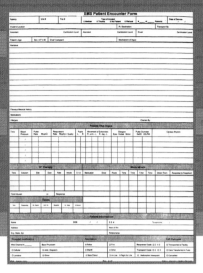

9 Documentation

CHAPTER OUTLINE

Prehospital Care Report

Principles of Documentation

Components of a Prehospital Care Report

Special Authorization Forms

Scenario

You respond to a 42-year-old woman who developed slurred speech while eating lunch in the cafeteria at her workplace. During your examination, you note drooping of the right side of her face and weakness of the right arm. She responds to your questions appropriately, but her speech is noticeably slurred. You provide basic care and transport the patient to the local stroke center. After your departure from the emergency department, the neurologist arrives and reviews your prehospital care report, looking for key information to help guide diagnosis and therapy. He discovers the following:

- The patient's signs and symptoms had started 90 minutes ago.
- The patient was alert on your arrival and became drowsy en route to the hospital.
- She had a history of high blood pressure.
- Her blood pressure was 180/100, with pulse 90 and regular.
- Physical exam revealed a left-sided weakness.
- She had no history of trauma.

After reviewing the information, the neurologist examined the patient and proceeded to order and review a computed tomography (CT) scan and began treatment for an ischemic cerebrovascular accident (stroke).

Documentation is an essential function that you will complete as an Emergency Medical Technician (EMT). The **prehospital care report (PCR)** documents all aspects of a given call and is a valuable part of a patient's record. It is also an important part of a legal record in the event of a lawsuit, which can occur years after the event. EMTs often view documentation as drudgery and a nonessential aspect of their work; however, a call report can be as useful as a well-applied splint in the care of the patient. Effective documentation includes the systematic collection of data from the dispatch phase through the transfer of the patient to the emergency department staff. Times, location, patient identifiers, assessment and treatment information, changes in condition, and other information should be carefully documented to ensure that it is readily accessible if the need arises (**Figure 9-1**).

Most importantly, the PCR is linked to patient assessment and care. A properly completed report carefully documents all findings in the scene size-up, initial (primary) assessment, focused (secondary) assessment (history and physical examination), and ongoing assessment or reassessment. Times should be as accurate as possible to reflect clearly the sequence of care and changes in the patient's condition from the time the call was received through arrival at the hospital.

Accuracy and honesty are essential when completing the PCR. When mistakes occur, they should be corrected as soon as possible using the appropriate correction methods. PCRs also document refusal of care and other legally sensitive information. Carefully documenting these events and securing the signature of a witness on the scene are critical.

As an EMT, you should take personal pride in the quality of your documentation, recognizing that it plays an essential role in the continuity of patient care, improvement of the emergency medical services (EMS) system, and the best protection against legal problems that may occur in the future.

LEARNING OBJECTIVES
- Describe the legal implications associated with the written report.
- Explain the rationale for gathering data in an EMS system.
- Explain the rationale for patient care documentation.

Prehospital Care Report

A Medical Record

The PCR has several distinct purposes. First and foremost, it is a medical record of prehospital care. It provides the physician with a history of the events that surrounded the patient's call for help. During the first critical hours of illness or injury, this information plays an important role in the decision-making process. The physician caring for the patient may review the PCR during several phases of hospital care, including actions in the emergency department (ED), operating room (OR), and intensive care unit (ICU). The mechanism of illness or injury, vital signs, chronology of signs and symptoms, and drugs or poisons found at the scene are all examples of data that may be lifesaving for a given patient. The scenario at the beginning of this chapter illustrates the importance of meticulous documentation. Many conditions exist for which the physician uses the PCR to evaluate changes in the patient's condition and formulate a working diagnosis.

A Legal Document

The PCR is a legal document and should include the following:
- Accurate times
- Status of the patient on arrival at the scene and during transport
- Emergency care provided
- Changes in condition up to arrival at the hospital
- Any unusual events that occurred during the call

The PCR is also a critical ingredient for protection from lawsuits. If a patient or family member suggests negligence on the part of the medical staff, a well-developed record is important in establishing the facts. Because most lawsuits do not occur until weeks, months, or even years after an incident, a record may provide the only means of recalling the details of a call. In addition, the document serves as evidence of the care given,

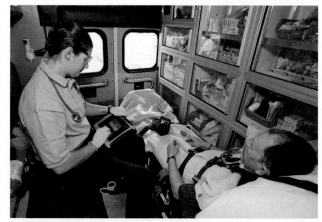

Figure 9-1 An EMT documents information about the call on an electronic prehospital care report (PCR).

which reinforces the need to document thoroughly all aspects of assessment and treatment, including pertinent objective and subjective information.

Continuous Quality Improvement

The PCR also promotes **continuous quality improvement (CQI).** These reports often are reviewed to evaluate the effectiveness of prehospital care. Audits of records rely on the validity and reliability of the documented data to evaluate properly the appropriateness of care. Many changes that occur in EMS systems are based on this type of review. Research in out-of-hospital care also depends on careful and accurate documentation. For example, to study strategies in resuscitation, when minutes can make the difference, documentation and synchronization of times are especially important to integrate dispatch, prehospital, and hospital data accurately.

The data collected on the PCR can be used at a later time for analyzing patient care to improve the local EMS system (EMSS). This may include both administrative and medical review. Typical CQI activities may include the following:

- A review of response and transport times
- Documentation of assessment and treatment
- Follow-up of patients who refused medical attention
- Other patient care issues

Some systems follow up with patients to determine their satisfaction and outcome of their care. CQI is constructive, not adversarial, and its success depends on the willful cooperation of all providers in an EMSS, especially you, the "eyes and ears" of the system in the field at the patient's side.

NEMSIS: National Quality Improvement and Research

Local data recorded on a PCR also have national CQT implications through an organization called the **National Emergency Medical Services Information System (NEMSIS).** In conjunction with national experts in EMS, NEMSIS defines what should be documented on a PCR and will ultimately serve as a national data collection center. This will allow for research that helps improve the practice of EMS. Almost all states have committed to following NEMSIS standards so that EMTs collect data in a uniform manner.

Continuing Education

Many EMS systems conduct *call review* as a primary means of continuing education (CE) for EMTs. In these sessions, EMTs are asked to present cases to a group of their peers and their physician medical director. The prehospital care is analyzed and critiqued to verify effectiveness of care and to identify areas needing improvement. This CE area is extremely valuable because it clarifies specific experiences for field personnel. The success of these sessions depends largely on the documentation clearly describing what occurred on a call.

Administrative Uses

Planning optimal distribution of ambulances, compiling annual reports, and billing are examples of how the PCR information is used. Always approach the record-keeping process in such a way so as to facilitate use of these data.

> **LEARNING OBJECTIVES**
> - Explain the rationale for patient documentation.
> - Explain the rationale for using medical terminology correctly.
> - Explain the rationale for using an accurate and synchronous clock so that information can be used in trending.

Principles of Documentation

The effectiveness of a PCR depends on the following four major factors:

1. Accuracy and honesty
2. Clarity
3. Chronology and trends
4. Completeness

Many forms used in EMS systems today are structured to facilitate adherence to these principles. Boxes that can be checked are often used to save time and allow for computer transfer of essential data. However, because no single form can account for all possible categories of information that should be recorded, narrative descriptions of the patient's status are important in almost all cases. As an EMT, you must be able to apply individual judgment in determining important entries. For example, if an unconscious patient vomits and aspirates while en route to the hospital, a clear notation of this event is essential to guide follow-up care. A check-box system cannot account for all these variables.

Accuracy and Honesty

You should make every attempt to be accurate and honest about the recorded data. An example of accuracy is recording the chief complaint in the patient's words, such as, "It feels like someone is stabbing me with a knife." EMTs who forget to record vital signs and create false values or repeat the previous values (without actually measuring vital signs a second time) are dishonest and may jeopardize the quality of patient care. Deliberate falsification can lead to revocation of your certification or license.

Although it is important to be accurate about times, diagnostic signs, treatments, and other entries, it may be impossible to be exact about certain data. For example, the time of arrival at the scene or the time of treatments must often be approximated because these times are documented during transport or after arrival at the hospital. In these cases, you should review times from dispatch through arrival at the hospital to develop the best possible approximation of data.

If an error occurs or if something is omitted, be honest and do not try to cover it up. Instead, document what happened and what steps were taken to correct the situation. Accuracy is also important for documenting unusual behavior or events. In many situations, you should describe your findings rather than make conclusions. For example, the recorded statement, "The patient was found drunk on the floor of the apartment," is too judgmental because it concludes that there was alcohol intoxication without definitive evidence. The same event could be recorded as, "The patient was found disoriented on the apartment floor with an alcohol-like smell on his breath." This statement more accurately reflects the actual observations rather than the conclusions you made at the scene.

Clarity

Ideally, a PCR is written for the reader. You should develop it clearly and legibly so that the data are easily understood. If your handwriting is not legible, print. Use black or blue ink. Any abbreviations or characters used to shorten a statement should be accurate. Be careful to spell words properly. Many words have different meanings when they are spelled incorrectly. Use abbreviations only if they are standard in your system (**Table 9-1**). When describing areas of pain or the location of wounds, you should be as exact as possible. Body diagrams are useful tools in achieving clarity. The location of wounds, fractures, and other injuries can be drawn on diagrams of the body. Some EMS systems provide diagrams on the PCR (**Figure 9-2**).

Chronology and Trends

The time relationships of response, assessment, treatment, transport, and arrival at the hospital are critical areas of documentation. They provide the physician with a history of events in the order they occurred. For example, if a patient exhibits signs of hypoxia and improves with oxygen therapy, the relationship of therapy to this improvement should be clearly noted. Conversely, if a patient's condition deteriorates, you should note the sequence of significant changes in the order they occurred. This allows you and the physician to identify progressive problems and effectiveness of therapy

more easily. Changes in the patient's condition continue to be analyzed in the hospital. By synchronizing system times, hospital staff can more accurately compare the prehospital and hospital phases of the patient's assessment, resulting in improved patient care. You can easily synchronize watches and clocks on a regular basis to ensure consistency of time documentation.

The recordings in **Figure 9-3** illustrate the importance of accurate entries. In this figure, signs consistent with internal bleeding are demonstrated. The patient's condition continued to deteriorate during transport, and emergency treatment became critical for survival. This example shows effective documentation of chronology, which is invaluable to the ED physicians in estimating the rate and severity of blood loss.

Completeness

Deciding which factors should be included in the PCR is probably the most difficult task. You should always record all assessment, treatments, and reassessment procedures in their chronological order. Include both pertinent positive findings and pertinent negative findings as you perform your focused history and physical examination (e.g., "Patient complains of severe, squeezing, left-sided chest pain but denies radiation"). Note events that affected treatment or transport. For example, record a prolonged extrication time to account for delay on the scene. If other EMS providers or first responders participated in the call, you also should document their role. Similarly, note treatment provided by laypeople, such as cardiopulmonary resuscitation (CPR) or first aid, before your arrival. Record the names and addresses of physicians, especially if definitive care such as drug therapy or defibrillation was administered at the scene. Some EMS systems request physicians providing critical

Table 9-1	Common Abbreviations and Symbols Used in Prehospital Care Documentation

Abbreviation/Symbol	Definition
♂	Male
♀	Female
ā	Before
BP	Blood pressure
c̄	With
c/o	Complaining of
CPR	Cardiopulmonary resuscitation
DOB	Date of birth
Hx	History
LLQ	Left lower quadrant (of abdomen)
LUQ	Left upper quadrant (of abdomen)
NTG	Nitroglycerin
O_2	Oxygen
PO, po	By mouth
Pt	Patient
Px	Physical examination
RLQ	Right lower quadrant (of abdomen)
RUQ	Right upper quadrant (of abdomen)
SL	Sublingual
SOB	Shortness of breath
Tx	Treatment
y/o	Years old

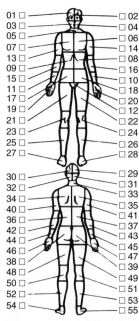

Figure 9-2 Example of a diagram on a PCR.

Patient Vital Signs															
Time	Blood pressure	Pulse rate	Rhythm	Respirations rate	Rhythm/quality	Pupils L	R	Movement of extremities R - arm - L	R - leg - L			Glasgow Eyes Verbal Motor			Pulse oximeter SaO2 O2LPM		Cardiac rhythm

Time	Blood pressure	Pulse rate	Rhythm	Resp rate	Rhythm/quality	L	R	R-arm-L	R-leg-L	Eyes	Verbal	Motor	SaO2	O2LPM	Cardiac rhythm
1427	110/70	90	Reg	20	Labored	N	N	Y Y	Y Y	4	5	6	97	12	
1432	110/70	96	Reg	24	Labored	N	N	Y Y	Y Y	4	5	6	98	12	
1437	106/70	98	Reg	24	Labored	N	N	Y Y	Y Y	4	5	6	98	12	

Figure 9-3 Vital signs trends. *Modified courtesy of HealthONE EMS, Englewood, Colo.*

treatment at a scene either to accompany the patient in the ambulance or to contact medical direction to transfer care to the EMSS.

Other unusual occurrences, such as belligerent or aggressive actions by the patient or the patient's relatives or friends, should be recorded. Avoid being judgmental or "editorializing" such events. Simply record the behavior and its implications regarding your treatment of the patient. You should also document if a family member rides in the ambulance.

Police or family members may occasionally remove valuables from the patient. You should document the person, shield number (in the case of police), and the property removed.

LEARNING OBJECTIVES
- Explain the components of a written report, and list the information to be included.
- Identify the various sections of the written report.
- Describe what information is required in each section of a written report and how it is entered.

Components of a Prehospital Care Report

Although each EMSS has its own version of a PCR, most records have common components. Formats include traditional records with check boxes and a narrative section, as well as new, computerized versions that might use an electronic clipboard or similar device. These include the following (**Figure 9-4**):
- Run data
- Patient data
- Special authorization forms

Run Data

The dispatch data (**run data**) usually consist of the call location, the date and time of the call, the crew names or numbers, the type of call, and the sequential times of response. Important times include the following:
- Time the call was received
- Time the unit responded
- Time the unit arrived on the scene
- Time the patient was reached
- Time the unit left the scene
- Time the destination was reached

- Time of transfer of care
- Time the unit returned to service

Most EMS systems use military time to document the phases of a call. Military time is a four-digit expression of time starting at 0000 (12 midnight) and running through 2359 (11:59 PM). For instance, 0700 means 7 AM, 1200 means 12 noon, and 1530 means 3:30 PM. Some forms may include route information, such as cross streets or major thoroughfares. A space may also be provided for a call identification number. When recording dispatch data, confirm the information if it is unclear, and repeat the location of a call if radio protocol permits. Most emergency communication systems strive to reduce the time spent on a given dispatch, so routine location confirmation may be inappropriate. If there is any doubt, however, confirm. If the address seems incorrect according to your knowledge of the area, note this to the dispatcher. The dispatcher frequently has a callback number to confirm questionable information while you respond to the scene. In many EMS systems, you may receive calls directly from the victim or bystander. Firmly direct the interview to ensure you receive the call location, the nature of the problem, and the callback number.

Patient Data

The **patient data** generally include the following:
- Name
- Gender
- Age
- Date of birth
- Patient's address

The patient's religion and name and telephone number of the next of kin may be included. Some systems include information about health insurance and assistance at the scene (e.g., police, physicians). Make a reasonable attempt to secure this information. Most systems discourage a search of personal property in the absence of police or in-hospital personnel. Time limitations may not allow gathering all this information at the scene or en route to the hospital if the patient is critically ill and requires constant attention. However, the PCR often becomes the primary source of basic patient data, especially if the patient becomes unconscious in the ambulance or on arrival at the hospital and has no personal identification. Contacting private physicians, locating patient records, and communicating with relatives are essential activities that may depend on your accurate collection of patient data.

Prehospital Care Report

Agency 00159	Unit # 04182	Trip # 423814	Type of incident □Medical ☒Trauma □No patient □Refusal	# _1_ of _1_ Patients	Date of service 10 / 11 / 08

Incident location Main St/Park Avenue, Plains, NY		Pt. destination Oakview	Transport by Life Star

Attendant E. Brown	Certification level EMT	Attendant	Certification level	Driver L. Smith	Certification level EMT

Patient's age 30	Sex □F ☒M	Chief complaint Chest and abdominal pain	Mechanism of injury MVC

Narrative 30 year old male involved in a front end motor vehicle collision into a tree. Law enforcement state, "30" ⊕ displacement of front axle, pt. unrestrained, deformity of steering wheel, and spidering of windshield." Pt. complains of SOB and chest/abdominal pain. Law enforcement state "pt. lost consciousness for 2 minutes." Pt. is alert on arrival of EMS. Assessment reveals contusions on the head, ① anterior chest and abdominal pain. Pt. denies pain in the pelvis or extremities. Slight ↓ in BP and ↑ in pulse during transport. Oxygen administered by nonrebreather at 12 lpm. Rapid extrication, in-line immobilization, and CISD applied. Pt. transported on spineboard.

Previous medical history None

Medications Pt. states "No medications"

Allergies NKDA   Charted by

Patient Vital Signs

Time	Blood pressure	Pulse rate	Rhythm	Respirations rate	Rhythm/quality	Pupils L	Pupils R	Movement of extremities R-arm-L	Movement of extremities R-leg-L	Glasgow Eyes	Glasgow Verbal	Glasgow Motor	Pulse oximeter SaO2	Pulse oximeter O2LPM	Cardiac rhythm
1427	110/70	90	Reg	20	Labored	N	N	Y Y	Y Y	4	5	6	97	12	
1432	110/70	96	Reg	24	Labored	N	N	Y Y	Y Y	4	5	6	98	12	
1437	106/70	98	Reg	24	Labored	N	N	Y Y	Y Y	4	5	6	98	12	

IV Therapy / Medications

Time	Solution	Site	Size	Rate	Initials	S/U	Medication	Dose	Route	Time	Time	Time	Time	Order from	Response to treatment

Total infused   cc   Response

Times

Tone	Responding	On scene	ALS on	Departed	Arr hosp	In service
1420	1420	1425		1436	1441	1501

Patient Information

Name John Doe	DOB 12 / 20 / 77	SS#	Telephone (444) 973-8672

Address 100 Main St.	Next of kin Susan Doe

City, State, Zip Plainview, NY 11987	Relationship Mother

Hospital notification	Assistance		Call outcome	
Med channel #_____	Base physician Dr. Schiavone	☒ Police □ Fire	Response code □2 ☒3	☒ Transported to facility
☒ Cellular	□ Amb dispatch	□ Sheriff □ Other	Transport code □2 ☒3	□ Care transferred in field
□ Landline	□ Other	□ State Patrol □ Air Life □ Flight for Life	□ Helicopter transport	□ Cancelled

Figure 9-4 Completed PCR. *Modified courtesy of HealthONE EMS, Englewood, Colo.*

Patient Assessment Data

During evaluation of the patient, you should attempt to record the following data:

- Critical signs and symptoms
- The chief complaint
- Vital signs
- Mental status
- Assessment of the skin

These conditions constitute the minimum dataset to be recorded for all patients (**Table 9-2**).

Making notes during critical care may not be possible. In these cases, you should make recordings during transport or at the first opportunity after arrival at the hospital.

Continuous reassessment findings of the patient should also be recorded to establish a record of improvement or deterioration of the patient's condition during transport. Some systems use a check-box format for recording assessment and treatment information. This format should not prevent you from making additional notes, when necessary, to cover contingencies not accounted for in the format. A narrative or "comments" section is often provided for this purpose. This is an area in which you may note findings from your focused (secondary) assessment (history and physical examination). Be sure to include pertinent positive and negative findings. Pertinent *positive* findings are those findings that *do* exist, such as "pale skin" or "deformed arm." Pertinent *negative* findings are expected findings that *do not* exist, such as "no sweating" or "no pain."

These assessment findings are a combination of subjective and objective findings. **Objective findings** are those that you see, such as a laceration or blue (cyanotic) lips. **Subjective findings**

Table 9-2	Minimum Dataset for Patient Assessment in Prehospital Care Report (PCR)

Data Element	Definition	Explanation or Comments
Chief complaint	Statement of problem by patient or other person	Use the patient's own words
Level of consciousness (AVPU)	*A*lert, responds to *v*erbal or *p*ainful stimuli, *u*nresponsive	In narrative, describe how the patient responds to verbal or painful stimuli
Systolic blood pressure	Patient's systolic blood pressure	If none, note 0/0
Skin perfusion	Patient's skin perfusion, expressed as normal or decreased	"Normal" is warm, pink skin "Decreased" is cool, pale, mottled, dusky skin
Skin color and temperature	Patient's skin color and temperature as seen and felt	Pink, pale, cyanotic, flushed, jaundiced, and cold or warm
Pulse rate	Patient's palpated or auscultated pulse rate expressed in number of beats per minute	The pulse rate is a component of various triage scoring systems and permits an assessment of the severity of illness.
Respiratory rate	Unassisted patient respiratory rate expressed as number of breaths per minute	If patient is not breathing and requires assisted ventilation, this data element should be coded as "000."
Time incident reported	Time when call is first received by Public Safety Answering Point or other designated entity	Provides start point of the EMS response and allows managers to assess the adequacy of EMS response, identify delays, and plan resources in a manner to provide expeditious EMS response
Time unit notified	Time when response unit is notified by EMS dispatch	Permits measurement of the actual responder response or delays; assists planning of communication resources for individual responders, and allows identification of system delays after the dispatch component of the EMS system
Time of arrival at patient	Time when response personnel establish direct contact with patient	Desirable in certain situations when there may be a significant delay between the time when a response unit arrives at the scene and the time when personnel can access patient. For example, if EMTs are prevented from approaching patient because of fire or adverse conditions, this time will be useful. Search and rescue operations will also note delays between arrival at the scene and actual patient contact.
Time unit left scene	Time when the response unit began physical motion from scene	Permits calculation of scene time by subtracting the time of arrival at scene from the time that the unit left scene
Destination/ transferred to	Healthcare facility or prehospital unit/home that received patient from EMS responder providing record	Allows reporting by destination facilities and allows linking when a patient is transferred between EMS responder agencies. "Not applicable" would be selected when there is no patient. It is anticipated that each region or state will codify its list of hospitals in an internally consistent manner, permitting reports by facility.

are those that the patient will report to you, such as difficulty breathing or chest pain.

To establish the chronology of assessment and care, also use this section to construct a summary of key assessments and treatments, including your ongoing assessments. This provides the physician with a concise account of the prehospital care.

REALWorld

When you start working clinically in EMS, you will quickly learn that it is very difficult to memorize variations in vital signs by age. However, distinguishing between normal and abnormal vital signs is critical to treatment. A "trick of the trade" is to attach a *pediatric vital sign chart* to the clipboard used to complete the PCR. Some systems provide these charts on the back of the PCR. Also, several tools (e.g., Broselow Tape) provide a system for estimating pediatric values by the size of the patient. Don't always rely on your memory; tools such as pediatric vital sign charts are invaluable. . . in the real world.

Patient Treatment Data

Every treatment given should be documented clearly in the PCR, and a time relationship should be established. If other providers intervened before your arrival, note their actions. Also note whether extraordinary factors prevented the timely application of treatment, such as difficulty in gaining access to the patient, weather conditions, or hazards to rescue personnel.

Treatment data also include the transportation method, time of transport, and notification of the hospital. Document whether the patient was taken to a trauma center or other specialty referral hospital. This information is of special importance if a closer hospital was bypassed.

Patient Disposition

The patient disposition information may include the following:
- Receiving hospital
- Special transport mode (e.g., helicopter)
- Rationale for facility selection (e.g., nearest facility, patient's choice, specialty hospital)
- Reason for not receiving a patient (e.g., refusal of medical aid)
- Final disposition of the patient at the hospital

A space may be provided for your signature and the signature of the receiving nurse or physician. Some states or regions may have special documentation requirements. Know what constitutes the minimum dataset in your region.

Table 9-3 summarizes the sections of a PCR.

EXTENDEDTransport

If transport times are long, reports can become long as well. With extended transports, the time between vital signs may lengthen. In some situations, it may be appropriate to do several small sets of documented assessments marked with time. For example, every 15 minutes, document the time, then document the reassessment of the patient, and then document changes in treatment. Multiple pages may be necessary to provide a complete and thorough report.

Table 9-3	Sections of a Prehospital Care Report
Data Items	**How Entered**
Run Data	
Identifying number	Often preprinted
Date	
Times	Military times using synchronized clocks
Service	
Unit	Unit number as assigned by EMS system
Crew	Identifying name or number as per local system
Patient Data	
Name	
Address	
Date of birth	
Age	
Gender (Sex)	Use check boxes as appropriate; fill in boxes completely, avoiding stray marks.
Nature of call	
Mechanism of injury	
Location of patient	
Treatment administered before arrival of EMT	
Chief complaint	
Signs and symptoms	
Baseline vital signs	Enter times of vital signs
SAMPLE history	Include positives and negatives (e.g., "no allergies")
Changes in condition	For every reassessment, record time and findings
Insurance information	If time and patient condition allow
Narrative Data Examination	
Focused (secondary) assessment (history and physical examination)	"Describe"; do not "conclude" Record important observations about the scene (e.g., suicide note, weapon)
State and local reporting requirements	Avoid radio code
Other patient information and data from the scene not included above	Use only standard abbreviations If sensitive information is documented (e.g., communicable information), note source of information Spell words correctly, especially medical terms; if unsure of spelling, use other words For every reassessment, record time and findings

---

LEARNING OBJECTIVES
- Define the special considerations regarding patient refusal.
- Discuss all state and/or local record-keeping and reporting requirements.

Special Authorization Forms

Treatment Refusal

Prehospital care reports often include authorization or treatment refusal forms. If a patient refuses medical aid or an aspect of care, such as oxygen therapy, you should obtain a signature of this refusal. The patient's signature should be accompanied by the signature of a witness, preferably a relative, friend, or police officer (**Figure 9-5**). You should first make every effort to convince the patient to accept treatment or transport. The refusal signature is of no value unless the patient has been clearly informed of the potential consequences of treatment refusal. One way to decide if a patient understands the consequences of refusing care is to ask the patient to state the possible consequences of refusing your care. For example, a patient who states, "I understand my chest pain may be a sign of a heart attack, and I could be at risk for sudden death if I don't let you bring me to the hospital, but I will not go," is making an informed refusal. In such cases, it is good practice to add the statement refusing treatment or transportation to the preprinted form before the patient signs it. Later, if the patient dies at home, you have good documentation that the patient was making an "informed refusal of medical attention" decision. The patient should be vigorously convinced to go to the hospital using family members and the physician at medical control, but in the end, it is the patient's decision.

Occasionally, a patient who refuses aid may also refuse to sign. This should be noted and the form signed by a witness, if possible, such as a family member, police officer, or bystander.

Ask the witness to include information such as a telephone number, address, or shield number (if a police officer) so that the witness can be identified and contacted later if needed.

Patients may also sign to select an institution that is beyond the closest receiving hospital. For example, they may have a critical illness but refuse transport anywhere but the hospital where their physician will meet them. Some systems have policies that cover these possibilities.

Case in Point

Two EMTs respond to a 58-year-old man complaining of "squeezing" chest pain. The history and physical exam are highly suggestive of a heart attack, and the patient has a very slow and irregular pulse. When the EMTs are ready to transport, the patient indicates that he does not want to go to the hospital. The EMTs explain that his condition is potentially serious and outline the possible cause of the signs and symptoms. The patient still refuses care. The EMTs then recruit the patient's daughter to convince him to go to the hospital. He still refuses. Finally, the EMTs contact the physician at medical control, who makes it clear to the patient that death is a likely outcome of his decision. Finally, the patient agrees to be transported. Shortly after his arrival in the emergency department, the patient goes into cardiac arrest but is successfully resuscitated by the physicians and nurses in attendance.

REAL*World*

Documentation of "refusal of care" is extremely important. However, strategies that convince patients to seek help result in much better outcomes. In the case cited, the patient clearly would have died if left untreated at the scene. An altruistic and understanding attitude toward these patients by the EMT is invaluable to ensure quality care. Thus the adage, "Treat every patient as if they were a family member." An unsympathetic provider may have prematurely given up on this patient and had him sign a release.

**REFUSAL OF TRANSPORT AND TREATMENT
PLEASE READ THIS DOCUMENT**

This form has been given to you because you have refused treatment or transportation to the hospital by Emergency Medical Service personnel. Your health and safety are our primary concerns. Even though you have decided not to accept our offer of treatment or transport to the hospital, please remember the following:

1. We recommend that you be evaluated and treated by a physician.

2. Your decision to refuse treatment and transport may result in delay, which may result in worsening of your condition.

3. Medical evaluation or treatment may be obtained by calling your personal physician or by going to any hospital's Emergency Department.

4. You may change your mind about transport. Please do not hesitate to contact us. We will not hesitate to return to assist you.

5. **Do not wait!** When medical treatment is needed, it is usually better to get it sooner than later.

DIAL 911
IF YOU NEED
EMERGENCY MEDICAL SERVICES

_____   _____
Attending EMS Personnel   Date/Time

_____   _____
Patient Signature   Witness Signature

Figure 9-5 "Refusal of treatment" form. *Modified courtesy of HealthONE EMS, Englewood, Colo.*

Table 9-4 lists the EMT response and documentation for patients refusing medical attention.

Special Situations and Incident Reporting

As an EMT, you must be familiar with documentation requirements for special situations and incident reporting. Because EMS systems may have different reporting forms and procedures, be sure you know what is expected in your region. Some common situations that occur everywhere include the correction of errors, exposure to infectious diseases, and on-the-job injury.

Most systems have guidelines and **special situation report** forms for certain circumstances that may arise. A special situation report may be used to document lost property, special incidents, and injury to the patient during treatment or transport, as well as to fulfill state and local reporting requirements. You should complete these reports in a timely manner to ensure proper medical or administrative follow-up. For example, communicable disease exposures should be documented and filed as soon as possible to ensure that any necessary treatment is rendered in time to make a difference. Be accurate and objective, and describe rather than conclude. Never "editorialize" about the incident, particularly when describing the behavior of

| Table 9-4 | Patient Refusal of Medical Attention: Response and Documentation |

Action	Explanation
Make an effort to persuade the patient to go to the hospital	
Ensure that the patient is able to make an informed and rational decision	The patient may be confused because of alcohol, drugs, illness, or injury. If there is doubt about the patient's competence, do not take a signature.
Inform patients why they should go to the hospital and what may happen if they do not go	To make an informed decision, the patient must know what you suspect to be the medical problem and the possible consequences of refusing treatment.
Consult medical direction as per local protocol	The physician may be able to convince the patient to go and assist you with patient disposition.
Document emergency assessment and treatment given, even if the patient still refuses	Your assessment is the basis of your decision making. Your treatment may have changed the patient's state of mind (e.g., giving glucose to a diabetic patient with hypoglycemia).
Have both the patient and a witness sign the patient refusal form	A witness would preferably be a family member or the police; if neither is present, a bystander.
If the patient refuses to sign, have a witness on the scene sign that the patient refused to sign the form	A family member or police officer would be most desirable; next would be a bystander.
Complete the PCR	Document all assessment conducted and treatment rendered. At times, the extent of the assessment or treatment allowed by the patient is limited because of refusal; if so, note this fact.
Document care that the EMT sought to provide	State that patient was offered immobilization or transport and refused.
In the narrative or comments section, document that the EMT explained to the patient the possible consequences of failure to accept care, including potential death	You may also add a statement to the refusal-of-care form before the patient and witness sign, such as: "I understand that my chest pain might be from heart disease and I could experience sudden death." Denial is common in those with many diseases, especially heart disease. Competent adult patients have a right to refuse care, but they must be fully informed of possible consequences to make a rational, informed decision.
Offer alternative methods of obtaining care	Even though the patient has signed a refusal-of-care form, you may suggest alternative methods of transportation (e.g., by family or friend) or that the patient see his or her personal physician rather than go to the emergency department.
State your willingness to return	Let the patient know that you will return and to call EMS if the condition persists or if symptoms change.

patients and bystanders. Some reports may be evidence in legal proceedings or obtained by reporters and others under "freedom of information" laws. Therefore, you should list only the facts and describe an objective and clear chronological sequence of the events. Submit the report and copies to the proper local authorities, as described in your policy and procedure manual. In certain situations, you may receive a copy for your own records.

Correction of Errors

Occasionally, you may make an error during completion of the PCR. Because the PCR is both a medical record and a legal document, correct the document in the accepted manner recommended in your EMSS. In general, if an error is discovered while the report is being written, simply draw a single line through the error, initial the error, and enter the correct information (**Figure 9-6**). Do not obliterate incorrect information; this may be confusing to the reader or interpreted as an attempt to cover up a mistake if the document is used in a legal proceeding.

Errors discovered after the report has been submitted should be corrected in a similar manner, with the date and time of correction noted. Draw a single line through the error, add the date and time of the correction, and initial the notation. If possible, use a different-colored ink (**Figure 9-7**). If information was omitted from the document, add a note with the correct information, including the date and time of the addition, and initial your entry.

Multiple-Casualty Incidents

During a disaster or a multiple-casualty incident, the time needed to treat and transport numerous patients may hamper your ability to complete the standard PCR. Because documentation remains important to the patient's care, most systems have special **triage tags** that allow for more limited, yet critical, notation about a patient's status (**Figure 9-8**). Triage tags may include basic patient-identifying data, major injuries, vital signs, triage status, treatment, and patient disposition. The triage tags are attached to the patient. These often have sections (fields) for reassessment findings, such as vital signs, to document trends or changes in the patient's condition. Even though the data you enter may be limited, make an attempt to input critical entries that may not be obvious or remembered. For example, vital

Prehospital Care Report

Agency 00159	Unit # 04182	Trip # 423814	Type of incident ☐Medical ☒Trauma ☐No patient ☐Refusal	# 1 of 1 Patients	Date of service 10 / 11 / 08

Incident location Main St/Park Avenue, Plains, NY	Pt. destination Oakview	Transport by Life Star

Attendant E. Brown	Certification level EMT	Attendant	Certification level	Driver L. Smith	Certification level EMT

Patient's age 30	Sex ☐F ☒M	Chief complaint Chest and abdominal pain	Mechanism of injury MVC

Narrative 30 year old male involved in a front end motor vehicle collision into a tree. Law enforcement state, "30" ⊕ displacement of front axle, pt. unrestrained, deformity of steering wheel, and spidering of windshield." Pt. complains of SOB and chest/abdominal pain. Law enforcement state "pt. lost consciousness for 2 minutes." Pt. is alert on arrival of EMS. Assessment reveals contusions on the head, ① anterior chest and abdominal pain. Pt. denies pain in the pelvis or extremities. Slight ↓ in BP and ↑ in pulse during transport. Oxygen administered by nonrebreather at 12 7pm. Rapid extrication, in-line immobilization, and CISD applied. Pt. transported on spineboard.

121pm pdd

Previous medical history None

Medications Pt. states "No medications"

Allergies NKDA   Charted by

Figure 9-6 Correction of errors that were discovered during charting. *Pt*, Patient; *SOB*, shortness of breath. *Modified courtesy of Health ONE EMS, Englewood, Colo.*

Prehospital Care Report

10-12-08 1300 hrs

Previous medical history Hx of hypertension and ~~angina~~ PBD Angina–hospital admission 2 yrs ago

Medications NTG, Inderal, Cardizem

Allergies Lidocaine   Charted by

Patient Vital Signs

Time	Blood pressure	Pulse rate	Rhythm	Respirations rate	Rhythm/quality	Pupils L	R	Movement of extremities R - arm - L	R - leg - L	Glasgow Eyes	Verbal	Motor	Pulse oximeter SaO2	O2LPM	Cardiac rhythm
0807	104|72	92	Reg	20	Regular								92	12	
0812	104|72	88	Reg	20	Regular								92	12	
0817	106|72	88	Reg	20	Regular								94	12	

IV Therapy / Medications

Time	Solution	Site	Size	Rate	Initials	S/U	Medication	Dose	Route	Time	Time	Time	Time	Order from	Response to treatment

Total infused   cc   Response

Times

Tone	Responding	On scene	ALS on	Departed	Arr hosp	In service
0801	0801	0806		0813	0818	0834

11-12-08 1300 hrs

Patient Information

Name Jane Brown	DOB ~~07 / 19 / 49~~ 07 / 19 / 60	SS#	Telephone (444) 786-1329

Address 417 Main Street	Next of kin Tyler Brown

City, State, Zip Plains, NY 11999	Relationship Spouse

PBD

Figure 9-7 Corrections of errors at a later time. *Modified courtesy of HealthONE EMS, Englewood, Colo.*

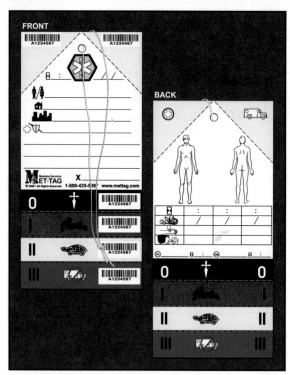

Figure 9-8 Triage tag. *Courtesy MET-TAG, Draper, Utah.*

signs can be forgotten if they are not immediately documented. Likewise, a patient may later become unconscious, and identification can be lost if not noted on the tag. Review your local multiple-casualty incident plan to become familiar with the standards for documentation in your region.

Documentation of Death

Some EMS systems permit EMTs to withhold resuscitative methods for victims of cardiac arrest if evidence of irreversible brain damage exists. For example, a patient with complete destruction of the brain or decapitation after an automobile collision may be left on the scene. Cases of obvious death must be recorded clearly. It is not sufficient to record "dead on arrival," "DOA," or other general statements. All factors that demonstrate irreversible or biological death must be noted. These include decomposition of the body, **rigor mortis** (muscle rigidity after death), or extreme **dependent lividity** (mottling of the dependent areas of the body caused by the gravitational pooling of the blood). You may also record time factors. However, time itself is never a reason to withhold resuscitation. An example of a well-documented instance of death follows:

The patient was found prone, with no pulse or respirations, with extreme dependent lividity and rigor mortis present. According to family members, the patient was last seen 2 days ago.

This documentation includes both evidence of clinical death (no pulse or breathing) and evidence of irreversible death (rigor mortis and dependent lividity).

Many individuals make end-of-life decisions and record their wishes in writing in the form of a **do not resuscitate (DNR) order.** If you discover that a patient who is in cardiac arrest has a DNR order, no attempts should be made to resuscitate the patient. In addition to documenting physical findings of death, you also must document the existence of the DNR, how the DNR was determined to belong to the patient, and if applicable, the number on the DNR.

Emotionally Disturbed, Minor, or Unconscious Patients

Whenever possible, minors should be accompanied by an adult relative or a teacher to facilitate consent for treatment, to help contact parents, and to be available to support the child until family arrives at the hospital. A family member or police officer should accompany unconscious patients if possible. They can help provide information and support at the hospital, as well as eliminate the chance of later allegations regarding missing property or improper behavior by the EMT. If circumstances prevent accompaniment, do not delay transport. In the case of the emotionally disturbed patient, the presence of a police officer is preferable, especially if the patient is acting irrationally. Most EMS systems have policies that define these issues clearly. In the case of school incidents, ask for the emergency contact data provided by parents.

Dying Statements

You may occasionally find yourself the sole witness to a dying patient's last words. These comments may have a legal or personal significance to family members and should be properly recorded. This is of particular importance in cases of suicide or trauma associated with criminal acts.

Homicide and Suicide

If you are the first person to arrive at the scene of a homicide or suicide, you must carefully document any significant findings. The position of the body, potential mechanisms of injury (e.g., empty bottle of sleeping pills), and other essential facts should be noted. Take care not to disturb the crime scene unnecessarily or move the body because this may be important in the investigation. You should report these and other criminal acts to the police at the appropriate time.

Electronic Patient Report

Technology is driving change in many ways in the field of EMS. Using electronic patient records is the most innovative aspect of documentation. Many systems are using electronic tablets and personal digital assistants (PDAs) to record the prehospital event **(Figure 9-9).** This technology has the following advantages:

- Ensures legibility because writing does not have to be deciphered by the hospital staff and others who use the PCR after the call
- Facilitates data collection for quality assurance, billing, research, and other activities
- Allows for relatively easy download of data into a personal computer (PC) for sharing with other departments
- Helps the provider navigate through the most important fields for a given call by providing sequential menus

Become familiar with the electronic patient record used by your system, to avoid inappropriate data entry or loss of critical data. As with any patient record, attention to detail is critical to quality.

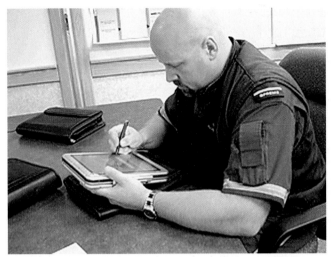

Figure 9-9 EMT completing an electronic patient care report.
Courtesy Grande Prairie Regional EMS. In Sanders M, McKenna K:
Mosby's paramedic textbook, *ed 3 revised, St Louis, 2007, Mosby-*
Elsevier.

Confidentiality

All information recorded on the PCR is confidential. Requests by bystanders or reporters should be directed to the police, physician, or administrative staff at the hospital. Certain conditions, such as communicable diseases, dog bites, and suspected child abuse, may warrant additional action, such as reporting the event to a specific agency.

Health Insurance Portability and Accountability Act

The Health Insurance Portability and Accountability Act of 1996 (HIPAA) is a set of rules to be followed by physicians, hospitals, and other U.S. healthcare providers. HIPAA helps ensure that all medical records, medical billing, and patient accounts meet certain consistent standards with regard to documentation, handling, and privacy. An important part of HIPAA regulations is the issue of privacy. Every patient is entitled to privacy. EMS providers must attend training in HIPAA regulations to ensure that the patient's privacy rights are not violated. This involves a broad spectrum of information on securing the patient's personal health information. For example, it would be inappropriate to leave a PCR in a location where it could be read by someone not directly involved in the care of the patient. Conversely, EMS

records can be used for quality assurance purposes. However, every attempt should be made to maintain privacy of the patient's name whenever it is not relevant to the review.

Scenario Follow-up

This case illustrates the compelling nature of good documentation. The treatment of ischemic stroke is "time dependent." If the symptoms had started more than 3 hours ago, some of the more aggressive treatments would not be appropriate for this patient. The physician relies on the information acquired by you as EMT at the scene to determine how long the patient experienced these symptoms. In this patient the weakness found on only one side was consistent with an ischemic stroke caused by a blood clot lodged in an artery of the brain. The patient received medication to break up the blood clot, and she was released to a rehabilitation facility for the physical therapy. One of the first documents read by the staff when the patient arrives is the prehospital care report. Clear documentation is indeed an essential part of patient care.

Summary

The prehospital care report (PCR) begins the patient's medical record and documents the first findings in the continuum of care that begins with the field treatment provided by you, the EMT. The PCR is reviewed continuously by ED physicians and nurses, physicians in the OR and ICU, and specialty physicians when patients require transfer to specialty receiving hospitals such as burn centers. The PCR is a record of what happened to the patient according to your documentation at the scene and the patient's condition and response to emergency care.

A minimum dataset for all patients notes the chief complaint, level of consciousness, vital signs, and critical times of the incident and patient encounter. When documenting findings from the focused (secondary) assessment (history and physical examination), you should include pertinent negative as well as positive findings that clearly describe which signs were present and which were not.

Documentation of special situations and incidents is done on separate forms as required by individual states or EMS systems. You should follow general guidelines in all documentation, including making timely, accurate, objective, and descriptive entries so that the events are clear to others caring for the patient.

The Bottom Line

Learning Checklist

✓ Prehospital care reports (PCRs) serve several functions, including that of patient record, legal document, continuous quality assurance and research data source, and educational and administrative data source.

✓ Sections of a PCR include run data (identification number, date, times, service, unit crew), patient data (age, gender, assessment/treatment, changes in condition, insurance information), and narrative (assessment/treatment, state/local reporting information, other patient information not previously included).

✓ Document special reporting circumstances with the appropriate regional or state form provided by your EMSS.

✓ Document death by recording physical findings such as decomposition, extreme dependent lividity, rigor mortis, or obvious lethal injuries (e.g., decapitation).

✓ Make corrections to errors on a PCR according to local practices. General rules for correcting errors include crossing out the error, providing corrected data, and initialing next to the correction. Errors that are recorded at a later time should also include the date.

✓ Carefully document patient refusal of care, including the signature of the patient and a witness at the scene.

✓ Document special circumstances or unusual events on the PCR.

✓ Triage tags and other time-saving methods may be used to document assessment and care in multiple-casualty incidents.

✓ Electronic reporting options increase legibility and facilitate data collection.

✓ The Health Insurance Portability and Accountability Act (HIPAA) is a set of rules that include protection of the patient's privacy.

Key Terms

Continuous quality improvement (CQI) Working toward the goal of optimal excellence in the services rendered to every patient; includes review of the PCR.

Dependent lividity Discoloration of body tissues in the lower or dependent areas of the body, caused by the collection of coagulated blood.

Do not resuscitate (DNR) order The end-of-life wishes recorded in writing by the patient before death, to stop any resuscitation attempts in case of cardiac arrest.

National Emergency Medical Services Information System (NEMSIS) National organization that defines what to document in prehospital care reports, setting standards with EMS experts, and ultimately to serve as data collection center to promote research.

Objective findings Physical signs that can be visualized by the EMT (e.g., pale skin, deformed extremity).

Patient data Identification information provided by the patient or by family or friends; includes the patient's name, gender, age, date of birth, and address.

Prehospital care report (PCR) The standardized patient record used in the EMS system.

Rigor mortis State of body stiffness caused by the depletion of proteins in muscles after death.

Run data The part of the documentation that records the location, type of call, and times related to the response.

Special situation report Special report used to document unusual occurrences, such as an injury to the patient during transport.

Subjective findings Symptoms reported by the patient but not seen by the EMT (e.g., headache).

Triage tag Special tag with more limited but critical information on a patient's status, attached to the patient in multiple-casualty incidents.

Review Questions

1. What are the national regulations that include rules pertaining to privacy called?
   a. NHTSA
   b. HIPAA
   c. NAEMT
   d. NAEMSP

2. Which of the following is a major advantage of an electronic patient record?
   a. Ease of data collection for CQI
   b. Accuracy of data entry
   c. Weight of record
   d. Confidentiality

3. You should confirm the correction of an error on a PCR by:
   a. Writing an explanation
   b. Initialing the new entry
   c. Making a completely new PCR
   d. Drawing an arrow

4. If an error is corrected at a later time on the PCR, you should:
   a. Write change in capital letters
   b. Date and time the correction
   c. Have a supervisor sign the form
   d. Rewrite the entire record

5. In a multiple-casualty incident, appropriate documentation usually includes:
   a. Completion of the standard PCR
   b. No documentation is necessary
   c. Major injuries and vital signs and field treatment
   d. Check box only on PCR

6. Which of the following is an important use of a PCR?
   a. Quality improvement
   b. Documentation of relatives' history
   c. Inventory management
   d. Documentation of equipment repair

7. An EMT failed to record the application of a splint to a swollen and deformed extremity. A year later he receives a notice of intent to sue. In all probability, this documentation omission:
   a. Is insignificant in subsequent legal investigations
   b. May be a basis for assuming that a splint was not applied
   c. Can be corrected by completing a new PCR
   d. Can be easily resolved by the EMT's recall 1 year later

8. Patient refusal of emergency medical care:
   a. Is an infrequent problem in EMS
   b. Should be documented by a witness whenever possible
   c. Is a patient's right, even if the patient is confused
   d. Should never be honored, even for competent adults

9. Insurance companies will reimburse ambulance companies based on the type and severity of patient injury or illness. This determination is made based on the report written by the EMT. How could incomplete documentation by the EMT affect reimbursement?
   a. Decreased reimbursement rates
   b. Overpayment for services
   c. No effect
   d. The EMT will be given the opportunity to redo the report.

For Further Review

In the Student Workbook

- Multiple-choice questions
- Fill-in-the-blank questions
- Case scenario questions
- Crossword puzzle

On Evolve

- Weblinks
- Lecture notes
- Exercises

Learning Objectives

Cognitive Objectives

- Describe the legal implications associated with the written report.
- Explain the components of the written report, and list the information to include.
- Identify the various sections of the written report.
- Describe what information is required in each section of a written report and how to enter it.
- Define the special considerations concerning patient refusal.
- Discuss all state and/or local record-keeping and reporting requirements.

Affective Objectives

- Explain the rationale for patient care documentation.
- Explain the rationale for gathering data in an EMS system.
- Explain the rationale for using medical terminology correctly.
- Explain the rationale for using an accurate and synchronous clock so that information can be used in trending.

Psychomotor Objectives

- Complete a PCR.

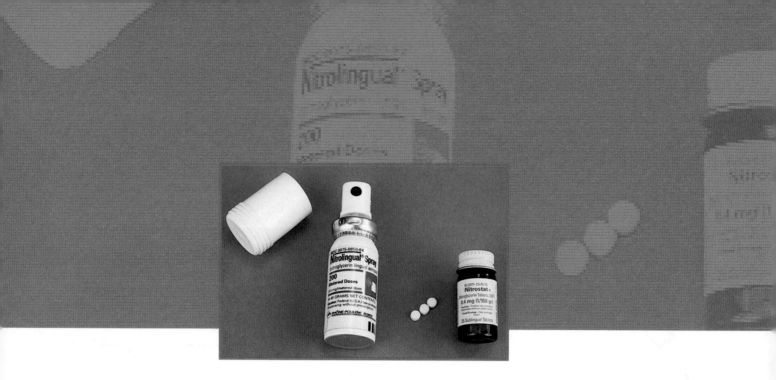

10 General Pharmacology

CHAPTER OUTLINE

Medications and the EMT

Assisting with a Prescribed Medication

Reassessment Strategies

Geriatric Considerations

Scenario

A 19-year-old woman with a history of food allergies has a tingling in her throat and shortness of breath after eating take-out food from a new restaurant. She sends her friend down the hall to pick up her medication for anaphylaxis. You arrive to find the patient near collapse by the table with severe respiratory distress, stridor, and hypotension. Her friend returns and advises you that the patient has a history of allergy to peanuts and almost died 2 years ago from a severe reaction. The friend hands you an autoinjector syringe of epinephrine, prescribed by the patient's allergist, which the friend has just retrieved from the patient's medicine cabinet. The patient is weak, struggling to breathe, and incapable of administering the drug herself. You immediately apply high-flow oxygen via nonrebreather mask and contact medical direction. You advise the physician of the patient's findings and that prescribed medication for her condition is available at the scene and has not expired. The physician orders you to assist the patient with an intramuscular injection of epinephrine. You inject the medication, initiate transport, and reassess the patient en route. After a few minutes, the patient's blood pressure begins to rise, and her breathing is less labored.

Pharmacology is the science that deals with the origin, nature, chemistry, effects, and uses of drugs. A **medication,** or **drug,** is any chemical compound that may be administered to a patient as an aid in the assessment, treatment, or prevention of disease or other abnormal condition. It may be used to relieve, control, or improve an abnormal condition. An emergency medical technician (EMT) carries certain medications on the ambulance, notably oxygen, **oral glucose,** aspirin, **activated charcoal,** and in some regions, injectable nerve agent antidotes. In addition, EMTs are trained to assist patients with the administration of certain common medications used to treat emergency conditions; these include **nitroglycerin, metered-dose inhalers** (bronchodilators), and **epinephrine.** To administer medications, an EMT should have a basic understanding of some principles of pharmacology, including actions of the drug, indications, contraindications, forms of medication, doses or quantities of drugs to be given, side effects, and how to monitor effectiveness.

REAL*World*

"Medication" has two meanings that are often used interchangeably. *Medication* is defined both as a medicine, drug, or remedy (noun) and as the act or process of "medicating" (verb), in which the drug or remedy is introduced into or applied to the body.

LEARNING OBJECTIVES

- Identify which medications will be carried on the unit.
- State the medications carried on the unit by the generic name.
- Identify medications that the EMT may assist the patient in administering.
- State by generic name the medications that the EMT can assist the patient in administering.
- Discuss the forms in which medications can be found.

Medications and the EMT

As an emergency care provider, an EMT administers some drugs to patients in the course of treating emergency conditions. The EMT typically carries the following medications on the EMS vehicle:

- Oxygen
- Aspirin (**Figure 10-1**)
- Oral glucose (**Figure 10-2**)
- Activated charcoal (**Figure 10-3**)

The EMT may also assist with the administration of three other medications that patients have in their possession that were prescribed for specific conditions requiring emergency care, as follows:

- Prescribed metered-dose inhaler (MDI) (**Figure 10-4**)
- Nitroglycerin (**Figure 10-5**)
- Epinephrine for injection (**Figure 10-6**)

In some EMS systems, medical direction may call for EMTs to carry epinephrine, nitroglycerin, or medications that can be inhaled for bronchodilation on their vehicles if a patient needs a drug and does not have personal medication readily available. For example, patients with anaphylaxis have had attacks and died because they did not have epinephrine available. In some states, legislation requires that EMTs and others, such as camp counselors, be trained and equipped to administer epinephrine for these severe allergic conditions. Similarly, medical direction might mandate stocking of ambulances with nitroglycerin and

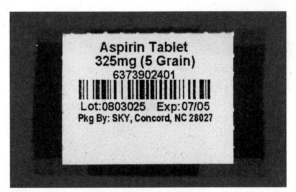

Figure 10-1 Aspirin. *From Guy J: Pharmacology for the prehospital professional, St Louis, 2009, Mosby-Elsevier.*

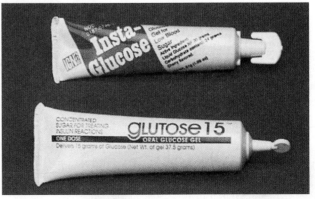

Figure 10-2 Oral glucose gel.

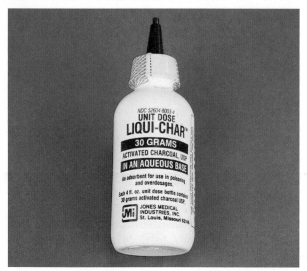

Figure 10-3 Activated charcoal.

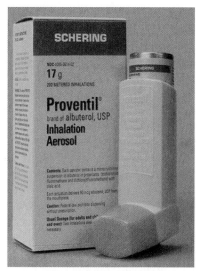

Figure 10-4 Metered-dose inhaler. *From McSwain N, Paturas J: The Basic EMT: comprehensive prehospital patient care, ed 2, St Louis, 2003, Mosby.*

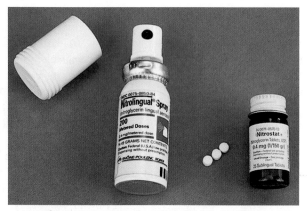

Figure 10-5 Nitroglycerin spray and tablets.

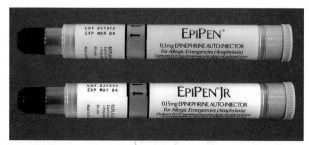

Figure 10-6 Premeasured doses of epinephrine for injection are packaged in the EpiPen and EpiPen Jr.

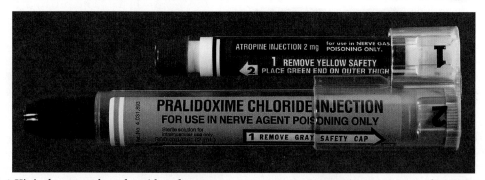

Figure 10-7 Mark 1 Kit is the prepackaged antidote for nerve agent exposure. It contains premeasured atropine and pralidoxime.

aspirin for patients with chest pain and inhaled medications for patients with asthma attacks. In some regions, EMTs may carry nerve agent antidotes on the ambulance (**Figure 10-7**).

Medication Names

Medications may have both a **generic name** and a **trade name.** The generic name is a simple form of the chemical name of the drug and may be listed in the *U.S. Pharmacopeia*, which is a government publication listing all drugs available in the United States. For example, epinephrine and nitroglycerin are

two generic names. The trade name is the brand name a manufacturer uses in marketing the drug. Although healthcare providers often use the generic name because they are referring to the medical properties of a drug, patients are often more familiar with the brand name because it is prominently displayed on the packaging of their medicine and promoted by the manufacturer to medical and laypersons. The EMT should become familiar with both the generic and the trade name of some common drugs that may be administered in prehospital care (**Table 10-1**).

| Table 10-1 | EMT Prehospital Medications | | |

Generic Name	Trade Names	Form	Prehospital Use
Oxygen		Gas	Low-oxygen states, shortness of breath, shock, chest pain, and other serious emergencies
Glucose, oral	Glutose Insta-Glucose	Gel	Altered mental status (suspected low blood sugar)
Activated charcoal	SuperChar InstaChar Actidose-Aqua Liqui-Char	Suspension	Suspected toxic ingestion

Prescribed inhalers
  Albuterol
  Metaproterenol
  Isoetharine
  Terbutaline
	
	Proventil, Ventolin
	Alupent, Metaprel
	Bronkosol, Bronkometer
	Brethaire
		Fixed-dose liquid: vaporized nebulizers or hand-held metered-dose inhalers
		Fine powder for inhalation
			Respiratory emergency for which patient has prescribed inhaler (e.g., asthma, chronic obstructive pulmonary disease)

Nitroglycerin	Nitrostat tablets Nitrolingual Spray	Compressed powders or tablets Sublingual spray	Chest pain in patients with known heart disease
Epinephrine	EpiPen, EpiPen Jr.	Liquid for injection	Anaphylaxis (severe allergic reaction)
Epinephrine hydrochloride	Adrenaline		
Aspirin	Bufferin, Bayer	Tablets	Suspected acute coronary syndromes
Atropine and pralidoxime	Mark 1	Liquid for injection	Nerve agent toxicity/antidote

Indications and Contraindications

The **indications** for use of a drug are the most common conditions in which the action of the drug is expected to benefit the patient. For example, a drug that dilates the bronchioles might be indicated for asthma, a condition in which bronchial constriction causes increased work of breathing.

Contraindications are conditions or situations in which a drug should not be used because it may cause harm to the patient. For example, the action or effect of nitroglycerin is dilation of the blood vessels. Because dilating the blood vessels can also decrease in blood pressure, nitroglycerin is contraindicated in a patient who has profound hypotension.

Case in Point

An EMT is evaluating a patient with a history of a myocardial infarction who is currently experiencing chest pain. It becomes apparent that the patient's chest pain is being caused by angina. The EMT has protocols to help the patient take his nitroglycerin. Nitroglycerin is indicated to help relieve pain caused by angina. After obtaining the patient's vital signs, the EMT discovers that his blood pressure is too low for the patient to receive nitroglycerin safely. In this case, nitroglycerin is contraindicated.

Medication Forms

Medications come in different forms, such as gas, liquid, and solid. Oxygen is a gas. Epinephrine for injection is a liquid. Drugs such as nitroglycerin may be in the form of a compressed powder (tablet) or as a spray or **aerosol** (a suspension of ultramicroscopic solid or liquid particles in air or gas) that is administered as a fine mist. Aerosol is the form used to deliver medications to the lungs. You should always look at the medication container and follow the instructions. For example, the instructions may advise you to shake the container before releasing the aerosol to make sure the medication is evenly dispersed. Activated charcoal is often packaged as a **suspension** of solid particles mixed in a liquid that must be shaken before the patient drinks it because the activated charcoal tends to settle to the bottom of the container. Oral glucose might be packaged as a **gel**, a viscous substance that is jellylike in consistency.

Dose

The **dose** is the quantity of a drug to be administered at one time. The dose, or the specified amount of medication, is usually expressed in the metric system. For example, the EMT delivers oxygen through a nonrebreather mask at a flow rate of 15 L/min so that the oxygen reservoir bag does not collapse when the patient inhales.

The metric terms for drugs used by the EMT are generally in grams or milligrams of weight. One gram (g) is equal to 1000 milligrams (mg). The EMT might administer 15 g of oral glucose to a patient to raise the patient's blood sugar. Nitroglycerin tablets or spray is usually given as a dose of 0.4 mg. Drugs administered as a liquid are typically administered in a measured weight such as grams (g), milligrams (mg), or micrograms (mcg) dissolved in a measured volume or capacity of fluid expressed in liters (L) or milliliters (mL); 1 L is equal to 1000 mL. When using an epinephrine autoinjector (EpiPen), for example, a premeasured dose of 0.3 mg of epinephrine is contained in 2 mL of total volume for injection into the muscle. See **Table 10-2** for further review of metric measures of weight and volume.

Table 10-2	Metric Weight Conversions		
Kilograms	**Grams**	**Milligrams**	**Micrograms**
1 kg	1000 g		
	1 g	1000 mg	
		1 mg	1000 mcg

Liters	**Milliliters**
1 L	1000 mL
0.5 L	500 mL
0.1 L	100 mL
0.01 L	10 mL
0.001 L	1 mL

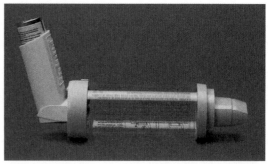

Figure 10-8 A child who is administered a bronchodilator from a metered-dose inhaler may benefit from inhaling the medication through a spacer, or extended tube, attached to the inhaler.

Drugs are administered as a **therapeutic dose,** or the amount necessary to provide the desired effect yet low enough to minimize side effects or toxic effects from too much of the drug. It is essential to administer the appropriate quantity of the drug carefully to avoid administering an overdose to the patient.

Most medications that the EMT administers (other than oxygen) are prepared in single-unit doses so they do not have to be measured by the EMT. For example, an MDI can deliver a *premeasured* or metered dose with each spray of the inhaler. The correct drug dose for the patient might be 2 puffs of the inhaler.

Predetermined measures of a drug dose minimize errors, but the EMT must still check the drug name and dose to confirm it is right for the patient according to local protocols and medical direction. The EMT may be asked to read to medical direction the name and dose of a patient's prescribed medication and therefore should be familiar with basic terms of weights and volumes in the metric system. The expiration date of a medication is also found on the label. Checking to make sure a medication has not expired is important because a drug can lose its potency and intended effect when it is used after the expiration date. Practice reading the labels shown in the accompanying figures and on medications used in your system to ensure you are comfortable with drug names, metric terms, and forms of medications.

REAL*World*

Children have less body mass than adults, and drug doses may need to be adjusted accordingly. It is important to know the child's weight. Often a dose is calculated as milligrams of drug per kilogram of body weight (mg/kg); there are 2.2 pounds in 1 kg.

Children may also have some difficulty in coordinating inhalation of a metered-dose inhaler. *Spacers,* or extension tubing, between the aerosol and the mouth are often used to ensure delivery of the medication when patients are just being introduced to MDIs or have difficulty coordinating delivery with inhalation (**Figure 10-8**). Adults also may use spacers.

Children may also be reluctant to take a medication, so gaining their cooperation and trust early is important. Be honest with them. Obtain the support of the child's parents. With medications such as activated charcoal, flavorings are sometimes added to make the slurry more palatable to children.

LEARNING OBJECTIVE
• Explain the rationale for the administration of medications.

Administration

Routes of drug administration used by the EMT include the following:
• Oral
• Sublingual
• Inhaled
• Injected

Oral

Oral administration requires swallowing by the patient, with the medication absorbed through the gastrointestinal tract into the blood. Glucose gel is given orally in prehospital care. Activated charcoal is also swallowed; its role is to bind other drugs or poisons that may have been swallowed, as in an overdose. This limits the absorption of the drug or poison from the stomach into the blood.

Sublingual

Sublingual administration (under the tongue) is used for nitroglycerin tablets or spray, where small particles of the drug can dissolve in the saliva and can be rapidly absorbed into the blood vessels in the mucous membranes. Nitroglycerin tablets are composed of compressed powder that dissolves when placed under the tongue. Nitroglycerin in spray form is a mist of small particles in a gas and can be administered under or directly onto the tongue.

Case in Point

You respond to a 48-year-old man with crushing substernal chest pain lasting 20 minutes and radiating to the left arm. You suspect acute coronary syndromes (ACS) and call medical control. You are instructed to give the patient 160 mg of aspirin and ask him to chew the tablet before he swallows. On arrival in the emergency department, the patient is rushed to the catheterization laboratory, where he undergoes angioplasty and has reperfusion through the blocked coronary artery.

Aspirin is given early in the treatment of ACS because it can decrease the risk of total coronary artery obstruction and increase the chance of survival.

Inhaled

Drugs administered in MDIs are intended to be inhaled into the lungs, where they are absorbed into the blood vessels, and also have local effects. For example, inhalation of bronchodilators causes the drug to be delivered directly to the intended site of action, the lower airways.

Injected

Some drugs are injected into the body. Epinephrine may be injected into the subcutaneous tissue just under the skin, into the muscle, or into a vein. EMTs usually use the **intramuscular (IM)** approach.

Other Routes

Other routes of drug administration an EMT will encounter include transcutaneous or transdermal, rectal, and intraosseous. *Transcutaneous*, or transdermal, means "through the skin" and is a common means of administering drugs such as nitroglycerin in a slow and sustained manner. Patients may wear a "patch" of nitroglycerin on their skin so that they can receive continuous absorption of the drug. Rectal administration of medication, often by suppository, is used when patients may be vomiting or for infants and young children. *Intraosseous*, or "through the bone," is another method of administering fluids and medications in emergency situations when it is difficult to establish an intravenous line; instead a metal needle is inserted through bone into the marrow.

Depending on the route of administration, the dose and the concentration of a medication required to achieve the desired therapeutic effect may vary. Thus, understanding *dose, form,* and *route* is important to ensure effective drug delivery.

Intravenous Lines

Emergency medical technicians usually are not responsible for establishing intravenous (IV) lines. In some EMS systems, EMTs may be responsible for transporting patients from one facility to another with an IV line in place. The EMT must be familiar with the basic principles of IV therapy and how to troubleshoot if a problem with the IV line develops during transport.

Purpose

Intravenous lines are established for a variety of reasons. IV lines are used to help maintain blood pressure by administering fluid into the vascular space. They are also used to administer drugs and to draw blood samples. An IV line is a sterile plastic catheter placed into a peripheral vein. The hub of the catheter is connected to the IV tubing, which is attached to the IV bag. The fluid contained in the IV bag is most often a dilute saltwater solution known as *normal saline* (NS). In some cases a dilute dextrose (sugar) solution may be used. **Table 10-3** lists the various components of a typical IV set. **Figure 10-9** illustrates the usual placement of an IV line.

Flow Rates

The rate of flow through the IV line can be adjusted based on the patient's needs. IV flow rates are measured in milliliters per hour (mL/hr) and can be adjusted using the sliding clamp on the IV tubing (**Figure 10-10**). Patients requiring large amounts of fluid will have their IV line set as "wide open" (WO). More often the IV line will be set at a slow rate designed to keep the catheter from clotting, referred to as "to keep open" (TKO) or "keep vein open" (KVO). **Box 10-1** illustrates the formula used to convert drops per minute (drops/min) to mL/hr delivered to the patient.

Complications

When the catheter pulls out or punctures the back wall of the vein, the fluid runs into the tissue rather than into the vascular space. This is known as *infiltration*. A blood clot, sheared piece of catheter, or air may travel from the IV site into the vascular space and lodge in the lungs, causing a pulmonary embolus. If the flow rate is not monitored appropriately, the patient may

---

Table 10-3	Components of an Intravenous (IV) Administration System

Component	Purpose	Comments
IV catheter or needle	Inserted directly into vein to administer medications or fluid to draw a blood sample.	Needles are used only occasionally as the primary access to the vein when insertion of a catheter is not possible. IV catheters are inserted with the use of a needle that is removed after placement of the device.
IV administration set	Set consisting of IV tubing, drip reservoir to measure flow, and connector that inserts into IV fluid bag. Along the tubing is a flow regulator, used to adjust rate of IV fluid administration, and one or two medication ports where medications can be injected or additional IV lines connected.	
Extension set	An additional length of IV tubing is often added to end of administration set to allow for easy replacement of administration set when needed.	
IV fluid	A variety of IV fluids are administered to the patient based on purpose of IV line. Common fluids include 5% dextrose and water (D_5W), normal saline (NS), and Ringer's lactate (RL) solution.	Dextrose or saline is generally used when the IV line is being used strictly for medication administration. Saline and RL are typically used for blood volume expansion caused by dehydration or bleeding. Many other types of fluids are available, depending on the patient's needs.

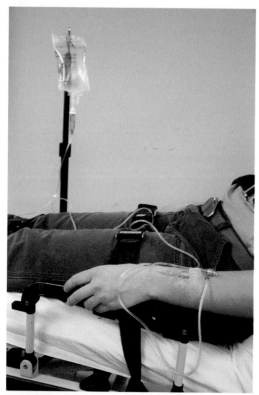

Figure 10-9 Typical IV line placement.

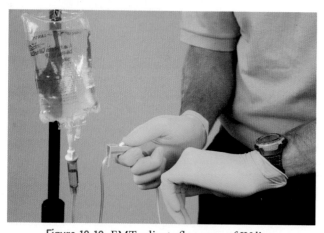

Figure 10-10 EMT adjusts flow rate of IV line.

receive too much fluid, resulting in fluid overload. In some cases the IV line may stop running. **Box 10-2** outlines general problem-solving steps.

Actions, Side Effects, and Drug Interactions

The *action* of a drug is the desired change or effect it has on the body or the target organ. The effect or action of supplemental oxygen is to increase the amount of oxygen in the blood and correct hypoxia (low oxygen state). The effect or action of oral glucose is to increase the glucose level in the blood.

Few drugs have only one effect on the body. Most drugs have side effects or other effects on the body in addition to the desired actions. These side effects may be undesirable or even detrimental. A drug that has the most beneficial action for the condition requiring treatment and the fewest side effects would

---

| **Box 10-1** | Calculating Drip Rate for an Intravenous Line |

Intravenous (IV) infusion sets vary in the volume delivered in relation to the number of drops per minute. Some administration sets deliver 1 mL for every 60 drops (microdrip) of fluid in the chamber. Other administration sets deliver 1 mL for every 10 drops (macrodrip) of fluid in the chamber. To apply the following equation, you must first know the type of administration set attached to the patient:

$$\text{Drops/minute} = \frac{\text{Volume to be infused} \times \text{Drops/mL (administration set)}}{60 \text{ (minutes)}}$$

Sample using a 10-drop/mL set when the physician orders 100 mL/hour of fluid:

$$\text{Drops/minute} = \frac{100 \text{ mL (per hour)} \times 10 \text{ Drops/mL}}{60 \text{ (minutes)}}$$

$$= 17 \text{ Drops/minute (rounded off)}$$

Sample using a 60-drop/mL set when the physician orders 100 mL/hour of fluid:

$$\text{Drops/minute} = \frac{100 \text{ mL (per hour)} \times 60 \text{ Drops/mL}}{60 \text{ (minutes)}}$$

$$= 100 \text{ Drops/minute}$$

NOTE: Patients who have an IV line in place for the purpose of fluid administration usually are regulated with a macrodrip.

| **Box 10-2** | General Problem-Solving Steps for IV Line Complications |

1. Note the position of the IV bag. If it is lower than the heart, it must be elevated to initiate flow using gravity.
2. Make sure that the flow regulator is in the open position and that there are no kinks in the IV tubing.
3. Make sure that the IV catheter is not kinked as a result of the position of the catheter in the patient's vein. For example, a catheter that is inserted at or near a joint may become obstructed when the elbow or wrist is flexed. If this is suspected, straighten the joint and observe for flow. An arm board can be placed at the joint to maintain it in the straightened position to prevent further obstruction.
4. If no flow is noted, lower the bag below the patient's heart and observe for blood return in the IV line. If no return is noted, check for signs of infiltration or clotted blood in the IV line.
5. If none of these maneuvers can clear the IV line, consult medical direction for guidance.

---

be the "drug of choice." At times, drugs are used despite significant side effects because the benefit of the drug outweighs the potential risks.

Knowledge of both the actions and the side effects of drugs administered in prehospital care is important so that you are aware of what to look for during ongoing assessment or reassessment. You will learn more about each drug in upcoming chapters. **Table 10-4** reviews the terms used in general pharmacology.

One drug might interact with another in an unwanted manner. For example, if nitroglycerin is given to a man taking

Table 10-4	Terms Used in General Pharmacology

Term	Definition
Generic name	Name of medication listed in *U.S. Pharmacopeia,* a government publication listing all drugs used in the United States
Trade name	Brand name; name a manufacturer uses in marketing the drug, often designated by the trademark symbol
Indication	Conditions for which a drug is considered effective
Contraindication	A situation in which a drug should not be used because its use may cause harm
Form	Physical property of drug as used for patient administration (gas, vapor, aerosol, liquid, powder, suspension, tablet)
Dose	Amount of drug delivered to a patient at one time
Route of administration	How a drug is introduced into the body: oral ingestion, sublingual (under the tongue), injection (e.g., intramuscular), inhalation, etc.
Action	Desired effect a drug has on a patient, body systems, or both
Side effects	Effects of a drug other than those for which the drug is used

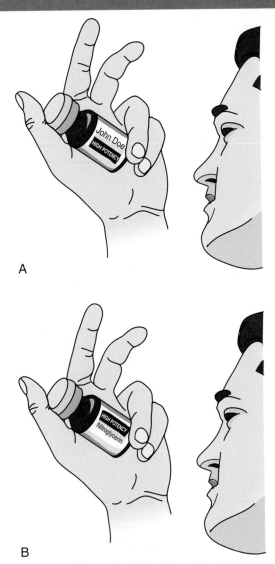

A

B

Figure 10-11 **A,** Make sure it is the *right patient* by looking at the label on the medication to verify it is for the patient you are treating. **B,** Check the name of the drug to be sure it is the *right drug* for the condition requiring treatment.

sildenafil (Viagra), unwanted hypotension from a **drug interaction** may result.

Assisting with a Prescribed Medication

General principles of assisting a patient with medication administration that promote patient safety are often remembered by following the "five rights": *right* patient, *right* drug, *right* dose, *right* route of administration, and *right* time. Although straightforward, take the time to review these five rights, which you will use to prevent mistakes in drug delivery (**Figure 10-11** and **Box 10-3).**

Check that the five rights are consistent with your local protocols, either online with medical direction or by your "standing orders."

Reassessment Strategies

A drug is administered to treat a condition. After drug delivery, the EMT will reassess the patient to check for anticipated effects and side effects of the drug and for a noticeable change in the condition for which the drug was administered. For example, if oxygen is given to a patient with altered mental status, rapid heartbeat, and cyanosis, during the ongoing assessment you would look for such changes as an improvement in mental status and a return of the heartbeat and skin color toward normal. As you become familiar with the other drugs you will administer, you will check for signs of their actions and side effects in your ongoing assessment or reassessment.

Document the time of drug administration, then document the times of your ongoing assessments, including vital signs, change in the condition for which the drugs were administered, and any anticipated effects or side effects from drug administration (see Table10-1).

Geriatric Considerations

Elderly patients tend to use multiple medications and may have more than one illness. They may have several medications and may not be sure why they are taking each one. The more medications they take, the more prone they are to adverse effects, drug interactions, and inadvertent overdose. Often the medications provide clues to the patient's chronic illness and current problems. Whenever possible, *transport the patient's medications to the hospital* to help hospital staff diagnose the condition and manage the patient's condition.

| Box 10-3 | "Five Rights" of Medication Administration |

1. Make sure this is the **right patient** by looking at the label on the medication to verify it is for the patient you are treating. If there is no label, verify with the patient that it is his or her medication. This is also a good time to check that the medication has not expired.
2. Check the name of the drug to be sure it is the **right drug** for the condition requiring treatment. For example, a patient with chronic obstructive pulmonary disease may have different medications in the form of metered-dose inhalers (MDIs). Also, check the form of the medication, and follow the instructions on the label. For example, if the form is a suspension, the directions might state to shake the container to disperse the medication uniformly within the container. With some MDIs and sprays, the directions might state to release "test sprays" into the air before administering a dose to a patient, particularly if the device has never been used or has not been used for some time.
3. Check the dose of the drug to be sure it is the **right dose** for the patient. For example, in some states, EMTs may carry epinephrine on the ambulance. For autoinjectors that deliver a premeasured dose of epinephrine, the dose in the adult EpiPen is twice the dose in the child-size EpiPen Jr.
4. Check to make sure the **right route of administration** is used for drug delivery. For example, nitroglycerin tablets are intended to be absorbed through the vessels in the mucous membranes under the tongue. If a patient swallowed the tablet, the absorption of this medication would be different than if it is allowed to dissolve under the tongue. You may encounter a patient who was prescribed sublingual nitroglycerin who has never actually taken it. You can assist by instructing this patient to leave the tablet under the tongue until it is fully dissolved and not to swallow it.
5. Drugs that can be repeated can only be delivered at set intervals; ensure it is the **right time** to administer the drug. After the administration of a drug, the EMT should note the time and then monitor the patient for changes. After the prescribed time for redosing, the EMT may readminister the drug as directed by the physician.

Scenario Follow-up

The young woman improved after administration of injectable epinephrine for her allergic reaction. Because she was at a restaurant in the mountains, however, the EMTs had a long transport time to the nearest hospital. Twenty minutes after her first medication, she began to wheeze, and her blood pressure fell. Epinephrine acts quickly, but it has a relatively short duration of action. The EMTs called medical control, who directed a repeat dose of epinephrine. Fortunately, these rural-based EMTs were prepared for long transports and had a second dose available. After administration of the epinephrine, the patient's breathing difficulty eased, and her blood pressure returned to normal. For a short time, she also had a rapid heart rate, a side effect of the epinephrine.

Summary

As an EMT, you may administer drugs or medications, including oxygen, activated charcoal, oral glucose, prescribed inhalers, epinephrine, nitroglycerin, aspirin, and nerve agent antidotes. You will carry some medications on the ambulance. Other medications may be prescribed by a physician and carried by the patient, who may need your assistance in administration because of the illness. Oxygen is administered early in the course of care according to assessment findings and "standing orders." Other medications are given according to local medical direction policy, either through standing orders or by direct online physician order. The EMT who administers drugs has the responsibility for knowing some basic information, including the indications, contraindications, dose, route of administration, effects, and side effects regarding the drug to be administered. In later chapters, you will learn necessary facts about each of the drugs that EMTs may administer in prehospital care.

The Bottom Line

Learning Checklist

✓ Activated charcoal, oral glucose, aspirin, and oxygen are among the drugs carried by an EMT unit, according to local emergency medical system protocols.

✓ Prescribed medications that a patient may carry and that the EMT may assist in administering include a prescribed inhaler, epinephrine, and nitroglycerin.

✓ Medication forms that an EMT may administer include compressed powders or tablets, liquids for injection, gels, suspensions, and fine powders or mists for inhalation.

✓ EMTs should be familiar with the indications (when to use a drug to treat a specific illness) and the contraindications (when a drug should be not used) of the drugs that they may administer or assist in administering.

✓ EMTs should be familiar with the dose, route, actions, and side effects of the drugs that they may administer or assist in administering.

✓ EMTs should be familiar with the "five rights" of drug administration: right patient, right drug, right dose, right route of administration, and right time.

✓ Children may need extra help with medication administration

Key Terms

Activated charcoal Residue of the distillation of organic materials (charcoal) that has been treated to increase its absorptive properties; used often to absorb ingested drugs and poisons.

Aerosol Medicinal particles suspended in a gas or in air.

Contraindication Any condition that renders a particular line of treatment improper or undesirable.

Dose Quantity of a substance to be administered at one time, as in a specified amount of medication.

Drug Any medicinal substance.

Drug Interaction Any effect seen when two or more drugs are administered or taken by a patient at the same time. Effects can be harmful.

Epinephrine Hormone secreted by the adrenal glands that increases sympathetic activity (e.g., heart rate and force of contraction of the heart, bronchodilation, and other effects); also called *adrenaline*.

Gel Gelatinous substance that is firm in consistency but contains much liquid.

Generic name Drug name not protected by a trademark that is usually descriptive of the chemical nature of the drug.

Indication Condition or disease for which a drug is expected to have a beneficial effect.

Intramuscular (IM) Within the muscular substance; route of drug administration.

Medication Drug or remedy for a certain condition.

Metered-dose inhaler (MDI) Method for delivering a medication through inhalation that allows a controlled, precise dose.

Nitroglycerin Medication that works to reduce the work of the heart by decreasing peripheral vascular resistance while improving blood flow to the myocardium by dilating the coronary arteries; usually placed under the tongue for absorption.

Oral glucose Form of glucose gel that is administered orally to patients with suspected hypoglycemia.

Route of drug administration Method through which a drug is administered to a patient, such as intramuscularly, orally, or intravenously.

Side effect Consequence other than the desired effect for which a substance is used.

Sublingual Under (beneath) the tongue.

Suspension Preparation of a finely divided, undissolved substance dispersed in a liquid vehicle.

Therapeutic dose Dose of a medication required to have the desired effect on a patient.

Trade name Trademarked name that a manufacturer uses in marketing a given drug; also called *brand name*.

Review Questions

Questions 1-6. Match the drug in column A with a condition in column B that is an indication for its use.

Column A
1. Nitroglycerin
2. Oral glucose
3. Activated charcoal
4. Inhalers
5. Epinephrine
6. Oxygen

Column B
a. Cyanosis
b. Overdose or poisoning
c. Asthma
d. Anaphylaxis (severe allergic reaction)
e. Chest pain
f. Suspected low blood sugar

7. Two puffs from a prescribed metered-dose inhaler are given to a patient with asthma. Which of the following effects would be considered the intended action of the drug?
a. Fast heart rate
b. Muscle tremors
c. Bronchodilation
d. Fast respiratory rate

8. A patient with severe chest pain is conscious with a blood pressure of 70 by palpation. He tells you he has prescribed nitroglycerin in his medicine cabinet. You call medical direction, and they advise you not to assist with nitroglycerin administration because of his blood pressure. Which of the following terms best describes low blood pressure with respect to not administering nitroglycerin in this scenario?
a. Action
b. Effect
c. Contraindication
d. Indication

9. You have a patient who weighs 220 pounds. What is his weight in kilograms?
   a. 120 kg
   b. 100 kg
   c. 12 kg
   d. 10 kg

10. One liter of water equals how many milliliters?
    a. 1,000,000
    b. 100,000
    c. 10,000
    d. 1000

11. One milligram of gold equals how many grams?
    a. 0.001
    b. 0.1
    c. 10
    d. 1000

Questions 12-16. Match the form of a drug in column B to the appropriate medication administered by the EMT in column A (there is one extra form):

Column A	Column B
12. Nitroglycerin	a. Suspension in pressurized aerosol unit
13. Oral glucose	b. Gel
14. Activated charcoal	c. Capsule
15. Metered-dose inhaler	d. Suspension
16. Epinephrine	e. Tablet or spray
	f. Liquid for injection

For Further Review

In the Student Workbook

- Multiple-choice questions
- Matching questions
- Fill-in-the-blank questions
- Case scenario questions
- Crossword puzzle

On Evolve

- Weblinks
- Lecture notes
- Exercises

Learning Objectives

Cognitive Objectives

- Identify which medications will be carried on the unit.
- State the medications carried on the unit by their generic name.
- Identify the medications the EMT may help administer to the patient.
- State by generic name the medications that the EMT can assist the patient in administering.
- Discuss the forms in which medications may be found.

Affective Objective

- Explain the rationale for administering medications.

Psychomotor Objectives

- Demonstrate general steps for assisting the patient with self-administration of medications.
- Read the labels and inspect each type of medication.

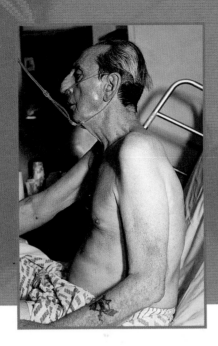

11 Respiratory Emergencies

CHAPTER OUTLINE

Scenario

A 48-year-old man called 9-1-1 because he had a sudden onset of shortness of breath. As you approach the patient, you note he is sitting bolt upright in a chair, struggling to breathe. He has audible wheezing, especially on exhalation. As you introduce yourself, he nods in response and speaks in short phrases between breaths. As you perform the initial (primary) assessment, you notice respirations at a rate of 30 breaths/min with accessory muscle use and a pulse rate of 120 beats/min. His skin is cool, pale, and clammy. Your partner administers high-concentration oxygen to the patient by a nonrebreather mask.

The patient's wife informs you that he had an acute asthma attack while working in the backyard about 30 minutes ago. He has had asthma attacks for several years and a history of allergy to common environmental agents. He had hoped that the attack would pass after he took 2 inhalations from his self-administered inhaler; however, he says the attack is worse than usual. The patient denies chest pain or other symptoms. You perform a focused (secondary) assessment with physical examination and confirm your previous findings and also note equal and bilateral noisy breath sounds with a high-pitched musical quality on exhalation.

You contact medical direction, then advise the physician of the findings and the type and dose of medication taken by the patient. You are directed to assist the patient with another administration of the metered-dose inhaler. You then place the patient on the stretcher in the sitting position and transport him to the hospital.

Respiratory emergencies are one of the most common reasons for emergency medical services (EMS) dispatch. Respiratory emergencies are also among the most life-threatening situations you may encounter as an emergency medical technician (EMT). Regardless of the cause, maintaining an open airway and ensuring adequate ventilation and oxygenation are the keys to effective management. Some patients with lower airway obstruction, such as asthma, may need medication to help open their airways to breathe effectively. You can learn to assist asthmatic patients with administration of their self-administered metered-dose inhalers as part of prehospital care.

This chapter discusses how to assess patients with difficulty breathing, allowing you to become familiar with questions used during the focused history that will assist in evaluation and the signs elicited during the physical examination associated with the chief complaint of shortness of breath.

LEARNING OBJECTIVES
- List the structures and functions of the respiratory system.
- State the signs and symptoms of a patient with breathing difficulty.
- Describe the emergency medical care of the patient with breathing difficulty.
- Describe the emergency medical care of the patient with respiratory distress.
- Establish the relationship between airway management and the patient with breathing difficulty.
- List the signs of adequate air exchange.

Anatomy and Physiology

Anatomy and physiology provide the basis for understanding assessment and treatment of illness and injury. The respiratory system is designed to deliver oxygen to the blood so it can be transported to the tissues of the body. For this to occur, a patent airway must exist from the nose and mouth to the alveoli. Muscles of respiration must move air effectively in and out of the body, and diffusion of gases across the alveolocapillary membrane must occur. The respiratory system also depends on the brainstem to monitor and control respiration through specialized nerves.

Airway

The airway begins at the nose and mouth as air enters and passes through the nasopharynx and oropharynx. The air continues through the upper airway, past the epiglottis, which protects the airway during swallowing, and down the trachea and into the two main bronchi, which direct the air into the right and left lungs. The bronchi subdivide into smaller and smaller bronchioles until they end in air sacs called alveoli, which lie next to the capillaries (**Figure 11-1**).

Alveolar-Capillary Exchange

At the alveolar-capillary junction, gas diffuses from high concentration (alveolar) to low concentration (capillary). Here the oxygen from the air diffuses into the blood, where it is carried by hemoglobin for delivery to the body. At the same time, the waste product carbon dioxide diffuses from the capillaries into the alveoli, where it is discharged into the atmosphere during expiration (**Figure 11-2**). Hemoglobin saturated with oxygen gives the blood its red color. In contrast, hemoglobin without oxygen is blue, which can produce the finding of cyanosis.

The movement of air into and out of the lungs is a result of the actions of the muscles of respiration. In essence, the muscles of respiration contract to expand the thoracic cavity during inspiration. By expanding the thoracic cavity, the pressure of air within the thorax falls with respect to the atmosphere, and air moves into the lungs. When the muscles of respiration relax, the natural elasticity (recoil) of the lungs and the chest wall causes a decrease in the size of the thoracic cavity. As the thoracic cavity decreases in size, it increases the pressure of the air in the lungs relative to the atmosphere, and air moves out through the mouth and nose.

Mechanics of Breathing

In normal quiet breathing, the principal muscle of respiration is the *diaphragm,* aided by the external intercostal muscles. Quiet inspiration occurs when the dome-shaped diaphragm contracts downward and flattens while the intercostals pull the ribs upward and outward. This action increases the anterior-posterior, superior-inferior, and lateral dimensions of the chest cavity. When more forceful breathing is needed, as during exercise or with respiratory disease, accessory muscles of respiration may be used during both inspiration and expiration. You should look for signs of accessory muscle use, such as prominent neck muscles or retractions above the sternum, below the rib cage, or between the ribs, during patient assessment. Because the chest

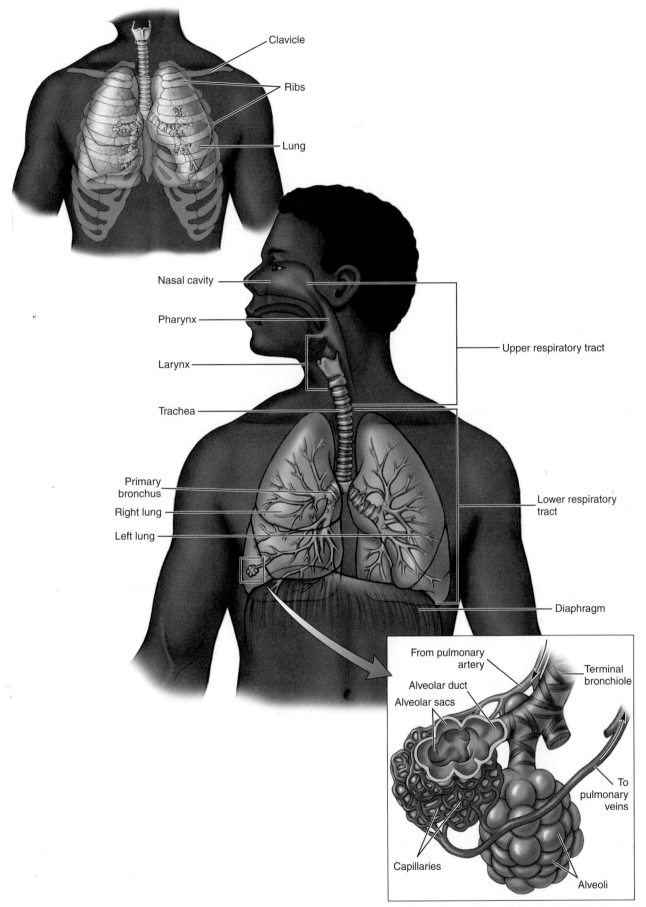

Figure 11-1 The respiratory system. *From Herlihy B, Maebius W: The human body in health and illness, ed 3, Philadelphia, 2007, Saunders-Elsevier.*

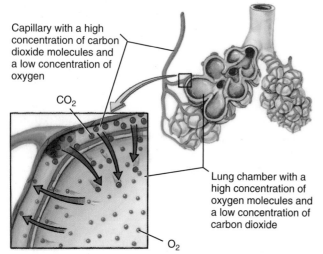

Figure 11-2 Diffusion of oxygen and carbon dioxide in the lungs.

wall of the infant and child is soft compared with the adult chest wall, signs of accessory muscle use are more obvious in the pediatric population.

Central Nervous System Controls

Breathing normally takes place without conscious control or voluntary effort. The central nervous system (CNS) is affected by the level of carbon dioxide and oxygen in the blood and adjusts the rate and depth of breathing accordingly to maintain these levels within a normal range. The rate of breathing (breaths per minute) normally ranges from 12 to 20 for an adult, 15 to 30 for children, and 25 to 50 breaths/min for infants. The tidal volume is the amount of air exchanged during one breath. The brain controls both rate and depth of breathing so that an adequate amount of air reaches the alveoli to ensure enough oxygen exchange to meet the body's need. The product of the number of breaths per minute multiplied by the tidal volume is called the *minute volume* (breaths/min × tidal volume = minute volume). The minute volume determines the adequacy of ventilation. If the minute volume is low, the patient will be poorly oxygenated and retain carbon dioxide.

As an EMT, you monitor the rise and fall of the chest and the rate of breathing. When chest rise is not visible or when the rate of breathing is too slow, you should consider the need for assisted positive-pressure ventilation to improve the minute volume and ensure adequate ventilation for the patient. Key to oxygen delivery to the blood is bringing adequate volumes of oxygenated air to the alveoli so that oxygen can diffuse across the alveolar capillary membrane into the blood, where it can be transported to the cells of the body.

Pathophysiology

Reviewing the anatomy and physiology of normal respiration helps you understand the problems that can occur, the significance of signs and symptoms, and the actions necessary to assist a patient.

The airway can be blocked at multiple points. In unconscious patients, the tongue may fall back and block the oropharynx,

producing a snoring sound. Manual opening of the airway or insertion of an oropharyngeal airway may be needed. The epiglottis can be swollen from infection, resulting in obstruction above the vocal cords. When this occurs, stridor or crowing (high-pitched sounds) may be heard during inspiration. This condition is of particular concern when the airway becomes completely obstructed by swelling of the epiglottis; a surgical opening in the airway may be needed, which can be done only by paramedics or physicians at the hospital. Gurgling can be a clue to wet secretions in the upper airway tract and an indication for suctioning to prevent aspiration of fluid into the lungs, where it would block diffusion of oxygen across the alveoli.

Inadequate breathing may occur when breathing is too shallow or when the respiratory rate is too slow. For example, if a patient's normal rate is 12 breaths/min and the tidal volume is 500 mL per breath, the minute volume is 6000 mL/min:

$$12\,\text{breaths/min} \times 500\,\text{mL/breath} = 6000\,\text{mL/min}$$

If a patient has taken an overdose of sleeping pills and the respiratory rate falls to 6 breaths/min with the same tidal volume, the minute volume is now 3000 mL/min, or half the patient's normal volume:

$$6\,\text{breaths/min} \times 500\,\text{mL/min} = 3000\,\text{mL/min}$$

Likewise, if breathing is very shallow and the tidal volume is 200 mL/min and the rate is 24 breaths/min, the minute volume is still lower than normal despite the increased rate of breathing:

$$24\,\text{breaths/min} \times 200\,\text{mL/breath} = 4800\,\text{mL/min}$$

These examples should help you understand how physiology and anatomy are used during assessment and treatment of patients. As you learn more about specific illnesses, you will appreciate how to focus your history and physical examination (secondary [focused] assessment) when you encounter different chief complaints.

Inadequate oxygenation can also occur when fluid, pus, or other material is present at the level of the alveoli. This can occur in patients with pneumonia or pulmonary edema (fluid buildup in the lungs as a result of heart failure). Fluid collecting in the alveoli or between the alveoli and capillaries can impair diffusion of gases across the alveolocapillary membrane, resulting in hypoxia. For these patients, you should increase delivered oxygen through the use of supplemental devices, such as a nonrebreather mask or nasal cannula (when a mask cannot be tolerated by the patient). If the patient exhibits signs of inadequate ventilation, oxygen is administered by positive-pressure ventilation.

> **REAL**World
>
> Management of positive-pressure ventilation in infants involves two key concerns. First, ventilation of the pediatric patient requires minimal volumes of air, which makes it easier to achieve adequate tidal volumes than in the adult patient. Second, however, infants and small children are more prone to complications such as gastric inflation and pneumothorax. In the real world, it is crucial to ventilate until you see visible chest rise, and no more. Carefully observe chest rise during each breath.

Table 11-1	Signs of Inadequate Breathing

Sign	Findings and Explanations
Respiratory rate	Outside normal ranges according to age Adult: 12-20 breaths/min Child: 15-30 breaths/min Infant: 25-50 breaths/min
Rhythm	Irregular
Quality	Breath sounds diminished or absent Chest expansion unequal or inadequate Increased effort of breathing Accessory muscle use (especially noticeable in infants and children)
Depth of breathing	Inadequate and shallow
Skin	Pale, cyanotic Cool and clammy
Retractions	Above clavicles, between ribs, and below the rib cage (especially noticeable in infants and children)
Nasal flaring	Especially noticeable in infants and children
Seesaw breathing	In infants and children, where abdomen and chest move in opposite directions
Agonel breathing	Occasional gasping breaths often seen just before death

Anatomic Considerations in Infants and Children

The airway of infants and children differs in important ways from that of the adult. The internal diameter of the child's airway is smaller at all levels: from the nose, mouth and pharynx, through the larynx and trachea, and extending through the bronchi and bronchioles. The tongue is large in relation to the airway and has a greater potential to cause obstruction.

The narrowest part of the pediatric airway is at the ring formed by the cricoid cartilage. In the adult airway, the vocal cords are the narrowest part of the airway. The cartilage that forms the larynx and trachea in the child is softer than the firm cartilage in the adult, an important fact to consider during opening of the pediatric airway.

Because the chest wall is softer, infants and children tend to depend more on the action of the diaphragm muscle for breathing.

The differences in the infant and child airway have practical implications in airway management. For example, the head position for opening the airway varies with age. For infants (<1 year), place the head in the sniffing, or neutral, position to avoid bending and kinking the soft trachea. For toddlers and small children (1-8 years), extend the neck slightly but do not hyperextend. The head of a child or infant is proportionately larger than in adults. It may be helpful to pad under the child's shoulders to maintain an airway. Because the tongue in children is relatively large, you must keep it from obstructing the airway. When inserting an oropharyngeal airway, use a tongue blade to displace the tongue, because rotating the airway in the usual manner may damage the soft tissues of the palate.

Table 11-2	Signs of Adequate Versus Inadequate Positive-Pressure Ventilation

Adequate	Inadequate
Chest rises and falls with each breath	No chest rise with breaths
Breathing rate is sufficient. Adults: about 12 breaths/min Infants/children: about 20 breaths/min	Breathing rate is too slow or too fast
Heart rate returns to normal with positive-pressure ventilation	Heart rate does not return to normal

Given the small caliber of the infant's airway, small obstructions such as swelling and mucus can result in significant blockage of airflow. Although 1 to 2 mm of airway edema in an adult is inconsequential, it is a significant obstruction in an infant.

Infants prefer to breathe through the nose. In fact, infants are considered *obligate nose breathers* (they must breathe through the nose because the oral cavity has limited room for air movement). Blockage of the nasal passages from mucus or swelling can significantly narrow the airway and increase an infant's work of breathing. If an infant has an upper respiratory tract infection, such as a common cold, and a disease of the lower airway, the blockage in the nasal pharynx may cause the baby to decompensate. Suctioning the baby's nasal passages with a bulb suction or soft catheter with low-to-medium suction may significantly improve the condition. Administration of humidified supplemental oxygen to the child may also help by loosening any encrusted mucus or secretions.

See Chapters 4 and 6 for further discussion of the anatomy and physiology of the respiratory system, signs of inadequate breathing, signs of adequate and inadequate artificial ventilation, and pediatric anatomic considerations. **Table 11-1** reviews the signs of inadequate breathing. **Table 11-2** reviews the signs of adequate and inadequate positive-pressure ventilation.

Assessing the Patient with Difficulty Breathing

Scene Size-up

Begin your assessment with the scene size-up. In general, make sure that the scene is safe for you, the patient, and any bystanders. If trauma is a contributing factor, consider the mechanism of injury and provide appropriate spinal immobilization. Be alert for a possible toxic environment, such as the presence of poisonous gases or other hazardous materials.

Consider the need for body substance isolation by using standard precautions and transmission-based precautions. For example, if suctioning and positive-pressure ventilation are needed and splashing is likely, wear protective eye gear, masks, and gloves. If tuberculosis or other airborne diseases are suspected, you should wear a high-efficiency particulate air (HEPA) respirator to protect against airborne transmission (see Figure 2-6).

Initial (Primary) Assessment

As you approach the patient, what is your general impression? Pertinent questions are as follows:

- Is there an obvious threat to life, such as respiratory arrest?
- Does the patient appear to be unconscious?
- In what position is the patient found?
- Does the patient speak in complete sentences, or is the patient struggling to catch his or her breath and speaking in short sentences?

Patient Position

The patient's position may provide the first clue to the seriousness of the problem. Generally, most patients who have shortness of breath prefer to be sitting bolt upright for unrestricted expansion of the diaphragm and chest wall (**Figure 11-3**). Children with upper airway obstruction may be found sitting upright and leaning forward with their weight distributed on the hands, the mouth open, the tongue protruding, and the chin thrust forward to maximize the diameter of the airway (sniffing position). This is sometimes called the **tripod position**. In general, patients should be supported and transported in the position that eases their work of breathing.

Patients in respiratory distress who are found lying down or who begin to fall back in a chair or bed from a sitting position may be tiring from the increased work of breathing or from lack

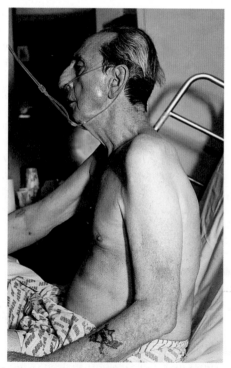

Figure 11-3 The position a patient assumes during scene size-up may be a clue to breathing difficulty. Note the bolt-upright position of this patient with emphysema and the pursed-lip (puckered-lip) breathing used to keep the bronchioles from collapsing during exhalation.

of oxygen. Patients who are weak as a result of respiratory difficulty may need assistance with positive-pressure ventilation.

Mental Status

As you introduce yourself to the patient, assess the mental status according to the AVPU (*a*lert, *v*erbal, *p*ainful, *u*nresponsive) criteria. Alterations in mental status that may be observed as a result of difficult breathing and hypoxia range from restlessness, agitation, and anxiety to lethargy or sleepiness and complete unresponsiveness. If you note any alteration in mental status or suspect low blood oxygen concentration, you should administer high-concentration supplemental oxygen and look closely at the adequacy of breathing and ventilation. The feeling of shortness of breath or difficulty breathing causes anxiety and agitation in most individuals regardless of whether oxygen delivery is actually impaired.

Airway

The inability to speak is a sign of a severe (or complete) airway obstruction. If foreign body obstruction is suspected, initiate the basic life support airway obstruction maneuvers. If another cause of airway obstruction is suspected (e.g., croup, epiglottitis, anaphylaxis), initiate rapid transport and provide positive-pressure ventilation, if needed, and other appropriate treatments (see Chapters 12 and 25).

Some patients may be clearly moving air, but as their shortness of breath and breathing efforts become more severe, they may have difficulty speaking. Like a runner who is out of breath, they have difficulty communicating because of the frequency of breaths and the increased effort associated with breathing.

Is the patient's breathing noisy? A variety of audible respiratory sounds indicate obstruction of the airway by the tongue, narrowing of the upper or lower airway tract, or fluid in the lungs. You might also note coughing if a patient is trying to clear a foreign body, phlegm, or secretions. A barking cough is heard with *croup*, a common viral infection of the upper airway tract in young children. *Stridor*, or crowing (like a rooster's crow), are high-pitched sounds that are usually heard on inspiration (but also may be heard on expiration) and are a sign of upper airway tract narrowing. Gurgling or wet sounds are generated by air moving through fluid in the airway. Snoring is usually associated with partial closure of the airway. A hoarse voice is a sign of swelling of the larynx. Depending on the circumstances, these sounds can be the first clue of the need for basic life support airway obstruction maneuvers, suctioning, and use of airway adjuncts such as an oropharyngeal or nasopharyngeal airway. When the obstruction cannot be relieved with basic maneuvers, rapid transport to the hospital for advanced airway maneuvers such as a cricothyroidotomy should be considered. In EMS systems with paramedics who can perform surgical airway maneuvers, an advanced life support (ALS) intercept should also be considered.

Wheezing, a high-pitched whistling noise associated with narrowed bronchioles, can sometimes be heard without a stethoscope. **Table 11-3** reviews various audible respiratory sounds and their possible significance.

Age-appropriate techniques and equipment should always be used. In patients with suspected head or neck trauma, take cervical spine precautions when caring for the airway.

Table 11-3	Noisy Breathing Sounds and Significance

Respiratory Sound	Description	Possible Significance
Stridor or crowing	High-pitched sound, usually heard on inspiration	Obstruction of upper airway from foreign body or swelling; swelling can be caused by allergic reactions or infections of epiglottis, larynx, or trachea
Audible wheezing	High-pitched whistling noise from narrowed bronchioles; usually heard on expiration	Caused by constriction or partial obstruction of lower airways
Gurgling	"Wet" sounds generated by air moving through fluid in airway	Caused by fluid in upper or lower airway from aspiration, near-drowning, or heart failure
Snoring	Low-pitched sounds, usually associated with partial closure of airway by tongue	Deep, unconscious states or other cases of partial obstruction of pharynx by tongue

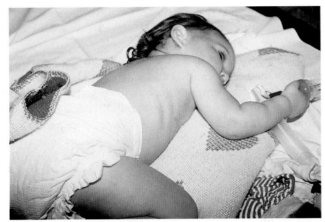

Figure 11-4 Note the retractions between the lower ribs in this child in respiratory distress.

Breathing

One of the most important decisions you will make as an EMT is whether a patient requires positive-pressure ventilation. When the patient is not breathing, the decision is obvious. In other respiratory emergencies, you must rely on your assessment. The criteria used to determine the need for positive-pressure ventilation include slow and irregular breathing, shallow breathing (evidenced by little or no chest rise), diminished breath sounds, seesaw breathing (infants and children), decreased level of consciousness, and other signs of severe hypoxia.

Rate and Depth of Respiration. During respiratory difficulty or distress, patients usually increase their rate and depth of breathing. For example, if part of the lung is collapsed, the amount of air that can exchange oxygen at the alveoli is diminished. Increasing the number of breaths per minute is one way the body works to maintain oxygenation of the blood.

Slow and irregular breathing may be a sign of respiratory fatigue and impending respiratory failure and should alert you to the need for positive-pressure ventilation. Slow and irregular breathing can be caused by many conditions. A long period of labored breathing can lead to muscular exhaustion and fatigue. Similarly, a stroke can damage the part of the brain that controls breathing. Slow and shallow breathing can be caused by an overdose of drugs that depress the CNS, such as heroin or barbiturates.

In addition to respiratory rate, you must evaluate the depth of breathing. Shallow breathing, as indicated by little or no chest rise or abdominal movement and poor airflow, suggests the need for positive-pressure ventilation. Even a patient who has rapid and shallow breathing may need assisted ventilation. A critical volume of air must enter the lungs each minute to ensure that enough oxygen passes into the circulation to meet the body's needs. This minute volume might be too low even if the respiratory rate is high.

You should assess the work of breathing by observing for any accessory muscle use in the neck, between the ribs or below the rib cage, or excessive movement of the abdomen (**Figure 11-4**). These are signs of increased work of breathing, and patients may become fatigued. Because breathing is usually done as an unconscious effort, the work of breathing is often taken for granted. Working to breathe against resistance, however, requires muscular effort and tires the body. For example, individuals with asthma must breathe through narrowed bronchioles, which requires greater effort with each breath. After prolonged, difficult, and labored breathing (dyspnea), a patient will become fatigued, the respiratory depth will diminish, and the respiratory rate can slow, a condition called **respiratory failure.**

The patient may feel sleepy, start to lie down, and have altered mental status. Patients who have tired after prolonged, labored breathing are in critical condition and need assisted ventilation.

The combination of an altered mental status, especially when the patient is sleepy or lethargic, with slow or shallow breathing suggests the need for positive-pressure ventilation.

Assisted Ventilation. When providing assisted ventilations to a patient with some respiratory efforts but inadequate ventilation, you should coordinate your efforts to amplify and enhance the patient's voluntary efforts rather than work against them. This is called *assisted positive-pressure ventilation.* If the patient has inadequate ventilation but a respiratory rate of more than 12 breaths/min, assisted ventilation should be timed to supplement the patient's own effort for at least one breath every 5 seconds. For example, if a patient has shallow respirations at a rate of 36 per minute, you would augment every third breath (every 5 seconds) during the patient's inspiratory phase. As the patient begins to inspire, gently squeeze the bag on the bag-mask device over 1 second until chest rise occurs.

If a patient's breathing is slow and shallow, additional assisted breaths should be added between the patient's own efforts to breathe. For example, a patient breathing 6 times a minute would receive an assisted breath at inspiration followed by an interposed breath 5 seconds later. With this approach, the patient will receive a total of 12 breaths/min that result in chest rise. Supplemental oxygen should be used whenever assisted ventilation is required (see Chapter 6).

Sometimes the situation will be confusing. Do you assist ventilation or just administer high-concentration oxygen? When this occurs, err on the side of assisted ventilation. If patients are alert enough to support their own ventilation, they will resist your attempts to ventilate and push the mask from their face. When this happens, apply high-concentration oxygen and closely monitor the effectiveness of the patient's own breathing attempts. Again, when in doubt, provide positive-pressure ventilation.

REALWorld

Always pay close attention to positive-pressure ventilation. When transporting a patient from the scene to the ambulance, it can be difficult to maintain a seal with a bag-mask or other ventilation device. The common mistake made by providers is to move too fast and not adequately control the airway and ventilation. Control your team, and move carefully enough to provide adequate ventilations. When moving down stairs, provide a few breaths and then quickly move to the next landing, and provide a few breaths before your next move. Remember, airway management and ventilation are critical to survival.

Circulation

When patients experience respiratory distress or other serious problems, the pulse rate may be increased or decreased as hypoxia progresses. Early in hypoxia, the heart beats faster in an attempt to compensate for the low oxygen content of the blood by increasing blood flow through the body. As the patient's condition persists, the heart itself may be receiving too little oxygen, fatiguing the organ and slowing the pulse rate. In the setting of respiratory failure, a slow pulse rate is an ominous sign.

Patients in severe respiratory distress may have cool, pale, and sweaty skin, a sign of adrenaline release. Adrenaline release occurs when the body is reacting to shock. Cyanosis, a bluish discoloration of the mucous membranes or skin around the lips, results from oxygen-depleted hemoglobin and is always an indication for supplemental oxygen and possibly positive-pressure ventilation.

After completing the initial assessment, you should consider the need for rapid transport or an ALS intercept. The call for ALS may be particularly important for patients with airway obstruction that is unrelieved by basic procedures or for patients who cannot be adequately ventilated with basic airway devices. When the need for ALS is identified, you should make the call early.

Focused (Secondary) Assessment

Obtain a SAMPLE history to help guide further treatment and to focus the physical examination.

SAMPLE History

Box 11-1 presents important questions for the medical patient with respiratory complaints. As you learn more about common illnesses and conditions that cause respiratory emergencies, such as those discussed later in this chapter, the line of questioning you choose will become more apparent in a given situation.

Remember to ask the OPQRST questions: *o*nset, *p*rovocation, *r*elieving factors, *q*uality of pain, *r*adiation, *s*everity, and *t*ime of symptoms.

Physical Examination

For responsive patients with no history of trauma, you should perform a physical examination directed by findings from the SAMPLE history and the initial assessment. Reassess the patient's mental status and skin condition. Check the head, neck, and chest for signs of respiratory distress, such as nasal flaring, accessory muscle use, and retractions. You should look at the neck for jugular vein distention and check for crepitation that may be caused by air leakage under the skin from damage to the lung or airways, particularly for patients who may have had a recent chest injury. Is the trachea midline? You may notice that the contour of the chest is barrel shaped (increased anterior and posterior diameter from chronic air trapping) in patients who have chronic obstructive lung disease (emphysema and chronic bronchitis).

Auscultate the lungs below the middle of the clavicles anteriorly and at the lung bases at the midaxillary line and posteriorly at the bases. Note whether the breath sounds are equal on both sides and are present in all four locations. While listening to the lungs, you may note abnormal sounds. For example, a patient with asthma might have high-pitched whistling or musical sounds (wheezes) heard on expiration. Expiration is usually longer than inspiration in a patient with asthma. Some asthmatic patients may have wheezing that is audible even without a stethoscope.

Another sound you might note is crackles or rales. *Crackles* are similar to the sound made when rubbing hair together near your ear. This sound is often caused by fluid in the airways. Crackles may be heard on one side only, as with pneumonia or an infection in one lung, or on both sides, which might occur with fluid in both lungs from congestive heart failure. Crackles are often positional in nature. For example, a patient who has been lying on the back may have crackles in the posterior lung area (see Chapter 12).

You might note that breath sounds are diminished on one or both sides. This could be caused by fluid in the lungs, collapse of a lung, or shallow breathing. As an EMT, you are not expected to interpret breath sounds, but you are expected to note their presence or absence at the four locations and whether they are equal on both sides.

Your examination might include other parts of the body, such as the abdomen or extremities, as you focus the physical examination based on the history and previous findings. For example, a patient may also complain of (or have noticeable) swelling of the ankles and lower extremities if the condition is heart failure, which often presents with difficulty breathing. Unresponsive patients should always receive a rapid head-to-toe physical assessment to ensure that key findings are not overlooked (**Box 11-2**).

Baseline Vital Signs

Record baseline vital signs, paying particular attention to the respiratory rate and pulse, and reevaluate the need for positive-pressure ventilation. During your ongoing assessment or reassessment, usually performed en route to the hospital, check for any changes in the patient's breathing.

Box 11-1   Collecting a SAMPLE History for Patients with Respiratory Complaints

Signs and Symptoms

- What is bothering you?
- Why did you call the ambulance?
- In addition to the chief complaint, are there other signs and symptoms bothering you?

Associated complaints may include weakness, cough (dry or sputum-producing), chest pain, leg swelling, fever, and chills. If there are associated complaints, establish the sequence of events, then develop the chief complaint and the history of the present illness more fully with the OPQRST mnemonic:

Onset: When did you first become short of breath? What were you doing when it first occurred? Were you exerting yourself, or were you at rest?

Provocation: Does anything make your breathing problem worse (e.g., increased activity, walking up stairs, change in position, lying down)?

Quality: Is there any associated pain? Where is the pain? Can you point to the area with one finger? How would you describe it? Is the pain made worse by breathing?

Radiation: Does your pain go anywhere, such as to your arm, neck, or jaw?

Severity: How severe is the shortness of breath (or the pain)? Can you rate it on a scale of 1 to 10 (with 10 being the worst you ever experienced and 1 being barely perceptible)? Patients with chronic respiratory problems such as emphysema might be able to compare their present condition with their usual status. For example, a man who can usually walk a block before becoming short of breath now becomes breathless walking across the room to the bathroom.

Time: How long have you had the shortness of breath and/or the pain?

Allergies

The allergy history may give important clues for patients with shortness of breath. For example, many patients with asthma have allergies. Exposures to the allergen, such as dust or pollen, can provoke attacks of asthma. Other patients might have anaphylactic reactions that result in respiratory distress as the chief complaint and the call for help (see Chapter 14).

Medications

- What medications are you taking?

Often the medication history gives clues to the underlying problem. Patients might say they are taking "heart medicine," or they may have an inhaler for asthma. If the medications are readily available, bring them to the hospital. You should refer to the medication as part of your history if you call medical direction. Patients with chronic lung disease may have oxygen at home. If so, note the delivery device and the dose (in liters per minute).

Pertinent Past Medical History

- Do you have any serious medical or surgical conditions for which you are receiving medical care or that have resulted in hospital admissions?

Common conditions that may be associated with a respiratory complaint include asthma, emphysema, bronchitis, tuberculosis, heart disease, and chronic renal failure. You are not looking for every condition or a life history. Keep this part of the history focused.

Last Oral Intake

- When was the last time you ate or drank?

Events Leading up to the Present Illness

If there are multiple complaints or associated complaints, establish a brief chronology or time sequence of the various complaints. For example, a patient might state that he had fever and chills for 2 days before he experienced shortness of breath.

LEARNING OBJECTIVES

- Recognize the need for medical direction to assist in the emergency medical care of the patient with breathing difficulty.
- State the generic name, medication forms, dose, administration, action, indications, and contraindications for the prescribed inhaler.
- Defend EMT treatment regimens for various respiratory emergencies.
- Explain the rationale for administering an inhaler.

Emergency Medical Care

Most patients with shortness of breath should receive high-concentration supplemental oxygen early in the course of care and assisted positive-pressure ventilation if breathing is inadequate. Patients with shortness of breath are priority patients for early transport. Most patients with shortness of breath prefer to remain in a seated position, but you should allow the patient to remain in a position of comfort. Reduce any unnecessary physical exertion on the part of the patient. Patients with shortness of breath who begin to tire and lie down should be closely watched for adequacy of breathing, because fatigue is a sign of respiratory failure and may require positive-pressure ventilation. Sometimes you may be unsure whether positive-pressure ventilation is needed. When in doubt, you should attempt positive-pressure ventilation. If the patient resists, continue with high-concentration supplemental oxygen by a nonrebreather mask and monitor the patient's condition closely. Patients with inadequate breathing may become agitated when you apply a positive-pressure device or an oxygen mask. They may feel that it interferes with their own breathing efforts and may try to push you away. In these cases, you may be able to administer oxygen by nasal cannula or by holding the mask near the patient's face.

Prescribed Inhalers

Patients who have shortness of breath and prescribed inhalers may benefit from administration of medication in the field. Patients often tell you they have asthma and may even be holding the medication in their hand.

Box 11-2 Signs and Symptoms of Difficulty Breathing

Shortness of breath
Restlessness
Increased pulse rate
Increased or decreased breathing rate
Shallow or slow breathing
Irregular breathing rhythm
Abdominal breathing (diaphragm only)
Noisy breathing
Stridor (crowing)
Audible wheezing
Gurgling
Snoring
Inability to speak
Skin color (cyanotic, pale, flushed)
Retractions
Use of accessory muscles
Coughing
Upright or tripod position
Unusual anatomy (barrel chest)

Table 11-4 Commonly Prescribed Inhalers

Generic Name	Trade Name
Albuterol	Proventil, Ventolin
Metaproterenol	Alupent
Pirbuterol	Maxair
Salmeterol*	Serevent*
Ipratropium†	Atrovent†
Levabuterol	Xopenex

*Salmeterol is a long-acting β_2-agonist indicated for long-term, twice-daily administration in the maintenance treatment of asthma or COPD or to prevent exercise-induced bronchospasm. Serevent should not be used to treat acute symptoms. Rather, patients should use an inhaled, short-acting β_2-agonist for acute symptoms.

†Ipratropium is a bronchodilator that works by a different mechanism than albuterol. It is usually prescribed for maintenance treatment of COPD. Ipratropium also comes combined with albuterol in an aerosol form called Combivent.

NOTE: Not all inhalers work the same or may be the drug of choice for acute prehospital treatment. Always check local medical protocols.

Most patients are capable of self-administering prescribed inhalers; as they become fatigued, however, they may need assistance. You must obtain certain key information to determine whether you should assist the patient with administration of the medication in the field. To do so, you should understand the general pharmacologic principles of prescribed inhalers (see Chapter 10).

Medication Name

Look at the name of the prescribed inhaler so that you can communicate the information to medical direction or compare it with your standing orders. **Table 11-4** presents some common generic and trade names of inhaled medications. You should note that not all inhalers are appropriate medications for acute attacks. Ask patients whether the respiratory problem they are experiencing is the same problem for which they are using the prescribed inhaler. Ask about the last dose and the number of treatments they have self-administered before your arrival. Assess the patient for signs or symptoms of a respiratory emergency. Communicate as directed in your EMS system protocol with medical control.

Actions and Side Effects

The intended action of a prescribed inhaler is dilation of the bronchioles. Most prescribed inhalers for asthma contain β-agonists, drugs that act on the *beta receptors* of the autonomic nervous system, similar to the receptors for epinephrine (adrenaline). Epinephrine causes the "fight or flight" reaction, which has many effects, including increased level of alertness, dilated pupils, rapid pulse, dilated bronchioles, and increased blood flow to skeletal muscles. Because prescribed inhalers are similar to epinephrine in action, the effect or action of the drug, namely bronchodilation, is also accompanied by other effects, such as those just listed. In particular, the side effects noted from prescribed inhalers may include:

• Rapid pulse
• Muscular tremors
• Nervousness

The fact that the inhaled drug is administered directly to the bronchioles tends to focus the effects on the respiratory tree and minimize other side effects. Because these drugs generally act selectively on the beta portion of the sympathetic nervous system, which increases heart rate and dilates the bronchioles, they are called *β-agonists*.

Indications

You should assist the patient with a self-administered inhaler in the following circumstances:
• When the patient exhibits signs and symptoms of respiratory distress.
• When the patient has a hand-held metered-dose inhaler (MDI) prescribed to the patient by a physician.
• When you are specifically authorized by medical direction.

Know your local protocols for medical direction regarding these devices (**Box 11-3**).

Contraindications

In general, do *not* assist with administration in the field in the following circumstances:
• The patient is unable to use the device (e.g., because of an altered mental status or inadequate ventilations). They are unable to inhale the medication.
• The patient has taken the maximum prescribed dose before your arrival. This may be a relative contraindication in that medical direction might order another treatment, depending on the prescribed medication and the individual patient.

Medication Form

As an EMT, you will assist patients in the use of hand-held **metered-dose inhalers (Figure 11-5)**. Inhalation therapy may also be delivered by a **nebulizer,** which administers medication as a mist by a home nebulizer or an oxygen administration

> **Box 11-3** Sample Protocol for Difficulty Breathing and Respiratory Distress

1. Perform initial (primary) assessment and focused (secondary) assessment (history and physical examination).
2. Ensure an open airway.
   Consider the need for:
   • Manual maneuvers (head-tilt/chin-lift, jaw thrust)
   • Suction
   • Oropharyngeal airway, nasopharyngeal airway
3. Ensure adequate ventilation.
   If ventilations are inadequate, as evidenced by respiratory rate, respiratory depth, mental status, or other signs of inadequate breathing, provide artificial ventilation at a rate of 12 breaths/min for adults and 20 breaths/min for children. Observe for chest rise.
4. Ensure adequate oxygenation.
   If ventilations are adequate but the patient has difficulty breathing or other signs of respiratory distress, administer oxygen by a nonrebreather mask.
5. Administer prescribed medication with orders from medical direction.
   If the patient has a prescribed inhaler, contact medical direction to determine the need for initial or follow-up administration.
6. Transport the patient in a position of comfort, usually the sitting position.
7. Perform ongoing assessment or reassessment.
   At least every 5 minutes, reevaluate the adequacy of breathing and document your findings.

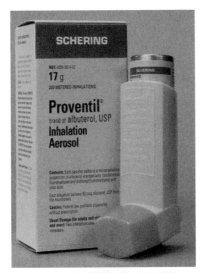

Figure 11-5 Hand-held metered-dose inhaler (MDI).

device; a liquid medication is aerosolized so it can be inhaled deep into the lungs.

Dosage

Medical direction orders the number of metered doses of the inhaler to give the patient. The dose delivered by an MDI is a *unit* dose, and you will usually be directed to assist the patient in administering 1 or 2 puffs of the aerosol.

> **Box 11-4** Administering a Prescribed Inhaler

1. Obtain an order from medical direction, either online or offline.
2. Check the expiration date of the inhaler.
3. Check to see whether the patient has already taken any doses.
4. Make sure that the inhaler is at room temperature or warmer.
5. Shake the inhaler vigorously.
6. Remove the oxygen mask from the patient.
7. Have the patient exhale deeply.
8. Have the patient place his or her lips around the mouthpiece of the inhaler.
9. Have the patient depress the hand-held inhaler as he or she inhales deeply.
10. Have the patient hold the breath for as long as comfortable so that medication can be absorbed.
11. Replace oxygen on the patient.
12. Allow the patient to breathe a few times, and repeat the dose per medical direction.
13. Use a spacing device if the patient has one. (A spacing device is an extension tube added to the mouthpiece that ensures more complete inhalation of the metered dose. It is used especially with children or new-onset asthmatic patients who have not yet experienced metered-dose inhalers.)

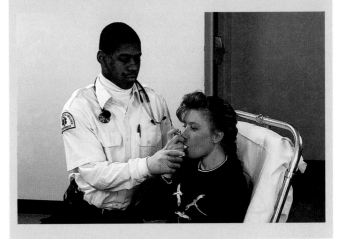

Administration

You should be familiar with administering prescribed inhalers because panic and anxiety often accompany shortness of breath. Key steps to effective administration include knowing the principles of drug delivery and getting the cooperation of the patient. For example, effective delivery of the drug to the lower airways depends on deep inhalation during aerosol delivery, followed by a short period of breath holding (**Box 11-4**). Infants and small children may require the use of a spacer device (**Figure 11-6**) because they cannot synchronize their inhalation with the spray of medication. By storing the medication in a space between the inhaler and the patient, all the medication is inhaled with the subsequent breaths. **Skill 11-1** outlines the steps in the administration of medication using a nebulizer.

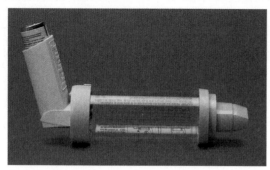

Figure 11-6 Spacer used for infants and small children to facilitate inhalation of medication.

EXTENDED*Transport*

Patients with asthma and other obstructive airway problems can become severely fatigued over time. During long transports, you must be diligent in monitoring vital signs and physical findings related to respiratory failure. Pay particular attention to mental status and respiratory rate and depth. When patients become lethargic or sleepy, or when respirations become shallow, you must consider the need for positive-pressure ventilation. An early decision to ventilate can make the difference between life and death.

Ongoing Assessment or Reassessment

To assess the effectiveness of the therapy, assess vital signs and repeat the secondary (focused) assessment (physical examination) as part of your ongoing assessment. Document the time of medication administration and the findings from your reassessment on the prehospital care report.

LEARNING OBJECTIVES

- Distinguish among the emergency medical care of the infant, child, and adult patient with breathing difficulty.
- Differentiate between upper airway obstruction and lower airway disease in the infant and child patient.

Infants and Children

Asthma is a common condition in children, and MDIs or home nebulizers (powered by an air pump to allow continuous medication flow from a hand-held device) may be present on the scene. It is important to note that asthma often manifests as coughing rather than wheezing. In very young children, inflammation and constriction of the bronchiole are called *bronchiolitis*. This condition may also be treated with MDIs or home nebulizers.

Treatment of children with inhaler therapy is similar to that of adults. Pediatric MDIs may have spacers to help ensure full delivery of the drug. Again, you should become familiar with the use of a spacer device so that you can assist children as appropriate.

When caring for infants and children with respiratory difficulty, distinguishing between lower and upper airway disease is

important. Upper airway problems, such as croup and epiglottitis, can cause sudden onset of respiratory distress and warrant special consideration. Signs of upper airway disease include stridor, usually on inspiration; patients with lower airway disease will have wheezing heard over the lungs, often during expiration.

Because the rib cage is softer and more movable (compliant) in children than in adults, retractions may be more evident. Cyanosis should be considered a danger sign in children because at this point their condition can deteriorate rapidly. See Chapter 25 for a more complete discussion of respiratory emergencies in infants and children.

Conditions That Cause Respiratory Emergencies

Patients with respiratory emergencies may have a new illness or a complication of a chronic respiratory condition. You will routinely encounter patients with conditions such as asthma, emphysema, chronic bronchitis, and heart failure who have complications of their chronic illness and call EMS because they are short of breath. Other conditions you may encounter include croup, epiglottitis, pneumonia, pneumothorax, and hyperventilation syndrome. The following descriptions of these conditions will help you understand some common presentations in prehospital care.

Case in Point

Two EMTs respond to a 68-year-old man complaining of difficulty breathing at home. His wife states that the problem started about 2 hours ago while the patient was watching TV. The patient has a history of high blood pressure, a heart attack 3 years ago, and COPD. He is taking atenolol, nitroglycerin, daily aspirin, and albuterol (inhaler).

On physical examination the EMTs note the patient is an extremely obese man who is lethargic and has rapid and shallow breathing. His blood pressure is 180/120, pulse 110 and regular, and respiratory rate 36 and very shallow. His lips and nail beds are cyanotic. Breath sounds are diminished bilaterally with faint wheezes throughout the lungs. He has severe pitting edema in his ankles.

The EMTs place the patient in the supine position on a stretcher and provide assisted ventilation at a rate of 12 breaths/min. Because the patient is breathing 36 breaths/min, they provide an assisted breath every third attempt by the patient. They suspect the patient is experiencing COPD and respiratory failure. En route to the hospital, his color improves, and his respirations increase in rate and quality.

Chronic Obstructive Pulmonary Disease

Chronic obstructive pulmonary disease (COPD) is a chronic respiratory condition that includes chronic bronchitis or emphysema. These terms describe two classic presentations of COPD. Both chronic bronchitis and emphysema are most frequently caused by long-term smoking, although a genetic disorder (α_1-antitrypsin deficiency) can also cause emphysema. Shortness of breath is the primary complaint of COPD patients. Patients with COPD can have classic signs and symptoms of either emphysema or chronic bronchitis, or of both. Bronchoconstriction is often a component of COPD, and patients may use inhaled bronchodilators.

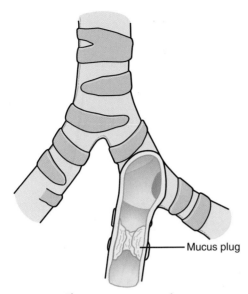

Figure 11-7 Mucus plug.

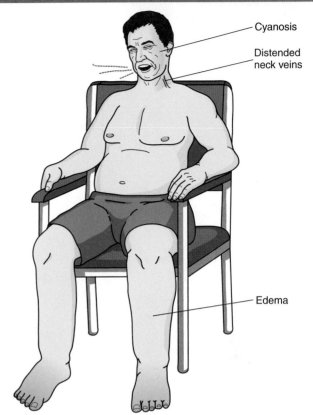

Figure 11-8 Chronic bronchitis is characterized by excessive mucus production, chronic productive cough, and cyanosis. Edema from right-sided heart failure manifests as swelling in the legs and abdomen and distended neck veins.

Chronic Bronchitis

Chronic bronchitis is defined as a condition in which a chronic productive (producing phlegm) cough is present for at least 3 months per year for at least 2 years. It is caused by smoking or exposure to environmental pollutants; long-term irritation results in a number of changes within the lung. Mucus-secreting glands become enlarged, and excessive mucus production causes plugging of the bronchi and bronchioles (**Figure 11-7**). The retained secretions also cause the characteristic productive cough. This harsh, phlegm-producing cough is especially active on waking in the morning.

The obstructed bronchi result in poorly ventilated alveoli. This in turn causes poorly oxygenated blood and cyanosis. The term *blue bloater* was coined to describe the patient's cyanotic skin color and puffy, edematous appearance. The edema that accumulates in the ankles, hips, or abdomen is the result of right-sided heart failure, which is a complication of COPD. Heart failure also causes distention of neck veins (**Figure 11-8**).

Auscultation of breath sounds may reveal wheezing and sometimes crackles from secretions or mucus and fluid throughout the airway.

A patient with chronic bronchitis may be found sitting bolt upright with a tissue in one hand and a cup nearby to collect the phlegm from the chronic cough.

Emphysema

Emphysema is a disease caused by destruction of the alveoli. With fewer alveoli, patients have less lung surface through which oxygen can diffuse into the blood. The muscular portion of the small bronchioles within the lung is also damaged. Bronchioles, in their normal condition, resist collapse when pressure rises within the chest during exhalation. However, the damaged bronchioles of patients with emphysema collapse during exhalation (**Figure 11-9**), and patients are left with a higher volume of air remaining in the lung. This is called *air trapping* and explains the characteristic barrel-chest appearance of the patient with COPD. The chest wall is gradually reshaped as the patient "breathes around"

the trapped air. To better appreciate the sensation of air trapping, take a full breath and release only a small amount of air. Now take another few breaths, never releasing beyond this point.

Because the airways tend to collapse during exhalation, patients with emphysema find that they breathe better when they exhale against a resistance, thus maintaining pressure within the airways. They make their own resistance to exhalation by exhaling against pursed lips (puckering), similar to breathing out through a straw.

To compensate for emphysema, the body may increase the number of red blood cells and amount of hemoglobin in the blood, which may result in a characteristic pink appearance to the skin. The combination of the pursed-lip breathing and the pink appearance has resulted in the name *pink puffer* to describe a finding in some patients with emphysema (**Figure 11-10**).

Chronic obstructive pulmonary disease has many presentations that often are very disabling and result in the use of oxygen at home. Patients often exhibit a mix of symptoms that characterize both emphysema and chronic bronchitis.

Daily activity for patients with COPD is usually limited, and small changes in their condition, including infections, can exceed the capacity of their lung function and cause them to seek emergency care. For example, a patient with COPD may be so limited that he or she can only walk short, level distances (e.g., to bathroom) at home and not up stairs. With a worsening of the condition, walking several steps may be the limit without severe shortness of breath.

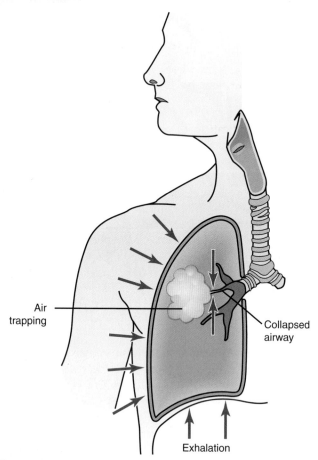

Figure 11-9 Air trapping occurs when the increased pressure in the thoracic cavity during expiration causes collapse of the small bronchioles, which are weakened by emphysema.

As an EMT, you should inquire if a patient with COPD uses home oxygen and determine the dose. Normal regulation for breathing is the amount of carbon dioxide in the blood. Because patients with COPD may retain and have very high levels of carbon dioxide, their brains may use the low oxygen (hypoxic) levels of the blood as the main drive to breathe. When administering supplemental oxygen to a patient with COPD, the hypoxic drive may be turned off by the increased oxygen in the blood, and the patient may experience hypoventilation or even respiratory arrest as a result. Therefore, you should be alert when treating COPD patients with supplemental oxygen. Oxygen should not be withheld for COPD patients in shock, with altered mental status, or in severe respiratory distress, but you should be prepared to monitor ventilations for signs of hypoventilation and to assist ventilations if necessary.

Respiratory Failure

Patients with emphysema and individuals with chronic bronchitis are subject to respiratory infections that can aggravate their condition. During these episodes, patients are subject to severe hypoxic states. The hypoxic state is caused by the further obstruction of the tracheobronchial tree by inflammation and swelling. In individuals who already have a decreased number of functional airways, any further deterioration can be life

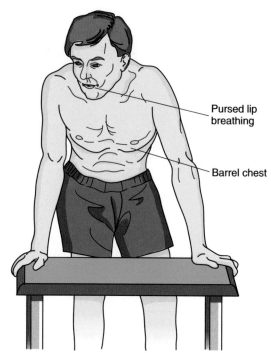

Figure 11-10 Patients with emphysema find they can breathe better if they exhale against resistance. They make this resistance by pursing their lips. To compensate for the loss of alveoli, the body produces more hemoglobin; thus the pink coloring of extra hemoglobin and the puffing sound from blowing against pursed lips.

threatening because they cannot deliver sufficient oxygen to the blood. When the respiratory system becomes so ineffective that it can no longer support life, these patients are said to be in a state of respiratory failure. At this point, your actions as an EMT are essential.

Case in Point

Two EMTs respond to a 16-year-old girl complaining of difficulty breathing. She states that the problem started about 1 hour ago while riding her bicycle. She has a history of asthma. She took 2 puffs on her metered-dose inhaler before the EMTs arrived.

On physical examination the EMTs note that the patient is alert and having severe difficulty breathing. Her blood pressure is 130/90, pulse 100 and regular, and respiratory rate 32 and labored. Breath sounds reveal wheezes throughout the lungs. She is exhibiting active accessory muscle use.

The EMTs place the patient in the upright position on a stretcher, assist in administration of an additional dose of her MDI, and attach her to a nonrebreather mask. En route to the hospital, her color improves, and her respirations decrease in rate and depth.

Asthma

Asthma is an obstructive respiratory disease that may occur suddenly and can affect both adults and children. Asthma is caused by constriction of the lower airways triggered by stress, infection, or allergy. The obstruction in the lower airways is the result of muscular contraction and spasm of the bronchioles (bronchoconstriction). It can be further complicated by the presence of secretions that contribute to blockage of the lower airways. The spasm and secretions reduce airflow to the alveoli and cause the patient to experience difficulty breathing (dyspnea). Protracted asthma (lasting years) can be a component of COPD. Most asthmatic patients can compensate for the narrowed airways by hyperventilation and can usually maintain adequate blood oxygen levels. However, if the attack does not improve with medications, which normally include prescribed inhalers, an asthmatic patient may become exhausted and enter respiratory failure. Steroids are medications taken orally and by inhaler that reduce inflammation and the severity and duration of asthma attacks.

An acute asthma attack is characterized by shortness of breath; the patient assumes the upright posture and uses accessory muscles to increase ventilation. The patient may be flushed and breathe forcefully. Wheezing and prolonged expirations may be audible, even without a stethoscope. As the work of breathing continues, the patient may become fatigued, leading to respiratory failure. With severe asthma attacks, patients become exhausted and may produce little airflow, have no wheezing, have difficulty speaking, and decreased breath sounds. Patients may need assisted ventilations during rapid transport to the hospital.

As noted earlier, bronchodilators, usually administered by MDI, are the main medications to treat asthma. In severe attacks, a more frequent treatment schedule than usually prescribed may be necessary. Look for the presence of such medication, and consult with medical direction regarding further administration before arrival at the hospital.

Pneumonia

Pneumonia is an inflammation of alveolar spaces caused by various types of infecting organisms or by aspiration of gastric contents into the tracheobronchial tree. The accumulating fluid is usually the result of the normal body defenses. The fluid may interfere with normal exchange of oxygen with blood.

Pneumonia may present in many ways depending on the underlying cause, but certain signs and symptoms are common. The disease often follows a pattern of upper respiratory tract infection (like the common cold), fever, and cough, with the production of thick, colored sputum (containing pus). In other cases, onset of cough, fever, and chills in either a previously healthy person or an immune-deficient patient (e.g., infected with HIV) can occur suddenly. Pneumonia caused by aspiration of stomach contents can follow unconscious states, including from excess alcohol and drug overdose.

Patients may complain of dyspnea (difficulty breathing), chills, headache, productive rusty-colored or bloody sputum, and pain that increases with breathing or coughing. The physical examination may reveal a fever. Breath sounds can include crackles and diminished sounds in local areas where the lung is infected.

Emergency care of the pneumonia patient is determined by the degree of distress. If the patient appears hypoxic but is ventilating adequately (as evidenced by adequate chest rise, respiratory rate, and an alert mental status), high concentrations of oxygen should be administered through a nonrebreather mask. Usually the patient will prefer to sit in the upright position to improve ventilatory efforts during transport. If signs of respiratory failure develop, including altered mental status (particularly sleepiness), minimal or no chest rise, diminished or absent breath sounds, or cyanosis, you should begin assisted ventilation with high-concentration supplemental oxygen. Although most patients with pneumonia are not contagious, some types of pneumonia are caused by contagious organisms; you should use droplet transmission precautions or airborne precautions as indicated.

Pulmonary Embolism

Blood clots that are released from the leg veins are the most common cause of pulmonary embolism. This can occur after surgery or in patients taking birth control medications. Fat emboli can also be released from long-bone fractures. As the clot is released, it travels up through the vena cava, into the right atrium and right ventricle, and then into the pulmonary artery. There the clot becomes lodged, obstructing blood flow to the lungs. The changes in lung circulation can cause severe hypoxia, sudden onset of difficulty breathing, and chest pain. When a large artery is involved, shock may result from obstruction of blood flow.

Patients typically complain of difficulty breathing and chest pain that increases with breathing. They may also cough up bloody sputum. The history may also reveal calf tenderness, recent history of surgery, prolonged bed rest, recent travel, use of oral contraceptives, and phlebitis (inflammation of leg veins).

The physical findings in a patient with pulmonary embolism are often normal. A rapid pulse and shock may be present in the worst cases. If there is significant obstruction of blood flow, the patient may exhibit signs of right-sided heart failure (see previous section). Signs of hypoxia, including cyanosis and altered mental status, may also be present.

High-concentration oxygen should be administered immediately. Treatment for shock should be provided as needed.

Hyperventilation Syndrome

A common respiratory problem is hyperventilation syndrome. These patients may feel as if they cannot breathe and may begin voluntarily to increase both the rate and the depth of breathing. This is often accompanied by anxiety. The increased minute ventilation that results from the increased rate and depth of breathing decreases the amount of carbon dioxide in the blood and changes the acidity of the blood. As a result, the patient may feel tingling around the mouth and fingers and dizziness. Sometimes the cause is an emotional event.

Patients experiencing hyperventilation syndrome usually have shortness of breath as their chief complaint. Frequently, the history of present illness reveals no other significant complaints. Patients often complain of tingling about the mouth and fingers, nausea, and a feeling of dizziness. In severe cases, the fingers and toes may go into a spasm, further frightening the patient.

Hyperventilation may be the suspected cause of a patient's respiratory distress, but it is best to make sure there is no underlying medical cause such as asthma or COPD. Supplemental oxygen will not hurt a patient who is hyperventilating and should be administered. The oxygen may help calm anxious patients and will treat patients with true respiratory distress while assessment and treatment continue. Calm reassurance is needed.

In the past, hyperventilating patients were sometimes asked to breathe into a paper bag. The rebreathing of expired air from a paper bag allowed the carbon dioxide concentration in their blood to return to normal more quickly. However, rebreathing from a paper bag also means that the patient breathes in more and more expired air. With every breath into the paper bag, the air in the bag has more carbon dioxide and less oxygen. This may cause some people to become hypoxic. Having a patient breathe more slowly through calm direction and reassurance also returns carbon dioxide levels to normal without the risk of breathing the lower oxygen in expired air.

Case in Point

Two EMTs respond to a thin, muscular 23-year-old man complaining of a sudden onset of difficulty breathing while at work at a construction site. He states that the difficulty breathing started suddenly 20 minutes ago associated with some chest pain, which worsens when taking a breath. The patient has no significant medical history.

On physical examination the EMTs note the patient is alert and in respiratory distress. His blood pressure is 120/80, pulse 96 and regular, and respiratory rate 28 and labored. Breath sounds are normal on the left side but significantly diminished on the right side. He is actively using his accessory muscles to breathe.

The EMTs place the patient in the sitting position on a stretcher and attach a nonrebreather mask. They suspect the patient has a spontaneous pneumothorax, given his physical findings and profile.

Spontaneous Pneumothorax

A spontaneous pneumothorax, or rupture of part of the lung, allows air to exit the lung and enter the space between the pleural lining of the chest cavity and the outer covering of the lung. When the lung ruptures and air enters the pleural space, the patient experiences a sudden onset of dyspnea and pleuritic chest pain. The lung may partially or totally collapse.

A spontaneous pneumothorax may occur in an otherwise-healthy patient who has congenital *blebs* (blisters on the lung wall) present since birth. For some reason, this event frequently occurs in thin, muscular young men and should be considered in patients complaining of dyspnea who fit this description. Breath sounds may be diminished or absent, depending on the degree of collapse when listening to the lung.

Key signs of spontaneous pneumothorax include sudden onset of the event and findings of diminished breath sounds on one side. It is very important to monitor the patient for progression of a simple pneumothorax to a *tension pneumothorax,* a condition that causes tension from the air in one chest cavity to compress the lung and heart to the other side. This may be recognized by absent breath sounds on one side, distended neck veins as the vena cava is collapsed, low blood pressure, and deviation of the trachea to the other side. Pneumothorax is discussed further in Chapter 22.

Croup and Epiglottitis

Croup and epiglottitis are two upper respiratory problems that occur primarily in children, although epiglottitis occasionally occurs in adults. Croup is a viral infection that causes swelling and narrowing of the upper airway, primarily at the level of the cricoid cartilage, just below the thyroid cartilage or Adam's apple. *Epiglottitis* is a bacterial infection that causes swelling of the epiglottis and can result in obstruction at the opening of the larynx.

Both conditions can lead to significant upper airway obstruction that can cause hypoxia and sometimes even a severe obstruction of the airway. The signs of croup and epiglottitis are similar, including fever, dyspnea, coughing, stridor or crowing, and signs of increased work of breathing (accessory muscle use and retractions). Both types of patients may assume the tripod position in an attempt to maintain an open airway.

Patients with epiglottitis may also complain of a sore throat, drooling, and difficulty swallowing caused by the pain of the inflamed epiglottis. Patients with croup may exhibit hoarseness of the voice. The management of these diseases includes administration of humidified oxygen, positioning, and positive-pressure ventilation, if needed. The specific management of croup and epiglottis is discussed in detail in Chapter 25.

Pertussis

Pertussis is a highly contagious bacterial infection of the respiratory system. It is transmitted through direct contact with the mucous membranes of the infected patient. Pertussis is commonly called "whooping cough." It is extremely common worldwide, with approximately 30 to 50 million cases per year and approximately 300,000 deaths (mostly children). There are approximately 5000 to 7000 cases in the United States each year.

The common symptoms include a high-pitched "whooping" cough that occurs in multiple spasms. In severe cases the patient may develop pneumonia, have fever, and exhibit signs of hypoxia. The treatment is primarily supportive, including the administration of oxygen by nonrebreather mask. Droplet precautions are important if you suspect pertussis, including gloves, eyewear, mask, and gown, particularly when suctioning or providing positive-pressure ventilation.

Scenario Follow-up

The opening scenario illustrates the importance of proper assessment of respiratory emergencies and coordination with medical control to manage a patient with respiratory distress. This patient had asthma and was found in acute respiratory distress, as confirmed by the history and physical findings, including use of accessory muscles and wheezing on auscultation. Administration of high-concentration oxygen and a metered-dose inhaler were important steps to open up the constricted bronchioles and ensure adequate oxygenation. These actions also helped prevent respiratory failure caused by muscle fatigue. Management of respiratory emergencies is a careful balance between preventing respiratory failure and arrest and treating the respiratory distress promptly when encountered.

Summary

Difficulty breathing is an anxiety-filled event for patients and families. Administration of oxygen and positive-pressure ventilations may be lifesaving therapy. Assisting certain patients with administration of prescribed inhalers can be of great value in the field. Such therapy is done in conjunction with an order from medical direction. As with other patients, the indication for treatment is based on assessment of the patient. When a patient shows signs of inadequate breathing, as evidenced by altered mental status, slow and irregular breathing, or other signs of respiratory failure, prompt actions can save the patient's life.

Skills

| **Skill 11-1** | *Administering Medication through a Nebulizer* |

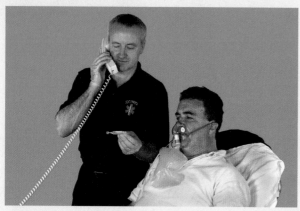

1. Check for allergies, and obtain an order from medical direction, either online or offline.

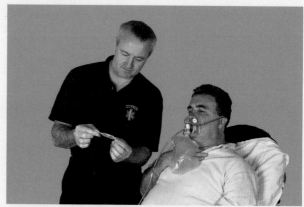

2. Check the medication *three times* for the following: correct medication, correct dose, correct patient, expiration date, loss of clarity or dislocation, and particulate matter.
- **First check:** When first selecting medication.
- **Second check:** After pouring medication into nebulizer.
- **Third check:** Before administering medication to the patient.

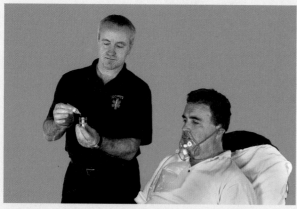

3. Pour contents of unit dose into nebulizer chamber.

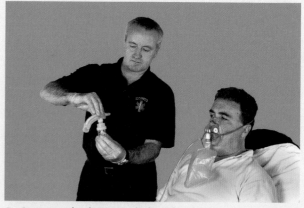

4. Screw top back onto nebulizer.

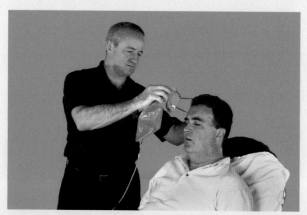

5. Remove the oxygen delivery device from the patient.

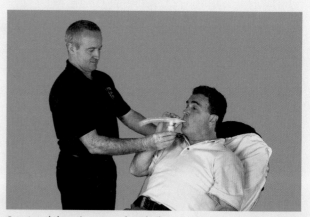

6a. In adult patient, attach nebulizer oxygen tubing to regulator and set at 6 L/min of flow. Instruct patient to breathe in and out through nebulizer mouthpiece.

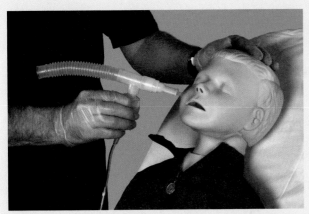

6b. In a young child, hold the mouthpiece at the opening of the patient's mouth and instruct the child to inhale normally *(blow-by technique)*.

7. Monitor patient and medication. Have the patient continue to breathe through the nebulizer until the medication is depleted, about 5 to 15 minutes.

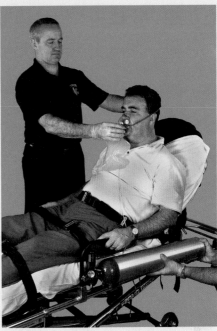

8. When nebulizer treatment is completed, reattach oxygen administration device.

Reevaluate the patient, and if appropriate, contact medical direction for additional treatment.

The Bottom Line

Learning Checklist

✓ Patients with respiratory emergencies typically have difficulty breathing, inadequate breathing, or respiratory arrest.

✓ Primary management of respiratory emergencies includes airway management, positive-pressure ventilation, administration of supplemental oxygen, positioning, and assisting patients in the administration of prescribed inhalers.

✓ Signs and symptoms of difficulty breathing include shortness of breath, restlessness, increased pulse rate, increased or decreased breathing rate, shallow or slow breathing, irregular breathing, abdominal breathing (diaphragm only), noisy breathing, crowing or stridor, audible wheezing, gurgling, snoring, inability to speak, pale or cyanotic skin, coughing, and tripod position.

✓ Signs of inadequate breathing include very slow and very rapid respiratory rates, shallow breathing evidenced by little or no chest rise, diminished or absent breath sounds, altered level of consciousness, seesaw breathing (infants and children), pale or cyanotic skin color, cool and clammy skin, and signs of increased work of breathing.

✓ Signs of increased work of breathing include accessory muscle use, retractions, and nasal flaring.

✓ Patients with dyspnea often sit bolt upright, supported by their hands in the tripod position.

✓ Management of the airway for the patient in respiratory distress may include clearing obstruction of the upper airway, suctioning, manual maneuvers to open the airway, and adjuncts to maintain a patent airway.

✓ Patients with respiratory distress should receive supplemental oxygen.

✓ Patient with signs of inadequate breathing should receive high-concentration supplemental oxygen and positive-pressure ventilation when needed.

✓ Patients with asthma and COPD may carry metered-dose inhalers (MDIs). You may have to assist these patients in administering the medication.

Key Terms

Asthma Obstructive respiratory disease with narrowing of the airways, usually precipitated by stress, infection, or an allergic response.

Chronic bronchitis Disease characterized by a productive cough for at least 3 months of the year for at least 2 consecutive years. Caused by inflammation of the bronchi with repeated attacks of coughing and sputum production.

Chronic obstructive pulmonary disease (COPD) Chronic respiratory condition that includes chronic bronchitis and emphysema; shortness of breath is the primary complaint; usually caused by smoking.

Emphysema Disease characterized by the destruction of alveoli and the loss of elastic recoil within the lung.

Metered-dose inhaler (MDI) Hand-held device for delivering medication through inhalation that allows for a controlled dose of the drug.

Nebulizer Device for producing a fine spray or mist that includes medication to be inhaled.

Respiratory failure The state that exists when the respiratory system becomes so ineffective that it can no longer support life.

Tripod position Position characterized by a posture that is upright and leaning forward with the head and neck thrust forward; associated with respiratory distress.

Review Questions

Questions 1-6. Indicate whether each of the following is generally associated with a or b:

1. Respiratory rate of 16 breaths/min
2. Active neck muscles
3. Cyanosis
4. Flaring of the nostrils
5. Seesaw breathing in children
6. Agonal breathing

   a. Adequate breathing.
   b. Respiratory distress or inadequate breathing.

7. You respond to a 16-year-old girl with difficulty breathing. She has a history of asthma. She is alert and speaking in short sentences and is exhibiting active accessory muscle use. Her vital signs are pulse 92 and regular, respirations 24 and labored, and blood pressure 140/80. Which of the following drugs is most likely prescribed for her condition?
   a. Albuterol
   b. Furosemide
   c. Prednisone
   d. Diazepam

8. Which of the following are appropriate actions when using a prescribed inhaler? (More than one answer may be correct.)
   a. Have patients hold their breath after administration.
   b. Spray the inhaler every 30 seconds until the breathing clears.
   c. Have patients seal their lips around the opening of the inhaler.
   d. Shake the inhaler vigorously several times before administration.

9. The primary effect of a prescribed inhaler is:
   a. Opening collapsed alveoli
   b. Dilating bronchioles
   c. Stimulating respiratory muscles
   d. Increasing the respiratory rate

10. After administering the prescribed inhaler, you perform a reassessment. Which of the following is a *likely* side effect of prescribed inhaler administration?

   a. Low blood pressure
   b. Rapid pulse
   c. Constriction of the pupils
   d. Dry skin

11. You respond to a 58-year-old man with difficulty breathing. He has a history of COPD. He is lethargic and has cyanotic lips and nail beds. His vital signs are pulse 120 and regular, respirations 36 and very shallow, and blood pressure 140/80. His breath sounds are barely audible in both lungs. Which of the following approaches is the appropriate management?

   a. Supplemental oxygen by nonrebreather mask
   b. Assisted ventilation with bag-mask
   c. Positive-pressure ventilation at 24 breaths/min
   d. Nasal cannula at 6 L/min

12. Which of the following signs is seen more often in children than in adults?

   a. Shortness of breath
   b. Retractions
   c. Increased respiratory rate
   d. Restlessness

13. You respond to a 3-year-old boy with difficulty breathing. He has had a fever for 24 hours and is making high-pitched sounds on inspiration. He is alert and agitated and is exhibiting active accessory muscle use. Which of the following conditions is the probable cause of this problem?

   a. Lower airway obstruction
   b. Fluid in the lungs
   c. Collapse of the alveoli
   d. Upper airway obstruction

For Further Review

In the Student Workbook

- Multiple-choice questions
- Matching questions
- Fill-in-the-blank questions
- Case scenario questions
- Skill check questions

On Evolve

- Chapter challenge
- Anatomy challenges
- Weblinks
- Exercises

Learning Objectives

Cognitive Objectives

- List the structures and functions of the respiratory system.
- State the signs and symptoms of a patient with breathing difficulty.
- Describe the emergency medical care of the patient with breathing difficulty.
- Describe the emergency medical care of the patient with respiratory distress.
- Establish the relationship between airway management and the patient with breathing difficulty.
- List signs of adequate air exchange.
- Recognize the need for medical direction to assist in the emergency medical care of the patient with breathing difficulty.
- State the generic name, medication forms, dose, administration, action, indications, and contraindications for the prescribed inhaler.
- Distinguish among the emergency medical care of the infant, child, and adult patient with breathing difficulty.
- Differentiate between upper airway obstruction and lower airway disease in the infant and child patient.

Affective Objectives

- Defend EMT treatment regimens for various respiratory emergencies.
- Explain the rationale for administering an inhaler.

Psychomotor Objectives

- Demonstrate the emergency medical care for breathing difficulty.
- Perform the steps in facilitating the use of an inhaler.

References

Guyton AC, Hall JE: *Textbook of medical physiology,* ed 11, Philadelphia, 2006, Saunders-Elsevier.

Haskell GH, Gausche-Hill M, American Heart Association: *Pediatric advanced life support,* ed 3, New York, 2007, McGraw-Hill.

Kovacs G, Law J: *Emergency airway management,* New York, 2008, McGraw-Hill.

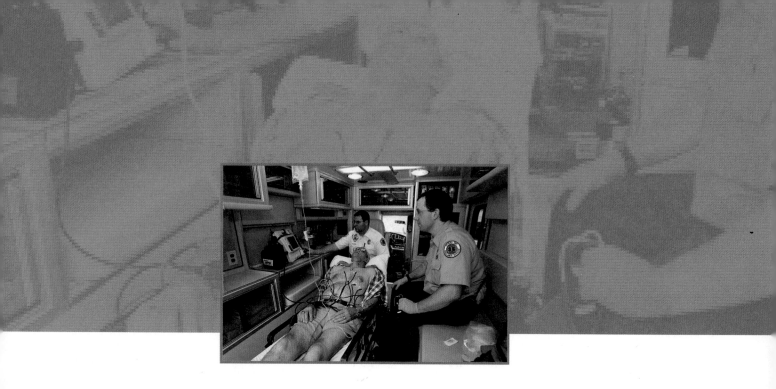

12 Cardiovascular Emergencies

CHAPTER OUTLINE

Chain of Survival

Anatomy and Physiology

Cardiovascular Disease

Acute Coronary Syndromes

Cardiopulmonary Resuscitation

Automated External Defibrillators

Skills

Scenario

You respond to the scene of a cardiac arrest. You enter the living room to find the police performing cardiopulmonary resuscitation (CPR) on a 52-year-old man. His wife states that he grabbed his chest and collapsed suddenly and that she immediately called 9-1-1. The total time from collapse to your arrival has been approximately 5 minutes, and CPR was begun 1 minute before your arrival.

You stop CPR briefly and assess the patient. The patient is not breathing, and there is no palpable pulse. You turn on the **automated external defibrillator (AED)** and connect the electrode pads. The AED analyzes the patient's electrocardiogram (ECG) rhythm and advises a shock. You clear the patient and press the shock button. The patient's muscles contract as the shock is delivered. You immediately perform 5 cycles of CPR over 2 minutes, stop, and allow the AED to reanalyze. The AED analyzes a second time, and you repeat the shock sequence of "all clear" and press the shock button. You immediately start CPR, monitoring the quality of compressions and minimizing interruptions to ensure adequate perfusion of vital organs, including the brain and heart.

After another 2 minutes and 5 cycles of CPR, you determine that the patient is moving and breathing. He makes weak, ineffective respiratory gasps, and you assist his breathing with a bag-mask. The patient gradually increases his own respiratory rate and shows signs of adequate ventilation. You administer high-concentration oxygen by a nonrebreather mask, and he exhibits some voluntary movement and opens his eyes.

Paramedics arrive at the door, and you give a quick report as you transfer care of the patient. They start an intravenous line and administer medications to help prevent recurrence of the lethal rhythm. The patient's wife, who has witnessed the entire scene, has tears in her eyes. As you look around the room, you realize that you have participated in the "chain of survival" that saved this patient's life.

LEARNING OBJECTIVES
- Define the role of the EMT in the emergency cardiac care system.
- Predict the relationship between basic life support and the patient experiencing cardiovascular compromise.
- Explain the rationale for early defibrillation.
- Explain why cardiac arrest does not occur in all patients with chest pain and why all do not need to be attached to an AED.
- Discuss the role of the American Heart Association in the use of automated external defibrillation.
- Discuss the fundamentals of early defibrillation.

More than 340,000 patients die each year from sudden cardiac arrest. Most of these deaths occur outside the hospital. For many patients, collapse from sudden cardiac arrest is their first sign of heart disease.

To prevent unnecessary deaths from heart disease, the American Heart Association (AHA) promotes the concept of the *chain of survival,* which includes early access to 9-1-1, early CPR, early defibrillation, and early advanced care (**Figure 12-1**). In the introductory case scenario, every component of the chain of survival worked to save a life. The patient had early access to emergency cardiac care when his wife witnessed the collapse and immediately called 9-1-1; police, acting as first responders, delivered early CPR; the emergency medical technician (EMT) applied early defibrillation; and paramedics arrived to provide advanced cardiac life support to help stabilize the patient's condition.

Chain of Survival

The chain of survival is designed to deliver CPR to perfuse the brain and heart during cardiac arrest, provide early defibrillation to restore a normal heart rhythm, and prevent subsequent cardiac arrest after successful resuscitation by providing advanced care. Most patients with a sudden onset of cardiac arrest have **ventricular fibrillation,** a useless quivering of the heart in which no circulation is possible. **Defibrillation,** which is the application of electrical shock through the chest wall to the heart, stops the quivering and allows the heart to establish a normal rhythm. Early defibrillation offers the best chance for survival in most patients with sudden cardiac arrest. For every minute that passes from the time of sudden cardiac arrest until defibrillation, the chance for survival decreases by 7% to 10% (**Figure 12-2**). If the patient's heart is defibrillated within 5 minutes, the chance for survival is approximately 50%. If defibrillation is delayed by 10 to 12 minutes, the chance of survival drops to approximately 2% to 5%.

Early access (recognizing the need for help and calling 9-1-1) is designed to deliver a **defibrillator** to the patient's side as quickly as possible. While the defibrillator is en route, CPR is used to sustain life by circulating oxygenated blood to the brain. However, CPR cannot reverse ventricular fibrillation; this can be achieved only by prompt defibrillation. *Early advanced cardiac care,* including drugs and advanced airway skills, supports the patient after defibrillation and is necessary to resuscitate patients who experience cardiac arrest from rhythms other than ventricular fibrillation. Defibrillation and advanced modalities administered by the EMT are performed under medical direction, usually by standing orders or written protocols. In some cases, review of calls by medical direction can be facilitated by the simultaneous documentation of care recorded in the defibrillator's medical control module.

REAL*World*

With the recognition that early defibrillation in conjunction with CPR offers patients in cardiac arrest the best chance of survival, there has been a push for **public access defibrillation (PAD).** Public access AED is when AED units are placed in public areas for use by any trained individual. AEDs can be found in hotels, airports, and schools. For example, the use of AEDs in Las Vegas casinos has resulted in a 60% survival rate of patients with sudden cardiac arrest. When patients received shocks within 3 minutes, the survival rate was greater than 75%. Public access AEDs are usually found next to other rescue equipment (e.g., fire extinguishers) and are marked with a heart and lightning bolt. In some cases, an EMT may arrive on scene to discover that a patient in cardiac arrest has an AED already in place and may have already received a shock. In the 1990s, the concept of early defibrillation was taken to a new level by encouraging the use of AEDs by trained laypersons.

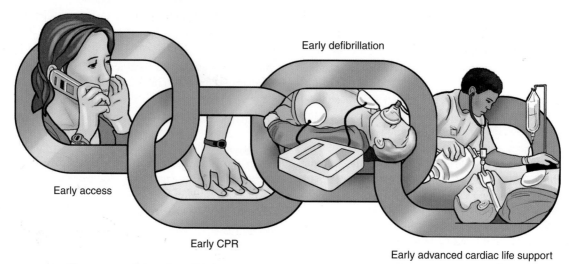

Figure 12-1 Chain of survival. *From Aehlert B:* ACLS study guide, *ed 3, St Louis, 2007, Mosby.*

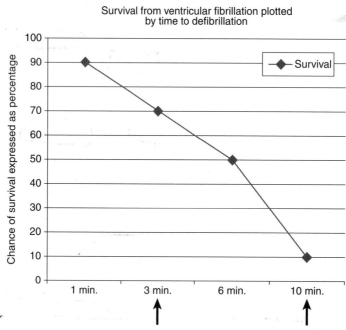

Survival from ventricular fibrillation plotted by time to defibrillation

Figure 12-2 Survival from sudden cardiac death caused by ventricular fibrillation is time sensitive. With every minute that passes, the chance for survival decreases by 7% to 10%. This graph clearly shows why methods to ensure early access to defibrillation, including EMS response time, first-responder programs such as police and fire personnel with AEDs, and public access defibrillation by laypersons, are so important to the patient in cardiac arrest. The arrow at the 3-minute interval shows that early defibrillation offers the patient a 70% chance for survival. The arrow after the 10-minute mark shows how late defibrillation offers the patient a 10% (or less) chance of surviving.

Not all patients with chest pain go into cardiac arrest. In fact, most do not. However, the patient with a heart attack will also benefit from the chain of survival. Because these patients are at high risk for sudden death, the chain of survival ensures that a defibrillator is brought to the patient's side in case ventricular fibrillation occurs. In addition, early treatment with oxygen, drugs, and advanced cardiac techniques can limit the damage to the heart and prevent cardiac arrest.

As an EMT, you will perform the following functions for the patient with chest pain or sudden cardiac arrest:

- Bring oxygen to the patient's side.
- Assist the patient with administration of prescribed nitroglycerin.
- Provide defibrillation when sudden cardiac arrest occurs.
- Request advanced life support (ALS) assistance at the scene.
- Provide prompt transportation for hospital-based treatment.
- Communicate assessment findings to healthcare providers at the hospital for timely administration of advanced care en route or at the receiving hospital.

You will encounter three major categories of patients with heart disease: (1) patients with ischemic chest pain, (2) patients with heart failure, and (3) patients who sustain sudden cardiac death.

LEARNING OBJECTIVE
• Describe the structure and function of the cardiovascular system.

Anatomy and Physiology

The circulatory system is the transport system of the body. It delivers oxygen and nutrients to the tissues and returns the waste products of metabolism (carbon dioxide and cellular wastes) to the lungs and kidneys for exhalation and excretion from the body.

The tissues of the body depend on an adequate supply of oxygen for survival. A compromise in circulation can lead to tissue damage or death. The most oxygen-sensitive tissues are those of the central nervous system (CNS) and the heart; therefore examination of these organ systems may reveal the earliest signs of inadequate oxygenation. Accordingly, rapid assessment of brain and circulatory function is given priority in the early part of every patient assessment. The EMT must be able to recognize the indicators of cardiovascular failure quickly and to administer prompt emergency treatment.

Proper functioning of the circulatory system depends on the following three components:

• Heart
• Blood
• Blood vessels

These components are interdependent. Oxygen and nutrients are transported in the blood. The vessels are the pathways that direct blood to the various cells of the body. The heart is the pump that provides the driving force necessary to keep the blood circulating.

Heart

The heart is responsible for generating blood flow to all parts of the body. The force must be sufficient to open the vessels so that blood can pass through and thereby perfuse the body's organs and tissues. When cardiac arrest occurs, blood flow ceases and the organs of the body become deprived of oxygen and begin to die.

The inner portion of the heart is divided into four chambers: right atrium, left atrium, right ventricle, and left ventricle.

The right atrium collects blood from the body through the inferior and superior venae cavae. This blood then flows down through the tricuspid valve and into the right ventricle (**Figure 12-3**). The right ventricle pumps blood through the lungs, where the hemoglobin in the red blood cells (RBCs) picks up oxygen across the alveoli and the blood releases carbon dioxide for exhalation from the body. Blood returning to the heart from the pulmonary circulation is now saturated with oxygen, and it collects in the left atrium. Blood then flows from the left atrium to the left ventricle through the mitral valve.

The left ventricle pumps oxygen-rich blood (and other nutrients) to the rest of the body, where it is needed for energy. Blood returning to the heart from the systemic circulation collects in the right atrium. Thus, blood is returned to the pulmonary circulation to begin the cycle once again. **Figure 12-4** shows how blood flows through both the pulmonary and the systemic circulation.

Conduction System

The heart has a conduction system composed of specialized tissues that "fire" or depolarize and transmit impulses that order the rhythmic contraction and relaxation of the heart's cells. The conduction system is anatomically designed so that the atria contract first, followed by the ventricles. For example, during ventricular relaxation, the atria contract and help fill the ventricles with blood. During ventricular contraction, the ventricles pump blood out through the arteries.

The conduction system starts with the firing of the sinoatrial node (the **pacemaker** of the heart, located in the right atrium) and depolarization of the atria (upper chambers of the heart). The sinoatrial node discharges, or fires, about 60 to 80 times a minute in an adult at rest and begins an electrical impulse that spreads through the atria and then down through the ventricles. This electrical event can be recorded on an electrocardiogram (ECG). Each part of the event is represented by a wave. The P wave represents the depolarization (movement of electrically charged ions across a cell membrane) of the atria. The QRS complex represents the depolarization of the ventricle. When abnormal heart rhythms occur, such as ventricular fibrillation, the shape and rate of these waveforms change and can be interpreted by a trained professional or through a computer analysis in specialized ECG devices or AEDs.

Cardiac Output

Cardiac output refers to the volume of blood pumped by the heart in 1 minute. It is calculated by multiplying the number of heartbeats per minute times the amount of blood pumped with each beat. The amount of blood ejected with each beat is referred to as the stroke volume.

$$\text{Heart rate (beats/min)} \times \text{Stroke volume (mL/beat)} = \text{Cardiac output (mL/min)}$$

Normally, the stroke volume is approximately 70 milliliters (mL) of blood. If the average heart rate is 70 beats/min, the cardiac output is calculated as follows:

$$70 \text{ beats/min} \times 70 \text{ mL/beat} = 4900 \text{ mL/min of cardiac output (mL/min)}$$
(or approximately 5 liters of blood per minute)

The amount of blood pumped out of the heart varies from minute to minute, depending on the changing needs of the body. Muscles require more oxygen during exercise and less during rest. If the heart rate is too slow or the volume pumped with each beat is decreased as a result of heart damage, cardiac output will decrease. This can cause weakness, low blood pressure, and other signs of shock.

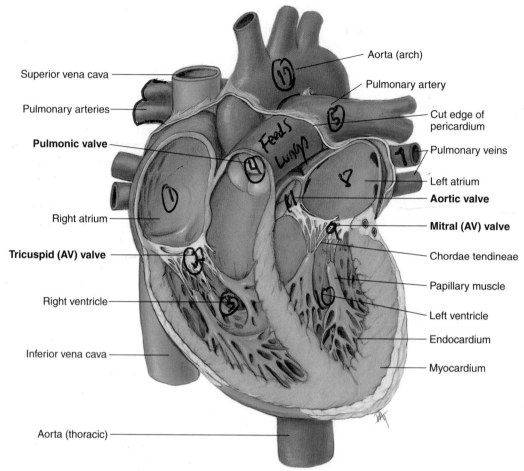

Figure 12-3 Internal view of the heart. *Modified from Jarvis C: Physical examination and health assessment, ed 3, Philadelphia, 2000, Saunders.*

Blood Vessels

The three major types of blood vessels are arteries, capillaries, and veins. Together these vessels form a branching network that directs the blood through every part of the body. The arteries direct blood flowing away from the heart. The veins direct blood returning to the heart. Capillaries are located between the arteries and veins. The capillaries are thin-walled vessels that come into close contact with the cells so that the exchange of oxygen, nutrients, and waste products between the blood and cells can occur.

The structure of vessels in the body has often been compared with a tree because of the continuous branching. The arterial system subdivides while branching until it reaches the size of the arterioles, whose diameter is approximately that of a hair. The capillary network begins beyond the arterioles and further subdivides to ensure close contact with the cells. The capillaries then start to reconnect, thereby forming the smallest veins, called venules. The venules begin to unite and form larger and still larger tubes, the veins, which ultimately connect with the inferior or superior vena cava and the pulmonary veins.

The major arteries where the pulse can be palpated at the skin's surface include the following (**Figure 12-5**):
- Carotid artery
- Radial artery
- Brachial artery
- Femoral artery
- Posterior tibial artery
- Dorsalis pedis artery

Blood Pressure

Blood pressure is the force exerted by the blood volume on the walls of the vessels. Blood pressure depends on the volume of blood within the vessels and the size of the vascular space. When blood is pumped into the arteries during ventricular contraction (systole), the amount of blood in the arteries increases and the pressure rises. The pressure measured during systole is the systolic blood pressure. As the heart relaxes (diastole) and the aortic valve closes, blood continues to move forward through vessels at a lower pressure. The pressure measured during diastole is the diastolic blood pressure.

Microcirculation

The entire circulatory system is designed to bring blood to the lungs and body tissues in order to deliver oxygen and other nutrients and remove carbon dioxide and other waste products to meet the body's needs. The capillaries are close to the body's cells, separated by a fluid that bathes them, called *interstitial fluid*. The capillaries are so narrow that RBCs must pass through them one at a time.

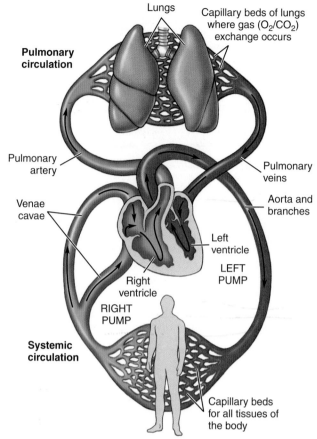

Figure 12-4 Pulmonary and systemic circulation. *From Herlihy B, Maebius N: The human body in health and illness, Philadelphia, 2000, Saunders.*

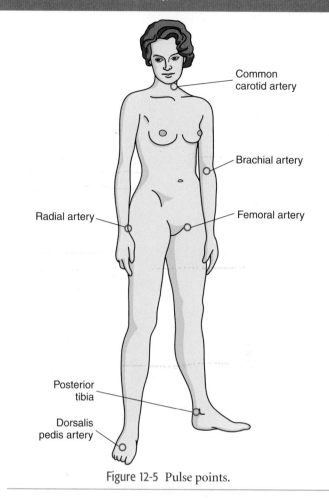

Figure 12-5 Pulse points.

Pores or openings in the wall of the capillaries allow small particles and water to pass into the interstitial fluid surrounding the capillary. Likewise, water and other particles can pass back into the capillary from the interstitial fluid. Normally, larger particles and RBCs cannot pass through the capillary walls. However, through special mechanisms, white blood cells (WBCs) can travel through to sites of infection. The natural forces that allow this movement of fluid and particles include diffusion, osmosis, and hydrostatic pressure.

Diffusion

Diffusion is a process in which particles move from an area of *higher* concentration to an area of *lower* concentration to reach a state of equilibrium. For example, if there were 100 particles of X on side A of a space and no particles of X on side B of a space, the particles would tend to move to side B until there were approximately 50 particles of X on both sides. This concept is best illustrated in the movement of oxygen (O_2) and carbon dioxide (CO_2) in the lungs and body tissues. When blood returns to the lungs, there are less O_2 particles and more CO_2 particles than in the alveoli of the lungs. Through the process of diffusion, CO_2 moves from the capillaries (where there is more) to the alveoli (where there is less), whereas O_2 moves from the alveoli (where there is more) into the capillaries (where there is less). Take a

moment and review Figure 4-22 in Chapter 4 to appreciate how this force works.

Capillary Blood Pressure and Osmosis

The continuous movement of fluid and particles from the capillaries into the interstitial fluid and back again is called *microcirculation*. The primary force that moves fluid and particle into the interstitial fluid is the blood pressure or *hydrostatic pressure* within the capillary. As the blood travels through the capillary, pressure is exerted on the walls of the capillaries. This hydrostatic pressure drives fluid and particles into the interstitial fluid. If this were the only force, there would be an imbalance, resulting in a disproportionate amount of fluid remaining in the interstitial space.

The primary force that brings fluid back into the capillaries is called *osmosis*. Osmosis is the process in which fluid moves from an area of *lower* concentration of particles to an area of *higher* concentration of particles. Large particles suspended in blood (e.g., plasma proteins) exert a "pulling force" on water. This pulling force draws fluid to the particles.

The primary particles in blood that exert this pulling force are large particles called *plasma proteins*. Because plasma proteins are predominantly found in blood, this creates a return of water movement to balance the effects created by hydrostatic pressure within the capillary. Essentially, hydrostatic

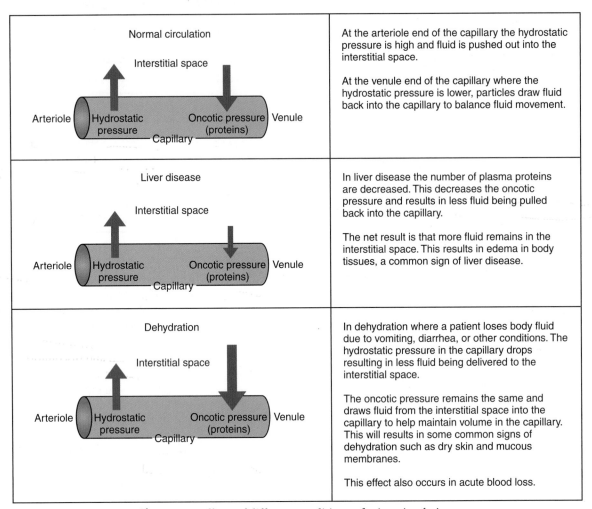

Figure 12-6 Effects of different conditions of microcirculation.

pressure moves fluid out of the capillary, and the osmotic pulling force, called *oncotic pressure,* pulls fluid back into the capillary. These pushing and pulling forces create a balance that ensures adequate fluid in both compartments. This is important, because too much or too little fluid in either compartment would result in potentially serious problems, including dehydration, hypovolemia, and fluid in the lungs (pulmonary edema).

Problems that disturb the fluid balance can occur in essentially the following two ways:

1. The pressure in the capillary can rise or fall, resulting in a net increase or decrease in fluid movement into the interstitial space.

2. The amount of proteins that reside in the capillaries can increase or decrease, resulting in a net increase or decrease in the amount of fluid movement back into the capillaries.

These scenarios can occur with different diseases or conditions, including liver disease, blood loss, heart failure, dehydration, and hypovolemia. Review the different scenarios in **Figure 12-6** to better appreciate implications of microcirculation, hydrostatic pressure, and osmosis.

Shock

Shock is a state of inadequate circulation in which vital tissues of the body are poorly perfused (hypoperfusion) and vital processes of the body fail. Shock results in diminished perfusion of blood through the capillaries and inadequate oxygenation of organs.

Shock or hypoperfusion can occur when any of the three parts of the circulatory system fails. For example, a low blood volume, which can occur from bleeding, may not fill the vascular space, and the blood pressure falls. If the blood vessels are too dilated, even a normal blood volume cannot fill the vascular tree, and pressure drops. If the heart muscle is damaged, blood is not propelled normally through the vessels, and again, blood pressure can decrease.

Whatever the cause, shock results in inadequate perfusion of the body's tissues, and if the state of shock is prolonged, injury and death to body cells result. The body may release epinephrine to compensate in an effort to increase blood pressure and shunt blood preferentially to more vital organs. Signs of epinephrine release may be found in addition to symptoms of hypoperfusion. **Table 12-1** presents signs and symptoms of inadequate circulation.

Patients with signs and symptoms of shock, regardless of the cause, are high-priority patients. Treatment of shock from cardiac damage *(cardiogenic shock)* is limited in prehospital care. Along with rapid transport to a hospital facility, important steps include securing an airway, ensuring the patient can breathe, and ensuring oxygenation.

Case in Point

Two EMTs respond to a patient with chest pain at his home. The patient states that the chest pain started approximately 30 minutes ago, accompanied by perfuse sweating, nausea, and dizziness. The EMTs quickly perform a focused history specific to the chief complaint of chest pain. They note that onset (30 minutes) was relatively recent and discover that the pain occurred while the patient was at rest. The pain radiated to the left arm and neck. The patient characterizes the squeezing pain as a "9" on a scale from 1 to 10, continuing unrelieved after taking one nitroglycerin tablet. The patient has a history of high blood pressure, angina, and diabetes. His prescribed medications include Acupril (blood pressure), nitroglycerin, and a diuretic.

On physical examination the EMTs note the patient is alert, pale, and sweaty. His blood pressure is 120/80 and pulse grossly irregular. The EMTs administer oxygen and assist in administration of a second nitroglycerin tablet and a chewable aspirin. They recognize that the patient is likely experiencing acute coronary syndromes and would benefit from therapies provided at the hospital ("clot busters" and angioplasty) and that he is also at high risk for sudden cardiac arrest.

The EMTs quickly transport the patient to the ambulance on a rolling cot stretcher. In the ambulance they prepare for a potential cardiac arrest by keeping the mouth-to-mask device, bag-mask, cardiac resuscitation board, and AED at the ready. On arrival at the emergency department, the patient experiences cardiac arrest and is successfully defibrillated back to a normal rhythm.

The appropriate attention to detail saved this patient's life.

Cardiovascular Disease

The leading cause of death in the United States is cardiovascular disease and its resulting complications. These diseases and complications include acute coronary syndromes (e.g., myocardial infarction, angina), heart failure, and sudden cardiac death.

Pathophysiology of Acute Coronary Syndromes

Arteriosclerosis

As with any other body tissue, the heart must have a continuous supply of oxygen. **Arteriosclerosis** is a progressive disease of the arteries that results in narrowing of the lumen of arteries because of deposits of fat and hardening of the arterial wall. *Coronary artery disease* (CAD) begins when fatty deposits accumulate in the walls of the coronary arteries, which carry blood to the heart itself. As more and more of these deposits accumulate, the internal diameter of the artery narrows, and less blood can flow through. This process is also known as "hardening of the arteries."

The accumulation of fatty deposits takes many years. During the early stages of the disease, there may be no symptoms. A person is completely unaware of what is taking place in the

Table 12-1	Signs and Symptoms of Inadequate Circulation
Sign or Symptom	**Cause/Explanation**
Weakness or altered mental status	Poor perfusion to muscles and brain
Anxiety and restlessness	Side effects of epinephrine release
Pale, cool, and clammy skin	Epinephrine release, reducing circulation to less vital organs (skin, gut) so that blood is redistributed to heart, lung, and brain
Rapid, weak pulse	Increased heart rate to compensate for failing circulatory system

body. As the arteries continue to narrow, however, less and less blood can pass through (**Figure 12-7**).

The first indication of CAD may occur under conditions of physical or emotional stress. At such times, the heart beats faster, and the heart muscle needs more oxygen than the obstructed coronary arteries can deliver. Pain and discomfort in the chest develop when insufficient oxygen is delivered to the heart. If the person stops to rest, the pain may disappear. This type of CAD, which causes pain after exertion or stress and is relieved by rest, is called angina pectoris (Latin for "chest pain").

Myocardial Oxygen Supply and Demand

Normally, oxygen delivered by blood flow through the coronary arteries matches the needs of the heart muscle. A mismatch occurs when an increase in the heart's work is not met with a corresponding increase in blood supply. For example, if a person has narrowed coronary arteries, the heart muscle may not receive adequate blood to meet the increased oxygen needs during stress or exercise. A mismatch can also occur when the heart's ordinary needs (at rest) are not met because of a blockage of blood flow through the coronary arteries. For example, a thrombus, or blood clot, can form in a coronary artery and severely limit or obstruct blood flow to part of the heart. When this happens, not enough oxygen is delivered, even at rest, to meet the needs of the myocardial tissue.

Myocardial Ischemia and Myocardial Infarction

Ischemia refers to a state of decreased blood flow to an organ or tissue, causing problems—but not permanent damage—if corrected. *Infarction* refers to a more severe obstruction resulting in necrosis or death of heart cells. Myocardial ischemia occurs when there is not enough blood flow to satisfy the oxygen needs of the myocardium. Myocardial ischemia that causes pain during stress or exertion but no permanent damage to the heart muscle is called *angina* or angina pectoris. **Myocardial infarction** is severe and sustained oxygen deprivation of the myocardium that results in the death of heart cells. This group of illnesses characterized by ischemia to heart tissue is known as acute coronary syndromes.

Because the consequences of ischemic heart disease include severe pump failure, life-threatening heart rhythms *(dysrhythmias)*, permanent damage to myocardial muscle, and

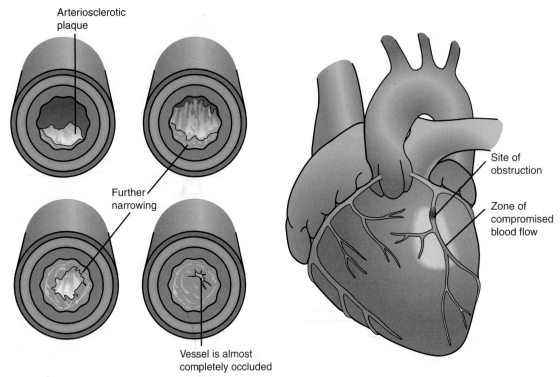

Figure 12-7 Progression of arteriosclerosis. An arteriosclerotic plaque forms on the lining of the vessel and projects into the lumen. As the plaque enlarges, it provides a rough surface that can lead to the formation of a thrombus that further narrows the vessel lumen. Eventually, the opening is too narrow to supply the heart's oxygen needs, and the surrounding tissue becomes ischemic or dies. *Modified from American Heart Association:* Health provider's manual for basic life support, *AHA, 1990.*

sudden death, patients with ischemic chest pain are treated with the highest priority.

LEARNING OBJECTIVES
- Describe the emergency medical care of the patient experiencing chest pain or discomfort.
- Discuss the position of comfort for patients with various cardiac emergencies.
- Establish the relationship between airway management and the patient experiencing cardiovascular compromise.
- Recognize the need for medical direction of protocols to assist in the emergency medical care of the patient with chest pain.

💿 Acute Coronary Syndromes

Cardiac patients may have many signs or symptoms, but the most common chief complaint is chest pain. After conducting an initial (primary) assessment, administering oxygen, and assessing ventilation, you should perform the focused (secondary) assessment (history and physical examination). Because patients with chest pain are priority patients, you might complete the focused assessment while en route to the hospital.

Scene Size-up

As always, ensure that the scene is safe, and take the appropriate body substance isolation precautions. Identify the mechanism of injury or illness; what was the patient doing when the discomfort began? During a call for chest pain or shortness of breath, patients may benefit from additional resources, such as an ALS response. Quickly consider the need for ALS, and notify dispatch early. For example, patients with an altered mental status or patients who appear to be in shock may benefit from early ALS because they may have an impending cardiac arrest or a serious treatable dysrhythmia.

Initial (Primary) Assessment

Form a general impression of the patient to identify the need for priority care. Identify the patient's chief complaint, age, and gender. Is there evidence of a life-threatening condition? For example, if the patient with chest pain has an altered mental status, you may need to prepare for an impending cardiac arrest. This would include having an airway kit and AED readily available on the scene.

Assess the mental status and the ABCs (airway, breathing circulation). If alert, the patient may prefer the sitting position. If the patient appears weak, the supine position may be more comfortable. Consider the need for management of the airway and ventilation. You should also note the rate, regularity, and quality of the patient's pulse and check for signs of poor perfusion. Again, in patients with chest pain, these signs and symptoms may suggest an impending cardiac arrest. Patients with chest pain should receive high-concentration supplemental oxygen. Patients with signs of shock or difficulty breathing should receive high-concentration oxygen by nonrebreather mask, and you should consider the need for positive-pressure ventilation.

Box 12-1 Collecting a SAMPLE History for Patients with Cardiac Complaints

Signs and Symptoms

- What is bothering you?
- Why did you call the ambulance?
- In addition to the chief complaint (i.e., chest pain), is there anything else bothering you?

    Associated complaints may include difficulty breathing, leg swelling, or pain in other locations. If there are associated complaints, establish the sequence of events. Then develop the chief complaint and the history of the present illness more fully with the OPQRST approach:

Onset: What were you doing when the pain (or other symptoms) began?

Provocation: Does anything make the pain (or other symptoms) better or worse? Have you had this pain (or other symptoms) before? Does it get better with rest? Do you take medication for it, such as nitroglycerin?

Quality: How would you describe the pain? Where is the pain? Can you point to the area with one finger? Is there any associated pain? Is the pain made worse by breathing?

Radiation: Does your pain go anywhere (such as to your arm, neck, or jaw)?

Severity: Describe the pain on a scale of 1 to 10 (with 10 being the worst pain you have ever experienced and 1 being hardly painful at all), and compare it with previous experiences (if appropriate).

Time: When did the pain (or other symptoms) first occur? How long have you had the pain (or other symptoms)?

Allergies and Medications

- Do you have any allergies? What medications are you taking? Bring the medications to the hospital if available.

Past Medical History

- Do you have any serious medical or surgical conditions for which you are receiving medical care or that have resulted in hospital admissions?

    Common conditions that may be associated with a cardiac complaint include heart disease, heart surgery, or chronic obstructive pulmonary disease. You are not looking for every condition or a life history. Keep this part of the history focused.

Last Oral Intake

- When was the last time you ate or drank anything?

Events Leading up to the Present Illness

If there are multiple complaints or associated complaints, establish a brief time sequence of events. For example, a patient might have first had pain in his chest, which then traveled down his arm before he started to become short of breath.

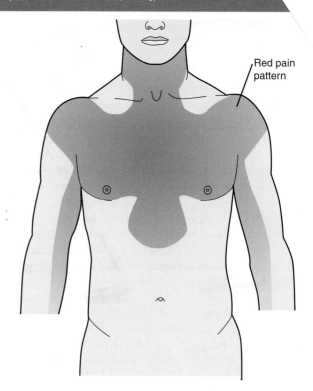

Red pain pattern

Figure 12-8 Possible pain patterns in ischemic chest pain. Pain may radiate from chest to neck, jaw, or arms, or it may be felt only as an ache outside the chest.

Sample history

during a SAMPLE history (see Chapter 7 and Table 7-6). Box 12-1 lists questions to ask when chest pain is the chief complaint.

Signs and Symptoms. Patients with **ischemic chest pain** usually complain of intense pain described as crushing, pressing, tight, viselike, heavy, aching, or constricting. Other descriptions may include burning or discomfort in the chest. The pain is usually located in the anterior chest and often radiates to the neck, jaw, either arm or shoulder (more often the left), or rarely to the back. At times, pain occurs just in the arm or jaw (**Figure 12-8**). Patients may describe the pain while placing a clenched fist across the chest. The pain usually lasts for several minutes, often more than 30 minutes, and may be relieved with rest or nitroglycerin (this drug may or may not be used to treat patients with angina). In a small percentage of patients, pain may not be the chief complaint. This is most likely to occur in women, older patients, or patients with diabetes. These patients might have shortness of breath, weakness, or altered mental status. Patients may also equate the pain with indigestion, located in the upper abdomen (epigastric region). Associated complaints may include the following:

- Nausea
- Vomiting
- Weakness
- Shortness of breath
- Palpitations
- Lightheadedness
- Sweating
- Dizziness
- Loss of consciousness

Focused (Secondary) Assessment

SAMPLE History

A patient may voluntarily elaborate on the nature of the chief complaint. Chest pain and shortness of breath are common. When evaluating pain or shortness of breath, remember the OPQRST mnemonic when asking about signs and symptoms

Allergies and Medications. Ask the patient if he or she has allergies and what medications are being taken; you should bring the medications to the hospital if they are available.

Pertinent Past Medical History. The patient may have a history of angina, heart attack, other heart disease, diabetes, or hypertension. The medication history may reveal cardiac or hypertensive drug therapy. If a patient has had a previous heart attack or a history of angina, inquire whether the present symptoms are similar to those experienced in the past.

A record of the last oral intake and events surrounding the chief complaint complete the SAMPLE history.

Physical Examination

The patient may be apprehensive, anxious, and fearful or may deny that the symptoms being experienced are serious. If the patient's mental status is altered or the patient is lethargic, drowsy, or cannot be aroused, these findings may indicate low cardiac output from associated heart failure or dysrhythmia. Examine the neck for jugular vein distention (indicating backup of blood returning to the heart) and use of accessory muscles of breathing.

Palpation is a valuable part of the physical examination. At times, the chest wall may be tender to palpation in an area where the patient complains of chest pain. You should interpret this tenderness with caution. Some patients might have had recent trauma in the tender area. Ask if they had a recent injury. Some patients with heart attack or myocardial infarction may describe tenderness of the chest when you palpate their chest, but their complaint of pain is separate and distinct from any chest wall tenderness.

Baseline Vital Signs

A range of vital signs may be encountered. Associated preexisting medical conditions (e.g., hypertension), the patient's psychological response to the chest pain, epinephrine release, and the extent and location of the infarction to the myocardium can all contribute to changes in the patient's vital signs. Rapid or slow pulses are common, as are variations in blood pressure. Some patients may have normal vital signs.

The patient's skin may appear pale and feel cool and sweaty. Listen to the lungs and note the presence of equal breath sounds as well as any abnormal sounds, such as rales. The patient's condition should be closely monitored en route to the hospital for changes in mental status or vital signs.

Ongoing Assessment or Reassessment

Cardiac patients are subject to a variety of complications. The patient should be continually reevaluated while en route to the hospital. Check vital signs and monitor the patient's mental status and the response to therapy. Check for continuation of pain and dyspnea as well as the rate, rhythm, and quality of the pulse. To avoid delay in the event of sudden cardiac arrest, the AED and mechanical aids for CPR (bag-mask, suction, backboard) should be readily available.

Transportation

Make a priority transportation decision for patients with chest pain. If a patient is having myocardial ischemia or a myocardial infarction, time to treatment with *fibrinolytic* (thrombus-dissolving) drugs or coronary interventions such as *angioplasty*

Box 12-2 Protocol for Responsive Cardiac Patient
1. Perform the initial (primary) assessment
2. Ensure an open airway and consider the need for:
• Manual maneuvers (head-tilt/chin-lift, jaw thrust)
• An oropharyngeal or nasopharyngeal airway
• Suction
3. Evaluate the adequacy of breathing and consider need for positive-pressure ventilation
4. Administer supplemental oxygen
5. Reduce activity and anxiety
6. Carry the patient to the ambulance in a position of comfort
7. Prioritize transport
8. Consider administration of nitroglycerin
9. Perform ongoing assessment en route to the hospital

(mechanically opening the blocked artery) is the most critical factor in preserving heart muscle and preventing death. Transportation should be rapid but quiet. Avoid the use of sirens whenever possible. Notify the hospital about the imminent arrival of a patient with suspected myocardial infarction to let staff prepare for timely intervention, especially if "clot buster" drugs or interventional therapy is needed.

Emergency Medical Care

Treatment of a cardiac patient is based on the "supply and demand" concept of oxygen. You should seek to reduce the work of the heart and enhance oxygen delivery to cells. As always, the first consideration is the ABCs (airway, breathing, circulation) of the initial assessment. **Box 12-2** reviews a sample protocol for the responsive cardiac patient.

Decreasing Body Oxygen Requirements

Limiting anxiety and any unnecessary activity reduces the need for oxygen. Psychological stress and fear can cause the release of epinephrine. One effect of epinephrine release is increased heart rate and force of the heart's contractions. Both these effects increase the heart's oxygen needs. You reduce energy requirements by carrying the patient to the ambulance. You increase oxygenation by administering supplemental oxygen.

When working to reduce the patient's oxygen requirements, always act in a professional manner. Be calm and reassuring and show the patient that you care. You should make the patient aware that treatment has begun. Act efficiently and quickly to address the patient's problems without displaying your own emotions.

During care of the cardiac patient, you may have to deal with *patient denial*. To deny that one's life may be in jeopardy is a common human response. Denial has led many victims of heart attack to delay seeking medical care and contributes to the high number of deaths that occur outside the hospital. Often you will find that a patient's relative or a bystander has made the call for help. The patient may feel better by the time you arrive and deny previous complaints. Dealing with denial is a true skill. You might ask the patient to describe the complaints in more detail. If you think that the patient has experienced ischemic chest pain, an honest response is to tell the patient that you cannot be sure whether there is a heart problem and inform the patient that the greatest risk lies in the next 2 hours. Advise the patient to accompany you to the hospital for evaluation.

Patients with compromised respiratory or circulatory systems should be carried to the ambulance in a position most appropriate for their condition. Patients who are alert or who are experiencing shortness of breath should be placed in a position of comfort. Patients struggling to breathe will usually prefer sitting up and resist a supine condition. Be ready to move them into a supine position if their respiratory status deteriorates and you need to provide positive-pressure ventilation. Place patients in the supine or recovery position if they are in shock or exhibiting signs of poor circulation and oxygenation to the brain, such as an altered mental status.

LEARNING OBJECTIVES
- List indications for the use of nitroglycerin.
- State contraindications and side effects for the use of nitroglycerin.
- Explain the rationale for administering nitroglycerin to a patient with chest pain or discomfort.

Nitroglycerin

Patients can live with ischemic heart disease for a long time. They learn to limit activity so that they will have fewer attacks of chest pain. They may take nitroglycerin to help relieve anginal pain when it occurs. Nitroglycerin is usually taken in the form of a pill that is placed under the tongue, where it is rapidly absorbed (**Skill 12-1**). Nitroglycerin is also available as a spray, administered under or onto the tongue.

Nitroglycerin dilates the larger veins, allowing more blood to pool in the dependent areas of the body and reducing blood returning to the heart. With less venous blood returning to the heart, there is less blood to pump with each contraction, decreasing cardiac output and heart work. With less work, less oxygen is required, and the blood supply to the heart now becomes adequate to meet the heart's oxygen demands. Because nitroglycerin dilates the vessels in the head as well, patients often complain of headaches, especially throbbing pain, after administration. Patients learn to sit or sometimes lie down when they place a nitroglycerin tablet under the tongue because of the dilation of veins. They may feel lightheaded if they continue to stand.

Nitroglycerin also dilates arteries, decreasing the resistance to blood moving out of the heart and thus further reducing the work of the heart. In addition, nitroglycerin dilates the coronary arteries to improve blood flow to the heart itself.

Many patients have nitroglycerin patches that they apply to their skin to help prevent anginal attacks. The skin absorbs the nitroglycerin slowly over several hours, giving the benefit of sustained action that helps prevent anginal attacks. However, nitroglycerin patches are not as useful for the treatment of acute anginal attacks (sudden and severe) because the dosing is too gradual. Generally, the presence of a nitroglycerin patch will not change the treatment you provide. You will still be advised to administer tablets or spray. However, if the patient is or becomes hypotensive, you may be directed to remove the patch and wipe the medication from the skin. Generally, nitroglycerin

Table 12-2	Pharmacology of Nitroglycerin
Generic name	Nitroglycerin
Trade name	Nitrostat (tablets), Nitrolingual (spray)
Indication	Ischemic chest pain (when patient has prescription)
Contraindication	Low blood pressure
Forms	Sublingual tablet and spray
Dosage, tablets	One tablet sublingual, if systolic blood pressure >100 mm Hg and authorized by medical direction Repeat in 3 to 5 minutes if no relief, up to a maximum of three doses
Dosage, sprays	One or two sprays (0.4-mg metered dose) under or onto tongue, as authorized by medical direction
Administration	See Skill 12-1
Actions	Dilates blood vessels; decreases work of heart
Side effects	Hypotension, headache, pulse rate changes (may increase in response to fall in blood pressure)
Reassessment strategies	Monitor blood pressure Ask patient whether pain is relieved Seek medical direction before readministration Record reassessment data

tablets and spray are also contraindicated if the patient's systolic blood pressure is less than 100 mm Hg. Nitroglycerin should also be avoided if the patient has recently taken Viagra or similar drug. Check your local protocols for clarification of this intervention. **Table 12-2** summarizes the pharmacology of nitroglycerin.

Aspirin

Many emergency medical services (EMS) systems have integrated the use of aspirin in their protocols to decrease the formation clots during acute coronary syndromes (ACS). Aspirin has specific anticlotting actions that complement the in-hospital clot-busting treatments, including fibrinolytic therapy and percutaneous coronary intervention (PCI) such as angioplasty. Early administration of aspirin has been proven to reduce mortality from ACS. The specific recommendation of the AHA guidelines for the EMS treatment of ACS states, "If the patient has not taken aspirin and has no history of aspirin allergy and no evidence of recent gastrointestinal bleeding, EMS providers should give the patient non-enteric aspirin (160-325 mg) to chew."

Before administering aspirin, you should carefully assess for the following contraindications:
- Is the person allergic to aspirin?
- Has the patient recently taken aspirin?
- Does the patient have a recent history of gastrointestinal bleeding?

If any of these contraindications is present, you should not administer aspirin, or you should contact medical direction for

Table 12-3	Pharmacology of Aspirin
Generic name	Aspirin
Trade name	Bayer Aspirin (many other brand names)
Indications	Antipyretic, analgesic, antiinflammatory, antiplatelet (primary EMS use)
Contraindications	Allergy to aspirin, recent history of gastrointestinal bleeding
Forms	Tablet
Dosage, tablets	Antiplatelet: one to four tablets, 160-325 mg, chewed
Administration	See Chapter 10
Actions	Inhibits actions of platelets (clotting mechanism)
Side effects	Gastrointestinal bleeding
Reassessment strategies	Routine monitoring of patient

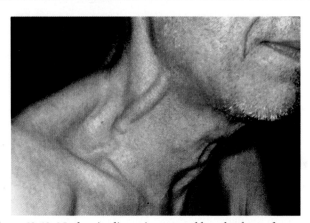

Figure 12-9 Pitting edema. *From Harkreader H, Hogan MA:* Fundamentals of nursing, *ed 3, St Louis, 2007, Mosby-Elsevier.*

further information. **Table 12-3** summarizes the pharmacology of aspirin.

Case in Point

Two EMTs respond to a 68-year-old woman complaining of difficulty breathing at her work. The patient states that the problem started while sitting at her desk about 15 minutes after eating a meal that was high in salt. The patient has a history of high blood pressure and had a heart attack 3 years ago. She is taking Inderal (propranolol), nitroglycerin, and daily aspirin.

On physical examination the EMTs note she is a markedly obese woman who is alert and in severe respiratory distress. Her blood pressure is 220/120, pulse 110 and regular, and lips and nail beds cyanotic. Her breath sounds are diminished, with crackles throughout the lungs. She has severe pitting edema in her ankles.

The EMTs administer oxygen via nonrebreather mask and place the patient in the sitting position on a stretcher. They suspect the patient is experiencing heart failure and acute pulmonary edema. While being transported to the ambulance, the patient becomes increasingly lethargic and sleepy. Her respirations slow to 8 breaths/min and shallow. The EMTs quickly place her in the ambulance and begin assisted ventilation using a bag-mask. En route to the hospital, her color improves, and her respirations increase in rate and quality.

Heart Failure

The heart can lose its ability to pump adequately for many reasons, but common causes include heart attacks and prolonged hypertension. In an acute heart attack, or myocardial infarction (MI), destruction of the heart muscle reduces the heart's power of contraction. This condition is referred to as **heart failure.**

History. Patients with heart failure will have a history or hypertension or signs of a recent MI such as chest pain. They may complain of shortness of breath, weakness, and limited activity increasing over several days or, in the case of MI, over several hours. The weakened heart cannot adequately pump blood out of the ventricles (right or left). With less blood pumped forward through the arteries, less oxygen is available to meet the needs of active muscles. Because the heart is not adequately pumping the blood out of the ventricles through the arteries, blood can

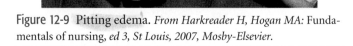

Figure 12-10 Neck vein distention caused by a backup of pressure from the right ventricle. *From Swartz MH:* Textbook of physical diagnosis, *ed 5, Philadelphia, 2006, Saunders.*

back up in the atria and venous system. As blood backs up in the venous system, it increases the pressure in the capillary beds and "leaks" out of the microscopically thin–walled vessels into the lungs (from backup from the left side of the heart) and into the body tissues (from backup from the right side of the heart). Fluid in the lungs causes breathing difficulty.

Physical Examination. Other signs of heart failure are noisy respirations, decreased breath sounds with or without crackles (rales) at the base of the lung fields, accessory muscle use, cyanosis, and swelling of the ankles and lower legs. When the plasma fluid from blood leaks out into the tissue, you may notice swelling of the soft tissues or edema. The effects of gravity often cause the fluid to accumulate in the dependent portions of the body, such as the ankles, legs, and lower back. Therefore a person sitting up will notice swelling of the feet, ankles, and lower legs (**Figure 12-9**). A patient who is bedridden might have swelling of the lower back. Massive tissue swelling can cause fluid accumulation in the abdomen *(ascites),* the lower back, and generalized or widespread body edema. Other signs of increased pressure in the veins include distended neck veins (**Figure 12-10**).

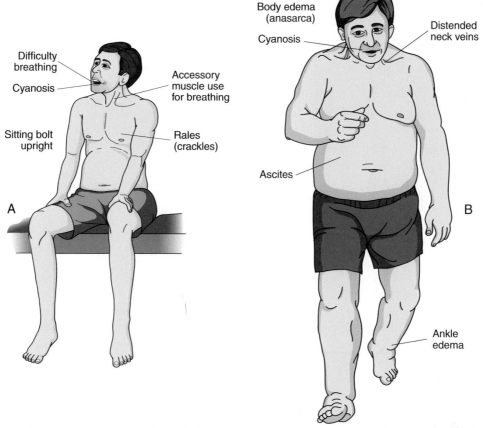

Figure 12-11 **A,** Signs of left-sided heart failure. **B,** Signs of right-sided heart failure.

REALWorld

What are the main differences between a novice and experienced EMS provider? As you progress through your EMS career, every patient encounter can improve your knowledge, instincts, and performance in the practice of prehospital emergency care. This assumes that you are always trying to sharpen your skills and knowledge by continuing the learning process both in the classroom and by the bedside. One such benefit of experience is referred to as *Augenblick* (German, "in the blink of an eye") diagnosis. This concept applied to clinical instinct refers to the increasing ability of medical providers to recognize quickly what is going with a patient within the first few seconds of an encounter. For example, when you walk into a residence at 3 AM and see an older patient with severe difficulty breathing, cyanosis, swollen ankles, and active accessory muscle use, you may immediately associate this with heart failure and acute pulmonary edema before you conduct your history and physical exam.

Augenblick diagnosis is a powerful tool for EMS providers. However, all tools must be applied carefully. In this case, you should follow-up Augenblick with a systematic history and physical examination to confirm your prehospital impression. Treatments should be based on clear data about the patient, not just instinct. The combination of Augenblick and a disciplined prehospital approach can help you fine-tune your assessment skills.

Figure 12-11 indicates the signs of left-sided and right-sided heart failure. These patients should be treated according to their chief complaints and assessment findings, which include respiratory difficulty and chest pain.

Treatment. Patients with left-sided heart failure are at risk for respiratory compromise from impaired movement of oxygen across the alveoli into the capillaries (the air sacs from which oxygen moves into blood are filled with fluid). Patients who have difficulty breathing should receive high-concentration supplemental oxygen administered by nonrebreather mask. Patients with inadequate breathing, as evidenced by signs such as altered mental status and poor air exchange, may require assisted positive-pressure ventilation with a bag-mask or other ventilation device. With fluid accumulating in dependent areas of the body, in some cases simply placing the patient in an upright position and allowing the legs to hang down may relieve the pulmonary congestion. Patients with congestive heart failure may also benefit from early ALS medications, such as nitroglycerin, *diuretics* (drugs that increase water loss through the kidneys and promote excretion of urine), and morphine.

Thoracic Aortic Dissection

Aortic dissection is a life-threatening emergency that occurs most frequently in men and persons over age 50. **Thoracic aortic dissection** is caused by a tear in the wall of the aorta that results in blood entering the inner lining of the vessel (**Figure 12-12**). The aorta begins to split (or *dissect*), forming a false passage. Dissections may be proximal or distal. *Proximal* dissections travel along the ascending aorta and sometimes include the descending aorta (**Figure 12-13,** *A*). *Distal* dissections travel along the descending aorta (**Figure 12-13,** *B*). The false passage

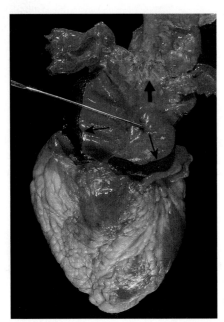

Figure 12-12 **A,** Internal view of the ascending aorta of patient who died from aortic dissection. The probe is showing a point where the lining of the aorta was torn. *From Kumar V et al:* Robbins and Cotran pathologic basis of disease, *ed 7, Philadelphia, 2005, Saunders.*

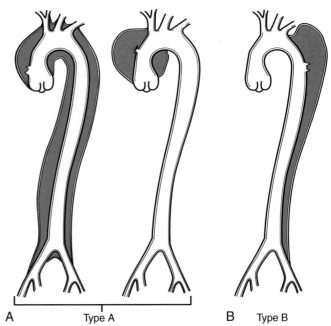

Figure 12-13 **A,** Proximal dissection of the aorta, *left,* involving only the ascending aorta, and *right,* involving both the ascending and the descending aorta. **B,** Distal dissection of the aorta, involving only the descending aorta. *From Kumar V et al:* Robbins and Cotran pathologic basis of disease, *ed 7, Philadelphia, 2005, Saunders.*

may block vessels along the way or even block passage of blood through the aorta. The dissection may also rupture the entire wall of the aorta, causing massive and often lethal hemorrhage. If the blood from the proximal dissection enters the pericardium, the patient may experience *pericardial tamponade,* a condition in which blood around the heart and aorta can result in poor venous return, profound shock, and death if untreated.

History. Thoracic aortic dissection typically presents with tearing, ripping, or searing chest pain that radiates to the back and continues down into the abdomen. Often the pain is difficult to differentiate from pain caused by acute coronary syndromes. The patient may also have complaints related to the occlusion of vessels blocked from the aorta. Because the branches of these vessels feed the head, neck, and arms, the patient may faint, exhibit signs of a stroke, or experience numbness in the arm caused by ischemia. The patient may have a history of hypertension or a known aneurysm.

Physical Examination. The physical findings related to thoracic aortic dissection are related to the mechanisms of injury: (1) occlusion of vessels, (2) hemorrhage, and (3) pericardial tamponade.

When vessels are occluded, circulation may be diminished or absent on one side of the body. This results in pulse differences in the neck or upper extremity. One pulse may be weaker than the other in the carotid and radial arteries, or one pulse may be absent on the affected side. The blood pressure may also vary from one arm to the other; small variances are normal. Motor or sensory changes (paralysis, weakness, or difference in sensation) may be caused by CNS injury related to occlusion to vessels supplying the brain.

To identify potential hemorrhage, check for a rapid pulse and other signs of adrenaline release. If the blood travels into the lining of the heart, symptoms will appear related to pericardial tamponade, including distended neck veins, narrowed pulse pressure (difference between systolic and diastolic pressure is less), and general signs of shock.

Treatment. The most important treatment for aortic dissection is immediate surgical intervention at the hospital. Therefore, the role of EMS providers is to deliver the patient to the most appropriate hospital as soon as possible while providing supportive care, including high-concentration oxygen or positive-pressure ventilation if needed. Treatment for shock should be provided as needed, including maintaining body temperature and elevating the legs to maintain cerebral perfusion.

Abdominal Aortic Aneurysm

An *aneurysm* is a localized abnormal dilation of a blood vessel or the heart. Aneurysms can occur in the brain, heart, aorta, and other blood vessels. **Abdominal aortic aneurysms** (AAAs) occur in the descending aorta and are a life-threatening emergency. If the aneurysm bursts, the patient can experience internal *exsanguination* (massive loss of blood volume) and die of profound shock (**Figure 12-14**).

History. An AAA typically presents with tearing, ripping, or searing abdominal or back pain that localizes to the back. The patient is usually older and may have a history of hypertension or a known aneurysm. Patients may have the sensation of needing to move their bowels.

Physical Examination. To identify potential hemorrhage, check for signs of poor perfusion; a rapid pulse, and other signs

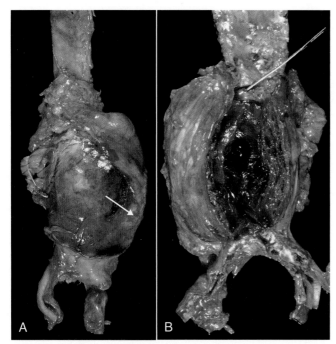

Figure 12-14 **A,** External view of abdominal aortic aneurysm (AAA) showing the point of rupture *(arrow).* **B,** Internal view of AAA showing the point of rupture and the clots that formed in the aneurysm before rupture. *From Kumar V et al:* Robbins and Cotran pathologic basis of disease, *ed 7, Philadelphia, 2005, Saunders.*

of adrenaline release (e.g., pale, cool, and sweaty skin). The patient may present with a rigid and distended abdomen with tenderness. On gentle examination of the abdomen, you may note a "pulsatile mass" generated by the bulging aneurysm. As with a thoracic dissection, the aneurysm may occlude one or both of the femoral arteries, resulting in a weak or absent femoral pulse. The combination of these signs and symptoms in association with the classic signs of shock are enough to maintain a high index of suspicion and to manage the patient accordingly.

Treatment. The most important treatment for AAA is immediate surgical intervention at the hospital. Once again, the role of EMS providers is to deliver the patient to the hospital as soon as possible while providing supportive care, including high-concentration oxygen or positive-pressure ventilation if needed. Treatment for shock should be provided as needed, including maintaining body temperature and elevating the legs to maintain cerebral perfusion.

Pulmonary Embolism

Blood clots that are released from the leg veins are the most common cause of **pulmonary embolism.** This can occur after surgery or in patients taking birth control medications. Fat emboli can also be released from long-bone fractures. As the clot is released, it travels up through the vena cava, into the right atrium and right ventricle, and then travels into the pulmonary artery, where it becomes lodged, obstructing blood flow to the lungs. The changes in lung circulation can cause severe hypoxia, sudden onset of difficulty breathing, and chest pain. When a large artery is involved, shock may result from obstruction of blood flow.

History. Patients typically complain of difficulty breathing and chest pain that increases with breathing. They may also cough up bloody sputum. The history may also reveal calf tenderness, a recent history of surgery, prolonged bed rest, recent travel, use of oral contraceptives, or phlebitis (inflammation of leg veins).

Physical Examination. The physical findings of a patient with pulmonary embolism are often normal. A rapid pulse and shock may be present in the worst cases. If there is significant obstruction of blood flow, the patient may exhibit signs of right-sided heart failure (see earlier discussion). Signs of hypoxia, including cyanosis and altered mental state, may be seen.

Treatment. High-concentration oxygen should be administered immediately. Treatment for shock should be provided as needed. Rapid transport is crucial because large pulmonary embolisms may cause cardiac arrest.

Cardiac Arrest

Cardiac arrest occurs when the patient's heart goes into a rhythm that does not generate blood flow. This may include **asystole** ("flatline"), where there is no electrical activity or contraction of the heart; **pulseless electrical activity,** where there is an organized electrical heart rhythm but no palpable pulse; or ventricular fibrillation. Ventricular fibrillation is the most common cause of sudden cardiac arrest in adults. Because time to defibrillation is the most critical treatment variable for survival from ventricular fibrillation, activation of the EMS system (EMSS), performance of CPR, and application of an AED are the most important actions taken for the victim of cardiac arrest. The EMT is trained to recognize the need for AED use to increase the patient's chance of survival.

Respiratory problems are the most likely cause of cardiac arrest in children, and attention should focus on providing ventilations. Although ventricular fibrillation is less common in children than in adults, it can occur. In general, AEDs designed for adults are not recommended for use on patients who are younger than 8 years or who weigh less than 55 pounds (25 kg), unless modified by special equipment. For example, some AEDs have special **electrode pads** (conductors used for electrical contact) and cables for children that modify the dose of defibrillation energy and make them suitable for infants and for children younger than 8 years. Check with your local EMSS to determine local treatment protocols and available equipment for cardiac arrest victims younger than 8 years.

REAL*World*

When an adult patient presents in sudden cardiac arrest, treatment focuses on effective CPR and use of an AED. Most sudden cardiac arrests in adult patients are a result of cardiac dysrhythmias such as ventricular fibrillation. In children, however, most cardiac arrests result from hypoxia. Although electrical therapy from an AED may be needed, the primary cause of the arrest is usually hypoxia from an obstructed airway. The EMT must work to ensure the airway is patent or open and the patient is being ventilated adequately.

Relationship to Basic Life Support. The EMT incorporates "chain of survival" strategies when approaching patients in cardiac arrest. Two-person CPR is the most common technique used at the scene of a cardiac arrest. One-person CPR is rarely performed by the EMT, but it may be needed while a partner is preparing an AED or during transport in the back of an ambulance. During ambulance transport, you should maintain a secure position, particularly during the performance of chest compressions. A "spotter" who physically helps to support the compressor during ambulance movement is invaluable in preventing injury.

The EMT must also consider the following important modalities and factors when applying CPR:

- Body substance isolation
- Use of AED
- Use of airway adjuncts
- Suctioning of the airway
- Use of a bag-mask, flow-restricted oxygen-powered ventilation device, or other equipment to provide enriched-oxygen delivery during CPR
- Techniques for lifting and moving patients who are in cardiac arrest
- Interviews with bystanders and family regarding the events leading up to the cardiac arrest

---

LEARNING OBJECTIVES
- Discuss the importance of CPR.
- Discuss the integration of CPR into other resuscitation procedures (e.g., AED use).
- Explain why changing EMTs every 2 minutes is so important during CPR.
- Discuss the importance of chest compressions that are hard, fast, and minimally interrupted.
- List the steps for one-person CPR and two-person CPR for the adult, child, and infant victim of cardiac arrest.

Cardiopulmonary Resuscitation

Cardiopulmonary resuscitation (CPR) is a sequence of actions that includes positive-pressure ventilation in combination with chest compressions. CPR is generally designed to provide temporary perfusion to vital organs (heart and brain) until an effective circulation can be restored. It is well recognized that CPR plays an important role in patients who have a collapse-to-treatment interval longer than 5 minutes. A heart that has not been perfused for periods greater than 4 to 5 minutes can significantly benefit from 2 minutes of CPR before defibrillation. In one study, patients in ventricular fibrillation who had CPR before defibrillation were six times more likely to survive than those without prior CPR.

Use of CPR can also resuscitate victims of *short-term* cardiac arrest caused by respiratory failure or respiratory arrest. This type of cardiac arrest is usually caused by conditions such as submersion, suffocation, infections, and trauma. In one study, pediatric submersion victims in cardiac arrest exhibiting occasional gasping breaths had a 90% chance of survival when CPR was performed immediately.

Most adult victims of cardiac arrest also require early defibrillation to restore an effective heart rhythm. CPR supplies temporary blood flow to vital organs and extends the resuscitation period until defibrillation and advanced care can be provided. When integrated in the chain of survival early by a bystander, CPR can double or triple the chances of survival for a cardiac arrest victim.

For CPR to have the greatest benefit, laypersons and EMTs must pay close attention to the following details:

1. **Activation of the 9-1-1 system by the layperson must occur quickly.** This will ensure the earliest possible response of EMS providers, a defibrillator, and advanced life support (ALS). In most resuscitation efforts, CPR provides perfusion to vital organs until the heart can be restored to a normal rhythm through defibrillation, medications, and other ALS measures. ALS may also be needed to prevent a subsequent cardiac arrest or to manage respiratory arrest in the postresuscitation period.

2. **CPR must be provided early.** CPR provided within a few minutes of collapse will extend the chances of survival. If laypersons or first responders can provide CPR within the first few minutes after collapse, and defibrillation follows within an additional few minutes, the chance for survival increases significantly. In a study of Las Vegas casinos, where CPR was provided in approximately 3 minutes and defibrillation in about 4½ minutes after collapse, the survival rate for witnessed ventricular fibrillation was approximately 60%. This rate compares to a national survival rate of about 5%.

3. **Rescuers must pay close attention to the administration of positive-pressure ventilation to yield the greatest benefit and prevent complications.** Ventilations must be delivered slowly (over a 1-second period with *sufficient volume to make the chest rise*). This will ensure adequate ventilation (removal of CO_2) and oxygenation while preventing gastric inflation, regurgitation, and aspiration.

4. **Compressions must be delivered with sufficient force and at the appropriate rate to maximize blood flow to the heart and brain.** During resuscitation efforts, the "compressor" should be closely monitored to ensure the consistent delivery of adequate chest compressions. This includes monitoring both the rate and the depth of compressions by direct observation and indirect measures of effective compression, such as a palpated pulse. When possible, compressors should switch places every 2 minutes (or 5 cycles of CPR) to prevent ineffective compressions from fatigue. It is critical that each compression is followed by a complete release of the chest wall.

Remember, effective CPR will significantly increase the patient's chance for survival. Too often the quality of CPR is ignored during resuscitation efforts while EMTs focus on defibrillation and ALS procedures.

Adult CPR

The performance of CPR includes opening the airway, assessing for breathing, assessing for a pulse, and performing chest compressions. This section reviews airway and ventilation issues and techniques discussed in Chapter 6 and integrates the performance of compressions. The AHA 2005 guidelines discourage the routine reassessment of a pulse by EMTs during performance of CPR or use of an AED. The guidelines advise that the pulse should be assessed by an ALS provider in conjunction with ECG monitoring. However, the current National EMS Education Standards include assessment of pulses by EMTs. This discussion incorporates the reassessment of a pulse during CPR and AED use, recognizing that EMS systems can select a strategy that best meets their needs. When an AED is used, reassessment of the pulse occurs before each defibrillation, which is immediately followed by 5 cycles of CPR. This allows time for the heart to recover fully and establish a functional, perfusing heart rhythm.

Context of CPR Education

The traditional method for teaching CPR starts with the assumptions that the person is outside the hospital and that EMS has not yet arrived at the scene. This approach ensures that the "chain of survival" strategy is completely addressed. It also shows the relationship between field evaluation of the victim and EMSS activation.

Assess Responsiveness and Activate EMSS

The first person at the scene of a collapsed victim should check for responsiveness (gently tap or shake the victim and shout, "Are you all right?"); if the victim is unresponsive (and you are acting outside the EMS environment), immediately activate the local 9-1-1 system. Again, time to defibrillation is the most important variable for victims of cardiac arrest caused by ventricular fibrillation. If alone, the person activates the EMSS and retrieves the AED if available. When responding as an EMS provider, one person can assess for responsiveness while the other person prepares the AED for use. The only exception to this rule involves cardiac arrest caused by *asphyxia* (e.g., from drowning, suffocation, toxic gas inhalation). In these cases, perform 5 cycles (2 minutes) of CPR before phoning 9-1-1. For these patients, CPR may be lifesaving and can restore normal breathing and circulation.

Airway

Place the unresponsive victim in the supine position on a firm surface. Often a CPR board or a long spine board is used to provide a firm surface over the mattress on the rolling cot stretcher. This helps to ensure effective compressions by resisting the movement or "give" that would be absorbed by the mattress.

If a spinal injury is suspected, log-roll the victim carefully while maintaining alignment of the spinal column (see Chapter 5).

In the unresponsive victim, the tongue and epiglottis may obstruct airflow through the pharynx. Open the airway using the head-tilt/chin-lift method, or if trauma is suspected, use the jaw thrust (see Chapter 6).

Breathing

Once the airway is opened, you should assess breathing by looking for chest rise and listening and feeling for air exchange at the mouth and nose. Victims who are unresponsive and breathing spontaneously can be placed on their side in the recovery position to prevent aspiration if vomiting occurs.

If the victim is not breathing or is breathing inadequately, provide two breaths while observing for chest rise. You must also be aware of *agonal breathing*, characterized by occasional, weak, and ineffective breaths and not to be confused with adequate spontaneous ventilation. If agonal breathing is present, positive-pressure ventilation is still provided.

Care must be taken not to breathe too forcefully or too rapidly because this will result in higher airway pressures. Higher airway pressures will force air into the esophagus, causing air to enter and build up in the stomach. This can result in gastric inflation, vomiting, and aspiration of stomach contents into the lungs. This situation can significantly complicate resuscitation efforts. Furthermore, hyperventilation and forceful ventilation can significantly decrease circulation. Hyperventilation reduces venous return to the heart.

Breaths should be delivered over 1 second with sufficient force to generate *visible chest rise.* This technique will provide a sufficient volume of air to ventilate the patient effectively while not causing high airway pressure that will cause gastric inflation. If available, ventilation options such as mouth-to-mask and bag-mask can be used to ventilate the patient.

Circulation

Again, when cardiac arrest occurs, there is a complete cessation of circulation and oxygenation to body tissues, including the heart and brain. Chest compressions create blood flow by creating changes in pressure within the thoracic cavity (thoracic pump mechanism) and directly compressing the heart between the sternum and the spine (cardiac pump mechanism).

Check for Pulse. Recognizing cardiac arrest is the first and most important step in establishing the need for the performance of chest compressions. EMTs determine cardiac arrest by checking for unresponsiveness, breathing, and a pulse. Care should be taken when checking for a pulse.

Studies have resulted in the following findings:
- Responders require too much time to evaluate a pulse; 50% of subjects required more than 24 seconds to find a pulse.
- When a pulse was absent, 10% of responders identified the pulse as present.
- When a pulse was present, 45% of responders identified the pulse as absent.
- The overall error rate was 35%.

Therefore the current guidelines for CPR recommend that laypersons check only for unresponsiveness and breathing rather than for a pulse to confirm cardiac arrest. Healthcare providers should check for unresponsiveness using breathing together with a pulse check. Assessment of the pulse is performed as follows:
1. After delivering two rescue breaths, maintain a head tilt, locate the larynx (Adam's apple) by using two or three fingers of your other hand, and slide your fingers in the groove between the larynx and the muscle at the side of the neck (**Figure 12-15**).
2. Palpate the carotid artery with your fingertips.
3. This should take no longer than 10 seconds and no less than 5 seconds.

- *If there is no breathing but a pulse is present,* provide rescue breathing at a rate of 10 to 12 breaths/min (one breath every 5 to 6 seconds)
- *If there is no pulse,* begin chest compressions **(Skill 12-2).**

Chest Compressions. Several studies have documented that a relatively rapid compression rate is needed to optimize blood flow and coronary and cerebral perfusion during CPR. Maintaining a rate of 100 compressions per minute is critical and should be monitored closely during resuscitation efforts. Studies have shown that use of audio tonal devices (e.g., metronomes) may be helpful in achieving this goal.

The CPR guidelines recommend a ratio of 30 compressions and 2 breaths for both one-person and two-person CPR for adults in cardiac arrest unless the airway is secured with an endotracheal (ET) tube or other ALS airway device. In these patients, continuous compressions can be performed. Ventilations are provided at a rate of 8 to 10 breaths per minute with interrupting chest compressions. Studies have demonstrated that coronary and cerebral perfusion can be improved by the performance of longer sets of continuous compressions.

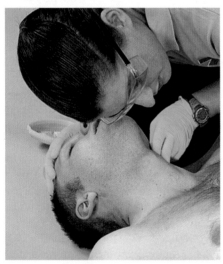

Figure 12-15 Pulse check. After delivering 2 rescue breaths, using two or three fingers of your other hand, slide your fingers in the groove between the larynx and muscles and the side of the neck.

Compress the sternum approximately 1½ to 2 inches (3.5-5 cm) in the adult victim. When possible, a second person should palpate a carotid or femoral pulse during the performance of compressions to determine effective force and depth. Release the pressure on the chest to allow blood to flow into the chest and heart. After each compression, you must release the pressure completely and allow the chest to return to its normal position. Keep your hands in light contact with the victim's sternum to maintain proper hand position. Effective cerebral and coronary perfusion has been shown to occur when 50% of the cycle is devoted to the chest compression phase and 50% to the chest relaxation phase.

During cardiac arrest, properly performed chest compressions can produce systolic arterial blood pressure peaks of 60 to 80 mm Hg, but diastolic blood pressure is low. Mean blood pressure in the carotid artery seldom exceeds 40 mm Hg. Again, cardiac output resulting from chest compressions is probably only one fourth to one third of normal and decreases during the course of prolonged conventional CPR.

After 30 compressions, provide 2 breaths. Continue the cycle of 30 compressions and 2 breaths for 5 cycles. Continuous and effective CPR is critical until the victim regains spontaneous circulation or until defibrillation is provided.

One-Person CPR

One or two persons can perform CPR. EMS providers must be flexible in their selection of techniques. When only two persons are available at the scene of a cardiac arrest, one-person CPR can be performed by one person (see Skill 12-2) while the other applies an AED and evaluates the quality of chest compressions. If there are more than two persons on the scene, including first responders (e.g., police, firefighters) or trained laypersons, two-person CPR can be performed.

Two- Person CPR

In two-person CPR, one person is positioned at the victim's side and performs chest compressions. The other person remains at the victim's head, maintains an open airway, monitors the carotid pulse for adequacy of chest compressions, and provides rescue breathing **(Figure 12-16)**. The compression rate for two-person CPR is 100 per minute. The compression/ventilation

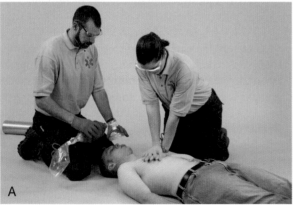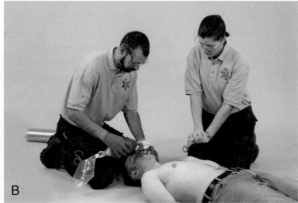

Figure 12-16 Two-person CPR. **A,** One person is positioned at the victim's side and performs chest compressions. The other person remains at the victim's head, maintains an open airway, monitors the carotid pulse for adequacy of chest compressions, and provides rescue breathing. **B,** The EMT providing compressions stops compressions to allow for 2 ventilations and then immediately resumes compressions.

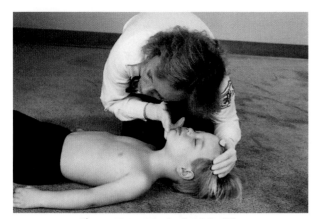

Figure 12-17 Head-tilt/chin-lift.

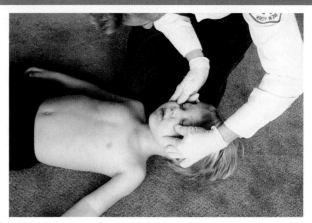

Figure 12-18 Jaw thrust. *From Chapleau W:* Emergency first responder, *St Louis, 2007, Mosby-Elsevier.*

ratio is 30:2, with a pause for 2 ventilations of 1 second each until the airway is secured with an advanced airway device (e.g., ET tube). Exhalation occurs between the 2 breaths and during the first chest compression of the next cycle. Every attempt should be made to change compressors every 2 minutes because fatigue will likely cause undercompression.

When performing CPR on a patient who has an ET tube in place, continuous-compression CPR is provided. Approximately 8 to 10 breaths are delivered each minute *without interrupting compressions.* Patients who have an ET tube in place are not subject to gastric inflation because each breath is directly delivered to the patient's trachea and air cannot enter the esophagus.

Infant and Child CPR

Cardiopulmonary resuscitation for infants and children incorporates the same principles and techniques as CPR for adults, with some modifications related to size and physiology. For the purposes of CPR, an *infant* is someone less than 1 of year of age, and a *child* is someone between 1 year of age and puberty. Puberty is identified by breast development in females and underarm or chest hair in males. When using an AED, a *child* is defined as someone between 1 and 8 years of age.

The causes of cardiac arrest differ significantly for infants and children compared with adults. Sudden cardiac arrest and the incidence of ventricular fibrillation are relatively rare in infants and children. Children sustain cardiac arrest principally from causes of respiratory failure and respiratory arrest, including traumatic incidents, submersion incidents, poisoning, choking, asphyxia, infectious disease, and other mechanisms that lead to hypoxia, cessation of breathing first, and, if left untreated, cardiac arrest. Because most infant and child arrests are caused by respiratory problems, the emphasis is on the early delivery of positive-pressure ventilation. For most pediatric prearrest conditions, early ventilation may prevent cardiac arrest.

Assess Responsiveness and Activate EMSS

As with an adult, the first person at the scene of a collapsed infant or child should check for responsiveness. Gently tap or shake the victim and shout, "Are you all right?" If the victim is unresponsive, you are acting outside the EMS environment,

and you have a second person assisting you, immediately activate the local 9-1-1 system and obtain an AED, if available. If you are alone and outside the EMS environment, perform 5 cycles of CPR before activating the EMSS. This approach recognizes that CPR may resuscitate the infant or child who has recently had a respiratory or cardiac arrest. The one exception is when a child suddenly collapses in your presence. In this case, activate the EMSS and retrieve the AED. This type of situation increases the likelihood that the child experienced sudden cardiac arrest as a result of ventricular fibrillation and would benefit from the use of an AED immediately.

Airway

The unresponsive victim should be placed in the supine position. If spinal injury is suspected, log-roll the victim carefully while maintaining alignment of the spinal column and placed on a firm surface (see Chapter 5).

Head-Tilt/Chin-Lift

- *Child.* Place one hand on the forehead and the index and middle fingers of your other hand on the bony part of the child's chin. The victim's head is then rotated slightly while simultaneously lifting the chin (**Figure 12-17**).
- *Infant.* Performed in the same manner as the head-tilt/chin-lift for the child, except the head is placed in the neutral (or sniffing) position, with padding placed under the torso.

Jaw Thrust. To perform the jaw thrust for the child or infant, grasp the angles of the victim's lower jaw with your index and middle fingers and lift with both hands while maintaining the head in a neutral position (without flexion or extension). As you lift the jaw, open the victim's mouth with your thumbs. If the jaw thrust does not adequately open the airway, the head-tilt/chin-lift should be used (**Figure 12-18**).

Breathing

Once the airway is opened, you should assess breathing by looking for chest rise and listening and feeling for air exchange at the mouth and nose. Infants and children who are unresponsive and breathing spontaneously can be placed on their side in the recovery position to prevent aspiration if vomiting occurs. If breathing is not present or is not adequate, begin rescue breathing by using methods discussed in Chapter 6, such as mouth-to-mask or bag-mask device.

Circulation

The evaluation of pulse and the performance of compressions differ slightly for the infant and child compared with the adult.

Check for Pulse. Assessment of pulse in the child and infant is performed as follows:

- *Child.* Maintain a head tilt, locate the larynx with two or three fingers of your other hand, and slide your fingers in the groove between the larynx and muscle at the side of the neck. Continue to palpate the carotid artery while you assess for breathing and coughing and scan the body for movement. This should take no longer than 10 seconds and no less than 5 seconds.
- *Infant.* While maintaining a head tilt, locate the brachial pulse point on the medial aspect of the arm halfway between the elbow and the armpit. Continue to palpate the brachial artery while you assess for breathing and coughing and scan the body for movement. Again, this should take no longer than 10 seconds.

If there is no breathing but there is a pulse of greater than 60 beats/min with signs of poor perfusion, provide rescue breathing at a rate of 20 breaths/min (1 breath every 3 seconds) and recheck the pulse every 2 minutes.

Chest Compressions. If pulse rate is less than 60 beats/min with signs of poor perfusion (pale skin, delayed capillary refill, unresponsiveness), begin chest compressions; see **Skill 12-3** for child and infant CPR. After 30 compressions, deliver 2 breaths. Continue the cycle of 30 compressions and 2 breaths for approximately 5 cycles, then switch EMTs. Continuous and effective CPR is critical until the victim regains spontaneous circulation or until defibrillation is provided.

One-Person or Two-Person CPR

One or two persons can perform CPR for the infant or child. The technique for two-person CPR in the infant and child remains the same as for the adult, with one person assuming the role of the "ventilator" and the other person the role of the "compressor."

In two-person pediatric CPR, one person is positioned at the victim's side and performs chest compressions. The other person remains at the victim's head, maintains an open airway, and provides rescue breathing. The compression/ventilation ratio is 15:2, with a pause for 2 breaths. Exhalation occurs between breaths and during the first chest compression of the next cycle. Make every attempt to change positions every 2 minutes to avoid undercompression caused by fatigue.

LEARNING OBJECTIVES
- Discuss the various types of AEDs.
- Discuss the procedures that must be taken into consideration for standard operation of the various types of AEDs.
- State the reasons for ensuring that the patient is pulseless and apneic when using the AED.
- List the indications for automated external defibrillation.
- List the contraindications for automated external defibrillation.
- Discuss the circumstances that may result in inappropriate shocks.
- Explain the considerations for interruption of CPR when using the AED.
- Discuss the advantages and disadvantages of AEDs.
- Summarize the speed of operation of automated external defibrillation.
- Discuss the use of remote defibrillation through adhesive pads.
- Discuss the special considerations for rhythm monitoring.
- List the steps in the operation of the AED.
- Explain the impact of age and weight on defibrillation.

Automated External Defibrillators

Automated external defibrillators (AEDs) are monitor/defibrillation devices designed to achieve the following goals:
- Monitor the patient's heart rhythm.
- Identify shockable versus nonshockable heart rhythms through computerized analysis of the waveforms.
- Advise the AED operator to initiate a defibrillation.

The most common and treatable cause of sudden death is ventricular fibrillation from ischemic heart disease. Most victims of sudden death experience this rhythm. In conditions such as heart attacks, the conduction system may lose control of the heart's cells. The cells in the heart have a property called *automaticity* (ability to generate an electrical impulse and discharge on their own); therefore, uncontrolled cells may act independently of the conduction system and of each other. This may result in the chaotic rhythm known as ventricular fibrillation. No effective synchronized contraction of the heart is possible, and no blood is pumped. The heart's pacemaker has lost control.

Electrically shocking the cells simultaneously and making all cells enter a rest period can stop the useless quivering of the heart in ventricular fibrillation. Once in a state of rest, the fastest cells to recharge are those that constitute the pacemaker of the heart. Because these cells recharge first, the goal of defibrillation is to allow the pacemaker to resume control of the heart's contraction.

The forced discharge, or *firing,* of the heart's cells can be accomplished by *defibrillation,* the external application of an electric shock that travels across the heart. Sufficient energy must be delivered to most of the heart cells to ensure successful defibrillation.

Many patients who receive early defibrillation can be saved. Without defibrillation, ventricular fibrillation deteriorates to cardiac standstill, or *asystole* (no contraction and no electrical activity). Resuscitation of patients with asystole is much less likely than in patients with ventricular fibrillation.

Evolution of Defibrillation Concept

Before the 1960s, patients who experienced cardiac arrest outside the hospital rarely survived. When they arrived at the hospital by ambulance, most were pronounced dead. In 1960 the technique of CPR was developed to provide artificial ventilation and circulation for victims of cardiac arrest until they could receive advanced care in a hospital setting. Advanced care consisted of defibrillation, specialized airway management (i.e., intubation), and drug therapy. Hospital experience clearly showed that the early application of both CPR and ALS (especially defibrillation) resulted in a higher patient survival rate.

With the development of portable defibrillators in the 1960s, application of defibrillation in the field became technologically feasible for saving critical minutes from the time of cardiac arrest to the application of defibrillation and other advanced skills. Studies of care rendered by paramedics and advanced EMTs documented the effectiveness of prehospital *advanced cardiac life support* (ACLS) systems. Survival rates of 43% were reported when victims of cardiac arrest from ventricular fibrillation received prompt CPR (within 4 minutes after collapse) and prompt ALS (within 8 minutes after collapse). However, these skills were practiced by a small number of EMS providers and therefore available to a minority of cardiac arrest patients. Training time for advanced EMT programs was lengthy. Learning heart rhythm recognition and pharmacology required additional training time for prehospital personnel. This prevented availability of advanced techniques in many areas, particularly where volunteers who were EMTs provided the bulk of the personnel.

Evaluation of the most important elements necessary to resuscitate the clinically dead patient highlighted the time that elapsed between the onset of cardiac arrest and the initiation of CPR and defibrillation. In the 1970s and early 1980s, Eisenberg, Copass, Cummings, and other scientific investigators from Seattle studied the performance of defibrillation by EMTs. Again, they noted an increase in the survival rate. Many other programs in urban, rural, and suburban settings have demonstrated the effectiveness of EMTs performing defibrillation.

REAL*World*

EMTs represent the largest group of providers of prehospital emergency care in the United States. With current training and availability of AEDs, the EMT routinely learns this skill as part of the national curriculum for the following reasons:

1. The most common and most treatable rhythm encountered early in cardiac arrest is ventricular fibrillation.
2. Defibrillation is the definitive treatment for ventricular fibrillation, and training can be accomplished in a short time with AEDs.
3. Time from cardiac arrest to defibrillation is the most important variable in the successful treatment of ventricular fibrillation.
4. EMTs are the most likely emergency medical personnel initially to encounter someone in cardiac arrest.

EMTs administer defibrillation under the authorization and orders of a physician who assumes responsibility for medical direction. Defibrillation is administered as part of an EMSS response in a "chain of survival."

Operation

Several brands of AEDs are available. They vary slightly in appearance and operational steps. Some AEDs are activated by pressing a button on the face of the device. Other devices automatically turn on when the case lid is opened. However, the differences in these devices are minor, allowing trained AED users to adapt easily to other devices without additional training.

In general, the energy of most AEDs is appropriate for patients age 8 years and older. Some specialized defibrillation electrode pads reduce the energy levels to 50 joules (J) for use with infants and small children. You should check with your EMSS to learn about the equipment used in your system and the AED protocols for adults and children.

Attaching Electrode Pads

Automated external defibrillators are attached to the patient by cables connected to monitoring defibrillation electrode pads. These pads are attached to the patient below the right clavicle on the right border of the sternum and 2 to 3 inches (5-7.5 cm) below the left armpit.

Analysis of Cardiac Rhythm

Automated external defibrillators evaluate the patient's cardiac rhythm and determine the presence of a rhythm for which a shock is indicated. When the AED interprets the rhythm as one requiring a shock, it charges capacitors within the device that hold the charge in preparation for delivery of the shock. Because the AED is portable, its function depends on the presence of properly charged defibrillator batteries.

Field tests of AEDs have demonstrated a high degree of accuracy both in correctly shocking ventricular fibrillation (or ventricular tachycardia) and in *not* shocking other rhythms that are not treated with defibrillation. Inappropriate delivery of shocks is rare. Mechanical errors are extremely rare with AEDs; more often the error is in *not* shocking a rhythm that might be helped by defibrillation rather than delivering a shock to the wrong rhythm. The chance of human error is minimized by not attaching the device to a patient unless signs of circulation are absent and by stopping patient movement before analyzing the rhythm.

Ventricular Tachycardia. Ventricular fibrillation is not the only rhythm that an AED may advise shocking. **Ventricular tachycardia** is a very rapid heart rhythm that may or may not produce a pulse or other signs of circulation. Often present in cardiac arrest, ventricular tachycardia may be the first abnormal rhythm resulting in pulselessness. Ventricular tachycardia can rapidly lead to ventricular fibrillation. **Figure 12-19** compares ventricular tachycardia, ventricular fibrillation, asystole, and a normal ECG.

Automated external defibrillators can recognize ventricular tachycardia and shock the patient's heart if the rate is higher than preset values. The computer analysis of the ECG rhythm is highly accurate. Because the AED is applied only to unconscious patients who have no signs of circulation, additional patient safety is ensured with respect to providing appropriate treatment if ventricular tachycardia is the underlying rhythm.

Interruption of CPR

Defibrillation is one of the few times when CPR is interrupted. Because CPR might interfere with rhythm analysis, and because the rescuer could receive a shock if there is patient contact, the following rules apply:

1. Stop chest compression and positive-pressure ventilation.
2. Do not touch the patient when the rhythm is being analyzed and the shocks are being delivered.

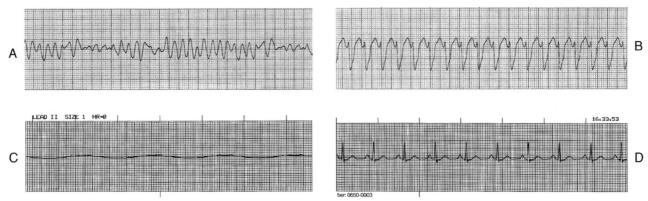

Figure 12-19 Electrocardiogram (ECG) tracings. **A,** Ventricular fibrillation **B,** Ventricular tachycardia (AED will shock faster versions of this rhythm). **C,** Asystole. **D,** Normal sinus rhythm.

During this period there is no patient contact, including assessing the pulse or performing CPR. Time to defibrillation is the most important predictor of successful resuscitation, and patient contact after the first two shocks would only delay analysis and defibrillation. After shocks, you should resume CPR for 2 minutes (5 cycles) starting with compressions, and then reassess the pulse. AEDs prompt you with a voice recording to check for a pulse (and airway and breathing) and advise you to perform CPR following a shock. The AED will often time CPR efforts for 2 minutes—to perfuse the heart and improve the chance of successful defibrillation—and then reanalyze the patient's rhythm. Two minutes of CPR is recommended before defibrillation if the patient has been in cardiac arrest for 5 minutes or longer.

Skill 12-4 outlines operation of the AED.

Advantages

Automatic external defibrillators offer many advantages. First, they are easy to learn to use, and memorizing the treatment sequence is simpler than remembering the steps of CPR. The device also allows rapid treatment of the patient. Because the device is used within an EMSS, medical direction and quality improvement are available, thus providing feedback to the EMT. The technology of the AED allows real-time recording of the rhythm, the shocks, and depending on the machine, even voice recording. The recording of information enhances quality improvement review and verification of skill competency. EMS systems routinely provide continuing medical education to ensure retention of AED skills.

The electrode pads designed for the AED have several advantages. First, they promote responder safety because the provider can stand clear of the patient during shocks. Second, the large electrode pads help maintain constant contact throughout resuscitation and enhance shock delivery through the chest wall surface, helping to deliver the current to the patient. In addition, some AEDs have screens that display the heart's rhythm or ECG, which enables continued use of the device by ALS providers to monitor rhythms during care after resuscitation.

> **LEARNING OBJECTIVES**
> - Differentiate between the single-person and multiperson care with an AED.
> - Explain the reason for pulses not being checked between shocks with an AED.
> - Discuss the importance of coordinating ACLS-trained providers with personnel using AEDs.
> - Discuss the importance of postresuscitation care.
> - List the components of postresuscitation care.
> - Define the function of all controls of an AED, and describe event documentation and battery defibrillation maintenance.

Resuscitation Attempts

When approaching a patient who appears unresponsive, put on your personal protective equipment if you have not already done so. While one of your team members performs the initial assessment, you should ensure the availability and preparation of the AED. If CPR is in progress on arrival, stop CPR and check for breathing and a pulse before attaching the device. If the pulse is absent, resume CPR until the AED electrode pads are attached. When the AED is at the patient's side, turn it on and attach the monitor-defibrillator electrode pads to the patient. Stop CPR and clear everyone from the patient. The device will then analyze the patient's rhythm. If a shock is advised, make sure everyone is clear of the patient by saying, "I'm clear, you're clear, everybody is clear," or simply "Clear," and check that no one is touching the patient or stretcher. While the machine is charging, it may emit a tone, a light indication, a voice-synthesized message, or a combination of similar signals. When the device is charged, you may then need to push the shock button. Some fully automated AEDs, designed mainly for laypersons, deliver the shock automatically without the need to push a button.

When the shock is delivered, you may note a generalized muscle contraction with some movement of the body. Immediately start 5 cycles of CPR, beginning with chest compressions. After 5 cycles of CPR, check a pulse and allow the AED to reanalyze. The AED will then reassess the patient's heart rhythm and determine whether a second shock is advised. If it is, the machine will charge. Ensure that everyone is clear, and push the shock button.

"No Shock Advised"

If at any time the rhythm analysis states, "No shock advised," you should perform 5 cycles of CPR, check a pulse, and reanalyze. If there is a pulse and a "no shock advised" message, you should assess breathing for adequacy and provide positive-pressure ventilation and supplemental oxygen as needed and transport the patient to ALS care. If no pulse is present, continue the pattern of CPR and rhythm analysis. If at any time a shock is advised, restart the defibrillation sequence.

Special Situations

While preparing to apply the AED, you must identify whether any of four situations is present that may change your approach to using the device, as follows:

- Hair on a man's chest interfering with the adherence of the pads.
- Patient lying in freestanding water.
- Patient wearing transdermal medication patches.
- Patient with an implanted pacemaker or cardioverter-defibrillator.

Hairy Chest

If a male victim has a hairy chest, the electrode pads may not adhere to the chest wall. The machine will usually provide a "check electrode" or similar message. If this occurs, press down firmly on the electrode pads. If the "check electrode" message persists, remove the pads; this also removes hair from the chest. If most of the hair is removed, open a new pack of electrodes and apply the new pads to the chest. If a large quantity of hair remains, quickly shave the area before you apply new pads, and continue the analysis process.

Water

Water is a good conductor of electricity and may represent a pathway of energy from the AED to the EMTs and bystanders treating the patient, resulting in shocks or burns. Water can also provide a direct path of energy from one electrode pad to the other (arcing) and decrease the effectiveness of the shock, because the energy moves *over* rather than through the chest. It is critical for the EMT to remove the patient quickly from freestanding water and wipe the chest wall dry before using the AED. If the situation involves a diving incident or other possible cause of spinal injury, the EMT should take care to maintain inline manual stabilization of the head and neck during movement of the patient.

Transdermal Medications

Common medication patches include nitroglycerin, nicotine, pain medication, and blood pressure medication. Placing an AED electrode pad on top of a medication patch may block the delivery of energy from the electrode pad to the heart and may cause small burns to the skin. Medication patches should be removed and the area wiped clean before attaching the AED electrode pad.

Pacemakers and Cardioverter-Defibrillators

Patients with abnormal heart rhythms may have medical devices implanted in the chest or abdomen that are wired directly to the myocardium. Pacemakers and **implanted cardioverter-defibrillators (ICDs)** create a hard lump beneath the skin of the upper chest or abdomen. The lump is about half the size of a deck of cards and usually has a small overlying scar. Placing an AED electrode pad directly over an implanted medical device may reduce the effectiveness of defibrillation. Do not place an AED electrode pad directly over an implanted device. Place an AED electrode pad at least 1 inch (2.5 cm) to the side of any implanted device.

Automated ICDs (AICDs) deliver a limited number of low-energy shocks directly to the myocardium. You might feel the current if it discharges while you touch the patient, but it should not be dangerous to you. If you encounter a patient with an AICD in cardiac arrest, the AED should be attached and standard operating procedures followed. If the patient collapses in your presence and the AICD is delivering shocks to the patient, allow the device to deliver its shocks while you prepare the AED and wait for 30 to 60 seconds for the AICD to complete the treatment cycle. Then use the AED as you would for any other patient.

> **LEARNING OBJECTIVE**
> - Discuss the standard of care for a patient with persistent or recurrent ventricular fibrillation and no available ACLS.

Persistent Ventricular Fibrillation

After you have completed a few to several sets of CPR and shocks on the scene, the patient may still remain in ventricular fibrillation (persistent ventricular fibrillation). These patients may be helped by ALS drug interventions, but advanced EMS providers are not always available. Some protocols might direct you to deliver further defibrillation shocks at the scene or during transport. While delivering shocks during transport, you must stop the vehicle so that movement does not interfere with rhythm analysis or jeopardize safety during delivery of shock.

Recurrent Ventricular Fibrillation

When circulation has returned after defibrillation, you should monitor the patient closely for recurrent ventricular fibrillation. Ideally, you should seek early hospital intervention with or without ALS intercept to help stabilize the patient with medication. When this is not available on the scene, protocols may suggest transport while closely monitoring the patient. You should leave the AED attached to the patient. If the patient is unresponsive, attend to breathing and make frequent checks for signs of circulation. If circulation is lost en route, stop the vehicle, analyze the rhythm, and deliver a shock if necessary.

When a conscious patient collapses and has absent signs of breathing and circulation en route to the hospital, the vehicle should be stopped and the AED applied; you should proceed as previously described. Patients most likely to benefit from defibrillation are those whose cardiac arrest is witnessed by EMS providers. The AED should be readily available on the ambulance in case cardiac arrest occurs. Because patients with chest pain are at higher risk for sudden cardiac death, be especially prepared to apply the AED to these patients if indicated.

Single EMT

In some situations, you are the only EMT at the scene when an AED needs to be used. This can occur in EMS systems that use single-EMT first-response vehicles and when your partner has not yet arrived at the interior location of a business, house, or apartment. In these situations, you should perform the initial assessment. After you confirm no breathing or signs of circulation, apply the AED. Initial assessment steps to this point include the following:

1. Check for responsiveness
2. Check for breathing
3. Deliver 2 breaths
4. Check for pulse

By including the initial 2 breaths, this sequence allows you to detect an obstructed airway. When an obstructed airway is present, your initial efforts should be devoted to clearing the obstruction before attaching the AED. This is a relatively rare event. In cardiac arrest patients, defibrillation is the priority treatment. As a single EMT, you should stop CPR and assume the role of defibrillator operator and follow the defibrillation protocol as previously described. Provide 5 cycles of CPR between defibrillations.

> **LEARNING OBJECTIVES**
> • Explain the importance of prehospital ACLS intervention if available.
> • Explain the importance of urgent transport to a facility with ACLS if not available in the prehospital setting.
> • Discuss the need to complete the "Automated Defibrillator: Operator's Shift" checklist.

Coordination with Advanced Life Support Personnel

Because of the widespread use of AEDs, paramedics, physicians, nurses, and other healthcare providers are familiar with their use. When paramedics arrive at the scene where you have already applied the AED, you should be ready to assist them with use of the AED and CPR. ALS personnel have medical authority at the scene after their arrival. However, they may ask you to operate the AED if continued analysis of rhythm for shock is indicated.

Local protocols generally cover the interaction of ALS personnel with basic life support providers. This includes notification for ALS intercept at the earliest time possible because of the added benefits of ALS measures for cardiac arrest patients.

The EMT can assist paramedics in many ways at the scene of patients in cardiac arrest. For example, the EMT might provide assisted ventilation with the bag-mask, continue compressions, or operate the AED. Cardiac patients who are not in cardiac arrest can be helped by smooth interaction between EMT and paramedic personnel. Time to definitive therapy is critical for the outcome of patients with myocardial infarction. In addition to advanced airway interventions and drug therapy, 12-lead ECGs, and advanced notification to hospitals, other common tasks benefit patients by saving time to definitive care. By cooperating with paramedics so that these tasks can be accomplished quickly and efficiently, the EMT contributes directly to the patient's outcome.

If an intercept with ALS is not possible, you should rapidly transport the patient to the closest facility where ACLS is available.

Postresuscitation Care

Patients who regain spontaneous circulation after cardiac arrest show varying responses and vital signs. Continue to monitor ventilations closely and administer positive-pressure ventilations as needed. You should give supplemental oxygen to the patient who is breathing adequately. Often a lapse occurs between return of circulation and return of spontaneous breathing and consciousness. This is particularly likely if the patient was in cardiac arrest for several minutes, because the brain requires time to recover from the hypoxia. Your handling of the airway and ventilation is critical. Patients whose hearts are defibrillated immediately after a witnessed cardiac arrest are more likely to have a rapid return of spontaneous ventilations and consciousness than those not defibrillated. Patients who have spent a longer time in cardiac arrest may require continued respiratory support and may have no return of consciousness in the prehospital setting. Again, care of the airway and ensuring ventilations are important factors in improving chances of survival after a pulse has returned.

Maintenance

The AED must be maintained to ensure readiness and prevent operational failure. Carefully follow the manufacturer's instructions and setup, and adhere to a regular schedule of maintenance, visual checks, and testing of delivered energy. Keep a log to record these maintenance functions. An "Automated Defibrillator: Operator's Shift" checklist is an effective tool to remind the EMT of all AED components requiring routine evaluation, and it can serve as documentation to verify these checks.

Battery maintenance varies according to the type of machine; however, all batteries in AEDs should be tested regularly to ensure an adequate charge. Backup batteries should be available in sufficient number to ensure that fresh batteries are at hand if needed.

> **LEARNING OBJECTIVE**
> • Explain the importance of frequent practice with the AED.

Training and Sources of Information

A variety of publications with additional information on automated external defibrillation are available to enrich your knowledge and skills on this subject. You should practice frequently to maintain your skill proficiency. Most systems require practice and evaluation to ensure competency in AED use.

LEARNING OBJECTIVES
- Explain the role medical direction plays in the use of automated external defibrillation.
- State why you should complete a case review after the use of the AED.
- Discuss the components to include in a case review.
- Discuss the goal of quality improvement in automated external defibrillation.

Medical Direction and Quality Improvement

Medical direction is an essential part of any EMT defibrillation program. Physicians must assume responsibility for the program. The essential components requiring medical direction include initial education, protocol development, continuing education, case and call review, and evaluation of prehospital outcomes.

Standing orders are used in EMT defibrillation programs. *Standing orders* are written protocols directing the actions of EMTs to save valuable time in administering advanced therapy for critically ill patients. Standing orders are especially important in conditions such as ventricular fibrillation, in which prompt application of defibrillation makes a difference in outcome.

REAL*World*

In the management of cardiac arrest, some medical providers may exercise a lack of "attention to detail." Chest compressions during CPR provide minimal blood flow compared with normal circulation. During chest compressions, only 20% to 30% of blood flow is generated to vital organs. Accordingly, small reductions in blood flow can make the difference between life and death. For example, if the responder undercompresses a patient, blood flow can drop significantly during performance of CPR. If the responder also interrupts CPR frequently and for relatively long periods while performing procedures such as ventilation and AED use, blood flow to the brain and heart can be further reduced. Eventually, this marginal blood flow can drop to levels that no longer achieve the desired result: perfusion of the heart and brain and restoration of a normal heart rhythm.

To achieve optimal results during resuscitation attempts, skills must be applied in the form of "cardiac choreography," with great attention to detail. Compressions must be consistently hard and fast. To achieve this, EMTs must take turns performing the physically fatiguing skill of chest compressions. They must also stay focused to ensure that the sternum moves 1½ to 2 inches and results in complete release during the upstroke. Ventilations should be delivered over 1 second each, with compressions resumed in the shortest possible time. During skills where CPR is stopped, such as the attachment of an AED, pads should be fully applied before stopping CPR to allow analysis. In short, procedural steps must be executed with the greatest care to ensure the best perfusion possible.

The medical director or designated representative must review every event in which an AED was used. Every incident in which CPR is performed must undergo a medical review to establish whether the patient was treated in accordance with professional standards and local standing orders. Whether ventricular fibrillation and other rhythms were treated appropriately with defibrillation and basic life support must be considered in each review. Other dimensions of performance that can be evaluated include command of the scene, safety, efficiency, speed, professionalism, ability to troubleshoot, completeness of patient care, and interactions with other professionals and bystanders.

The process is performed by review of the written report, solid-state memory modules of information about each use of the device, and voice tape recorders (attached to some AEDs). The latter two methods are innovative approaches to event documentation, record keeping, and data management incorporated into AEDs. Case reviews that use all three approaches appear to offer the most complete information. Particular requirements or constraints in some systems, however, may dictate various combinations of these approaches rather than all three. Innovations in event documentation, such as digital voice recordings, annotated rhythm strips, and other microprocessor-based approaches, offer even more options.

Scenario Follow-up

The resuscitation of victims of cardiac arrest can be the most rewarding type of encounter in EMS, literally restoring life to a clinically dead patient. As shown in this chapter's scenario, being effective at resuscitation requires precise actions. Cardiac arrest must be carefully confirmed by assessment of responsiveness and breathing and palpation of a carotid pulse. When cardiac arrest is confirmed, you must immediately start CPR. CPR must be performed in a precise manner with compressions that are hard and fast and minimal interruption. Remember: *chest compressions are the only time during CPR that the brain and heart are being perfused.*

The AED must be used as soon as possible to increase the patient's chances of survival. In this scenario, the time from collapse to your arrival was relatively short, about 5 minutes, which increased the likelihood that the heart would respond to a shock. As a rule, the chance of survival decreases by 7% to 10% with each minute that passes. The implementation of bystander CPR doubles or triples the chance of survival.

This scenario illustrates the importance of each link in the "chain of survival." As an EMT, you play a critical role in educating the public, responding in a timely manner, performing CPR, and defibrillating a patient to restore a normal heart rhythm. You will be better prepared to prevent cardiac arrest by effectively managing patients with acute coronary syndromes and heart failure, knowing that cardiovascular emergencies are particularly important because cardiovascular disease is by far the most common cause of death in the United States.

Summary

Patients with chest pain are at high risk for cardiac arrest. Time to advanced care is important because early intervention can reduce the risk of death and limit the damage from heart attacks. As an EMT, you can assist patients in several ways. Assessment and communication of findings allow for early preparation by medical direction and receiving hospitals. Oxygen and assistance with prescribed nitroglycerin are early intervention options in the field, as is the automated external defibrillator (AED), if cardiac arrest occurs en route.

Defibrillation is a dramatic intervention that has saved the lives of many victims of cardiac arrest. Because EMTs are the largest group of medically trained personnel first to reach emergency patients, EMT defibrillation can be crucial. The chance for survival decreases by 7% to 10% with every minute that passes. Learning to use an AED is not difficult, and the steps should be performed as a "reflex action." You should regularly attend skill updates to retain your skills and review equipment operation and protocols when conducting maintenance checks. Defibrillation is conducted as part of an EMSS, under medical direction and according to protocols. Awareness of local protocols helps the EMT notify and interact with ALS personnel at the earliest opportunity. Continuing medical education and quality improvement efforts enabling feedback to the EMT are greatly enhanced by the AED's documentation features.

Skills

Skill | 12-1   *Administering Nitroglycerin*

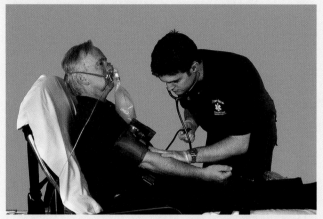

1. Perform a focused (secondary) assessment of the cardiac patient. Take a blood pressure reading (systolic blood pressure must be greater than 100 mm Hg to administer drug).

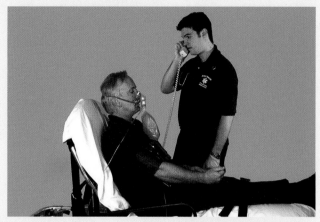

2. Question the patient regarding administration of the last dose and effects of the medication, and ensure that patient understands the route of administration. Contact medical direction if there are no standing orders. Obtain an order from medical direction either online or offline.

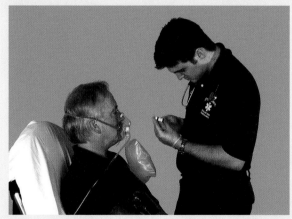

3. Ensure the right medication, right dose, and right route; that the medication is not expired; and that the patient is alert.

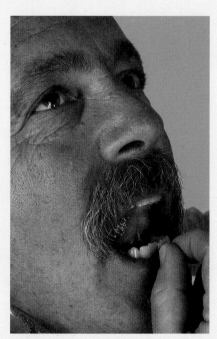

4. Ask the patient to lift the tongue, and place the tablet or spray under the tongue, or have the patient self-administer the medication. Have the patient keep the mouth closed, with the medication under the tongue (without swallowing).

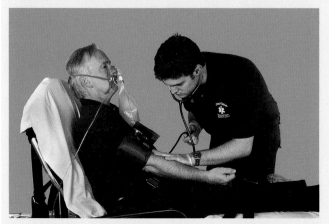

5. Recheck blood pressure within 2 minutes. Record activity and times. Perform reassessment.

Skill | 12-2   *One-Person CPR*

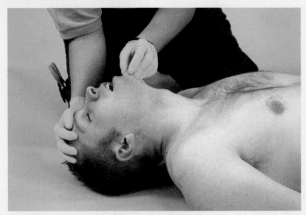

1. Check for unresponsiveness. Open the airway with the head-tilt/chin-lift or jaw thrust maneuver.

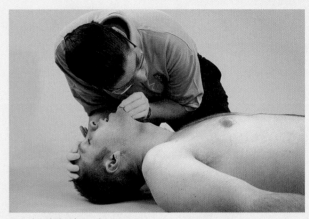

2. Check for breathing.

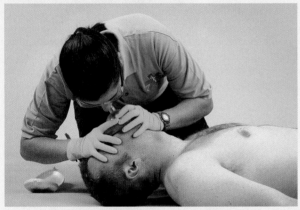

3. If not breathing, begin rescue breathing with 2 initial breaths and 1 breath every 5 to 6 seconds.

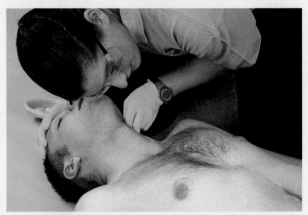

4. Check for a carotid pulse (no more than 10 and no less than 5 seconds). If there is no pulse, begin chest compressions.

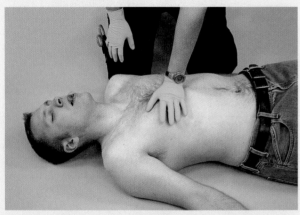

5. Locate proper hand position. Place hand at midnipple line.

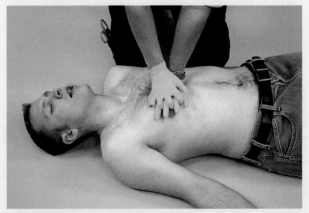

6. Perform external chest compressions at a rate of 100 compressions per minute with a compression/ventilation ratio of 30:2.

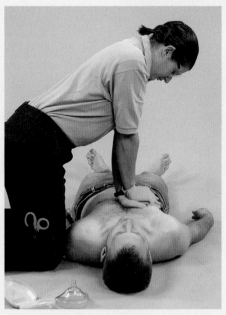

7. Depress the chest 1½ to 2 inches with each compression. Perform 5 complete cycles of 30 compressions and 2 ventilations. Reevaluate after 5 cycles of compressions and ventilations.

Skill | 12-3   *Child and Infant CPR*

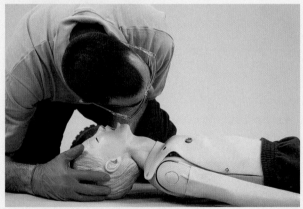

1. Check for responsiveness. Open the airway with a head-tilt/chin-lift or jaw thrust maneuver. For a child, tilt the head slightly; for an infant, place the head in the neutral position, with padding placed under the torso. Check for breathing.

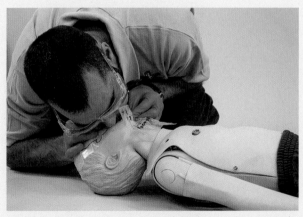

2. If not breathing, begin rescue breathing with two initial breaths sufficient to make the chest rise.

Continued

Skill | 12-3 *Child and Infant CPR—cont'd*

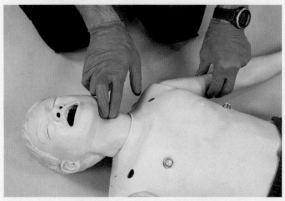

3. Check for pulse. If there is no pulse, or if pulse rate is less than 60 beats/min with signs of poor perfusion, begin chest compressions.

CHEST COMPRESSIONS ON A CHILD

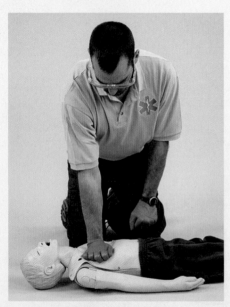

4. Perform 30 external chest compressions at a rate of 100 compressions per minute. Depress the chest one-third to one-half the depth of the child's chest diameter (front to back). Perform approximately 5 cycles of 30 compressions and 2 breaths. Reassess after 5 cycles of 30 compressions and 2 ventilations.

CHEST COMPRESSIONS ON A INFANT

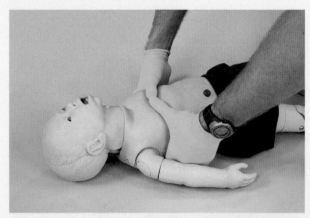

Place two fingers on the lower half of the sternum just below the nipple line, or use the two-handed thumb-encircling technique.

At one-third to one-half the depth of the infant's chest diameter, perform 30 external chest compressions at a rate of 100 compressions per minute.

Skill | 12-4 *Operating an Automated External Defibrillator (AED)*

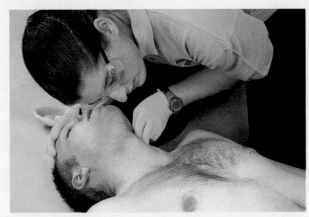

1. Take infection control precautions. Check for responsiveness. Open airway. Check for breathing in and provide 2 breaths. Check for a pulse (pulse absent).

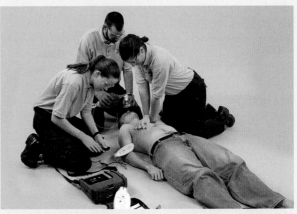

2. Begin CPR. Position the AED close to the victim. Turn on the AED by pressing the power switch or lifting the top of the case.

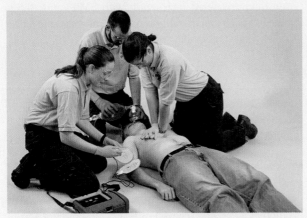

3. Prepare to place the AED pads on the patient's chest while CPR is in progress.

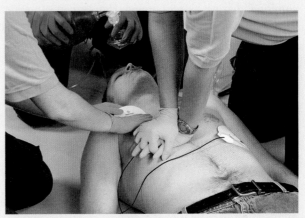

4. Attach electrode pads to the patient at the right sternal border, below the clavicle and 2 to 3 inches below the left armpit.

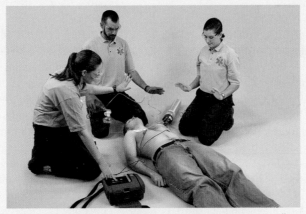

5. Clear the patient, and press the analyze button or allow the machine to analyze automatically after attaching the pads. If shock advised, confirm that everyone is clear, and press the shock button. Immediately resume CPR, starting with chest compressions.

The Bottom Line

Learning Checklist

✓ Arteriosclerosis is a progressive narrowing of the arteries that results in the development of acute coronary syndromes, including angina pectoris and myocardial infarction.

✓ Ischemic chest pain typically occurs in the center of the chest and may radiate to the neck, jaw, or arms. Patients may also complain of abdominal pain or indigestion.

✓ Angina pectoris is chest pain that is usually caused by increased oxygen demands on the heart (e.g., stress, exertion, exercise) not met by the oxygen supply and that is relieved by rest and nitroglycerin.

✓ Myocardial infarction (MI) is defined as death of heart muscle caused by blockage or occlusion of a coronary artery.

✓ Signs and symptoms of MI may include ischemic chest pain, sweating, pale and cool skin, shortness of breath, nausea, vomiting, dizziness, and fainting. However, many patients may not experience chest or other common symptoms. This is more common in women, diabetic patients, and elderly persons.

✓ Victims of MI may deny their symptoms and refuse treatment. EMS providers should make every attempt to convince patients with signs of heart disease to go to the hospital for evaluation.

✓ Place patients with chest pain or shortness of breath in the position of comfort.

✓ EMTs may assist patients with prescribed nitroglycerin with administration of the tablets or spray.

✓ Nitroglycerin administration may be repeated every 3 to 5 minutes, up to a total of three doses, if the systolic blood pressure is greater than 100 mm Hg.

✓ Heart failure is a condition resulting from a damaged or weak heart muscle that is caused by severe MI, chronic hypertension, and other causes.

✓ Patients with heart failure may exhibit shortness of breath; noisy breath sounds (left-sided heart failure); swelling of the ankles, lower back, or abdomen; or distended neck veins (right-sided heart failure).

✓ Cardiac arrest is caused by heart rhythms that result in no blood flow, including asystole, pulseless electrical activity, or ventricular fibrillation/ventricular tachycardia.

✓ Effective, early cardiopulmonary resuscitation (CPR) with a compression/ventilation ratio of 30:2 increases survivability of a cardiac arrest event.

✓ CPR is most effectively performed by two persons but can be done by one person.
  Interruptions in CPR should be limited and kept short, typically no longer than 10 seconds.

✓ Ventricular fibrillation is a useless quivering of the heart that results in no blood flow.

✓ The only effective treatment for ventricular fibrillation is electric shock with a defibrillator.

✓ An automated external defibrillator (AED) is a computerized device that recognizes shockable versus nonshockable heart rhythms and advises the operator to deliver an electric shock when appropriate.

✓ AED electrode pads are placed on the right upper chest, below the clavicle on the right border of the sternum and on the left chest 2 to 3 inches below the armpit.

✓ The operation of an AED involves four distinct steps: (1) turning the device on; (2) attaching the electrode pads; (3) clearing the patient and allowing the device to analyze; and (4) when advised, clearing the patient and pushing the shock button.

✓ Most AEDs can safely be used on persons older than 8 years. Special patches allow AED use on infants and children.

✓ Continual training on CPR and AED use is crucial if the EMT is to remain proficient.

✓ Smooth, coordinated interaction with EMTs and ALS personnel (e.g., paramedics, flight nurses) increases the patient's chance of survival in all cardiac events.

Key Terms

Abdominal aortic aneurysm Localized abnormal dilation of the descending arota that becomes a life-threatening emergency on rupture.

Acute coronary syndromes Group of diseases (e.g., myocardial infarction, angina) characterized by ischemia of heart tissue.

Angina pectoris Temporary chest pain caused by lack of blood flow to the heart to meet the oxygen needs; usually caused by exertion or stress and relieved by rest.

Arteriosclerosis Progressive disease of the arteries that results in narrowing of the lumen caused by deposits of fat and hardening of the arterial wall.

Asystole Cardiac standstill, or an absence of any cardiac rhythm; "flatline."

Automated external defibrillator (AED) Defibrillation that interprets the patient's ECG rhythm and automatically initiates or advises defibrillation as needed.

Defibrillation External application of an electric shock across the heart of sufficient energy to convert ventricular fibrillation into an organized rhythm.

Defibrillator Device capable of delivering an electric shock to reverse an otherwise-lethal cardiac rhythm.

Electrode pads Adhesive pads that transmit electrical signs from the body through cables to detect the heart's electrical activity and in turn transfer electrical energy from the defibrillator to the body.

Heart failure Condition resulting when destruction of the heart muscle reduces the heart's power of contraction.

Implanted cardioverter-defibrillator (ICD) Automated device implanted in a patient's chest that delivers a number of low-energy shocks directly to the myocardium; also called *automated ICD (AICD)*.

Ischemia Insufficient blood supply to an area.

Ischemic chest pain Characteristic pain resulting from inadequate blood supply to the myocardium.

Myocardial infarction Severe and sustained oxygen deprivation of the myocardium resulting in the death of heart cells; commonly known as a "heart attack."

Pacemaker Group of cells in the heart that initiates the electrical impulses of the heart. Also, a mechanical device implanted to control certain dysrhythmias or provide a backup should the heart's natural pacemaker fail.

Public access defibrillation (PAD) Strategy of placing AEDs in public places such as airports and encouraging their use by trained laypersons.

Pulmonary embolism Obstruction of the pulmonary artery, often caused by a blood clot from leg veins.

Pulseless electrical activity Condition in which the heart has an organized electrical rhythm, but there is no palpable pulse.

Thoracic aortic dissection Tear in the wall of the aorta that causes the vessel to split (dissect), forming a false passage; proximal and distal types.

Thrombus A clot that develops within a blood vessel.

Ventricular fibrillation Chaotic quivering of the heart resulting in cardiac arrest.

Ventricular tachycardia Rapid dysrhythmia (100-200 beats/min) that may or may not be capable of producing a pulse.

Review Questions

1. A 68-year-old man has collapsed in the presence of his co-workers. Place the following actions taken by the lay rescuer in the correct order:
   a. Phone the local EMSS and send someone to retrieve an AED (if available)
   b. Check for responsiveness
   c. Check for breathing
   d. Start CPR

2. A 72-year-old woman is complaining of severe difficulty breathing. She has a history of high blood pressure. Her vital signs are pulse 88 and regular, blood pressure 180/110, and respirations 26 and labored. Her breath sounds reveal crackles (rales) in the bottom of her lung fields. What is the likely cause of her difficulty breathing and crackles?
   a. Cardiac arrest
   b. Pulmonary edema
   c. Heart failure
   d. Allergic reaction

3. How would you explain why cardiac arrest victims collapse into a state of unconsciousness following the start of ventricular fibrillation?
   a. Irreversible damage to the brain
   b. Diminished perfusion of blood to the brain
   c. Respiratory distress
   d. Damage to the aorta and major vessels

4. Ischemic chest pain often includes which of the following characteristics?
   a. Radiation to the back
   b. Sharp and intermittent quality
   c. Radiation to the left arm
   d. Increased amount with breathing

5. You respond to a 60-year-old woman with "squeezing" chest pain. She is pale, sweaty, and has shortness of breath. Her blood pressure is 140/90 and pulse 96 and regular. List three medications that you can administer as an EMT, assuming there are no complications or contraindications.

6. List two reasons why *early* defibrillation is so critical to the survival of patients with ventricular fibrillation and sudden cardiac arrest.

7. Why should you never touch a patient during the analysis of an AED?
   a. A movement could affect the AED's ability to interpret the rhythm
   b. The EMT could be shocked
   c. The AED could read the EMT's heart
   d. It could cause the AED to arc

8. Why is performing 5 cycles of CPR so important after a defibrillation?
   a. It helps to disperse the electricity from the AED
   b. It allows the AED time to reset
   c. It keeps all EMTs busy
   d. It allows the heart to perfuse and improves the chances of a successful defibrillation

9. If the first rhythm analysis with an AED reads "no shock advised" and the patient has no pulse, you should:
   a. Perform a chest thump and then analyze the rhythm
   b. Transport immediately with CPR en route
   c. Perform CPR for 5 cycles and reanalyze
   d. Defibrillate three times before transport

10. What should you do if a patient who was resuscitated and has an AED attached becomes unresponsive and pulseless during transport?
    a. Stop the ambulance and analyze the rhythm
    b. Continue with CPR
    c. Analyze the rhythm while en route
    d. Stop the ambulance, perform 1 minute of CPR, and then analyze the rhythm

11. As a single EMT with an AED, you encounter a pulseless patient who collapsed approximately 8 minutes ago. What should you do first?
    a. Perform 2 minutes of CPR
    b. Prepare the patient for immediate transport
    c. Wait for ALS
    d. Shock immediately

12. What should you do if you find a patient in cardiac arrest in a puddle after being removed from a pool?
    a. Apply a shock to the patient on the ground
    b. Move the patient to a dry surface, dry the chest, and attach the AED
    c. Hold an umbrella over the patient and apply shock
    d. Wipe the ground dry around the patient

13. What should you do after successful restoration of a pulse after defibrillation?
    a. Check for breathing and provide positive-pressure ventilation if necessary.
    b. Refrain from moving the patient until ALS crews arrive.
    c. Remove the AED.
    d. Administer self-prescribed nitroglycerin if available.

For Further Review

In the Student Workbook

- Multiple-choice questions
- Matching questions
- Short-answer questions
- Case scenario questions
- Skill check questions

On Evolve

- Anatomy challenge
- Weblinks
- Lecture notes
- Exercises

Learning Objectives

Cognitive Objectives

- Define the role of the EMT in the emergency cardiac care system.
- Predict the relationship between basic life support and the patient experiencing cardiovascular compromise.
- Explain the rationale for early defibrillation.
- Explain why cardiac arrest does not occur in all patients with chest pain and why all do not need to be attached to an AED.
- Discuss the role of the American Heart Association in the use of automated external defibrillation.
- Discuss the fundamentals of early defibrillation.
- Describe the structure and function of the cardiovascular system.
- Describe the emergency medical care of the patient experiencing chest pain or discomfort.
- Discuss the position of comfort for patients with various cardiac emergencies.
- Establish the relationship between airway management and the patient with cardiovascular compromise.
- Recognize the need for medical direction of protocols to assist in the emergency medical care of the patient with chest pain.

- List indications for the use of nitroglycerin.
- State contraindications and side effects for the use of nitroglycerin.
- Discuss the importance of CPR.
- Discuss the integration of CPR into other resuscitation procedures (e.g., AED use).
- Explain why changing EMTs every 2 minutes is so important during CPR.
- Discuss the importance of chest compressions that are hard, fast, and minimally interrupted.
- List the steps for one-person CPR and two-person CPR for the adult, child, and infant victim of cardiac arrest.
- Discuss the various types of AEDs.
- Discuss the procedures that must be taken into consideration for standard operation of the various types of AEDs.
- State the reasons for ensuring that the patient is pulseless and apneic when using the AED.
- List the indications for automated external defibrillation.
- List the contraindications for automated external defibrillation.
- Discuss the circumstances that may result in inappropriate shocks.
- Explain the considerations for interruption of CPR when using the AED.
- Discuss the advantages and disadvantages of AEDs.
- Summarize the speed of operation of automated external defibrillation.
- Discuss the use of remote defibrillation through adhesive pads.
- Discuss the special considerations for rhythm monitoring.
- List the steps in the operation of the AED.
- Explain the impact of age and weight on defibrillation.
- Differentiate between single-person and multiperson care with an AED.
- Explain the reason for pulses not being checked between shocks with an AED.
- Discuss the importance of coordinating ACLS-trained providers with personnel using AEDs.
- Discuss the importance of postresuscitation care.
- List the components of postresuscitation care.
- Define the function of all controls on an AED, and describe event documentation and battery defibrillator maintenance.
- Discuss the standard of care for a patient with persistent or recurrent ventricular fibrillation and no available ACLS.
- Explain the importance of prehospital ACLS intervention if available.
- Explain the importance of urgent transport to a facility with ACLS if not available in the prehospital setting.
- Discuss the need to complete the "Automated Defibrillator: Operator's Shift" checklist.
- Explain the importance of frequent practice with the AED.
- Explain the role medical direction plays in the use of automated external defibrillation.
- State why you should complete a case review after the use of the AED.
- Discuss the components to include in a case review.
- Discuss the goal of quality improvement in automated external defibrillation.

Affective Objectives

- Defend the reasons for obtaining initial training in automated external defibrillation and the importance of continuing education.
- Defend the reason for maintenance of AED.
- Explain the rationale for administering nitroglycerin to a patient with chest pain or discomfort.

Psychomotor Objectives

- Demonstrate the assessment and emergency medical care of a patient experiencing chest pain or discomfort.
- Demonstrate the application and operation of the AED.
- Demonstrate the maintenance of an AED.
- Demonstrate the assessment and documentation of patient response to the AED.

- Demonstrate the skills necessary to complete the "Automated Defibrillator: Operator's Shift" checklist.
- Perform the steps in facilitating the use of nitroglycerin for chest pain or discomfort.
- Demonstrate the assessment and documentation of patient response to nitroglycerin.
- Practice completing a prehospital care report for patients with cardiac emergencies.

References

American Heart Association: Guidelines for cardiopulmonary resuscitation and emergency cardiovascular care. Part 4. Adult basic life support, *Circulation*112(suppl IV):19-34, 2005.

Aufderheide TP, Pirrallo RG, Yannopoulos D, et al: Incomplete chest wall decompression: a clinical evaluation of CPR performance by EMS personnel and assessment of alternative manual chest compression-decompression techniques, *Ressuscitation* 64(3):353-362, 2005.

Lurie KG, Mulligan KA, McKnite S, et al: Optimizing standard cardiopulmonary resuscitation with an inspiratory impedance threshold valve, *Chest* 113(4):1084-1090, 1998.

Safer P, Escarrag LA, Elam JO: A comparison of mouth-to-mouth and mouth-to-airway methods of artificial ventilation with the chest-pressure, arm-lift methods, *N Engl J Med* 258:671-677, 1958.

Wik L, Kramer-Johansen J, Myklebust H, et al: Quality of cardiopulmonary resuscitation during out-of-hospital cardiac arrest, *JAMA* 293:299-304, 2005.

Yannopoulos D, McKnite S, Aufderheide TP: Effects of incomplete chest wall decompression during cardiopulmonary resuscitation on coronary and cerebral perfusion pressures in a porcine model of cardiac arrest, *Resuscitation* 64(3):363-372, 2005.

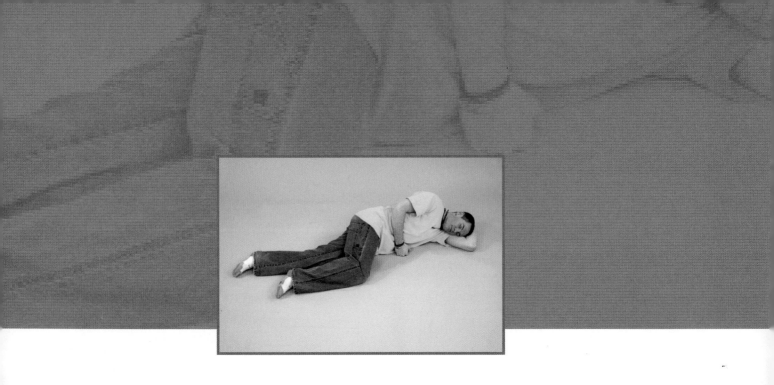

13 Altered Mental Status

CHAPTER OUTLINE

Anatomy and Physiology

Causes of Altered Mental Status

Diabetic Emergencies

Seizures

Stroke

Emergency Medical Care for Patients with Altered Mental Status

Chronic Neurologic Diseases

Skills

Scenario

You are called to a grocery store where the store's security office has reported a 45-year-old man wandering the aisles, picking up groceries as if to eat them, and acting bizarrely. You find the man in an aisle and identify yourself. The patient is sitting up and breathing adequately but not answering your questions. His skin is clammy, and his pulse is 120 beats/min. During the focused (secondary) assessment (physical examination), you notice a necklace with a MedicAlert tag identifying the patient as a diabetic. The patient is able to swallow. According to your protocol, you administer one tube of oral glucose between the patient's cheek and the gum and transport the patient. Ten minutes later, en route to the hospital, the patient begins to speak and tells you that he had taken his insulin but had skipped a meal.

An alteration in a person's mental status is a common reason people call for emergency medical care. An altered mental status can range from mild confusion and abnormal behavior to deep coma, a condition in which the patient is totally unresponsive to verbal or painful stimuli. An altered mental status indicates a problem either originating in the brain, such as a stroke, or affecting the brain, such as hypoglycemia, poisoning, or hypoxia. Some forms of altered mentation represent a medical emergency requiring rapid assessment and intervention on the part of the emergency medical technician (EMT). Other forms are chronic conditions to be noted by the EMT but do not require emergency treatment, such as dementia or Alzheimer's disease.

Problems with the brain take high priority in emergency care because the brain controls consciousness, sensation, motor ability, and vital functions. The general goals of prehospital care for patients with altered *central nervous system* (CNS) function are as follows:

- Ensuring adequate ventilation and circulation.
- Administration of supplemental oxygen and, if needed, glucose.
- Assessment and treatment of the underlying cause.
- Assessment and treatment of other problems.
- Considering the possibility of trauma (and if trauma exists, supporting the spine).

On finding an alteration in mental status, the EMT must immediately assess the adequacy of ventilations because control of vital functions such as breathing and circulation may be compromised. For example, with an overdose of a CNS depressant (e.g., opioid, barbiturate), a patient may at first appear sleepy or lethargic, then gradually enter a more depressed and unresponsive state (coma). Continued depression of the CNS can affect the ability to breathe, and the patient may hypoventilate and enter respiratory arrest. In fact, a common cause of death from overdose is failure of the respiratory system.

Respiratory problems are also the first concern for patients with conditions such as stroke or seizures. Loss of control of the musculature may allow the tongue to fall back into the pharynx, blocking the airway. Loss of a reflex action, such as the ability to gag or to clear the airway, places the patient at risk for aspiration of any secretions or vomit into the lungs. In fact, all patients who are unresponsive are subject to complications from airway obstruction, aspirations, and respiratory failure.

One way to categorize alteration of mental status is by using the **AVPU** mnemonic (*a*lert, *r*esponsive to *v*erbal stimuli, responsive to *p*ainful stimuli, and *u*nresponsive). However, healthcare providers use many terms to describe an alteration in mental status that you should be familiar with, such as the following:

- *Lethargy.* Sluggishness or sleepiness. The patient is easily aroused but drifts into a sleepy state without continued stimulation.
- *Confusion.* An inability to maintain a coherent stream of thought or action.
- *Delirium.* An agitated and confused state.
- *Stupor.* A state of lessened responsiveness. The patient can be aroused, but more stimuli are required than for the lethargic patient. In addition, with arousal the stuporous patient does not reach a normal level of consciousness and function. For example, speech may be slurred or garbled, and motor ability may be sluggish and uncoordinated.
- *Semicoma.* A condition of unconsciousness or lack of awareness of the environment from which the patient may be aroused.
- *Coma.* A lack of responsiveness to the environment. The patient is unconscious and cannot be aroused by external stimuli.

Although these terms are often used to describe a patient's condition, their use has certain disadvantages. For example, the same patient may be described as "semicomatose" or "stuporous" by different observers. Furthermore, an EMT will have difficulty in assessing changes in a patient's condition by using these terms alone. For this reason, most authorities recommend using more precise descriptions of a patient's ability to respond to stimuli. This is the reason that such methods as AVPU or the Glasgow Coma Scale are used by emergency medical services (EMS).

Some patients devolve by degrees from an alert state to a coma, as might happen with the gradual but continued absorption of a toxic drug or chemical. Other patients may suddenly become comatose because of a condition such as a generalized seizure or a burst blood vessel within the brain. The history of the event is therefore important for determining whether the change in mentation is acute or sudden in onset or has occurred gradually.

Conscious and alert patients also may experience degrees of intellectual and memory function. You can quickly determine whether a patient is oriented to the environment. A confused patient may not be aware of the time of day, the date, or even the year. Similarly, a patient may not be aware of the immediate surroundings. Less frequently, patients may not be aware of their own name. As often happens with patients who have a concussion, loss of memory can also occur. Patients may not be able to remember the immediate events preceding or following their injury.

Case in Point

You are called to the Northpoint Nursing Home for an elderly patient who has fallen and is unable to walk. On arrival, you notice a patient on the floor in the dining room, and his right leg appears shortened and externally rotated. The aide tells you he cried out in pain as soon as he fell and has been complaining about hip pain. During your assessment you ask the patient, "What is your name? Do you know where you are? And what is today's date?" He answers correctly to his name and place, but for date he tells you a month and year in the past.

The aide tells you this is not unusual for Mr. Johnson. One of his medical problems is Alzheimer's disease. You note on your record this past medical history and that he is "Alert and Oriented x2," to person and place.

REAL_World_

Some may look at a geriatric patient with an altered mental status and assume the change in mentation is because of age. It is important to know that a change in mentation is not considered a normal part of aging. Elderly patients presenting with abnormal speech, thoughts, or actions must be assumed to have a medical condition and must be evaluated and transported for treatment.

Anatomy and Physiology

The nervous system is the controlling organ of the body. It is the center of consciousness and the location of intellectual, emotional, and behavioral functions that make up much of the characteristics of personality and human behavior. It receives and interprets stimuli from the internal and external environment, and it directs and regulates other organs and tissues. Some of the brain's activity is conscious or willful, but much of it is unconscious or involuntary in response to the external and internal environment.

Central Nervous System

The central nervous system (CNS) is composed of the brain, brainstem, and spinal cord. The brain is the central computer. It processes sensory input from sensory nerves and organizes responses that are then transmitted back to the body by outgoing motor nerves. Sensory input includes sight, hearing, smell, taste, and touch. Temperature, pain, vibration, pressure, and tickle are all variations of touch or feeling. Special receptors in the ear and special nerve pathways relay input concerning balance and equilibrium. The brain receives input about the oxygen and carbon dioxide content of the blood as well as about the body's circulatory and nutritional status. All this information is processed at incredible speeds, as evidenced by your reaction to a startling noise or noxious taste or odor. So much information is received by the brain at any one time that people are ordinarily conscious of only about 1% of the sensory input.

Brain

The largest and most superior portion of the brain is called the _cerebrum_. The _cerebrum_ is _divided_ down the middle into right and left halves called _hemispheres_. Generally, the right hemisphere controls the left side of the body, and vice versa.

The hemispheres are further subdivided into different _lobes_ or sections that have specific and distinct functions. The lobes are named by their location with respect to the overlying skull bones; for example, the _frontal_ lobe is the area responsible for intellectual functions and motor control of skeletal muscles. The _occipital_ area is the center for receiving and processing visual stimuli, and the _temporal_ area receives smell and hearing signals. **Figure 13-1** shows the distribution of functions in the brain.

The _brainstem_ is the lower part of the brain. Nerve centers in the brainstem monitor and direct respiratory and circulatory function. Damage to certain parts of the brainstem can result in abnormal breathing patterns or cessation of breathing.

The _cerebellum_ is an outpocketing of the brain located behind or posterior to the brainstem. It is primarily concerned with coordination of movement and balance.

Blood Supply of the Brain

The brain has a very rich blood supply to meet its metabolic needs. The main blood supply to the brain is provided through the carotid arteries, which provide 80% of the blood supply to the brain. The remainder of circulation to the brain occurs through the vertebral arteries that feed the brainstem, then connect to the basilar artery, which then joins the carotid arteries in the center of the brain. From this point, all regions of the brain are fed through multiple arterial networks. Each area has its own blood supply, which explains the damage and physical findings that can occur when a particular artery is blocked with a blood clot. For example, if an artery supplying the occipital lobe in the posterior cerebrum was blocked, the patient might experience visual disturbances or even blindness. **Figure 13-2** illustrates major arteries supplying circulation to the brain.

Sensitivity to Deprivation of Oxygen and Glucose

The brain is extremely sensitive to deprivation of oxygen and glucose. For example, when blood flow ceases to the brain and oxygen delivery stops, unconsciousness follows within 5 to 10 seconds. If the brain is completely deprived of oxygen, as in cardiac arrest, biological death (irreversible brain death) of the brain can occur within 4 to 6 minutes. Thus, early application of cardiopulmonary resuscitation (CPR) and defibrillation are critical to survival.

The brain also relies on a constant supply of glucose to serve its metabolic needs. It cannot store glucose for future use. When deprived of glucose, a patient may exhibit an altered mental status that ranges from simple confusion to combativeness to coma. Patients who are exhibiting "psychiatric symptoms" or appear to be drunk must be carefully evaluated, because these symptoms may be related to glucose deprivation caused by medications used to treat diabetes or other causes of hypoglycemia.

Causes of Altered Mental Status

Altered mental status has many causes. CNS problems may have a structural or a metabolic origin. This basic understanding helps the EMT appreciate physical findings that may provide a rationale for treatment in the prehospital or hospital phase of

care. When damage to part of the structure of the CNS occurs, part of the brain is disrupted while other parts are left intact. A metabolic problem, such as low levels of blood glucose or blood oxygen, affects all parts of the brain.

Structural Causes

The most common structural problem encountered by the EMT is a **stroke** or **cerebrovascular accident (CVA).** When the blood supply to part of the brain is disrupted, that portion of the brain fails to function from lack of oxygen. Because only part of the brain has been damaged, the patient may have findings on the physical examination that are one-sided (unilateral) or *asymmetrical.*

Many victims of stroke also have an altered mental status. The presence of asymmetrical motor and sensory findings in the medical patient with an altered mental status should suggest a structural condition such as a CVA. Another possibility to consider is whether the patient has a history of recent head trauma. The patient could have an expanding blood clot originating from a head injury that occurred a week or a month earlier.

Case in Point

You are assessing an elderly man whose speech is difficult to understand. The family states that the patient is not acting normally. The patient appears to understand when spoken to and can follow simple commands. When asked to hold up both arms, the patient can only hold up his right arm. This unilateral (one-sided) weakness suggests the patient had a CVA (stroke).

Metabolic Causes

Most patients with altered mental status have metabolic conditions. These conditions usually originate outside the CNS. Although metabolic conditions can affect brain function by many different mechanisms, they tend to affect both sides of the brain equally. Therefore the physical findings are generally two-sided (bilateral) and diffuse rather than one-sided and localized.

The sources of metabolic problems may be external or internal **(Table 13-1).** Examples of external problems include the following:

- Poisoning (see Chapter 15)
- Overdoses and alcohol abuse (see Chapter 15)
- Environmental conditions such as hypothermia (abnormally low body temperature) and hyperthermia (abnormally high body temperature) (see Chapter 16)
- Infectious organisms that invade the CNS

Examples of internal problems include the following:

- All respiratory or circulatory conditions that result in hypoxia or hypoperfusion of the brain
- Diabetic states (especially those causing low blood sugar)
- Failure of the liver or the kidneys, which causes a buildup of toxic substances

Figure 13-3 illustrates the motor-sensory findings in patients with structural versus metabolic problems.

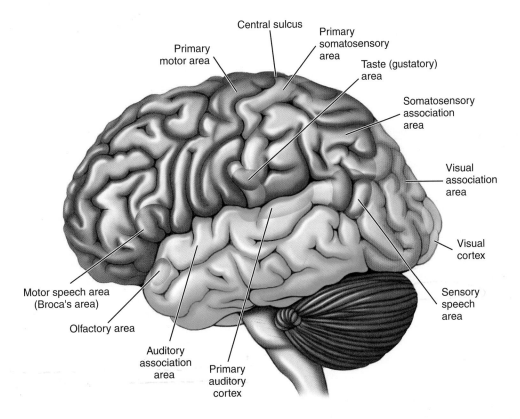

Figure 13-1   Anatomy of the brain. Different parts of the brain have different functions, such as vision, hearing, speech, motor control, and sensation. *From Herlihy B, Maebius N:* The human body in health and illness, *Philadelphia, ed 3, 2007, Saunders.*

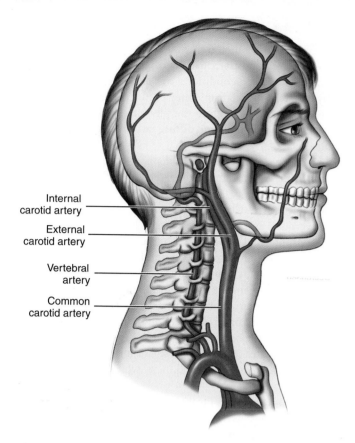

Figure 13-2 Blood supply of the brain. When an individual artery is blocked, the part of the brain distal to the flow is compromised. Blockage of different arteries leads to different stroke syndromes, such as loss of speech, loss of motor control on one side, or loss of sensation on one side. *From Herlihy B, Maebius N: The human body in health and illness, Philadelphia, ed 3, 2007, Saunders.*

LEARNING OBJECTIVE
- Identify the patient taking diabetic medications with altered mental status and the implications of a diabetes history.

Diabetic Emergencies

Physiology

Diabetes is a disease caused by an inadequate secretion of the hormone **insulin.** Insulin helps regulate the use and storage of glucose. **Glucose** is a sugar molecule (a type of carbohydrate) used by the cells for energy. Glucose is absorbed into the blood after a person eats food. As the blood glucose level increases, insulin is secreted to move glucose into the cells, where it is used for energy or stored for future use.

The body depends on glucose for its basic energy needs. However, most cells can also use other sources of fuel, such as fats, if the supply of glucose is low. The brain is unique in that it depends almost exclusively on glucose. When the brain is deprived of glucose, brain function is altered and unconsciousness, seizures, and brain cell death can occur.

Table 13-1	Causes of Altered Mental Status*	
	Metabolic	
Structural	**External**	**Internal**
Stroke	Poisonings	Hypoxia
Recent head trauma	Overdoses	Hypotension
	Hypothermia or hyperthermia	Diabetic states
	Infections	Organ failure

*Psychiatric conditions may cause altered mental status. Always consider metabolic and structural causes in all patients before attributing a change in mental status to a psychiatric cause.

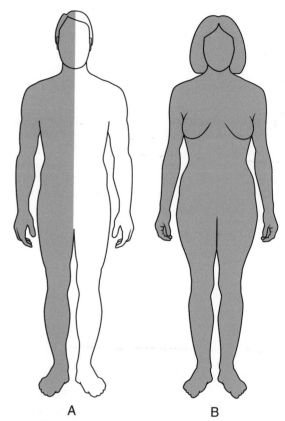

A   B

Figure 13-3 **A,** Structural injuries result in one-sided or asymmetrical signs, such as the inability to move the left arm or leg but with normal movement on the right side. **B,** Metabolic conditions affect all portions of the brain equally and result in bilateral physical findings.

Many complications of diabetes are associated with a blood sugar level that is too low or too high. Two life-threatening conditions faced by diabetics that require emergency care are **hypoglycemia** (low blood glucose level or insulin shock) and **diabetic ketoacidosis (DKA)** (high glucose level).

Glucose Metabolism

Insulin. Insulin is produced within specialized cells in the pancreas. As the glucose level in the blood increases after a meal, the body secretes insulin to cause movement of the glucose

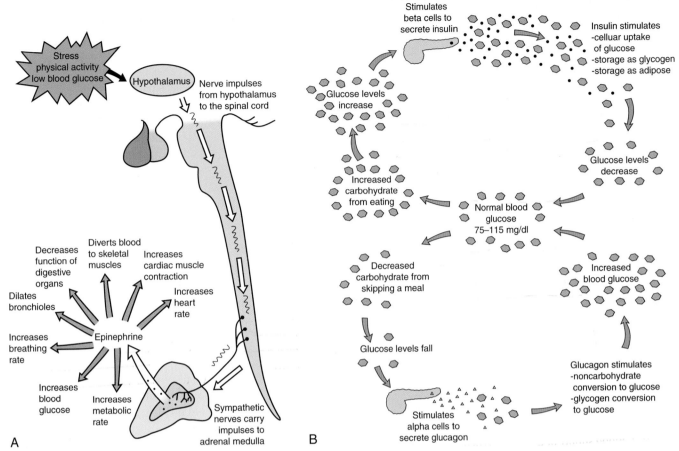

Figure 13-4 **A,** Epinephrine effects and control of its secretion. **B,** Effects of insulin and glucagon. *From Applegate E:* The anatomy and physiology learning system, *ed 3, Philadelphia, 2006, Saunders.*

and other food products into cells for immediate use as fuel and for storage for future needs. Some glucose is stored in the liver and muscle as a larger molecule called *glycogen* (composed of multiple glucose molecules). Some glucose is converted to fat, where it is stored for future use. As glucose moves into the cells, the blood glucose level falls, and insulin secretion is reduced.

The body uses both glucose and fats for fuel. After meals, glucose may be the main fuel used throughout the body. Between meals, fats are used. The brain, however, must continue to have an adequate supply of glucose because it cannot burn fats for its energy needs.

Glucagon. To ensure an adequate supply of blood glucose between meals, the hormone **glucagon** causes stored forms of glucose to be released and glucose to be synthesized from other molecules. Glucagon is secreted when the blood glucose level starts to fall. Glucagon causes glycogen to convert back to glucose molecules, which then enter the blood. It also can cause cells to make glucose from other molecules. The actions of insulin and glucagon maintain a relatively constant blood level of glucose after eating and between meals (**Figure 13-4, B**).

Glucagon is released when use of glucose is increased (e.g., during exercise) or when intake of glucose from meals is reduced (e.g., fasting). For example, muscles consume the blood's glucose during exercise; the blood glucose level starts to decrease, which activates the release of glucagon. Glucagon, in turn, releases stored glucose from glycogen and makes glucose

from other molecules to maintain the glucose needs of muscles and the brain.

Glucagon can be injected and is used to treat hypoglycemia. Many diabetic patients have glucagon emergency kits in their homes that can be used by family members if they become unable to swallow because of altered mental status from hypoglycemia, an abnormally low blood glucose level. You may encounter this medication when you arrive at the home of an unconscious diabetic patient. In some states, glucagon is administered by EMTs.

Epinephrine. Epinephrine, released during stress or exercise, also has a glucagon-like effect. In hypoglycemia, epinephrine causes further release of glucose from the liver. During stress, epinephrine increases the supply of both energy sources—glucose and fat (fatty acids)—to provide fuel for the fight-or-flight reaction.

Signs of epinephrine release, such as pale and cool skin, rapid pulse, sweating, and a normal or slightly elevated blood pressure, can be noted in patients with hypoglycemia (**Figure 13-4, A**).

Classification of Diabetes

In diabetic patients the pancreas does not secrete an adequate amount of insulin. If untreated, patients would have inappropriately high concentrations of blood glucose and abnormal metabolism. The two general classifications of diabetes are as follows:

- Insulin-dependent (type 1)
- Non-insulin-dependent (type 2)

Insulin-Dependent Diabetes

Patients who have a severe or absolute lack of insulin require treatment with insulin, which must be injected on a daily basis. Insulin is available in different forms, which vary according to time of onset, peak effect, and duration of action.

Diabetic patients must also be careful to balance their food intake with their medication. For example, if they take insulin and do not eat, their blood glucose level will drop too low. If they overeat or do not take insulin, their blood glucose level will rise too high. Other factors that can affect the balance between glucose and insulin are illness and exercise. Infections and fever may increase the body's insulin requirement. Exercise increases glucose requirements. Patients with diabetes learn to adjust their food intake and insulin injections accordingly. They must test their blood for glucose on a regular basis to make the appropriate adjustments in food intake and insulin. Blood testing may be performed with a glucometer, which gives a numeric result. EMTs in some EMS systems carry and use glucometers to test whether low blood glucose is a problem for a patient.

Non-Insulin-Dependent Diabetes

Patients in whom diabetes develops later in life may not require insulin injections. This type of diabetes is referred to as non-insulin-dependent diabetes. Some patients can control their blood glucose level by diet alone. Others require oral medications to stimulate the pancreas to secrete more insulin **(Table 13-2)**.

Table 13-2	Oral Agents Used for Diabetes*
Generic Name	**Brand Name**
Chlorpropamide	Diabinese
Glimepiride	Amaryl
Glipizide	Glucotrol
Glyburide	DiaBeta
Glyburide/metformin	Glucovance
Metformin	Glucophage
Pioglitazone	Actos
Repaglinide	Prandin
Rosiglitazone	Avandia
Tolazamide	Tolinase
Tolbutamide	Orinase

*This table shows only a partial listing.

REALWorld

Non-insulin-dependent (type 2) diabetes once was considered an "adult-onset" disease. It is now associated with obesity and poor diet. The increased incidence of childhood obesity and inactivity has resulted in an increase in pediatric onset of type 2 diabetes.

LEARNING OBJECTIVES
- Identify the patient taking diabetic medications with altered mental status and the implications of a diabetes history.
- Establish the relationship between airway management and the patient with altered mental status.
- Explain the rationale for administering oral glucose.

Hypoglycemia

Hypoglycemia (an abnormally low blood glucose level) is the most common and treatable problem among diabetic patients encountered in prehospital care. The major signs and symptoms are related to an altered mental status caused by the brain's need for glucose and signs of epinephrine release.

Although hypoglycemia can occur for other reasons, it usually occurs as a result of too much insulin, too little food, or a combination of these factors. (A patient who is vomiting would be at risk for too little food intake.)

Situations that may result in hypoglycemia include (1) unusual exercise or physical exertion without extra food intake and (2) a person who takes insulin in the morning (or oral medications that stimulate insulin release) and then forgets to eat breakfast or lunch. Some diabetic patients are particularly prone to hypoglycemia, and no identifiable predisposing factor may be noted. Hypoglycemia tends to occur suddenly. Hypoglycemia also can occur in patients who do not have diabetes, such as malnourished individuals (e.g., alcoholics) or infants with poor glycogen supplies.

The signs of altered mental status are extremely variable. Hypoglycemic patients can be mistaken as psychotic or intoxicated because they may display combativeness, hostility, and bizarre behavior. Patients may be described by friends or co-workers as acting unusual or not "like themselves."

The patient may progress from an agitated, anxious, and excited state to a sleepier or more lethargic state with less spontaneous conversation, disturbances in judgment, and confusion. Further deterioration may result in seizures or coma. If untreated, severe hypoglycemia leads to brain death.

Other Signs

Certain signs and symptoms may precede alterations in mental status **(Table 13-3)**. Early signs may include the following:
- Hunger
- Nausea
- Uneasiness
- Weakness
- Increased salivation

As the blood glucose level dips lower, sympathetic nervous system and epinephrine responses become apparent. Related signs and symptoms include the following:
- Rapid pulse
- Cold, pale, clammy skin
- Dilated pupils
- Increased nervousness, trembling, and excitability

Table 13-3	Signs and Symptoms Related to Hypoglycemia*

Mental Changes	Early Signs†	Sympathetic Nervous System Signs‡
Lethargy	Hunger	Rapid pulse
Less spontaneous speech	Nausea	Pale, cool skin
	Weakness	Sweating
Bizarre behavior	Uneasy feeling	Dilated pupils
Agitated, anxious, excitable, combative, or hostile behavior	Salivation	Trembling
		Excitability
Confusion		
Seizures		
Coma		

*Changes can be confused with a psychiatric or intoxicated patient. In some cases, only signs and symptoms of altered mental status may be present.
†Not always elicited or present.
‡With lowered blood glucose level.

REALWorld

The signs and symptoms seen with hypoglycemia are similar to those seen with alcohol intoxication. Therefore it is important for EMTs to do a thorough evaluation of the patient to ensure appropriate treatment, rather than just assuming they are dealing with "just a drunk."

Diabetic Ketoacidosis

Some diabetic patients are seen by EMS for problems related to a blood glucose level that is too high and an insulin level that is too low. When the body lacks insulin, it burns fats rather than glucose for fuel, and glucose does not move into the cells but accumulates in the blood. This presentation tends to occur more slowly than hypoglycemia. The odor of fatty acids, which resembles acetone or nail polish remover, may be on the patient's breath. The patient may breathe deeply and quickly to compensate for the increased acidity of the blood caused by the abnormal metabolism. When the blood glucose level is very high, some glucose is filtered into the urine, pulling water with it, resulting in increased urination and leaving the patient dehydrated, dry, and thirsty. In extreme situations, the patient may be unresponsive. This condition is referred to as diabetic ketoacidosis (DKA). Often an infection or other stressful event may be associated with this crisis. You may obtain a history that the patient has been "spilling sugar" in the urine or showing high blood glucose levels.

LEARNING OBJECTIVES

- State the steps in the emergency medical care of the patient taking diabetic medicine with an altered mental status and a history of diabetes.
- State the generic and trade names, medication forms, dose, administration, action, and contraindications for oral glucose.
- Evaluate the need for medical control in the emergency medical care of the diabetic patient.

Management of Diabetic Emergencies

Because diabetes is so prevalent, hypoglycemia as a cause of altered mental status must always be considered.

Glucose Administration

Because a lack of glucose causes brain cell death, EMTs administer supplemental glucose to patients with an altered mental status when hypoglycemia is suspected as a cause of altered mental status, especially if they cannot immediately measure the *blood glucose level* (BGL). Following such a regimen allows treatment of patients with hypoglycemia if the history is unavailable, and at the same time it does no harm to those who have normal or elevated BGLs. In some areas and systems, EMTs are allowed to use glucometers to evaluate a patient's BGL (**Skill 13-1**). If this skill is allowed, the EMT should check the BGL before administering the glucose. This establishes a baseline value for the hospital and helps confirm the suspicion of hypoglycemia. EMS systems may also use intravenous (IV) glucose or intramuscular (IM) glucagon; however, high-concentration **oral glucose** solutions or gel may be administered to patients who are capable of swallowing (**Figure 13-5**). Table 13-4 reviews the pharmacology of oral glucose.

As a rule, you should never administer an oral medication or substance to an unconscious patient or a patient who is not able to swallow (e.g., with secretions pooling in mouth). **Skill 13-2** reviews the steps in administering oral glucose.

In some states, EMTs may administer glucagon if a patient is unconscious and unable to swallow glucose (**Table 13-5** and **Skill 13-3**).

Table 13-4	Pharmacology of Oral Glucose

Generic name	Oral glucose (unit dose)
Trade name	Multiple brand names available
Indication	Altered mental status from suspected low blood glucose level for patients not unconscious and able to swallow
Contraindications	Unresponsive Unable to swallow
Form	Gel, in toothpaste-type tube
Dose	Usually one tube is unit dose; check local protocols "Glucose 15" is 15 g designed for unit dosing.
Route of administration	Oral, and have patient swallow Between cheek and gum (see Skill 13-2)
Actions	Increases blood glucose level
Side effects	None when given properly May be aspirated if given to patients without a gag reflex
Reassessment strategies	Reassess mental status If patient loses consciousness or has a seizure during reassessment, remove tongue depressor from patient's mouth

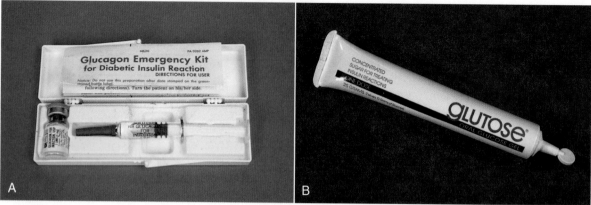

Figure 13-5 **A,** Glucagon for intramuscular (IM) injection. Diabetic patients have home kits for emergency treatment of hypoglycemia when they are unable to swallow glucose. **B,** Multiple forms of glucose gels (and tablets) are on the market. The American Diabetes Association recommends that diabetic patients always carry some item containing 15 g of glucose to treat low blood sugar level (BSL). The general rule is to swallow the unit dose of 15 g, wait 15 minutes, and check BSL. If still low, swallow another unit dose.

Case in Point

You respond to a call for an unconscious 47-year-old man living on a farm in a small town. You find him lying on his couch, and his wife tells you he has insulin-dependent diabetes and she suspects he is having another episode of hypoglycemia. She has checked his blood glucose with their home glucometer, and the level is 30, dangerously low. Usually he knows when his sugar is low and drinks orange juice, but today he is unresponsive. They have an emergency glucagon kit, but the wife says it has expired, and she didn't want to use it.

There are no signs of trauma, and the patient is breathing adequately and has a strong pulse. There are secretions in his mouth. You place him in the recovery position as your partner phones medical control for orders. You carry glucagon and are trained to use it. You are instructed to give 1 mg of glucagon intramuscularly. You place the patient in the ambulance and begin transport to the hospital, which is 45 minutes away. About 10 minutes en route, the patient begins to wake up. When he is able to speak and swallow, you give him oral glucose. By the time you reach the hospital, the patient is fully alert.

LEARNING OBJECTIVES

- List the signs and symptoms of a grand mal seizure, including tonic, clonic, postictal, and aura.
- Explain the management of a patient with seizure.

Seizures

A **seizure** is defined as a temporary alteration in behavior caused by abnormal electrical activity in the brain.

Seizures have many causes. Several of the causes of altered mental status previously mentioned can result in seizures. A scar on the brain or its covering from previous head trauma is one identifiable cause. Other causes may include drug or alcohol withdrawal, eclampsia (toxemia of pregnancy), trauma, infections, fever, poisonings, hypoglycemia, and hypoxia. Many other patients have a history of seizures for which no cause can be found (idiopathic). Patients often take an anticonvulsive drug,

such as phenobarbital, phenytoin (Dilantin), carbamazepine, valproic acid, or other medications, to prevent seizures from recurring. If they stop taking these medications, they are prone to convulsions.

The results of this abnormal electrical activity depend on which portions of the brain are stimulated. The most dramatic seizures are those that involve the motor cortex, resulting in spasmodic contractions of the skeletal muscles. However, some types of seizures affect only the cognitive, or thinking, portion of the brain.

Types of Seizures

Grand Mal Seizures

A **grand mal seizure** is the type most people think of when they hear terms such as "convulsion." A grand mal seizure usually has the following three phases:

- Tonic
- Clonic
- Postictal ("after seizure")

During the *tonic phase*, all voluntary muscles are in a state of sustained contraction. This usually results in extension of the body and the extremities. This phase lasts for up to 30 seconds. During this phase, ventilation can be compromised because of the sustained contraction of the respiratory muscles.

The tonic phase is followed by the *clonic phase*, characterized by intermittent contractions and relaxation of the skeletal muscles, which causes rapid jerking movements. During this period the patient may be injured by striking surrounding objects. The clonic phase lasts from a few seconds to a few minutes. Again, the spasms of contraction and relaxation interfere with ventilation, and the patient can become cyanotic. These spasms may be followed by a short period (up to 30 seconds) of flaccid paralysis while breathing is slowly reestablished. The patient may urinate while in the tonic phase and may bite the tongue during the clonic phase.

The final phase of a seizure is the *postictal phase*, when the patient shows a depressed level of consciousness and confusion.

Table 13-5	Pharmacology of Glucagon
Generic name	Intramuscular glucagon
Trade name	Glucagon Emergency Kit for Low Blood Sugar (see Skill 13-3)
Indication	Hypoglycemia
Contraindications	Allergy to the product or additives
Medication form	Stored as a powder that is reconstituted with supplied diluent and then mixed and injected intramuscularly
Dosage	1 mg for adults One-half adult dose (0.5 mg) for children <44 lb (20 kg)
Administration	Intramuscular injection in arm or thigh
Actions	Increases blood glucose Glucagon acts on liver glycogen, converting it to glucose
Side effects	Patients occasionally may have nausea and vomiting or a rapid heart rate
Reassessment strategies	Look for return of consciousness When patient is able to swallow, give oral glucose

The patient slowly awakens but may feel confused and drowsy and may fall asleep for a short period. Afterward the patient may complain of headache, some muscle aching, and perhaps a sore tongue.

Some seizures originate in one specific part of the brain, producing early warning signs particular to the site of origin. Some patients may become aware of strange smells, visual or auditory sensations, or motor events in only one part of the body. These sensations or activities may herald the onset of a generalized convulsion. These preliminary events are referred to as an *aura*.

Focal Seizures

Some patients have focal seizures that do not generalize or involve the entire brain. These may cause seizure movements that affect only a portion of the body or may manifest as an alteration in mental status with bizarre behavior.

Status Epilepticus

A rapid succession of seizures without an intervening period of consciousness or a prolonged seizure is called **status epilepticus.** This can be life threatening because of sustained respiratory compromise.

Febrile Seizures

The term **febrile seizure** is used to describe a seizure in a child between 6 months and 6 years of age that is precipitated by a rapidly rising high temperature in the setting of an infection. Febrile seizures occur in up to 5% of children.

Case in Point

You are called to the home of a 6-year-old child who is convulsing. You find a girl lying on her bed looking dazed and calling for her mother. The child is talking, her color is pink, and her skin feels very warm. The mother tells you her daughter has been home from school for 2 days with a fever and sore throat. Today her temperature was over 101° F. As the mother was giving her acetaminophen, the child rolled her eyes back, her muscles tensed, and she began to shake violently for 2 to 3 minutes; this had never happened before. During this time the mother told her older child to call 9-1-1 for help.

Petit Mal Seizures

A petit mal seizure involves brief lapses of attention and awareness lasting from 10 to 20 seconds. These are more common in childhood but sometimes persist into adulthood. Petit mal seizures can occur many times a day. The patient may suddenly stare, with the eyes turned upward or to the side and eyelids fluttering. The episode is always brief, lasting only seconds, and the patient can continue or return to previous activities as if nothing happened.

REAL*World*

Children with petit mal seizures may have low grades in school. Their teacher may report they are not paying attention and are not focused. Some children have been misdiagnosed as having attention deficit disorder (ADD).

Management of Seizures

The general goals of management of seizures are the same as those for any patient with altered mental status. However, patients with seizures also require some special interventions.

Airway Compromise

After a grand mal seizure, the patient may need assistance in establishing an airway. The patient may have a short period of flaccid paralysis or significant depression of the nervous system. If no gag reflex is present, an oropharyngeal or nasopharyngeal airway may have to be inserted to keep the tongue from obstructing the airway. As the patient's reflexes return, this airway must be removed to prevent gagging, which may induce vomiting.

If the seizure does not stop within 5 minutes, or if seizures recur without a return of consciousness (status epilepticus), respiratory compromise becomes the major concern. High-concentration supplemental oxygen should be given and, if possible, assistance with positive-pressure ventilation. However, because of the intensity of the muscle contractions, only small and inadequate tidal volumes may be delivered by positive-pressure

---

| **Box 13-1** | Sample Protocol for Seizures |

Management of Patient with Active Seizure

1. Protect the patient from harm, remove hazards from the patient's immediate area, and avoid unnecessary physical restraint.
2. Ensure that the patient's airway is open. Do not force the patient's mouth open or force an oral airway device or any other device into the patient's mouth if it is clenched tightly during the seizure. A nasal airway may be used.
3. Suction the airway as needed. Avoid stimulation of the posterior pharynx during suctioning because this may cause vomiting.
4. Administer high-concentration supplemental oxygen, and provide positive-pressure ventilation if necessary.
5. Transport immediately, keeping the patient warm.
6. Obtain and record the vital signs, and report en route as often as the situation indicates.
7. Record all patient care information, including the patient's medical history and all treatment provided, on a prehospital care report.

Management of Patient after Seizure

1. Ensure that the patient's airway is open and that breathing and circulation are adequate.
2. Suction the airway as needed. Avoid stimulation of the posterior pharynx during suctioning because this may cause vomiting.
3. Administer high-concentration supplemental oxygen.
4. Treat injuries sustained during the seizure.
5. Be prepared for additional seizures.
6. Obtain and record the vital signs, and repeat en route as often as the situation indicates.
7. Transport, keeping the patient warm.
8. Record all patient care information, including the patient's medical history and all treatment provided, on the prehospital care report.

breathing. The patient is at risk for death or brain damage from ventilatory failure.

In EMS systems in which prehospital advanced life support exists, paramedics may be called on to administer drugs that can eliminate seizure activity within minutes. This is recommended only when the estimated time of arrival of the paramedics is less than the transport time to the hospital and when it is consistent with local protocols.

Psychological Aspects for Patients with Seizures

Patients who have recurrent seizures may be very sensitive to the perceptions of those around them after they have recovered from an attack. The reliability of information solicited during the history may be affected by the refusal of the epileptic patient to acknowledge the disease in the presence of co-workers or friends. Concern for this sensitivity can be shown by clearing crowds away from the patient and creating a relatively private environment before conducting an interview.

Box 13-1 summarizes the management of a seizure patient.

💿 Stroke

Stroke (CVA) is the third leading cause of death in the United States and the leading cause of brain injury in adults. Each year approximately 500,000 Americans have a stroke, almost one fourth of whom die. Recent developments in stroke therapy, including early administration of thrombolytic or fibrinolytic drugs (clot-busting medications), are part of the search for effective treatment for victims of stroke. However, some of these medications require administration within 3 hours of symptom onset to be effective. EMS plays a critical role in the early recognition of stroke and rapid transport to a hospital that is prepared to expeditiously assess and treat the patient.

As with ischemic heart disease, stroke is a part of arteriosclerotic disease, characterized by progressive narrowing of the arteries within the brain. When the narrowing obstructs flow, patients may become symptomatic because reduced blood flow causes oxygen deprivation to parts of the brain. Stroke may also occur when a weakened artery in the brain ruptures.

Transient Ischemic Attack

A **transient ischemic attack (TIA)** is a reversible episode of focal neurologic dysfunction (functional failure in a part of the brain) that typically lasts a few minutes to a few hours. The symptoms may be the same as a stroke. If the symptoms completely resolve within 24 hours, the event is then classified as a TIA. However, EMS providers are not usually able to make a distinction between a TIA and a stroke unless the symptoms are gone on arrival at the scene. A history of TIAs is a significant indicator of stroke risk. Approximately one fourth of patients presenting with stroke have had a previous TIA. In addition, approximately 5% of patients with a TIA will have a stroke within 1 month if untreated.

Acute Stroke

A stroke is a permanent neurologic impairment caused by a disruption in blood supply to a region of the brain. Strokes can be classified as either ischemic or hemorrhagic (Figure 13-6).

Approximately 75% of strokes are *ischemic*, resulting from complete occlusion of an artery that deprives the brain of essential nutrients. These occlusions are caused by blood clots that develop within the brain artery itself (cerebral thrombosis) or clots that arise elsewhere in the body and then migrate to an artery in the brain where they become lodged and obstruct blood flow (cerebral embolism).

Hemorrhagic strokes are caused by either rupture of an artery with bleeding onto the surface of the brain (*subarachnoid* hemorrhage) or bleeding into the tissue of the brain (*intracerebral* hemorrhage). The most common cause of a subarachnoid hemorrhage is an aneurysm. Hypertension is the most common cause of intracerebral hemorrhage.

Although both forms of stroke can be life threatening, ischemic stroke rarely leads to death within the first hour, whereas hemorrhagic stroke can be fatal at onset. Even among those who survive the first few hours after a stroke, brain injury progresses quickly and can lead to permanent disability. The classification of stroke as ischemic or hemorrhagic is important because hospital-based management of the two is quite different.

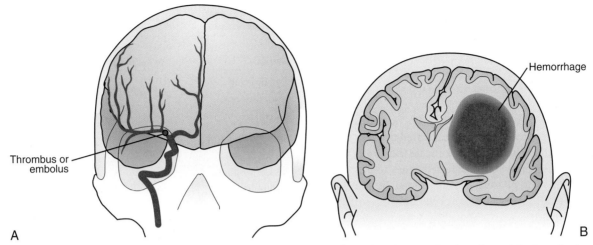

Figure 13-6 **A,** Thrombosis. As a result of the loss of the smooth inner surface, clots form at the site of arterial sclerosis. A stroke caused by an embolus occurs when a small clot from the heart or a central vessel comes loose and travels to a vessel within the brain, where it becomes lodged. **B,** Hemorrhage. A hemorrhagic stroke results from a rupture of a vessel within the brain. Symptoms of the hemorrhagic stroke tend to be more abrupt and more severe than other types of stroke.

Patients with ischemic strokes may be treated with clot-busting or thrombolytic (fibrinolytic) medication if they arrive at the hospital within a few hours of symptom onset. Thrombolytic medication is not indicated for patients with hemorrhagic stroke and, in fact, would worsen intracerebral bleeding. Hospitals caring for stroke victims use computed tomography (CT) to detect whether hemorrhage is the cause of stroke and then determine treatment options. The EMS role is to detect signs of stroke and make transportation decisions to bring patients to a hospital where they get timely care.

Assessment of Stroke Patients

Initial (Primary) Assessment

Airway obstruction may be a major problem in acute stroke if the patient is unconscious or has an altered mental status. The most common cause of airway obstruction in the unconscious patient is occlusion by upper airway structures such as the tongue. You should perform a head-tilt/chin-lift or jaw thrust as indicated. Constantly assess the patient's airway, oxygenation, and ventilation and support these as needed with positive-pressure ventilation, administration of oxygen, or both measures.

Focused (Secondary) Assessment

Stroke should be suspected in any patient with sudden loss of neurologic function or alteration in consciousness. The symptoms of stroke outlined in **Box 13-2** occasionally occur alone or in any combination. The findings can be most severe at the beginning and change as the stroke progresses. Headaches (often described by the patient as "the worst headache of my life"), disturbances in consciousness, nausea, and vomiting are more likely with hemorrhagic strokes than with ischemic strokes.

The EMS providers can greatly assist the chances of patient eligibility for beneficial treatment by identifying the possibility

---

Box 13-2 Signs and Symptoms of Stroke

- Alteration in consciousness (coma, stupor, confusion, seizures, delirium)
- Intense or unusually severe headache of sudden onset or any headache associated with decreased level of consciousness or neurologic deficit; unusual and severe neck or facial pain
- Aphasia (incoherent speech or difficulty understanding speech)
- Facial weakness or asymmetry (paralysis of the facial muscles, usually noted when the patient speaks or smiles); may be on the same side as limb paralysis or on the opposite side
- Incoordination, weakness, paralysis, or sensory loss of one or more limbs; usually involves one half of the body, particularly the hand
- Ataxia (poor balance, clumsiness, or difficulty walking)
- Visual loss (monocular or binocular); may be a partial loss of visual field
- Dysarthria (slurred or indistinct speech)
- Intense vertigo, double vision, unilateral hearing loss, nausea, vomiting, photophobia, or phonophobia

---

of stroke, transporting the patient to a stroke center (a hospital capable of timely evaluation of stroke patients and of giving specialized therapy for stroke), and notifying the stroke center before arrival. You should incorporate awareness of these time-critical factors into prehospital assessment and management.

Focused History. Quickly interview the conscious patient for chief complaint and symptoms such as headache, dizziness, nausea, vomiting, weakness, seizure, and difficulty speaking. If possible, establish the time of onset of signs and symptoms of stroke; this timing will have important implications for potential therapy. The onset of symptoms is viewed as time "0," and eligibility for thrombolytic therapy can be related to that time.

Try to be as accurate as possible. Because of the stroke, the patient may not be able to communicate well. You should interview family members or friends at the scene regarding when the patient was last seen to be completely normal and other information that will give the receiving hospital the best estimate of the time of onset of symptoms. Include questions to complete a SAMPLE history.

Focused Physical Examination. As an EMT, you must identify stroke rapidly. Two stroke scales that are used to assess patients are the **Cincinnati Prehospital Stroke Scale (Box 13-3)** and the **Los Angeles Prehospital Stroke Screen (Figure 13-7).**

Another important physical examination finding to assess is the patient's level of consciousness. The **Glasgow Coma Scale (GCS)** is frequently used to score the patient's response to simple stimuli (voice, pain) by assessing verbal and motor responses and eye opening (**Table 13-6** and **Box 13-4**). Although this scoring system was initially designed for victims of head injury, it is a well-known, reproducible scoring system and reliable when applied to patients with stroke.

These focused examinations can help quickly identify a stroke patient who requires rapid transport to the hospital and can give more precise descriptions of the patient in the prearrival notification to the receiving hospital. Once stroke is suspected, time in the field should be minimized. The presence of acute stroke is an indication for rapid transport because of limited time to institute therapy, which must be provided in the emergency department (ED) of the receiving hospital. A more extensive examination or institution of supportive therapies can be accomplished en route to the hospital and in the hospital ED.

Check vital signs to detect abnormalities and changes. Disturbances of vital signs are common after stroke. Abnormal respirations often occur in comatose patients and may indicate serious brain dysfunction.

| Table 13-6 | Glasgow Coma Scale—Total |

Variable	Points Assigned to Response	Notes
Eye Opening		
Spontaneous	4	
To voice	3	
To pain	2	
None	1	
Verbal Response		
Oriented	5	
Confused	4	*Patient's best response*
Inappropriate words	3	Arouse patient with voice or painful stimulus.
Incomprehensible sounds	2	
None	1	
Motor Response		
Obeys command	6	
Localizes pain	5	
Withdraw (pain)	4	*Patient's best response*
Flexion (pain)	3	Arouse patient with voice or painful stimulus.
Extension (pain)	2	
None	1	
TOTAL SCORE	3-15	

Stroke patients are often hypertensive, a major risk factor of stroke. Hypotension is rarely caused by stroke, so other causes should be considered.

Management of Stroke Patients

General emergency therapy of stroke patients focuses on maintaining airway patency, breathing, and oxygenation and the transport decision. Because of loss of muscle tone and paralysis, upper airway occlusion can occur and present as noisy, obstructed breathing. In more extreme cases the patient will develop a bluish discoloration around the lips and in the nail beds (cyanosis). Open the airway in such patients (head-tilt/chin-lift) and, if breathing is absent or inadequate, initiate rescue breathing or positive-pressure ventilation with a pocket mask or a bag-mask and administer supplemental oxygen.

Recognition of stroke and prehospital assessment should occur as quickly as possible to minimize field time. Unless the patient requires prehospital stabilization, initiation of patient transport should be prioritized. EMS systems should be aware of all receiving hospitals' capability to evaluate and treat stroke victims and implement transport destination policies consistent with local protocols.

Early notification of ED personnel has always played a critical role in emergency cardiovascular care and trauma systems because it enables hospital personnel to prepare for the imminent arrival of a seriously ill or injured patient. It plays an equally

| Box 13-3 | Cincinnati Prehospital Stroke Scale |

- Facial droop (Have patient show teeth or smile.)
  Normal—both sides of face move equally.
  Abnormal—one side of face does not move as well as the other side.
- Arm drift (patient closes eyes and holds both arms out straight for 10 seconds)
  Normal—both arms move the same or both arms do not move at all.
  Abnormal—one arm does not move or one arm drifts down compared with the other.
- Abnormal speech (Have the patient say, "You can't teach an old dog new tricks.")
  Normal—patient uses correct words with no slurring.
  Abnormal—patient slurs words, uses the wrong words, or is unable to speak.

Interpretation

If any of these three signs is abnormal, the probability of a stroke is 72%.

Modified from Kothari RU et al: Cincinnati Prehospital Stroke Scale: reproducibility and validity, *Ann Emerg Med* 33:373-378, 1999.

Los Angeles Prehospital Stroke Screen (LAPSS)

1. Patient name: _____   _____
                        (Last name)   (First name)

2. Information/History from:
   [   ] Patient
   [   ] Family member   _____   _____
   [   ] Patient   (Name)   (Phone)

3. Last known time patient was at baseline or deficit free and awake:

   _____   _____
        (Military time)   (Date)

SCREENING CRITERIA

	YES	UNKNOWN	NO
4. Age >45	[ ]	[ ]	[ ]
5. History of seizures or epilepsy **absent**	[ ]	[ ]	[ ]
6. Symptom duration less than 24 hours	[ ]	[ ]	[ ]
7. At baseline, patient is not wheelchair bound or bedridden	[ ]	[ ]	[ ]
8. Blood glucose between 60 and 400	[ ]	[ ]	[ ]
9. Exam: **LOOK FOR OBVIOUS ASYMMETRY** (right versus left) in **any** of the following:	[ ]	[ ]	[ ]

	Normal	Right	Left
Facial smile/grimace	[ ]	[ ] Droop	[ ] Droop
Grip	[ ]	[ ] Weak grip	[ ] Weak grip
		[ ] No grip	[ ] No grip
Arm strength	[ ]	[ ] Drifts down	[ ] Drifts down
		[ ] Falls rapidly	[ ] Falls rapidly

Based on exam, patient has only unilateral (and not bilateral) weakness:

YES	NO
[ ]	[ ]

10. Items 4, 5, 6, 7, 8, 9 all YES's (or unknown)—LAPSS screening criteria met:

YES	NO
[ ]	[ ]

11. If LAPSS criteria for stroke met, call receiving hospital with a "code stroke." If not, then return to the appropriate treatment protocol. (Note: The patient may still be experiencing a stroke even if the LAPSS criteria are not met.)

Figure 13-7 The Los Angeles Prehospital Stroke Screen. (For more information, contact Charles S. Kidwell, MD, Department of Neurology, UCLA Medical Center, Reed NRC, 710 Westwood Plaza, Los Angeles, CA 90095, or e-mail ckidwell@ucla.edu.)

Box 13-4   Administration of Glasgow Coma Scale

One method of objective assessment of mental status used by emergency medical service (EMS) and hospital personnel is the Glasgow Coma Scale (GCS). This method assesses the three parameters of eye opening, verbal response, and motor ability.

Although the GCS was designed initially for patients with head trauma, it is also useful for evaluating and describing the neurologic status of all unresponsive patients because of its reliability. It enables healthcare personnel at all levels to "speak the same language."

The GCS is intended for use with patients with an altered mental status. Patients range from individuals who are well oriented and able to obey commands to patients who are deeply comatose and unable to respond to any stimuli. Accordingly, stimuli are applied sequentially, starting with verbal questions and commands and followed by administration of painful stimulus if there is still no response.

The patient's status is then scored according to set criteria within the three general parameters. There are four possible eye responses, five possible verbal responses, and six motor response criteria. The best score is 15, and the most unresponsive patient receives a score of 3.

To apply a pain stimulus, you should apply pressure to the patient's nail bed. Another technique used by many EDs and prehospital personnel is to pinch the skin over the patient's forearms, shoulder, or trapezius to administer a painful stimulus. The pain stimulus should be applied to both sides of the body, since there may be a sensory deficit on one side. A score of 1 is the lowest score for each component of the GCS.

Eye Opening

If the patient's eyes are open on your arrival or open spontaneously without being stimulated, the patient receives a score of 4. If the eyes open on verbal command, "Open your eyes!" the score is 3. If the eyes open following painful stimuli, the score is 2. If the eyes do not open in response to pain, the score is 1.

Verbal Response

The alert and oriented patient receives the highest score of 5. A patient who is confused but able to respond in a conversational manner receives a score of 4. A patient who cannot maintain a conversation and gives inappropriate responses to questions posed by the examiner receives a score of 3. This patient may respond in a disorganized fashion with exclamatory or profane language. However, the key in distinguishing the confused from the inappropriate response is whether the attention of the patient can be maintained. The confused patient will converse with the examiner, and the patient's attention can be maintained. The patient with inappropriate responses will drift off and will not answer the examiner's questions without repeated verbal stimulation. This patient has a more depressed mental status than the patient who is confused.

The patient who responds with incomprehensible sounds and moaning and no recognizable words receives a score of 2. The patient who does not respond verbally at all receives a score of 1.

Motor Response

The score of 6 is given to a patient who obeys verbal commands, such as "Move your arms," by making the appropriate movement. (It is assumed that the patient has no fractures or other wounds of the extremities that would affect motor function.) The GCS is concerned with brain function, not the status of any other components necessary for movement.

For example, a patient with a spinal injury that leaves the legs paralyzed would receive a score of 6 if he or she is able to move an arm in response to a verbal command. This is evidence that the brain is intact. The fact that the patient's legs cannot move is a result of damage to a lower structure, in this case the spinal cord.

The other possible scores are elicited after application of painful stimuli. If a patient can localize the pain, a score of 5 is given. Localizing pain is an attempt by the patient to reach to or to remove the source of a painful stimulus For example, if the left shoulder is pinched as a painful stimulus, a patient might reach a hand up toward the examiner's fingers.

If the patient does not reach up for the examiner's hand but rather pulls away from the pain stimulus, the patient is said to "withdraw." A *withdrawal* response is given a score of 4.

Some patients respond with flexion of one or both arms in response to pain. This is called a *decorticate* response and indicates that the higher brain centers are damaged. The *flexion* response receives a score of 3.

With deeper coma or more extensive brain damage, a patient may respond to pain with the extension of both the arms and the legs. The extension of the arms is quite characteristic. The shoulders rotate internally, and the wrists flex. This response is also known as a *decerebrate* response. It indicates that the entire upper brain is functionally separate from the brainstem and the rest of the nervous system. The extension response receives a score of 2. The lowest score of 1 is given if no response is observed from verbal or painful stimuli.

A patient's status is graded according to the best response that would give the patient the highest score. The response need not be bilateral; that is, if the patient could not move one side but responded on the other side with a flexion response, the motor score would receive a grade for the flexion that was observed. You should remember to apply a painful stimulus to each side.

You should always describe the patient and record your findings according to the subcomponents of the score. Your records may have space for the score, such as follows:

    Glasgow Coma Scale: Verbal (1-5) _____, Motor (1-6) _____, Eyes (1-4) _____; Total Score _____

critical role in patients with stroke. In addition to standard information, you should communicate the results of your special assessments, such as the Cincinnati Prehospital Stroke Scale, the GCS, and the estimated time of symptom onset. In most hospitals this notification shortens the time needed to evaluate the patient and provide critical interventions.

Take the time to review the prehospital stroke management algorithm (**Figure 13-8**), which summarizes the assessment and management of the stroke patient in the prehospital phase of care.

Emergency Medical Care for Patients with Altered Mental Status

Initial (Primary) Assessment

The initial (primary) assessment recognizes the role of the CNS in directing vital functions with the initial check for responsiveness. As always, identifying and treating life-threatening conditions take precedence. All unconscious patients are at risk for airway obstruction, and manual techniques and mechanical airway devices should be used to ensure the patency of the airway. Establish the need for ventilatory support because airway and ventilatory compromise represent the greatest threat to life in the prehospital phase. Assess the possibility of head trauma during this phase, and use appropriate airway-opening techniques and early immobilization of the spine if indicated. You should always think about hypoxia and hypoglycemia when you see a patient with altered mental status. If there is any chance of hypoxia, administer supplemental oxygen. If hypoglycemia is suspected, administer glucose (or glucagon). If allowed, a glucometer should be used to determine the actual BGL.

Focused (Secondary) Assessment

The focused (secondary) assessment (history and physical examination) provide the rationale for prehospital treatment and early transport decisions. Furthermore, early hospital therapy is often determined on the basis of prehospital findings and clues. A systematic approach that always includes key questions maximizes information gathering in a timely manner. For example, always obtaining a medication history and bringing the patient's medications to the hospital provide important information to the hospital staff.

Focused History

With medical patients the history is often the primary rationale for treatment. A patient may have no positive physical findings other than an altered mental status. In such a case, a history of diabetes provides the rationale for administering glucose. Certain key areas for questioning provide much valuable information. The time from the patient's last normal level of function to the present condition should be ascertained. You may have to rely on family and bystanders, depending on the patient's mental status.

The presence of associated complaints, the chronology of events, and a history of similar past experiences are invaluable in identifying the underlying cause. A patient may present with a deterioration of consciousness and have a history of recent head injury. This chronology might point to the possibility of bleeding within the skull. Similar past experiences are especially helpful in identifying chronic or recurrent conditions, such as hypoglycemia and seizures.

A history of diabetes is essential to elicit in the patient with an altered mental status. Even if a history of psychiatric disease is given, you should never assume that an alteration in mental status is caused by the psychiatric disorder. Many medical problems can result in depressed, agitated, and combative states with bizarre behavior. The possibility of an overdose or poisoning should not be overlooked.

Epilepsy is another condition to ask about. A seizure may not have been witnessed. Patients in the postictal phase have depressed mental function, and you may encounter a wide range of findings.

You should obtain an allergy history (see Chapter 14). If the patient's condition changes, it may not be possible to question the patient later.

Questioning witnesses about the pattern, activity, and duration of any seizures that are described is important. Did the patient have a focal seizure initially (limited activity in one area of the body) that evolved into a grand mal seizure? This information may aid the physicians in determining the cause of the seizure. The last meal taken is of particular interest if hypoglycemia is suspected.

Vital Signs

The character of the pulse and the blood pressure should be noted. Is there evidence of adequate perfusion? Are breathing patterns abnormal? Are there signs of epinephrine release?

Check the temperature to assess the possibility of infectious causes, hyperthermia, or hypothermia. At times an alteration in temperature may be the result of CNS disease, whereas at other times it may point to the condition.

Case in Point

You respond to a man found lying on the sidewalk in a residential neighborhood. A bystander called on her cell phone and is still at the scene. The man is lying on his side, unable to get up, and begins to vomit. You smell alcohol and wonder if the patient has had too much to drink. The patient is breathing adequately and has a good pulse. His eyes are closed, and when you apply painful stimuli, he withdraws from pain, moans, and opens his eyes. You begin a head-to-toe survey, and when you palpate his scalp, you notice a small, soft lump on his right occipital area. You notice blood on your gloved finger that touched this wound.

You wonder if the patient fell. As you search for identification, you notice he has no wallet. Your differential now includes possible robbery and a blow to the head. You make a transport decision and alert the trauma center for a man with altered consciousness and a GCS score of 8. At the hospital it is shown that the blood alcohol level did not account for the change in consciousness. The CT scan of the brain showed an injury, which was the real problem.

Most EMS systems can relate incidents in which the smell of alcohol led to "being drunk" as the reason for a patient's altered mental status, and further assessment stopped, with the real cause initially going unnoticed. Adhering to a structured assessment when serious conditions are encountered helps reveal problems not initially apparent, which can be lifesaving to the patient.

Prehospital Stroke Management Algorithm

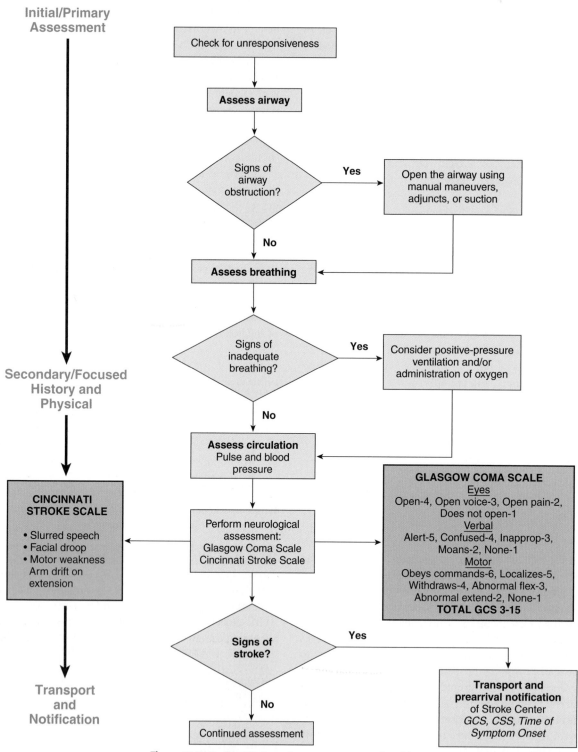

Figure 13-8 Prehospital stroke management algorithm.

Focused Physical Examination

Check skin color and moisture to help identify hypoxia (cyanosis) and hypoperfusion (pale and clammy). Warm, hot, dry skin suggests heat stroke. Note abnormal smells on the breath, such as the odor of alcohol. A fruity odor suggests diabetic acidosis. Check pupils as you would check the patient with a head injury; note size, equality, and reactivity to light. Check the patient for motor and sensory function in the same manner as you would check the patient with a head injury. Check both sides of the body, looking for equal strength and sensation on each side. As with the patient with head injuries, you should periodically re-evaluate the vital signs and the mental status and record your

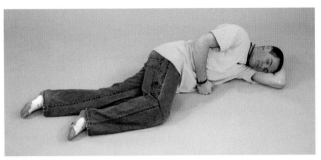

Figure 13-9 Transport medical patients who are unresponsive or who have an altered mental status in the recovery position to avoid aspiration in the event of vomiting.

findings. Look for MedicAlert tags, and ask about previous hospitalizations or whether the patient is under a physician's care. You may uncover significant past illness or conditions that still require treatment. Bring the patient's current medications to the hospital.

If stroke is suspected, use a prehospital stroke scale to determine status. If time and circumstances permit, perform a detailed physical examination in patients in whom the focused examination does not give a clear picture of the problem to make sure other clues are not overlooked.

LEARNING OBJECTIVE
- Establish the relationship between airway management and the patient with altered mental status.

Management

Airway Compromise

The most treatable and one of the most common hazards faced by patients with altered mental function is airway compromise. Obstruction caused by the tongue or the inability to clear secretions can place the patient in jeopardy. Airway patency is achieved through a combination of appropriate manual airway techniques and mechanical airway devices. Check for the presence or absence of a gag reflex in all unconscious patients. If the gag reflex is absent, use an oropharyngeal or nasopharyngeal airway. Secretions and vomit should be cleared from the airway with a combination of suctioning and proper positioning. You should routinely place all nontraumatic unconscious patients with adequate ventilations in the recovery position in recognition of these concerns (**Figure 13-9**).

Ventilation and Supplemental Oxygen

All patients with altered mental status should be assumed to have inadequate oxygen delivery to the brain until proven otherwise. Supplemental oxygen is indicated, and the respiratory rate and depth must be carefully assessed to identify the need for positive-pressure ventilation. If doubt exists about the adequacy of ventilations, assist the patient. Administer supplemental oxygen to patients who are agitated or combative if it is tolerated.

Glucose should be considered for patients with altered mental status caused by diabetes or from an unknown cause. Follow local protocol.

Transport Decisions

Certain findings in a patient dictate an early transport decision. The decision to transport must be considered as part of the patient's treatment. As with uncontrollable internal hemorrhage, certain CNS disorders require early hospital treatment.

EXTENDED *Transport*

When transporting a patient with an altered level of consciousness, it is important to remember that patients may change during transport, especially if transport is long, such as from a rural area. Patients who were hypoglycemic and received oral glucose with a resulting increase in mentation may deteriorate during a long transport. The body will quickly use the glucose given to the patient, who will once again present with an altered level of consciousness. Another dose of glucose may be required during transport. If a patient had a seizure and presented postictally to the EMT on scene, the patient may experience another seizure during a long transport. The EMT is then faced with protecting the patient from physical harm and controlling the airway in the confines of the ambulance. If a patient experienced a hemorrhagic stroke, the bleed in the brain may cause the brain to herniate or push through the hole in the base of the skull. This herniation may cause the patient to lose the ability to breathe. The EMT must be prepared to control the airway and appropriately ventilate the patient.

During an extended transport, patients need to be continually monitored for changes in their presentation. The EMT must be prepared to treat any change in the patient. The driver may need to pull safely to the side of the road and join the EMT in the back to help with patient care. The EMT should always consider the possibility of rendezvousing with an advanced life support (ALS) service, either ground or air, to provide more advanced care.

Ongoing Assessment or Reassessment

Any changes in the patient's condition that occur during your care should be noted. Is the patient's mental status improving or deteriorating, or does it remain the same?

In addition to repeating your assessment of vital signs, you should repeat the neurologic assessment scales used in your region, such as AVPU, GCS, or stroke scale. Did the therapy you instituted (e.g., oxygen, glucose) make any difference?

Box 13-5 provides a sample protocol for the emergency medical care of the patient with altered mental status.

Chronic Neurologic Diseases

You will encounter patients who have chronic neurologic disease. Chronic diseases can have adverse effects on the ability to remember, function intellectually, move, swallow, and breathe. For some patients, the chronic disease may result in the need for your assistance; for example, the difficulty in swallowing may lead to choking. In other patients the disease may be part of the patient's background and medical history.

Box 13-6 describes common chronic neurologic diseases.

Box 13-5 Sample Protocol for Altered Mental Status

1. Perform an initial (primary) assessment and focused (secondary) assessment (history and physical examination).
2. Ensure that the patient's airway is open and that breathing and circulation are adequate. Suction as necessary.
3. Administer high-concentration supplemental oxygen.
4. Obtain and record the vital signs, including determining the patient's level of consciousness.
5. If the patient is unresponsive or responds only to painful stimuli, transport immediately, keeping the patient warm.

6. Check for a history of diabetes.
7. If the patient is conscious, has a gag reflex, and is able to drink without assistance, provide glucose or a sugar solution (if available) by mouth, transport, and keep the patient warm.*
8. Repeat and record the vital signs, including the level of consciousness, en route as often as the situation indicates.
9. Perform an ongoing assessment en route to the hospital.

*Local protocols may include testing blood for glucose concentration and administering intravenous glucose or intramuscular glucagon, or both.

Box 13-6 Degenerative Neurologic Diseases and Cerebral Palsy

Alzheimer's Disease*

Also called: AD

Alzheimer's disease (AD) is the most common form of dementia among older people. *Dementia* is a brain disorder that seriously affects a person's ability to carry out daily activities.

AD begins slowly. It first involves the parts of the brain that control thought, memory, and language. People with AD may have trouble remembering things that happened recently or names of people they know. Over time, symptoms worsen. Patients may not recognize family members or may have trouble speaking, reading, or writing. They may forget how to brush their teeth or comb their hair. Later on, they may become anxious or aggressive, or wander away from home. Eventually, they need total care. This can cause great stress for family members who must care for them.

AD usually begins after age 60. The risk goes up as people age. The risk is also higher if a family member has had the disease.

No treatment can stop AD. However, some drugs may help keep symptoms from worsening for a limited time.

Amyotrophic Lateral Sclerosis†

Also called: ALS, Lou Gehrig's disease

Amyotrophic lateral sclerosis (ALS) is a nervous system disease that attacks nerve cells called neurons in the brain and spinal cord. These neurons transmit messages from the brain and spinal cord to the voluntary muscles, those that can be controlled, as in the arms and legs. At first, this causes mild muscle problems. Some people notice:
- Trouble walking or running
- Trouble writing
- Speech problems

Eventually, people lose strength and cannot move. When muscles in the chest fail, the person cannot breathe. A ventilator can help, but most people with ALS die from respiratory failure.

ALS usually strikes between age 40 and 60, with men affected more often than women. No one knows what causes ALS. It can run in families, but usually it strikes at random. There is no cure. Medicines can relieve symptoms and in some patients can prolong survival.

Parkinson's Disease

Also called: PD, paralysis agitans, shaking palsy

Parkinson's disease (PD) is a disorder that affects nerve cells, or neurons, in a part of the brain that controls muscle movement. In PD, neurons that make a chemical called dopamine die or do not work properly. Dopamine normally sends signals that help coordinate body movements. No one knows what damages these cells. Symptoms of PD may include:
- Trembling of hands, arms, legs, jaw, and face
- Stiffness of the arms, legs, and trunk
- Slowness of movement
- Poor balance and coordination

As symptoms worsen, PD patients may have trouble walking, talking, or doing simple tasks. They may also have problems such as depression, sleep problems, and trouble chewing, swallowing, or speaking.

PD usually begins around age 60, but it can start earlier. It is more common in men than in women. There is no cure for PD. A variety of medicines sometimes alleviate symptoms dramatically.

Cerebral Palsy†

Also called: CP

Cerebral palsy (CP) is a group of disorders that affect a person's ability to move and to maintain balance and posture. The disorders appear in the first few years of life. Usually these disorders do not worsen over time. People with CP may have difficulty walking. They may also have trouble with tasks such as writing or using scissors. Some have other medical conditions, including seizure disorders or mental impairment.

CP occurs when the areas of the brain that control movement and posture do not develop correctly or sustain damage. Early signs usually appear before 3 years of age. Babies with CP are often slow to roll over, sit, crawl, smile, or walk. Some infants are born with CP; others develop it after birth.

There is no cure for CP, but treatment can improve the lives of these patients. Treatment includes medicines, braces, and physical, occupational, and speech therapy.

From http://www.nlm.nih.gov/medlineplus/degenerativenervediseases.html. Accessed August 2007.
*From National Institute on Aging.
†From National Institute of Neurological Disorders and Stroke.

Scenario Follow-up

The patient acting bizarrely in the grocery store was being detained by the guard when you arrived. The guard told you he thought initially the man was trying to shoplift and then thought that he might be "crazy." Abnormal behavior can be seen because of metabolic problems, including low blood glucose. Your attention to detail and careful assessment and the resulting treatment showed this patient's "altered mental status" was caused by hypoglycemia.

Summary

Patients with neurologic emergencies who present with altered mental status deserve a close look for two treatable and common causes: hypoxia and hypoglycemia. Causes of altered mental status often encountered by EMS include diabetic emergencies, seizures, and stroke. Diabetic emergencies include hypoglycemia and hyperglycemia. Hypoglycemia is managed with oral glucose in patients who can still swallow. Seizures most often require routine management that protects the patient from further injury, but at times ventilation is compromised. Early recognition of signs of stroke is important because timely treatment may minimize brain damage.

Skills

| Skill | 13-1 | *Blood Glucose Monitoring* |

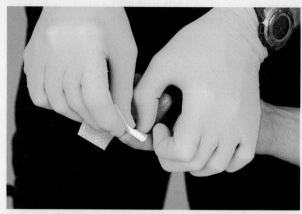

1. Gather all equipment, and explain the procedure to the patient. Prepare the patient's finger with an alcohol pad.

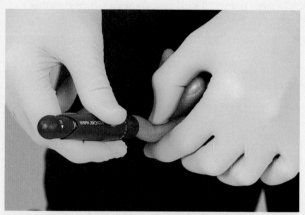

2. Holding the patient's finger securely, use a lancet to puncture the tip of the finger. Dispose of the needle in a sharps container.

4. Dress the wound as needed, and document results.

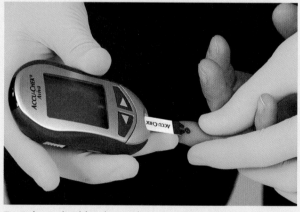

3. Culture the blood sample on a test strip, and record the reading from the monitor.

Skill | 13-2   *Administering Glucose*

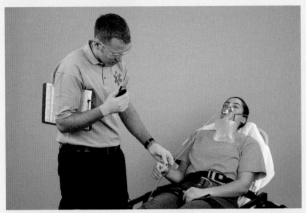

1. Obtain an order from medical direction either online or offline. Check for altered mental status or a history of diabetes. Make sure that the patient is conscious and can swallow. Remove the oxygen mask.

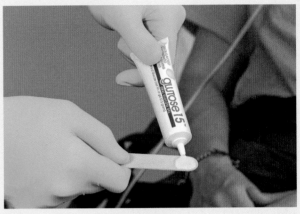

2. Place glucose on tongue blade.

4. Perform ongoing assessment.

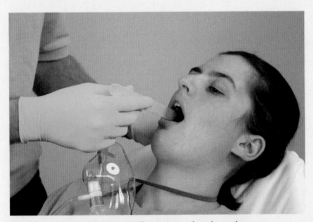

3. Administer oral glucose between cheek and gum.

Skill | 13-3   *Administering Glucagon from Glucagon Emergency Kit*

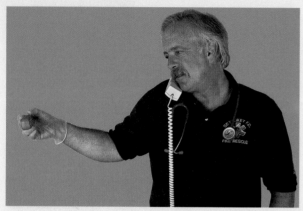

1. Obtain the order from medical direction, either online or offline.

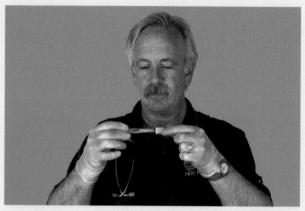

2. Obtain the patient's prescribed emergency kit or the kit carried on the ambulance. Check the following:

- Prescription is written for the patient, or there is local protocol for administration
- Dose is correct
- Medication has not expired

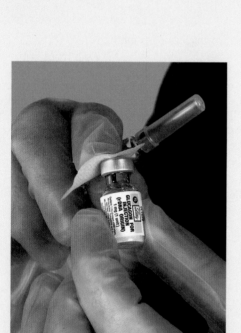

3. Remove the flip-off seal from the bottle of glucagon, and wipe the rubber stopper on the bottle with an alcohol swab.

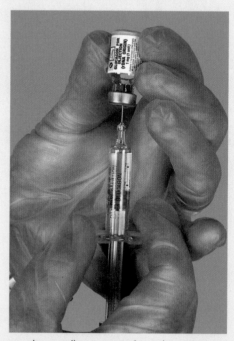

4. Remove the needle protector from the syringe, and inject the entire contents of the syringe into the bottle of glucagon. Do not remove the plastic clip from the syringe. Remove the syringe from the bottle.

Skill | 13-3   *Administering Glucagon from Glucagon Emergency Kit—cont'd*

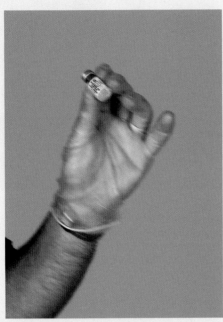

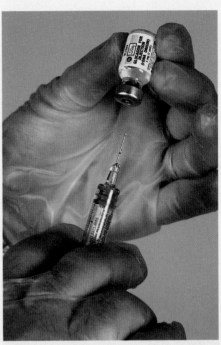

5. Swirl bottle gently until glucagon dissolves completely. Glucagon should not be used unless the solution is clear and of a waterlike consistency.

6. Using the same syringe, hold the bottle upside down, and making sure that the needle tip remains in the solution, gently withdraw all the solution (1-mg mark on syringe) from the bottle.

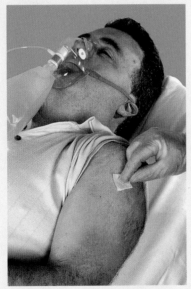

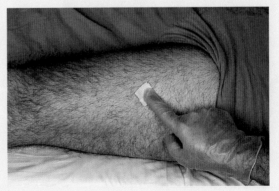

7. Cleanse the injection site on the patient's arm or thigh with an alcohol swab.

Continued

Skill | 13-3 — *Administering Glucagon from Glucagon Emergency Kit—cont'd*

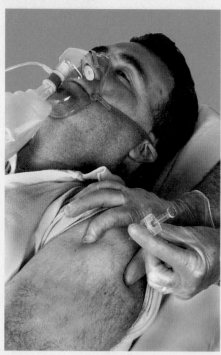

8. If injecting in the arm, go two fingerbreadths below the tip of the acromion (lateral tip of shoulder) and insert the needle at a 90-degree angle under the cleansed injection site. Inject the entire contents (for children <44 lb, inject half). Apply light pressure at the injection site, and withdraw the needle.

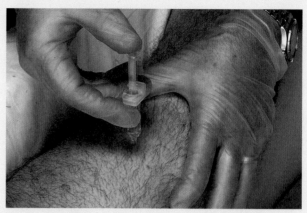

9. If injecting in the thigh, with the patient in the supine position, cleanse the injection site on the anterolateral aspect of the middle third of the thigh. Insert the needle at a 90-degree angle as for the arm injection.

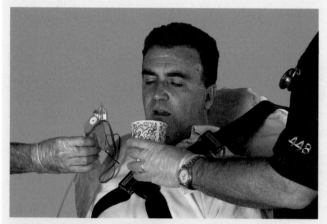

10. Place the patient in the recovery position.

11. As soon as the patient awakens, administer a glucose-rich solution, such as a regular soft drink or fruit juice. If you have not arrived at the hospital and the patient has not awakened within 15 minutes, contact medical direction for administration of an additional dose (as per local protocol).

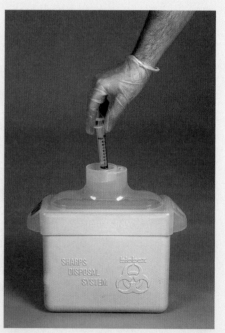

12. Reevaluate the patient frequently during transport, and monitor airway and ventilation. Dispose of injector in a biohazard (sharps) container. Record activity and time.

The Bottom Line

Learning Checklist

✓ Altered mental status may be caused by either structural conditions (injury or damage to an area of the brain) or metabolic problems (affect entire brain, such as hypoxia or hypoglycemia), as well as psychiatric causes.

✓ Structural conditions (e.g., stroke, head injury) are characterized by "one-sided" signs such as paralysis, facial droop, and weakness on one side of the body.

✓ Metabolic conditions (e.g., diabetes, hypoxia) affect both sides of the brain equally and are primarily recognized on the basis of altered mental states and history.

✓ Diabetes is a disease caused by a partial or total lack of insulin production.

✓ The two major diabetic emergencies are hypoglycemia and diabetic ketoacidosis.

✓ Signs and symptoms of hypoglycemia include alteration of mental status (anxiety, confusion, combativeness, bizarre behavior, coma); rapid pulse; pale, cool, and clammy skin; dilated pupils; and seizures.

✓ Symptoms of high blood glucose include increased urination and thirst and general lethargy.

✓ Thrombolytic therapy represents a treatment for acute stroke that may limit disability if given within a few hours of symptom onset.

✓ Treatment for acute stroke is time sensitive, making education of at-risk patients, early prehospital recognition, rapid assessment, and prompt transport to a stroke center with prearrival notification imperative.

✓ A transient ischemic attack (TIA) and stroke present with acute neurologic disability. If symptoms completely resolve within 24 hours, the event is classified as a TIA. TIAs are a substantial risk factor for stroke.

✓ Approximately 75% of strokes are ischemic and therefore possibly eligible for treatment such as thrombolytic therapy.

✓ Patients with hemorrhagic stroke are not eligible to receive thrombolytic therapy and, in general, appear more seriously ill and have a more rapid course of deterioration than those with ischemic stroke.

✓ Laypersons should be educated to call 9-1-1 immediately when experiencing or recognizing symptoms of a possible stroke, to facilitate rapid assessment and transport to a stroke center.

✓ The goals of prehospital management of suspected stroke are (1) support of vital functions: initial (primary) assessment and management, (2) rapid identification of stroke: focused (secondary) assessment (history and physical examination), (3) rapid transport to a stroke center, and (4) prearrival notification of the stroke center.

✓ For patients with suspected stroke, the prehospital focused (secondary) assessment and prehospital notification should include the best estimate of the time of symptom onset and assessment (e.g., Cincinnati Prehospital Stroke Scale, Glasgow Coma Scale).

✓ A grand mal seizure usually has three phases: tonic (all voluntary muscles in state of sustained contraction), clonic (intermittent contractions and relaxation of skeletal muscles, causing rapid jerking movements), and postictal (depressed level of consciousness and confusion).

✓ Management of a patient with seizure centers on protecting the patient from harm, assisting with airway and ventilation, and giving supplemental oxygen as needed.

✓ Hypoxia and airway compromise are often associated with seizure activity, and aggressive care is needed.

✓ Alcohol can mimic and hide several causes of altered mental status, so the EMT must be diligent to assess other potential causes of the patient's signs and symptoms and not assume the patient is "just drunk."

Key Terms

Altered mental status Any change from normal in a patient's mental state; alterations can range from mild confusion and abnormal behavior to deep coma, a condition in which the patient is totally unresponsive to verbal or painful stimuli.

AVPU Mnemonic to help EMTs remember the level of patient responsiveness: **A** wake, patient is awake and responds without stimuli; **V**erbal, patient responds to verbal stimuli; **P**ain, patient requires some form of tactile or painful stimuli to generate a response; **U**nresponsive, patient is unresponsive to any form of stimulation.

Cerebrovascular accident (CVA) Blockage or disruption of blood flow in an artery feeding the brain; also called a *stroke.*

Cincinnati Prehospital Stroke Scale Type of screening device used to rapidly identify stroke patients.

Diabetes Disease that results from the failure of the pancreas to produce sufficient amounts of insulin.

Diabetic ketoacidosis (DKA) Condition resulting from a relatively prolonged insulin deficiency in which the blood glucose level rises and fatty acids are produced in the blood.

Febrile seizure Seizure in a child that is caused by a rapidly rising body temperature.

Glasgow Coma Scale (GCS) Assessment of a patient's level of consciousness according to the patient's best eye movement, response to voice, and motor movement.

Glucagon Substance secreted by the pancreas that can cause stored forms of glucose to be released and glucose to be made from other molecules.

Glucose Sugar molecule (carbohydrate) in a form that is used by the cells for energy.

Grand mal seizure Seizure that involves three phases: tonic (sustained contraction of all voluntary muscles), clonic (intermittent contractions and relaxation of skeletal muscles), and postictal (depressed level of consciousness and confusion).

Hypoglycemia Abnormally low blood glucose (sugar) level.

Insulin Hormone produced by the pancreas necessary for glucose metabolism.

Los Angeles Prehospital Stroke Screen Screening device used to rapidly identify stroke patients.

Oral glucose Form of glucose gel that is administered orally to patients with suspected diabetic emergencies.

Seizure Temporary alteration in behavior caused by abnormal electrical activity in the brain.

Status epilepticus Rapid succession of seizures without an intervening period of consciousness or a prolonged period of continuous seizures.

Stroke Usually sudden onset of symptoms caused by blockage or disruption of blood flow in an artery feeding the brain; also called *cerebrovascular accident* (CVA).

Transient ischemic attack (TIA) Temporary loss of brain function caused by diminished blood supply to part of the brain; completely resolves within 24 hours.

Review Questions

1. During the medication history, you might identify someone as a diabetic patient by which of the following medications?
   a. Albuterol
   b. Metformin
   c. Adrenaline
   d. Ativan

2. Which of the following would most likely cause a patient with insulin-dependent diabetes to become hypoglycemic?
   a. Too little insulin, too much food
   b. Too much exercise, too little food
   c. Too little insulin, too little food
   d. Too little exercise, too much food

3. What should the EMT do before administering oral glucose?
   a. Check that the patient can swallow
   b. Check for urine glucose
   c. Check the insulin level
   d. Place the patient supine

4. For patients who are unresponsive, which of the following is a key element of airway management?
   a. An oropharyngeal airway might be needed to keep the tongue from obstructing the airway.
   b. Suction as long as needed.
   c. Placing the patient face-down will help bring the tongue away from the pharynx.
   d. Unresponsive patients rarely have trouble protecting their own airway.

5. Which of the following is considered routine management of patients with seizures?
   a. Remove hazards from immediate area of the patient.
   b. Force an airway into the patient's mouth to prevent tongue biting.
   c. Restrain the patient's extremities.
   d. Administration or oral glucose to stop the seizure.

6. Which of the following represent two common causes of altered mental status that must always be considered by the EMT?
   a. High blood pressure and rapid pulse
   b. Low blood oxygen and low blood glucose
   c. High blood oxygen and high blood glucose
   d. Normal blood oxygen and high blood glucose

7. Which of the following is *true* as it pertains to the general pharmacology of oral glucose as administered by the EMT?
   a. Indication—altered mental status in a diabetic patient or a patient with a low blood glucose level
   b. Contraindication—none if hypoglycemic
   c. Generic name—glucagons
   d. Action—increases epinephrine secretion

8. Glucose is given under medical direction, usually by which of the following methods?
   a. An online order or standing order
   b. The patient's personal physician
   c. Visual inspection of insulin prescription
   d. Administration of patient's prescribed oral glucose gel

9. Which of the following does *not* support the routine administration of glucose to patients with altered mental status who have a diabetic history?
   a. A prolonged low blood glucose level can cause damage to nerve cells.
   b. Giving oral glucose to patients with a normal or high blood glucose level is not harmful.
   c. Altered mental status is always caused by a low blood glucose level in diabetic patients.
   d. There is little danger of complications if given to patients who can swallow.

10. You respond to an unconscious 55-year-old woman. Family members state that she was complaining of being dizzy and nauseated and was having difficulty speaking and moving her left arm and leg before collapsing and becoming unconscious. The patient is supine on the living room floor and is cyanotic with snoring respirations. What is the most likely cause of the snoring respirations and cyanosis?
    a. Respiratory arrest
    b. Obstruction of the airway by the tongue
    c. Cardiac arrest
    d. Swelling of the vocal cords

11. You respond to a 78-year-old man who is having difficulty speaking; his right arm drifts downward, and he has a facial droop. These three symptoms comprise which of the following?
    a. Glasgow Coma Scale
    b. Cincinnati Prehospital Stroke Scale
    c. Kent Emergency Scale
    d. French Scale

12. An 86-year-old man is noted by family to be slurring his words and having difficulty walking, with weakness in the left arm and leg. He has a history of a TIA 1 month ago. What is the most likely cause of his symptoms?
  a. Hemorrhagic stroke
  b. Ischemic stroke
  c. Subarachnoid hemorrhage
  d. Cerebral hemorrhage

13. You assess a patient who opens his eyes only in response to pain, moans incomprehensibly, and extends his limbs in response to pain. What is the Glasgow Coma Scale score for this patient?
  a. 4
  b. 5
  c. 6
  d. 7

14. When transporting a suspected stroke patient to the stroke center, you contact the center to communicate the estimated time of symptom onset, the Cincinnati Prehospital Stroke Scale score, and the Glasgow Coma Scale score. The benefit of this communication is to allow the stroke center to do which of the following?
  a. Calculate the patient's risk of dying
  b. Assess bed availability
  c. Estimate the chances of full recovery
  d. Mobilize resources to reduce time to treatment

For Further Review

In the Student Workbook

- Multiple-choice questions
- Matching questions
- Fill-in-the-blank questions
- Short-answer questions
- True/false questions
- Case scenario questions
- Crossword puzzle

On the Website

- Anatomy challenges
- Weblinks
- Lecture notes
- Exercises

Learning Objectives

Cognitive Objectives

- Identify the patient taking diabetic medications with altered mental status and the implications of a diabetes history.
- State the steps in the emergency medical care of the patient taking diabetic medicine with an altered mental status and a history of diabetes.
- State the generic and trade names, medication forms, dose, administration, action, and contraindications for oral glucose.
- Evaluate the need for contact with medical control in the emergency medical care of the diabetic patient.
- List the signs and symptoms of a grand mal seizure, including tonic, clonic, postictal, and aura.
- Explain the management of a patient with seizure.
- Establish the relationship between airway management and the patient with altered mental status.

Affective Objectives

- Explain the rationale for administering oral glucose.

Psychomotor Objectives

- Demonstrate the steps in the emergency medical care for the patient taking diabetic medicine with an altered mental status and a history of diabetes.
- Demonstrate the steps in the administration of oral glucose.
- Demonstrate the assessment and documentation of patient response to oral glucose.
- Demonstrate how to complete a prehospital care report for patients with diabetic emergencies.

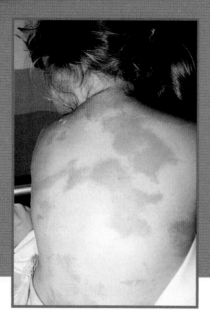

14 Allergies

CHAPTER OUTLINE

Allergic Reactions
Assessment
Management
Skills

Scenario

You respond to a 38-year-old man who was stung by a bee while working in his yard. Your scene size-up and initial (primary) assessment find the man lying on a chaise lounge chair complaining of weakness and difficulty breathing. He is pale and sweaty and exhibits signs of stridor and use of accessory muscles of breathing. His respiratory rate is 32 breaths/min, and his pulse rate is 140 beats/min. His blood pressure is 60/40 mm Hg. He has severe swelling of the face, lips, and tongue. You also note raised red blotches over his chest and abdomen. His wife tells you that he had an allergic reaction to a bee sting a year ago, and his doctor prescribed an epinephrine injection pen, which he has never used. You and your partner administer high-concentration supplemental oxygen by a nonrebreather mask, place the patient on a wheeled stretcher with legs elevated, and prepare him for transport while you contact the physician at medical direction. You receive an order to administer the epinephrine injection in the thigh. You transport the patient to the hospital and perform ongoing assessment en route.

Allergies are a common problem, and signs and symptoms can range from simple nasal congestion to *anaphylaxis,* a life-threatening condition that can result in death within minutes. Both allergy and anaphylaxis are conditions in which an *antibody-antigen reaction* results in the release of substances that can cause leakage of fluid in tissues, swelling, and a variety of other responses by body systems, including respiratory, circulatory, gastrointestinal (GI), and skin reactions. An *antigen* is a substance that is recognized as foreign to the body. An *antibody* is a protein that combines with an antigen. Antibodies usually are helpful in fighting infections and neutralizing toxins. Antibody-antigen reactions take place constantly and are part of the body's normal defense against foreign materials and infection.

The essential difference between a simple allergic reaction and anaphylaxis is the extent and scope of the reaction. Simple allergic reactions tend to be local and relatively mild responses. For example, an individual allergic to pollen may exhibit nasal congestion, sneezing, and coughing without any other responses. Another example is a person who develops an allergic rash when using a new laundry detergent. An anaphylactic reaction, however, affects the body systemically, involving multiple body systems.

> **LEARNING OBJECTIVE**
> - Describe the mechanisms of allergic response and the implications for airway management.

Allergic Reactions

An allergic reaction is an antibody-antigen reaction gone "haywire," in which the effects are detrimental rather than protective. The reaction of an antigen with an antibody causes the release of chemicals such as histamine. Histamine causes blood vessels to dilate, capillaries to leak, and lung tissue to constrict. An allergic reaction develops when this response occurs in an exaggerated manner.

Allergic reactions can be localized or systemic. Local reactions affect only one area or body system. For example, persons allergic to a laundry detergent may break out in hives where their clothes touch their skin, but nowhere else. These reactions tend to be less severe than systemic reactions unless the system affected is the respiratory system. More severe responses can result in profound dilation of blood vessels; the blood pressure will fall, resulting in shock. With plasma leakage from the capillaries, swelling of the skin, face, mouth, tongue, and other airway structures can occur.

Anaphylaxis can involve multiple body systems, leading to shock, swelling of tissues, constriction of the bronchioles, airway obstruction, or a combination of these symptoms. This multisystem response is referred to as being *systemic.* The most common manifestations of an anaphylactic reaction involve the skin and the respiratory, circulatory, and GI systems. The onset of this reaction can be extremely rapid and can result in death within minutes. Patients with anaphylaxis need immediate treatment to reverse the effects of the reaction, maintain an open airway, and stabilize the cardiovascular system.

As an EMT, you can help in the management of anaphylaxis by quickly recognizing the signs and symptoms, establishing a patent airway, and ensuring adequate ventilation. You may also be able to assist some patients who have previously been diagnosed with anaphylaxis and carry an *epinephrine autoinjector* pen. In some states, EMTs carry epinephrine in the ambulance to treat patients with anaphylaxis. **Epinephrine** is a potent drug that can block the effects of histamine and slow the anaphylactic process.

Common Agents That Cause Anaphylaxis

Although multiple agents can provoke anaphylaxis, the most common are as follows:

- Certain drugs
- Foods
- Insect bites

Penicillin, cephalosporins (e.g., cephalexin [Keflex]), tetracycline, and nitrofurantoin are examples of antibiotics that have caused anaphylactic reactions. Some dyes used for radiographic contrast studies can cause an anaphylaxis-like response, as can antiinflammatory drugs such as aspirin and indomethacin (Indocin).

Foods that often cause anaphylaxis in sensitized individuals include nuts, shellfish, eggs, chocolate, cottonseed oil, grains, and beans. Food preservatives, such as sulfites, have also been implicated.

Insect stings, especially from yellow jackets, honeybees, wasps, and hornets, have also been associated with anaphylaxis. Honeybees leave their stingers in their victims, which can cause continued exposure. Fire ants, seen in the southern United States, can cause anaphylaxis.

Some individuals become sensitized to latex. This is of particular concern to healthcare providers and patients because of the widespread use of gloves when following standard precautions. The reaction is usually an irritation of the skin in contact with the latex. However, latex antigens can be airborne and carried by the powder in many gloves. If someone has latex allergy, exposure to the powder may lead to irritation of the eyes and nose, asthma, or even anaphylaxis. You may encounter patients with known latex allergies who are concerned about the type of gloves you are wearing. Special latex-free gloves are available and are often supplied as an alternative. As an EMT, you should be aware of the content of the gloves you use.

Anaphylactic Reactions

As mentioned, when antigens react with the preformed antibodies in an anaphylactic reaction, specialized cells are activated to release histamine and other chemical substances. The actions of agents such as histamine explain many of the signs and symptoms seen in anaphylaxis. These actions include the following:

- The constriction of bronchial smooth muscle in the airway results in decreased airflow and difficulty breathing. Constriction of smooth muscle in the GI tract causes abdominal cramps, vomiting, and diarrhea.
- Increased permeability (ability of fluid and particles to move through a membrane) of capillaries causes leakage of plasma and protein, resulting in edema (swelling) and loss of blood volume.
- Dilation of the arterial vessels results in decreased resistance in blood vessels and a fall in blood pressure.
- Dilation of the venous system causes venous pooling of blood, which in turn causes decreased venous return and decreased cardiac output and hypotension.
- Increased mucus secretions in the respiratory tree and GI tract further contribute to respiratory and GI problems and also explain some of the symptoms seen in more localized allergic reactions (e.g., nasal congestion, sneezing).

Anaphylactic reactions vary significantly from patient to patient according to their degree of hypersensitivity to the antigen, the amount of antigen absorbed or injected, and the route of exposure. The following occur in the most severe cases:

- Upper airway swelling and acute bronchospasm lead to upper and lower airway obstruction and respiratory failure.
- Vasodilation and hypovolemia cause circulatory collapse. In circulatory collapse the cardiovascular system can no longer generate the pressure needed to distribute blood adequately to vital organs. This condition is known as *shock* and is the primary complication of an anaphylactic reaction and may cause death.

REAL*World*

Allergic reactions tend to increase in severity with repeated exposure to the causative agents. A person may be stung by a wasp for the first time and experience a localized reaction such as swelling and hives around the site. The second time this person is stung, the patient may rapidly progress into anaphylactic shock. Some people can become so sensitive that even indirect exposure can cause a reaction. Based on this, many elementary schools do not allow peanut butter for lunch or any product with peanuts brought into the school.

LEARNING OBJECTIVE
- Recognize the patient experiencing an allergic reaction.

Assessment

Scene Size-up and Initial (Primary) Assessment

You should take appropriate body substance isolation precautions and ensure that the scene is safe. Pay close attention to the ABCs (airway, circulation, breathing) because patients with anaphylaxis may have airway obstruction caused by swelling of the upper airway. If the airway is totally occluded, rapid access to advanced life support (ALS) is critical to the patient's survival; endotracheal intubation or a surgical airway, such as a cricothyroidotomy, may be needed to restore adequate ventilation. This may include calling for an ALS intercept or transporting the patient to the local hospital, depending on local protocols. Also, check for signs of poor perfusion, and treat the patient for shock.

Focused (Secondary) Assessment

Focused History

Some patients may know they are hypersensitive to a particular substance and can help you with this history. Some patients may wear identification bands and may carry medication to block or counteract the anaphylactic response. A medication typically prescribed to patients with anaphylaxis is an autoinjector containing epinephrine (see later discussion). Other patients may be unaware of their hypersensitivity, and the present allergic reaction may be their first. You may connect the onset of symptoms with a recent history of a significant exposure, such as the following:

- Administration of a drug
- Ingestion of a particular food
- An insect sting

Some anaphylactic symptoms occur almost immediately after antigen contact. However, the route of administration affects the speed of onset (e.g., injection is usually faster than ingestion). For example, intravenous injection of a drug may result in a more rapid onset of symptoms than an ingestion of a food allergen.

Physical Examination

Skin and General Signs. Common signs of an anaphylactic reaction involve several body systems. A feeling of warmth often precedes the reaction. The patient may present with the following signs:

- Tingling of the face, extremities, and upper chest
- Itching and generalized flushing of the skin
- **Urticaria (hives):** raised, red patches of skin (Figure 14-1)
- **Angioedema:** a condition that results from vasodilation and causes hives and swelling of the face, lips, tongue, and airway (Figure 14-2)
- Nasal congestion, sneezing, and itching around the eyes
- Headache
- Abdominal pain
- Sense of impending doom

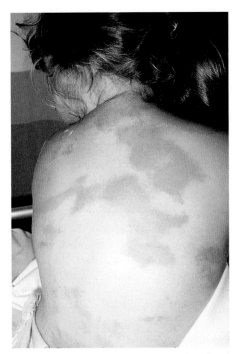

Figure 14-1 Urticaria (hives). Raised, red, itchy blotches on the skin are obvious in this young girl with an allergic reaction. Although urticaria may be seen with anaphylaxis, it is most often seen without any signs of anaphylaxis.

Respiratory Signs. The airway may become narrowed, causing dyspnea, tightness of the throat, hoarseness, and stridor. Other generalized signs of respiratory distress may also be present, including cyanosis, use of accessory muscles of breathing, and suprasternal and intercostal retractions. Wheezing and noisy breathing may be auscultated or heard at the patient's mouth from bronchoconstriction and mucus secretion. Breath sounds may be absent or diminished because of hypoventilation. The patient may ultimately present with complete airway obstruction and respiratory failure. This can be the result of total airway closure or exhaustion from the increased work of breathing. At this point, positive-pressure ventilation may be lifesaving.

Cardiovascular Signs. The cardiovascular signs associated with an anaphylactic reaction can change and are primarily related to dilation of the vessels and leakage of fluid through the capillaries. Diffuse dilation of blood vessels may initially cause a generalized "pink" appearance as a result of increased blood flow to the skin. This phase may be short lived as the cardiovascular system fights to maintain pressure and perfusion in an enlarging vascular space. Fluid loss, occurring through leakage of the capillaries, further limits the cardiovascular system's attempts to maintain the blood pressure.

As with other types of shock, the body will attempt to compensate by an increase in the pulse and respiratory rate. The skin becomes pale and sweaty as the cardiovascular system attempts

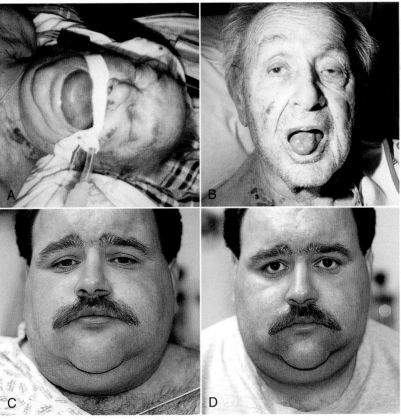

Figure 14-2 **A,** This patient had an anaphylactic reaction, probably to a medication, with rapid swelling of the tongue and cardiac arrest from hypoxia. Intubation around the tongue and administration of epinephrine restored his airway and allowed for resuscitation. **B,** The patient later awoke and was discharged from the hospital. **C,** Different patient with anaphylaxis and hives and swelling of the face and lips before treatment. **D,** Same patient as in *C* after treatment with epinephrine, antihistamines, and steroids. *A and B photos courtesy Lester Kallus, MD.*

| Box 14-1 | Symptoms and Signs of Anaphylaxis |

Symptoms
Anxiety
Itching
Sneezing, coughing, wheezing, runny nose
Hoarseness
Loss of voice, fainting
Sense of impending doom
Tightness in throat
Tingling feeling
Itchy, watery eyes

Signs
Hives
Hypotension, rapid pulse
Wheezing, difficulty breathing
Facial, pharyngeal, and laryngeal edema
Stridor and noisy breathing
Cardiac or respiratory arrest
Flushing of skin
Swelling of face, neck, hands, feet, and tongue
Rapid, labored breathing
Decreased mental state
Cramping, abdominal pain, vomiting, diarrhea

---

to maintain adequate circulation. The patient may ultimately become hypotensive and show signs of decreased brain perfusion, including an altered mental status ranging from agitation to lethargy to coma.

Box 14-1 summarizes assessment findings in patients with anaphylactic shock.

LEARNING OBJECTIVES
- Describe the emergency medical care of the patient with an allergic reaction.
- State the generic and trade names, medication forms, dose, administration, action, and contraindications to the epinephrine autoinjector.
- Explain the rationale for administering epinephrine with an autoinjector.
- Evaluate the need for medical direction of the emergency medical care of the patient with an allergic reaction.
- Differentiate between the general category of those patients having an allergic reaction and those patients having an allergic reaction and requiring immediate medical care, including immediate use of an epinephrine autoinjector.

Management

The patient with an anaphylactic reaction requires the immediate administration of epinephrine, which blocks the effects caused by the antigen-antibody reaction. The primary goals of

prehospital care of the anaphylactic patient include airway management, ventilation and oxygenation, support of circulation, administration of epinephrine (according to local protocol), and rapid transport.

Lifesaving Medications

The definitive treatment for anaphylactic shock is the injection of epinephrine and other drugs to combat the reaction. The patient who carries an anaphylactic kit should self-administer the medication(s) as quickly as possible. The EMT may assist patients in administering epinephrine according to state and local protocols. Some states permit the use of epinephrine for patients who do not have a prescribed autoinjector, such as first-time cases of anaphylaxis. Check the local protocols.

Epinephrine is usually administered subcutaneously or intramuscularly at a dose of 0.3 mg. The pediatric dose is 0.01 mg/kg.

The EpiPen autoinjector is a preloaded syringe for self-administration containing 0.3 mg of epinephrine. **Table 14-1** summarizes the pharmacology of the EpiPen. The pediatric version, EpiPen Jr., contains 0.15 mg of epinephrine. These syringes are intended for intramuscular (IM) injection. The lateral portion of the thigh is the injection site to avoid intravenous (IV) or intraarterial injection (**Figure 14-3**).

The onset of action of epinephrine is rapid; effects are seen minutes after injection. The clinical effects of the drug may peak 15 to 20 minutes after injection and then begin to diminish. Some patients may initially show improvement after the epinephrine injection, but then their condition deteriorates. These patients may benefit from a second injection, and you should consult medical direction. The prescribed autoinjector now comes as a double kit, recognizing that patients may need a second injection before they reach a hospital.

Case in Point

You are part of EMS on site at a festival at a state park when you are called to care for an 8-year-old boy with shortness of breath. The child is exhibiting accessory respiratory muscle use, and you hear stridor as you approach the patient. He speaks in short sentences, and auscultation reveals wheezing on both sides. He has a red, blotchy rash over his face and trunk. His mother tells you that he unknowingly ate foods with peanut oil, and he is highly allergic to peanuts.

The boy's lips are swelling, and his tongue is protruding from his mouth. The mother retrieves the epinephrine autoinjector from the car, which he has been prescribed but has never used.

You contact medical control and are directed to give one dose, 0.15 mg, intramuscularly into the midlateral thigh. You then begin transport. The boy begins to breathe easier, and the swelling of his tongue and lips recedes. His blood pressure is normal. The hospital is 30 minutes away.

Twenty minutes later, the boy starts to exhibit signs of respiratory distress. He has audible stridor and visible chest wall retractions and accessory muscle use. You contact medical control and are directed to administer a second dose of epinephrine, again 0.15 mg by autoinjector, into the midlateral thigh of the other leg. As you arrive at the hospital the boy again begins to breathe easier, and the pulse oxygen is 98% when breathing oxygen through a nonrebreather mask.

Table 14-1	Pharmacology of Epinephrine of EpiPen Autoinjector

Generic Name	**Epinephrine**
Trade name	Adrenalin, EpiPen
Indications for use	Three criteria must be met (unless otherwise directed by local protocol):
	1. Patient exhibits assessment finding of an allergic reaction.
	2. Medication is prescribed for this patient.
	3. Medical direction authorizes use for this patient.
Contraindications	None when used in a life-threatening situation.
Form	Liquid administered through automatic injected needle and syringe system (autoinjector)
Dose	One adult autoinjector (0.3 mg)
	Pediatric (0.15 mg) for patients <30 kg (66 lb)
Route of administration	Midlateral aspect of thigh (see Skill 14-1)
Actions	Dilates the bronchioles; constricts the blood vessels
Side effects	Increased heart rate, pallor, dizziness, headache, nausea, vomiting, excitability, and anxiousness
Reassessment strategies	Transport
	If patient's condition continues to worsen, as evidenced by the following:
	Decreasing mental status
	Increasing breathing difficulty
	Decreasing blood pressure
	Contact medical direction for:
	Repeat dose of epinephrine
	Treatment for shock (hypoperfusion)
	Preparation to administer basic life support (CPR, automatic external defibrillation)
	If patient's condition improves, provide supportive care as follows:
	Oxygen
	Treatment for shock (hypoperfusion)

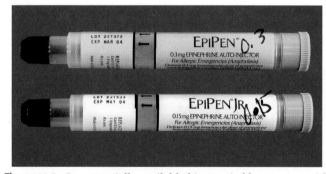

Figure 14-3 Commercially available kits carried by persons with a history of anaphylaxis: EpiPen and EpiPen Jr.

Some prescribed regimens also include administration of an oral antihistamine. Diphenhydramine (Benadryl) is a potent antihistamine that can help block the release of histamine from the cells and thus reduce the effects of allergic reactions. Once the reaction has taken place and airway symptoms or shock are present, however, antihistamines are of less value than epinephrine. If no medication is available at the scene, or even if it has been injected, rapid transport is essential because anaphylaxis can progress quickly, and the patient may need another dose of medication. **Skill 14-1** demonstrates the administration of epinephrine with an autoinjector.

> **LEARNING OBJECTIVE**
> • Establish the relationship between the patient with an allergic reaction and airway management.

EXTENDED *Transport*

When transporting a patient who has experienced an anaphylactic reaction, the EMT needs to be aware that the administration of an EpiPen is not the "cure" for the patient's condition. The drug opens the lungs and helps increase blood pressure. The anaphylactic reaction may still be in progress. When the epinephrine wears off, the patient can quickly deteriorate once again, going into shock and becoming hypoxic. The EMT crew must be prepared to administer a second dose of the autoinjector for this potential deterioration. The patient's EpiPen may contain two doses, or the patient may have two EpiPen units that should be brought with the patient. Some EMS systems allow ambulances staffed by EMTs to carry EpiPen. When considering time of transport, ALS rendezvous or a faster mode of transportation such as helicopter might be necessary.

Respiratory Support

Complete Airway Obstruction

If the patient is exhibiting signs of complete airway obstruction from swelling, rapid transport to advanced life support is essential. Because airway obstruction procedures (abdominal and chest thrusts and finger sweeps) are of no value, rapid transport is the main priority. These patients may require intubation or a surgical airway to establish a patent airway.

Positive-pressure ventilation with high-concentration supplemental oxygen should be attempted during transport in an effort to deliver lifesaving amounts of air. In some patients the airway closure may be so complete that adequate ventilation may not be possible.

Respiratory Distress or Failure

High-concentration supplemental oxygen through a nonrebreather mask should be administered to all patients who are exhibiting signs of respiratory distress. Patients who are hypoventilating, as evidenced by decreased respiratory rate, minimal or no chest excursion, or altered mental status, should receive assisted ventilation with 100% oxygen. Remember to coordinate rescue breaths with the patient's attempt to inspire.

Cardiovascular Support

Patients who are exhibiting signs of shock should be placed in the supine position with the legs elevated and should be treated according to local protocol. This should include rapid transport to the hospital because the patient needs medication and may require invasive procedures to secure the airway or stabilize the cardiovascular condition. You may also consider an ALS intercept. As with all patients in shock, prevent the loss of body heat to conserve energy and decrease the cardiovascular workload.

Vital signs should be recorded every 5 minutes, or more often when circumstances permit. Do not allow the patient to take anything by mouth except prescribed medications that may help reduce the effects of anaphylaxis.

Box 14-2 summarizes the management of anaphylaxis.

Case in Point

You are dispatched for a "difficulty breathing" call at a summer camp. On arrival you find a 20-year-old counselor in obvious respiratory distress. He had been well all day and developed shortness of breath when playing basketball after dinner. He first attributed his shortness of breath to playing basketball, but it persisted and worsened even as he sat down to rest. A fellow counselor was so concerned that he called an ambulance.

The patient is able to answer questions but is using accessory muscles of breathing and has warm, flushed skin. Pertinent findings are wheezing in both lungs and appearance of raised, blotchy, red lesions on the skin. SAMPLE history reveals he is allergic to peanuts and has been prescribed an EpiPen. He denies eating any nuts. You administer supplemental oxygen and check other vital signs, which include a respiratory rate of 32 breaths/min, pulse of 120 beats/min, and blood pressure 130/86 mm Hg.

Many fellow camp counselors are standing nearby; when the cook hears the patient is allergic to peanuts, he informs you and the patient that peanut oil was used in preparing the evening meal. Another counselor runs to the man's cabin and retrieves his EpiPen from his medicine cabinet. The history and physical examination are consistent with anaphylaxis. You contact medical direction and report the findings and are ordered to assist the patient with administration of his epinephrine as soon as possible and to be ready to administer the second dose of the autoinjector. As you perform your ongoing assessment en route, you note less accessory muscle use and wheezing and the blotchy lesions on the skin are beginning to fade. The patient's respiratory rate is 26 breaths/min, pulse is 110 beats/min, and blood pressure is 136/88 mm Hg on repeat vital signs. You continue to administer supplemental oxygen and continue your ongoing assessment as you transport the patient to the hospital.

Box 14-2 Sample Protocol for Anaphylaxis

1. Perform initial (primary) assessment, and ensure that the patient's airway is open and that breathing and circulation are adequate.
2. Administer high-concentration supplemental oxygen, and consider need for positive-pressure ventilation.
3. Perform focused (secondary) assessment (history and physical examination) and note the following:
   - History of allergies, what patient was exposed to, how the patient was exposed, what effects, progression, and intervention.
   - Assess baseline vital signs, and collect SAMPLE* history.
   - Assess for shock. If shock is present, keep patient warm and place in supine position with legs elevated 8 to 12 inches.
4. Determine if patient has been prescribed epinephrine; if so, contact medical direction for order (or follow standing orders).
5. Assist in administration of epinephrine, if necessary.
6. If patient does not have an autoinjector, transport immediately.
7. If cardiac arrest occurs, perform cardiopulmonary resuscitation (CPR).
8. Reassess and record vital signs in 2 minutes.

*Signs and symptoms, Allergies, Medications, Pertinent past history, Last oral intake, Events leading to current illness/injury (anaphylaxis).

Scenario Follow-up

The 38-year-old man stung by a bee responded to the injection of epinephrine, with an increase in blood pressure to 100/70 mm Hg and less-labored respirations. Epinephrine constricts the blood vessels and dilates the bronchioles, raising blood pressure and making it easier to breathe. Epinephrine has a short duration of action, and more doses may be necessary. The patient also received steroids and antihistamines at the hospital, where he was observed for several hours before discharge home. Hypotension and severe bronchoconstriction and swelling, with obstruction of the upper airway, can cause death. Early treatment with epinephrine can be lifesaving to many such patients.

Summary

The prehospital management of severe allergic reactions requires rapid identification of signs and symptoms of anaphylaxis and administration of epinephrine. The key signs and symptoms that indicate the need for treatment include general signs of an allergic reaction (e.g., hives, itching, coughing, sneezing) accompanied by signs of respiratory distress, airway obstruction, or shock.

When prescribed epinephrine is available at the scene, coordination with medical direction and rapid administration of epinephrine will help reverse the life-threatening effects of anaphylaxis, including airway obstruction and shock (hypoperfusion). Additionally, management of the patient's airway and treatment for shock provide support during transport to advanced life support or hospital interventions.

Skills

Skill | 14-1   *Administering Epinephrine with an Autoinjector*

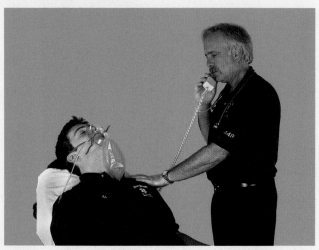

1. Obtain order from medical direction either online or offline.

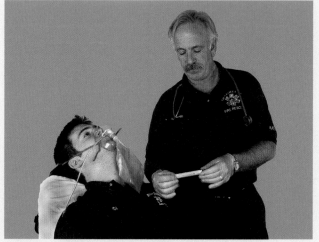

2. Obtain patient's prescribed autoinjector. Check the following:
- Prescription is written for the patient experiencing allergic reactions.
- Dose is correct.
- Medication has not expired.
- Medication is not discolored (if it can be seen).

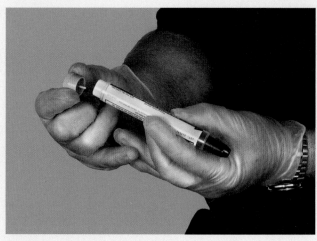

3. Remove the safety cap from the autoinjector.

Continued

Skill | 14-1   *Administering Epinephrine with Autoinjector—cont'd*

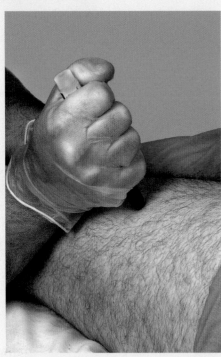

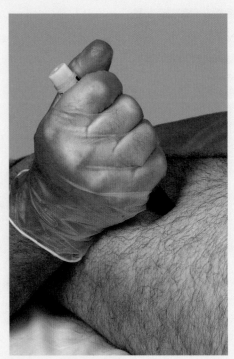

4. Place the tip of the autoinjector against the anterior lateral portion of the patient's thigh midway between the waist and the knee. The manufacturer recommends injection through clothing when the clinical situation requires immediate action.

5. Push the injector firmly against the thigh until the injector activates. Hold the injector in place until the medication is injected. Dispose of injector in a biohazard (sharps) container. Record activity and time.

The Bottom Line

Learning Checklist

✓ Allergies and anaphylaxis are conditions in which an antibody-antigen reaction results in the release of substances that can affect the skin and the respiratory, circulatory, and gastrointestinal systems.

✓ Anaphylaxis is an antibody-antigen reaction gone "haywire," in which the effects are detrimental rather than protective.

✓ Anaphylaxis is often caused by drugs (e.g., antibiotics), foods (e.g., nuts, shellfish, eggs, chocolate, cottonseed oil, grains, beans), and insect bites (e.g., bees, yellow jackets, wasps).

✓ General signs and symptoms of anaphylaxis include tingling of the face, extremities, and upper chest; itching and generalized flushing of the skin; urticaria or hives; angioedema; nasal congestion, sneezing, and itching around the eyes; headache; abdominal pain; and a sense of impending doom.

✓ Cardiovascular signs of anaphylaxis include early signs (flushed skin, rapid pulse) and late signs (pale, cool, clammy skin; hypotension; altered mental state).

✓ Respiratory signs of anaphylaxis include dyspnea, tightness of the throat, hoarseness, stridor, cyanosis, use of accessory muscles of breathing, retractions, wheezing and noisy breathing, and signs of complete airway obstruction (inability to speak or cough), respiratory failure (hypoventilation), and respiratory arrest.

✓ The EMT may assist in the administration of epinephrine prescribed by the patient's physician with an autoinjector. In some areas, EMTs may carry epinephrine on the ambulance to treat patients who may not have their medication with them or who are having their first episode of anaphylaxis.

✓ Epinephrine is administered at a dose of 0.3 mg to adults and 0.15 mg to children intramuscularly with an autoinjector.

✓ Rapidly transport patients with anaphylaxis who develop complete airway obstruction to advanced life support capabilities because a surgical airway (e.g., cricothyroidotomy, tracheostomy) may be needed to restore adequate ventilation.

Key Terms

Anaphylaxis Allergic condition in which an antibody-antigen reaction results in a release of substances that can cause shock, bronchoconstriction, and airway obstruction.

Angioedema Condition that results from vasodilation and causes hives and swelling of the face, airway, and other tissues.

Epinephrine Potent drug that can block the effects of histamine and slow the anaphylactic process.

Urticaria Raised, red patches of skin; also called **hives**.

Review Questions

1. Which of the following is a sign often seen with an allergic reaction?
   a. High blood pressure
   b. Tremors
   c. Hives
   d. Dry nose and eyes

2. Which of the following foods is a common cause of a severe allergic reaction?
   a. Fruits
   b. Soft drinks
   c. Nuts
   d. Ice cream

3. Where should the epinephrine autoinjector be injected?
   a. Biceps muscle
   b. Anterior lateral thigh
   c. Lateral arm
   d. Lower thigh

4. Which of the following are the most common life-threatening complications of an allergic reaction?
   a. Vomiting and dehydration
   b. Abnormal heart rhythms and brain damage
   c. Kidney failure and hypertension
   d. Airway obstruction and shock

5. Which of the following is a common side effect of epinephrine?
   a. Respiratory arrest
   b. Sleepiness
   c. Hives
   d. Rapid pulse

6. The EpiPen medication is injected into the patient's muscle by doing which of the following?
   a. Pushing a button on the top of the pen
   b. Propelling a plunger at the top of the pen
   c. Pressing the pen firmly against the leg
   d. Twisting the top of the pen

7. A 46-year-old woman complains of shortness of breath, which she has never experienced and which came on suddenly. Which of the following is consistent with a diagnosis of anaphylaxis?
   a. She traveled on a plane for 12 hours and has a swollen left leg.
   b. Listening to the lungs reveals absent breath sounds on the right side.
   c. She has stridor, bilateral wheezing, and an itchy rash.
   d. Listening to her lungs reveals rales bilaterally.

8. A 25-year-old man tells the EMT he has been stung by a wasp. The patient was stung once before and developed a rash and had mild shortness of breath, but he never consulted a physician; the symptoms resolved without treatment. How should the EMT expect the patient to respond to this event?

    a. It should be the same as the first time.

    b. It will be less severe.

    c. It will be more severe.

    d. It depends on the time of year.

For Further Review

In the Student Workbook

- Multiple-choice questions
- Matching questions
- Short answer questions
- Case scenario questions

On Evolve

- Anatomy challenges
- Weblinks
- Exercises

Learning Objectives

Cognitive Objectives

- Describe the mechanisms of allergic response and the implications for airway management.

- Recognize the patient experiencing an allergic reaction.
- Describe the emergency medical care of the patient with an allergic reaction.
- State the generic and trade names, medication forms, dose, administration, action, and contraindications for the epinephrine autoinjector.
- Evaluate the need for medical control in the emergency medical care of the patient with an allergic reaction.
- Differentiate between the general category of those patients having an allergic reaction and those patients having an allergic reaction and requiring immediate medical care, including immediate use of epinephrine autoinjector.
- Establish the relationship between the patient with an allergic reaction and airway management.

Affective Objectives

- Explain the rationale for administering epinephrine with an autoinjector.

Psychomotor Objectives

- Demonstrate the emergency medical care of the patient experiencing an allergic reaction.
- Demonstrate the use of an epinephrine autoinjector.
- Demonstrate the assessment and documentation of patient response to an epinephrine injection.
- Demonstrate proper disposal of equipment.
- Demonstrate completing a prehospital care report for patients with allergic emergencies.

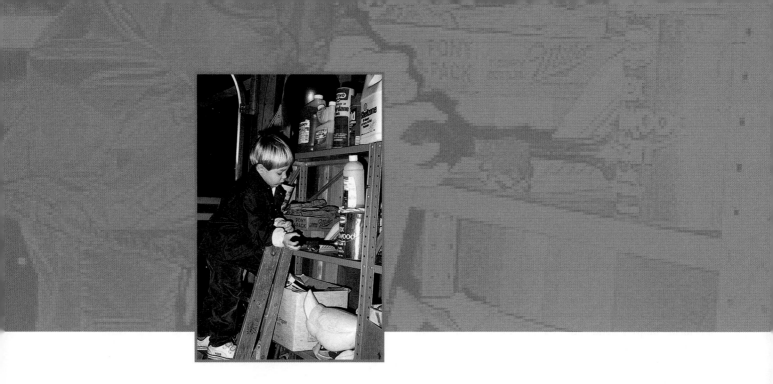

15 Poisoning and Overdoses

CHAPTER OUTLINE

Scenario

You and your partner arrive at a park after receiving a call for an unconscious man. You see a crowd gathered around a person lying on the sidewalk. You do not detect any personal threat, and you put on your gloves as you approach the patient. You ask the bystanders to stand back and note a young man who appears to be in his teens and who is unresponsive, with blue lips and slow, shallow respirations with a regular pulse. There is no sign of trauma. You begin positive-pressure ventilation with high-concentration oxygen and note an improvement in the patient's color. He remains unresponsive to voice or painful stimuli. As you continue ventilation, his friends approach and ask if he will be all right. They tell you they had bought some "heroin" to snort in the park and didn't realize how strong it was. As you are preparing the patient for transport, the paramedics arrive and review your findings. They ask you to continue ventilations as they administer naloxone to counteract a possible overdose of heroin. Within a minute, the patient begins to take some deep breaths and to move and open his eyes.

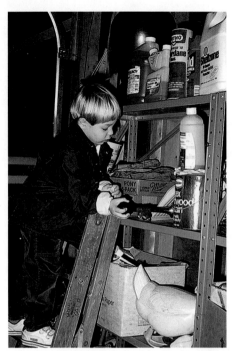

Figure 15-1 Hazardous household materials can be found in homes and garages in reach of curious toddlers. Substances commonly available include insecticides, antifreeze (ethylene glycol), and windshield washing fluid (methanol), all of which can be very toxic if ingested.

As an Emergency Medical Technician (EMT), you may encounter many patients with poisoning or overdose. First, you must be careful to take appropriate precautions for self-protection. Look closely for signs of threats to life, and provide life support as indicated. For many patients, maintaining an airway and providing positive-pressure ventilation and supplemental oxygen will be lifesaving, as in the case above. Gather clues from the scene that help identify the substance involved, and bring these to the attention of the emergency department (ED) or poison center staff. In some cases when a substance has been ingested, you will administer activated charcoal to limit absorption from the stomach. Although the number and types of substances involved in poisoning and overdose are many, basic principles of assessment and management can guide your response.

A **poison** is defined as a substance that usually kills, injures, or impairs an organism through its chemical action. **Toxicology** is the study of poisons. The effects of a poison are said to be **toxic,** and poisons are often referred to as *toxins.*

Overdose is a term applied to self-administration of drugs, taken in excess or in combination with other agents, to the point at which poisoning occurs. In this sense, poisoning is a matter of degree. For example, a medication that is beneficial at one dose may be detrimental or even lethal when taken in excess. An overdose can involve therapeutic drugs, alcohol, or illegal drugs, often called "recreational" drugs. Patients, particularly elderly patients who take a number of medications, may become confused at times and unintentionally take excess medications or a combination of medications that proves harmful.

A poisoning may be unintentional, such as when a child ingests household products or medications, thinking that these are food or candy. A poisoning can also be intentional, such as a suicide attempt or murder. Poisoning can also occur from plants or from insect, snake, and arthropod (including spiders) venom. Poisoning that occurs by venom is referred to as *envenomation.*

Incidence

According to the American Association of Poison Control Centers (AAPCC), more than 2 million poisonings occur each year, resulting in thousands of deaths. These numbers are only estimated because many overdoses may go unreported. Many of the unintentional poisonings occur in children younger than 5 years. Toddlers who put everything into their mouths may unintentionally ingest household products, unsecured pills, or other agents (**Figure 15-1**).

In adolescent and older age groups, suicide is often attempted by poisoning, usually by ingestion. Recreational drug users and addicts may cause an overdose by injecting drugs of unknown strength purchased illegally or by using combinations of different drugs; as illustrated in the opening scenario, adolescents who experiment with drugs are particularly prone to adverse events. Industrial incidents account for a significant number of poisonings. Snakes, certain insects, arthropods, and sea creatures can cause poisoning through injection of their venom.

More than 250,000 potentially poisonous drugs and commercial products currently exist.

Poison Control Centers

Because of the number of poisonings each year and the extensive number of potentially toxic products, poison control centers (PCCs) have been established in regions throughout the United States. PCCs provide information on toxins, management of poisoning victims, and antidotes. A regional PCC is accessible by phone at all times to physicians, emergency medical services (EMS) personnel, and the public. The national toll-free telephone number available in the continental United States that reaches the regional PCC is 800-222-1222.

Poison control centers can provide the following services:

- *Access to experts in toxicology.* PCCs are staffed 24 hours a day and have consultants who can be reached by phone.
- *Emergency response coordination.* Within a region, PCCs can provide advice to patients at home, refer people to area hospitals with poisoning care capabilities, and advise EMTs, physicians, and nurses on immediate and long-term treatment.

In some regions, EMTs in the field consult poison control centers to determine whether a patient needs ED care. Patients who have nontoxic exposures may be safely left at the scene, whereas those who need hospital follow-up benefit from early PCC consultation. Integration of PCC advice in prehospital decision making should be in accordance with policies established by your medical director.

Case in Point

You are dispatched to care for a 2-year-old child for a possible poisoning. When you arrive, the mother, who has no transportation, tells you she called 9-1-1 when she found her son with crayons in his mouth, two partially eaten.

The toddler is in no distress, and activity, respiratory rate, and pulse are normal for his age. You look at the box of crayons and call medical control, which conferences your call with the poison control center. The PCC verifies your information and informs you that the child has a nontoxic ingestion, and further care is not necessary. Medical control directs that transport is not necessary, and you reassure the mother that what the child chewed and swallowed is nontoxic. She thanks you for your help. You leave to prepare for the next call.

LEARNING OBJECTIVES

- List various ways in which poisons enter the body.
- List signs and symptoms associated with poisoning.
- Discuss the emergency medical care for the patient with a possible overdose.
- Describe the steps in the emergency medical care for the patient with suspected poisoning.
- Establish the relationship between the patient with poisoning or overdose and airway management.

Types of Exposure

Poisons can enter the body through the gastrointestinal (GI) tract (ingestion), the airway (inhalation), or the skin (absorption) or by injection (including envenomation).

Ingestion

The most common route of entry of poisons into the body is ingestion (swallowing) through the GI tract. Ingestion includes the suicidal patient who takes all the pills in the medicine cabinet, the street alcoholic who drinks methanol (wood alcohol, windshield washer solution) in place of ethanol, and the toddler who roams into the garage and drinks from an open bottle of antifreeze (ethylene glycol) or insecticide.

Inhalation

Carbon monoxide (CO) is the most frequently inhaled toxin. Other toxic gases, such as cyanide, phosgene, and nitrous dioxides, may be inhaled in industrial or agricultural incidents or with smoke from fires. When rescuing victims of poisoning by inhalation, EMTs must be particularly careful to take protective measures to avoid exposure to themselves and others. Glue sniffing, freebasing cocaine, and smoking crack are other examples of poisoning by inhalation.

Absorption

Some poisons can be absorbed through the skin. Common examples include insecticides, such as organophosphates. Corrosives, such as acid and alkali, usually damage the skin itself. Hydrofluoric acid (used in the cleaning of building surfaces and the manufacture of computer chips) can chemically burn the skin *and* be absorbed into the circulation. Cocaine, when snorted through the nose, is absorbed by the membranes in the nasopharynx.

Injection

Injected poisons (drugs injected intravenously) that are self-administered can include an overdose of opioids that a drug addict injects when "shooting up" or an overdose of insulin that a diabetic patient inadvertently administers. Bee stings and venomous snake bites are other examples. Poisons injected directly into the bloodstream have the fastest onset of action.

Assessment

Caring for poisoned patients is a challenge that is often very rewarding. As an EMT, you should be open-minded because so many different substances can be toxic. If you are, you will learn more about emergency medical care and the human body and give better care to your patients.

Poisonings require that you be a good detective and maintain a high level of suspicion. Poisons are not always obvious and may be suspected in individual cases and situations in which several individuals suddenly become ill. *Clues that are not evident to ED staff may be available to EMTs. A good scene assessment is imperative.*

You should look for patterns of multiple exposures to help identify poison epidemics in a community. For example, when many people in a building have symptoms such as headaches, nausea, and loss of consciousness, CO poisoning may have occurred through a common ventilation system. Do not put yourself in jeopardy if the possibility of ongoing hazardous exposure exists; you should always take appropriate scene safety precautions.

Case in Point

In 1982, several people died from cyanide-laced acetaminophen (Tylenol) capsules in the Chicago area. The mass poisonings were discovered in part by alert EMTs who overheard two ambulance radio transmissions that described young patients inexplicably struck down by what appeared to be central nervous system and cardiac problems. With the SAMPLE history, they noted all patients had recently ingested Tylenol. Their observations led authorities to examine the Tylenol in those victims' homes, which tested positive for cyanide.

Emergency medical technicians provide critical historic information from the scene. When possible, containers of medications and toxic agents should be brought to the hospital. You should report any noticeable odors that may give a clue to toxin identification (**Table 15-1**). Search for clues of trauma. Because so many potentially toxic agents exist, any information gathered from the scene is especially important in terms of hospital evaluation.

Remember to treat *the patient,* not the poison. The clinical condition of the patient, rather than the specifics of the overdose, is the first priority in almost all cases. Establish adequacy of breathing, maintain and protect the airway, and give positive-pressure ventilation as needed. Management consists mainly of supportive care. Most poisoned patients who arrive alive at a hospital that is capable of treating the poisoning will survive, even if they are unresponsive on arrival.

Some toxins, such as cyanide and nitrites, may require timely administration of an antidote for the patient to survive. However, the number of such cases is few, and even in these situations, careful attention to oxygenation and ventilation is the primary principle.

Scene Size-up

Survey the scene with care to protect yourself and bystanders from inadvertent poisoning. Toxic gases and toxins that are absorbed through the skin can be as dangerous to the EMT as to the patient (see Case in Point). You should take precautions to ensure that you do not enter a toxic environment without adequate protection. Only trained rescuers should remove a patient from a toxic environment. Be careful not to contaminate your skin inadvertently with a toxin that can be absorbed.

Decontamination of the patient should begin as early as possible by competently trained and equipped personnel. You should be wearing protective gear so you do not become contaminated yourself by splashes or direct skin contact. Eye exposure and skin contamination call for immediate action to remove the toxin. For example, after exposure to corrosives, the eyes should be flushed with lukewarm water for at least 20 minutes and preferably until the eyes can be checked in the ED. Contaminated clothing should be removed and contaminated skin flooded with water (or soap and water) as soon as possible to remove any remaining toxins and minimize contact with the body. For some exposures, such as caustics or corrosives, the irrigation should continue for 20 minutes or longer. If the skin is contaminated with a powder, brush it off before irrigation. Training in hazardous material operations is invaluable for your own safety and that of your patients. Follow local protocols.

Case in Point

This case report illustrates the importance of scene size-up and personal protection to reduce the risk of secondary contamination when caring for victims contaminated with toxic chemicals. Consider what happened to these ED staff members when a patient was brought in without being decontaminated in the field. Note that they did not follow decontamination procedures recommended by the PCC.

ED staff members caring for patients contaminated with toxic chemicals are at risk for developing toxicity from secondary contamination. This report describes three cases of occupational illnesses associated with organophosphate toxicity caused by exposure to a contaminated patient and underscores the importance of using personal protective equipment (PPE) and establishing and following decontamination procedures in EDs.

Patient 1

On April 11, a 40-year-old man intentionally ingested approximately 110 g of a veterinary insecticide concentrate. The insecticide contained 73% naphthalene, xylene, surfactant, and 11.6% phosmet (an organophosphate). On clinical examination at a local hospital ED approximately 20 minutes after the ingestion, the patient had profuse oral and bronchial secretions, vomiting, bronchospasm, and respiratory distress. He was intubated for airway management and ventilation. He received 4 g of pralidoxime and 22 mg of atropine during the next 24 hours to control secretions. The patient's condition improved over a 9-day period, and he was transferred to a psychiatric facility.

The patient was brought to the ED by a friend, not by EMS, and the friend subsequently developed symptoms that required treatment. ED personnel exposed to the patient had symptoms within an hour of his arrival. The staff noted a chemical odor in the department and contacted the regional PCC, which recommended decontaminating the patient's skin and placing gastric contents in a sealed container to minimize evaporation; however, no decontamination was performed.

Healthcare Provider 1

A 45-year-old ED nursing assistant providing care to patient 1 developed respiratory distress, profuse secretions, emesis (vomiting), diaphoresis (sweating), and weakness. She had contact with the patient's skin, respiratory secretions, and vomit. She was admitted to the hospital and required intubation for 24 hours to support respiration. After medical management and serial doses of atropine and pralidoxime for 7 days, her respiratory function improved, and she was discharged after 9 days of hospitalization.

Healthcare Provider 2

A 32-year-old ED nurse had diaphoresis, confusion, hypersalivation, nausea, and abdominal cramps while caring for patient 1. Although she did not have skin contact with the patient's secretions or emesis, she had shared his breathing space. After treatment with 10 mg of atropine and pralidoxime over the next 12 hours, her symptoms resolved.

Table 15-1	Examples of Diagnostic Odors*

Odor	Possible Substance
Acetone (sweet, fruity)	Ethanol, isopropyl alcohol, diabetic ketoacidosis
Alcohol	Alcohol, isopropyl alcohol
Disinfectants	Phenol, creosote
Eggs (rotten)	Hydrogen sulfide
Garlic	Parathion, malathion (organophosphate insecticides)
Tobacco (stale)	Nicotine
Wintergreen	Methyl salicylate

*You might notice a particular odor from the patient or at the scene that could be of diagnostic value to the physician. Some odors are obvious, such as ammonia; others may be helpful clues for the physicians or poison control center staff who help in the care of the patient.

Healthcare Provider 3

A 56-year-old nurse providing care for patient 1 was admitted to the hospital with dyspnea, confusion, and headache. Although she did not have skin contact with secretions or emesis from patient 1, she had shared his breathing space. She was given 6 mg of atropine without relief of the dyspnea. As a possible result of excessive atropine, she experienced hallucinations. Her condition improved overnight, and she was discharged.

Follow-up

During the incident in this report, healthcare providers were exposed to a patient contaminated with an organophosphate insecticide. These healthcare providers were not wearing appropriate respiratory or skin PPE while caring for the patient. As a result, three healthcare workers developed symptoms consistent with organophosphate intoxication and required treatment. This was the third episode reported during 2000 to the Georgia Poison Center of nosocomial (occurring in healthcare environment) poisoning of ED staff involved in the care of patients who had intentionally ingested a concentrated organophosphate mixed with xylene and other hydrocarbon solvents. Similar incidents have occurred elsewhere.

Depending on the extent of the contamination, healthcare workers caring for chemically contaminated patients should use level C protection (full face mask and powered/nonpowered canister/cartridge filtration respirator) or level B protection (supplied air respirator or self-contained breathing apparatus). The type of canister/cartridge should be appropriate to the agent; if the agent cannot be identified, an organic vapor/HEPA filter is recommended. To prevent dermal absorption, chemical barrier protection appropriate to the contaminant is needed; latex medical gloves are of little protection against many chemicals. In addition to the need for surface decontamination of patients, body fluids also must be contained to prevent dermal and inhalational exposure. To limit distant spread of the contaminant, the ED's ventilation exhaust should be directed away from the hospital's main ventilation system.

EDs may have to care for persons contaminated with chemicals resulting from self-inflicted contamination, industrial incidents, and terrorist events. To protect healthcare providers caring for these patients, EDs should adhere to existing guidelines and decontamination protocols, train staff in the use of PPE, and maintain adequate quantities of antidotes.

EMTs need to take appropriate protections to prevent secondary contamination from toxic chemicals. Only personnel who are properly equipped and trained should undertake decontamination.

NOTE: Although this is an extreme example in that the patient ingested a large amount of concentrated poison, it clearly illustrates the need for rescuers to take precautions.

From Nosocomial poisoning associated with emergency department treatment of organophosphate toxicity—Georgia, 2000, *MMWR* 49(51): 1156, 2001. http://www.cdc.gov/mmwr/preview/mmwrhtml/mm4951a2.htm.

Initial (Primary) Assessment

What is your general impression? Does evaluation of the scene and other findings indicate the patient has any traumatic injury? Overdoses can lead to falls. This information is important for both field and hospital evaluation, particularly with patients who are unconscious or have an altered mental status. Conversely, in clear-cut cases of trauma, you should not overlook the possibility that the patient may also be a victim of poisoning or, more likely, could be experiencing the effects of an alcohol or drug overdose.

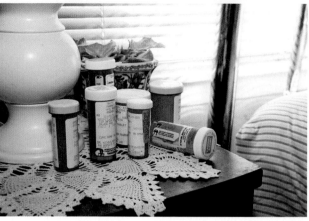

Figure 15-2 Obtain information from pill, medication, or other container and bring it to the hospital to identify the substance and help estimate the possible dose ingested.

Is the patient awake and responsive, or does the patient require verbal or painful stimuli before response? Because most deaths occur from respiratory depression, check the airway and adequacy of breathing and intervene if necessary. If necessary, you should remove fragments of tablets, pills, or capsules from the mouth or upper airway tract during your initial assessment with a gloved hand, taking care not to injure yourself. The possibility of a cervical spine injury should be considered in any unconscious patient, and if indicated, you should protect and support the patient's cervical spine. Check pulse and skin for signs of perfusion.

Patient History

Because of the many types of poisons, history taking is especially important. Available clues, such as empty pill bottles or containers, are invaluable to hospital personnel and the poison control center in an attempt to identify the substances (**Figure 15-2**). The following information must be sought:

- What is the poison?
- How was it taken? Was it ingested, inhaled, absorbed, or injected?
- When was it taken?
- How much was taken? Over what time period?
- What evidence supports the history? For example, are there any empty pill bottles, commercial products, or plant samples?
- Were any interventions attempted (e.g., vomiting, dilution, activated charcoal, syrup of ipecac [medication used to induce vomiting], or antidote)?
- What is the weight of the patient?

These critical questions should be asked of the patient, family, or others present at the scene. In many cases, multiple agents may have been taken.

At times, the history may be unreliable. A suicidal patient may want to hide knowledge of the toxin to hinder treatment. A distraught patient who has taken multiple agents (e.g., everything in the medicine cabinet) may not have stopped to consider or read what the medications were. Household products not stored in their original containers may be difficult to identify.

Focused (Secondary) Assessment

After the initial assessment, you should assess and reassess the points shown in **Box 15-1** during your examination of the patient. You should review the mental status and, if the patient is unconscious, use the AVPU method of assessment (alert, verbal, painful, unresponsive). If the patient is awake but has an altered mental status, make sure the patient can swallow to see whether the patient can protect the airway before you administer anything by mouth. Patients who have no ability to swallow their secretions should be transported with diligent attention to protecting the airway and ensuring adequate ventilations.

Some poisons present a classic clinical picture that may be obvious on examination. For example, the patient with an opioid overdose often has an altered mental status (with lethargy to coma), shallow and slow respirations, and pinpoint pupils **(Figure 15-3)**. There may be fresh or old needle marks over the veins ("tracks"), indicating intravenous (IV) drug use. A patient with organophosphate poisoning has secretions coming from many sites—sweating, drooling, urinating, defecating, vomiting, and tearing—as well as weakness, difficulty breathing, and possibly a slow heart rate and constricted pupils. As an EMT, you will gradually learn about different clinical effects of various poisons. It is important to document findings noted during the physical examination to help time the onset of drug effects and to chart the progression of signs as the toxic agent is further absorbed or eliminated.

Always look for signs of injury as well. The poisoned patient may have had a fall or other traumatic incident. The injury may be the cause of the patient's altered mental status, not any alcohol or drugs the patient may have also consumed. Without this information, definitive treatment may be delayed. Perform a detailed assessment of the unconscious patient or the patient who has been injured to make sure you do not miss any findings.

LEARNING OBJECTIVES

- State the generic and trade names, indications, contraindications, medication form, dose, administration, actions, side effects, and reassessment strategies for activated charcoal.
- Recognize the need for medical direction in caring for the patient with poisoning or overdose.
- Explain the rationale for administering activated charcoal.
- Explain the rationale for contacting medical direction early in the prehospital management of the poisoning or overdose patient.

Box 15-1 — Sample Protocol for a Poisoning or Drug Overdose Patient

Special Assessment Considerations

1. Survey the scene; note especially:
   - Hazardous situations
   - Remnants of the poison or drug
   - Containers and drug paraphernalia
   CAUTION: **Take precautions not to contaminate self or others.**
2. Determine age and weight of the patient.
3. Attempt to determine the drug or poison:
   - How was it taken?
   - How long ago was it taken?
   - How much of the substance was taken?
4. Determine the patient's present signs and symptoms, such as injection sites, skin color, breath odor, and burns to mouth.
5. Assess need for advanced life support assistance.
6. If possible, bring the product or substance and container with the patient to the hospital.

Patients Who Are Conscious

1. Remove the patient from any hazards.
2. Maintain ABCs (airway, breathing, circulation).
3. Administer high-concentration supplemental oxygen.
4. Assist ventilations as necessary.

Swallowed Poisons

1. If possible, contact the poison control center or EMS medical direction for instructions on treatment, which may include the administration of milk, water, or activated charcoal.
2. Transport, keeping the patient warm.
3. Obtain and record the vital signs and repeat as necessary.

Inhaled Poisons

1. Ensure that the scene is safe for entry. If the danger of poisonous gases, vapors, or sprays or a low-oxygen environment is present, it may be necessary to obtain assistance from trained rescue personnel.

2. Remove the patient to fresh air.
3. Ensure that the patient's airway is open and that breathing and circulation are adequate.
4. Administer high-concentration supplemental oxygen.
5. Transport, keeping the patient warm.

Injected Substances

1. Look for track or needle marks. Treat as ingested poison, except for use of activated charcoal.
2. If a bite or sting:
   - Remove jewelry from the affected area if swelling begins.
   - Place the injection site lower than the patient's heart if possible.
   - If the injury is from a snake, implement a procedure for snakebite.

Absorbed or Surface Contact Substances

1. Remove the patient from the source as soon as it can be done safely.
2. Remove all contaminated clothing.
3. Rinse the affected area thoroughly with saline, sterile water, or plain water for 20 minutes.

Patients Who Are Unconscious or Who Have Altered Mental Status

1. Ensure that the patient's airway is open and that breathing and circulation are adequate. Suction as necessary.
2. Administer high-concentration supplemental oxygen.
3. Transport, keeping the patient warm and in the recovery position if appropriate.

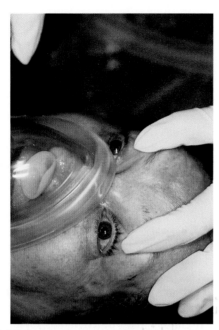

Figure 15-3 Note the pinpoint pupils in this unresponsive patient who has a nasopharyngeal airway and is receiving positive-pressure ventilation after an opioid overdose. The classic signs of opioid overdose are depressed mental status, depressed respirations, and constricted pupils.

Table 15-2	Pharmacology of Activated Charcoal
Generic name	Activated charcoal
Trade name	Actidose-Aqua; Actidose with sorbitol; Liqui-Char*
Indication	Toxic ingestions
Contraindications	Altered mental status Inability to swallow Acid or alkali ingestion
Forms	Premixed in water, frequently available in plastic bottles containing various amounts of activated charcoal (e.g., 15 g, 25 g, and 50 g)
Dose	Adults and children: 1 g/kg of body weight
Route of administration	Oral (see Skill 15-1)
Actions	Binds certain poisons and prevents absorption into the body. Most effective if given shortly after the ingestion
Side effects	Black stool (takes on color of charcoal) Some patients may vomit, especially those who have ingested poisons that cause nausea; if patient vomits, repeat dose one time
Reassessment strategies	Watch for vomiting Watch for deterioration caused by poisoning

*Liqui-Char and Actidose with sorbitol are premixed combinations of activated charcoal and sorbitol used to treat ingestions. Sorbitol is added as a sweetener and cathartic (hastens transit time through gastrointestinal tract and evacuation of bowels).

Management

As with all patients, you should continue to ensure an open airway and provide any needed ventilation with supplemental oxygen to poisoned patients. Then, regardless of the type of poison or the route of exposure, treatment for poisoning has two major goals: prevent further absorption and treat the signs and symptoms.

Prevent Further Absorption

In addition to basic life support (BLS), the main aspect of prehospital treatment for poison ingestions is preventing further absorption of the poison into the body. The means to prevent absorption depends on the type of exposure. For example, in ingestions, prevention of absorption may be accomplished by administering activated charcoal or diluting the body's poisonous contents. These maneuvers are appropriate for the alert patient who can swallow. If in doubt, you should check for the ability to swallow before you consider giving anything by mouth. The drowsy or unconscious patient must have other treatment rendered in the hospital setting, and prehospital management focuses on BLS.

Activated charcoal is an absorbent material that binds most toxins. It keeps toxins within the GI tract until they are eliminated, thereby reducing absorption into the body. The dose of charcoal is usually 1 g/kg body weight (about 50 g for adults). It comes premixed as a thick liquid in the form of a souplike slurry. Because of time factors, the premixed solution is preferred for field use. Sweeteners may be added to make it more palatable to children. There is almost never any harm resulting from administering activated charcoal if patients can swallow and are alert enough to protect the airway. To be effective, however, it generally should be given to patients who have ingested toxins less than an hour before administration of charcoal. **Table 15-2** reviews the pharmacology and administration of activated charcoal (**Skill 15-1**).

Induction of vomiting is another means of removing toxins that are still in the stomach. Some patients may induce vomiting at home with syrup of ipecac; however, this method is not widely recommended today, except for certain ingestions, such as plants. The induction of vomiting may be contraindicated for certain drugs or poisons (e.g., caustic agents, most hydrocarbons) or certain patients (e.g., infants, patients with coma or no gag reflex).

Treat Signs and Symptoms

Certain signs and symptoms of poisoning may respond to medical treatment. For a few poisons, an **antidote,** a remedy that counteracts a poison, may be available. Most antidotes are administered in the hospital setting; however, oxygen, the antidote for CO poisoning, is routinely administered by EMTs. Naloxone, an antidote for opioids (e.g., heroin, morphine, methadone), can be administered intravenously, intramuscularly, or atomized intranasally by advanced-level providers such as paramedics. Atropine is also carried by advanced-level providers and may be necessary to treat patients with organophosphate poisoning.

Other patients may require supportive drug therapy that counteracts the *effects* of a poison. In fact, "true" antidotes are available for only a few drugs and poisons. The major treatment for the poisoned patient is supportive care, which is initiated, as indicated, by the EMT. The methods for achieving these treatment goals vary with the type of poisoning; however, general principles guide the handling of ingestions, inhalations, skin exposures, and injections.

See **Box 15-1** for a summary of the management of a poisoning or overdose patient.

Transport Patient

Unconscious patients or patients with deteriorating mental status should be transported with care to protect the airway and continuously assessed for the need for respiratory support. The left lateral recumbent position (recovery position), with the head down, may be used during transport to protect the airway from vomit or secretions.

Emotions and the Poisoned Patient

Patients who have taken an overdose or who have been poisoned may have many types of reactions. Patients may have altered mental status from the emotional events surrounding an overdose or from the physical effects of the drugs. The patient may be agitated, despondent, uncooperative, and difficult.

Suicidal patients may be extremely depressed and despondent. They may have left a note. Some patients may have taken the overdose in an area where they are likely to be found. Other patients may purposely hide any toxic products to prevent discovery, or they may take an overdose in an area where it is unlikely that they will be discovered.

Parents may feel guilty about a child having found and ingested toxic substances around the home.

Emergency medical technicians themselves may experience feelings of hopelessness when caring for a patient who has abused drugs. On the other hand, EMTs may feel a sense of identity with patients of similar age who have attempted suicide.

As an EMT, you must maintain a professional approach in assessing and managing poisoned patients to minimize the potential for emotional responses that interfere with care. At all costs, you should avoid antagonizing the patient. Be careful not to "label" patients. Express to patients that your first and foremost priority is to deal with the poisoning. In this way, you are more likely to gain the cooperation of the patient, family, and bystanders. Patients who are antagonized are less receptive to treatment and transportation to the hospital. Psychiatric consultation is obtained in the hospital setting for patients who have intentionally poisoned themselves.

Patients Who Refuse Medical Attention

Some patients may refuse medical care. They may insist that they want to die and be left alone. These patients must not be abandoned. Encourage them to accompany you to the hospital. Call police, if necessary, to place these patients in protective custody. Patients cannot be presumed to be acting in their best interest if they are suicidal or if the drug or poison has altered their mental status and judgment.

Ingested Poisons

History and Physical Examination

In most cases, poisons are ingested. As an EMT, you should suspect poisoning from either the history or the physical examination. A patient may give a history of poisoning before signs or symptoms occurred, or signs of poisoning might be noted on examination. These signs are varied and cover all extremes. For example, the pupils could be constricted or dilated, the heart rate fast or slow, or the mental status agitated or depressed. Seizures or coma may occur. The blood pressure may be high or low and the skin dry or moist. Alterations in body temperature, both increased and decreased, are typically encountered from both drug effects and exposure. A patient may have nausea, vomiting, diarrhea, and abdominal pain. You should be prepared to see extremes in many different organ systems. The key is to include poisoning as a possible explanation for a patient's signs and symptoms.

> **REAL**World
>
> Pediatric patients can be a greater concern than other age groups in regard to poisoning and overdose. In addition to the difficulty obtaining a history of what and how much the pediatric patient ingested, many pills are labeled as "one-pill killers" regarding ingestion by children. In other words, just because a child ingested only one or two pills does not mean the situation should not be considered critical.

As with most medical patients, the history may help clarify the chief complaint. The following points should be covered while the history is gathered:

- Ask patient or bystanders what the patient may have taken.
- Establish the time that the ingestion occurred. Were all the pills taken at once, or did the patient take more and more of a substance at repeated intervals? Some patients may inadvertently take a toxic level of analgesics (pain killers) by repeatedly taking medication beyond the prescribed dosage.
- How much did the patient take? How many pills from each bottle? How many ounces of a liquid substance?
- As evidence, bring along the containers of any substance ingested. Obtain the pill container or the bottle with any identifying marks, and bring it to the hospital. Prescription bottles have identifying information that may help establish the amount and strength of any medication that was possibly ingested.
- In the case of commercial products, it is important to bring the container. Again, the possible amount ingested can be estimated. Check the contents on the label for toxic effects. If the ingredients are not listed, call the poison control center, medical direction, or manufacturer to obtain this information. Obtaining the brand name alone is inadequate. Companies invest large sums of advertising dollars to achieve brand loyalty among customers. Ingredients may change, but the

company may continue to use the same brand name. Whenever possible, the container should be brought to aid identification.

- Has the patient vomited or instituted home treatment since the ingestion? Vomit could be brought to the hospital for possible analysis.

Is there evidence from the physical findings that a poisoning has occurred? Remember, with some substances it takes time for the effects of poisoning to become evident. The suicidal patient who calls for help hours after taking a bottle of acetaminophen may have no symptoms when you arrive. Acetaminophen can destroy the liver, but there may be few signs in the first 24 hours; without hospital treatment, however, the effects may be delayed and fatal. Other patients may have alterations in consciousness or other physical complaints related to the onset of toxicity. As you obtain the history and perform your physical examinations, note pertinent positive and negative findings. Pupil size, skin condition, and presence or absence of breath odors should be recorded.

EXTENDED*Transport*

When EMTs transport a patient who has overdosed or ingested a poison, they must be conscious of gastric absorption times. When ingested, a substance will not have an effect until it is absorbed into the bloodstream from the GI tract. Many prescription medications are "time release," preparations, resulting in a slower absorption. At the start of transport the patient may be stable but 30 minutes later may be in cardiac arrest.

Types of Ingested Poisons

Sedative-Hypnotics and Antianxiety Agents

Commonly prescribed agents include **sedatives**, which are calming and reduce activity and excitement; **hypnotics**, which induce sleep; and antianxiety agents. In general, the most severe toxic effects of these drugs are respiratory depression and depression of mental status (from relaxation through stupor to coma). Death is usually caused by respiratory depression. When these drugs are used in combination with alcohol, the effects of the depressants on mental status and respiration are greatly increased.

Opioids

Opioids (narcotics) are a special class of central nervous system (CNS) depressants. These drugs alter the perception of pain. A patient may feel pain, but it does not "hurt." In excess, opioids cause depressed mental status and coma and depress respirations. Most opioids cause pinpoint pupils. The patient with depressed respirations, a depressed mental status, and pinpoint pupils displays the classic signs of opioid overdose. Intravenous users of opioids such as heroin may have track marks or scarring over veins from previous injections.

Opioid is a term for drugs with opium-like or morphine-like activity. These drugs include natural derivatives of opium (morphine and codeine), semisynthetic opioids such as heroin and oxycodone (Percocet, Oxycontin), and synthetic opioids such as methadone and meperidine (Demerol). Opium and its derivative-type drugs are used to soothe pain and usually produce a feeling of well-being and drowsiness; if used continuously, opiates can result in addiction, and excessive dosage can be fatal.

In medical practice the word *narcotic* usually refers to opioid-type drugs. However, the term is confusing because it has different lay, legal, and medical definitions. The *Merriam-Webster Dictionary* has defined narcotic as "a drug that in moderate doses allays sensibility, relieves pain, and produces profound sleep but that in poisonous doses produces stupor, coma, or convulsions." This dictionary includes alcohol as a narcotic. The legal definition of narcotic can also include drugs such as cocaine, which is quite different pharmacologically because cocaine stimulates, rather than depresses, the CNS. Because of the range in definitions for the word "narcotic," *opioid* is the term preferred by toxicologists to describe medications derived from opium and other drugs with opium-like effects.

Naloxone (Narcan) is an *antidote* to an opioid overdose that rapidly reverses respiratory and mental depression. Paramedics frequently use naloxone as an agent in the field for opioid overdose.

Stimulants

Stimulants include amphetamines, methylphenidate (Ritalin), amphetamine derivatives such as methylenedioxymethamphetamine (MDMA), cocaine and its altered forms (e.g., "crack"), and phencyclidine (PCP).

Stimulant overdoses cause excitability and can induce seizures. Fast heart rates, hypertension, and chest pain can occur. Patients who are taking cocaine may call EMS because they experience ischemic chest pain; they may not initially reveal the history of cocaine use. Behaviorally, patients can be anxious, delirious, and paranoid. Psychotic and violent behavior is possible. Sudden death can result from acute cardiac dysrhythmia.

Cocaine is often inhaled (or smoked) as crack or "freebased." PCP is usually smoked. Amphetamines may be taken as pills, injected, or smoked as "ice." Cocaine overdose can occur from ingestion when drugs are swallowed to avoid detection during an arrest or when drug transporters swallow balloons or condoms filled with cocaine. In the latter case the condoms may burst, releasing massive amounts of cocaine to be absorbed by the intestine.

After assessing the need for cardiorespiratory support, *be conservative*. The major problems in the prehospital setting may be behavioral and psychological. To gain compliance, reassure the patient. Be nonthreatening, and offer as calm an environment as possible. Maintain verbal contact with the patient. You should not be judgmental. Avoid restraints, if possible, because these patients are often in a hyperactive state and strain against restraints, which can cause elevations in body temperature and the breakdown of muscle tissue (rhabdomyolysis) from hyperactivity and severe muscle strain. Stimulant overdose can cause myocardial infarction, bleeding in the brain, and convulsions, with subsequent coma and respiratory depression.

Alcohol

Alcohol is the most frequently abused drug. It has a depressant effect on mental status and respirations when taken in high doses. When taken in combination with depressant drugs, alcohol adds to the respiratory and mental status depression. The mixture of alcohol with other drugs is responsible for a

Box 15-2 CAGE Alcoholic Assessment Tool

C—Does the patient feel the need to "cut back" on his drinking?
A—Does the patient feel **a**nnoyed with criticism about her drinking?
G—Does the patient feel **g**uilty about his drinking?
E—Does the patient need an "**e**ye opener"?

large number of severe overdoses and deaths. Alcohol slows reflexes and suppresses inhibitions. It causes uncoordinated movements and unpredictable behavior.

Acute alcohol intoxication by itself can be lethal because it can cause coma and even respiratory failure. Some patients choke on their own vomit. Deaths occur in adolescents who are unfamiliar with alcohol and drink excessive amounts, causing extremely high blood alcohol levels.

Over time, alcohol will affect every organ system in the body. It can cause the brain to shrink and, coupled with frequent falls, can result in brain bleeds. Alcohol can cause the heart to become ineffective and can destroy the liver, resulting in cirrhosis.

A patient experiencing *withdrawal* from alcohol can be as great a concern to the EMT as the patient who is intoxicated with alcohol. Withdrawal can cause a condition known as **delirium tremens ("DTs")**. Patients experiencing the DTs may have tremors, weakness, and nausea. Severe cases can result in hallucinations, seizures, cardiovascular collapse, and death.

An assessment tool used to assess the chronic alcoholic is called CAGE (**Box 15-2**).

Physical findings in a chronic alcoholic may include slender extremities with a distended abdomen. They may have bruises at different stages of healing caused by frequent falls. Their skin may have a yellow tint known as **jaundice,** caused by the failing liver.

Management of alcoholic patients is to treat them symptomatically. In other words, the EMT should treat the signs and symptoms that are found. Open wounds should be dressed. Oxygen should be given to patients who are short of breath, and these patients should be transported for treatment of both their acute condition and their chronic condition.

Case in Point

You arrive at the home of an elderly man who was found unarousable by his neighbor on his couch. The patient moans and withdraws on both sides to painful stimuli. The vital signs are within normal limits. You are gathering more history when the son, alerted by the neighbor, calls the house. As you speak to him about his father's condition, the son tells you his father has been depressed ever since his wife died and has been drinking alcohol heavily. You relay this information to the hospital when you present your findings to the physician and nurse on arrival. They add this to their differential diagnosis.

Prescription Drugs

Patients who are suicidal may take any available medications. Drugs prescribed for circulatory and respiratory ailments can cause a wide range of symptoms. Of particular concern are alterations in heart rate and rhythm, changes in blood pressure, and dysrhythmias.

Analgesics

Over-the-counter (OTC) pain relievers such as salicylates (aspirin) and acetaminophen can cause death from overdose. Salicylates, acetaminophen, and nonsteroidal antiinflammatory drugs (NSAIDs) such as ibuprofen (Motrin, Advil) are widely available and often used.

Few if any symptoms may be present early after the overdose. An aspirin overdose only increases the respiratory rate initially but later can lead to coma. Acetaminophen overdoses cause mild GI discomfort (including nausea and vomiting) and malaise or no symptoms at all during the first 24 hours. After 48 hours, evidence of liver damage can appear with high doses. All patients with acetaminophen or aspirin overdose should receive further evaluation to determine whether treatment is necessary.

Commercial and Industrial Products

Ingestion of hydrocarbons, caustics, insecticides, and other household products is most often seen in children, particularly toddlers, and despondent or psychotic adults.

Caustics include both acids and alkalis. *Acid* products include toilet bowel cleaners, bleaches, metal cleaners, and battery acid. *Alkalis* are found in drain cleaners (lye, Drano) and Clinitest tablets (used by diabetics to test their urine for sugar). Chemistry laboratories and industrial sites are sources of caustic exposure (usually spills).

Caustics can be diluted by having the alert and conscious patient drink one or two glasses of water or milk. Induced vomiting should be avoided after ingestion of acids or alkalis because it reexposes the esophagus to a second passage of a substance that causes chemical burns. Follow your local protocols when treating caustic ingestions.

Methanol and Ethylene Glycol

Methanol and ethylene glycol can initially cause signs of mild inebriation (or no findings at all), but if left untreated can lead to coma and death. *Methanol* is found in "dry gas," in windshield washing solution, and as a fuel for warming food (Sterno). *Ethylene glycol* is most commonly found as antifreeze. Patients who ingest either of these substances experience severe acid formation in the blood when these products are broken down. Formation of the acid breakdown products can be delayed by administering *ethyl alcohol* ("drinking alcohol"), which interferes with the metabolism of these poisons into toxic byproducts.

In an attempt to "blow off," or eliminate, excess acid, the methanol-poisoned or ethylene glycol–poisoned patient may hyperventilate. Patients poisoned with methanol or ethylene glycol need hospital care and, in severe ingestions, dialysis.

Insecticides

Insecticides may contain substances called *organophosphates*. Organophosphates cause an overstimulation of secretions, bronchoconstriction, and muscle weakness. In excess, they cause death by respiratory muscle paralysis and/or pulmonary

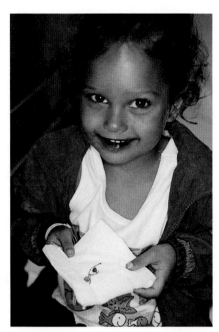

Figure 15-4 A young girl brings a sample of the mushrooms she ate to the hospital to help identify them. She has been given activated charcoal (note the color of her lips) pending the identification of the mushrooms. These mushrooms were not harmful.

The most severe type of food poisoning is _botulism,_ which may begin as a flulike illness with double vision, difficulty moving the eyes and swallowing, and then descending (from head to toe) weakness, paralysis, and respiratory arrest. Management requires respiratory support, positive-pressure ventilations, and use of an antitoxin.

Poisonous _mushroom_ consumption can cause GI disturbances, hallucinations, and delirium. Symptoms of some of the more toxic mushrooms are often delayed, and the patient may not associate the illness with the mushroom. In most cases, care is supportive. It is extremely important to bring any available mushrooms or even mushroom fragments found at the scene to the hospital to help with identification (**Figure 15-4**).

Plants

Many common household and wild plants can cause adverse effects on the GI, circulatory, and neurologic systems. In addition, some plants can cause severe skin and mucous membrane irritation. One common household plant, the _dieffenbachia,_ can cause severe irritation and swelling in the mouth if ingested. Chewing the crystals in the leaf feels like biting into ground glass. Management centers on keeping the airway open. In general, care is supportive, and the plant should be transported to aid in identification.

Inhaled Poisons

Rescue Considerations and Precautions

Victims of toxic gas must always be approached with consideration for the safety of the rescuers. Rescuers are of no use to a patient if they become incapacitated as well. In many cases, EMTs and rescuers have succumbed to the same toxic gases or fumes that claimed the initial victims. Rescuers should avoid inhalation of fumes. Only trained rescuers should enter a contaminated area or a closed space, and they should be equipped with adequate protection, such as a self-contained breathing apparatus (SCBA).

Victims of inhalation should be removed from the toxic environment to fresh air as soon as possible and given necessary ventilatory support and humidified supplemental oxygen.

A frequently encountered and lethal poisonous gas is carbon monoxide. CO is found in fires, charcoal burners, vehicle exhaust fumes, and inadequately ventilated stoves and home heaters (**Figure 15-5**). Management includes administration of 100% oxygen. In severe cases, the patient may also require hyperbaric oxygen treatment if available. Other patients may inhale vapors or gases from containers to seek a "high" or to commit suicide. Bring available containers, if appropriate, with the patient to the hospital.

Poisonous Gases

The greatest concern in toxic gas exposure is **asphyxiation,** or death from lack of oxygen. Gases can cause asphyxiation by simply displacing the oxygen in the air, by causing chemical actions within the body, or by irritating the respiratory tract.

oversecretion, as well as bronchoconstriction. In addition, there is an outpouring of secretions from most body openings, including vomiting, salivation, sweating, lacrimation (tearing), urination, and diarrhea. The patient usually has small pupils and a slow heart rate. The slow heart rate is notable because these patients often have respiratory distress, a situation in which increased heart rate is expected to compensate for respiratory compromise. In severe cases, patients require the antidotes _atropine_ and _pralidoxime._ Prehospital treatment centers on providing supplemental oxygen and ventilatory support. Rapid transport is indicated in severe cases because administration of atropine can be lifesaving.

Organophosphates may also be absorbed through the skin. When toddlers accidentally drink a solution containing organophosphates, they may spill these substances on their clothing. Contaminated clothing should be removed and the skin should be flushed and washed with soap and water. A garlicky odor may be noted but is often accompanied and masked by a hydrocarbon smell. Be careful to wear protective clothing if contamination is possible to avoid becoming poisoned yourself.

Food Poisoning

Food poisoning can be caused by bacteria, toxins produced by bacteria, and viruses. It is caused by improperly cooked or canned foods and by contamination of food with fecal bacteria by food handlers. Food poisoning is often suspected when two or more persons become ill after eating the same food. Typical symptoms include abdominal pain, nausea, vomiting, and diarrhea (sometimes bloody).

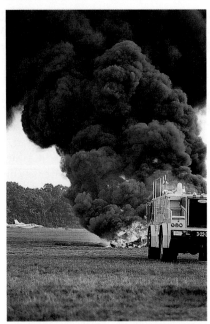

Figure 15-5 Fires produce carbon monoxide and many other poisonous gases. A history of the main substances under combustion is often helpful to poison control center and hospital personnel in deciding what gases might have been created in the fire.

Case in Point

To illustrate the hazards of toxic gas, consider the following reports from the Centers for Disease Control and Prevention (CDC) of farm workers who entered manure pits, where they were overcome by the low-oxygen environment. This is a repeated scenario in gas poisonings, where a would-be rescuer enters the same toxic space to save the first victim, only also to become a victim.

In June and July 1989, a total of seven farm workers in two separate incidents died after they were asphyxiated by methane gas in manure pits. Brief reports follow.

Ohio

On June 26, 1989, a 31-year-old male dairy farmer and his 33-year-old brother died after entering a 25-foot-square by 4-foot-deep manure pit inside a building on their farm. A pump intake pipe in the pit had clogged, and the farmer descended into the pit to clear the obstruction. While in the pit, he was overcome by lack of oxygen and collapsed. His brother apparently saw him collapse and entered the pit in an attempt to rescue him. The brother, too, was overcome and collapsed inside the pit. Four hours later, another family member discovered the two men, and the local fire department was called to rescue them. The coroner's report attributed the cause of death in both cases to "drowning" caused by loss of consciousness from methane asphyxia.

Michigan

On July 26, 1989, five farm workers in one family died after consecutively entering an outdoor manure pit on a farm. The pit measured 20 feet × 24 feet × 10 feet deep. The victims were a 65-year-old male dairy farmer, his two sons (ages 37 and 28), a 15-year-old grandson, and a 63-year-old nephew. The index victim, the 37-year-old son, initially entered the pit by ladder to replace a shear pin on an agitator shaft. While attempting to climb out of the pit, he was overcome and fell to the bottom of the pit. The grandson then entered the pit to attempt rescue. He, too, was

overcome and collapsed. One by one, the nephew, the younger son, and the dairy farmer entered the pit in attempts to rescue the others, were overcome by lack of oxygen, and collapsed. A carpet installer working at the farm then entered the pit as a rescuer and was overcome; however, he was rescued by his assistant and subsequently recovered. Finally, the owner of a nearby business arrived with two additional workers and, using a rope, extricated the five victims from the pit. When paramedics arrived, they began cardiopulmonary resuscitation. The nephew was pronounced dead at the scene, and the other four victims were transported to the emergency department of a nearby hospital. The dairy farmer and his younger son were pronounced dead on arrival at the hospital; the 37-year-old son died 1 hour after reaching the ED. The grandson was transferred by helicopter to a major trauma center but died within 6 hours of his removal from the pit. The medical examiner attributed the cause of death to methane asphyxia.

Follow-up

Acute traumatic occupational deaths in the United States are monitored by the Division of Safety Research, National Institute for Occupational Safety and Health (NIOSH), CDC, through the National Traumatic Occupational Fatalities (NTOF) file. For 1980 through 1985, the NTOF data file includes 16 work-related deaths that involved asphyxiation of workers in manure pits (or similar waste tanks) on farms. These deaths resulted from nine separate incidents in nine different states. Five of these episodes resulted in multiple fatalities. Because NTOF only includes deaths of workers 16 years of age or older that are clearly identified as work related, these 16 deaths represent the minimum number of asphyxiation fatalities that occurred during this period among U.S. farmers, farm family members, farm workers, and others working in manure pits.

A farm manure waste pit is a confined space, defined by NIOSH as a space that "by design has limited openings for entry and exit; unfavorable natural ventilation which could contain or produce dangerous air contaminants; and which is not intended for continuous worker occupancy." Manure pits are fermentation tanks where raw animal wastes undergo anaerobic bacterial decay. This bacterial action generates methane, hydrogen sulfide (H_2S), and other gases. Methane is a colorless, odorless, and flammable gaseous hydrocarbon. It can displace oxygen in confined areas, resulting in an oxygen-deficient atmosphere. H_2S is a highly toxic, colorless gas that, at concentrations of 300 parts per million (ppm) or greater, can cause unconsciousness, respiratory failure, and sudden death. If these gases are not properly vented from a tank or other confined space, an oxygen-deficient or toxic atmosphere may be created. In industrial settings, the Occupational Safety and Health Administration (OSHA) limits permissible peak exposures to H_2S to a ceiling of 50 ppm (for 10 minutes or less); NIOSH recommends a ceiling of 10 ppm (for 10 minutes or less). No OSHA permissible exposure limit for methane exists. OSHA exposure standards are not enforceable on farms with 10 or fewer employees.

That episodes such as those described here can result in multiple fatalities is a major concern. Fatal incidents resulting from entry into manure pits often involve more than one victim; the deaths of any additional workers occur during rescue attempts conducted without use of appropriate equipment or safety precautions. Investigations performed by NIOSH as part of the Fatal Accident Circumstances and Epidemiology Project show that approximately 43% of deaths related to confined spaces involved co-workers or other persons attempting to rescue the initial victim(s).

NOTE: Rescuers can fall victim as easily as the family members and co-workers. *Do not enter* a confined space where toxic gas is suspected unless you are appropriately trained and equipped to do so.

From Epidemiologic notes and reports fatalities attributed to methane asphyxiation manure waste pits—Ohio, Michigan, 1989, *MMWR* 38(33): 583-586, 1989.

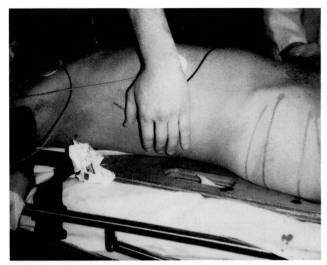

Figure 15-6 Red discoloration of the skin in a patient with carbon monoxide (CO) poisoning who was just resuscitated. (Compare color of normal hand.) The pink-red color of the skin, which is a late finding of CO poisoning, is caused by CO binding to hemoglobin, which turns the blood a bright-red color.

Simple Asphyxiants

Simple asphyxiants include gases such as methane and carbon dioxide (CO_2). When present in high quantities, these gases displace or dilute the oxygen in the air, rendering the victim hypoxic (see Case in Point).

Carbon Dioxide. CO_2 is heavier than air and collects in poorly ventilated areas (e.g., mine shafts, ship holds).

Small Hydrocarbon Molecules. Methane, ethane, and propane are made up of small hydrocarbon molecules that have no color or odor to warn the victim. (When used commercially, such as in gas stoves, *mercaptans* are added to give a warning odor). These gases can collect in closed spaces where leaks are present. A potential for explosion exists if a spark occurs, which can be caused by simply turning on an electric light switch in a room where these gases have collected.

Chemical Asphyxiants

Chemical asphyxiants attach to molecules in the body that are essential to respiration. Carbon monoxide binds to hemoglobin, decreasing oxygen delivery to the tissues. Cyanide and hydrogen sulfide alter the cells' ability to use oxygen. Whether the cell does not receive oxygen, or when it cannot use the oxygen, the result is the same: cell death.

Carbon Monoxide. CO exposure is expected at all fires. Most deaths from fires are caused by smoke inhalation and CO poisoning. CO is also present in engine exhaust; it is odorless and colorless. CO binds to hemoglobin and affects its ability to transport and deliver oxygen to the tissues as well as the tissues' ability to use the oxygen (**Figure 15-6**). Because of this impairment, the patient with CO poisoning may have a pink-red skin color. CO gives little warning regarding its lethal effect. Early on, a victim may have headache and nausea, often attributed to a flulike illness. Judgment is disturbed, coordination and motor ability are impaired, and victims may collapse on exertion.

With judgment and movement impaired, victims become lost and disoriented or do not have the power to flee the toxic environment. If concentrations in the atmosphere are high, fatal inhalations can occur in less than 1 minute.

Carbon monoxide poisoning is managed by administration of 100%-concentration oxygen. In extreme cases, the patient may require treatment in a hyperbaric chamber.

Cyanide. Cyanide is found in industries such as electroplating, photography, metallurgy, and metal cleaning. It is used as a fumigant on cargo ships. Cyanide is also used as a chemical agent. Some fires, particularly those that involve burning polyurethanes, produce cyanide.

Cyanide acts rapidly and affects the ability of the body to use oxygen. Clinical symptoms are nonspecific. The patient may initially have increased heart and breathing rates. Later the breathing may slow and the heart rate may decrease. Treatment with high-concentration oxygen is needed, and administration of an antidote in severe cases.

Many industries have cyanide antidote kits available for use. The nitrite-thiosulfate kit includes an ampule of amyl nitrite, which can be administered at the scene by trained personnel. Patients with cyanide poisoning need rapid transport to a hospital setting, where more nitrites and sodium thiosulfate can be given intravenously. During transport, provide high-concentration supplemental oxygen to the patient.

Hydrogen Sulfide. Hydrogen sulfide (H_2S) is a gas that smells like rotten eggs. It is used in such industries as petroleum and rubber processing. The gas also results from the decay of organic matter. Exposure can occur in sewers, animal-rendering plants, tanneries, fertilizer plants, and farming. Because of the characteristic odor, victims usually flee from exposure. Over time, however, the nose can become insensitive to the smell, leaving workers exposed to increasing levels in the environment. Treatment includes administration of high-concentration supplemental oxygen.

Irritant Gases

Irritant gases cause inflammatory damage to the airway and bronchoconstriction. They react with water in the airway to cause toxic reactions to the mucosa.

The most soluble agents, such as ammonia, sulfur dioxide, and hydrogen chloride, react almost immediately, causing tearing, coughing, and an uncomfortable sensation in the nose and throat. Victims are impelled to flee if they are able, and an EMT would have warning signs of danger. Unless the irritant gases are inhaled in extreme concentrations, such as in a closed space, or by an unconscious victim, damage is usually confined to the upper airway. Closure of the upper airway is of greatest immediate concern.

By contrast, irritating gases with low solubility, such as phosgene and the nitrogen oxides, are less likely to react immediately in the upper airway. As a result, the warning irritation may not be present, and victims, unaware that they are in danger, often inhale these agents over a longer period. Similarly, because the gases are not consumed by reaction with the water in the upper airway, they enter the lower airway, where damage can occur over hours to days. Severe symptoms develop some time after the patient has been removed from the smoke or gas exposure.

Organophosphates

The spraying of fields and gardens with insecticides can result in inhalation of organophosphates. When these substances are inhaled, the victim may first experience visual problems and difficulty breathing from bronchoconstriction and excessive pulmonary secretions before the onset of the other symptoms. The threat of spraying organophosphates as an act of war or terrorism has led to training of first responders in their recognition and the use of antidotes atropine and pralidoxime.

Absorbed Poisons

The skin is damaged by corrosive and caustic agents that can cause severe chemical burns. With these patients, you should look for a history of exposure, liquid or powder on the patient's skin, burns, itching, irritation, and redness. Caustic agents should be flushed from the skin with copious amounts of water after contaminated clothing is removed. Gently and thoroughly irrigate the eyes with water for at least 20 minutes, beginning at the scene and continuing en route to the facility. If the agent is a dry powder (e.g., dry lime), brush it off the skin before flushing with water.

The skin is a large organ, and many agents can be absorbed through it into the body. Insecticides are an example of a systemic toxin that can be absorbed. Toxic agents should be washed off the skin by flooding it with water and then washing with soap and water (irrigation). Contaminated clothing should be removed and placed in a secure container for proper handling to prevent exposure to others. Call the local poison control center to help identify the agent and the best course of management in the field. The EMT must wear protective clothing to avoid contamination with the toxic substance by direct contact or splashes.

Injected Poisons

Injections cause the most rapid onset of drug effects. Injection emergencies are often self-administered overdoses; however, bites and stings can result in injections of venom through the skin as well (see Chapter 16).

Heroin, amphetamines, and cocaine are commonly injected drugs. Findings and management are the same as if the drugs were ingested or inhaled, except no attempt is made to prevent absorption because the drugs are already in the blood.

Drugs of Abuse

Drug abuse is one of the greatest problems in modern society. Both illegal and legal drugs can be abused. Some familiarity with problems of drug abuse and "street" drugs is useful in managing these patients, who are frequently encountered by EMS personnel.

Drug or substance abuse involves the repeated self-administration by ingestion, inhalation, or injection for a sense of well-being or a "high" (**Figure 15-7**). As a person continues to use a drug, tolerance to the drug effects develops. Tolerance means that larger and larger doses are required to reach the same feeling of well-being. The drug abuser may begin to mix different substances to seek a unique or different high, or sense of euphoria. A person becomes dependent on a drug when the sense of well-being cannot be sustained without drug administration. This dependency can

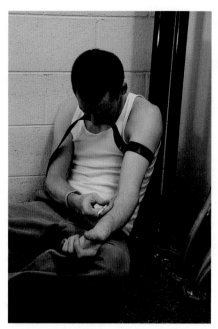

Figure 15-7 Injecting heroin into a vein produces effects in 7 to 8 seconds. Injection into muscle or under the skin can produce effects in 5 to 8 minutes. Addicts may inject themselves up to four times a day.

be psychologic or physical. Physical and psychologic withdrawal symptoms can occur if the person stops using the drug. Ultimately the person may become addicted, a condition manifested by compulsive behavior concentrated on obtaining the drug.

The most commonly abused drug is alcohol. Withdrawal from prolonged drinking can cause shakes, tremors, and seizures. In severe cases the "DTs" can result, with the patient experiencing hyperactivity, increased respiratory and pulse rates, increased temperature, and hypertension. The patient may have hallucinations and typically sees insects crawling nearby. Delirium tremens is a medical emergency and can cause death if untreated.

Other drugs of abuse include heroin, cocaine, lysergic acid diethylamide (LSD), phencyclidine (PCP, "angel dust"), ecstasy, and many prescription drugs. The drug effects vary widely. Heroin causes lethargy, coma, and respiratory depression. Cocaine (especially crack), PCP, and amphetamines can cause hyperexcitable states with extremes of behavior, often violent, and seizures.

> ## REAL*World*
>
> The Drug Abuse Warning Network (DAWN) reports that drug abuse typically begins in the eighth grade. These children begin experimenting with accessible chemicals found around the home (e.g., paint) and glue. EMTs doing a scene assessment may be looking for pipes and needles when they should be checking for rags with gasoline or tubes of glue.

The EMT's contact with patients who are abusing drugs often occurs when they have taken an overdose, have a behavioral emergency, or are experiencing trauma complicated or caused by a drug overdose. Many patients deny drug involvement, making it difficult to gather a reliable history. The EMT often has to treat psychological and physical manifestations simultaneously. **Tables 15-3 to 15-8** list some commonly abused drugs, their street names, how they are taken, and the associated signs and symptoms.

Table 15-3	Commonly Abused Drugs: Cannabinoids			
Substance Name	**Street Names**	**How Taken**	**Intoxication Effects**	**Potential Health Consequences**
Hashish	Boom, chronic, gangster, hash, hash oil, hemp	Swallowed, smoked	Euphoria, slowed thinking and reaction time, confusion, impaired balance and coordination	Cough, frequent respiratory infections; impaired memory and learning, increased heart rate, anxiety, panic attacks; tolerance, addiction
Marijuana	Blunt, dope, ganja, grass, herb, joints, Mary Jane, pot, reefer, sinsemilla, skunk, weed	Swallowed, smoked	Same as for hashish	Same as for hashish

From National Institute of Drug Abuse. www.niha.gov/DrugPages/DrugsofAbuse.html.

Table 15-4	Commonly Abused Drugs: Depressants			
Substance Name	**Commercial and Street Names**	**How Taken***	**Intoxication Effects**	**Potential Health Consequences**
Barbiturates	*Amytal, Nembutal, Seconal, phenobarbital* Barbs, reds, red birds, phennies, tooies, yellows, yellow jackets	Injected, swallowed	Reduced pain and anxiety; feeling of well-being; lowered inhibitions; slowed pulse and breathing; lowered blood pressure; poor concentration; sedation, drowsiness	Fatigue; impaired coordination, memory, judgment; respiratory depression and arrest; addiction; depression, unusual excitement, fever, irritability, poor judgment, slurred speech; dizziness
Benzodiazepines (other than flunitrazepam)	*Ativan, Halcion, Librium, Valium, Xanax* Candy, downers, sleeping pills, tranks	Swallowed	Reduced pain and anxiety; feeling of well-being; lowered inhibitions; slowed pulse and breathing; lowered blood pressure; poor concentration; sedation, drowsiness	Fatigue; impaired coordination, memory, judgment; respiratory depression and arrest; addiction; dizziness
Flunitrazepam†	*Rohypnol* Forget-me pill; Mexican valium; R2, roche, roofies, roofinol, rope, rophies	Swallowed, snorted	Reduced pain and anxiety; feeling of well-being; lowered inhibitions; slowed pulse and breathing; lowered blood pressure; poor concentration	Fatigue; impaired coordination, memory, judgment; respiratory depression and arrest; addiction; visual and gastrointestinal disturbances, urinary retention, memory loss for time under drug's effects
GHB†	*Gamma-hydroxybutyrate* G, Georgia home boy, grievous bodily harm, liquid ecstasy	Swallowed	Reduced pain and anxiety, feeling of well-being, lowered inhibitions; slowed pulse and breathing; lowered blood pressure; poor concentration	Fatigue; impaired coordination, memory, judgment; respiratory depression and arrest; addiction; drowsiness, nausea/vomiting, headache, loss of consciousness, loss of reflexes, seizures, coma, death
Methaqualone	*Quaalude, Sopor, Parest* Ludes, mandrex, quad, quay	Injected, swallowed	Reduced pain and anxiety, feeling of well-being, lowered inhibitions; slowed pulse and breathing; lowered blood pressure; poor concentration; euphoria	Fatigue; impaired coordination, memory, judgment; respiratory depression and arrest; addiction; depression, poor reflexes, slurred speech

From National Institute of Drug Abuse. www.niha.gov/DrugPages/DrugsofAbuse.html.
*Taking drugs by injection can increase the risk of infection through needle contamination with staphylococci, HIV, hepatitis, and other organisms.
†Associated with sexual assaults.

Table 15-5	Commonly Abused Drugs: Dissociative Anesthetics			
Substance Name	**Commercial and Street Names**	**How Taken***	**Intoxication Effects**	**Potential Health Consequences**
Ketamine	*Ketalar SV* Cat, Valiums, K, Special K, vitamin K	Injected, snorted, smoked	Increased heart rate and blood pressure, impaired motor function At high doses: delirium, depression; respiratory depression/arrest	Memory loss, numbness; nausea, vomiting
PCP and analogs	*Phencyclidine* Angel dust, boat, hog, love boat, peace pill	Injected, swallowed, smoked	Increased heart rate and blood pressure, impaired motor function; possible decrease in blood pressure and heart rate, panic, aggression, violence	Memory loss, numbness; nausea, vomiting; loss of appetite, depression

From National Institute of Drug Abuse. www.niha.gov/DrugPages/DrugsofAbuse.html.
*Taking drugs by injection can increase the risk of infection through needle contamination with staphylococci, HIV, hepatitis, and other organisms.

Table 15-6	Commonly Abused Drugs: Hallucinogens			
Substance Name	**Commercial and Street Names**	**How Taken**	**Intoxication Effects**	**Potential Health Consequences**
LSD	*Lysergic acid diethylamide* Acid, blotter, boomers, cubes, microdot, yellow sunshines	Swallowed, absorbed through mouth tissues	Altered states of perception and feeling; nausea; increased body temperature, heart rate, blood pressure, loss of appetite, sleeplessness, numbness, weakness, tremors	Chronic mental disorders, persisting perception disorder (flashbacks)
Psilocybin	Magic mushroom, purple passion, shrooms	Swallowed	Altered states of perception and feeling; nausea, nervousness, paranoia	Same as for LSD

From National Institute of Drug Abuse. www.niha.gov/DrugPages/DrugsofAbuse.html.

Table 15-7	Commonly Abused Drugs: Opioids and Morphine Derivatives			
Substance Name	**Commercial and Street Names**	**How Taken***	**Intoxication Effects**	**Potential Health Consequences**
Codeine	*Empirin w/Codeine, Fiorinal w/Codeine, Robitussin A-C, Tylenol w/Codeine* Captain Cody, Cody, schoolboy With glutethimide: doors & fours, loads, pancakes and syrup	Injected, swallowed	Pain relief, euphoria, drowsiness; less analgesia, sedation, and respiratory depression than morphine	Respiratory depression and arrest, nausea, confusion, constipation, sedation, unconsciousness, coma, tolerance, addiction
Fentanyl	*Actiq, Duragesic, Sublimaze* Apache, China girl, China white, dance fever, friend, goodfella, jackpot, murder 8, TNT, Tango and Cash	Injected, smoked, snorted	Pain relief, euphoria, drowsiness	Same as for codeine
Heroin	*Diacetylmorphine* Brown sugar, dope, H, horse, junk, skag, skunk, smack, white horse	Injected, smoked, snorted	Pain relief, euphoria, drowsiness, staggering gait	Same as for codeine
Morphine	*Roxanol, Duramorph* M, Miss Emma, monkey, white stuff	Injected, swallowed, smoked	Pain relief, euphoria, drowsiness	Same as for codeine
Opium	*Laudanum, Paregoric* Big O, black stuff, block, gum, hop	Swallowed, smoked	Pain relief, euphoria, drowsiness	Same as for codeine

From National Institute of Drug Abuse. www.niha.gov/DrugPages/DrugsofAbuse.html.
*Taking drugs by injection can increase the risk of infection through needle contamination with staphylococci, HIV, hepatitis, and other organisms.

Table 15-8 Commonly Abused Drugs: Stimulants

Substance Name	Commercial and Street Names	How Taken*	Intoxication Effects	Potential Health Consequences
Amphetamine	*Adderall, Biphetamine, Dexedrine* Bennies, black beauties, crosses, hearts, LA turn-around, speed, truck drivers, uppers	Injected, swallowed, smoked, snorted	Increased heart rate, blood pressure, metabolism; feelings of exhilaration, energy, increased mental alertness; rapid breathing; hallucinations	Rapid or irregular heartbeat; reduced appetite, weight loss, heart failure; tremor, loss of coordination; irritability, anxiousness, restlessness, delirium, panic, paranoia, impulsive behavior, aggressiveness, tolerance, addiction
Cocaine	*Cocaine hydrochloride* Blow, bump, C, candy, Charlie, coke, crack, flake, rock, snow, toot	Injected, smoked, snorted	Increased heart rate, blood pressure, metabolism; feelings of exhilaration, energy, increased mental alertness; increased temperature	Rapid or irregular heartbeat; reduced appetite, weight loss, heart failure; chest pain, respiratory failure, nausea, abdominal pain, strokes, seizures, headaches, malnutrition
MDMA (methylenedioxy-methamphetamine)	*DOB, DOM, MDA* Adam, clarity, ecstasy, Eve, lover's speed, peace, STP, X, XTC	Swallowed	Increased heart rate, blood pressure, metabolism; feelings of exhilaration, energy, increased mental alertness; mild hallucinogenic effects, increased tactile sensitivity, empathic feelings, hyperthermia	Rapid or irregular heartbeat; reduced appetite, weight loss, heart failure; impaired memory and learning
Methamphetamine	*Desoxyn* Chalk, crank, crystal, fire, glass, go fast, ice, meth, speed	Injected, swallowed, smoked, snorted	Increased heart rate, blood pressure, metabolism; feelings of exhilaration, energy, increased mental alertness; aggression, violence, psychotic behavior	Rapid or irregular heartbeat; reduced appetite, weight loss, heart failure; memory loss, cardiac and neurologic damage; impaired memory and learning, tolerance, addiction
Methylphenidate	*Ritalin* JIF, MPH, R-ball, Skippy, the smart drug, vitamin R	Injected, swallowed, snorted	Increased heart rate, blood pressure, metabolism; feelings of exhilaration, energy, increased mental alertness; increase or decrease in blood pressure, psychotic episodes	Rapid or irregular heartbeat; reduced appetite, weight loss, heart failure; digestive problems, loss of appetite, weight loss

Continued

Table 15-8 Commonly Abused Drugs: Stimulants—Cont'd

Substance Name	Commercial and Street Names	How Taken*	Intoxication Effects	Potential Health Consequences
Nicotine	Bidis, chew, cigars, cigarettes, smokeless tobacco, snuff, spit tobacco	Smoked, snorted, taken in snuff and spit tobacco	Increased heart rate, blood pressure, metabolism; feelings of exhilaration, energy, increased mental alertness; tolerance, addiction	Rapid or irregular heartbeat; reduced appetite, weight loss, heart failure; additional effects attributable to tobacco exposure: adverse pregnancy outcomes, chronic lung disease; cardiovascular disease, stroke, cancer
Anabolic steroids	Anadrol, Oxandrin, Durabolin, DepoTestosterone, Equipoise Roids, juice	Injected, swallowed, applied to skin	No intoxication effects	Hypertension, blood clotting and cholesterol changes, liver cysts and cancer, kidney cancer, hostility and aggression, acne†
Inhalants	Solvents (paint thinners, gasoline, glues), gases (butane, propane, aerosol propellants, nitrous oxide), nitrites (isoamyl, isobutyl, cyclohexyl) Laughing gas, poppers, snappers, whippets	Inhaled through nose or mouth	Stimulation, loss of inhibition; headache; nausea or vomiting; slurred speech, loss of motor coordination; wheezing	Unconsciousness, cramps, weight loss, muscle weakness, depression, memory impairment, damage to cardiovascular and nervous systems, sudden death

From National Institute of Drug Abuse. www.niha.gov/DrugPages/DrugsofAbuse.html.
*Taking drugs by injection can increase the risk of infection through needle contamination with staphylococci, HIV, hepatitis, and other organisms.
†Other potential health consequences of anabolic steroids by age/gender:
Adolescents: Premature stoppage of growth.
Men: Prostate cancer, reduced sperm production, shrunken testicles, breast enlargement.
Women: Menstrual irregularities, development of beard and other masculine characteristics.

Scenario Follow-up

After the patient has been safely transported to the hospital and his care turned over to the ED staff, you discuss the case with the paramedics. You all note that the findings of depressed respirations, depressed mental status, and pinpoint pupils, clues you gathered during your patient assessment, are classic for an opioid overdose. Positive-pressure ventilation with high-concentration oxygen was essential to prevent this patient, with slow respirations and signs of low oxygen concentration throughout his body, from further deterioration and possible cardiac arrest. The advanced life support (ALS) intercept allowed for early administration of naloxone, an antidote that reversed the effects of the heroin.

Summary

The primary goals in the prehospital management of poisoning are to prevent injury to EMS personnel and bystanders, provide cardiorespiratory support to the patient, prevent further absorption of the poison, and gather information to aid in identifying the poison to assist hospital and poison control center personnel. For ingested poisons, administration of activated charcoal may prevent further absorption. Poisons that are absorbed through the skin should be washed off the patient (dried powders are brushed off first), and patients should be quickly removed from environments that contain toxic gases. When possible, document the type and quantity of poison, time of exposure, and how the patient was exposed (ingestion, inhalation, injection, skin exposure). The EMT should bring pill bottles, substance containers, and other sources to the hospital to help identify the toxin whenever possible. Remember to treat the patient, not the poison. Perform an organized patient assessment and provide lifesaving treatment as needed. The poison control center and medical direction are essential resources for prehospital personnel and should be consulted for guidance whenever possible.

Skills

Skill | 15-1 **Administering Activated Charcoal**

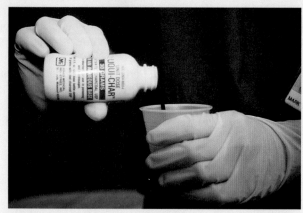

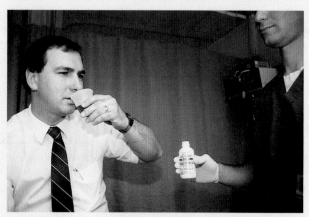

1. Obtain an order from medical direction either online or offline.

2. Shake the container thoroughly. Select or measure proper amount of solution per medical direction.

3. Obtain patient cooperation to drink the solution. The solution is black and "chalky," and patients may be reluctant to drink it. Cover the solution, and provide a straw to aid ingestion, especially with children. (A sweetener or flavoring may be added in some systems.)

Reshake the solution if the patient takes a long time to drink it, because the charcoal will settle to the bottom.

Record activity and time.

The Bottom Line

Learning Checklist

✓ Poisons can enter the body by ingestion, inhalation, injection, and absorption.

✓ Scene size-up is used to anticipate hazards to EMS personnel and bystanders from exposure to the toxin or secondary contamination. Prevent secondary contamination by using appropriate personal protective equipment, having trained rescuers remove patients from a toxic environment, and decontaminating the victims.

✓ Signs and symptoms of poisoning can present as extreme stimulation or inhibition of most organ systems (e.g., fast or slow heart rate, dry or moist skin, coma, or seizures), depending on the toxin involved.

✓ Emergency medical care for patients with poisoning or overdose focuses on preventing injury to EMS personnel or bystanders, ensuring an adequate airway, providing ventilations and oxygenation, preventing further absorption, and gathering evidence of the poisoning.

✓ During the history, important questions to ask include the following:
  ✓ What substance is involved?
  ✓ How much was involved?
  ✓ Over what period did the poisoning occur?
  ✓ What interventions were performed before your arrival?
  ✓ What is the patient's weight?

✓ With substances on the skin, prevent further absorption by removing contaminated clothing while protecting yourself from contamination, brushing any powder off the patient before irrigation, and irrigating the skin with clean water or soap and water for at least 20 minutes (continuing en route to the facility if possible).

✓ At scenes of possible inhaled exposures, have trained rescuers remove patients from the poisonous environment.

✓ For patients with inhaled toxins, removal to fresh air and administration of supplemental oxygen are indicated.

✓ Under medical direction, administer activated charcoal to prevent absorption of ingested poisons at an approximate dose of 1 g/kg body weight.

✓ Contraindications to activated charcoal include altered mental status, inability to swallow, and ingestion of acids and alkalis.

✓ Consider ALS intercept for victims of opioid and organophosphate overdose because lifesaving antidotes may be carried by advanced life support personnel.

✓ Opioid overdose may be recognized by the classic presentation of depressed mental status, depressed respirations, and pinpoint pupils.

✓ Organophosphate overdose may be recognized by overstimulation of secretions (salivation, sweating, tearing, vomiting, diarrhea, urination, pulmonary secretions), bronchoconstriction, and muscle weakness.

Key Terms

Activated charcoal Residue of the distillation of organic materials (charcoal) that has been treated to increase its adsorptive properties and binds most toxins; often used to absorb ingested drugs and poisons.

Antidote A remedy that counteracts a poison.

Asphyxiation Lack of oxygen or excees of carbon dioxide causing unconsciousness and often death.

Delirium tremens ("DTs") Shakes, tremors, and seizures accompanied by hyperactivity; increased respiration, pulse, and temperature; hypertension; and sometimes hallucinations associated with drug withdrawal.

Hypnotic Frequently prescribed agent that induces sleep.

Jaundice Yellow color to the skin caused by liver failure.

Opioid Narcotic agent with opium-like or morphine-like effects.

Overdose Result of drug being taken in excess or in combination with other agents to the point where poisoning occurs.

Poison Substance that, on ingestion, inhalation, absorption, or injection, may cause structural damage or functional disturbance.

Sedative Frequently prescribed agent with calming effects.

Stimulant Drug that causes excitability and can induce seizure with overdose; can be prescription (e.g., amphetamines) or street (e.g., PCP) drug.

Toxic Poisonous.

Toxicology The study of poisons.

Review Questions

1. Which of the following is the most common route by which a poison may enter the body?
   a. Ingestion
   b. Inhalation
   c. Absorption
   d. Injection

2. You would expect the pupils of a patient who injected heroin to be:
   a. Dilated and unequal
   b. Dilated and equal
   c. Normal and equal
   d. Constricted and equal

3. Which of the following is most important in the treatment of a poisoned patient?
   a. Administering activated charcoal
   b. Transporting in the recovery position
   c. Taking an accurate blood pressure
   d. Ensuring an open airway and breathing

4. Which of the following would be least effective in preventing aspiration of vomit in the overdose or poisoned patient?
   a. Placing patient in the recovery position
   b. Inserting an oropharyngeal airway in all patients
   c. Assessing mental status and ability to swallow before administering charcoal
   d. Having suction equipment readily available

5. Which of the following is a correct part of the pharmacologic description of activated charcoal?
   a. Dose: 3 g/kg body weight
   b. Indication: ingested poisons or overdoses
   c. Action: melts certain poisons and speeds absorption into the body
   d. Side effects: fruity breath

6. Which of the following rationales *best* explains the reason for early prehospital contact with medical direction in cases of poisoning?
   a. Some poisons may necessitate early administration of antidote by advanced life support intercept or hospital.
   b. Compilation of poison statistics is essential for prevention of injury.
   c. Administration of oxygen and positive-pressure ventilation should be done only with medical direction.
   d. The recovery position may be warranted and ordered by medical direction.

7. Which of the following is an essential step in administration of activated charcoal?
   a. Placing the patient supine
   b. Shaking the premixed form of the drug
   c. Checking the gag reflex after administration
   d. Measuring 50 g for all patients

8. A patient drank 1 g/kg of activated charcoal and then vomited shortly afterward. Which of the following may be ordered by medical direction?
   a. Repeat the dose of activated charcoal
   b. Administer the universal antidote
   c. Repeat at twice the dose of activated charcoal
   d. Administer medication to induce further vomiting

9. Which of the following questions would be least important to ask when treating the effects of an overdose?
   a. What was ingested?
   b. How much was ingested?
   c. Why was it ingested?
   d. When was it ingested?

10. A patient is found unresponsive with infrequent respirations (6 breaths/min), and pinpoint pupils. The mouth and skin are dry. Given this presentation, what actions are most likely to be of benefit to this patient?
    a. Maintain the airway, ventilate the patient with supplemental oxygen, and call for ALS intercept to give an antidote for nerve agents.
    b. Maintain the airway, ventilate the patient with supplemental oxygen, and call for ALS intercept to give an antidote to opioids.
    c. Maintain the airway, ventilate the patient with supplemental oxygen, and call for ALS intercept to treat cocaine overdose.
    d. Maintain the airway, ventilate the patient with supplemental oxygen, and call medical control to give glucose gel.

For Further Review

In the Student Workbook

- Multiple-choice questions
- Matching questions
- Fill-in-the-blank questions
- Short-answer questions
- Case scenario questions

On Evolve

- Weblinks
- Lecture notes
- Exercises

Learning Objectives

Cognitive Objectives

- List various ways in which poisons enter the body.
- List signs or symptoms associated with poisoning.
- Discuss the emergency medical care for the patient with a possible overdose.
- Describe the steps in the emergency medical care for the patient with suspected poisoning.
- Establish the relationship between the patient with poisoning or overdose and airway management.
- State the generic and trade names, indications, contraindications, medication form, dose, administration, actions, side effects, and reassessment strategies for activated charcoal.
- Recognize the need for medical direction in caring for the patient with poisoning or overdose.

Affective Objectives

- Explain the rationale for administering activated charcoal.
- Explain the rationale for contacting medical direction early in the prehospital management of the poisoning or overdose patient.

Psychomotor Objectives

- Demonstrate the steps in the emergency medical care for the patient with possible overdose.
- Demonstrate the steps in the emergency medical care for the patient with suspected poisoning.
- Perform the necessary steps required to provide a patient with activated charcoal.
- Demonstrate the assessment and documentation of patient response.

References

American Association of Poison Control Centers, 2006. www.aapcc.org/Annual %20Reports/06Report. Accessed 2008.

Chudler EH: Neuroscience for kids. http://faculty.washington.edu/chudler/neurok.html. May 2008. *Drug identification bible, 2008*, Grand Junction, Colo, Amera-Chem.

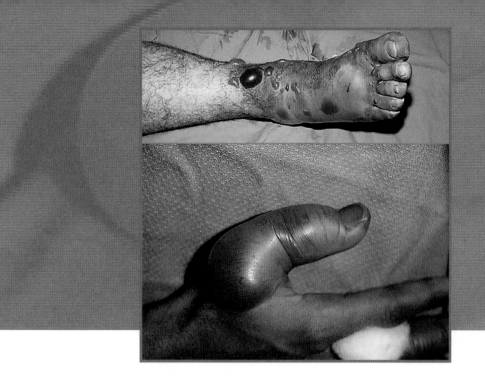

16 Environmental Emergencies

CHAPTER OUTLINE

Scenario

You are dispatched to the home of an unconscious elderly man. It is another hot, humid day during a heat wave. The man's son states that his father has been in bed with the flu; since he had the chills last night, the son covered him with blankets and closed his window. The home has no air conditioning. The temperature in the bedroom is stifling. The patient is unresponsive to pain, is breathing, and has a pulse and hot, dry, flushed skin. The remainder of the focused (secondary) assessment (history and physical examination) reveals a pulse of 120 beats/min, respirations of 20 breaths/min, and a blood pressure of 100/60 mm Hg. The patient's lips and mouth are dry, and breath sounds are normal. You administer oxygen and transfer the patient to the air-conditioned ambulance. You loosen and remove his clothing, keep the skin moist by applying water with wet towels, fan aggressively, and apply cold packs to the neck, groin, and armpits. You inform the receiving hospital that your patient is unresponsive and has a suspected heat emergency.

Thermoregulation

The body maintains a relatively constant internal temperature even when the temperature of the outside environment fluctuates greatly. Although 98.6° F (Fahrenheit) or 37° C (Celsius) is generally regarded as the normal body temperature, some variation occurs with daily activity and from person to person. The range of normal deviation of the body's central core temperature is from 96.4° F to 99.8° F (35.8° C to 37.7° C). With strenuous exercise, the core body temperature can increase to 104° F (40° C). At night when the body is at rest, the temperature may drop to 96.4° F (35.8° C). Variations from normal body temperature beyond this range are not well tolerated. If the temperature is too low or too high, the body can lose its ability to regulate temperature, which can cause extreme changes in temperature and even death (**Figure 16-1**).

The body's maintenance of a normal temperature is a continuous process that is accomplished through the careful regulation of heat production and heat loss. In most parts of the world, the outside temperature is less than the body's normal temperature. Therefore, heat must be generated internally to maintain a temperature of 98.6° F (37° C). Normal metabolism, or the chemical changes in living cells by which energy is provided for the vital processes (e.g., breathing) and activities of daily living, gives off heat as a byproduct. Increased metabolism, as occurs with exercise, greatly increases heat production. Heat is distributed throughout the body by the cardiovascular system and is lost primarily through the skin, the organ that is in greatest contact with the outside environment (**Figure 16-2**). The *hypothalamus* (temperature control center in the brain) regulates the many factors involved with the production of heat and its loss or conservation.

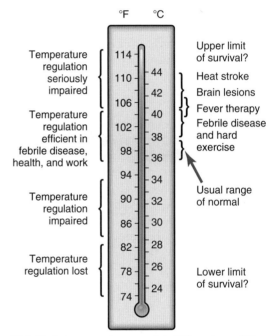

Figure 16-1 Body temperatures under different conditions.
From DuBois EF: Fever, Springfield, Ill, 1948, Charles C Thomas.

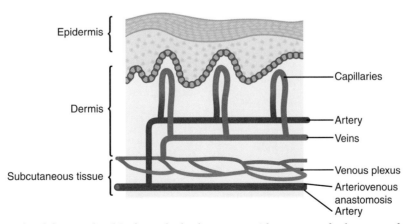

Figure 16-2 Skin circulation. Blood flow to the skin from the body core provides a means for heat transfer with the outside environment, making the skin an effective heat "radiator" system. A high rate of blood flow (when vessels dilate) causes heat to be conducted from the body core to the skin, whereas low blood flow (when vessels constrict) would decrease heat conduction from the core to the skin.

Core Temperature

Most references to body temperature indicate the temperature of the body *core,* or the temperature within the skull, the thorax, and the abdominal-pelvic cavities. The body's regulatory processes maintain this core temperature within narrow limits. A greater variance occurs between the temperatures within the body shell and the outer layers of the body (e.g., skin, soft tissues) and the extremities. At room temperature, for example, a gradual reduction from the core temperature occurs as the temperature of the muscle, subcutaneous tissue, and skin is sampled (**Figure 16-3).** Also, various regions of the body's shell have different temperatures as the distance from the heart and trunk increases.

The body's temperature is usually measured by oral or rectal thermometers, with the rectal temperature generally being 1° F (⅝° C) greater than the oral temperature. As an emergency medical technician (EMT), you can get a sense of the patient's temperature by placing the back of your hand on the patient's skin, such as on the abdomen of a patient suspected of having a heat or cold emergency.

Heat Production

All metabolic processes within the body generate heat. The metabolic activity necessary to maintain cellular functions at rest is called the *basal metabolism,* and it provides a constant supply of heat. In comfortable environments the basal metabolism generates more than enough heat to maintain the core temperature. The metabolic rate can be increased by hormones under the influence of the central nervous system. Muscular activity can greatly increase heat production. Shivering is a form

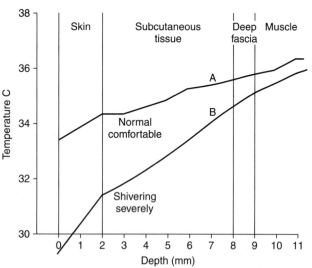

Figure 16-3 Range of temperature in the forearm. *A,* Under warm conditions when the patient is comfortable. *B,* Under cold conditions that lead to shivering. Observe the difference in temperatures from the deeper structures in the body to the outer layers in the extremities. A normal body temperature of 37° C refers to the body core because a normal temperature of the forearm could be 34° C. The extremities are most likely to be affected by cold injuries such as frostbite. *From Bazett HC, McGlone B: Temperature gradients in the tissues of man, Am J Physiol 82:415, 1927.*

of involuntary forced muscular activity that increases heat production when the body is exposed to cold. In fact, the heat generated by basal metabolism and muscular activity could cause the core temperature to increase to dangerous levels if the excess heat is not released to the environment through the skin. Heat is also gained from the environment when the temperature outside exceeds body temperature.

> **LEARNING OBJECTIVE**
> • Describe the various ways that the body loses heat.

Heat Loss

The five primary ways that heat can be lost from the body are as follows (**Figure 16-4**):
- Radiation
- Conduction
- Convection
- Evaporation
- Breathing

Under normal conditions, most heat loss occurs through radiation (60%). Evaporation accounts for approximately 22%, and conduction to the air accounts for about 15% of heat loss. Smaller amounts of heat are lost through direct conduction to objects, breathing, and urine and feces.

Radiation

Radiation is the transfer of heat in the form of infrared heat rays. All objects, including the human body, radiate heat rays. At 70° F (21° C), which is average room temperature, the body radiates heat to objects in the environment. When the environmental temperature exceeds body temperature, for example, on a 102° F day, more heat from radiation is gained by the body than is lost.

Conduction

Conduction is the transfer of heat to objects in direct contact with the body. Sitting on a chair that is cooler than body temperature results in the loss of heat from the body to the chair. As the temperature of the chair becomes heated from body heat, the transfer ceases.

The conduction of heat is influenced by the heat transfer properties of the materials in direct contact with the body. For example, water conducts heat much faster than air does. Compared with air, the transfer of heat is 5 times greater with wet clothing and 25 times greater with immersion in cold water.

The air immediately surrounding the body is heated by conduction. Air is a poor conductor of heat, however, and once the air immediately surrounding the body is heated, it insulates the body from further heat loss unless air movement is significant.

Convection

Heat is first conducted to the air immediately surrounding the body. **Convection** then takes place: heat is carried away by air currents, removing the warmed air and replacing it with cooler air. Wind velocity influences heat loss by convection. The wind chill factor is a familiar reference to the chilling effects that wind can add to environmental temperatures (**Figure 16-5**).

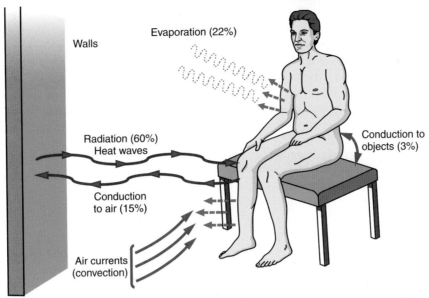

Figure 16-4 Mechanism of heat loss from the body (assumes an unclothed person in a room at normal temperature). *Adapted from Guyton AC, Hall JH: Textbook of medical physiology, ed 11, St. Louis, 2007, Saunders.*

Temperature (°F)																		
Calm	40	35	30	25	20	15	10	5	0	−5	−10	−15	−20	−25	−30	−35	−40	−45
5	36	31	25	19	13	7	1	−5	−11	−16	−22	−28	−34	−40	−46	−52	−57	−63
10	34	27	21	15	9	3	−4	−10	−16	−22	−28	−35	−41	−47	−53	−59	−66	−72
15	32	25	19	13	6	0	−7	−13	−19	−26	−32	−39	−45	−51	−58	−64	−71	−77
20	30	24	17	11	4	−2	−9	−15	−22	−29	−35	−42	−48	−55	−61	−68	−74	−81
25	29	23	16	9	3	−4	−11	−17	−24	−31	−37	−44	−51	−58	−64	−71	−78	−84
30	28	22	15	8	1	−5	−12	−19	−26	−33	−39	−46	−53	−60	−67	−73	−80	−87
35	28	21	14	7	0	−7	−14	−21	−27	−34	−41	−48	−55	−62	−69	−76	−82	−89
40	27	20	13	6	−1	−8	−15	−22	−29	−36	−43	−50	−57	−64	−71	−78	−84	−91
45	26	19	12	5	−2	−9	−16	−23	−30	−37	−44	−51	−58	−65	−72	−79	−86	−93
50	26	19	12	4	−3	−10	−17	−24	−31	−38	−45	−52	−60	−67	−74	−81	−88	−95
55	25	18	11	4	−3	−11	−18	−25	−32	−39	−46	−54	−61	−68	−75	−82	−89	−97
60	25	17	10	3	−4	−11	−19	−26	−33	−40	−48	−55	−62	−69	−76	−84	−91	−98

Wind (mph)

Frostbite Times   ▨ 30 minutes ▧ 10 minutes ▢ 5 minutes

Effective 11/01/01

Figure 16-5 Wind chill factor. *Data from National Weather Service and National Oceanic and Atmospheric Administration, US Department of Commerce.*

For example, on a day when the thermometer registers 30° F, a 20-mph wind makes the temperature feel like 17° F.

Evaporation

Evaporation is the loss of heat that occurs when moisture vaporizes on the body's surface. The rate of evaporation depends on the temperature, movement of air, and humidity (relative water content in the air for a given temperature). When the humidity is high, less perspiration evaporates. When humidity nears 100%, little heat is lost by evaporation. When perspiration runs off the body instead of evaporating, no cooling occurs. In addition, evaporation from clothing is less efficient than sweat evaporating directly from the skin.

Air movement replaces the air immediately surrounding the skin, which has become more saturated with water vapor from evaporation, with "less humid" air. This enhances evaporation; wind currents are particularly important on humid days. Air can hold more water vapor as the temperature rises.

The importance of evaporation in heat loss cannot be overemphasized, because when the environmental temperature approaches or exceeds body temperature, evaporation is the only mechanism for the body to lose heat and maintain a "normal" temperature.

Breathing

Inhaled air is heated or cooled to body temperature. The body loses heat when inhaled air is cooler than body temperature because it gives off heat to the air as it passes through the respiratory tract on its way to the lungs. The body gains heat when the inhaled air is warmer than body temperature because the air is cooled by giving off heat to the respiratory tract on its way to the lungs. The respiratory tract is able to cool hot, dry air effectively because the moist respiratory tract is a much more potent conductor of heat than is air and is able to cool the air somewhat before it reaches the lungs. This explains why the lungs are less likely to be burned by inhalation of hot, dry air in fires but may be injured by inhalation of steam.

> ### REAL*World*
>
> Environmental conditions have a great influence on how body heat is lost. The environmental temperature, wind velocity, and humidity all affect the ability of the body to lose or conserve heat. We feel comfortable on a hot day when the humidity is low because it is easier for evaporation to occur. A fan or wind currents add to the comfort level by replacing the heated and moist air immediately around the body with cooler and drier air. This promotes heat loss by conduction and evaporation. Conversely, high humidity and no wind velocity on a hot day make it harder for the body to lose heat.

As an EMT, you should obtain the following information when encountering patients who are exposed to the environment:
- What is the source and duration of exposure?
- Has the patient lost consciousness?
- Are heat effects localized or general?

Mechanisms of Control

If you think of the brain, the cardiovascular system, and the skin working together to regulate body temperature, you can understand why patients have certain symptoms during heat and cold emergencies in addition to the signs you encounter during your assessment.

Brain

The brain, specifically the hypothalamus, sets the body's thermostat and regulates temperature by its influence on the metabolic rate (heat production), the cardiovascular system (heat distribution), and the skin (heat loss). When the hypothalamus senses an increase in body temperature, it increases heat loss by directing vasodilation of skin vessels. This brings heat to the surface of the body where it can be lost by radiation, conduction, and convection. Heat loss can also occur through sweating, which speeds evaporation.

Cold body temperatures cause the hypothalamus to increase the metabolic rate and the production of heat. Other receptors in the skin and spinal cord cause shivering (to increase heat production), inhibit sweating, and cause vasoconstriction of skin vessels (to prevent heat loss).

Cardiovascular System

The cardiovascular system brings heated blood from the body core to the skin and extremities. When more heat must be lost, the skin vessels dilate to allow more blood to be in contact with the skin so that heat can be lost through radiation, conduction, and convection. This vasodilation is accompanied by an increase in the cardiac output. Conversely, when heat must be conserved, the skin vessels undergo vasoconstriction to reduce heat loss to the environment.

Vasodilation and vasoconstriction of the skin's blood vessels can result in great changes in blood flow through the skin. Under resting conditions, about 5% of the cardiac output flows through the skin. For a 70-kg man with a cardiac output of approximately 5 L/min, this represents 250 to 300 mL of blood flow per minute through the skin. The transfer of heat between the skin and the environment then takes place according to thermal gradients (from hot to cold) and the various mechanisms of heat exchange.

Under heat stress, when the skin vessels are dilated, the blood flow to the skin can increase to 3000 mL/min, resulting in a large increase in cardiac output to deal with heat loss alone. With so much of the blood now flowing to the skin, the blood volume left to circulate through the rest of the body is reduced. At such a point, blood flow may be insufficient to meet additional needs of muscular activity, and efforts to run or walk may lead to a feeling of exhaustion. Most individuals usually do not feel like undertaking strenuous activity on a hot, humid day.

In cold conditions, when the vessels in the skin have undergone vasoconstriction, blood flow can be reduced to 30 mL/min, allowing less heat transfer to the cold environment.

Skin

The skin is the interface between the external and internal environments and therefore has a primary role in heat regulation. In addition to its protective role as a barrier to infection and foreign elements, the skin and its subcutaneous fat serve as a layer of insulation. Vasoconstriction and vasodilation of blood vessels within the skin influence the exchange of core body heat with the environment. Heat loss is also regulated by the skin through evaporation of perspiration and changes in the flow of blood to the skin. Evaporation is influenced by stimulation of sweat glands within the skin.

Behavioral Regulation

Behavioral regulation is the conscious process of making changes to adapt to alterations in temperature. For example, a person may put on a coat in cold temperatures and seek shade on a hot day outside. Several medical conditions may alter this ability, subjecting patients to extremes of temperature.

> **LEARNING OBJECTIVES**
> - List the signs and symptoms of exposure to cold.
> - Explain the steps in providing emergency care to a patient exposed to cold.

Cold Emergencies

Exposure to cold can cause local injuries, such as frostnip and frostbite, as well as a lowered core body temperature, resulting in hypothermia and death.

Exposure to either below-freezing environments for short periods or above-freezing environments for longer periods can result in local cold injury. **Frostbite** and **frostnip** involve freezing of the water between and within body cells, resulting in ice crystal formation. "Trench foot" is a localized cold injury that occurs without ice crystal formation.

Hypothermia is defined as a core body temperature lower than 95° F (35° C). Hypothermia occurs when the body's ability to produce heat and regulate heat loss is unable to prevent loss of heat to the environment. Severe stresses, such as immersion in icy water, can overwhelm the body's ability to produce heat and regulate heat loss, and death may result within minutes. Patients with a compromised ability to generate heat or prevent heat loss, such as young infants, elderly persons, or intoxicated patients, may become hypothermic at room temperature.

In general, if a patient with a cold emergency can reach the hospital in less than 2 hours, transport is the recommended priority. Prehospital care is mainly directed toward preventing further heat loss, protecting the injured parts, and providing rapid transport.

Case in Point

Two EMTs respond to a call about an "unconscious" patient in an apartment building. On arrival they discover an unresponsive 55-year-old man, found by his neighbor, with a large scalp laceration and a pool of blood surrounding him on the floor. The laceration is not actively bleeding. The patient is unresponsive to verbal and painful stimuli and has a blood pressure of 80/60 mm Hg, respiratory rate of 12 breaths/min, pulse of 80 beats/min, and a smell of alcohol on his breath. His skin is pale, cool, and dry. Assessment findings lead to treatment of hypovolemic shock.

Further assessment and treatment in the hospital confirm the assessment of shock caused by blood loss from a scalp laceration and reveal a core body temperature of 31° C (88° F). The EMTs note that the temperature in the apartment where they found the patient was normal. Blood analysis shows that the patient had a significantly high blood alcohol level.

This case illustrates that extreme environmental temperatures are not necessary to cause hypothermia. The patient was intoxicated with alcohol (resulting in vasodilation and unconsciousness). Combined with shock, this left him unable to maintain body temperature, even though he was in a 70° F (21° C) apartment. Radiation and conduction to both air and the floor exceeded the heat production from his metabolism, which was compromised by hypovolemic shock and malnutrition (from his alcoholism). The hypothermia might explain why his pulse was "normal" rather than rapid in the presence of hypovolemic shock.

Physiologic Response to Cold

Normally the body produces more than sufficient heat to maintain body temperature. In temperate climates, more than 90% of the average body heat generated during daily activities must be lost (see earlier discussion on mechanisms of heat production and heat loss). Clothing, buildings, and heating-cooling systems make it much easier to live in cold (and temperate) climates than in the past.

When faced with cold, the body's thermoregulatory centers respond by increasing heat production and decreasing heat loss. Early responses to cold include an increase in the metabolic rate to generate more heat and vasoconstriction to reduce heat loss. Shivering occurs if these measures are inadequate.

Shivering is the involuntary contraction of small groups of muscles, which can generate great amounts of heat. It begins when the temperature of the body's central core is around 95° F (35° C). Shivering may continue for a few hours until the body's energy stores are depleted. Malnourished individuals and those with insulin shock (hypoglycemia from too much insulin) may deplete their energy stores in a shorter time. Shivering begins involuntarily but is stopped with physical activity and purposeful movements, such as walking. Certain drugs, such as phenothiazines, barbiturates, and alcohol, may suppress or inhibit the shivering response. Shivering usually stops when the body temperature dips below 87.8° F (31° C) and muscle rigidity is noted. Once shivering stops, the body temperature may drop precipitously.

When the core body temperature falls to 92° F (34° C), amnesia and slurred speech may appear, signs that the central nervous system is affected. Alterations in mental status progress through irrational behavior, stupor, and coma as the temperature continues to drop.

A vicious cycle that inhibits escape develops with cold exposure. As the body temperature decreases, mentation is affected and judgment may be disturbed. At the same time, the ability to use the hands is impaired as the extremities succumb to local cold injury; clumsiness of hand movements progresses to stiffness of the limbs and muscular rigidity as the temperature drops. The inability to build a shelter or move to a safer environment leaves the victim subject to further exposure, more extensive freezing injuries to body surface parts and the extremities, and lowering of the core body temperature. Once shivering stops, the body temperature drops more rapidly. Muscles become rigid, and the patient is eventually unable to undertake voluntary movements and lapses into coma. Cold effects on the heart result in depression of the pacemaker, dysrhythmias, and clinical death.

Cold has a direct effect on the rate of metabolism and therefore on oxygen needs. Metabolism decreases 6% for every centigrade degree that the body's temperature drops. The corresponding decrease in oxygen requirements increases the time from clinical death (onset of cardiac arrest) to biological death (irreversible brain death), and patients have had full neurologic recovery after prolonged periods of cardiac arrest caused by hypothermia. Therefore, continued resuscitation efforts are recommended while attempts are made to raise the body temperature.

Hypothermia

Depending on the type of exposure, cold injuries may take minutes or hours to occur. The temperature of the outside environment and the type of exposure (air or water immersion) are important variables.

Acute Immersion

Acute immersion in icy water can result in death within 15 minutes; rarely can someone survive for more than 1 hour. At water temperatures of 60° F (15.5° C), exposure of 6 hours is the upper limit for most people. Because water is such a good conductor of heat, swimming instructors and others who spend prolonged periods in the water require water temperatures of 89° F to 90° F (32° C) to be comfortable.

Cold Exposure

Subacute Exposure. Exposure to cold air results in longer survival times than does submersion in water of the same temperature. However, if clothing becomes soaked, it offers little insulation value, reducing the time until cold injury occurs. Similarly, wind chill plays a significant factor in tolerance.

Chronic Exposure. Hypothermia over hours or days can occur, usually in compromised individuals. Such factors as disease and drug intoxication, which alter heat production, the ability to retain heat, or the ability to escape a dangerous environment, make a person susceptible to hypothermia. Shock can compromise heat production and compensatory actions. (see earlier Case in Point).

Predisposing Factors

Heat loss by radiation is proportional to the temperature difference between the environment and the body. Exposure of body parts, such as a bare head, increases radiation loss. Conductive heat loss is increased by contact with water, ice, snow, metal, and other objects that conduct heat faster than air. Convection heat losses are greater when the victim cannot find shelter from the wind or is improperly clothed. Wet clothing provides little insulation. Evaporative heat losses can occur with wet clothing or after sweating from exertion.

Age. Persons at the extremes of age are most susceptible to cold injuries. Older people may have difficulty fleeing a cold environment, generating heat by muscular activity, and regulating body temperature. A newborn has less fat tissue for insulation and inefficient shivering and thermoregulatory mechanisms. After a field delivery, the newborn must be kept warm. Infants have proportionately larger heads and a greater skin surface area relative to body weight than do adults, so they lose heat and moisture through the skin more easily. Infants and very small children are also at risk because they cannot care for themselves by adapting to changes in environmental conditions by adding or removing clothing or seeking shelter.

Medical Conditions. Certain medical conditions can affect the ability to generate heat and regulate temperature. These include diseases causing malnutrition, infections of the blood, endocrine diseases (diabetes, hypoglycemia), shock, head injury, and brain disease. Conditions affecting the skin, such as burns, also predispose the patient to hypothermia. In patients with spinal cord injuries, vessels in large areas of skin may not be able to undergo vasoconstriction, increasing heat loss.

Drugs and Alcohol. Drugs or poisons that can predispose the patient to hypothermia include benzodiazepines, tricyclic antidepressants, general anesthetics, narcotics, organophosphates, carbon monoxide, barbiturates, and phenothiazines. Alcohol causes vasodilation, which decreases the insulating property of the skin. It can also suppress shivering, disturb central thermoregulation, and interfere with judgment.

Signs and Symptoms. Patients with hypothermia can display various signs and symptoms depending on the core body temperature. Most standard thermometers measure ranges of temperature from 94° F to 106° F and cannot measure lower temperatures. *Hypothermic thermometers,* which are used in hospitals, can measure the lower readings. In the field, you can reach beneath the patient's clothing and palpate the abdomen.

| Table 16-1 | Levels of Hypothermia |

Temperature		Signs and Symptoms
°C	**°F**	
Mild		
35	95	Shivering begins
34	93.2	Amnesia
33	91.4	Poor muscular coordination
Moderate		
32	89.6	Stupor
31	87.8	Shivering stops
30	86	Irregular heart rhythms
29	85.2	Further loss of consciousness Pupils dilate
28	82.4	Ventricular fibrillation possible
27	80.6	Loss of voluntary motion
Severe		
26	78.8	Unresponsiveness to pain
24	75.2	Significant hypotension
22	71.6	Ventricular fibrillation likely

Modified from Danzl DF: Accidental hypothermia. In Marx J, Ockberger R, Walls R, editors: *Rosen's emergency medicine: concepts and clinical practice,* ed 5, St Louis, 2002, Mosby.

If the abdomen is cold to the touch, it is likely that the patient is experiencing generalized hypothermia. In general, the hypothermic patient feels cold to the touch, has a decreased level of consciousness, has decreased motor ability, and tends to have depressed vital signs. Shivering, seen with mild stages, ceases as the temperature falls below 88° F (31° C) and is replaced by muscular rigidity (**Table 16-1**).

Mild Hypothermia (89.6° F to 95° F; 32° C to 35° C)

The earliest stage of hypothermia can be noted by cool, flushed, or pale skin; shivering; difficulty in speech and movement; and amnesia. Vital signs may be normal.

Moderate Hypothermia (80.6° F to 89.6° F; 27° C to 32° C)

As the body temperature drops, the patient becomes stuporous. Shivering stops and is replaced with muscular rigidity and gradual loss of voluntary motion. Cardiac output drops, pulse and respirations become depressed, and pupils dilate. Skin may be pale or cyanotic. The pulse may become irregular from the development of dysrhythmias or abnormalities in the heart's conduction system. As the temperature approaches 82.4° F (28° C), ventricular fibrillation may develop.

Severe Hypothermia (<80.6° F; <27° C)

With severe hypothermia, the cerebral blood flow is one third of normal, and the patient is unresponsive to pain. Cardiac output is greatly depressed, and significant hypotension is noted. Cardiac arrest is likely.

Management

Management of hypothermia is determined primarily by the time required to transport the patient and the degree of hypothermia. The goals of prehospital management are to reduce further heat loss and to transport the patient rapidly but gently to a medical facility, where active rewarming can be initiated. Gentle handling is required because of the risk of dysrhythmias; modification of cardiopulmonary resuscitation (CPR) techniques may be needed. Active external rewarming is not usually undertaken in the field.

Patients can sustain long periods of hypothermia and still make a full recovery. The greatest risk is from ventricular fibrillation, which is resistant to treatment until the body is rewarmed. Because a depressed pulse may be adequate to meet the reduced oxygen needs of the cold patient, you should take care to avoid maneuvers that may precipitate dysrhythmias and ventricular fibrillation. These maneuvers include rough handling, stimulation of the gag reflex, overventilation, unnecessary cardiac compressions, and active external rewarming. Once CPR is initiated, however, it should be continued until the patient is rewarmed. Full recovery has been reported after prolonged periods (>3 hours) of CPR.

Reduce Further Heat Loss

In all hypothermic patients, further heat loss should be avoided. This is accomplished by carefully replacing wet clothes with dry clothes or blankets, using sleeping bags or other insulating devices, and protecting the patient from the wind.

Resuscitation Techniques

The respiratory rate and pulse may be severely depressed in the hypothermic patient. Supplemental oxygen should be given along with ventilatory assistance. Respiratory rates of 2 to 3 breaths/min have been observed. If ventilatory assistance is needed, be careful to avoid hyperventilation. Sudden hyperventilation can result in rapid changes in the acidity of the blood and may lead to dysrhythmias in the hypothermic patient. Any necessary airway devices should be inserted carefully to avoid stimulating a gag reflex because this also may cause dysrhythmias and ventricular fibrillation.

Careful assessment of pulses must be undertaken before cardiac compressions are initiated. Assess pulses for 30 to 45 seconds before starting CPR. Peripheral pulses may be particularly difficult to palpate because of vasoconstriction and associated frostbite. The patient's pupils may be dilated and unresponsive to light because of hypothermia, and the blood pressure may not be measurable. Extra care is needed because unnecessary cardiac compressions given to a hypothermic patient with a depressed, slow, and barely perceptible heartbeat may precipitate ventricular fibrillation. For all arrests, attach the automated external defibrillator (AED). If shock is advised, provide one shock and then continue CPR. In hypothermia where the temperature is below 86° F (30° C), current guidelines recommend withholding further shocks until the temperature can be raised above this level of profound hypothermia.

Active Rewarming Techniques

Active rewarming techniques involve application of heat internally or externally. In general, most active rewarming techniques are not recommended in the field.

Internal techniques that are applied in the hospital setting include the following:
- Instillation of warmed intravenous fluids
- Peritoneal dialysis with warmed fluids
- Hemodialysis
- Instillation of heated fluids in the gastrointestinal tract
- Administration of warmed, humidified oxygen

In the hospital, rewarming procedures are guided by the patient's core temperature. In the field, such monitoring is not possible. Therefore the recommended active rewarming techniques are limited to administration of warm, humidified oxygen and application of local heat to the large superficial vessels. Warm fluids containing sugar can be given to the conscious patient who is capable of drinking.

In restricted circumstances, immersion in a tub of hot water (98.6° F to 105° F [37° C to 40.6° C]) or application of warmed blankets or hot-water bottles to the body's "shell" may be necessary. These techniques are not recommended for all patients because of the possibility of complications from *rewarming shock.* This term describes the effects of extremity and shell rewarming before the core temperature can be raised. Many factors contribute to rewarming shock. Active thawing of the extremities can result in vasodilation of peripheral vessels and an increase in the size of the circulatory system before the heart has a chance to warm and increase the cardiac output. In addition, movement of cold blood from the extremities to the core can further decrease the core temperature. Because of these complexities, active rewarming outside the hospital should be considered only in limited and extraordinary circumstances. In such cases, risks to the patient, availability of shelter and equipment, and eventual evacuation and movement of the patient all need to be considered, with input from medical direction.

Transport

Transport of the patient to a medical facility should be undertaken as soon as possible. The patient must be handled gently, and a rough ride should be avoided.

EXTENDED *Transport*

When transport of a patient with a frostbite injury is extended, care must be taken to avoid additional injury. If there is any chance of the extremity being refrozen, it is better *not* to rewarm and to leave the extremity frozen until arrival at the hospital.

Prevention

Emergency medical technicians who attempt rescue missions in cold environments must be conscious of hazards and take appropriate precautions based on principles of heat loss. Clothing must provide adequate insulation and protection from wind and moisture, and layering is recommended to allow the EMT to adapt to changes in environmental temperature and heat production from physical exertion. Wet clothing should be removed because it provides little insulation and speeds heat loss from evaporation. Heat loss through radiation can be reduced by covering the body, particularly the head. Avoid contact with conductors of heat, such as metal, snow, and water. Alcohol

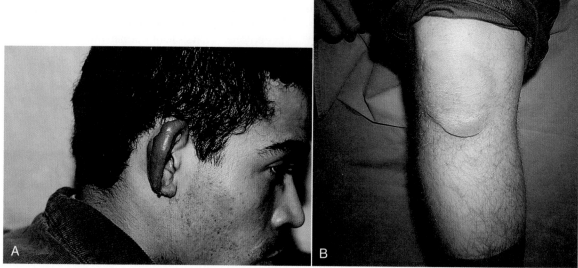

Figure 16-6 A, Minor superficial frostbite of the ear. Note blister formation one day after thaw. **B,** Superficial frostbite of the knee from kneeling to change a tire, 12 hours after thawing. Contact with the ground accelerates heat transfer by conduction, resulting in local cold injury. *From Auerbach P:* Wilderness medicine, *ed 5, St Louis, 2007, Mosby.*

intake should be avoided because of its vasodilatory effect and its ability to suppress shivering.

Do not smoke when attempting a rescue mission in a cold environment because nicotine is a potent vasoconstrictor and therefore affects the thermoregulatory responses of blood vessels. Take along food that is high in carbohydrates to sustain heat production. Keep moving, which will also generate heat. Knowing your physical abilities is important because your body temperature may drop rapidly if you become fatigued, and you may be unable to continue rescue activities. Seek shelter before hypothermia clouds your judgment and hampers your motor abilities.

Local Cold Injuries

Cold injuries tend to occur in the extremities and exposed ears, nose, chin, and cheeks, where there is a relatively large surface area for a small volume of tissue. These injuries tend to be localized and sharply demarcated, and they gradually progress from superficial to deep with continued exposure. The process is progressive. Vasoconstriction of the extremities in response to cold leaves less heat to warm the superficial parts. The water in the superficial tissues freezes, and the vasoconstriction becomes more intense, which results in still less blood flow and freezing of deeper tissues. The entire area may become frozen. The ice crystals that form can cause damage to cellular structure, but in many cases recovery is possible after proper rewarming. You should never rub or massage frostbitten parts because this can cause additional damage to the cells.

Rewarming causes marked vasodilation of the area, resulting in a marked flushed coloring. Swelling results from capillary leakage. If blood clots form in small vessels, they can affect the local circulation and cause areas of reduced blood flow. For example, areas where venous blood flow is obstructed, causing poor capillary return, may appear bluish or purplish.

These areas may alternate with areas of arterial vasoconstriction, which appear pale or gray, causing a mottled skin appearance.

Frostnip

Frostnip is a completely reversible cold injury caused by intense vasoconstriction to cold exposure. Frostnipped areas first appear as a sudden blanching of the skin. Loss of feeling and a sensation of cold occur in the affected area, leaving the victim unaware of the process. The skin does not become hardened. The area can be warmed by applying firm pressure with a hand or other warm body part or by blowing warm breath on the area. On rewarming, the area may be red, and a tingling sensation may be noted.

Superficial Frostbite

If unrecognized, frostnip can lead to superficial frostbite, or the freezing of water within the upper layers of skin. With superficial frostbite the skin appears white and waxy and is firm to the touch, but the tissues beneath the skin are soft and resilient.

After thawing, the skin may appear flushed or mottled, with alternating patchy red-purple and blanched areas. Edema may be present, and blisters can form in the area after 1 to 24 hours. The area is usually painful (**Figure 16-6**).

Deep Frostbite

With deep frostbite, the freezing extends throughout the dermis and can involve subcutaneous tissues, muscle and tendons, neurovascular structures, and possibly even bone. The skin becomes white, feels frozen, and resists depression. It is difficult to gauge the extent of deep frostbite.

An area of deep frostbite that has partially thawed may appear mottled and blue or gray. A line of demarcation usually separates injured from healthy tissue (**Figure 16-7**).

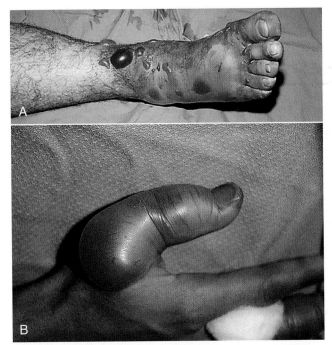

Figure 16-7 **A,** Deep frostbite. Swelling and blister formation 24 hours after frostbite injury in area covered by a tightly fitting boot. **B,** Deep frostbite. One day after thawing. *From Auerbach P:* Wilderness medicine, *ed 5, St Louis, 2007, Mosby.*

Management of Frostbite

Optimal management for frostbite requires well-controlled but rapid rewarming, a technique that in most cases should not be undertaken in the field. Active rewarming, properly done, may be time-consuming and can delay assessment of hypothermia and evacuation from the area, and the potential complications that follow thawing are best handled in the hospital. Furthermore, any body part that is thawed must be carefully protected from refreezing. Thawing and refreezing of the affected part is worse than remaining frozen for the same amount of time. The frostbitten part, whether frozen or thawed, must be handled carefully to avoid any further trauma.

The injured area should be protected from further heat loss, use, or traumatic injury. Cover the injured part to protect from further cold injury by insulating the area with layers of clothing and blankets. Protect the area from moisture, and remove wet clothing and any jewelry.

If an area has thawed, do not break the blisters; instead, cover them with sterile dressings. If the hands or feet are involved, separate the fingers and toes with small, folded dressings. Handle the area with care, and do not allow the patient to walk on an affected lower extremity. You may splint the affected limb. Avoid exposure of the area to direct dry heat, as from a fire. You should administer supplemental oxygen and pay careful attention to assess the patient for hypothermia and other injuries and to prepare for evacuation from the scene.

In wilderness situations or in other extraordinary circumstances in which transport may be significantly delayed, the rapid rewarming technique may be advisable in the field. In rare situations when transport may be delayed so long that slow thawing would take place, rapid thawing can be performed if conditions permit, and the part can be kept from refreezing. When a victim must walk out of a wilderness or other area, it is best if the attempt is made on the frozen extremity and not on a thawed or partially thawed one.

Case in Point

Two men trapped in a winter storm are located the next day. You are part of a rural EMS wilderness rescue team and are the first medical provider to reach the men. You find them in a cabin deep in the woods. They tell you that they followed a stream to the cabin, and one of the men slipped through the ice, soaking both his feet. They continued for another 2 hours until they found shelter. They were able to make a fire and tried to warm themselves through the night. As you examine the man's feet, you note swelling, discoloration, and blister formation from the ankle down on both feet. The men are eager to leave for home. Looking at the man's feet, you advise them to stay in place as you confer with the rescue team about available evacuation strategies, to minimize walking on the affected limbs.

Rapid rewarming is used in the emergency department (ED) or when field transport is delayed and facilities permit. Be sure to know and follow your local protocols. The steps for rapid rewarming include the following:

1. Immerse the affected part into a basin of water large enough to accommodate the part without it touching the walls of the container.
2. Preheat the water temperature to about 105° F (40.6° C) and maintain between 104° F and 108° F (40° C and 42° C). If the water temperature is too hot, the part may be harmed, and lower temperatures are not as effective. If no thermometer is available, water that is at 43.3° C can be estimated as the temperature that causes only slight discomfort. Water at 44.4° C is uncomfortable to most people.
3. Keep the water circulating to keep an even temperature. A whirlpool-type tub is ideal; otherwise, stir the water continuously as it is added.
4. Anticipate that the patient will feel pain on thawing. The process is complete when the part is again soft and color and sensation are present.
5. Dress the area with sterile dressings. Do not break any blisters. Place folded sterile dressings between toes and fingers before covering a foot or hand.

The thawed part must be protected from refreezing. The rapid rewarming process can take from 20 to 40 minutes.

Trench Foot or Immersion Foot

Prolonged exposure (10-12 hours) to above-freezing temperatures and dampness, generally below 50° F (10° C), can result in cold injury to the extremities, particularly if they are wet. This condition is called "trench foot," or *immersion foot,* and was a common cold injury in wartime when soldiers stood for long periods in cold, wet trenches. Trench foot causes damage to the small vessels and nerves and occurs in stages. The limb may have a different appearance, depending on when the EMT encounters the patient.

In response to the cold, the vessels in the extremity undergo vasoconstriction, causing paleness or blueness and diminished pulses as well as further lowering of the extremity's temperature. After a prolonged period of vasoconstriction, ischemic changes occur, including damage to small vessels and nerves, with capillary leakage, associated edema, and decreased or absent sensation. Thus, early in the encounter, the foot may appear cold, swollen, pale, or blue, with diminished pulses and sensation.

This phase is followed by an increase in circulation to the area, as if to make up for the period of prolonged vasoconstriction and ischemia. This increased circulation makes the foot appear hot, red, and dry. Pulses may be bounding, and the limb is extremely painful because of the cold and ischemic injury. Ulcers and gangrene can follow.

Patients who have had immersion foot injuries may have pain and discomfort in response to cold and weight bearing for a prolonged period after the injury. In contrast to frostbite, injury results without ice crystal formation. Management consists of keeping the extremity warm, dry, and protected from weight bearing and further injury.

LEARNING OBJECTIVES
- List the signs and symptoms of exposure to heat.
- Explain the steps in providing emergency care to a patient exposed to heat.

Heat Emergencies

General types of heat-related conditions and heat emergencies (**Table 16-2**) are as follows:

- *Heat rash.* A red rash with small bumps, usually found at the neck, under the arms, and in the groin, caused by blocked sweat glands.
- *Heat cramps.* Muscular cramps that occur during strenuous exertion and from excessive loss of body fluid through perspiration.
- *Heat exhaustion.* Inability of the cardiovascular system to keep up with stresses imposed by a hot environment. Heat exhaustion rarely causes death.
- *Heat syncope.* A transient loss of consciousness resulting from the blood vessels dilating to compensate for excessive heat.
- *Heat stroke.* A complete failure of the thermoregulatory system that results in extreme increases in core body temperature and damage to cells as well as changes in mentation. Heat stroke is associated with a high mortality rate.

Predisposing Factors

Factors that predispose a person to heat-related illnesses include the following:

- Climate
- Exercise and acclimation
- Age
- Preexisting illness
- Drug and alcohol use

Table 16-2	Heat Emergencies	
Condition	**Signs and Symptoms**	**Treatment**
Heat cramps	Muscular cramps after exercise	Cool environment Fluid replacement Stretch affected muscle
Heat exhaustion	Weakness or exhaustion Dizziness, faintness Skin moist, pale (or pink), may be cool Vital signs normal or tachycardia, orthostatic hypotension, elevated temperature (102 °F [38.8° C])	Cooling efforts Cool environment Fanning Loosen or remove clothing Fluids Supine position (legs elevated)
Heat stroke	Altered mental status Hot, dry skin (may be moist) Elevated body temperature (usually >104° F [40° C])	Aggressive cooling measures (wet sheets, fanning, ice to vessels of neck, armpits, groin) Rapid transport Oxygen

Climate

As previously mentioned, temperature, humidity, and wind velocity all play a large role in heat illness. The outside temperature relative to the body temperature determines whether heat is lost by radiation and conduction or whether heat is gained. *High humidity* decreases the rate of evaporation because the air is already saturated with water. Mortality rates from heat emergencies increase threefold during heat waves.

Exercise and Acclimation

Muscular activity greatly increases heat production. For example, the temperature of an athlete may rise to 104° F (40° C). On hot, humid days, dissipation of increased heat is more difficult. Many heat emergencies occur among high school football players early in the season when the weather is still warm and among military recruits who are unaccustomed to strenuous exercise.

As an individual trains, sweating begins early and increases in amount. In fact, the amount of sweat can increase from 1 to 3 L/hour. Water replacement should be available on hot days during strenuous exercise (e.g., football practice, marathon race). Otherwise, a person may become relatively hypovolemic. Sweat contains salt, and the amount of salt in sweat decreases as a person trains. Replacement of water is the most important factor in maintaining an adequate blood volume. Salt is usually adequately replaced by diet, and supplemental electrolyte solutions are not usually needed unless there has been a sustained period of activity accompanied by decreased food intake or repeated days of sustained sweat loss.

Awareness of the hazards of excessive exercise on hot, humid days has led to the institution of training programs that introduce gradual increases in the amount of daily exertion, supply a liberal amount of water, and encourage the wearing of loose, nonocclusive clothing, which promotes rather than inhibits evaporation.

Age

The very old and the very young populations are at increased risk for heat emergencies. The tendency of some parents to wrap infants in occlusive clothing, even though the outside temperature is hot, places infants at increased risk. Newborns in particular are at great risk because they have a poor thermoregulatory mechanism and sweating capability during the first days of life.

Because infants and some older patients lack mobility, they may remain in dangerous environments during heat waves. Examples include an infant left in a vehicle or a bedridden, debilitated patient without air conditioning.

Case in Point

A young mother is driving with her 3-month-old daughter when she remembers she has no formula left for the next feeding. Passing the supermarket, she decides to run inside. Her infant is sleeping, so she leaves her in the car seat and locks the doors, leaving the windows open just a crack.

Inside the store, the mother notices a sale on formula and asks the stock boy to get her a carton from the back and bring it to checkout counter. As she waits, she picks up other items from the aisles near the counter. Time passes quickly; before she knows it, 20 minutes has elapsed.

As she hurries from the store to her car, she sees lights and hears sirens. Police are gaining access to her vehicle. The temperature is 98° F. Her daughter's shirt is drenched, but her face is pink and dry. She does not respond to verbal cries to arouse her.

Infants and young children left unattended in a car are subject to heat emergencies. A car's windows act like a greenhouse, trapping sunlight and heat. The National Highway Traffic Safety Administration (NHTSA) stated in a 2004 report that approximately 25 children a year die as a result of being left or becoming trapped in hot vehicles. Cars parked in direct sunlight can reach internal temperatures of 131° F to 172° F (55° C to 78° C) when the outside temperature is 80° F to 100° F (26.6° C to 37.7° C). Even outside temperatures of 60° F to 70° F (15° C to 21° C) can cause a car temperature to rise well above 110° F (43.3° C). When the outside temperature is 83° F (28.4° C), even with the window open 2 inches (5 cm), the temperature inside the car can reach 109° F (42.7° C) in only 15 minutes. Within the first 10 minutes, the temperature in an enclosed vehicle will rise an average of 19° F, or 82% of its eventual 1-hour increase. In warm weather, a vehicle can warm to dangerous, life-threatening levels in only 10 minutes. Very young children (≤4 years) are particularly susceptible to hyperthermia.

REAL World

According to the Medical College of Wisconsin, children's bodies have greater surface area–to–body mass ratio, so they absorb more heat on a hot day (and lose heat more rapidly on a cold day). Further, children have a considerably lower sweating capacity than adults, so they are less able to dissipate body heat by evaporative sweating and cooling.

Preexisting Illness

Heart disease and dehydration compromise the cardiovascular response to heat. *Obesity* can inhibit heat loss because of the increased insulating effect of the excess subcutaneous fat. In addition, obese individuals require more muscular effort to perform everyday activities because of their greater weight. Thus they generate more heat because of their obesity and have a more difficult time transferring this heat to the environment because their fat acts as insulation.

A fever places an individual at increased risk of heat illness, as do fatigue and lack of sleep. *Parkinson's disease*, with its constant muscle tremors and increased heat production, is another condition that predisposes an individual to heat illness. Patients with an altered mental status may be at increased risk because of an inability to take appropriate precautions.

Alcohol and Drugs

Amphetamines and cocaine can increase heat production, whereas other drugs (e.g., some tranquilizers, antihistamines) can affect the hypothalamus and inhibit sweating. Diuretics can result in dehydration and affect cardiovascular function. Drugs affecting mental function and judgment, such as narcotics, tranquilizers, and alcohol, can interfere with the ability to take appropriate precautions in hot environments.

Heat Rash

A heat rash is a painful red rash with small bumps, usually found under the arms, in the groin, and around the neck. It is caused by sweat trapped in the sweat glands and can be seen at any age but is more common in young persons. Heat rash is not an emergency but can interfere with the body's ability to compensate for increased heat production, resulting in more serious conditions.

Heat Cramps

Heat cramps are painful muscular contractions of heavily exercised muscles. According to one theory, heat cramps may be induced during excessive exercise or hard work because of a disproportionate loss of fluid and sodium through excessive sweating.

Signs and Symptoms

Patients with heat cramps may give a history of muscle cramping in heavily used muscles during or immediately after exertion. The individual usually experiences a period of excessive sweating.

Management

Management of heat cramps consists of moving the patient to a cooler environment and replacing fluid and electrolyte losses with an electrolyte fluid solution (e.g., sports drink) or water.

Immediate relief of cramping is best accomplished by stretching the cramped muscle.

Heat Exhaustion

Heat exhaustion is caused by the cardiovascular system's inability to respond to the demands for increased blood flow to the skin while still maintaining flow to the muscles and other organs. For the patient in a hot environment, the blood vessels to the skin vasodilate, and blood flow to the skin increases to lose the heat. In addition, if there has been a period of sweating and volume loss, the patient may be mildly hypovolemic. A previously dehydrated patient is more prone to this condition. Some individuals may not be able to maintain cardiac output great enough to meet the simultaneous demands of the skin, skeletal muscles, and other body organs.

Signs and Symptoms

The patient with heat exhaustion is usually in a hot environment and may have had a period of recent exertion. The skin is usually moist. Because of inadequate blood flow to the skin, the body temperature may be elevated. Because of inadequate blood flow to the skeletal muscles, the patient may complain of weakness or exhaustion. Inadequate blood flow to other organs can result in multiple complaints, such as dizziness, a feeling of faintness, nausea, and headache.

Because blood flow may be inadequate, the skin can appear gray or cold, but it sometimes appears pink. Vital signs may be normal, or *orthostatic hypotension* (fall in blood pressure when the supine patient stands) and tachycardia may be present. The body temperature may be normal or mildly elevated, up to 102° F (38.8° C).

Management

When the patient is moved to a cooler environment (which decreases the demand for blood flow to the skin) and given modest amounts of fluids (1-2 L), heat exhaustion is usually relieved. Therefore, management is directed toward reducing body temperature by placing the patient in a cooler environment and loosening or removing clothing that may be interfering with heat loss. A fan may speed the cooling process.

Place the patient in a supine (with legs elevated) position to ensure perfusion of vital organs. Fluid replacement can be accomplished with oral or intravenous fluids (a balanced electrolyte solution or even plain water).

Heat Syncope

Heat syncope is a transient loss of consciousness caused by dilation of the blood vessels. As the body is exposed to excessive heat, the blood vessels move to the surface of the skin and dilate to radiate heat from the body. Because this dilation occurs quickly, the patient will pass out.

Signs and Symptoms

Patients with heat syncope have a history of being exposed to high temperatures and report a short loss of consciousness. They are awake, but weak and dizzy on standing. Their skin is hot and diaphoretic. Their pulse rate is increased and blood pressure lower than normal.

Management

Treatment of heat syncope includes keeping the patient cool and supine. Oxygen may be administered as needed. Transport the patient for further evaluation.

Heat Stroke

Heat stroke is a life-threatening emergency. The mortality rate for untreated heat stroke is 80%. The primary and most important measure is to lower the body temperature. The following signs and symptoms are the classic triad for heat stroke:

• Altered mental status
• Elevated body temperature (>104° F [40° C])
• Hot, dry skin (However, many patients will have moist skin at the time of collapse.)

Heat stroke can occur in people of all ages. It results from a failure of the heat regulatory mechanism to respond to heat stress. Once the heat regulatory mechanisms are lost, the temperature quickly rises to dangerous levels. When the core body temperature rises to 107° F (41.6° C), direct damage to cells occurs, particularly to the cells in the brain and those lining the blood vessels. As mentioned earlier, situations that can lead to heat stroke include the athlete running in a marathon race on a hot, humid day; the debilitated, elderly patient with a fever who is covered with blankets in bed in a hot environment; and patients with preexisting conditions or who have taken drugs that inhibit sweating, increase metabolism, or affect cardiovascular performance and mental status.

Heat stroke is classically characterized by hot, dry skin. The importance of evaporation as a heat loss mechanism is underscored by this common finding. On hot, humid days, evaporation may represent the major (and only) existing means to dissipate heat from the body. Again, once this mechanism is lost, the internal body temperature increases rapidly to dangerous levels. However, many individuals are still sweating at the time of collapse from heat stroke. The temperature may not be measured at collapse and may be noted to be lower on arrival at the hospital after cooling measures have been applied. It is better to consider the possibility of heat illness as a cause of collapse for any patient on a hot, humid day or after vigorous exertion, whether the skin is moist or dry.

Signs and Symptoms

Heat stroke is characterized by an altered mental status, ranging from confusion to coma; high body temperature (≥104° F [40° C]); and hot, dry skin. The skin may be moist, however particularly in younger individuals who have undertaken strenuous activities, and dry skin should never be an absolute criterion for considering heat stroke.

Because of the increased blood flow to the skin resulting from vasodilation, most patients appear pink or flushed. Occasionally, however, a patient does not have adequate cardiac output to meet the increased demands of the skin, and the skin may appear ashen. The heart rate may be increased, as well as the respiratory rate. Some patients may be hypotensive. Seizures can occur.

Management

Lowering the body temperature of the patient with heat stroke is the highest priority. Efforts to reduce body temperature are more aggressive with heat stroke than with heat exhaustion or syncope. For patients with *heat exhaustion,* more passive efforts are often adequate, such as fanning, moving the patient to a cooler area, and removing restrictive or insulating clothing. Sheets or towels moistened with cool water can be applied, and air can be circulated by fans or by fanning to promote evaporation. For patients with *heat stroke,* these efforts are supplemented by applying ice packs to areas with large superficial blood vessels, such as the neck, armpits, and groin. Oxygen should be provided, and the patient should be quickly transported to the hospital.

The application of ice to all parts of the body in the field is controversial, as is immersion in ice-water baths. Although rapid lowering of body temperature is essential to successful treatment, it is important to follow local protocols, which may call for rapid transport to a hospital to initiate an ice bath. In the field, such aggressive measures present an additional problem. Patients with heat stroke have lost the thermoregulatory mechanism and can become hypothermic if overcooled. In hospitals, active cooling is stopped when the temperature reaches 102° F (38.8° C) to avoid this problem. This requires that a rectal temperature be obtained and monitored with a special probe that gives an accurate core body temperature.

> **LEARNING OBJECTIVES**
> • Recognize the signs and symptoms of water-related emergencies.

Drowning and Submersion Episodes

Approximately 4000 people drown in the United States each year. This number is estimated as many of the cases go unreported. **Drowning** is defined as respiratory impairment from submersion or immersion in a liquid medium. Not all persons who experience a drowning episode will die. Some persons will require immediate cardiopulmonary resuscitation by the EMT and others will die later due to complications associated with the drowning episode. Because of these complications all victims of a drowning episode should be transported for evaluation.

Typical drowning victims may have overestimated their endurance, been intoxicated, or may have fallen into the water and were unable to swim. The sequence of events often follows a pattern that includes panic, swallowing of water, and aspiration of water into the lungs. Sometimes, when water comes into contact with the vocal cords, the muscles spasm and close the glottis (entrance of the larynx) and initially prevent water from entering the lungs. The effects of water entering the lungs vary according to the type of drowning—salt water or fresh water—but this has no practical significance in terms of

resuscitation techniques. Whether a drowning episode occurs in salt water or fresh water, the major problem is *lack of oxygen.* Hypoxia results in unconsciousness and, ultimately, cardiac arrest.

The time to cardiac arrest may vary, particularly in cold water. Cold water can cool the core temperature and the basal metabolism and lessen the body's need for oxygen. In addition, patients may benefit from a response called the *mammalian diving reflex.* This mechanism slows metabolism, resulting in decreased oxygen consumption and redistribution of blood to more vital organs—brain, heart, and lungs. Both body cooling and the diving reflex are believed to be partly responsible for successful resuscitation after submersion for long periods, especially in cold water.

Management of Submersion Episodes

The first concern in a **submersion episode** is protection of the rescuers. A submersion episode is defined as any submersion requiring field care and transport to a hospital for treatment or observation. If possible, attempt to rescue the patient with a flotation device or a boat. Priority is given to the ABCs (airway, breathing, circulation). If the patient is unresponsive but breathing adequately, place the patient in the recovery position and administer supplemental oxygen. If breathing is inadequate, establish a patent airway. If necessary, you should begin suctioning and administer positive-pressure ventilation. High-concentration oxygen should be administered (100% if possible).

There is a distinction between clearing the airway and clearing the lungs of water. As with any other foreign substance, water in the upper airway should be removed by drainage or use of suction. Repeated suction may be necessary as fluids are expelled during positive-pressure ventilation. In addition, the patient may vomit and require suctioning. Vomiting is common; approximately 80% of submersion patients who receive CPR vomit. Most water will be absorbed into the central circulation during administration of positive-pressure ventilation.

The water swallowed during a submersion episode occasionally causes gastric distention and interferes with ventilation efforts. This is characterized by difficulty in the delivery of positive-pressure ventilation. These patients should be placed on their side and firm, gentle pressure applied to the epigastrium. Have suction ready to clear the airway if water is expelled. If no pulse is felt, cardiac compressions should be initiated. If the patient is in cardiac arrest, place the patient on a dry surface and towel-dry the chest wall before attaching the electrode pads of the AED.

Many drownings occur in shallow water as a result of diving incidents. If spinal injury is suspected, the patient should be removed from the water with alignment of the spine maintained. A long spine board or other floatable surface (e.g., surfboard) can be used to ensure proper immobilization during the rescue. The jaw thrust without head tilt maneuver should be used for these patients. In general, you should always suspect a spinal injury unless the patient was seen floundering or calling for help before submersion and the circumstances do not indicate a diving injury.

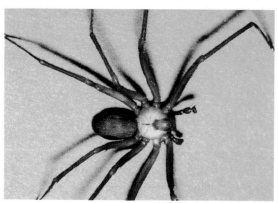

Figure 16-8 Brown recluse spider. *From Auerbach P: Wilderness medicine, ed 5, St Louis, 2007, Mosby.*

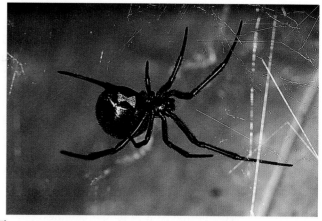

Figure 16-9 Mature female Western black widow spider. *From Auerbach P: Wilderness medicine, ed 5, St Louis, 2007, Mosby.*

> ### *LEARNING OBJECTIVE*
> • Discuss the emergency medical care of bites and stings.

Animal Bites and Stings

The most severe reaction to bites and stings is *anaphylaxis.* Other effects are usually local. Before swelling occurs, be sure to remove constricting clothing and jewelry. Watch for signs of allergic reaction and treat accordingly (see Chapter 14).

When an anaphylactic reaction is caused by a bite or sting, additional measures may be necessary to slow absorption. A constricting band should be placed above the bite or sting on an extremity. This band should be tight enough to restrict venous return but loose enough so that arterial flow is not obstructed. Check distal pulses. If the stinger or venom sac is present, remove it as quickly as possible. The manner of removal, whether scraping with the edge of a plastic card or pinching between thumb and forefinger and pulling out, is not important. The most important factor is not to delay removal because venom continues to be injected after the sting. Once the stinger is removed, you should place an ice pack over the bite or sting to cause vasoconstriction and further reduce the rate of absorption.

Insect and Spider Bites

Brown Recluse Spider

The bite of the brown recluse spider, which is found primarily in the southern United States but exists nationwide, can cause local *necrosis* (death of a portion of tissue) around the bite (**Figure 16-8**). This spider has a dark band on its back shaped like a violin. The venom causes local pain and then spreads from the bite site to the surrounding skin. Many patients are not aware that they have been bitten until they notice a painful red spot, sometimes with a central blister. The center darkens, the surrounding area blanches, and the outermost ring turns reddish, in some cases leading to a bull's-eye appearance. Few individuals have systemic reactions, which consist of fever, chills, and weakness and, in the worst cases, problems with the breakdown of blood cells and clotting mechanisms. The treatment for systemic complaints is hospital based.

Black Widow Spider

The black widow spider is more common and is found throughout the United States (**Figure 16-9**). The female has a characteristic shiny black body with a red hourglass shape on the abdomen. The venom contains a neurotoxin, and in severe cases it can cause weakness and respiratory depression. The usual symptoms are pain at the site of the bite, abdominal pain, and lower-extremity weakness. Slight swelling and faint bite marks may occur at the site of the bite. Rigidity and tenderness of the abdominal muscles occur in addition to fever, chills, rigidity, and spasms of other large muscle groups. Antivenin is available for severe cases. The need for antivenin in all but the most extreme cases has been questioned. Small children and debilitated adults are believed to be most susceptible to severe consequences. Black widow spider bite should be treated similar to snakebite. You should immobilize the extremity as if it were fractured and avoid unnecessary movement.

Fire Ants

Fire ants, found in the southern part of the United States, can inflict multiple stings if encountered in the loose mounds of dirt that they inhabit. Each sting can cause a small, circumscribed, elevated lesion, which produces pus in 6 to 24 hours. Care is supportive.

Ticks

Ticks are small parasites that live off the blood of mammals and birds. They attach themselves to their host by a harpoon-type structure at their mouth and are difficult to remove. Ticks are responsible for the spread of many diseases, including Lyme disease, Rocky Mountain spotted fever, tularemia, equine encephalitis, and Colorado tick fever. Treatment is supportive. Do not attempt to remove the tick. Assess the patient for signs of transmitted disease, such as muscle aches or headache.

Scorpions and Tarantulas

Scorpion stings, primarily occurring in the southwestern United States, cause local pain but are rarely fatal. Systemic effects can occur with scorpion stings. In addition to *paresthesias,* or unpleasant tingling feelings both at the site of envenomation and at distant sites, patients with severe reactions may have problems with vision and swallowing and slurred speech, as well as excess salivation and involuntary jerking and shaking of skeletal muscles. Prehospital care is supportive. For severe cases an antivenin is sometimes used.

Tarantulas usually cause local pain at the bite site, occasionally followed by redness and swelling. Local wound care and elevation and immobilization of an extremity may help control pain.

Bees and Wasps

Wasps and bees are flying insects that attack humans only in defense. Typically the insect is accidentally stepped on or the nest is disturbed. Bees are drawn to sweet beverages and will crawl into the container, stinging the drinker in the mouth or throat. Bee and wasp stings are painful and cause local irritation with a red, inflamed appearance. In some cases the stinger will break off in the patient's skin. The primary concern with these stings is systemic allergies and anaphylactic reactions, which must be treated aggressively (see Chapter14).

Snakebite

Venomous snakes in the United States include the pit viper (rattlesnake, cottonmouth, copperhead) and coral snake (**Figure 16-10**). The *pit viper* bite causes local necrosis; in severe cases, systemic effects occur, and death may result. Definitive care requires the use of antivenin. The bite of the *coral snake* causes no local necrosis. The nervous system is affected when the poison is absorbed. The onset of effects may be delayed up to 12 hours after envenomation. The systemic effects from coral snake bites can lead to respiratory paralysis and death. Because of the different actions of pit viper and coral snake venom, it is important from the outset to distinguish the type of snake, determine whether envenomation took place, and apply treatment accordingly.

Antivenin is available to treat severe envenomation. Controversy exists as to the best field therapy. It is generally agreed that because *coral snakes* kill by systemic effects and do not damage the tissues at the bite site, methods to delay absorption from the wound are a principal aim of treatment. Conversely, because *pit viper* bites are apt to cause local tissue damage, many experts do not recommend attempts to contain the venom at the bite site, where it can lead to more severe necrosis. Concentration of pit viper venom in an extremity may cause loss of the entire limb.

Pit Vipers

Recognition. Pit vipers can be distinguished from nonpoisonous snakes by their elliptical pupils, the "pit" (heat sensor) between the eyes and nostril, fangs, and the single row of plates on the tail. The bite is noted by the presence of fang marks at the bite site (**Figure 16-11**). The fangs are needle-sharp and inject the venom. Other common symptoms of a pit viper bite are swelling, pain, and redness at the site.

Coral Snakes

Recognition. Coral snakes are found in the southern United States. They are distinguished by their red, yellow, and black bands. The red and yellow bands on the coral snake are next to each other, thus the saying: "Red on yellow, kill a fellow; red on black, venom lack." This saying is useful to help distinguish the North American coral snake from nonvenomous lookalikes such as the king snake.

Coral snakes have tiny fangs that are close together, and their bite marks are more noteworthy than their fang marks. A drop of blood may be expressed after envenomation, confirming that fangs entered the skin. Often the coral snake holds onto and "chews" the victim for a few seconds and must be pulled off. Victims have described this sensation as similar to "pulling off Velcro." Early signs and symptoms may be mild, and usually only minimal redness and swelling are present at the bite site. In contrast, pit viper bites are marked by early pain and swelling at the site.

Management

Definitive snakebite treatment involves early antivenin administration.

When approaching the snakebite victim, do the following:
1. Move out of range of the snake. Although the rattlesnake's maximum speed is about 3 mph (human walking speed), it can strike at a speed of 8 feet per second and reach distances of approximately one-half its body length.
2. Observe the approximate size of the snake; the larger the snake, the greater the potential envenomation.
3. Look for presence of fang marks or small puncture wounds that may or may not be teeth marks. Pain is an early symptom, followed by swelling. Blood may continue to ooze from the fang marks, and ecchymosis may be noted both near and away from the bite.
4. Have the patient rest. Remove any jewelry, and immobilize the extremity as you would for a fracture.
5. If swelling is present, make a small mark at its edge so that any changes are evident on later evaluation.
6. Transport the patient to the closest hospital that is able to care for snakebites.

   If possible, bring the dead snake (or have it brought) to the hospital for identification. Do not handle the dead snake directly, not even the decapitated head, because reflex actions of the snake can cause envenomation.
7. For coral snake bites, many experts recommend application of a "loose" elastic bandage above or around the bite site to slow systemic absorption until antivenin can be given. If a constricting bandage is applied proximal to the wound, it should allow one finger to enter beneath it and not obliterate distal pulsations (**Figure 16-12**).

Most authorities recommend against using ice and cutting the wound and sucking out the venom. Learn and follow local protocols.

Exotic poisonous snakes may be kept as pets. Pet owners or friends are often bitten when they are intoxicated and handle

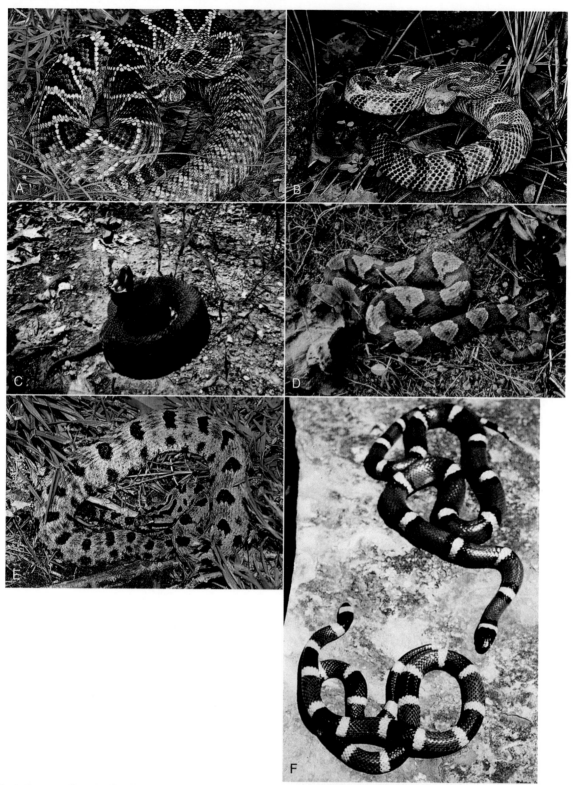

Figure 16-10 A, Eastern diamondback rattlesnake is the largest pit viper in the United States and can reach 6 feet in length. **B,** Timber rattlesnake is a large, dangerous snake of the eastern United States. **C,** Cottonmouth water moccasin exhibiting its threat display. The snake is most often found around standing water sources in the southeastern United States. **D,** Southern copperhead has markings that make it almost invisible when lying in leaf litter. **E,** Western pygmy rattlesnake is one of the smaller rattlesnake species of North America, generally less than 2 feet in length. **F,** Comparison of Texas coral snake with harmless Mexican milk snake. Coral snake *(bottom)* has contiguous red and yellow bands, whereas the milk snake has its red and yellow bands separated by black. Carefully noting the markings on a snake, such as these colored bands, may help in subsequent identification. *From Auerbach P:* Wilderness medicine, *ed 5, St Louis, 2007, Mosby.*

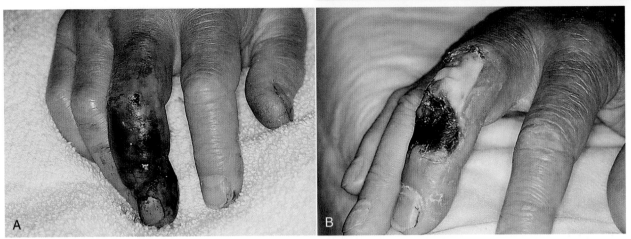

Figure 16-11 Pit viper bite. **A,** Soft tissue swelling and early necrosis after red diamond rattlesnake bite to the long finger (day 2). **B,** Seven weeks later. Note the degree of necrosis (death of tissue). *From Auerbach P:* Wilderness medicine, *ed 5, St Louis, 2007, Mosby.*

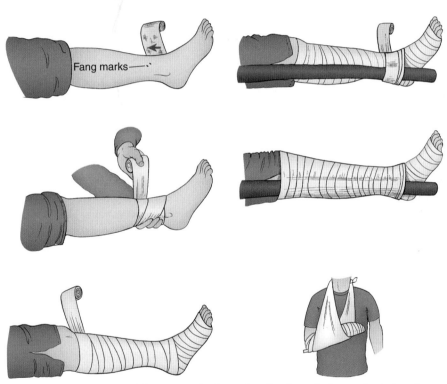

Figure 16-12 Australian compression and immobilization technique. Application of a loose elastic bandage around and above snakebite to minimize absorption of the venom. Roll a broad elastic bandage over the bite, and continue up the extremity as if treating a sprain. Splint the extremity and keep it at heart level. This technique may be useful for coral snake bites. *From Auerbach P:* Wilderness medicine, *ed 5, St Louis, 2007, Mosby.*

these snakes carelessly. Because keeping venomous snakes is illegal, persons bitten in this way may hide the true history.

Marine Animals

Certain sea animals can also cause stings and punctures. Stinging animals include the jellyfish, the Portuguese man-of-war, anemones, and species of coral. Treatment consists of flooding the affected area with sea water (never fresh water) and washing with acetic acid 5% (vinegar) or isopropyl alcohol. Another recommendation is to apply shaving cream, sand, or talcum powder to the area and then scrape it off to remove any remaining tentacles and nematocysts, which cause the stinging. Avoid washing the area with fresh water because this may cause the nematocysts to release more "stingers."

Punctures can occur from cone shells, urchins, stingrays, and spiny fish. Treatment consists of immobilizing the affected area and soaking it in water as hot as the patient can tolerate for 30 to 90 minutes. Be careful to avoid water that could cause heat injury; check it with your hand. The toxin introduced into the wound should be inactivated by the hot water.

LEARNING OBJECTIVES
• Describe the pressure laws associated with diving emergencies.
• Explain the steps in providing emergency medical care to a patient suffering from a diving incident.

Diving Emergencies

Incidence

Recreational "scuba" diving has become a popular sport over the last 20 years. The Divers Alert Network (DAN) estimates that 9 million certified divers reside in the United States. Diving is a relatively safe sport, with an estimated 900 to 1000 divers treated for dive-related injuries and 90 dive-related deaths each year.

Risk Factors

Divers who are not properly trained or certified are at an increased risk for injury. Other factors that increase risks are being in poor shape and not allowing enough time between dives. The use of drugs or alcohol may also put a diver at risk.

Prevention

SCUBA. SCUBA stands for "self-contained underwater breathing apparatus." The term *scuba* is used to identify state-of-the-art diving equipment designed to protect the diver (scuba suits, tanks, and regulators).

DAN. A not-for-profit organization that provides emergency medical advice and assistance for underwater diving injuries, DAN underwrites a wide range of research, education, and training programs that promote safe diving. The group offers assistance 24 hours a day, 7 days a week for injured divers. DAN also offers insurance for members that will cover treatment for dive-related injuries.

Physiology

Pressure Laws

Most dive injuries are associated with the pressure changes occurring as the diver descends and ascends. A brief review of pressure laws can help you better understand these injuries. Specific injuries are discussed later.

Boyle's Law. Boyle's law states that at a constant temperature, the volume of a gas is inversely proportional to the pressure exerted on it. In application, Boyle's law states that gas contained within a container, such as the lungs, intestines, or ears, will condense or expand based on the atmospheric pressure. As altitude increases, atmospheric pressure decreases, allowing gases to expand. People experience this law when they travel through mountains or fly in an airplane and have their ears "pop" as the altitude increases or decreases.

Henry's Law. Henry's law states that the pressure of a gas dissolved in a liquid is directly proportional to the partial pressure of that gas above the solution, or the mass of a gas that dissolves in a volume of liquid is proportional to the pressure of the gas. In application, Henry's law states the higher the pressure surrounding the body, the more gas will be absorbed. The human body functions well at normal atmospheric pressure. As the body is exposed to higher pressures, as in diving, more of the gases in our bodies, such as oxygen and nitrogen, will dissolve and will be absorbed, resulting in toxic levels.

Dalton's Law. Dalton's law states that the total pressure exerted by a mixture of gases is equal to the sum of the pressure of each of the different gases making up the mixture. In application, if oxygen created 20% and nitrogen 80% of the pressure, as a person dives, inserting pressure on the body, Henry's law states that the pressure and solubility of the gases increase, and Dalton's law states that the ratio of gases will remain 20:80.

Dysbarism

Dysbarism is a generalized term used to describe the physiologic changes seen when a person is exposed to pressure changes. The majority of the body is water and is not affected by pressure changes. Areas of the body filled with air, such as hollow organs and the lungs, have the greatest potential to be affected. As gases contract and expand, structures can be stretched or can collapse, causing pain and shortness of breath.

Decompression Sickness

As the body descends to depths, gases in the body are dissolved as described by Henry's law. If the diver ascends too quickly, the gases may form bubbles as the pressure on the body decreases. These bubbles can become trapped within the bloodstream, stretching vessel walls and disrupting clotting functions. This is known as *decompression sickness,* sometimes called "the bends." Signs of decompression sickness range from pain and itching to shortness of breath, shock, and death.

Treatment for all the conditions discussed here is first symptomatic, maintaining the ABCs. Second, the patient should be transported to a hospital with a *hyperbaric oxygen chamber* (HBO). These specialized chambers pressurize the patient and allow gases to return to their normal status.

Barotrauma

Air-filled chambers in the body are most susceptible to pressure changes. As a diver descends, the pressure placed on the body compresses areas such as the ears and lungs. While descending, divers must stop to equalize the pressure in their ears. As noted, people flying in an airplane or driving in the mountains often describe a "popping" in their ears. On the ascent, the ears and lungs are again susceptible to pressure. If a diver ascends too quickly, the pressure in their ears may increase, causing them to rupture, or may cause a pneumothorax if the pressure increases too quickly in the lungs.

Arterial Gas Embolism

If the lungs are damaged during ascent as just described, the diver is at risk for an arterial gas embolism. If the alveoli are damaged, air may be drawn into the arterial circulatory system. The air will move as an embolism, becoming potentially deadly. Signs of an arterial gas embolism include shortness of breath, seizure, paralysis, and weakness. Most cases present within 10 minutes of surfacing from the dive.

Nitrogen Narcosis

Nitrogen narcosis is also known as "raptures of the deep." As a diver descends, nitrogen in the body is affected as described in Dalton's law, dissolves in the bloodstream, and works as a narcotic drug. Nitrogen narcosis usually causes problems while the diver is at depth. Divers have been reported to forget to surface, take off their breathing apparatus, or otherwise act illogically.

> **LEARNING OBJECTIVES**
> - Describe the types of high-altitude illnesses.
> - Explain the steps in providing emergency medical care to a patient suffering from a high-altitude illness.

Altitude Illness

Incidence

High-altitude illnesses are seen in men and women with equal frequency. The less severe forms (e.g., acute mountain sickness) have been reported in 15% to 40% of skiers traveling from low to high altitude. The more severe types (e.g., high-altitude pulmonary edema) occur less frequently, in about 1% to 2% of patients at altitude.

Physiology

Altitude illness occurs when a person rapidly ascends to a higher altitude. At higher altitudes there is less atmospheric pressure, which can affect pressure gradients within the body. When pressures within the body or surrounding the body are changed rapidly, fluid may be forced across membranes, resulting in swelling. Other factors can increase the severity of the fluid shifts, such as dehydration, alcohol consumption, and age.

Types

High-Altitude Cerebral Edema

High-altitude cerebral edema (HACE) is the swelling of the brain following rapid ascent to altitude. Signs of HACE can mimic a stroke. Patients may present with a headache and alterations in vision and hearing. Their level of consciousness will change rapidly, from anxious and combative to unresponsive and eventually unconsciousness. They may have systemic neurologic deficits, such as weakness or paralysis, which tend to be bilateral rather than unilateral, as seen in a stroke. Nausea and vomiting may also occur, causing airway concerns.

High-Altitude Pulmonary Edema

High-altitude pulmonary edema (HAPE) is fluid pushed into the alveolar spaces as a person ascends rapidly to a high altitude. This is a life-threatening situation because the person is rapidly becoming hypoxic, with signs and symptoms of extreme shortness of breath. Patients may have a productive cough and cyanosis. Breath sounds will reveal bilateral rales and rhonchi or coarse crackles. Patients may develop an altered level of consciousness, ranging from anxiousness to unconsciousness.

Acute Mountain Sickness

Acute mountain sickness (AMS) is not as severe as HAPE or HACE. AMS can initially resemble the flu. Patients may present with body and muscle aches, headaches, and nausea. They may become lethargic.

Treatment

Treatment for all altitude illnesses is similar. First, the airway must by monitored and controlled. High-flow oxygen, suction, and airway adjuncts must be used as necessary. The primary focus of treatment is to bring the patient to a lower altitude. If advanced life support (ALS) personnel are available, they may be able to provide pharmacologic assistance, but this provides only temporary relief. The focus remains a rapid descent to a lower altitude.

> **Case in Point**
>
> A 54-year-old Florida resident goes on a ski trip in the Colorado mountains with his college buddies. He has a late first night "catching up" with friends and consumes much more alcohol than his usual intake.
>
> After arriving at the ski area the next morning, the man, excited to begin skiing, immediately jumps on the lift to the peak run at the top of the mountain. As he reaches the peak, he begins to develop extreme shortness of breath. Ski patrol officers recognize his distress and call for EMS to meet them at the bottom of the mountain.
>
> On physical assessment of the patient, the EMTs discover extreme shortness of breath with bilateral pulmonary edema. They quickly place the patient on a nonrebreather oxygen mask and prepare him for transport. They maintain the suction unit and bag-mask at their side in the event the patient should become worse. The EMTs recognize the signs of HAPE and know the patient needs to be transported to a lower altitude quickly.

Scenario Follow-up

At the hospital the patient was found to have a core temperature of 106° F (41° C). The ED physician was pleased with your evaluation of the scene and recognition of the heat-related emergency. The ED began aggressive cooling and rehydration procedures. As the patient's temperature dropped the ED staff was diligent in monitoring all body systems such as cardiac, renal, and neurogenic. The patient eventually regained consciousness and was released from the hospital 10 days postadmission with no deficits.

Summary

Heat and cold emergencies are frequently encountered by EMTs and range from minor local cold injuries or heat cramps to severe generalized hypothermia or heat stroke. Often the assessment that a patient is ill from extremes of temperature is suspected from the environment and the scene size-up. At other times, the EMT must maintain a high index of suspicion because patients may have had heat or cold exposure in less-than-extreme conditions. Knowledge of how the body deals with maintaining a constant temperature, including generating heat from metabolism and muscular activity and mechanisms of heat loss, is helpful. Risk factors such as extremes of age, underlying medical conditions, and drug and alcohol ingestion should be considered during evaluation. Treatment of heat emergencies is directed at rapid reduction of body temperatures and restoration of depleted fluids. Treatment of cold emergencies is aimed at preventing further heat loss and injury to local parts and rapid transport to a hospital environment, where active rewarming can be initiated. Because cold decreases metabolism, patients with a low body temperature may benefit from prolonged resuscitation efforts.

Drowning and submersion episodes are extreme environmental emergencies. The safety of the rescuer is the first concern. Associated cervical spine injuries should be suspected and the patient treated accordingly. Management of cardiopulmonary arrest is essentially the same as for all patients. Victims of cold-water drowning may be resuscitated even after sustained periods of immersion.

Bites and stings from insects, snakes, and marine animals can cause local pain and irritation or generalized allergic or toxic effects. Be alert for signs of allergic reaction and treat accordingly. Severe toxic reactions may require the use of antidotes, which are available in regional hospitals or through poison control centers.

For altitude illnesses (e.g. HACE, HAPE, AMS), treatment focuses on a rapid descent to a lower altitude.

The Bottom Line

Learning Checklist

✓ The five ways that heat can be lost from the body are *radiation* (transfer of heat from a warmer to cooler environment), *conduction* (transfer of heat from an object in contact with the body), *convection* (loss of heat from air currents around the body), *evaporation* (loss of heat through evaporation of water from the body's surface), and *breathing* (loss of heat through exhaled air).

✓ Shivering is an involuntary mechanism that the body uses to produce heat.

✓ Shivering is a sign of mild hypothermia and stops when the body temperature is lower than 87.8° F (31° C). *stops*

✓ Signs of mild hypothermia include shivering, amnesia, and poor muscle coordination.

✓ Signs of moderate hypothermia include stupor and loss of consciousness, cessation of shivering, irregular pulse, dilated pupils, and loss of voluntary motion.

✓ Signs of severe hypothermia include unresponsiveness to pain, significant hypotension, and cardiac arrest from ventricular fibrillation.

✓ General care of the hypothermic patient includes gentle handling, removal of wet clothing, keeping the patient warm, protecting the patient from wind, and providing warm, high-carbohydrate drinks to the conscious patient who has an intact gag reflex.

✓ Continue resuscitation for patients with hypothermia until the patient has been warmed.

✓ Check a suspected hypothermia patient's pulse for 30 to 45 seconds before administering CPR because the pulse may be blunted, slow, and difficult to detect.

✓ If a hypothermic patient goes into cardiac arrest, apply shocks up to three times with an automated external defibrillator (AED). Withhold additional shocks if the temperature is below 86° F (30° C) until the body is rewarmed above this temperature.

✓ Internal active rewarming techniques include warmed intravenous fluids, warmed humidified oxygen, peritoneal dialysis, hemodialysis, and instillation of heated fluids into the gastrointestinal tract.

✓ Internal active rewarming techniques may be needed to rewarm the hypothermic patient at the hospital. These techniques are rarely used in prehospital care.

✓ Severe vasoconstriction of the superficial areas of the body that occurs from hypothermia can lead to frostbite.

✓ Three types of local cold injuries are frostnip, superficial frostbite, and deep frostbite.

✓ Frostnip is a type of local cold injury characterized by pale, cold skin that loses sensation and becomes red and itchy on warming.

✓ Superficial frostbite is characterized by freezing of the upper layer of skin while the deep skin remains soft. Signs include white, waxy skin that is hard on the surface and soft below.

✓ Deep frostbite is characterized by freezing of the upper and deeper layers of skin. It appears white, feels frozen, and resists depression.

✓ Treatment of a mild or moderate frostbitten extremity includes removing jewelry, applying a dressing to the affected part, removing wet clothing, covering the part, and preventing further exposure to moisture. Do not rub or massage the part.

✓ Rapid rewarming is a technique in which the affected part is placed in 105° F (40.6° C) water until warmed. This technique is used at the hospital and possibly in the field when transport is delayed.

✓ There are three types of heat emergencies: heat cramps, heat exhaustion, and heat stroke. Two other heat-related illnesses are heat rash and heat syncope.

✓ Heat cramps are muscular cramps caused by strenuous exertion and excessive loss of body fluids and electrolytes.

✓ Move patients with heat cramps to a cooler environment, and provide water or a dilute electrolyte solution.

✓ Heat exhaustion is caused by the cardiovascular system's inability to provide blood flow to the skin while maintaining flow to skeletal muscle and other organs.

✓ Signs of heat exhaustion include weakness or exhaustion, faintness, pale skin (sometimes pink), rapid pulse, hypotension when sitting (or normal vital signs), headache, and nausea.

✓ Move patients with heat exhaustion to a cooler environment, loosen or remove clothing that may interfere with heat loss, place in the supine position (with legs elevated), provide 1 to 2 L of water to drink, and fan to increase the rate of cooling.

✓ Heat stroke is caused by failure of the body's heat loss mechanisms and the development of extremely high temperature (above 104° F [40° C]).

✓ Signs of heat stroke include altered mental status; hot, dry skin (may be moist); rapid pulse and respiratory rate; hypotension; and seizures.

✓ Treatment of heat stroke includes moving the patient to a cooler environment; administering high-concentration oxygen; cooling with a sponge or wet towels (and fanning); placing ice packs in the armpits, groin, and back of neck; and rapidly transporting to the hospital.

✓ When rescuing a drowning victim, rescuer safety is a priority. When possible, throw flotation devices to the victim or use a boat to remove the victim from the water.

✓ If a submersion patient is unresponsive and breathing adequately, provide supplemental oxygen and place the patient in the recovery position.

✓ Management of a submersion patient in cardiac arrest includes establishing an airway, providing rescue breathing and chest compressions if needed, and use of an AED for ventricular fibrillation. Provide up to three shocks with an AED for the patient who is severely hypothermic (temperature <86° F [30° C]).

✓ Spider bites may result in serious but rare complications such as bleeding disorders and can present with fever, chills, and weakness (brown recluse) or muscular rigidity (black widow).

✓ Prehospital care of insect bites includes supportive care, cleaning of the site, removing the stinger, and immobilizing the extremity.

✓ Poisonous snakes in the United States include pit vipers (copperheads, rattlesnakes) and coral snakes.

✓ Management of poisonous snake bites includes immobilizing the affected part with a splint, marking the edges of the swollen area to note changes later, and transporting to an appropriate hospital.

✓ Coral snake bites may also require the application of an elastic bandage around the bite and the limb, as if wrapping a sprain, to limit absorption of the venom, if directed by local protocols.

✓ Stings from marine animals (e.g., jellyfish, anemones) should be flooded with sea water (not fresh water) and rinsed with vinegar or alcohol. Punctures from cone shells, urchins, stingrays, and spiny fish are treated by immobilizing the area and soaking with hot water to inactivate their toxin.

✓ Diving emergencies include decompression sickness, barotrauma, arterial gas embolism, and nitrogen narcosis. Treatment is symptomatic (ABCs) followed by transport for hyperbaric treatment.

✓ Rapid ascent to an altitude can result in life threatening conditions such as cerebral edema and pulmonary edema. Treatment for altitude illnesses consists of airway management and rapid descent to a lower altitude.

Key Terms

Acute mountain sickness (AMS) General weakness, lethargy, and cognitive changes following a rapid ascent to a high altitude.

Conduction Transfer of heat to objects (including air) in direct contact with the body.

Convection Transfer of heat through the movement of air currents.

Drowning Respiratory impairment from submersion or immersion in a liquid medium.

Evaporation Loss of heat when moisture vaporizes on the body's surface.

Frostbite Injury to the skin caused by prolonged exposure to cold; liquid content of the skin cells freezes; may be superficial or deep.

Frostnip Completely reversible superficial cold injury caused by intense vasoconstriction that affects only the topmost portions of the skin.

High-altitude cerebral edema (HACE) Cerebral edema following a rapid ascent to a high altitude.

High-altitude pulmonary edema (HAPE) Pulmonary edema following a rapid ascent to a high altitude.

Hypothermia Abnormal and dangerous condition in which the body temperature falls below 95° F (35° C) and the body's normal functions are impaired; usually caused by prolonged exposure to cold.

Radiation Transfer of heat by infrared heat rays. Heat rays are radiated by the body and other objects in the environment. If the temperature of the body is greater than the temperature of the surroundings, heat is lost from the body.

Submersion episode Any submersion into water that requires field care and transport to a hospital for treatment or observation.

Review Questions

Questions 1-5. Match the description of heat loss in column B with the mechanism in column A.

Column A

1. Conduction
2. Evaporation
3. Convection
4. Radiation
5. Breathing

Column B

a. Transfer of heat by infrared rays from objects in a warmer environment to objects in a cooler environment.
b. Transfer of heat to objects in direct contact with the body.
c. Loss of heat as cool air passes through the respiratory tract.
d. Loss of heat when moisture vaporizes on the body surface.
e. Heat carried away by air currents.

6. Which of the following is *true* about shivering?
   a. It causes sweating.
   b. It is a voluntary activity.
   c. It may stop at low body temperature.
   d. Drugs and alcohol do not affect it.

7. Which of the following is a sign of local cold injury?
   a. Normal sensation
   b. Pink skin at the injury
   c. Skin possibly firm or frozen to touch
   d. Full range of motion

8. What is the most important treatment of a patient with hot, dry skin and altered mental status resulting from heat exposure?
   a. Administration of fluids.
   b. Rapid cooling of body temperature.
   c. Keeping the head elevated.
   d. Giving salt tablets.

9. Management of the submersion patient may include:
   a. Routine use of abdominal thrusts.
   b. Placing the patient on the left side to facilitate drainage from the upper airway.
   c. Vigorous deep suctioning of the lungs.
   d. Routine stomach emptying.

10. An EMT arrives at the parking lot of a pond and is asked to prepare for rescue of a potential drowning victim who has fallen through the ice. The EMT discovers his gloves and winter hat have been left behind. The temperature is −10° F, with 15-mph wind. How long being exposed to these conditions might lead to frostbite?
  a. 5 minutes
  b. 10 minutes
  c. 30 minutes
  d. 120 minutes

For Further Review

In the Student Workbook

- Multiple-choice questions
- Matching questions
- Short-answer questions
- True-false questions
- Case scenario questions
- Crossword puzzle

On Evolve

- Weblinks
- Lecture notes
- Exercises

Learning Objectives

Cognitive Objectives

- Describe the various ways that the body loses heat.
- List the signs and symptoms of exposure to cold.
- Explain the steps in providing emergency medical care to a patient exposed to cold.
- List the signs and symptoms of exposure to heat.
- Explain the steps in providing emergency care to a patient exposed to heat.
- Recognize the signs and symptoms of water-related emergencies.
- Discuss the emergency medical care of bites and stings.
- Describe the pressure laws associated with diving emergencies.
- Explain the steps in providing emergency medical care to a patient suffering from a diving incident.
- Describe the types of high-altitude illnesses.
- Explain the steps in providing emergency medical care to a patient suffering from a high-altitude illness.

Psychomotor Objectives

- Demonstrate the assessment and emergency medical care of a patient with exposure to cold.
- Demonstrate the assessment and emergency medical care of a patient with exposure to heat.
- Demonstrate the assessment and emergency medical care of a patient experiencing a water-related emergency.
- Demonstrate completing a prehospital care report for patients with environmental emergencies.

References

Divers Alert Network: *Report on decompression illness and diving fatalities: DAN's annual review of recreational scuba diving injuries and fatalities based on 1998 data,* Durham, NC, 2000, DAN.

Federal Emergency Management Agency, US Fire Administration: *Emergency incident rehabilitation,* FA-114, July 1992.

Idris AH, Berg RA, Bierens J, et al: Recommended guidlines for uniform reporting of data from drowning: the "Utstein Style," *Circulation* 108: 2565, 2003. http://www.emedicine.com/med/topic1956.htm.

http://www.nhtsa.dot.gov/people/injury/enforce/ChildrenAndCars/index.htm. August 2007.

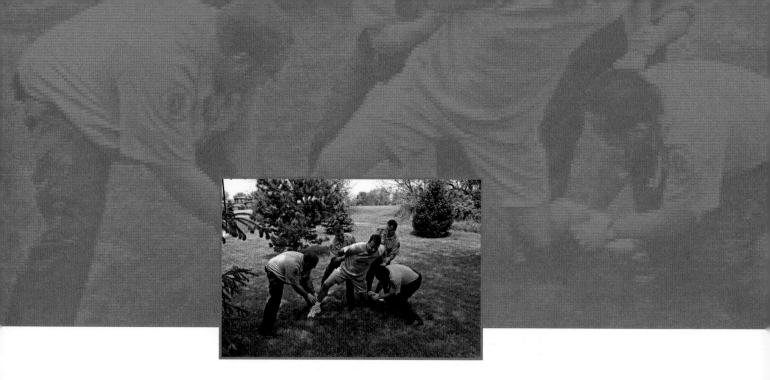

17 Behavioral Emergencies

CHAPTER OUTLINE

Scenario

You respond to a high-priority dispatch for a "male overdose." Police are already on the scene. As you enter the house, you note that the 16-year-old patient is acting strangely and appears intoxicated, confused, and angry. He is uncooperative with police officers. His mother, who called for help, tells you that he recently broke up with his girlfriend and since then has been distraught and depressed and talking about suicide. Today he has apparently been drinking large quantities of alcohol, as well as ingesting pills taken from the bathroom cabinet. You note two empty medication bottles on the floor near the patient, one for generic acetaminophen and the other a prescription antidepressant.

You observe that the patient becomes agitated and combative when approached and is refusing evaluation and threatens to harm you if you attempt to touch him; he is refusing to be interviewed, examined, or transported. You maintain a distance as you identify yourself and speak to him in a calm, reassuring voice, being direct and respectful. Despite all attempts to calm this agitated patient and provide medical care for this potentially unstable overdose, the patient continues to refuse any assessment or treatment.

After performing a thorough mental status examination, you ascertain that the patient lacks judgment and insight into his condition and clearly lacks the capacity to refuse care and transport. You confer with online medical direction, the patient's mother, and police, and all agree that restraint is necessary to ensure the safety of the patient and crew during transport. Using effective restraint techniques, you, your crew, and the police restrain the patient in the supine position, allowing frequent reassessment of the patient's airway and vital signs, monitoring for signs of clinical instability from the overdose. By appropriately restraining the patient, you are able to recognize and manage the respiratory depression that develops en route to the hospital.

The Emergency Medical Services Act of 1973 outlined seven disease-specific categories around which emergency medical services (EMS) systems would be designed. Because the U.S. government recognized the seriousness of "behavioral emergencies," they were included as one of the categories.

Behavior is defined as the manner in which a person acts or performs, including any or all of the person's physical and mental activities. A **psychobehavioral disorder** is any of various forms of behavior that are considered inappropriate by members of the social group to which an individual belongs. Psychobehavioral disorders include *thought disorders* (psychosis, schizophrenia), mood disorders (depression, bipolar disorder), *anxiety disorders* (panic attack, obsessive-compulsive disorder), personality disorders, addictive disorders (substance abuse, eating disorders), organic brain syndromes (delirium, dementia, drug intoxication/withdrawal), and risks for suicide and homicide. A **behavioral emergency** exists whenever an individual demonstrates actual or threatened/potential behavior of a violent, aggressive, or assaultive nature. It may arise from a variety of personal and situational factors, may manifest verbally or physically, and may result in harm to the individual and others.

Box 17-1	Common Causes of Behavior Alteration

Low blood sugar level
Low blood oxygen level
Hypoperfusion/inadequate blood flow to brain (e.g., shock, stroke)
Head trauma
Mind-altering substances
Psychogenic cause, resulting in psychotic thinking, depression, or panic
Excessive cold (hypothermia)
Excessive heat (hyperthermia)
Meningitis/encephalitis
Seizure disorders
Toxic ingestion, overdose
Withdrawal of drugs or alcohol
Polypharmacy (multiple medications causing interactions; especially in elderly)

Factors that may alter a patient's behavior, leading to violence or other inappropriate action, can be caused by situational stresses and emotional extremes, psychiatric problems, alcohol and other drugs, and medical conditions such as lack of oxygen, low blood glucose, toxic ingestion, hypoperfusion, infection, head trauma, and electrolyte imbalance (**Box 17-1**).

Caring for patients with behavioral disorders is an area of medicine that is highly subjective, especially for providers not specifically trained in psychiatry or psychology. Therefore the standards and guidelines for prehospital care are necessarily general in nature.

Probably no other area of medicine requires more careful judgment and experience or presents a greater danger of displaying an inappropriate bias or reacting negatively to patients than behavioral disorders. This area also may involve a high risk of personal injury for patients, family members, bystanders, and EMS providers. This chapter introduces one of the most complex areas that you will encounter as an emergency medical technician (EMT).

Behavioral emergencies can be generally categorized by the type of behavior displayed, such as depression, rage, anxiety, or an attempt at suicide, or by the cause of the behavior, such as psychosis, hypoglycemia, or head trauma. Behavioral emergencies do not always occur in isolation; often an emotional component is superimposed on an acute medical illness.

This chapter discusses the magnitude of the problem of psychobehavioral disorders, types and causes of behavioral emergencies, and evaluation and treatment.

LEARNING OBJECTIVES
- Define psychobehavioral disorders and behavioral emergencies.
- Explain the rationale for learning how to modify your behavior toward the patient with a behavioral emergency.

Scope of the Problem

The medical profession often focuses its greatest attention on diseases and conditions that are understandable, measurable, and treatable, such as heart attacks and pneumonia. Because your EMT training emphasizes medical and traumatic conditions, you may view heart attacks as "real" problems and behavioral conditions as "lesser" problems and not as important. This is not true, however, and behavioral emergencies present a great challenge and require much professionalism and compassion.

Morbidity and mortality statistics suggest that psychobehavioral disorders are of major significance. An estimated 26.2% of the U.S. population is affected by mental disorders during a given year. Depression affects 14.8 million Americans, schizophrenia 2.4 million, bipolar disorder 5.7 million, and panic disorder 6 million.

Healthcare providers may tend to discount symptoms in people who are difficult, demanding, angry, agitated and panicky, intoxicated, or "crazy." This is a normal human reaction, but it can lead to dangerous medical judgments. Many physical diseases present with behavioral manifestations, and many behavioral problems present with physical complaints. You must maintain your focus to evaluate and treat and not to judge, discount the potential seriousness of a complaint, or become angry with a noncompliant patient. This can be difficult when caring for a patient who is aggressive, abusive, or irrational. It is a natural tendency to discredit the importance of symptoms in people who are emotionally distraught. The interaction between you and the patient often occurs in a highly charged atmosphere, where a person is intensely concerned about his or her well-being, anxiety levels are high, and multiple distractions in the environment can interfere with successful care of the patient.

As you learn about behavioral emergencies, you should focus on the following principles in every case:

1. Maintain the safety of yourself, others, and the patient.
2. Always consider the possibility of an underlying medical cause, and especially consider whether the patient may need oxygen or glucose.
3. If the patient does not want to go to the hospital, ask if there is a need for care or transport against the patient's will. Generally, this is done only when there is a reasonable belief that the patient will harm self or others.
4. When patient restraint is necessary, do so in a manner that minimizes any harm to the patient, EMT, and others and allows you to monitor the patient en route. Restraining the patient must also be done in accordance with local laws and protocols. Always try to involve law enforcement professionals to assist in patient restraint.
5. Maintain a professional and nonjudgmental attitude and demeanor at all times.

LEARNING OBJECTIVES
- Discuss the general factors that may cause an alteration in a patient's behavior.
- State the various reasons for psychologic crises.

Types of Behavioral Disorders

Situational Reactions

Situational reactions are emotional responses to circumstances, such as a sudden illness, a death in the family, or another difficult personal experience. These behaviors are mechanisms to cope with stress and conflict. These behaviors take many forms and include the following:
- Anger
- Anxiety
- Denial
- Withdrawal

The EMT needs to show great sensitivity to communicate successfully with a patient experiencing such emotional stress. An *angry* patient may become argumentative, belligerent, and combative. It is imperative that the EMT remain respectful and calm, using dialogue and displaying body language that conveys compassion and sincerity. Always be professional, and never engage in an argument with a patient.

Anxiety manifests as increased nervousness, tension, pacing, hand wringing, and trembling. The patient may actually express this feeling to the EMT by saying, "I'm scared."

A person may show *denial* in a number of ways. For example, "He can't be dead," or "I just had a little chest pain; nothing's wrong with me," are expressions of denial.

The EMT may arrive at a scene where someone has been killed and find the victim's friend sitting there, refusing to talk or interact with the EMT; this behavior is *withdrawal.*

Psychogenic Crises

Psychogenic crises are behavioral changes from emotional responses that result in potentially unstable, dangerous patient manifestations. These include the following:
- Bizarre thinking and behavior
- Acute psychosis and paranoia
- Panic
- Agitation
- Danger to self (self-destructive behavior, suicide attempt)
- Danger to others (threatening behavior, violence)

The acutely psychotic patient has a distorted perception of reality and displays bizarre thoughts and behavior. *Hallucinations* are abnormal sensory perceptions that occur while a person is awake and conscious and are unrelated to outside events; the person sees, hears, smells, or feels things that do not exist. A *delusion* is something that a person believes to be true or real but that is actually false or unreal. These irrational beliefs defy normal reasoning and remain firmly set in the person's mind even when overwhelming proof is presented to dispute them.

A person with **paranoia** feels threatened by the immediate environment and may believe that "someone is out to get me" (a persecutory delusion). Such a patient might suspect that the oxygen you administer is a gas that is going to put the patient to sleep or that you are going to steal the patient's wallet. A person may also feel panic or sudden, overpowering fright.

REALWorld

If a patient tells you that he is hearing voices, you should not tell him that he is not hearing voices. Instead, you should tell the patient that you believe he is hearing voices, but that you cannot hear them. Do not pretend to hear the voices. As a follow-up, you should ask the patient what the voices are telling him. Knowing what the patient believes he is being told may help you understand the patient's behavior.

Panic is a sudden, overwhelming anxiety of such intensity that it produces terror and physiologic changes. The patient usually presents with uncontrolled hyperventilation and a sensation of shortness of breath, dizziness or faintness, palpitations or pounding heart, trembling or shaking, sweating, choking, numbness or tingling, chest pain or discomfort, and fear of dying.

You might observe the patient with *agitation* crying uncontrollably and beating her fists repeatedly against a wall or throwing herself to the ground. The agitated patient usually manifests abnormal vital signs, such as a rapid heart and respiratory rates and elevated blood pressure from adrenaline surging in her body.

Personality Disorders

Personality disorders are character traits that interfere with a person's ability to function successfully in work or personal relationships. A person with a personality disorder is characteristically manipulative and likes to shift the responsibility and blame for events onto other people. The individual typically does not perceive that he or she has a problem, although those around such a person certainly do. Such patients tend to be self-centered and selfish. They are "takers" rather than "givers"; they demand attention; and they view themselves as kind, generous, and receptive.

As an EMT, you may encounter this type of person at the scene of a motor vehicle crash. Having sustained only minor injuries, such a patient will still demand the EMT's time and attention and remain indifferent to the EMT's attempt to stabilize a more seriously injured person.

These patients can be trying and difficult to satisfy. There is no simple trick to dealing with them. You should avoid becoming angered by their behavior. Ignoring or belittling a patient's demands only angers the patient. Be positive with the patient, but establish limits in a professional manner. For example, saying, "There's nothing seriously wrong with you; we have to take care of the other patient," will be interpreted by the patient as, "We don't care about you; leave us alone." Instead, try saying, "I see that you've hurt [your ankle]; we will try to take care of it as soon as we've made sure that the other patient will be okay." This shows that you are aware of the patient's injury and concerned about it, even if you cannot focus on it immediately.

LEARNING OBJECTIVES
- Discuss the characteristics of an individual's behavior that suggest the patient is at risk for suicide.
- Discuss the general principles of an individual's behavior that suggest the patient is at risk for violence.
- Discuss methods to calm patients with a behavioral emergency.

Depression and Suicide

Depression affects at least 8.9% of the U.S. population, with up to 14.8% of adults experiencing at least one episode of "clinical depression" at some time during their lives. It is the leading cause of disability in the United States. Depression is the most common mental disorder in elderly patients.

Suicide is the eleventh leading cause of death in the United States, homicide ranks fifteenth. Approximately 32,400 people kill themselves each year. Notably, a large percentage of these suicide victims sought medical attention before the suicide. In many people, suicidal intentions and depression can be readily treated—if the diagnosis is made.

Individuals with depression experience a variety of symptoms, including the following:
- Loss of sleep, appetite, and sex drive
- Loss of pleasure in normally satisfying activities
- Sadness and tearfulness
- Guilt
- Hopelessness
- Thoughts and expressions of death or suicide
- Physical symptoms

The depressed patient may describe feelings of sadness, profound feelings of guilt, or both emotions. Such an individual may express hopelessness, a key complaint that points to a significant risk for suicide. The person may hide feelings effectively. It is critical to assess all patients with a potential behavioral emergency for suicide risk (**Box 17-2**). Truly suicidal patients frequently seek medical attention for physical symptoms before taking their lives, but do not express their depression directly. If you, as an EMT, see a patient whose symptoms are difficult to attribute to a medical problem, consider suicide or depression as a possible explanation.

According to statistics, successful suicide attempts are more likely to be made by patients with some of the following qualities:

Box 17-2 Suicide Risk Factors and Signs/Symptoms

Ideation or defined lethal plan of action (verbalized and/or written)
Alcohol and substance abuse
Purposelessness
Anxiety; agitation; unable to sleep or sleeping all the time
Feeling trapped; "no way out"
Hopelessness
Withdrawal from friends, family, and society
Anger; aggressive tendencies
Recklessness; engaging in risky activities
Dramatic mood changes
History of trauma or abuse
Major physical illness (e.g., cancer, congestive heart failure)
Previous suicide attempt
Job or financial loss
Relational or social loss
Easy access to lethal means
Lack of social support; sense of isolation

- Male gender
- Older than 40 years (although teens and young adults are also at high risk)
- Single, widowed, or divorced status
- Socially isolated
- Unemployed
- Psychiatric history
- Recent loss of significant loved one
- Previous suicide attempt
- Alcoholism or drug abuse
- Impulsive behavior
- Chronic or terminal illness
- Loss of job or status
- History of impending arrest or imprisonment

Other characteristics include unusual gathering of articles that can cause death, such as purchase of a gun or a large volume of pills, and verbalizing a defined lethal plan of action. Although women attempt suicide more frequently than men, men are more often successful.

A person about to commit suicide does not always show signs of sadness or depression. In fact, severely depressed patients who decide to end their lives often feel better once the decision is made because they know that the period of suffering is going to end. Be careful with the patient who says, "Nobody cares for me," or "I'll never be better." Be suspicious of "accidents" that could have occurred on purpose.

Sometimes patients make a *suicide gesture,* in which they do not really intend to kill themselves, to receive attention or for other motives. It is difficult to distinguish between a gesture and a real suicide attempt. Therefore, you should always assume that the attempt was real. Also, patients who make a suicide gesture sometimes accidentally take enough drugs or other substances to kill themselves.

REALWorld

Making the determination of a suicide gesture versus an actual suicide attempt is difficult and should not be attempted by the EMT. All suicide attempts should be considered by the EMT as serious, and patients should be transported for evaluation and treatment by a more trained psychiatric clinician. Just because a suicide attempt is not lethal does not mean that the act should not be taken seriously.

Assessment

When evaluating possibly suicidal patients, you should determine the following:

- Is the patient in an unsafe environment or with unsafe objects in hand?
- Has the patient displayed self-destructive behavior during initial (primary) assessment or before the emergency response?
- How does the patient feel?
- Is the patient a threat to self or others?
- Is there a medical problem?
- Is there trauma involved?
- Has the patient had suicidal tendencies in the past?
- What interventions have occurred (past hospitalizations—medical or psychiatric)?

Management

During the scene size-up, you should always look for any threats to personal safety. For example, does the patient have a gun? Is the patient in a garage filled with exhaust fumes? Take appropriate precautions. For example, if the patient has a gun, call police before entering the scene, and keep at a safe distance out of range.

Look for possible injuries or evidence of overdose or poisoning, and provide emergency medical care, as needed, to support the patient. If an overdose may have occurred, bring medications or drugs found at the scene to the medical facility. Calm the patient, and do not leave the patient alone. Restraint may be necessary, and the patient may need to be transported against his or her will. Consider the need for law enforcement.

Psychosis

The psychotic patient has disordered thoughts, distorted perceptions of reality, hallucinations, and inappropriate responses to the environment. Such a person is generally awake and alert, oriented to time and place, but may have bizarre thoughts or may hear voices commanding the performance of certain acts. An example of psychosis would be the idea that the U.S. president has sent the patient on a secret mission, or that the devil has captured the patient's family. Communication with such a patient is difficult; the patient often is out of control and speaks incoherently or in a rambling manner that makes little sense. Often the patient history must be obtained from bystanders, friends, or family members.

Organic Brain Syndromes

Agitated Delirium

Delirium is an acute confusional state in which a change in mental status occurs suddenly, fluctuates over 24 hours, alters consciousness, disturbs thinking and attention, and results in changed behavior. Delirium is not a "disease," but rather a *syndrome* with multiple causes that result in a similar constellation of symptoms. Main symptoms include clouding of consciousness, fluctuating levels of consciousness, difficulty maintaining or shifting attention, disorientation, and hallucinations. In elderly patients, delirium often is the presenting symptom of an underlying illness. Clues from the history and physical examination often suggest that the delirium is caused by a direct physiologic consequence of a general medical condition, an intoxicating substance, medication use, or more than one cause.

Delirium is considered a "medical emergency." If delirium is not recognized, it can lead to permanent disability or death.

Delirium is common in the United States and more often affects older persons; it is found in 14% to 56% of hospitalized elderly patients. In patients who are admitted to the hospital with delirium, mortality rates are 10% to 26%. As many as 80% of patients develop delirium at the time of death. Delirium is extremely common among nursing home residents.

Patients with delirium may have an increased state of arousal and psychomotor abnormalities such as tremor and agitation. This is called *agitated delirium*, which is observed in patients in a state of alcohol withdrawal or intoxication with phencyclidine (PCP), amphetamine, or lysergic acid diethylamide (LSD). Patients experiencing acute alcohol withdrawal are shaky (tremors), agitated, and confused and have a rapid heart rate and blood pressure. The patient may also develop hallucinations (typically visual), seizures, and possibly delirium tremens ("the DTs"). Delirium tremens is a life-threatening form of alcohol withdrawal, with a 35% mortality rate. Patients intoxicated with PCP can be extremely violent, agitated, and dangerous and should be approached with caution. PCP is usually smoked. Cocaine is often inhaled as crack or "freebased." Amphetamines are taken as pills, injected, or smoked as "ice." These stimulant drugs are especially dangerous for the EMT because they can induce irrational and violent behavior. After assessing the need for basic life support, be conservative.

A person with a behavioral disorder caused by medical illness, injury, toxicologic problem, or drug ingestion may present with various changes in mental status or behavior. You must look for underlying medical reasons for a patient's altered behavior, particularly if it is a recent change and the patient has no psychiatric history. You should consider hypoglycemia and hypoxia as possible causes of acute changes in behavior, knowing that as an EMT, you can administer glucose, oxygen, or both.

Other Organic Brain Syndromes

Hypoglycemia is a common medical problem presenting as a behavioral disturbance. Hypoglycemic patients are often confused, combative, and disoriented; the untrained observer often suspects they have a psychiatric disturbance. Hypoglycemia also causes a variety of illnesses and toxic ingestions. At times the term *organic brain syndrome* is used to include nonpsychiatric reasons for changes in behavior and mentation.

Organic brain syndrome can be acute in onset or can occur slowly over a longer period. People with medical causes of behavioral disorders typically have disordered thoughts, are disoriented to place and time, are confused, have difficulty with attention, experience varying levels of alertness, and may be incontinent. Asking the patient where he or she is, what day it is, and simple questions such as the name of the president of the United States can help determine whether the patient is oriented. Remember, your goal as an EMT is not to diagnose the problem but to provide a valuable history to the emergency physician at the hospital and sometimes help make a determination of the need for transport to the hospital against the patient's will. The latter judgment is often made on the basis of answering the question, "Is the patient a hazard to self or others?"

Auditory hallucinations, as when the patient hears voices that say to do certain things (e.g., commit suicide), are common with medical and toxicologic syndromes and psychoses. *Visual*, *tactile* (touch), or *olfactory* (smell) hallucinations almost always have organic causes. An example of a visual hallucination would be a patient who sees a monster next to him; a tactile hallucination would be the person having an adverse reaction to LSD ("bad trip") and feels spiders crawling under the skin.

The many causes of organic brain syndrome include primary problems with the brain, such as tumor, trauma, infections, or degeneration (e.g., senile dementia). It can also be caused by such conditions as hypoglycemia, shock, and drug intoxication. Distinguishing between psychosis and organic brain syndrome is often difficult. It is generally safer to assume that the cause is "organic" until proved otherwise.

To gain compliance and cooperation, reassure the patient, be nonthreatening, and offer as calm an environment as possible. Maintain verbal contact with the patient. Do not be judgmental. Avoid restraints, if possible, because these patients are often in a hyperactive state and fight against restraints, which can cause elevated body temperature and sudden, severe breakdown of muscle tissue (rhabdomyolysis) from hyperactivity and severe muscle strain. There may also be accumulation of metabolic waste products at the cellular level (metabolic acidosis). Also, be cognizant of the cardiovascular stresses on the patient caused by the body's release of adrenalin, which can cause heart attack in older patients with heart disease and hypertension.

Other patients with long-standing dementia, such as Alzheimer's disease, may exhibit behavior that is detrimental to their own safety. Because these problems are slower in onset and occur over a longer time, the family or caregiver can help you with the history.

Case in Point

An 80-year-old widower is found wandering the streets, and police dispatch an ambulance because the man is confused and agitated and displays disordered thoughts. The man is having visual hallucinations and sees his dead wife walking in the neighborhood.

The EMTs arrive, and the man is initially uncooperative with attempts at evaluation. Their approach to the man is calm and respectful, and the man allows them to interview and examine him. During the interview he discloses that he has no previous history of depression or psychiatric problems, but he thinks he was recently hospitalized. He agrees to be transported to the hospital.

Further assessment at the hospital reveals that the patient's change in behavior and mental status is an *agitated delirium*, the result of a fever and urinary tract infection, as well as the interactions between multiple new medications prescribed for the patient at his previous hospitalization 1 week earlier. After the offending medications were discontinued and the patient's infection was treated, the patient ceased to be confused and agitated. He returned home several days later, functioning well.

Violent Behavior

Violent or disruptive behavior may overlap with any of the behaviors previously discussed. A variety of medical and psychological problems can ultimately cause patients to lose control and to strike out at the environment, endangering themselves and others. In general, violent behavior occurs in response to a person's overwhelming inner fear or frustration about his or her situation or surroundings. Violence can often be prevented by helping the person deal with the stresses or causes of the feelings of frustration and helplessness.

Recognition of impending violence is vital. First, make sure you do not put yourself in jeopardy; then assess what can be done to prevent an outburst. Leave yourself an escape route. Although you may defend yourself if necessary, it is a better practice to avoid such a situation by recognizing the potential for violence and preplanning. You may recognize a potentially violent patient by the following signs:

- Angry voice
- Pressured speech
- Pacing; quick, irregular movements; tense muscles
- Expressions of violence
- Psychiatric history of emotional disturbances
- Drug intoxication
- Situational frustration
- Threatening posture or movements
- Presence of heavy or threatening objects

Psychotic patients can become violent if they feel threatened or have been subjected to prolonged questioning that they perceive as inappropriate. For example, a drug-intoxicated individual may suddenly and unexpectedly become violent. A patient subjected to delays in treatment or unsupportive remarks or who is scared by illness may react with anger or violence. A variety of toxins, drugs, alcohol, and metabolic abnormalities (e.g., low blood sugar, thyroid problems) can manifest as violent behavior. Again, you should look for clues in the environment, such as syringes, empty pill bottles, fire (possible inhalation of carbon monoxide), and signs of trauma.

Pediatric Behavioral Emergencies

Behavioral emergencies in the pediatric population pose some unique diagnostic and management challenges to the EMT, particularly in the context of consent/refusal of transport and in behavioral disorders more often seen in childhood and adolescence than in adults. As with adults, however, pediatric patients present with acute changes in behavior that may be a consequence of medical illness or substance abuse.

Suicidal behavior is perhaps the most urgent of pediatric behavioral emergencies. The rate of suicide among adolescents in the United States has tripled since the 1950s and now ranks as the third leading cause of death for this age group. In addition to completed suicides, suicidal ideation and suicide attempts are prevalent problems. In 2004, more than 5000 U.S. children and adolescents committed suicide. An additional 171,870 cases of nonfatal self-injuries were reported. In 2007, 14.5% of U.S. high school students reported having seriously considered killing themselves. The EMT must assess for present and past thoughts of suicide, prior self-destructive behavior, and current stressors. Even young patients may have a history of conduct disorder, antisocial behaviors, and substance abuse.

Young patients with *autism spectrum disorders* (ASDs) have difficulty with social interactions, language, and communication. Providing medical services to these individuals in a prehospital setting requires special consideration to improve compliance and facilitate a better outcome. Informed consent is an important concern when a child or adolescent psychiatric patient requires transport to the emergency department (ED). This requires a review with the patient and/or the guardian of the risks, benefits, and alternatives to the recommended

assessment and treatment. The situation is most often straightforward when the parent or guardian agrees to the assessment and subsequent recommendations. When there are disagreements between parents, the parent does not support the assessment, or a legal guardian cannot be found, the process may require the involvement of law enforcement professionals. Consent or assent by a minor to medical or psychiatric procedures varies by state. Parental involvement in mental health decisions is standard procedure and is not considered a deterrent to seeking treatment.

Violent behavior among children and adolescents is a growing problem, evident perhaps in the increasing incidence of fatal school violence. The pediatric patient's clinical presentation may include factors that predispose to violent behavior. Substance abuse, for example, is related to violence. The admission rate to the ED for substance-related illnesses or injury is as high or higher for older adolescents than the rate for adults. Aggressive behavior may be a symptom of an underlying disorder or disability. Concurrent psychiatric disorders, including schizophrenia, bipolar disorder, and major depression, escalate the risk of violence, particularly when the patient experiences delusions involving threat of harm. Hyperactive children develop conduct and antisocial disorders in adolescence if the problem is not addressed in childhood and is allowed to progress to more disruptive and dangerous behaviors. Patients with *attention deficit hyperactivity disorder* (ADHD) also act impulsively without consideration for safety. These children and adolescents are also considered *labile*, with wide fluctuations in mood and response. The result is frequently an individual prone to violence.

Child abuse of either a physical or a sexual nature should be considered in the course of any behavioral evaluation. Situations involving obvious or even suspected child abuse must be reported to appropriate state and local agencies. Failure to do so is considered a criminal offense and may lead to civil liability.

Case in Point

Emergency medical technicians are dispatched to a child hurt at a public playground and encounter an 8-year-old boy lying on the ground, rocking back and forth in pain. The child is awake and alert but not interactive or communicative. When the EMTs approach the boy to check for a likely ankle fracture, the patient screams and pushes them away, refusing any attempt at evaluation or treatment. He is in the park without a parent or guardian, having fallen off his bicycle, which he rode to the park alone. He was not wearing a helmet, and because the EMTs cannot examine him, they cannot exclude a head injury as the cause of his behavior.

A nearby adult recognizes the boy and informs you that he has autism. The police are at the scene and are unsuccessful in trying to reach the boy's parents. The EMTs confer with online medical direction and the police, and all agree that restraint and transport are necessary to ensure that the patient receives appropriate medical treatment for his deformed ankle and to ensure the safety of the patient and crew during transport.

The EMTs use appropriate methods to calm the agitated boy and provide safe, effective restraint. The patient is uneventfully transported to the ED for treatment of a seriously fractured ankle. When the boy's parents arrive at the ED and hear what happened, it is clear that they are appreciative of the care that the EMTs provided to their injured son.

Geriatric Behavioral Emergencies

Behavioral emergencies in elderly patients can be secondary to numerous factors, such as depression and suicide, behavioral disturbance caused by underlying organic conditions, substance abuse, elder abuse, and medication-induced adverse effects.

Depression is the most common psychiatric disorder in elderly patients and can lead to diminished motivation and lack of cooperation. The risk of depression in elderly persons increases with other illnesses and when the ability to function becomes limited. Estimates of major depression in older people living in the community range from less than 1% to about 5%, but rises to 13.5% in those who require home health care and to 11.5% in elderly hospital patients.

Older adults are at greater risk for *suicide* than other population groups, with elderly persons committing approximately 16% of all suicides. About 75% of older adults who committed suicide had been in the office of a primary care provider within the previous 30 days; approximately one-third had been in their provider's office within the last week of life.

Most conditions presenting as behavioral emergencies in this age group stem from an underlying organic cause. Comorbid medical conditions such as urinary tract infections, pneumonia, head injury, and thyrotoxicosis are among the illnesses that can cause delirium and agitation that may be mistaken for functional impairment.

The geriatric population is particularly susceptible to adverse drug reactions because in addition to age-related drug metabolism changes, they often have multiple coexisting medical conditions, increasing their use of polypharmacy.

The EMT must always consider *elder abuse and neglect* and must be attentive and observant during the scene survey and patient assessment to identify it. The American Medical Association (AMA) defines elder abuse and neglect as an act of omission that results in harm or threatened harm to the health or welfare of an elderly person. It may take many forms, including physical abuse, psychological abuse, caregiver neglect, self-neglect, and financial exploitation. It is estimated that over 2 million older adults are mistreated each year in the United States. Despite an increased incidence and awareness, elder abuse and neglect is still underreported.

> **LEARNING OBJECTIVE**
> - Discuss the special considerations for assessing a patient with behavioral problems.

Approach to the Patient with a Behavioral Emergency

Scene Size-up

For many reasons, the scene size-up is the most important aspect of assessment of the patient with a suspected behavioral emergency. Patients with aggressive or violent behavior can represent a serious threat to the safety of EMS personnel. Determining the mechanism of injury or nature of illness is important because the clues to organic and other causes of behavioral disorders may only be present at the scene of the emergency. Failure to identify these clues may cause delayed diagnosis at the hospital and harm to the patient.

At the scene of the behavioral emergency, you should be prepared to identify potential causes of the presenting problem. Some indicators may be obvious, such as aggressive or bizarre behavior. Patients may have open bottles of medication, syringes, or track marks on their arms. Evidence of suicide attempts may be obvious, such as a patient who is threatening to jump from a height. In such cases, you should be prepared to call for additional police resources, which may include a suicide intervention team.

Scene Safety

When responding to a suspected psychobehavioral disorder, you should have a heightened sense of awareness regarding potential dangers. If you are advised that there is a violent patient on the scene, you should await the arrival of the police before entering the area. If people on the scene are in danger, you should direct them to evacuate to a safe area, if this is possible without endangering yourself or your partner. Remember, your first priority is to prevent further injury, to yourself or others.

Environmental dangers may exist at the scene of a behavioral emergency. Patients may attempt suicide with gas exhaust or carbon monoxide from their vehicle. In these cases, you should use precautions to protect yourself and others. Open doors for ventilation, turn off the gas or vehicle engine, and quickly remove the patient and bystanders from the scene. You should be prepared to administer high-concentration oxygen or positive-pressure ventilation. If the patient is within a closed space, do not enter if you suspect gas fumes as the cause without proper protection; you must avoid becoming a victim yourself.

Initial (Primary) Assessment

The priority in the initial (primary) assessment is the identification of threats to life and treating the ABCs (airway, breathing, circulation). Is the patient responsive and breathing, with signs of circulation? Ensure a patent airway, and consider the need for positive-pressure ventilation and oxygen. Assess for trauma, control bleeding, and assess the need for cardiopulmonary resuscitation (CPR). Monitor vital signs closely, particularly looking for signs of hypoperfusion, hypoxia, hypoglycemia, and skin temperature alterations.

Critical to the assessment of the behavioral emergency patient is the mental status examination. Formulate a general impression by observing the patient's appearance from a distance. The patient's attire and hygiene are important factors, as well as the condition of the patient's living quarters. Does the patient appear disheveled, with poor hygiene? Is the patient living in squalid conditions? This potentially significant information must be conveyed to the hospital staff because it may represent unsafe living conditions, to which the patient cannot be discharged.

Assess the patient's mood as anxious, depressed, elated, or agitated, and describe the patient's alertness and distractibility. Observe for any abnormal *psychomotor activity* (physical gesture resulting from mental processes and a product of the psyche). The *agitated* patient may display psychomotor activities such as pacing, wringing of hands, and inability to sit still, whereas the *depressed* patient usually displays slowing of movements such as eye blinking. Describe the patient's language, specifically speech patterns and content. The *psychotic* patient usually talks with "pressured" (rapid, frenzied) speech, whereas the *delirious* patient may have incoherent, garbled, or unintelligible speech. The depressed or suicidal patient may display a "poverty" (restriction in amount) of speech, usually slow and monotone.

An essential component of the mental status examination is the patient's thought content and processes. Evaluate for disordered thoughts (do the thoughts make sense?), delusions (possess special powers, believe they are some other person), hallucinations (visual, auditory, olfactory, tactile), and any unusual worries or fears (paranoia). Assess the patient's judgment, concentration, memory, orientation (person, place, time), and intellectual functioning. Is the patient suicidal or homicidal?

Establish Rapport and Communication

Obtaining a history at the scene of a behavioral disorder requires a careful and measured approach. Your actions may contribute to calming the patient or igniting the situation. The EMT must utilize *therapeutic* interviewing techniques, such as engaging in active listening, being supportive and empathetic, limiting interruptions, and respecting the patient's territory by limiting physical touch.

Avoid threatening actions, statements, or questions, and always approach the patient slowly and purposefully. Use a calm, understanding approach. Identify yourself, and inform the patient that you are there to help. Tell the patient what you are doing, and ask questions in a calm, reassuring voice. Involve trusted family members and friends. Always maintain a comfortable distance, especially if the patient is agitated, potentially violent, or fearful of your presence. Avoid any unnecessary physical contact, and call for additional help if needed. Use good eye contact, and lower or reduce distressing stimuli in the environment. Acknowledge that the patient seems upset, and restate that you are there to help.

Respond honestly to the patient's questions, and allow the patient to tell you what happened without being judgmental. Tell the truth, and do not lie to the patient. Show that you are listening by rephrasing or repeating part of what is said, and acknowledge the patient's feelings. Do not "play along" with auditory or visual hallucinations or agree with disturbed thinking. Do not threaten, challenge, or argue with a disturbed patient, and do not make any quick moves. Treat patients with respect, and do not belittle or threaten them.

Box 17-3 outlines methods to establish rapport and to calm the patient with a behavioral emergency.

Focused (Secondary) Assessment

Patient History

If the patient is unresponsive, refuses to communicate, or is incoherent, collect a history from family or bystanders and perform a rapid assessment. Collect a SAMPLE history, noting signs and symptoms that may suggest an organic cause of the behavior (**Box 17-4**). Note allergies and medications that may indicate an illness, or a drug reaction that may explain the condition. Has the patient been exposed to drugs, toxins, or sustained trauma? Is any aspect of the past medical history pertinent, including

---

Box 17-3	Methods to Calm Patients with a Behavioral Emergency

1. Acknowledge that the patient seems upset and restate that you are there to help.
2. Inform the patient about what you are doing.
3. Ask questions in a calm, reassuring voice.
4. Maintain a comfortable distance.
5. Encourage patients to state what is troubling them.
6. Do not make quick moves.
7. Respond honestly to the patient's questions.
8. Do not threaten, challenge, or argue with disturbed patients.
9. Tell the truth; do not lie to the patient.
10. Do not "play along" with visual or auditory disturbances of the patient.
11. Involve trusted family members or friends.
12. Be prepared to stay at scene for a long time; always remain with the patient.
13. Avoid unnecessary physical contact. Call additional help if needed.
14. Use good eye contact.
15. Avoid threatening postures.
16. Keep other assessment techniques in mind.
    a. Always try to talk the patient into cooperation.
    b. Do not belittle or threaten patients.
    c. Be calm and patient in your attitude.
    d. Do not agree with disturbed thinking.
    e. Be reassuring.
    f. Avoid arguing with irrational patients.
    g. Lower distressing stimuli, if possible.
    i. Treat patient with respect.
    j. Protect the patient and yourself.

---

a behavioral disorder? If so, is the behavioral disorder chronic or acute? Is the patient wearing a Medic-Alert tag? Does the patient have a medical disorder that may explain the behavior, such as diabetes or electrolyte disturbances? Could a recent family event or other situation have caused emotional distress? If there has been a sudden change in the patient's behavior, when did it occur? What events occurred at the same time?

Physical Examination

Use caution when examining patients who may become violent, and respect their space. If patients refuse further examination, respect their wishes. During the physical examination, assess the patient's mental status and check to see if the patient is oriented to person, place, and time. Search for obvious evidence of medical causes of the illness. Can you smell alcohol or other substances on the patient's breath? Look for abnormal physical findings that may suggest an organic cause of the behavior, such as signs of hypoglycemia, hypoxia, drug overdose, or stroke. For example, a patient with a sudden change in behavior who is sweating, has a rapid pulse, and has a history of diabetes should be considered to have hypoglycemia and should be given glucose.

LEARNING OBJECTIVE

- Discuss special medicolegal considerations for managing behavioral emergencies.

| Box 17-4 | Collecting a SAMPLE History for Patients with a Behavioral Emergency |

Signs and Symptoms

Questions to ask the patient or to ascertain from the surroundings include:

- What is bothering you?
- Why did you call the ambulance?
- How do you feel? Are you in any pain?
- Have you harmed yourself? Is there a threat to either the patient or to others?
- Does the patient answer questions appropriately? How does the patient relate to you?
- Did these feelings come on suddenly, or have you been feeling them for awhile?

Medications and Allergies

Determine if the patient is taking any medications or has any allergies.

- Have you taken your medication? When was the last time? Can you show it to me?
- Has the patient been exposed to any poisons or drugs?
- Is the patient wearing a Medic-Alert tag?

Medications may point to either a psychiatric history or a medical history that could explain the behavior. The patient may have a medical disorder such as diabetes or electrolyte disturbances.

Pertinent Past Medical History

- Have you been seeing anyone about this?
- Have you been in the hospital before?

Last Oral Intake

- When was the last time you ate or drank anything? What was it? Hypoglycemia can cause an altered mental status.

Events Leading up to the Present Illness

- How long have you felt this way?
- Is there anything that happened that triggered these feelings?
- Has there been a trauma?
- What were you doing just before the ambulance was called?

Try to establish a chronology of events leading up to the behavioral emergency.

Transport and Patient Restraint Decisions

The management of emotionally or mentally disturbed patients represents an area of high legal risk for EMTs. When emotionally disturbed patients consent to care, legal problems are greatly reduced. However, emotionally disturbed patients often resist treatment and refuse transport. They may threaten EMTs and others.

To provide care without a patient's consent, you must show a reasonable belief that the patient is a threat to self or others. Ideally, you should contact medical direction to obtain input and guidance before restraint and transport. It is especially helpful to have law enforcement personnel assist restraining and removing these patients from the scene. Generally, such actions are taken to prevent the patients from injuring themselves or others around them. In such circumstances, many state and local governments permit the police to remove the patient under the concept of "protective custody."

If conditions permit, the patient's family or physician should be contacted to encourage the patient to submit to care. With violent and suicidal patients, however, this may not be possible. In these situations, EMS providers and police enter into close collaboration, particularly when the patient is violent. You should work together with medical direction, the police, and the patient's family to convince the patient to go to the hospital. At times, the police may not think they are justified to restrain a person under their interpretation of the law. In these cases, you must act in your role as a healthcare provider and in the best interest of the patient. In cases where medical judgment must decide what is best, it is often helpful to think what you would expect of medical professionals if the patient were a member of your own family. Many EMS systems have formal policies that involve medical direction in dealing with these situations, and you should be familiar with your local policy.

Because these patients are often transported against their expressed wishes, charges of "false imprisonment" and "battery" are sometimes brought in relation to restraint and transport or an injury sustained during the restraining process. **Battery** is the act of physically touching someone without the person's expressed consent. Therefore, it is important that as an EMT, you use "reasonable force." Reasonable force depends on what force was necessary to keep the patient from injuring self or others. The reasonableness is determined by looking at all circumstances involved and varies from case to case, considering the following factors:

- Patient's size and strength
- Type of abnormal behavior
- Patient's gender
- Patient's mental state
- Method of restraint

Some patients may appear calm after a period of combativeness and aggression and then suddenly threaten or cause injury to themselves or others. EMS personnel may use reasonable force to defend against an attack by emotionally disturbed patients. *Stay alert at all times.*

When forcible removal is necessary, take care not to harm the patient. Soft restraints are preferred. The use of handcuffs is discouraged because injury can occur when patients struggle. Special leather restraints with padding are often used because these provide strength to secure the patient to the stretcher while minimizing the chance of injury.

Patients may also make false accusations about unnecessary force and sexual misconduct. When possible, have same-sex attendants (if a same-sex EMT is available) with the patient, or call for help and have a third-party witness present, especially during transport.

Precise documentation is essential to record the circumstances that warranted the use of restraints and removal against the patient's will. Rather than using subjective words or phrases, specifically describe the patient's behavior or statements, such as, "The patient tried to strike the EMT during medical care," or the patient stated, "I am going to kill myself the first chance I get."

Restraining Patients

When using restraints, have police present, if possible, and use their help. Obtain approval from medical direction according to your local policies. Guidelines include the following:

1. *Be sure to have adequate help.* In general, aim to have at least four persons simultaneously approach the patient, with one assigned to each limb. If there are enough people to overwhelm the patient, the mere presence of a group may allow the violent patient to give up and cease resisting.

2. *Plan your activities.* Estimate the range of motion of the patient's arms and legs, and stay beyond this range until necessary.

3. *Act quickly.* Once you have made your decision to restrain the patient, act quickly, using only the force necessary.

4. *Communicate.* Have one EMT talk to the patient throughout the process.

5. *Restrain the patient.* Once the patient is subdued, place the patient on the stretcher, securing with multiple straps. *Never* secure a patient facedown, because you must ensure access to the airway at all times. The National Association of EMS Physicians recommends the face-up position if a patient must be transported restrained. Not only does the face-up position allow easier access to the patient if medical care is necessary en route, but some mental health experts also prefer it because patients perceive it as less demeaning. Careful ongoing monitoring of a restrained patient's respiratory status, circulation, and general condition is essential.

6. *Secure the patient.* Secure each limb to the stretcher with padded restraints. Securing the torso and legs with other straps may be necessary in agitated patients. Avoid unnecessary force.

7. *Adjust as necessary.* If the patient is spitting, cover the patient's face with a surgical mask. However, observe for any obstruction of the airway or breathing.

8. *Reassess frequently.* Reassess breathing and circulation frequently, especially circulation distal to the restraints, and document your actions and indications for use of restraints.

Skill 17-1 reviews the steps that should be taken in restraining a patient.

Case in Point

In medicine, patients are restrained for their protection and the protection of others. Tying a person down may seem inhumane or abusive, but if they are truly a threat, they must be restrained. Allowing patients to hurt themselves by not restraining them can make the EMT liable for their injury.

Scenario Follow-up

When you arrive at the hospital, you are ventilating the patient with a bag-mask, and a nasopharyngeal airway (NPA) is in place because the patient gagged on the oropharyngeal airway (OPA). The restraints are easily removed by the hospital staff, allowing for detailed assessment. The patient is treated using gastric lavage to empty the contents of his stomach. Because of the complete history obtained on the scene and the concise report given to the physician, the patient is able to receive the antidote for the medications involved in his overdose. The patient survives and is referred to an inpatient psychiatric counseling center.

Summary

EMTs respond to many situations involving behavioral emergencies. Some result from medical problems, intoxication, or injuries; some are related to psychiatric disorders; and others may be caused by extreme reactions to emotional events. EMTs must first ensure their own safety, attempt to identify the underlying cause, and transport the patient in a safe, effective manner. The EMT should be alert to the possibility of hypoglycemia, hypoxia, and other medical problems as a cause and provide treatment if appropriate. In most cases, however, treatment is limited in the field. Be honest with patients, and be their advocate. Work with medical direction and law enforcement officials when restraint and transport against the patient's will is necessary.

Skills

Skill | 17-1 *Restraining a Patient*

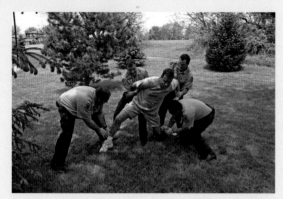

1. Plan your activities; estimate the range of motion of the patient's arms and legs, and stay beyond this range until necessary. Organize a sufficient number of personnel to restrain the patient safely. Once you have made your decision to restrain the patient, act quickly, using only the force necessary. Have one EMT talk to the patient throughout the process.

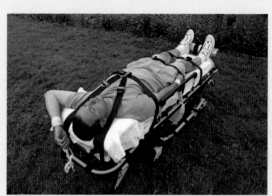

2. Once the patient is subdued, place on the stretcher and secure the patient faceup. The faceup position allows easier access to the patient if medical care is necessary en route and is preferred by mental health experts because it is perceived as less demeaning by patients. Secure each limb to the stretcher with padded restraints. Securing the torso and the legs with other straps may be necessary in agitated patients. Once restrained, careful and ongoing monitoring of the patient's respiratory status and general condition is essential. Reassess initial impressions and respiration and circulation frequently, and document your actions and indications for use of restraints. If possible, have someone of the same sex (family member, police officer, EMT) accompany the patient to the hospital to prevent accusations of impropriety.

Stoy W et al: *Mosby's EMT-basic textbook,* ed 2 rev, St Louis, 2007, Mosby.

The Bottom Line

Learning Checklist

✓ A behavioral emergency is any situation in which the patient exhibits abnormal behavior that is unacceptable or intolerable to self, family, or community.

✓ Behavioral emergencies leading to violence or other inappropriate action can be caused by extremes of emotion, a psychological condition, or a medical condition such as lack of oxygen, low blood glucose, toxic ingestion, or electrolyte imbalance.

✓ Behavioral emergencies may be caused by situational reactions, personality disorders, depression, or suicidal ideation and present with demonstrations of anger, paranoia, panic, agitation, denial, or withdrawal.

✓ Signs of depression include loss of sleep, appetite, and sexual drive; loss of pleasure in normally satisfying activities; sadness and tearfulness; guilt; hopelessness; thoughts of death or suicide; and physical symptoms.

✓ Risk factors of suicide include male gender; over age 40; single, widowed, or divorced status; social isolation; unemployment; psychiatric history; recent loss of a loved one; previous suicide attempt; alcoholism or drug abuse; impulsive behavior; chronic or terminal illness; loss of job or status; and history of impending arrest or imprisonment.

✓ Using a calm, understanding approach can be helpful when dealing with a violent or uncooperative patient.

✓ When approaching a patient with a behavioral disorder, you should introduce yourself, involve family members and friends, maintain a comfortable distance, avoid physical contact, use good eye contact, acknowledge that the patient is upset, and restate that you are there to help.

Key Terms

Anxiety Fearful emotional state characterized by increased nervousness, tension, pacing, hand wringing, and trembling.

Battery The act of physically touching someone without that person's expressed consent.

Behavior The manner in which a person acts or performs, including any or all of one's physical and mental activities.

Behavioral emergency Any situation in which the patient exhibits abnormal behavior that is unacceptable or intolerable to self, family, or community.

Delirium Acute confusional state marked by an altered mental state resulting in changed behavior.

Depression Condition characterized by loss of pleasure, deep sadness, feelings of hopelessness, difficulty sleeping, loss of sex drive, and feelings of guilt.

Panic Sudden, overwhelming anxiety of such intensity that it produces terror and physiologic changes.

Paranoia Condition in which a patient feels unduly threatened by the environment and those in contact with the patient.

Psychobehavioral disorder Any of various forms of behavior that are considered inappropriate by members of the social group to which an individual belongs.

Review Questions

1. What is the term for a situation in which a person exhibits abnormal behavior that is unacceptable or intolerable to self, family, or community because of emotional, medical, or psychological causes?
   a. Psychiatric emergency
   b. Psychosis
   c. Behavioral emergency
   d. Neurosis

2. Which of the following is a cause of altered behavior that can be reversed by the EMT?
   a. Stroke
   b. Head trauma
   c. Hyperglycemia
   d. Hypoxia

3. Which patient profile contains the most risk factors for suicide?
   a. A recently retired 65-year-old man whose wife just died.
   b. A 20-year-old woman who was fired from her job and has a history of diabetes.
   c. A 15-year-old boy who just broke up with his girlfriend and occasionally "smokes weed."
   d. An 80-year-old grandmother with heart disease whose grandchild is ill with cancer.

4. Which of the following best describes "reasonable force" as it pertains to restraining patients?
   a. Everyone who is on scene should help restrain the patient.
   b. The EMT closest to the patient's size should restrain the patient.
   c. The least amount of force, allowing for the safe restraint of a patient.
   d. Use all means available to restrain the patient.

5. Which of the following is the best example of how to communicate with a patient hearing voices?
   a. "You are not hearing voices."
   b. "I hear the voices as well."
   c. "I believe you can hear them, but I cannot hear them."
   d. "You just think you are hearing the voices; they are not real."

6. Which of the following is *not* a sign of potential violence?
   a. The patient's verbal threats of harm
   b. Quick, irregular movements and tense muscles
   c. A history of aggression
   d. The patient's tearfulness

For Further Review

In the Student Workbook

- Multiple-choice questions
- Short-answer questions
- True-false questions
- Case scenario questions

On Evolve

- Weblinks
- Lecture notes
- Exercises

Learning Objectives

Cognitive Objectives

- Define psychobehavioral disorders and behavioral emergencies.
- Discuss the general factors that may cause an alteration in a patient's behavior.

- State the various reasons for psychological crises.
- Discuss the characteristics of an individual's behavior that suggest the patient is at risk for suicide.
- Discuss the general principles of an individual's behavior that suggest the patient is at risk for violence.
- Discuss methods to calm patients with a behavioral emergency.
- Discuss the special considerations for assessing a patient with behavioral problems.
- Discuss special medicolegal considerations for managing behavioral emergencies.

Affective Objectives

- Explain the rationale for learning how to modify your behavior toward the patient with a behavioral emergency.

Psychomotor Objectives

- Demonstrate the assessment and emergency medical care of the patient experiencing a behavioral emergency.
- Demonstrate various techniques to safely restrain a patient with a behavioral problem.

References

American Foundation for Suicide Prevention. http://www.afsp.org/index.cfm?fuseaction=home.viewpage&page_id=050FEA9F-B064-4092-B1135C3A70DE1FDA.

Centers for Disease Control and Prevention, National Center for Injury Prevention and Control: Web-based Injury Statistics Query and Reporting System (WISQARS): www.cdc.gov/ncipc/wisqars.

Centers for Disease Control and Prevention, National Center for Injury Prevention and Control: Web-based Injury Statistics Query and Reporting System (WISQARS [online]), 2005, (accessed January 31, 2007). Available from URL: www.cdc.gov/ncipc/wisqars.

Centers for Disease Control and Prevention: Youth Risk Behavior Surveillance—United States, 2007. Surveillance Summaries, June 6, *MMWR* 57(No. SS-4), 2008.

Hybels CF, Blazer DG: Epidemiology of late-life mental disorders, *Clinics in Geriatric Medicine,* 19:663, 2003.

Kessler RC, Chiu WT, Demler O, Walters EE: Prevalence, severity, and comorbidity of twelve-month DSM-IV disorders in the National Comorbidity Survey Replication (NCS-R), *Archives of General Psychiatry,* 62(6):617, 2005.

Murray, CJL, Lopez, AD, eds: *The global burden of disease: A comprehensive assessment of mortality and disability from diseases, injuries, and risk factors in 1990 and projected to 2020.* Cambridge, MA, 1996, Harvard University Press, Harvard School of Public Health, on behalf of the World Health Organization and the World Bank.

Office of Applied Studies: *Results from the 2004 National Survey on Drug Use and Health: National findings* (DHHS Publication No. SMA 05-4062, NSDUH Series H-28), Rockville, MD, 2005, Substance Abuse and Mental Health Services Administration.

Regier DA, Narrow WE, Rae DS, et al: The de facto mental and addictive disorders service system. Epidemiologic Catchment Area prospective 1-year prevalence rates of disorders and services, *Archives of General Psychiatry,* 50(2):85, 1993.

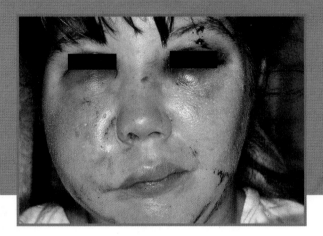

18 Abuse and Assault

CHAPTER OUTLINE

Domestic Violence
Types of Abuse and Recognition
Approach to the Suspected Victim of Domestic Violence or Abuse

Scenario

You and your partner respond to the report of 22-year-old pregnant female complaining of abdominal pain. You arrive at a small, well-kept apartment to find the young woman sitting on the couch, crying. She has a bruised right eye and is holding her abdomen. Police officers are on the scene with you. When you ask what happened, her answers are vague. She says something about being clumsy and falling down. The police officers tell you they responded to a noise complaint. After additional questioning, the patient finally states that her husband struck her in the face and then kicked her in the abdomen when she fell to the ground.

> **LEARNING OBJECTIVES**
> - Discuss the incidence of domestic violence.
> - Describe the categories of abuse.
> - Describe the cycle of violence.
> - Identify the profiles of the the at-risk partner/spouse, the at-risk elder, and the at-risk child.

Domestic Violence

In the last four decades, the family home in the United States has been extensively documented as one of the most common locations for the infliction of psychological, emotional, physical, sexual, and economic abuse, that is, **domestic violence.** For many women, children, and elderly persons, the home is far from a secure environment, but rather a hellish setting that includes neglect, beatings, rapes, and a wide variety of psychological and emotional abuse that takes a tremendous toll on the fabric of our society. In fact, domestic abuse may be appropriately cited as a fundamental cause of many societal problems, including **assault,** murder, robbery, drug and alcohol abuse, and almost any type of pathology present in U.S. culture.

The most common targets of domestic (or family) violence include children, wives or intimate partners, younger or female siblings, adolescents, elderly persons, and gay and lesbian couples. The most common unifying characteristic of the abuse is *emotional and physical dominance over the abused individual.* Children and women are the most frequently targeted victims in society because of the ability of a male spouse or parent to assert physical and emotional dominance over the often physically weaker or economically dependent individual.

As an emergency medical services (EMS) provider, you play a critical role in the identification and referral of individuals who are suspected of having sustained abuse. You are in the unique position of entering the home where evidence of abuse or neglect may be present; you therefore have the ability to gather information not available to other healthcare professionals. Many states require that healthcare professionals, including EMS providers, report abuse to the proper authorities, such as the police, state department of health, child protective services, or the hospital.

Because you may have a legal responsibility to report abuse, you should be familiar with the types of abuse, the common targets, the signs and symptoms of abuse and neglect, and the appropriate actions to take when abuse is identified or suspected. In some situations this may include asking direct questions of suspected abuse victims. This can be an uncomfortable process, but if you handle it appropriately, you can save someone's life. The first step to identification and referral of abused patients to the appropriate authorities is acquiring knowledge on the scope and nature of the problem.

Historical Perspective

Historical factors have provided the foundation for current acts of domestic violence and abuse. Physical disciplining of children and female spouses was a normal cultural practice dating back to biblical times and is still prevalent in many cultures worldwide.

In 753 BC, King Romulus of Rome established "laws of chastisement" that defined wives as possessions, holding husbands liable for the crimes of their wives. Constantine had a young wife boiled alive when she became inconvenient. The phrase "rule of thumb" is derived from the husband's right to beat his wife with a stick no larger than the thickness of his thumb. This law was upheld in U.S. courts until the late 1800s. In 1864 a Mississippi court allowed corporal (physical) punishment of a wife.

Corporal punishment of children continues to receive the support of many parents. The rationalizations that parents give for this behavior are often rooted in their personal experiences as a child. Social surveys have indicated the corporal punishment is extremely widespread, with as many of 84% to 97% of parents reporting the use of physical punishment on their children.

The current protections for abused women, children, and elderly persons originated in the 1960s, when discussion of "wife battering" first appeared in the medical literature. The first battered-women's shelter was not opened until 1971 in London, England.

Historically, spousal abuse of men has been noted, but women are much more often the victims of physical, sexual, psychological, economic, and emotional abuse. Women are less likely to report violence because of fear of retribution or because they love the spouse or intimate partner and often assume the blame for provoking the incident. Women are also reluctant to communicate to family members or friends because of the shame of being abused, especially in higher socioeconomic circles. Abusers also tend to isolate their victims from friends and family, effectively cutting away their lifelines along with their self-esteem.

Violence among gay and lesbian couples is another form of domestic abuse that may be underreported because of the bias of society against nontraditional couples.

Role of EMS

A call to 9-1-1 clearly represents a common access point for the most seriously abused victims. In fact, EMS providers are often the only medical personnel to encounter the victims of domestic violence, because these patients frequently refuse medical attention at the scene and are not transported to the local hospital for evaluation. Evidence suggests that victims of domestic violence are more likely to refuse medical transport to the hospital, therefore placing themselves at risk for continued abuse.

Consequently, police and EMS providers are often the only "safety net" for the victim of domestic violence. Unfortunately, they are often poorly prepared to assume this critical role.

Prevalence

Domestic and family violence are widespread in the United States and around the world. Domestic violence is not confined to any one socioeconomic, ethnic, religious, racial, or age group.

Violence against Women

Women are more likely to be assaulted, injured, raped, or killed by a male partner than by any other type of assailant. Statistics from the U.S. Department of Health and Human Services (DHHS) Administration for Children and Families show that 22% of all violence against women by a single offender is committed by an intimate partner—a husband, ex-husband, boyfriend, or ex-boyfriend. Accurate information on the extent of domestic violence is difficult to obtain because of extensive underreporting. However, it is estimated that as many as 4 million cases of domestic abuse against women occur annually in the United States. Some studies estimate that up to one fourth of all hospital emergency department (ED) visits by women result from domestic violence.

Domestic violence tends to follow a pattern referred to as the **cycle of violence (Figure 18-1)**. The cycle begins with the woman attempting to be perfect for her husband or boyfriend. This is known as the *tension phase*. Unfortunately, the man will become angered by something she did or did not do, such as cleaning the house or spending too much money. He will strike out with some form of verbal or physical abuse and then leave. This is known as the *violence phase*. After a time, he will calm down and return to apologize, offering flowers or other gifts, always with the promise that "it will never happen again." This is known as the *honeymoon phase,* or "wine and roses phase." The promise to stop the abuse is usually accompanied with a caveat such as, "You need to clean better or shop more frugally." This leads the woman to believe the abuse was her fault, and she works at being more perfect, starting the cycle over. Typically, over time, the phases intensify and occur more quickly. The violence increases in amount and severity.

Pregnant Women. Pregnant women are at increased risk for physical violence inflicted by partners. From information gathered in public and private healthcare settings, the Centers for Disease Control and Prevention (CDC, 2006) estimates that violence directed toward women during pregnancy ranges from 4% to 8%. An American Medical Association (AMA, 2001) study of mothers of newborns showed that women with unwanted pregnancies were more likely to experience physical violence. Homicide is a leading cause of death in pregnant women. The types of injuries seen in pregnant women are often different; pregnant women are more likely to be struck in the abdomen, whereas nonpregnant women are more frequently struck the face or other parts of the body. Abused women are less likely to seek prenatal care, putting themselves and their unborn child at even greater risk.

Child Abuse

Children are a common target group for family violence. According to DHHS, approximately 2.4 million children are abused each year in the United States. A parent or parents may abuse one or all of their children. Children whose mothers are victims of wife battery are twice as likely to be abused than those whose mothers are not victims of abuse. Children who witness violence in the home have many of the same symptoms as children who are directly abused.

Elder Abuse

The elderly population is also vulnerable to mistreatment in the form of physical assault, psychological or emotional abuse, sexual abuse, financial manipulation, and neglect. The most likely perpetrators of elder abuse are persons well acquainted or in continual contact with the dependent individual, including family members or nonfamily members who become caregivers, spouses or significant others, or professional caregivers.

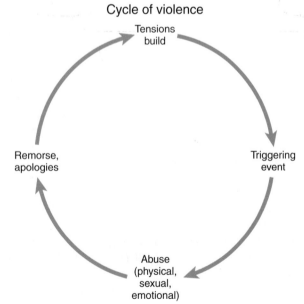

Cycle of violence

Tensions build

Triggering event

Abuse (physical, sexual, emotional)

Remorse, apologies

Figure 18-1 The cycle of violence. *Modified from Crisis Support Network, Pacific County, Wash; and Walker LE:* The battered woman, *New York, 1979, Harper & Row.*

> **REAL**World
>
> If EMTs are suspicious of geriatric abuse taking place in a nursing home, they have an obligation to report their suspicions. Every state has an **ombudsman** designated to investigate reports of institutional abuse. EMTs can find their state's ombudsman by going to http://www.ltcombudsman.org/static_pages/ombudsmen.cfm and clicking on their state.

Elder abuse is common throughout the United States, with approximately 1 million known cases occurring annually. Most cases of abuse are committed in residential rather than institutional settings. The majority of elder abuse victims are women; in a 1996 study, 67.3% of the victims were female. Types of elder abuse include neglect, physical abuse, exploitation, emotional abuse, and sexual abuse. The most common victim of elder abuse is an older woman with some chronic illness or disability, and the most common perpetrators are adult children, other family members, and spouses.

LEARNING OBJECTIVES
- Discuss examples of child abuse and neglect (maltreatment).
- Discuss examples of elder abuse.
- Discuss examples of partner/spousal abuse.
- Describe the characteristics associated with the following:
  - The typical abuser of a partner/spouse
  - The typical abuser of elderly persons
  - The typical abuser of children
  - The typical assailant of sexual assault
- Discuss examples of sexual assault.
- Discuss the assessment and management of the abused patient.
- Identify community resources that assist victims of abuse and assault.

Types of Abuse and Recognition

Evidence strongly suggests that abuse is associated with several known variables and conditions. Abuse by a caregiver can be fueled by the perpetrator's need to control another person; dependency; such factors as stress, ignorance, frustration, and desperation; or an inability to provide adequate care. Other potential variables include the environment in which the patient lives and the financial relationship, if any between caregiver and patient.

Domestic and family violence encompasses all acts of violence within the context of family or intimate relationships. It is an issue of increasing concern because it has a negative effect on all family members. Because most victims and perpetrators of domestic violence are likely to hide or deny the problem, your first role as an EMS provider is to identify signs or symptoms of violence, abuse, or neglect. Performing a physical assessment and patient history to clarify suspicions is critical to identifying suspected abuse.

The clues to abuse that follow are exhaustive and would be of little value if you were expected to review the list each time you had a suspicious encounter. More appropriately, you are expected to *recognize* these situations when they present themselves. You may also develop a "consciousness" when encountering trauma in women, children, and elderly persons that serves as a trigger in unusual or suspicious circumstances.

These circumstances may take many forms. Not all injuries are related to abuse, and it is also your responsibility to exercise good judgment in not overreporting suspected incidents of domestic and family violence. Medical direction can be invaluable in advising you when situations and clues are marginal or ambiguous.

Physical Abuse

Physical abuse refers to any physical injury inflicted on another person, including beatings, sexual assault, food or water deprivation, and inappropriate use of physical restraint. Physical abuse is usually recurrent and escalates in both frequency and severity. Most assaults on women do not result in death but do result in physical injury and severe emotional distress. Although the most obvious signs of domestic violence, physical injuries are frequently not reported by women and may go unrecognized by the professionals mandated to take action.

Signs of Physical Abuse

You should be aware of the numerous signs of physical abuse during your focused (secondary) assessment of a trauma patient (history, physical examination), especially when the patient is young, a woman, or an elderly patient (**Figure 18-2**). General signs include the following:
- Multiple bruises in different stages of healing
- Patterned bruises
- Black eyes, lacerations, and welts
- Defensive injuries to the arms
- Broken bones and bone fractures
- Burns
- Cuts or open wounds
- Sprains, dislocations, and internal injuries
- Broken eyeglasses
- Signs of restraint

REALWorld

Some cultures believe in "coining," or *cao gio* (pronounced "gow yaw"). This is a practice of rubbing heated oil on the chest, back, or shoulders of an ill child. The person then vigorously rubs a coin in a linear manner until a red mark is seen. It is believed that this allows the illness to be released from the body. The marks made from coining have been mistaken for abuse.

Other key clues may indicate abuse. For example, multiple calls to a person's home should raise a high index of suspicion. Being "prone to accidents" is a common "red flag" for domestic or family violence. Conversely, persons who wait to seek medical help for serious injuries may indicate a basic fear of discovery. In these cases the abuser may prevent the victim from calling EMS because of fear of arrest or loss of control.

You should also note injuries that do not match the story presented during the history. For example, a patient who says that she "fell down the stairs" but has a beltlike bruise on her back or neck might raise suspicion and lead you to inquire about physical abuse. Patients who are physically abused may also have injuries on many different areas of the body, especially areas that are less likely to be hurt, such as the face, throat, neck, chest, abdomen, and genitals. You may encounter wounds that are shaped like teeth, hands, belts, and cigarette tips, or a burn with a clear line of demarcation consistent with submersion in boiling water. An infant with burns only on the buttocks and feet but not the thighs should arouse suspicion; if the infant fell into hot water, the thighs would also be burned (knees drawn up to escape the pain).

Some general and nonspecific behaviors that may be associated with abuse include chronic use of alcohol or drugs, depression, and suicide attempts. These signs may not be helpful as a primary means for identifying abuse, but they may be triggers for raising your index of suspicion, leading to specific questions

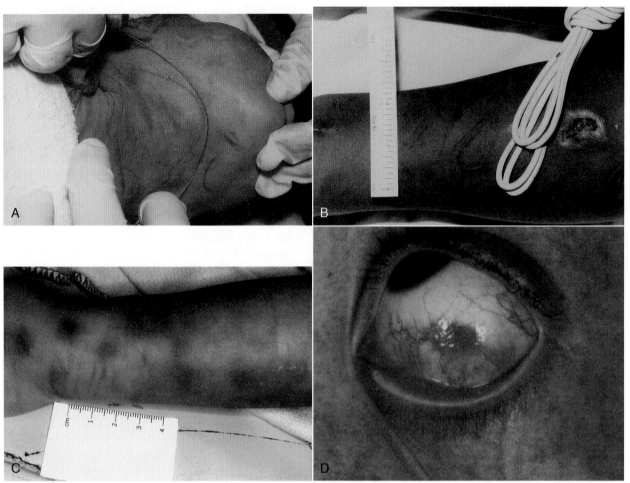

Figure 18-2 Images of abuse. **A,** Multiple ligature marks from wire. **B,** Contusions resulting from assault with electrical cord. **C,** Mutiple subtle fingertip contusions. **D,** Petechial hemorrhage from attempted strangulation. *A and B courtesy Dr Elizabeth Balraj, Cuyahoga County Coroner, Cleveland, Ohio; C courtesy Dr. Lisa Kohler, Summit County Medical Examiner, Akron, Ohio; D courtesy The Dove Program, Summa Health System, Akron, Ohio. In Polsky SS, Markowitz J:* Color atlas of domestic violence, *St Louis, 2004, Mosby.*

during the history, or they may support your suspicions when specific signs are also present.

Psychological and Emotional Abuse

Psychological abuse is often underestimated, trivialized, and at times difficult to define. Abused women report that psychological abuse is as damaging as physical battering because of its impact on the victim's self-image. It often precedes or accompanies physical abuse, but psychological abuse may occur by itself.

Emotional abuse represents a method of control that may consist of verbal attacks and humiliations, including repeated verbal attacks against the victim's worth as an individual or role as a parent, family member, co-worker, friend, or community member. The verbal attacks often emphasize the victim's vulnerabilities.

An abuser may repeatedly tell his victim that she is stupid, crazy, or insane and may often belittle her by calling her names. The woman is constantly reminded of her dependence on him for survival. The purpose of the verbal abuse is to destroy the woman's self-confidence, increase the perpetrator's feelings

of superiority, and maintain his control of her behavior and attitude.

Isolation occurs when perpetrators try to control the victims' time, activities, and contact with others. Perpetrators may accomplish this through interfering with supportive relationships, creating barriers to normal activities, such as taking away the car keys or locking the victim in the home, and lying or distorting what is real to gain psychological control.

Abusers often use manipulation of important possessions, such as children or pets, to coerce victims to behave in the way the abusers want. An abuser may threaten to abuse the family's children, actually abuse the children, or force the woman to watch or participate in the abuse. Many abused women are not allowed by their abusers to work outside the home and may not have any access to money. Even if a woman does work outside the home, she may have to give her paycheck to her partner to prevent an assault. Most abusers are very jealous of any relationships their partners may have. If an abused woman does work outside the home, her partner may often accuse her of having affairs with her co-workers. Often this is the cause of many quarrels and fights that lead to injuries and assaults. The victim may feel safer if she does not work.

Victims of emotional or psychological abuse may not be ready or able to communicate their fears. A typical victim may want to seek help but is afraid to ask. One such patient, when asked by a physician why she did not report incidents of abuse sooner, responded, "I was ready to talk, but they never asked."

Signs and Symptoms

Although the visible signs of emotional abuse can be difficult to find, this type of abuse leaves hidden scars that manifest in numerous behavioral ways. Patients may exhibit insecurity, poor self-esteem, destructive behavior, angry acts (e.g., fire setting, animal cruelty), withdrawal, poor development of basic skills, alcohol or drug abuse, and suicide. Difficulty in forming relationships and an unstable job history are possible results of emotional maltreatment.

Sexual Abuse

Sexual abuse is a form of violence in which the victim is forced to have sexual intercourse with the abuser or take part in unwanted sexual activity. It consists of a range of behaviors that may include pressured sex when the victim does not desire sex, coerced sex by manipulation or threat, physically forced sex, or *sexual assault* accompanied by violence. Victims may be forced or coerced to perform a type of sex they do not desire or at a time they do not want it. For some battered victims, this sexual violation is profound and difficult to discuss.

The Rape Abuse Incest National Network (RAINN) reports that one in six women and one in 33 men will be involved in a rape or attempted rape. Sexual assaults perpetrated on men account for 10% of all sexual assaults. Young, unmarried, separated, or divorced women and nonwhite women are the most frequent victims of **rape** and attempted rape. Black women have higher rates of rape than white or Hispanic women. An estimated 72% of cases involve someone the victim knows, and 60% are unreported.

Extreme sensitivity must be used with victims of sexual abuse. In addition to the physical injuries, a sexual abuse victim may sustain psychological injuries, which can become worse after insensitive treatment by healthcare providers. If the assault is recent, an effort should be made to preserve evidence. Patients should be encouraged not to bathe, shower, urinate, defecate, douche, brush their teeth, or change clothes until they have been examined in a hospital. Victims may not be receptive to this advice because they feel unclean and violated and may want to wash away all traces of the incident.

Many hospitals now have sexual abuse teams that are specially trained in treating these patients. A female rape victim may reject treatment by a male emergency medical technician (EMT). If this is the case and a female EMT is available, she could care for the patient. Conversely, gentle, supportive care rendered by a male EMT may be beneficial to the patient and ease her posttraumatic adjustment period. Physical assessment by either gender may be difficult for the victim because she was recently violated. Assessment and care should focus on assessing and treating life-threatening injuries. Injuries should be treated as needed but with awareness that evidence should be preserved when possible.

REAL*World*

Victims of sexual abuse commonly feel embarrassed, ashamed, and alone. The treatment they will need extends far beyond the ambulance and emergency department. The EMT should be prepared to offer abuse victims support line contact numbers. Two national groups are the National Domestic Violence Hotline at 1-800-799-SAFE (7233) and the National Sexual Assault Hotline at 1-800-656-4673.

Economic Abuse

Economic abuse may include control and access to the victim's resources, such as time, transportation, food, clothing, shelter, insurance, and money. The perpetrator may interfere with the victim's ability to become self-sufficient and insist that he or she control all the finances. This type of abuse is prevalent in elderly persons. It may involve theft or misuse of an elder's funds, property, or assets. Examples of this include stealing an older person's money or possessions, forging the older person's signature, cashing checks without authorization, and misusing guardianship or power of attorney.

Examples of financial abuse include, but are not limited to, the following:
- Changes in banking practice
- Unauthorized automated teller machine (ATM) withdrawals
- Addition of names to a bank signature card
- Sudden changes in a will
- Disappearance of funds or possessions
- Unpaid bills despite adequate financial resources
- Inadequate care despite adequate financial resources
- Relatives suddenly claiming rights to an elder's possessions
- Sudden transfer of money to a relative or nonfamily member

When a victim reports such abuses to you during an EMS call, you should report it to the hospital staff so that the appropriate follow-up can occur at the hospital.

Case in Point

While caring for an elderly woman complaining of weakness and lethargy, you notice that her room is sparsely decorated. She reports that she lives with her son and his family and that this is her space. She says that when she moved in 6 months ago, her son would not let her bring most of her personal belongings, telling her she would not need them. This may be a sign of geriatric abuse in the form of neglect or economic coercion.

Neglect

Neglect is also a common type of abuse found in the elderly population as well as in childhood. **Neglect** is defined as the failure to fulfill duties and obligations. This can include failure to pay for necessary care and failure to provide food, water, shelter, medicine, clothing, and other necessities for daily living.

Indicators of neglect include the following:
- Untreated wounds
- Poor personal hygiene

- Untreated medical conditions
- Unsanitary living conditions
- Harmful living conditions
- Failure to thrive
- Weight loss
- Constant demand for attention from the EMT

LEARNING OBJECTIVES
- Describe priorities for crew safety at the scene of possible domestic violence or abuse.
- Discuss the legal aspects associated with abuse and assault situations.
- Discuss the documentation associated with abused and assaulted patients.

Approach to the Suspected Victim of Domestic Violence or Abuse

When entering a scene where abuse may have occurred, the EMT has safety concerns, especially in the case of physical abuse. Remember that abuse is an effort to gain control. If the perpetrator believes the EMT is threatening that control, he may turn and physically assault the EMT. Scene safety is of the utmost importance.

Identification of abuse requires a systematic and measured approach in the prehospital phase of care. Once again, abused patients may not be willing to step forward and report the problem for fear of retribution by the abuser. You must create a safe environment as you collect your history to encourage victims of abuse to communicate cases of abuse to you and other authorities. To be cooperative and honest, the patient must first be assured that the ambulance and ED will provide protection from the abuser before volunteering information. If necessary, you should attempt to separate the patient from the suspected abuser so that the interview is objective. Expressing the need for patient privacy during the performance of the patient assessment can often accomplish this goal.

To gain the confidence of the patient, your style of communication must be calm, caring, and reassuring. The patient must feel that you are a person he or she can trust. Questions in the history should be nonthreatening. Questions should be asked in plain language and framed in a nonthreatening and nonjudgmental manner. The setting should be private and comfortable; when possible, the interview should occur without others being present, particularly the suspected abuser. Keep in mind that with abuse victims, volunteering information is the exception rather than the rule. Moreover, chief complaints may be evasive, vague, or completely unrelated to the issue at hand. Direct questions such as, "Did he hit you?" may deliver a more accurate picture of the situation than, "Is there anything you would like to tell me?"

Clues can be subtle. Suspicions should be raised, for example, if a victim's story is rehearsed, if the individual appears fearful or tentative, or if she is unable to sustain eye contact or is excessively cautious in presenting information. Frequent hospitalizations, surgeries, claimed or apparent disabilities, and transfusions are also vital clues that may imply recurrent abuse.

In some situations the patient may state directly that she was abused. In other cases she may minimize complaints and directly deny abuse. Patients may describe a cause of injury that is inconsistent with wounds or bruises found on the body or may say they fell or were injured by a stranger. Delayed access to EMS should raise your index of suspicion.

The information you gather surrounding the occurrence of an injury is extremely important, but it would be unwise to undertake an investigation. Careful observation without accusation or confrontation allows you to transport the patient to a hospital with the least amount of delay. This is in the patient's best interest, and once at the hospital, you can relay your suspicions and observations to the emergency physician.

As you obtain the history, the following should alert you to possible abuse:
- Repeated calls at the same address
- A story not consistent with the injury
- Changes in the history, depending on who is giving it
- Witnesses giving contradictory histories
- Patient reluctant to give a history
- Delay in obtaining medical attention
- Timing of the injury not consistent with clinical findings
- Spouse's or parent's response not appropriate to the severity of the injury
- Obvious alcohol or drug use by the patient or partner
- Patient afraid to discuss how the injury occurred
- Conflicting stories
- Fresh burns

You should pay particular attention to the environment, the sanitary state of the home, and any evidence of a struggle and determine especially the following:
1. Time of the incident
2. Presence of a witness
3. History of recent illness
4. Condition of the patient's clothing (e.g., cleanliness or presence of blood or dried secretions)

The abused victim may respond in various ways. The patient may be overly friendly or withdrawn or may display inappropriate responses, such as to pain. You should also be concerned about the child who is "too good."

Reporting Requirements

Reporting laws vary from state to state. In your local area, you may not be legally mandated to report abuse; however, you are morally and professionally responsible to set an investigation in motion if you suspect abuse. All the laws are written so that one can report suspicions and be protected from litigation for false accusations. Those who are mandated to report suspected abuse (e.g., EMS providers, physicians, nurses), however, would be held legally responsible for failure to report a suspicion and can be subject to prosecution for failure to report.

Case in Point

In 1987, Lisa Steinberg, an illegally adopted girl, was beaten to death by her father after years of physical abuse and neglect. Joel Steinberg waited 12 hours before summoning emergency aid. Lisa died 3 days later. A lawsuit was successfully brought against the city of New York by her natural mother for failing to protect the girl. A student teacher had reported bruises in various stages of healing to Lisa's teacher, who failed to report them to the authorities. Police and child welfare workers had visited the apartment but also failed to act.

By taking the initiative to follow your suspicions and report them to the authorities, with careful and objective documentation of your findings, you can help alleviate the problem of abuse. Your actions might even prevent another senseless death like that of Lisa Steinberg.

Scenario Follow-up

Abdominal pain associated with pregnancy is a common complaint. The crucial actions in this scenario were determining the underlying cause of the abdominal pain. Scenes, statements, and patient histories that do not make sense are all triggers for the EMT to consider some underlying issue. This patient fit the profile for abuse: young, female, and pregnant, with a nondescript recounting of events. Also, remember that the police responded for a noise complaint.

Summary

Domestic violence or abuse transcends age group, race, socioeconomic status, and gender. It is a societal disease kept secret based on power and fear and is the source of many EMS calls. The EMT on the scene is often the one person who can evaluate the sights and sounds and recognize the signs of abuse. EMTs have a legal and moral obligation to report suspected abuse to the appropriate authorities. EMS providers may not be able to stop the abuse and correct the situation on one call, but they can put the process in motion, helping the victim over the long term.

The Bottom Line

Learning Checklist

✓ Abuse affects persons of all races, ages, and socioeconomic status and both genders.

✓ Most assault victims are women, although men can fall victim to assault as well.

✓ Only an estimated 40% of rape cases are reported.

✓ Abuse can be physical, psychological, emotional, financial, or sexual.

✓ Abuse stems from the assailant's need to establish and maintain control.

✓ EMTs have moral, ethical, and often legal obligations to report cases of abuse.

✓ Signs of abuse include the following:
  ✓ Repeated calls at the same address
  ✓ A story not consistent with the injury
  ✓ Changes in the history, depending on who is giving it
  ✓ Witnesses giving contradictory histories
  ✓ Patient reluctant to give a history
  ✓ Delay in obtaining medical attention
  ✓ Timing of the injury not consistent with clinical findings
  ✓ Spouse's or parent's response not appropriate to the severity of the injury
  ✓ Obvious alcohol or drug use by the patient or partner
  ✓ Patient afraid to discuss how the injury occurred
  ✓ Conflicting stories
  ✓ Fresh burns

✓ In some cases, direct questioning may be the best form or history taking when dealing with victims of assault.

✓ Calls involving abuse present safety concerns for EMS personnel.

✓ Domestic violence usually follows a cycle: tension phase, violence phase, then honeymoon phase ("wine and roses" phase).

Key Terms

Assault The willful attempt to harm someone.

Cycle of violence Repeated phases of tension, violence, and "honeymoon" brought on by the victim's desire to be perfect and the perpetrator's anger.

Domestic violence Physical, emotional, psychological, sexual, or other forms of abuse perpetrated on a person in domestic relationship; the goal is usually to exert dominance or control.

Economic abuse Financial exploitation of a person by another to gain control.

Emotional abuse Emotional injury inflicted on a person by another to demonstrate power.

Neglect Failure to fulfill duties and obligations and to provide for the necessities for daily living.

Ombudsman An official, usually appointed by the government, who is charged with representing the interests of the public by investigating and addressing complaints reported by individual citizens.

Physical abuse Physical injury inflicted on a person by another to demonstrate power.

Rape Unwanted penetration of the genitalia.

Sexual abuse Unwilling or unlawful touch of genitalia, which may include rape.

Review Questions

1. Which of the following most likely suggests child abuse of a 5-year-old boy?
   a. Bruises on knees at different stages of healing
   b. Cut on the chin scabbed over
   c. Bruises on the back of the legs
   d. Multiple abrasions on the elbows

2. In the cycle of violence, which phase poses the most potential danger for EMS?
   a. Tension phase
   b. Violence phase
   c. Honeymoon phase
   d. There is no danger for EMS

3. An EMT is called to treat an elderly patient with dementia who is a poor history giver. The EMT is concerned the patient is being abused but is not sure. How should the EMT proceed?
   a. Report suspicions to the proper authorities.
   b. Investigate and report the alleged abuse only when the EMT has enough evidence.
   c. Confront the caregiver directly with the accusation.
   d. Do nothing; if it is abuse, a person more involved in the case will contact the authorities.

4. When taking a history from a patient who is a victim of domestic violence, which of the following questions may best elicit a history of the events?
   a. "Is there anything you want to tell me?"
   b. "Is there a secret you would like to share?"
   c. "Did your partner hit you?"
   d. This information is not important to EMS.

5. In an attempt to inform a victim of domestic violence that options are available to help the victim leave or improve the situation, which of the following statements would be best?
   a. "Why do you stay with that jerk?"
   b. "Why do you let him hit you?"
   c. "You are a fool for staying in this relationship."
   d. "Let me share some resources that can help you."

6. Which of the following most suggests neglect of an elderly patient?
   a. Bedsores that appear infected
   b. Bruises consistent with falling
   c. Altered state of consciousness
   d. Soiled clothes

7. When dealing with a victim who has been raped, why is it important not to let the person bathe or shower?
   a. The victim may change her mind about reporting.
   b. The victim may wash away evidence.
   c. Time is crucial if an arrest is to be made.
   d. EMS cannot be on the scene that long.

8. When assessing a conscious rape victim who has been assaulted, which of the following describes the best method of assessment?
   a. Cut away the patient's clothes, and perform a detailed physical assessment.
   b. EMS does not perform assessment of rape victims.
   c. Only assess arterial bleeding.
   d. Ask first if the patient is hurt or bleeding.

For Further Review

In the Student Workbook

- Multiple-choice questions
- Short-answer questions
- True-false questions
- Case scenario questions

On Evolve

- Weblinks
- Lecture notes
- Exercises

Learning Objectives

Cognitive Objectives

- Discuss the incidence of domestic violence.
- Describe the categories of abuse.
- Describe the cycle of violence.
- Identify the profiles of the at-risk partner/spouse, the at-risk elder, and the at-risk child.
- Discuss examples of child abuse and neglect (maltreatment).
- Discuss examples of elder abuse.
- Discuss examples of partner/spousal abuse.
- Describe the characteristics associated with the following:
  - The typical abuser of a partner/spouse
  - The typical abuser of elderly persons
  - The typical abuser of children
  - The typical assailant of sexual assault
- Discuss examples of sexual assault.
- Discuss the assessment and management of the abused patient.
- Identify community resources that assist victims of abuse and assault.
- Describe priorities for crew safety at the scene of possible domestic violence or abuse.
- Discuss the legal aspects associated with abuse and assault situations.
- Discuss the documentation associated with abused and assaulted patients.

Affective Objectives

- Demonstrate sensitivity to the abused patient.
- Value the behavior of the abused patient.
- Attend to the emotional state of the abused patient.
- Recognize the value of nonverbal communication with the abused patient.
- Attend to the needs for reassurance, empathy, and compassion with the abused patient.
- Listen to the concerns expressed by the abused patient.
- Listen to and value the concerns expressed by the sexually assaulted patient.

Psychomotor Objectives

- Demonstrate the ability to assess an abused partner/spouse, elderly person, and child.
- Demonstrate the ability to assess a sexually assaulted patient.

References

Centers for Disease Control and Prevention: Pregnancy risk assessment monitoring (PRAMS), February 2006, www.cdc.gov/pram/.

Gorbien M, Eisenstein A: Elder abuse and neglect: an overview, *Clin Geriatr Med* 21(2):279, 2005.

Horan I, Cheng D: Enhanced surveillance for pregnancy-associated mortality—Maryland, 1993-1998, *JAMA* 285:1455, 2001.

Rape Abuse Incest National Network (RAINN), www.rainn.org.

Straus MA, Stewart JH: Corporal punishment by American parents: national data on prevalence, chronicity, severity, and duration, in relation to child and family characteristics, *Clin Child Family Psychol Rev* 2:55, 1999.

US Department of Health and Human Services; Administration for Children and Families; Administration on Children, Youth, and Families, National Center on Child Abuse and Neglect, www.hhs.gov.

US Department of Justice, Bureau of Justice Statistics: Victim characteristics, Dec 19, 2007, www.ojp.usdoj.gov/bjs/intimate/victims.htm.

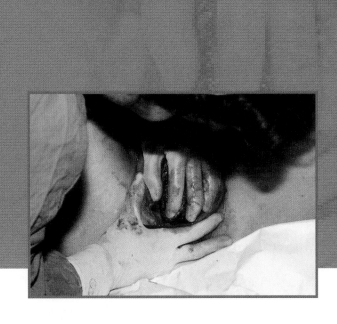

19 Obstetrics and Gynecology

Scenario

You respond to find a 27-year-old woman who is in labor on her living room couch. She appears very uncomfortable and cannot speak during her contraction, but when it subsides, she tells you that her contractions started a few hours ago and were short and sporadic. Now they are coming every 2 minutes, lasting a minute or more, and she feels an urge to move her bowels. The water sac has not yet broken. You now must visually examine her so you can decide whether to transport or prepare for immediate delivery.

You take appropriate personal precautions by putting on a gown, mask, goggles, and gloves. During the next contraction, you see the perineum bulge, and there is a sudden pop as the water sac breaks, drenching the couch. As the contraction peaks, the baby's head starts to crown. As the contraction subsides, the head recedes into the birth canal. You offer calm reassurance to the mother as you and your partner quickly lift her to the stretcher.

You open the obstetrics kit and place one drape from the kit on her abdomen and another under her hips at the entrance of the birth canal. Another contraction comes, and the mother cannot resist the urge to push as the head starts to crown. You apply gentle counterpressure to the crown of the head with your left hand while supporting the perineum and rectum with a sterile 4 × 4–inch gauze sponge in your right hand, actions to prevent an explosive delivery. The head is then smoothly delivered from the birth canal.

There is blood on the baby's face, and you wipe it with another sterile gauze sponge while supporting the head with your other hand. You suction the baby's mouth and then the nose with a bulb syringe. Next, you explore to see if the umbilical cord is wrapped around the newborn's neck; it is not, so you tell the mother to go ahead and push. Delivery of the shoulders and the rest of the baby proceeds so quickly that you barely have time to catch the slippery newborn by the feet with your right hand as you hold him firmly by the back of his neck with your left hand. You cradle him in your left arm close against your body at the level of the vagina and wipe his purple face clean of blood and mucus before suctioning his mouth and then each nostril with a bulb syringe. He starts to scream in protest and turns a bright pink as he cries. You clamp and cut the cord and gently place him on the drape on his mother's abdomen.

Your partner, who has recorded the time of delivery, continues care of the newborn. He dries the baby and wraps him in a clean, dry towel for warmth before handing him back to the mother. Because the infant is crying, has a heart rate greater than 100 beats/min, is pink in color, and is moving vigorously, your partner determines that the infant has an Apgar score of 15 and does not need further care. He will simply keep him warm and observe for any problems that might develop.

While your partner cares for the baby, you remove the soiled linen from under the mother, place a clean towel under her, and cover her with a warm blanket. The placenta has not delivered, but there is minimal bleeding; you decide to proceed to the hospital. An emergency physician supervises the delivery of the placenta shortly after your arrival.

Few calls are as rewarding as those in which you are able to assist in the delivery of a normal healthy baby. On the other hand, few calls are as devastating as those in which an infant dies, especially if the death was preventable. Although childbirth has transpired without intervention since the beginning of time, measures can be undertaken to make the process safer for both the mother and the infant. In rare instances in which resuscitation of the newborn is necessary, it must be initiated rapidly, or the baby may sustain irreversible brain damage or death.

Remembering that there are two patients is a crucial element in caring for a pregnant patient, whether she is bleeding, in labor, or a trauma victim. As a general rule, the best treatment for the unborn baby is dynamic management of the mother, with special attention to the tasks of maintaining vital signs and oxygenation. This chapter prepares you to assist in normal and abnormal deliveries, care for the newborn, and aid the patient with other obstetric or gynecologic emergencies.

LEARNING OBJECTIVES
- Explain the rationale for understanding the implications of treating two patients (mother and baby).
- Identify the following structures: uterus, vagina, fetus, placenta, umbilical cord, amniotic sac, and perineum.

Anatomy and Physiology

During the 40 weeks of pregnancy, the uterus provides a home for the developing unborn baby, or **fetus.** The uterus is a hollow organ with thick, muscular walls located in the pelvic cavity, behind the urinary bladder (**Figure 19-1**). About 3 inches (7.5 cm) long and only about 2 inches (5 cm) at its widest part before pregnancy, this amazing organ can expand enormously during pregnancy, as can the rest of the birth canal through which a baby must travel to be born. The first part of the journey out of the uterus is through the *cervix,* which is the lowest segment of the uterus. The cervix protrudes into the *vagina,* the lower part of the birth canal. The exit from the birth canal, including the area between the vagina and the anus, is the **perineum.** Despite its ability to stretch during childbirth, the perineum is often torn as the baby emerges. The area around the opening to the urethra, which is at the anterior outside edge of the birth canal, can also be damaged during childbirth, especially if the birth is not well controlled.

Attached to the side of the uterus are the female sex glands, or *ovaries.* Ovaries are responsible for housing and maturing the eggs and for producing estrogen and progesterone, hormones that are vital to menstruation and pregnancy. Because the ovaries function as hormone producers, they are classified as *endocrine* glands.

Arising from the upper outer walls of the uterus above the ovaries are two trumpet-shaped structures called the *fallopian tubes.* The length of these tubes varies from about 3 to 6 inches (7.5-15 cm). At the end closest to the ovary, they each contain fringelike projections that help to sweep the mature egg from the ovary into the tube. Muscular contractions of the tubes and gently swaying *cilia* (hairs), which line the tubes, speed the egg on its way to the uterus. The uterus, fallopian tubes, and ovaries have an extensive blood supply from the uterine and ovarian arteries, vessels that descend primarily from the aorta.

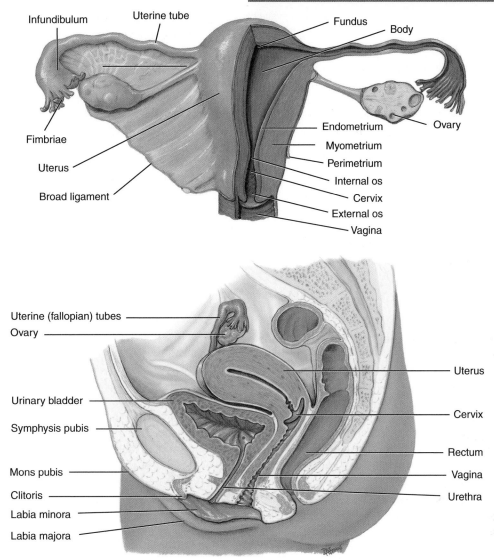

Figure 19-1 Anatomy of the female reproductive system. *From Applegate, EJ*: The anatomy and physiology learning system, *ed 3, St. Louis, 2006, Saunders.*

Approximately every 28 days an egg is released from the ovaries. The egg is drawn into the fallopian tubes and begins to move toward the uterus. In preparation to receive the egg, the blood supply to the uterus increases, and the walls of the uterus thicken. If the egg is fertilized by a sperm cell, the fertilized egg will implant on the wall of the uterus, and fetal development will begin. If the egg is not fertilized, the female body will discard the egg, extra blood, and tissue. This cycle is known as **menstruation,** or the *menstrual cycle.* The onset of menstruation is known as **menarche** and occurs at about age 12 to 14 years and will continue approximately every 28 days until age 40 to 60, when menstruation ceases, known as **menopause.**

REAL*World*

Young girls may have irregular menstrual cycles. They may report having a period one month and then missing their period for 3 months. This needs to be taken into consideration when assessing a female patient. In some cases, missing a period may suggest that the patient is pregnant, whereas in other situations it may be a normal variant for that patient.

Pregnancy

Implantation of the embryo in a pregnant woman occurs about 7 days after fertilization, usually in the upper segment of the uterus. By this time, the single cell has multiplied into a sphere containing hundreds of cells. The outermost cells eventually develop into the **placenta,** a vascular organ of pregnancy that serves as an exchange area. Nutrients and oxygen from the mother's blood are delivered to the fetus, and waste products such as carbon dioxide cross from the fetus to the mother's circulation. *Afterbirth* refers to the placenta and fetal membranes after they are expelled following the baby's birth.

Growing from the fetal side of the placenta and completely encasing the baby is the *amniotic sac,* which is a double-layered membrane. The membranes contain the developing fetus and 16 to 32 ounces (at term) of a clear, watery liquid known as *amniotic fluid.* The fetus floats in this fluid, which cushions it against injury and also helps it maintain a constant body temperature. If at any time during the later days of pregnancy or

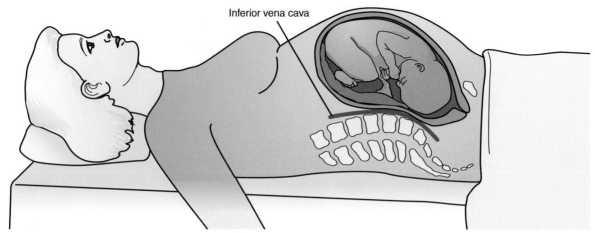

Figure 19-2 Supine hypotensive syndrome of pregnancy. The vena cava is occluded by the weight of the fetus. *Adapted from Burroughs, A: Bleier's Maternity Nursing, ed 5, Philadelphia, 1986, WB Saunders (out of print).*

labor the fetus is deprived of oxygen, his or her bowels may empty into this fluid, giving the fluid a greenish tinge. The color of the fluid may range from yellow to "pea soup" green, depending on the amount of feces, called **meconium,** discharged into the amniotic fluid. Meconium-stained fluid alerts you that the baby is, or has been, stressed. Because meconium-stained fluid contains solid fecal particles, it may cause respiratory distress if the baby aspirates it into the lungs at birth. Approximately 20% of the babies who pass meconium before delivery have some type of respiratory distress.

The life of the fetus depends on uninterrupted, two-way blood flow between the placenta and the fetus by the **umbilical cord.** About 1 inch (2.5 cm) wide and 22 inches (55 cm) long at term, the umbilical cord contains three blood vessels surrounded by a clear, protective gelatin. The largest vessel is the umbilical vein, which carries oxygenated and nourishing blood to the fetus. There are also two umbilical arteries, which carry waste products away from the fetus to the placenta. This is one of two instances in which oxygenated blood is carried by a vein while an artery carries waste products. The only other place this occurs is in the pulmonary circulation.

Physiologic Changes of Pregnancy

Women undergo massive physiologic changes during pregnancy that affect your treatment of the pregnant patient. Understanding the type and extent of these changes is an essential aspect of your training as an emergency medical technician (EMT).

Cardiovascular Changes

Plasma volume during pregnancy is increased by up to 50%. This raises the cardiac output from 5 L/min to about 7 L/min. At the same time, the red blood cell volume increases by only 18% to 32%. This dilution of the blood is often referred to as *physiologic anemia of pregnancy.* The heart rate increases 15 to 20 beats/min, and the blood pressure becomes lower than normal. Thus, some of the classic symptoms of shock (hypotension and tachycardia) are normal in pregnancy and may confuse the EMT treating the patient.

When hypovolemia occurs in a pregnant woman, a self-protective measure causes constriction of the uterine arteries that supply blood to the fetus, redirecting blood to her major organs. This compensatory mechanism occurs long before an observer notes a change in the mother's vital signs. Once the traditional signs of hypovolemic shock appear in the mother, it may be too late to save the fetus.

The position of the patient can intensify the effects of hypovolemia. When a pregnant woman lies in the supine position, the bulk of the fetus compresses the vena cava against the spinal column (**Figure 19-2**). By late pregnancy, total occlusion of the inferior vena cava may occur when the mother is supine. Compression of the vena cava inhibits venous return of blood to the heart, causing a decrease in cardiac output. This is known as supine hypotension syndrome. The well-known method of treating shock by positioning the patient supine and elevating the legs is ineffective in the pregnant woman because it does not relieve the compression of the vena cava caused by the baby.

Case in Point

A pregnant woman is having her hair washed at a salon. Shortly after reclining in the chair, the woman becomes unconscious. When EMS personnel arrive, they find her unconscious, supine in the chair. The simple act of lifting the woman to a stretcher and placing her on her left side relieves the compression on the vena cava, restoring cardiac return, cardiac output, and thus consciousness to the patient.

Many pregnant women cannot tolerate lying supine without fainting or at least feeling dizzy, regardless of whether blood loss has occurred. It is essential to transport a pregnant patient on her left side (**Figure 19-3**). In severe trauma cases, in which stability of the cervical spine and airway management take precedence, and you must keep the patient supine, place pillows or a wedge under the right side of the long spine board.

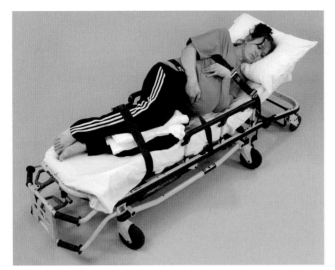

Figure 19-3 Position of choice for transporting a pregnant patient.

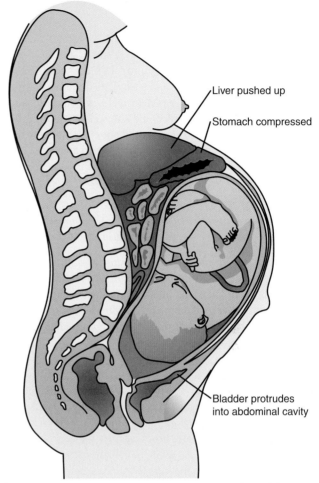

Liver pushed up

Stomach compressed

Bladder protrudes into abdominal cavity

Figure 19-4 Anatomic changes in pregnancy. *Adapted from Burroughs, A:* Bleier's Maternity Nursing, *ed 5, Philadelphia, 1986, WB Saunders (out of print).*

Pulmonary Changes

The respiratory rate remains the same or may increase slightly during a normal pregnancy, but the tidal volume increases by 50%. Oxygen consumption is greatly increased because of the high fetal demand for oxygen. Shortness of breath or the inability to fully expand the lungs is common, especially in late pregnancy or with twin gestations, because the bulk of the fetus causes upward displacement of the diaphragm. This elevation of the diaphragm reduces the capacity of the lungs and makes the pregnant patient more prone to hypoxia. The effect is even more exaggerated when she is supine. Progesterone also relaxes the diaphragm, often causing a feeling of air hunger. If a pregnant patient is having difficulty breathing while lying on her left side, she can be transported sitting up. Oxygen should always be administered in cases of blood loss, trauma, or dyspnea.

Gastrointestinal Changes

Progesterone, the hormone of pregnancy, has a slowing effect on the digestive tract. The rate of gastric emptying is decreased, and food remains in the stomach for a much longer time; the pregnant uterus also physically crowds the abdominal contents. Progesterone also causes some relaxation of the sphincter between the stomach and the esophagus, so an increased risk of vomiting by the pregnant patient always exists. Even if the patient has not eaten for several hours, you must assume that the stomach is full. Acid reflux, vomiting, and indigestion are common complaints during pregnancy, and aspiration is a major concern in an unconscious pregnant patient.

Genitourinary Changes

The urinary bladder, formerly located within the bony pelvis, becomes an abdominal organ in the second and third trimesters of pregnancy (**Figure 19-4**). Compression of the bladder between the uterus and the abdominal wall and stretching of the urethra cause an annoying sense of fullness, an inability to empty the bladder completely, and the need to urinate frequently. These changes make the bladder more susceptible

to injury from both blunt and penetrating trauma. The bladder is no longer protected from injury by the bony pelvis. Furthermore, the fullness of the bladder and its poor ability to empty may cause a "burst balloon" type of rupture when blunt trauma occurs.

Bladder infections during pregnancy are common and may cause premature labor. The patient may have flank pain or suprapubic pain, either continuous or in waves (contractions). The usual primary signs of bladder infection—frequency of urination and a constant urgency to void—are already familiar to the pregnant woman. Increased fluid intake and treatment of the bladder infection with antibiotics often relieve the premature labor caused by the infection.

The uterus itself, while shielding the abdominal contents from injury as it grows, becomes more susceptible to injury as it leaves the bony pelvis. In fact, as pregnancy progresses, a penetrating wound to the abdomen almost always involves the uterus, with or without its contents. The uterus in turn acts as a protective barrier for other organs.

Blood flow to the uterus during pregnancy is greatly enhanced. This increased vascularity is serious cause for concern if the uterus is injured. Pelvic fractures, always a severe cause of blood loss, are especially dangerous at this time.

Psychological Changes

Psychological changes vary from person to person but do occur during pregnancy. The hormonal changes associated with being pregnant can cause seemingly unprovoked changes in mood, such as spontaneous crying and unexplained feelings of anxiety. Pregnant women may begin to feel self-conscious about the change in their appearance and the weight gain. Early in the pregnancy, they may be concerned about losing their baby. Later in the pregnancy, they may be concerned about the delivery and their ability to care for the child later.

Childbirth

Stages of Labor

If delivery is not imminent, every attempt should be made to transport the mother to the hospital for delivery. Understanding the three stages of labor and knowing the signs of approaching or imminent delivery will help you decide whether to transport the patient to the hospital or prepare for an immediate delivery at the scene.

First Stage

The first stage of labor is the period that begins with the first **contraction** and ends when the cervix is fully dilated. During this stage, the powerful uterine muscles contract intermittently, pressing the baby down against the cervix, causing the cervix to thin and then open. It can take 14 hours or more of labor to dilate the cervix for a woman's first pregnancy. Subsequent labors tend to be much shorter. Women may experience irregular contractions of short duration throughout their pregnancy, increasing as they approach their delivery date. These are known as **Braxton Hicks contractions** and serve to strengthen the uterus, preparing it for delivery.

Labor contractions are timed from the beginning of one contraction to the beginning of the next contraction. In early labor, contractions are usually felt as mild and irregular cramps in the lower abdomen over the pubic bone and sometimes in the lower back. Toward the end of the first stage, the contractions become more painful, longer, and closer together. They may be 2 to 3 minutes apart and last as long as 90 seconds, so that the patient seems to be having a nearly continuous contraction. Contractions toward the end of the first stage of labor are usually so painful that the mother cannot walk or talk during a contraction. She may begin to shiver and perspire. Blood and mucus from the cervix, called "bloody show," may be seen. The amniotic sac may break at any time during labor or even before the onset of labor; therefore, rupture of the membranes or leaking of fluid is not necessarily an indication of impending birth.

Second Stage

The second stage of labor, or "pushing stage," begins when the cervix is fully dilated and ends with the birth of the baby. This stage usually takes an hour or more with the first baby but can occur very rapidly with subsequent births because the soft tissues of the pelvic floor have already been stretched and resistance is less. Many patients giving birth to their second or third child can deliver within a matter of minutes once the cervix is dilated. During the second stage of labor, pressure on the rectum by the fetal head as it descends causes an intense urge to push.

Third Stage

The third stage of labor begins with the delivery of the baby and ends with delivery of the placenta. After the baby has been born, the uterus is greatly reduced in size, and the surface area for attachment of the placenta to the uterine wall is comparatively reduced. The placenta is literally squeezed off the uterine wall. By contracting strongly into a hard ball, the uterus slows the flow of blood from the open blood vessels that were previously supplying the placenta.

Mechanics of Labor

Because humans walk upright, the shape of the human pelvis resembles a bent tin can. The passage of the fetus through the tight pelvic cavity during childbirth usually follows the same route, placing the fetus in a consistent series of positions. Visualizing this sequence of events provides a clearer understanding of childbirth and helps you anticipate the five major positions the newborn will assume as he or she emerges from the birth canal (**Figure 19-5**).

Flexion

The baby's head becomes flexed (chin on chest) as it meets resistance entering the pelvic canal. This move presents the smallest possible diameter of the head to the pelvis. The smaller the mother's pelvis, the more the baby's head must flex.

Internal Rotation

The entrance into the pelvis is a different shape than the exit. It is natural for the baby to follow the path of least resistance, squeezing the largest part of its head through the part of the outlet with the largest diameter. Therefore, although the head is usually facing one of the mother's sides when it first enters the pelvis, it must now turn 90 degrees as it descends into the pelvic outlet. By the time this internal rotation is completed, the baby is usually facing the mother's anus.

Extension

The baby's head, which was greatly flexed before and throughout internal rotation, must rise upward in extension as it emerges from under the symphysis pubis until it is completely born, after which it drops down toward the mother's anus if not supported.

Figure 19-5 The mechanics of childbirth refer to the movements that the fetus must make to negotiate the changing diameters of the female pelvis. **A,** Descent, engagement, and flexion. **B,** Internal rotation. **C,** Extension. **D,** Extension complete. **E,** External rotation. **F,** Expulsion. *From Murray SS, McKinney ES:* Foundations of maternal-newborn nursing, *ed 4, St Louis, 2006, Saunders.*

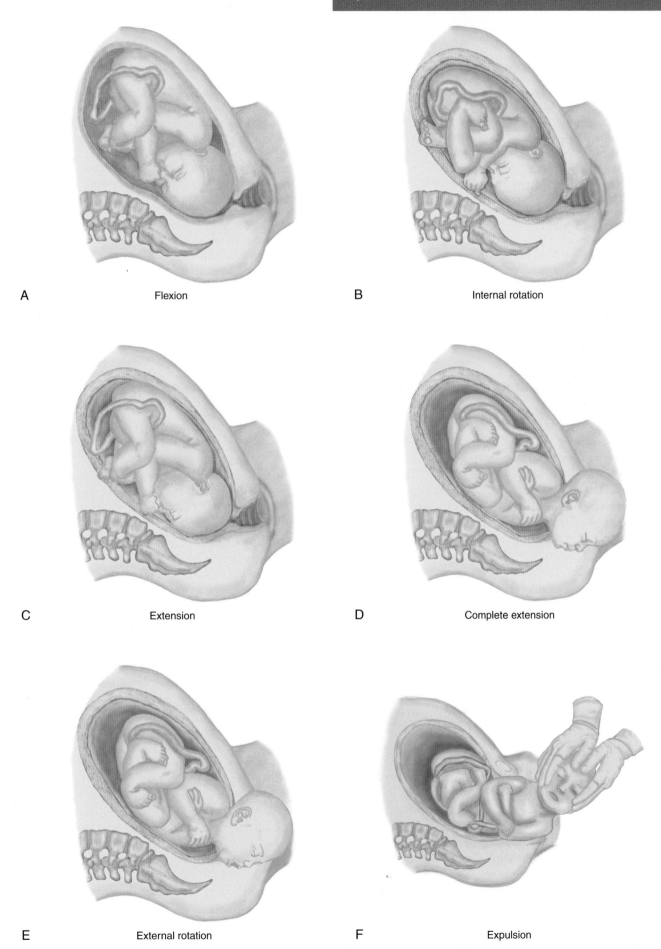

A   Flexion

B   Internal rotation

C   Extension

D   Complete extension

E   External rotation

F   Expulsion

| **Box 19-1** | Focused History Questions for Pregnant Patients with Possible Imminent Delivery |

- **Is this your first pregnancy?**

  If this is the first pregnancy, it will typically take an hour or more of hard pushing to deliver the baby, even after the cervix has been fully dilated. Women who have given birth before often will have short and unpredictable labors.

- **If you have had other children, how long were the previous deliveries? Did you deliver by cesarean section or have a normal vaginal delivery?**

  There is more risk involved for a woman who had a cesarean delivery. A laboring woman with a previous cesarean birth should be transported immediately, if possible.

- **What time did your contractions begin, and how far apart are they?**

  Contractions are closer together as labor progresses and eventually about 2 to 3 minutes apart and regular. Find out when the patient started to have regular contractions. A patient having her first baby and irregular contractions 10 minutes apart is probably in very early labor.

- **Has your water broken? If yes, what color was the fluid?**

  Remember that meconium-stained fluid may indicate an increased risk for the baby.

  Do not be surprised if the patient is not sure whether or not her membranes have broken. Fullness and pressure on the bladder often cause urinary incontinence. Rupture of the membranes may occur with a huge gush of fluid or as a tiny trickle, or a small amount may be expelled with each contraction. The membranes may rupture

before labor or may need to be ruptured at the time of delivery. Rupture of the membranes alone is not a sign of active labor.

- **Do you have an urge to move your bowels?**

  As the baby's presenting part moves down into the pelvic canal, it begins to put pressure on the nerves of the rectum. This creates an intense urge to move the bowels. If this is occurring, delivery is usually near, although a first-time mother may have a strong urge to push for an hour or more before delivery.

- **Have you had bleeding or a bloody show?**

  "Bloody show" is normal, especially toward the end of labor. If the membranes have ruptured, the bloody show may appear excessive as it mixes with amniotic fluid. However, excessive bleeding or passing large blood clots is abnormal.

- **When is your due date?**

  If the baby is more than 2 weeks early, notify the hospital to prepare for a possibly premature baby.

- **Have you had any problems with this pregnancy? Do you have any medical problems? Do you take any medications?**

  Diabetic mothers, for example, should be transported immediately because rapid intervention may be required. Because of fetal exposure to high levels of glucose during the diabetic mother's pregnancy, the baby is often large, and the delivery can be complicated.

- **When was your last oral intake?**

  Do not allow the patient to eat or drink, and recall that pregnant women have a slow gastrointestinal system and are more prone to aspiration.

External Rotation

After the head is born, it must realign with the shoulders, which have internally rotated so that one shoulder points upward (the anterior shoulder) and the other is down near the mother's anus. The head will now rotate to either the left or the right to stay in line with the body. At the completion of external rotation, the baby will be facing the inside of one of the mother's thighs.

Expulsion

After the head is born, the anterior shoulder is delivered first to avoid impaction behind the pubic bone. The posterior shoulder is then delivered. The rest of the body follows rapidly because it is much smaller in diameter then either the head or the shoulders.

> **LEARNING OBJECTIVE**
> - List indications of an imminent delivery.

Normal Delivery

Assessment of the Patient in Labor

The initial role of the EMT assessing a patient in labor is to decide whether to transport the mother to the hospital or to prepare for immediate delivery at the scene. You should ask specific questions in obtaining a focused patient history to determine whether the birth is imminent (**Box 19-1**).

A rapid oral history often is sufficient to ensure that transportation can safely proceed without a visual inspection of the

perineum. However, a visual examination is needed in the following situations:

- The patient cannot walk or talk during the contractions.
- The patient is in so much pain that she cannot answer you and appears to be pushing.
- The patient complains of an urge to push or tells you that the baby is coming.

Even though great urgency surrounds your decision to perform a visual examination, you must provide privacy for the patient, especially if you are in a public place. The patient must also consent to a physical examination. A calm voice, a respectful attitude, and an assurance that you intend to preserve her dignity can facilitate the necessary trust between you and the patient.

The visual examination involves checking for the distention or bulging of the perineum that occurs as the fetus begins to stretch the soft tissues of the vulva (**Figure 19-6**). The inside wall of the rectum may also be visible as the sphincter is stretched open by the tremendous pressure on the perineum. If a visual examination is indicated, it should always be performed during a contraction because the fetus will recede, disappearing between contractions until crowning occurs. *Crowning* is the protrusion of the largest diameter of the fetal head through the opening of the birth canal. After crowning, the fetus no longer recedes during contractions, and birth of the head will occur shortly. You should prepare for delivery at the scene if crowning or bulging of the perineum occurs.

As the presenting part descends into the pelvis, pressure is exerted on the rectum, and the mother has an intense urge to

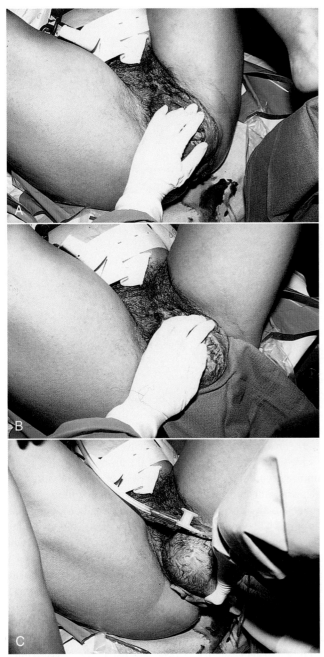

Figure 19-6 **A,** Distention of the perineum with part of the baby's head visible during contraction. Because the head may recede between contractions, the mother should be checked for crowning during a contraction. **B,** Crowning is complete, and the head has begun to extend upward toward the pubic bone. Once crowning has occurred, the presenting part no longer recedes between contractions. **C,** The baby's head is born and drops down toward the mother's anus. *From Murray SS, McKinney ES:* Foundations of maternal-newborn nursing, *ed 4, St Louis, 2006, Saunders.*

move her bowels. As the presenting part fills the pelvic cavity, any fecal material in the mother's rectum is expelled. Never allow a laboring mother who feels an urge to move her bowels to go to a toilet.

Box 19-2 indicates the signs and symptoms indicating that delivery is imminent and should be handled at the scene.

Box 19-2	Signs and Symptoms of Imminent Delivery

1. Crowning is evident.
2. The EMT notices "bloody show."
3. Contractions are strong, less than 2 minutes apart, and last 60 to 90 seconds.
4. The patient feels the need to have a bowel movement.
5. The patient has a strong urge to push or tells you "the baby is coming."

Managing Delivery at the Scene

When you deliver a baby at the scene, you probably will have little or no time to prepare yourself or the patient. If possible, you should lift the patient onto the stretcher and move her into the ambulance (or at least try to lift the mother onto the stretcher for delivery). This serves two purposes. First, the ambulance is a perfect place to provide privacy if the mother is about to deliver in a public place. Second, if complications arise or the delivery does not occur as rapidly as thought, you are ready to transport. If the head delivers and you are unable to deliver the shoulders, it is much more awkward to transfer the mother onto the stretcher with the infant's head hanging out of the birth canal. If you prepare a patient for delivery but she does not actually deliver within 10 minutes, you should transfer her to the hospital.

> **LEARNING OBJECTIVE**
> • Establish the relationship between body substance isolation and childbirth.

Personal Protection

Childbirth puts the EMT at risk for exposure to communicable diseases from body substances. For example, harmful viruses (e.g., hepatitis, HIV) are present in the blood and, to a lesser extent, amniotic fluid of infected patients. Blood, feces, and other body fluids are abundant at most deliveries. Therefore, every attempt should be made to isolate and contain these substances. This is accomplished by use of personal protective equipment (PPE) when assisting in childbirth or handling the newborn. PPE for childbirth includes gloves, a face mask with eye protection or separate goggles, and a fluid-resistant gown. Many obstetrics kits contain only a plastic apron, which is insufficient coverage to protect against the extensive body fluid exposure in childbirth.

With practice, it only takes a few seconds to put on protective clothing. The mask and gown are applied first, followed by the gloves, which are pulled up over the cuffs of the gown. When removing the soiled clothing after delivery, you should remove the gown and gloves as if they were a single article of clothing by turning the gown inside out (**Figure 19-7**). This prevents the contaminated side of the gown from contacting your skin. You should dispose of PPE with other contaminated material in appropriate containers and wash

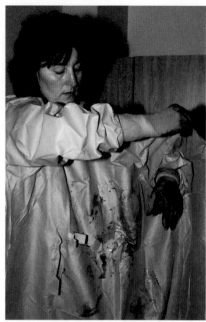

Figure 19-7 Proper removal of soiled garments. Remember not to touch unprotected parts of your body with soiled articles.

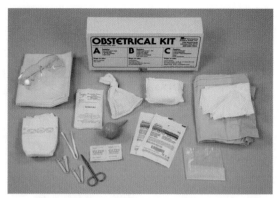

Figure 19-8 Contents of an obstetrics kit.

LEARNING OBJECTIVES
• List the steps to assist in the delivery.
• Describe care of the baby as the head appears.
• Describe how and when to cut the umbilical cord.
• Discuss special considerations with meconium.

your hands with antibacterial soap. Proper handwashing is the single best method of preventing the spread of disease-causing organisms.

LEARNING OBJECTIVES
• Identify and explain the use of the contents of an obstetrics kit.
• Outline the steps in the predelivery preparation of the mother.

Preparing the Mother for Delivery

The mother should be positioned on the stretcher in a semi-sitting position with her knees bent and legs spread apart to prepare her for delivery. She will feel less exposed if you keep a sheet over her abdomen and thighs. You should unwrap the obstetrics kit at the foot of the bed between the mother's legs (**Figure 19-8**). The kit usually contains several cord clamps (or hemostats) and bandage scissors (or a scalpel) to clamp and cut the umbilical cord. Kits with scissors are preferable because they are safer and easier to use in the event of a tight cord around the newborn's neck. The kit should also include a rubber bulb syringe for suctioning the infant's mouth and nostrils, sterile gloves, a fluid-resistant apron or gown, at least four towels, a dozen 4 × 4–inch gauze sponges, a baby blanket, sanitary napkins, and two large plastic bags for waste materials and the placenta. While you are opening the obstetrics kit, your partner should offer encouragement and moral support to the mother. If you are in a public place and have not had time to move the patient inside the ambulance, your partner can assign a person to create as much privacy as possible.

You should place two of the towels from the kit on the mother's abdomen and another towel on the stretcher beneath her buttocks. The newborn will be placed on the towels on the mother's abdomen, and the towel under her hips will absorb body fluids and waste.

Delivering the Baby

The Head

Delivery of the head can often be slowed and controlled by applying gentle pressure on the back of the baby's head with one hand while supporting the perineum with the other hand (**Figure 19-9**). This prevents an explosive delivery, which can cause excessive tearing of the perineum. If the amniotic sac has not yet ruptured, you should tear it with your fingers and spread the membranes away from the baby's face to minimize fluid aspiration and create an airway. Once the baby's head is born, you should support it with your left hand while you wipe the blood and fluid from the baby's face with a 4 × 4–inch gauze sponge. Next, while still supporting the head with your left hand, use a bulb syringe in your right hand to suction first the mouth and then the nose before the infant has a chance to take a breath. The mouth should be suctioned first because suctioning the nose may cause the baby to gasp and aspirate the large clog of secretions that is often present in the mouth. Meconium fluid is particularly dangerous to the infant and can act like cement if it is aspirated into the newborn's lungs, leading to severe respiratory problems.

To apply suction with a bulb syringe, compress the bulb between your thumb and fingers before placing the open tip into the mouth or nose. After the tip of the syringe is in the opening to be suctioned, gradually release the compression on the bulb until it is reinflated, then remove it to discard the mucus. Be very careful not to compress the bulb after you have placed the syringe into the baby's mouth or nose, or the mucus will be blown farther into the airway instead of removed.

REALWorld

As the mother pushes and the baby moves down the birth canal, the pressure placed on the intestines may cause the mother to have a bowel movement. If this occurs cover the feces with a clean sheet or towel and continue with the delivery. You must remain focused on the delivery process to avoid an explosive delivery tearing the mother's perineum and be ready to clear the child's airway once the head has delivered.

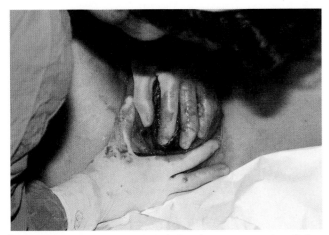

Figure 19-9 Delivery of the baby's head. Prepare to give slight counterpressure against the head while you support the perineum with your right hand. You may place a gauze sponge over the mother's anus to support the rectum and keep fecal material away from the infant's face. *From Al-Azzawi F:* Childbirth and obstetric techniques, *ed 2, St Louis, 1999, Mosby.*

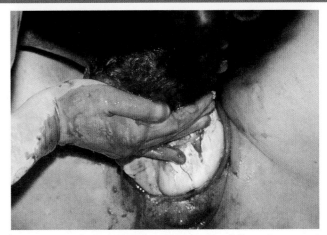

Figure 19-11 Lift the baby's head upward to deliver the posterior shoulder. *From Al-Azzawi F:* Childbirth and obstetric techniques, *ed 2, St Louis, 1999, Mosby.*

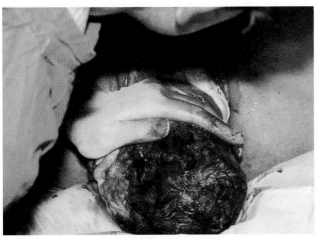

Figure 19-10 If the baby's shoulders do not deliver spontaneously, give gentle downward traction until the anterior shoulder appears. *From Al-Azzawi F:* Childbirth and obstetric techniques, *ed 2, St Louis, 1999, Mosby.*

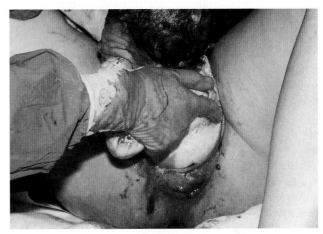

Figure 19-12 Slide your hand along the emerging body and prepare to catch the baby's feet. *From Al-Azzawi F:* Childbirth and obstetric techniques, *ed 2, St Louis, 1999, Mosby.*

After suctioning and before allowing the mother to push again, check the newborn to see if one or more loops of cord are around the neck. If a loose cord is around the neck, you may attempt to slip it over the baby's head. You should never pull too hard or jerk the cord roughly because it may tear and cause severe blood loss from the infant. If the cord is wrapped too tightly to slip free easily, you will need to clamp and cut the cord before delivery of the shoulders. Place two clamps close together on the cord, about 1 inch (2.5 cm) apart, and cut the cord between the clamps. Be sure to cut between these clamps. Unwrap the loop(s) of cord from around the neck, and proceed with the delivery.

The Shoulders

After the head is born, continue to support it as it rotates externally to the left or right; delivery of the shoulders and then the body should follow easily. If the shoulders do not deliver spontaneously, tell the mother to push while you hold the

baby's head in both hands and give gentle downward traction to guide the anterior shoulder under the pubic bone (**Figure 19-10**). When the anterior shoulder is visible, lift the head upward to deliver the posterior shoulder (**Figure 19-11**). Once the upper body is born, maintain your grip around the back of the neck to support the baby's head with your left hand while you slide your right hand along the emerging body and prepare to catch the feet (**Figure 19-12**). These manipulations are always carried out gently, without twisting the baby's neck. Pulling too hard on the head and neck if the shoulders do not deliver easily can cause permanent injury and paralysis of the infant's arm. If force is necessary for delivery, the mother should supply it by pushing harder. Ask her to inhale deeply, hold her breath, and bear down as if moving her bowels. Her chin should be flexed on her chest while pushing, and all pushes should be long and steady. The most effective pushing is done during a contraction so that the force of the uterus is working for you.

Your partner should record the exact time of delivery while you remove blood and mucus from the newborn's face with gauze from the obstetrics kit. While holding the baby in a neutral position at the level of the vagina, suction the mouth and then

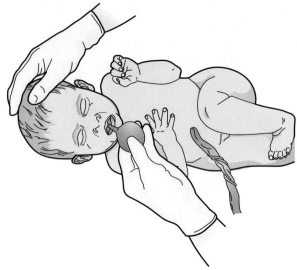

Figure 19-13 Hold the baby in a neutral position at the level of the vagina, suction the mouth, and then suction the nose with a bulb syringe.

each nostril one more time to clear the airway **(Figure 19-13)**. Raising the infant too high above the vagina before clamping the cord may cause the baby to lose too much blood by gravity through the cord. Holding the baby too far below the vagina before clamping the cord may cause the baby to have too much blood. Remember to compress the bulb before putting it in the newborn's mouth to prevent blowing mucus farther into the mouth. Aim the suction tip at the inside of the infant's cheek instead of the back of the throat. Deep suctioning in the back of the throat can cause apnea and bradycardia in the newborn.

Cutting the Cord

While still holding the infant at the level of the vagina, clamp the cord about 1 inch (2.5 cm) from the infant's abdomen. Place a second clamp 2 inches (5 cm) away from the first clamp. Once the cord is clamped, you can place the infant on the towel on the mother's abdomen. Cut the cord between the two clamps **(Figure 19-14)**. You should examine the stump of the infant's cord to make sure that the clamp is secure and there is no bleeding.

Your partner should take over care of the newborn while you continue with third-stage care of the mother. If you are the only trained person at the scene, your first priority at this time is to care for the newborn.

LEARNING OBJECTIVES
- Discuss the steps in the delivery of the placenta.
- List the steps in the emergency medical care of the mother after delivery.

Third-Stage Care of the Mother

The third stage of labor begins with delivery of the baby and ends with delivery of the placenta. After the baby is born, the uterus continues to contract every 2 or 3 minutes, but the contractions are relatively painless. When the placenta is still attached to the

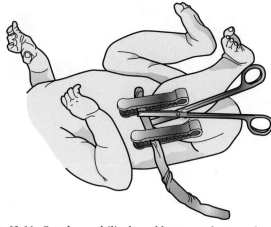

Figure 19-14 Cut the umbilical cord between the two clamps. Place the first clamp approximately 1 inch from the infant's abdomen and the second clamp 2 inches from the first (about four fingerbreadths from the newborn's abdomen).

---

uterine wall, the uterus is round and hard during contractions but flat between contractions. Once the placenta has separated from the uterine wall, the uterus should assume a constant round, hard shape. The placenta will now slide down the birth canal, often accompanied by a gush of blood. As the placenta descends toward the vagina, you will also see a lengthening of the umbilical cord that was attached to the baby.

If the placenta has not delivered by the time the baby is wrapped and the mother has been cleaned and made comfortable for transport, proceed to the hospital. The placenta may not deliver for some time. If you do note signs that the placenta has separated from the wall of the uterus, such as lengthening of the umbilical cord, contraction of the uterus into a raised globular shape, and a gush of blood from the vagina, you should ask the mother to bear down. Have a basin or plastic bag ready to receive the placenta and an expected gush of blood after the placenta is expelled. The weight of the placenta as it is expelled should be enough to extract the membranes.

You should never pull on the umbilical cord or the placenta; doing so may tear the cord or cause some of the tissue to be retained inside the uterus. Not all placentas are formed normally. Occasionally the placenta has more than one lobe **(Figure 19-15)**, or the cord may not be well implanted into the placenta **(Figure 19-16)**. A retained piece of placenta or a torn cord could cause severe hemorrhage. Save the placenta in the bag provided in the obstetrics kit because the obstetrician or emergency physician may want to examine it.

After delivery of the placenta, you should be able to palpate the uterus as a solid wall of muscle at the level of the umbilicus (mother's belly button). If the uterus fails to contract into a hard ball and a large amount of vaginal bleeding occurs, you should gently massage the uterus. This is done by placing one hand on the top of the uterus near the mother's umbilicus and the other hand above the pubic bone to support the lower part of the uterus **(Figure 19-17)**. You should continue to massage the uterus with a kneading motion until the bleeding is minimal and the uterus is firm. Normal childbirth can cause as much as a 500-mL blood loss, but the excess plasma volume

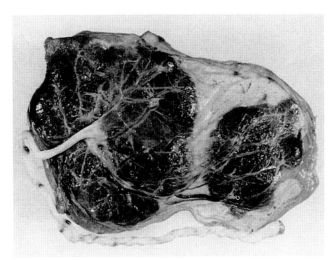

Figure 19-15 Never pull on the umbilical cord to deliver the placenta. The placenta may be abnormal, with an extra lobe. (See Figure 19-16.) *From Beischer NA, Mackay EV: Obstetrics and the newborn: an illustrated textbook, ed 2, Philadelphia, 1986, WB Saunders/Bailliere Tindall.*

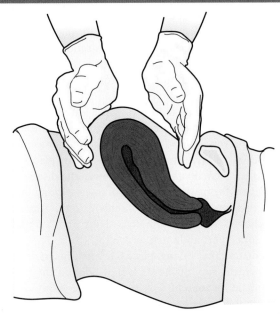

Figure 19-17 Massage the uterus to maintain contraction after delivery and prevent or stop postpartum hemorrhage.

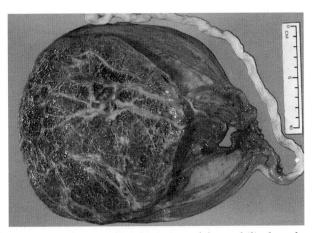

Figure 19-16 The area of implantation of the umbilical cord into the placenta may also be abnormal. Pulling on this cord could cause a massive hemorrhage, and you would not be able to do anything to control the bleeding if the cord should break inside the birth canal. *From Beischer NA, Mackay EV: Obstetrics and the newborn: an illustrated textbook, ed 2, Philadelphia, 1986, WB Saunders/Bailliere Tindall.*

knees together and straighten her legs, and then cover her with a warm blanket. It is normal for women to shake in the immediate postdelivery period. This is a physiologic response to the shock the body has undergone, hormonal changes, and the tremendous amount of energy expended during childbirth. If the mother plans to breast-feed and the baby is healthy and has not required resuscitation, she can nurse the baby at this time. When the infant suckles, an important hormone is released into the mother's circulation that contracts the uterus, preventing postdelivery bleeding. Early breastfeeding can also restore the infant's blood glucose supply, which may have been depleted in the stress of delivery and the effort to stay warm.

You should never leave the mother alone at this time, with or without the baby. She is weak and tired from blood loss and the strain of delivery, and postpartum hemorrhage is most likely to occur in the first hour after birth. If the hospital is some distance away, check every 15 to 30 minutes to confirm that the uterus remains contracted below the umbilicus and that bleeding is minimal. If the uterus relaxes, massage the uterus until it contracts.

LEARNING OBJECTIVE
- Summarize neonatal resuscitation procedures.

Resuscitation and Care of the Newborn

It is best if a second EMT assumes care of the baby immediately after the cord is clamped and cut. Childbirth entails two patients, and both patients require the full attention of a caregiver. The EMT who delivered the baby should attend to the mother.

The four main objectives in newborn care are as follows:
1. Providing warmth for the infant.
2. Continuously evaluating the infant's respirations, heart rate, and color.

of pregnancy allows the mother to tolerate this blood loss well. If uncontrolled bleeding or signs of hypovolemia are present, administer oxygen to the mother and treat her for shock. Once the baby is delivered, concern about compressing the vena cava is no longer a factor, and the mother can be transported in the supine position.

If the placenta delivers, the bleeding appears to be controlled, and the uterus remains firm, or if the placenta does not deliver within a few minutes, you should prepare the mother for transport to the hospital. First, remove the soiled towel from beneath her and replace it with a clean towel. Then gently place a sanitary pad on the perineum, which will be painful now and may have some lacerations. Ask the patient to bring her

3. Responding to the above criteria by providing stimulation, an airway and adequate ventilation through proper positioning, suctioning, and the administration of oxygen and positive-pressure ventilation as needed.

4. Providing cardiac compressions for a heart rate less than 60 beats/min.

If meconium-stained fluid is present, you must thoroughly suction the mouth and nose before stimulating the infant to breathe, to prevent aspiration of the meconium into the lungs. Otherwise, as soon as the newborn has been placed on the mother's abdomen, dry the baby vigorously and discard the wet towel, placing the newborn on a clean towel. Drying the infant helps to prevent heat loss and stimulates respirations. If the mother chooses, she may support her baby from the underside of the drapes on her abdomen.

Immediately after drying, place the infant in a neutral position (hyperextension of the neck is avoided in the newborn) and stimulate by rubbing the infant's back. As the newborn cries, more fluid may be brought up from the lungs. Remove the secretions by turning the infant's head to the side and suctioning the inside of the cheek with the bulb syringe.

Most infants cry briskly by this time and can simply be wrapped in a warm towel for transport, taking care to cover the head. The greatest heat loss can occur through the infant's head. When a newborn becomes chilled, metabolism must speed up to increase heat production. This requires a large amount of oxygen and glucose. The newborn's supply of glucose is limited compared with that of an adult or even an older baby. As the supply of glucose becomes exhausted, the blood glucose level decreases rapidly, and the baby becomes hypoglycemic. In this state, brain damage may occur because brain tissue depends on glucose to function. At the same time, oxygen is quickly burned and exhausted by the excessive metabolic effort exerted to keep warm. The oxygen needs of the infant accelerate, and the infant develops acidosis. Chilling a newborn who has not established good respirations makes a critical situation even worse.

Some infants require further resuscitation immediately after birth. The longer you wait to resuscitate, the longer it will take for the infant to breathe independently, and the higher the level of resuscitation that will be required, eventually involving drugs and intubation. For this reason, resuscitation should be initiated without delay. Any resuscitation started by the EMT that lasts longer than a few minutes should be continued en route to the hospital.

About 5% to 10% of all infants will require some resuscitation measures at birth. The initial evaluation of the infant, which determines the amount and type of resuscitation required, is based on three criteria that are always evaluated in the following order:

- Respirations
- Heart rate
- Color

Respirations

The initial steps of drying, positioning, suctioning, and stimulating a newborn should not take more than a few seconds. The next step is to evaluate the respirations. The best initiation of respiration in a newborn is to cry loudly. The alveoli of a fetus

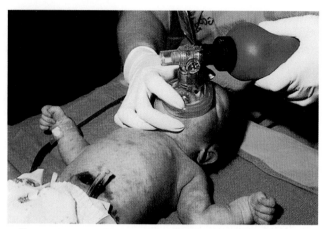

Figure 19-18 Positive-pressure ventilation of a newborn.

are filled with fluid. Most of this fluid is forced through the walls of the alveoli into the circulation when the infant takes the first few breaths of life, expanding the lungs completely for the first time. For this important event to occur, the baby must cry vigorously. Weak, slow, or gasping respirations are not sufficient to expand and drain the lungs and oxygenate the infant.

If the baby is still not breathing sufficiently to expand the lungs after the initial stimulation, you must immediately begin positive-pressure ventilation with a bag-mask device of an appropriate size for a newborn (no larger than 750 mL). An oxygen reservoir should be attached to provide close to 100% oxygen. Use a clear mask because it allows you to observe secretions; it should fit tightly enough to form a seal over the infant's mouth, nose, and chin without touching the eyes (**Figure 19-18**). Anatomically shaped masks with a cushioned rim are preferred because they allow a tight seal without placing undue pressure on the infant's face.

The rate of positive-pressure ventilation in a newborn is 40 to 60 breaths/min. Newborn lungs hold only 20 to 30 mL of air, so only fingertip compression of the bag is needed for adequate chest rise. If you do not detect chest rise, you should try to reposition the mask and the infant (into a neutral position) and suction the mouth. Increasing the force of compression of the bag is a last resort but may be required if all other steps have failed to initiate an adequate chest rise. Most infants will respond with only a few seconds of positive-pressure ventilation.

If the infant starts to cry or breathe well, you should proceed to the next step of checking the heart rate.

Heart Rate

If the infant is breathing well at birth, or after you have ventilated a nonbreathing infant for 15 to 30 seconds, you should check the heart rate. The heart rate is listened to (or palpated) for only 6 seconds, and the number of beats is multiplied by 10. (If you hear 9 heartbeats in 6 seconds, the heart rate is 90 beats/min. If you hear 14 heartbeats in 6 seconds, the heart rate is 140 beats/min.)

If the heart rate is less than 100 beats/min, or if the infant is still not breathing, positive-pressure ventilation should be continued for another 30 seconds. After an additional 30 seconds of ventilation, check the heart rate again. If the heart rate is less than 60 beats/min, begin chest compressions.

You should always accompany chest compressions with positive-pressure ventilation. It is best if there are two persons involved in the resuscitation—one to ventilate and one to perform the compressions. To begin chest compressions, draw an imaginary line between the infant's nipples. Encircle the infant's chest with both hands, and place both thumbs over the sternum just below this imaginary nipple line. Compress the sternum one third of the anterior-posterior depth of the chest at a rate of 120 compressions per minute. Breaths are interposed after every third compression. With compressions and ventilations coordinated at a total rate of 120 events per minute, 30 breaths and 90 compressions will be delivered per minute.

If you are the sole resuscitator, you may find it easier to compress with the alternative method of using two fingers at a right angle to the chest to compress while supporting the infant's back with the other hand.

After 30 seconds of chest compressions and positive-pressure ventilation, you should again check the heart rate. If the heart rate is still less than 60 beats/min, ventilations and chest compressions should be continued. You must proceed to the hospital while continuing your resuscitation because the infant now requires measures beyond your scope of practice.

If the heart rate is greater than 60 beats/min but still less than 100 beats/min, you should discontinue chest compressions but continue ventilation. Positive-pressure ventilation should always be continued until the heart rate is greater than 100 beats/min. If the heart rate is greater than 100 beats/min and the baby is breathing adequately, you may discontinue positive-pressure ventilation but continue to administer oxygen. Free-flow oxygen is administered to the newborn at a flow rate of 5 to 7 L/min by a face mask or by holding the oxygen tubing ½ inch from the infant's nose and cupping your hand around it.

Never withdraw oxygen suddenly from an infant you have resuscitated.

Color

If the infant is now breathing adequately and has a heart rate greater than 100 beats/min, check the baby's color. The newborn should be pink except for a slight normal cyanosis of the hands and feet. A bluish discoloration of the face on an otherwise crying, healthy infant with a pink body and pink mucous membranes is called a "pressure face" and is not true cyanosis. Oxygen is not needed. Cyanosis resulting from poor air exchange, hypothermia, or blood loss causes a blue, pale, or mottled skin tone. Dark-skinned babies may appear gray when cyanotic. The mucous membranes inside the mouth will be blue. If the infant is pale or cyanotic, oxygen should be delivered as close to 100% as possible until the infant is pink. If the infant remains cyanotic despite a trial of free-flow oxygen, give 15 to 30 seconds of positive-pressure ventilation, followed by continued free-flow oxygen.

Oxygen in high concentrations is not harmful to the newborn in a short-term situation, and you should be prepared to administer oxygen to every newborn if necessary. The newborn does not need oxygen if he or she cries vigorously, has a heartbeat greater than 100 beats/min, and has good color immediately after birth. If the cry is weak, or the infant is cyanotic, or the heartbeat is less than 100 beats/min, you should adminis-

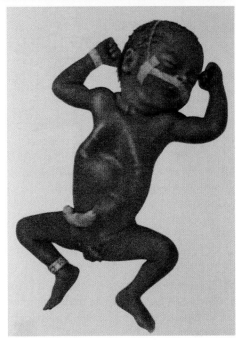

Figure 19-19 Sternal retractions, a sign of respiratory distress in the newborn. *Courtesy Ross Laboratories, Clinical Education Aid No. 5, 1985.*

ter positive-pressure ventilation with 100% oxygen without delay.

The infant's skin color should be observed continuously while you proceed to the hospital. If the baby turns pink and remains pink, you can slowly withdraw the oxygen. Color is the major indicator of respiratory distress in the newborn, but you should observe the infant carefully for a worsening condition and look for other signs of respiratory distress. Signs of respiratory distress in the newborn include the following:

- Nasal flaring
- Sternal retractions (**Figure 19-19**)
- Respiratory grunting

A respiratory grunt is similar to a weak, complaining cry during each exhalation. If any of these signs of respiratory distress is present, administer oxygen so that the infant's condition does not worsen as you proceed to the hospital.

Apgar Score

The **Apgar score** is a system used to evaluate a newborn rapidly in five specific areas. Although the Apgar score reveals nothing about specific birth defects or injuries the infant may have sustained during the birthing process, it provides the person receiving your report with an overview of how well the newborn adapted to life outside the uterus in the first 5 minutes after birth. The score is performed at 1 minute after birth and is repeated 5 minutes after birth. Named after Virginia Apgar, the word "Apgar" is also an acronym for the five criteria valuated. As shown in **Table 19-1,** the areas evaluated are *a*ppearance (color), *p*ulse (heart rate), *g*rimace (vigorous cry on stimulation), *a*ctivity (extremities should have good tone and should be flexed and moving), and *r*espirations.

	Points Assigned		
Criterion	**0**	**1**	**2**
Appearance (color)	Blue	Pink with blue extremities	Completely pink
Pulse (heart rate)	Absent	Less than 100 beats/min	More than 100 beats/min
Grimace (response to stimulation)	No response	Grimace	Vigorous cry
Activity (flexion of extremities)	Limp	Some flexion of extremities	Flexed limbs
Respirations	Not breathing	Weak respirations	Crying

TABLE 19-1 Apgar Scoring Chart

Most healthy newborns have a 1-minute Apgar score of 9, with 1 point deducted for cyanosis in the extremities only. Babies are often completely pink by the time 5 minutes have passed so that the 5-minute Apgar score is often 10. A score below 7 is poor and means that the baby required some type of resuscitation effort. A baby with a score of 8 to 10 was crying spontaneously soon after birth and needed minimal assistance of any type from you. The Apgar score is a retrospective event; because resuscitation must begin immediately after birth, thereby not allowing an Apgar score to be measured, resuscitative decisions are not based on the Apgar score.

Case in Point

Assessing an infant after birth, the EMT discovers that the newborn has blue extremities and a pink chest, a pulse (heart rate) of 78 beats/min, and a weak respiratory effort. The muscle tone is flaccid, and the infant only whimpers when stimulated. The EMT assigns the newborn an Apgar score of 4 and begins to ventilate with a bag-mask. The newborn responds quickly, becoming more responsive, and turns pink. The heart rate increases to 140 beats/min, and the baby begins to cry. After 5 minutes the EMT reevaluates and determines the newborn has an Apgar of 9. Then EMT ensures that the baby is warm and transports to the emergency department.

LEARNING OBJECTIVES
- Describe the procedures for abnormal deliveries: breech birth, prolapsed cord, and limb presentation.
- Differentiate the special considerations for multiple births.
- Discuss special considerations for a premature baby.

Special Circumstances in Childbirth

Premature Infant

An infant who weighs less than 5½ pounds (2.5 kg) or is born before 37 weeks' gestation is considered *premature*. The younger the gestational age, the more likely the baby will have respiratory and other problems. The respiratory problems occur because of insufficient pulmonary surfactant in the lungs of a premature infant to keep the lungs expanded. *Pulmonary surfactant* prevents the small alveoli from collapsing on exhalation. Because heat regulation is also underdeveloped in a premature infant, special care must be taken to maintain a warm environment. You should turn on the ambulance heater or turn off the air conditioner (if summer), and wrap the infant in several blankets. The mother's body heat can be used by placing the infant on the mother's chest, skin to skin, and covering both of them with blankets to prevent heat loss.

You should not allow *very premature* babies (<34 weeks' gestation) to nurse. They cannot coordinate sucking, breathing, and swallowing and are susceptible to aspiration. You should handle premature infants extremely gently because they are more susceptible to intracranial hemorrhage and other injuries. The blood volume of a very premature infant is only a few ounces, so even a slight loss of blood can lead to shock.

You should always communicate to the hospital that you are transporting a premature baby so equipment can be prepared to care for the infant.

Shoulder Dystocia

Occasionally, the head is born spontaneously, but the shoulders become wedged in the mother's pelvis. If gentle downward traction fails to release the anterior shoulder, suction the baby's mouth and transport the mother and infant immediately while supporting the baby's head. This complication illustrates why the mother should deliver on the ambulance stretcher instead of on her own bed or a couch, because it is extremely difficult to move the patient while the baby's head is protruding.

Breech Delivery

A possible impediment to the baby's movement through the birth canal may be an abnormal presentation of the infant. The presenting part of the baby is the lowermost part that first enters the pelvis. For example, in a *vertex presentation* the baby's head is sharply flexed with the chin on the chest, and the occipital, or vertex, portion of the head is the first part of the body to enter the pelvis. Vertex is the most desirable and most common presentation.

In a **breech presentation** the buttocks are lowermost in the pelvis. In a *frank breech* the buttocks are the presenting part. If one or both of the feet or arms enter the pelvis first, it is termed

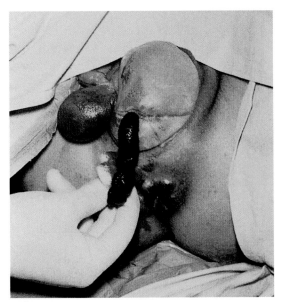

Figure 19-20 Breech delivery. Do not attempt delivery at the scene unless the full frank breech is showing. *From Beischer NA, Mackay EV:* Obstetrics and the newborn: an illustrated textbook, *ed 2, Philadelphia, 1986, Bailliere Tindall.*

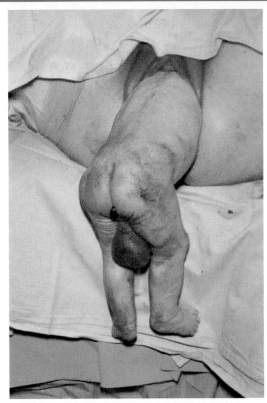

Figure 19-21 Breech delivery. Allow the breech to deliver unaided to the level of the baby's scapula or nipple line. *From Beischer NA, Mackay EV:* Obstetrics and the newborn: an illustrated textbook, *ed 2, Philadelphia, 1986, Bailliere Tindall.*

a *limb presentation.* When the baby is lying transverse in the uterus, there may be a *shoulder presentation,* in which case the baby cannot be delivered vaginally even if the cervix is fully dilated.

Rarely, you may have to assist in the delivery of a breech presentation. Unless the entire buttocks are clearly visible and about to emerge, transport this patient immediately on her left side with the hips elevated (**Figure 19-20**). You should administer high-concentration oxygen to the mother while in transport.

Several adverse events may complicate a breech delivery. Breech labors are usually longer than vertex labors because the buttocks do not make as good a wedge to dilate the cervix. Also, because the buttocks are not as large as the head, they may emerge before the cervix has fully dilated, leaving the head entrapped within the uterus. This is most common in premature babies because the premature head is proportionately much larger than the body.

Large amounts of thick meconium are common in a breech delivery, but the meconium is often expelled because of the pressure on the baby's abdomen and is not necessarily a sign that the fetus has been stressed.

Once the uterus has been partially emptied of the baby's body in a frank breech, the placenta may separate prematurely from the contracted uterus before the head has been expelled, also cutting off the baby's oxygen supply.

It is almost always necessary to assist somewhat in the delivery of a breech presentation. This assistance is given only after the baby's body has been partially delivered; a woman with a baby in any other breech position should be rushed to the hospital. It is easiest if the mother scoots down to the edge of the stretcher so that her buttocks are almost hanging off the end and her legs are flexed sharply. Allow the weight of the baby's body to bring about delivery up to the scapula (shoulder blades) without interfering (**Figure 19-21**).

All breech deliveries should be slow and controlled. External rotation of the shoulders must occur for the shoulders and arms to be born. Once one of the baby's armpits is visible, the body should be either lifted or pulled down to deliver the arms in whatever sequence they appear (**Figure 19-22**). To facilitate delivery of the anterior arm, apply downward traction; for the posterior arm, lift up the body.

After the shoulders and arms have been delivered, the body should rotate so that the back is again facing upward. If the baby's head is not delivered spontaneously at this point, you must flex the baby's chin onto the chest before you can move the head through the curved plane of the pelvis (**Figure 19-23**); otherwise, you can cause a severe neck injury or head trauma. While supporting the baby's body on your forearm, place the fingers of your left hand into the vagina. Locate the baby's mouth and place your fingers on either side of the nose and flex the baby's face by pressing on the maxilla. At the same time, apply slight pressure on the back of the baby's head with the fingers of your other hand. Once the baby's head is flexed, you can apply gentle downward traction to complete delivery of the head. It may also help if your assistant applies gentle suprapubic pressure to keep the baby's head flexed. At this point, the body should be lifted upward until the face and the rest of the head are born.

If you are unable to accomplish a breech delivery within 3 minutes, transport the mother to the hospital while you provide an airway for the baby. Exposure of the baby's body to the cooler outside environment as well as the forces of delivery

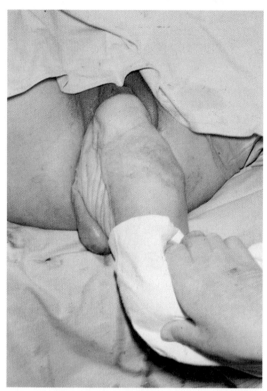

Figure 19-22 Breech delivery. Meconium makes the baby slippery, so use a towel. Upward traction has already delivered the posterior shoulder. Downward traction is used to deliver the anterior shoulder. *From Beischer NA, Mackay EV: Obstetrics and the newborn: an illustrated textbook, ed 2, Philadelphia, 1986, Bailliere Tindall.*

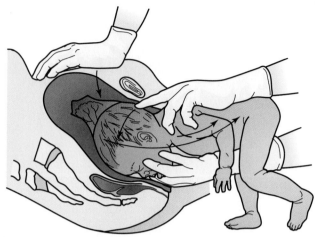

Figure 19-23 Breech delivery. The baby's head must be flexed (chin on chest) to deliver.

may stimulate spontaneous respirations while the baby's face is still pressed up against the vaginal wall. To provide an airway, place your hand in the vagina with your palm facing the baby's face and form a V under the nose, pushing the vaginal wall away from the face. This maneuver alone may provoke delivery of the head. If not, elevate the mother's buttocks to relieve pressure on the umbilical cord, on which the baby's body is resting, and continue to provide an airway. Administer high-concentration oxygen to the mother, and notify the hospital so that an obstetrician will be standing by.

Complications that may affect a breech-delivered infant include the following:
- Prolapsed cord
- Premature separation of the placenta
- Meconium aspiration
- Fractured clavicle
- Nerve damage with paralysis to one or both arms
- Head and neck injury, such as intracranial hemorrhage

Limb Presentation

In rare situations, you may be faced with a **limb presentation.** The small foot, leg, or arm can dangle out of the vagina when the cervix is only a few centimeters dilated. As an EMT, you should immediately recognize that this is an extreme emergency, and you should not attempt delivery in the field. Instead, you should position the mother on her left side, elevate her

hips, and provide high-concentration oxygen. You should not attempt to replace the dangling limb.

Prolapsed Cord

Occasionally the umbilical cord slips down past the presenting part of the fetus into the vagina. This complication, called a **prolapsed cord,** occurs most often in an abnormal birth, such as a breech or shoulder presentation (**Figure 19-24**). It may also occur when the membranes rupture early in labor before the baby's head is fully descended into the pelvis, allowing the cord to slip past the head into the vagina. Once the cord has prolapsed, it may be crushed between the baby and the pelvic bones or the vaginal wall, cutting off all or part of the fetal blood supply.

If you see a prolapsed cord, elevate the mother's hips with pillows, or place her in a knee-chest position. You should also attempt to elevate the presenting part of the baby (not the cord) by applying pressure to it with a gloved hand (**Figure 19-25**). This position and elevation of the presenting part should ease compression of the cord by the presenting part. Continue to elevate the presenting part, and administer high-concentration oxygen as you rush to the hospital. Rapid transport is vital, as is notifying the hospital so that preparations for an emergency cesarean delivery can be made.

Multiple Births

If you are expecting a multiple delivery in the field, always call for assistance. Because more than one resuscitation effort may be required, you must anticipate the need for extra equipment and personnel.

Several factors make the delivery of twins more risky than a normal delivery. First, twins are more likely to be born prematurely. You have no way of knowing whether the second twin is in a breech position, even if the first twin was born in a vertex position. The first twin may be born rapidly, but a long waiting period may ensue before the second twin appears. After the first twin is born, the second twin is in more danger because the uterus has decreased in size and the placenta may separate, cutting off oxygen to the second twin or causing hemorrhage through the placenta or the umbilical cord.

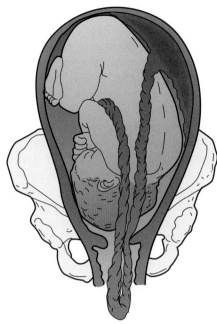

Figure 19-24 Prolapsed cord.

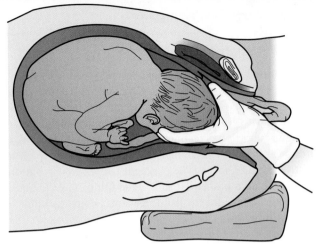

Figure 19-25 Elevate the presenting part of the baby in the event of prolapsed cord.

If both twins are born rapidly, pass off the first one to your partner, and care for the second twin yourself, unless a third trained person is available to care for the second infant while you attend to the mother. You will need two obstetrics kits or extra clamps for the second umbilical cord. You should record the times of delivery for each twin on the call report and keep track of which twin was born first. Never wait more than 10 minutes for the second twin to be born. Provide support for the mother, and resuscitate the babies as needed.

Postpartum Hemorrhage

Defined as blood loss greater than 500 mL after delivery, postpartum hemorrhage can be divided into two categories: early and late. *Early postpartum hemorrhage* occurs within the first 24 hours after delivery and is most often caused by *uterine atony* (failure of uterus to contract after delivery), which may be caused by retention of placental tissue. Early hemorrhage may also be caused by genital lacerations, although these are usually self-controlled or managed easily with pressure applied by a gauze pad. Uterine rupture or coagulation defects (blood-clotting problems) may also be responsible.

Uterine inversion, in which the uterus actually turns inside out, and *uterine prolapse* (prolapsed uterus), in which the supporting structures of the uterus fail, causing the uterus to dip out of the vagina, can both cause massive blood loss. Uterine prolapse occurs more often in older women who have had multiple births and in whom the structures that normally hold the uterus in place have become abnormally stretched and weakened. Uterine inversion may be precipitated by excessive traction on the cord while delivering the placenta or by bearing down too hard during the second stage of labor. This is one of the reasons that you are reminded never to pull on the cord and to be gentle in all maneuvers. A delivery in which the mother is standing upright and with no one to "catch" the baby can also cause this serious complication.

After delivery the normal uterus contracts firmly into a hard ball at or just below the level of the umbilicus. This strong contraction of the uterus is necessary to stop the bleeding from the raw placental site. When part of the placenta or any other matter, such as part of the membranes, is retained within the uterus, the uterus may fail to contract and fills with blood. The larger the uterus becomes as it fills with blood, the less able it is to contract and thus stem the flow of blood; consequently the condition worsens.

Massive bleeding from the vagina is the classic symptom of postpartum hemorrhage, and signs of shock quickly follow. On palpation the uterus is either poorly defined or resembles a soft, boggy mass, often above the level of the umbilicus. The uterus should be massaged until it becomes firm and hard. Note that the uterus is supported with one hand to prevent prolapse as it is massaged by the other hand. The mother may complain that this causes an uncomfortable feeling in her bladder, in which case you should tell her to go ahead and void because a full bladder interferes with uterine contraction. If bleeding is severe, treat the patient for shock.

Late postpartum hemorrhage usually occurs 6 to 10 days after delivery, and the most common cause is retained placental tissue. It may also be caused by infection, coital (sexual) trauma, or rupture of the episiotomy wound. The *episiotomy* is an incision made in the perineum by the physician to make delivery of the baby easier and to prevent a jagged laceration, which may be more difficult to repair. You should treat all cases of postpartum hemorrhage with uterine massage and your local shock protocol.

In rare situations, you may be able to control the bleeding. In postpartum hemorrhage, this can sometimes be accomplished through uterine massage. In cases of perineal trauma or postdelivery wound separation, direct pressure with a soft sanitary pad may help. You should not place packing or dressings inside the vagina.

LEARNING OBJECTIVES
- Identify predelivery emergencies.
- Differentiate the emergency medical care provided to a patient with predelivery emergencies from a normal delivery.

Predelivery Emergencies

Vaginal Bleeding

Vaginal bleeding in pregnancy has several possible causes, including preterm labor, *abruptio placentae* ("placental abruption," separation of placenta from uterine wall before delivery), *placenta previa* (growth of placenta over cervical opening), and threatened abortion. Treatment of severe vaginal bleeding, regardless of the cause, is similar and focuses on the prevention and treatment of shock. The pregnant patient who is bleeding should be placed on her left side. In addition, while the upper body is kept dependent or flat, the woman's hips should be elevated with pillows to relieve pressure on the cervix. Pressure on the cervix can cause uterine contractions and worsen vaginal bleeding if the bleeding is related to labor. Administer oxygen and monitor vital signs.

When reporting vaginal bleeding as you deliver your patient to the receiving hospital, it may be helpful to the diagnosis if you can describe the color of the blood (dark or "port wine"–colored blood as opposed to bright-red blood), determine the absence or presence of clots, and try to be specific about the amount of blood (e.g., "scant pink stain noted on pad," "soaked two sanitary pads with bright-red blood and several dark-red clots").

Threatened Abortion or Stillbirth

An **abortion** or *miscarriage* is the loss of a pregnancy before 20 weeks' gestation. After 20 weeks, it is termed a *stillbirth*. The earliest age of viability or gestational age that an infant is able to survive outside of the womb is currently about 23 weeks. As the management of very premature babies has advanced through the use of new technology, the age of viability has also changed. You may have difficulty distinguishing between an abortion, a stillbirth, and a very premature infant who requires resuscitation. If in doubt as to whether a premature infant is viable, you should attempt resuscitation. A term infant with a tight cord around the neck may appear to be stillborn at birth: limp, pale, and blue. Again, resuscitation should be initiated unless definite signs indicate that the infant has been dead for some time, such as *maceration*, a softening and sogginess of the skull and tissues, with peeling away of the skin.

The loss of a substantial amount of blood or leaking of amniotic fluid in the first trimester is a sign of threatened abortion. You may be able to aid the patient somewhat by elevating her hips to reduce stress on the cervix and the contractions that pressure on the cervix may stimulate.

In the event of a stillbirth or abortion, you should respect any religious requests by the parents. Be sensitive to their individual needs. When confronted with a stillborn or deformed infant, the parents may feel guilt and might even question you as to what they did to cause this condition. You may need to assure the parents repeatedly that they have not contributed to this situation and should not blame themselves. In deference to the parents' feelings, you should treat the body of a stillborn baby with the same gentle care you would provide to a living infant. Wrapping the baby in a blanket and, when appropriate, offering it to the parents to see and hold may help them to work through their grief at having lost a child.

Ruptured Uterus

Uterine rupture occurs when a weakening of the uterine wall causes the uterus to split open. Women who have had a previous cesarean birth or other uterine surgery, women who have had multiple births, and women who are carrying more than one fetus (e.g., twins) are at greatest risk for rupture of the uterus. The abdominal pain caused by a ruptured uterus is acute, and the patient may describe a sensation that "something has just given way." Once the uterus has ruptured, contractions cease entirely because the torn uterus cannot contract. You may be able to palpate the fetus beneath the thin abdominal wall. Vaginal bleeding is usually present, and signs of shock follow shortly. The mortality rate for both fetus and mother is high. The mother may have an *amniotic fluid embolism* when amniotic fluid is released into the maternal circulation through the rupture in the uterus. This serious complication resembles a pulmonary embolism, with the major symptoms of dyspnea, chest pain, cyanosis, and shock.

Rapid transport for immediate surgery is the only hope for both fetus and mother in the case of a ruptured uterus. Again, as with any pregnant patient who is not about to deliver immediately on the scene, place the patient on her left side, administer high-concentration oxygen, and transport rapidly.

REALWorld

Many women experience "morning sickness" after they become pregnant. Morning sickness can present with nausea and vomiting. Some pregnant women experience hyperemesis (excessive vomiting); in severe cases, women can experience weight loss and dehydration. These patients should be transported for evaluation and rehydration.

Preeclampsia and Eclampsia

Preeclampsia, also known as *toxemia,* is a condition of unknown cause that occurs during pregnancy. As many as 1 in 10 pregnancies are affected by preeclampsia, the second leading cause of maternal death in the United States. As the toxemia worsens, seizures occur, and the disease is called *eclampsia.* The three main symptoms of preeclampsia are as follows:

1. Elevated blood pressure (>140 mm Hg systolic or >90 mm Hg diastolic)
2. Protein in the urine
3. Edema

A patient with preeclampsia often has a "puffy look" from facial edema (**Figure 19-26**). As the disease progresses to potential seizures, the woman may complain of headache and dizziness (from elevated blood pressure and rupture of cerebral blood vessels), blurred vision or other visual disturbances (from retinal edema), and epigastric pain (caused by hemorrhages beneath liver capsule). Signs of pulmonary edema may be seen. The blood pressure increases so greatly that stroke, renal failure, and abruptio placentae can occur. The patient who becomes eclamptic will have a seizure (**Figure 19-27**).

The only "cure" for eclampsia or preeclampsia is delivery of the baby. Care of the preeclamptic patient includes providing a quiet, dark environment to avoid stimulating seizures. Use

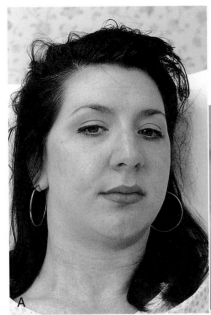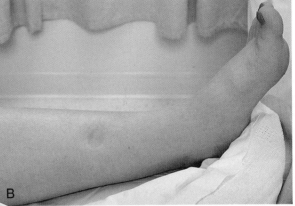

Figure 19-26 Generalized edema is a possible sign identified with preeclampsia, although it may occur in normal pregnancy and pregnancy complicated by another disorder. **A,** Facial edema may be subtle. **B,** Pitting edema of lower leg. *From Murray SS, McKinney ES: Foundations of maternal-newborn nursing, ed 4, St Louis, 2006, Saunders-Elsevier.*

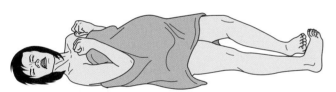

Figure 19-27 Eclampsia: convulsions or seizures. *From Lowdermilk DL, Perry SE: Maternity and women's health care, ed 9, 2007, St Louis, Mosby.*

of sirens and lights should be avoided. Speak in a soft voice, avoiding any unnecessary jostling or noise. An airway and suction should be available in case a seizure begins. Aspiration is a risk because most pregnant women have food in their stomachs hours after eating. If seizures occur, oxygen should be administered because the fetal oxygen supply is diminished during the seizure. As with any patient more than 5 months pregnant, the mother should be transported in the left lateral recumbent position. If pulmonary edema is present, the patient may be more comfortable in the full upright position with oxygen administration.

Trauma in Pregnancy

Motor vehicle crashes, the most common cause of trauma for all patients, are responsible for the majority of traumatic injuries in pregnant women. The injury is less severe if the mother is wearing a seat belt, especially one with a shoulder restraint. A lap belt alone is better than no seat belt, but it cannot prevent the violent flexion of the body that can greatly increase intrauterine pressure. This sudden increase in pressure can cause a burst-balloon type of uterine rupture, abruptio placentae, and fetal death.

Pelvic fractures and blunt and penetrating wounds to the abdomen are usually serious injuries, but they are even more dangerous to the pregnant patient. Broken ribs or pelvic bones may cause uterine lacerations that result in substantial blood loss.

Premature labor is a common complication of trauma in pregnancy. The uterine stimulation caused by blunt trauma to the abdomen may precipitate labor contractions and premature rupture of the membranes. Abruptio placentae is likely to follow any severe trauma, whether caused by motor vehicle injury, blunt trauma, or a fall. The extent of the "placental abruption," rapidity of treatment, and age of the fetus determine the fetal outcome.

When treating the pregnant trauma victim, recall the physiologic changes of pregnancy and how they affect your particular patient. Remember to assume that the stomach is full. This means that an emesis basin or suction for an unconscious patient should be at hand. ***You are treating two patients, and fetal outcome is determined by maternal outcome.*** It is especially important to prevent shock, which is devastating to the fetus. Spinal precautions and the initial ABCs (airway, breathing, circulation) take priority, followed by hemorrhage control and oxygen administration. Use the pregnant transport position, which can be lifesaving for the fetus. If spinal precautions are indicated, place a wedge of folded towels or a pillow under the right side of the spine board to keep it tilted to the left side. This will displace the weight of the fetus from the vena cava almost as well as when you place the victim on her left side. The uterus can also be manually displaced toward the left side by pushing against the right side of the uterus with your flat palm.

Thermal injuries are managed in the same way as for a nonpregnant patient. Again, you must remember that you are caring for two patients, and the best care you can provide for the fetus is to preserve the health of the mother.

REAL*World*

Pregnancy can place great stress on a relationship. Many women who are victims of domestic violence report the first incident of abuse occurred when they became pregnant. Several states report murder as a leading cause of death in pregnant women.

LEARNING OBJECTIVE
• Discuss the emergency medical care of a patient with a gynecologic emergency.

Gynecologic Emergencies

Vaginal Bleeding and Ectopic Pregnancy

Patients who present with vaginal bleeding severe enough to call an ambulance are often pregnant, even if they are unaware of the pregnancy. Your major objectives when treating the patient with vaginal bleeding are (1) estimating the blood loss, (2) treating the blood loss with oxygen and positioning *(shock protocol)*, and (3) minimizing the exposure of emergency personnel by isolation of body substances.

Ectopic pregnancy, a pregnancy that occurs outside the uterine cavity and a leading cause of death in women of childbearing age, is one cause of vaginal bleeding that may be seen by emergency personnel. Ectopic pregnancies may occur in the cervix, ovaries, or abdominal cavity, but 90% of all ectopic pregnancies occur within the fallopian tubes and are called *tubal pregnancies.* As the tubal pregnancy expands, the tube eventually ruptures and bleeds heavily into the abdominal cavity. Symptoms of ectopic pregnancy usually begin when the patient is 4 to 6 weeks pregnant.

The symptoms of ectopic pregnancy often include a history of *amenorrhea* (absence or cessation of menstrual periods) and a positive pregnancy test result, even though the pregnancy is not in the uterus. The abdomen may be swollen, and the patient may or may not tell you that she suspects or even knows that she is pregnant. Vaginal bleeding, if present, is usually light. A sudden onset of poorly localized lower abdominal pain occurs and may radiate to the shoulder area. Sometimes the pain is only felt in the shoulder. The severe shoulder pain is *referred pain* caused by bleeding into the peritoneal cavity, which irritates the diaphragm. Some vaginal or rectal pain may be present. Occasionally, nausea and vomiting may occur; ectopic pregnancy is often mistaken for appendicitis.

REAL*World*

During your assessment of a female patient with abdominal pain, she states that she cannot be pregnant because she uses birth control. No one method of birth control is 100% effective. The possibility of pregnancy must be considered in any female patient of childbearing age who is sexually active.

A patient with an ectopic pregnancy may have lost a large amount of blood and should be treated for shock if symptoms of hypovolemia are present. Occasionally a cyst on one of the ovaries ruptures, causing symptoms similar to a ruptured ectopic pregnancy. Severe shoulder pain in a woman of childbearing age who has no history of injury to the shoulder should alert you to the possibility of an ectopic pregnancy or a ruptured ovarian cyst. Both conditions can be life threatening because of the potential blood loss.

Rape

Extreme sensitivity must be used with rape victims. In addition to the physical injuries sustained by a rape victim, psychologic injuries can be worsened by improper treatment from healthcare providers. In an effort to preserve evidence, patients should be encouraged not to bathe, shower, urinate, defecate, douche, brush their teeth, or change clothes until they have been examined in a hospital. Victims may not be receptive to this advice because they feel unclean and violated and may want to wash away all traces of the incident.

Many hospitals now have rape teams specially trained in treating patients who have been raped. A female rape victim may reject treatment by a male EMT. If this occurs and a female EMT is available, she should care for the patient. Conversely, gentle, supportive care rendered by a male EMT may be beneficial to the patient and ease her posttraumatic adjustment period.

Rape victims often have injuries other than the psychologic trauma. Injuries should be treated as needed, but with awareness that evidence should be preserved when possible. (See also Chapter 18.)

Perineal Injuries

The perineum is one of the most vascular areas of the body, and perineal injuries can be painful and involve substantial loss of blood. Perineal injuries may result from a wide range of causes, from rape to straddling a boy's bicycle. Snow skiing and the popular sport of gymnastics are also responsible for perineal injuries in girls and women of all ages. Lacerations or hematomas may occur, and often associated bladder or urethral injury occurs with a painful spilling of urine onto the injured site. Bleeding should be controlled, if necessary, with direct pressure; an ice pack applied to the site may also slow the bleeding and provide some pain relief.

Scenario Follow-up

This case illustrates the appropriate steps to managing an uncomplicated delivery, including the correct personal protection (gloves, gown, eyewear) to avoid contact with blood and body fluids. The most important action taken during this call was careful decision-making regarding delivering the baby versus transport. The frequency of contractions, water breaking, and significant crowning of the baby's head all indicated an imminent delivery. The EMTs carefully prepared the delivery field and provided gentle counterpressure to avoid an explosive delivery. Care was taken to manage the baby's airway after delivery of the head. The EMTs maintained the newborn's body temperature after delivery and cut the umbilical cord. These are the most important steps needed to provide safe delivery of a newborn.

Summary

Treating patients with obstetric or gynecologic problems entails special considerations. First, because of the abundant blood supply to the female organs, you must consider the possible consequences to patient outcome if bleeding continues unchecked. Second, you must attempt in every situation to maintain the patient's privacy. The anxiety of being exposed in public can help create an uncooperative patient. Even though you are wearing a uniform, remember you are a stranger to this patient, and she may be hesitant to allow you to treat her. Providing privacy from a crowd, if present, helps in this regard. A calm, supportive person, if present, may be a great help by simply holding the patient's hand, offering encouragement, and helping her to breathe properly so that you can manage the medical treatment.

When encountering patients with obstetric problems, remember the basics and treat symptomatically: control bleeding when possible, treat shock with proper positioning, and administer oxygen. Become familiar with the normal delivery process and common complications. Practice neonatal resuscitation on a mannequin until you are able to perform the steps quickly and accurately. If you doubt whether you can manage a situation, proceed to the hospital while providing whatever support you can to the patient. Emotional support in crisis situations may be as beneficial to patient outcome as any other treatment you might provide.

The Bottom Line

Learning Checklist

✓ Remember that there are two patients to care for with a pregnancy. As a general rule, the best therapy for the unborn baby is dynamic management of the mother, with special attention paid to the tasks of maintaining vital signs and oxygenation.

✓ The uterus is a hollow organ with thick, muscular walls located in the pelvic cavity behind the urinary bladder. The uterus provides a home for the developing fetus.

✓ The placenta is a vascular organ that exchanges nutrients and oxygen between the mother and the baby.

✓ The amniotic sac is a double-layer membrane that contains the developing fetus and 16 to 32 ounces (at term) of amniotic fluid. The fetus floats in this fluid, which cushions it against injury and also helps it maintain a constant body temperature.

✓ Meconium is the early feces of the fetus. Meconium-stained fluid should alert you that the baby is, or has been, stressed.

✓ Many pregnant patients cannot tolerate lying supine without fainting or feeling dizzy. It is essential to transport a pregnant patient on her left side. This position displaces the uterus off the vena cava.

✓ Labor proceeds through three stages. The first stage begins with the first contraction and ends when the cervix is fully dilated. The second stage ("pushing stage") begins when the cervix is fully dilated and ends with the birth of the baby. The third stage begins with the delivery of the baby and ends with the delivery of the placenta.

✓ The initial role of the EMT assessing a patient in labor is to decide whether to transport the mother to the hospital or to prepare for an immediate delivery at the scene.

✓ The focused patient history should include questions such as: Is this your first pregnancy? How long were any previous deliveries? Did you have any problems, such as a cesarean section? What time did your contractions start, and how far along are they? Has your water broken? Do you have an urge to move your bowels? Have you had any bleeding or bloody show? When is your due date? Have you had any problems with this pregnancy? Do you have any medical problems? Do you take any medications? When was your last oral intake?

✓ A visual inspection of the perineum is needed if the patient cannot walk or talk during the contractions, if the patient is in so much pain she cannot answer you and appears to be pushing, or if the patient complains of an urge to push or tells you that the baby is coming.

✓ It is important to provide privacy for the patient during a visual examination.

✓ Personal protective equipment for childbirth includes gloves, face mask with eye protection or separate goggles, and fluid-resistant gown.

✓ An obstetrics kit usually contains several cord clamps and bandage scissors or a scalpel to clamp and cut the umbilical cord. It should also contain a rubber bulb syringe, sterile gloves, a fluid-resistant apron or gown, at least four towels, a dozen 4 × 4–inch gauze sponges, a baby blanket, sanitary napkins, and two large plastic bags for waste materials and the placenta.

✓ Delivery of the head can often be slowed and controlled by applying gentle pressure on the back of the baby's head with one hand while supporting the perineum with the other hand. This helps to prevent an explosive delivery.

✓ If the amniotic sac has not yet ruptured, you should tear it with your fingers and spread the membranes away from the baby's face to minimize fluid aspiration and to create an airway.

✓ Once the baby's head is born, you should support it while you wipe the blood and fluid from the baby's face with a 4 × 4–inch gauze sponge. Then you should suction first the mouth and then the nose before the infant has a chance to breathe.

✓ After suctioning, check to ensure the umbilical cord is not looped around the neck. If there is a loose cord around the neck, attempt to slip it over the baby's head. If the cord is wrapped tightly, you will need to clamp and cut the cord before delivery of the shoulders.

✓ After the baby's head is born, you should support the baby as it rotates and the rest of the body is delivered.

✓ Once the baby is born, you should remove blood and mucus from the baby's face and mouth. Holding the baby in a neutral position at the level of the vagina, suction the mouth and then each nostril to clear the airway.

✓ While holding the baby at the level of the vagina, clamp the cord about an inch from the infant's abdomen. Do this by placing two clamps approximately 2 inches (5 cm) apart and cutting the cord between the two clamps.

✓ After delivery of the baby, remember that the placenta must still deliver. If the placenta has not delivered by the time the baby is wrapped and the mother cleaned and made comfortable for transport, proceed to the hospital.

✓ If the uterus fails to contract into a hard ball after delivery and there is copious bleeding from the vagina, you should gently massage the uterus. Place one hand on the top of the uterus near the mother's umbilicus and the other hand above the pubic bone to support the lower part of the uterus.

✓ It is best if a second EMT takes over care of the baby immediately after the cord is clamped and cut. There are two patients, and both patients require the full attention of caregivers.

✓ The four main objectives in newborn care are to keep the newborn warm; continuously evaluate the infant's respirations, heart rate, and color; provide an airway and adequate ventilation though proper positioning, suctioning, and the administration of oxygen and positive-pressure ventilation as needed; and provide cardiac compressions for a heart rate less than 60 beats/min.

✓ If the infant does not begin to breathe with initial stimulation, you should provide positive-pressure ventilation with 100% oxygen at a rate of 40 to 60 breaths/min.

✓ If the infant is breathing well at birth, or after ventilating for 15 to 30 seconds, check the heart rate. If the heart rate is less than 100 beats/min or if the infant is still not breathing, continue positive-pressure ventilation for another 30 seconds. If the heart rate is less than 60 beats/min, you should begin chest compressions.

✓ After 30 seconds of chest compressions and positive-pressure ventilation, again check the newborn's heart rate. If the heart rate is still less than 60 beats/min, continue to ventilate and perform chest compressions. If the heart rate is between 60 and 100 beats/min, discontinue chest compressions and continue to ventilate. If the heart rate is greater than 100 beats/min and the baby is breathing adequately, discontinue ventilation but continue to administer oxygen.

✓ Signs of respiratory distress in a newborn include a bluish discoloration, nasal flaring, sternal retractions, and respiratory grunting.

✓ The Apgar score evaluates five criteria: *a*ppearance, *p*ulse, *g*rimace, *a*ctivity, and *r*espirations. The Apgar score is evaluated at 1 and 5 minutes after birth.

✓ A premature infant weighs less than 5½ pounds (2.5 kg) or is born before 37 weeks' gestation. Premature babies will likely have respiratory and other problems.

✓ Rarely, you will need to assist in the delivery of a breech presentation. Unless the entire buttocks are clearly visible and about to emerge, transport the mother immediately on her left side with the hips elevated. You should administer high-concentration oxygen to the mother while in transport.

✓ A prolapsed cord (umbilical cord slips down past presenting part of fetus into vagina) occurs most often in an abnormal birth (e.g., breech or shoulder presentation) but also occurs when the membranes rupture early in labor. If you see a prolapsed cord, you should elevate the mother's hips with pillows or place her in a knee-chest position. You should attempt to elevate the presenting part of the baby (*not the cord*) by applying pressure to it with a gloved hand.

✓ If multiple births in the field are expected, always call for assistance because more than one resuscitation effort may be required. You will also need multiple sets of equipment, one for each patient.

✓ Postpartum hemorrhage is defined as a blood loss greater than 500 mL after delivery. If bleeding occurs, you should massage the uterus until it becomes firm and hard. If bleeding is severe, treat the patient for shock.

✓ Vaginal bleeding caused by perineal trauma or postdelivery wound separation may be controlled by direct pressure with a soft sanitary pad. You should not place packing or dressings inside the vagina.

✓ An abortion or miscarriage is the loss of a pregnancy before 20 weeks' gestation. After 20 weeks it is termed a stillbirth. The earliest age of viability that the infant is able to survive outside the womb is currently about 23 weeks.

✓ Preeclampsia, or toxemia, occurs in as many as 1 in 10 pregnancies in the United States. The three main symptoms are an elevated blood pressure, protein in the urine, and edema. The only cure for preeclampsia is delivery of the baby.

✓ An ectopic pregnancy occurs outside the uterine cavity and is a leading cause of death in women of childbearing age. Vaginal bleeding is generally light, and the sudden onset of poorly localized lower abdominal pain may radiate to the shoulder area. Nausea and vomiting may be present. A patient with an ectopic pregnancy may have lost a large amount of blood and should be treated for shock if signs of hypovolemia are present.

Key Terms

Abortion Loss of a pregnancy before 20 weeks' gestation.

Apgar score System of quickly evaluating an infant's heart rate, respiratory effort, muscle tone, reflex irritability, and color at birth. The score is determined at 1 minute and repeated at 5 minutes after birth.

Braxton Hicks contractions Weak, irregular contractions of the uterus felt intermittently throughout pregnancy, serving to strengthen the uterus in preparation for delivery.

Breech presentation A birth in which the buttocks are the presenting part.

Contraction Cramps that occur in the lower abdomen over the pubic bone and sometimes in the lower back during labor.

Fetus Developing baby in the uterus (major structures outlined) from about 9 weeks after fertilization until delivery.

Limb presentation When one of the baby's extremities is the presenting part of the birth.

Meconium Substance that makes up the first stool of a fetus or newborn.

Menarche Onset of menstruation occurring around age 12 to 14 years.

Menopause Cessation of menstruation occurring around age 40 to 60.

Menstruation The 28-day cycle involving release of the egg and preparation of the uterus for pregnancy; also called *menstrual cycle.*

Perineum The pelvic floor.

Placenta An organ of pregnancy through which nutrients and waste products are exchanged between mother and fetus. *Afterbirth* refers to the expelled placenta and fetal membranes following the baby's birth.

Prolapsed cord Slipping of the umbilical cord down past the presenting part of the fetus into the vagina.

Umbilical cord Structure that connects the fetus to the mother, allowing the exchange of nutrients and waste products; contains three blood vessels surrounded by a clear, gelatinous substance.

Review Questions

1. In resuscitation of the newborn, which of the following evaluations is the basis for your actions?
   a. Pulse, grimace, and muscle tone
   b. Respirations, heart rate, and color
   c. Blood pressure, pulse, and temperature
   d. Apgar score

2. You respond to a 30-year-old woman who is in active labor. On examination you note that a leg is protruding from the birth canal. Which of the following is the appropriate action to manage this patient and baby?
   a. Apply gentle downward traction on the leg until you can grasp the other leg, then help with the delivery as you would in any breech birth.
   b. Attempt to replace the leg in the vagina.
   c. Elevate the patient's hips, give oxygen, and transport rapidly.
   d. Reach into the uterus and turn the baby to a vertex position.

3. Which of the following is *true* in regard to a premature infant?
   a. Low Apgar score
   b. High Apgar score
   c. Increased birth weight
   d. Lower risk of complications

4. A newborn is flaccid and does not respond to stimulation after delivery. The baby shows no signs of ventilation or a cry, and pulse rate is 120 beats/min. At what rate should you ventilate this baby?
   a. 120 breaths/min
   b. 40 to 60 breaths/min
   c. 30 breaths/min
   d. 15 to 20 breaths/min

5. An infant is breathing at birth with a heart rate of 90 beats/min. After you have dried, positioned, suctioned, and stimulated the newborn by rubbing the back, you should:
   a. Check the color.
   b. Initiate positive-pressure ventilation.
   c. Ask the mother whether she would like to nurse the baby.
   d. Shake the baby.

6. If the mother bleeds excessively after delivery of the placenta, you should:
   a. Pack the vagina with gauze.
   b. Massage the uterus until it is firm.
   c. Apply ice to the perineum.
   d. Have the mother drink hot liquid.

7. After the infant's head is born, and before proceeding with the delivery, you should:
   a. Suction the mouth and nose.
   b. Check for a cord around the neck.
   c. Perform both a and b.
   d. None of the above.

8. Green or yellow amniotic fluid indicates the presence of:
   a. Bloody show
   b. Meconium
   c. Crowning
   d. Imminent delivery

9. The rate and depth of cardiac compressions for a newborn are:
   a. 1 to 2 inches at 100 compressions/min
   b. ½ to ¾ inch at 100 compressions/min
   c. One-third the anterior-posterior depth of the chest at 120 events (90 compressions and 30 breaths) per minute
   d. 1 to 2 inches at 120 compressions/min

10. The best way to protect yourself from communicable disease is to:
    a. Ask the mother for her hepatitis and HIV status before performing the delivery.
    b. Wear personal protective equipment and wash hands thoroughly after each call.
    c. Use only disposable obstetrics kits.
    d. Wash the patient's perineum before delivery.

For Further Review

In the Student Workbook
- Multiple-choice questions
- Fill-in-the-blank questions
- Short-answer questions
- Case scenario questions
- Crossword puzzle

On Evolve
- Anatomy challenge
- Weblinks
- Lecture notes

Learning Objectives

Cognitive Objectives
- Identify the following structures: uterus, vagina, fetus, placenta, umbilical cord, amniotic sac, and perineum.
- List the indications of an imminent delivery.
- Establish the relationship between body substance isolation and childbirth.

- Identify and explain the use of the contents of an obstetrics kit.
- Outline the steps in the predelivery preparation of the mother.
- List the steps to assist in the delivery.
- Describe care of the baby as the head appears.
- Describe how and when to cut the umbilical cord.
- Discuss special considerations with meconium.
- Discuss the steps in the delivery of the placenta.
- List the steps in the emergency medical care of the mother after delivery.
- Summarize neonatal resuscitation procedures.
- Describe the procedures for abnormal deliveries: breech birth, prolapsed cord, and limb presentation.
- Differentiate the special considerations for multiple births.
- Discuss special considerations for a premature baby.
- Identify predelivery emergencies.
- Differentiate the emergency medical care provided to a patient with predelivery emergencies from a normal delivery.
- Discuss the emergency medical care of a patient with a gynecologic emergency.

Affective Objectives

- Explain the rationale for understanding the implications of treating two patients (mother and baby).

Psychomotor Objectives

- Demonstrate the steps to assist in the normal vertex (cephalic) delivery.
- Demonstrate necessary care procedures of the fetus as the head appears.
- Demonstrate postdelivery care of the infant.
- Demonstrate how and when to cut the umbilical cord.
- Attend to the steps in the delivery of the placenta.
- Demonstrate postdelivery care of the mother.
- Demonstrate the procedures for abnormal deliveries: breech birth, prolapsed cord, and limb presentation.
- Demonstrate the steps in the emergency medical care of the mother with excessive bleeding.
- Demonstrate completing a prehospital care report for patients with obstetric/gynecologic emergencies.

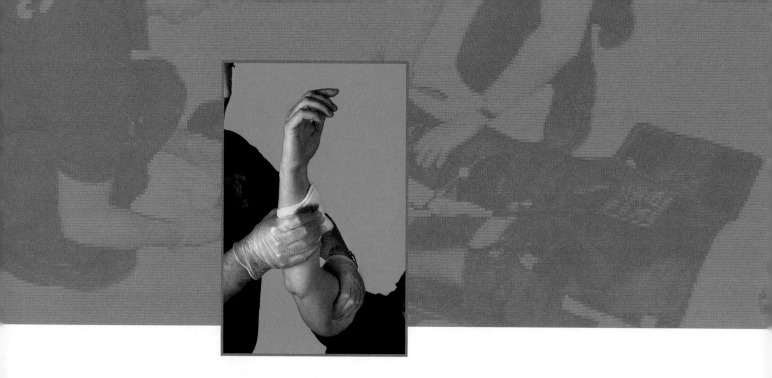

20 Bleeding and Shock

CHAPTER OUTLINE

Scenario

A 22-year-old man has been stabbed by an unknown assailant who has fled. On your arrival, police are present and have secured the scene. You approach the patient with gloves on and note that he is alert and bleeding from a wrist wound. You quickly control the bleeding with your gloved hand and a sterile dressing by using direct pressure while your partner applies a pressure bandage over the site. During the initial (primary) assessment and the focused (secondary) assessment (patient history, physical examination), you note a stab wound in the right upper quadrant of the abdomen. No other signs of injury are present. The patient is anxious, agitated, and has a weak pulse of 120 beats/min. His skin is pale, cool, and clammy. The blood pressure is 100/80 mm Hg. Respirations are 24 breaths/min and shallow. Breath sounds are equal on both sides.

You administer high-concentration oxygen and initiate rapid transport with the patient's legs elevated, covering him to maintain body temperature. En route you reassess the patient and notify the trauma center of the impending arrival of a victim of a stabbing with penetrating injuries to the wrist and abdomen and signs of hypovolemic shock.

Trauma is the leading cause of death in the United States for persons between ages 1 and 44 years. Loss of blood volume accounts for many of these deaths. Control of bleeding is the fundamental and most important treatment to save a life when there is excessive blood loss. For external bleeding, the emergency medical technician (EMT) learns skills to stop blood loss in the field and prevent further loss during transport. When internal bleeding is present, the EMT must maintain a high index of suspicion, actively look for signs and symptoms of blood loss, and initiate prompt transport to a hospital where internal bleeding can be controlled.

Direct pressure is the most important action you will take to control external bleeding. Bleeding that is not controlled by direct pressure alone may be better controlled by elevation or by using a **pressure point,** compressing an artery proximal to the wound. A **tourniquet,** or constricting band placed *proximal* to a wound on an extremity, can be used to control bleeding not controlled by direct pressure or other means. A tourniquet should be used only as a last resort when other methods have failed.

Internal bleeding can result in a range of signs and symptoms that will alert you to significant blood loss and **shock,** a state of profound depression of the vital processes of the body caused by inadequate perfusion of the vital organs with blood. By recognizing these signs and symptoms and taking prompt action to control bleeding and treat for shock, you will be able to assist patients with both traumatic and medical causes of bleeding and help reduce the risks for death and serious disability.

LEARNING OBJECTIVE
- Describe the structure and function of the circulatory system.

Anatomy and Physiology

The three major components of the circulatory system are as follows:

- Blood
- Heart
- Blood vessels

These components function together to perfuse the body with blood. The circulatory system brings nutrients to the cells, returns waste products to the organs for elimination, distributes various nutrients among the body's organs, and helps the body regulate temperature.

The blood is made up of liquid (plasma) and cellular components. The cellular components include red blood cells (RBCs), which transport oxygen; white blood cells (WBCs), which combat infection; and platelets, which help control bleeding.

The heart is made up of four chambers: two atria (receiving chambers) and two ventricles (pumping chambers). The left ventricle is the pump for circulation to the body, ejecting blood with each beat into the aorta, which carries it to major artery branches, distributing it to all parts of the body. The right ventricle pumps blood throughout the pulmonary arteries to the lungs, where the blood picks up fresh oxygen and unloads carbon dioxide for exhalation into the atmosphere.

The two circulations function at the same time. The blood vessels distribute the blood to all parts of the body and the lungs. The arteries carry blood away from the heart. The veins carry blood back to the heart. The arteries branch outward like a tree into smaller and smaller vessels that end in capillaries. The capillaries are one cell thick and close to body cells and the alveoli in the lungs for the exchange of gases, nutrients, and waste products. The capillaries connect with the smallest branches of the venous system, which join together until they end in the major veins, which return blood to the heart.

Cardiac Output

Each part of the circulatory system plays its own crucial role in delivering blood throughout the body. This dynamic system responds to the body's changing needs. For example, the heart rate can change in response to the level of activity. Usually the heart rate is between 60 and 100 beats/min. This rate can increase during exercise or stress and can decrease during sleep or relaxation. Similarly, when increased blood flow is needed, the heart can beat more forcefully, ejecting more blood with each beat. The amount of blood pumped out of the heart with each beat is called the *stroke volume*. The amount of blood pumped by the heart each minute is called the *cardiac output* (stroke volume × number of beats/min). An average stroke volume of 70 mL per beat multiplied by a heart rate of 70 beats/min generates a cardiac output of 4.9 L/min. An exercising adult with a stroke volume of 100 mL per beat and a heart rate of 150 beats/min would have a cardiac output of 15 L/min. The cardiac output varies to meet the body's needs.

The smaller blood vessels (arterioles) are not all open at one time. Rather, they open and close, depending on the needs of local tissues. During exercise, the muscles require more blood flow. After a meal the gastrointestinal (GI) tract needs increased flow. With exposure to cold temperature, skin vessels constrict, limiting heat loss by radiation. When some vessels are dilated, others are constricted. Although the average adult body contains 5 to 6 L of blood, there is not enough blood to fill all the vessels of the body at one time.

Blood Pressure

When an organ is perfused with blood, adequate oxygen and nutrients are delivered to meet its needs, and waste products are removed. To *perfuse* (flow through) the vessels in an organ, the blood must be propelled with a force called **blood pressure**. Blood pressure is the force exerted by the blood volume on the walls of the vessels. Both the volume of blood being circulated (cardiac output) and the size of the overall *vascular space* (size of the total space within the arteries, veins, and capillaries) determine the blood pressure. When blood is pumped into the arteries during ventricular contraction *(systole)*, the amount of blood in the arteries increases and the pressure rises. The pressure measured during systole is the systolic blood pressure. As the heart relaxes *(diastole)*, blood continues to move forward through lower pressure vessels (arterioles, capillaries, and veins), and the amount of blood volume remaining in the arteries decreases and the pressure falls. The pressure measured during diastole is called the diastolic blood pressure **(Figure 20-1).**

The normal systolic blood pressure for adults is estimated by calculating 100 mm Hg plus the patient's age (up to 140 mm Hg for adult men). The diastolic blood pressure is from 65 to 90 mm Hg in normal individuals. In general, the blood pressure is from 8 to 10 mm Hg lower in women.

In children, the blood pressure increases with age and shows considerable variation. Experts consider a systolic blood pressure of 70 mm Hg plus twice the child's age (in years) as the lower limit for systolic blood pressure in children older than 2 years.

The amount of blood ejected into the vessels is a function of the cardiac output. If the size of the vascular space remains the same, an increase in cardiac output results in an increase in blood pressure. Conversely, a decrease in the cardiac output leads to a decrease in blood pressure. A decrease in cardiac output can occur after severe bleeding, resulting in a fall in blood pressure.

Vascular Space

The size of the vascular space can also vary and is determined by the internal diameter of the vessels and the number of vessels that are open at a given time. If the amount of blood pumped into the vessels (cardiac output) remains the same, constriction of the vessels (decreased vascular space) will lead to an increase in blood pressure. Less space is available for the same amount of blood, and the pressure increases. Conversely, dilation of the vessels (increase in the vascular space) leads to a decrease in blood pressure, if the amount of blood available to occupy the vascular space remains the same.

The relationships among the volume of blood pumped by the heart per minute (cardiac output), the size of the vascular space, and blood pressure help explain how changes in blood pressure occur and the compensatory mechanisms used by the body to maintain blood pressure.

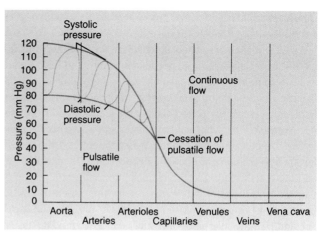

Figure 20-1 Blood flow in arteries and arterioles is pulsatile. The maximum pressure is created during ventricular contraction (systole). The lowest pressure occurs just before the next pulse wave (diastole). Blood flow in the capillaries, venules, and veins is not pulsatile. *Modified from Solomon EP, Phillips GA:* Understanding human anatomy and physiology, *Philadelphia, 1987, Saunders.*

If a part of the circulatory system fails, blood pressure decreases and **hypoperfusion** (inadequate blood flow through the organs) can result. Loss of blood volume, as occurs with bleeding, can lead to hypoperfusion and **hypovolemic shock** (shock caused by very low blood volume). The most life-threatening cause of hypovolemic shock is rapid and profuse bleeding, or **hemorrhage.** Recognition and control of bleeding are essential skills that must be mastered.

Normal Tissue Perfusion

Blood flow normally matches the body's energy requirements on an organ-by-organ basis. Blood perfuses the tissues in sufficient quantity to meet each organ's oxygen needs. When the tissues need more oxygen, the arterioles open up and permit more blood flow through the area. When the tissues have sufficient oxygen, the arterioles close.

Effects of Epinephrine

The body's response to crisis, real or imagined, is accompanied by a release of the hormone epinephrine. Epinephrine prepares the body to meet many challenges ("fight or flight" reaction), from simply hearing a strange noise in the dark to facing life-threatening danger. Epinephrine is released even during athletic competition.

A similar release occurs if an individual is injured and severely bleeding, is in respiratory distress, or is severely ill. When epinephrine is discharged, the following changes occur:

1. *Cardiac output is increased.* Both heart rate and force of contraction are increased.
2. *Blood flow to the brain is increased.* Alertness is needed to meet the challenge. This may be accompanied by apprehension and anxiety.
3. *The pupils dilate.*

4. *Blood flow is redistributed.* Blood is shunted away from less vital organs, especially the skin and digestive tract. The skin is pale, cool, and clammy, and it may become increasingly sweaty. A person may complain of nausea or "butterflies" in the stomach. The blood has been sent to the brain, heart (which is doing increased work), and muscles on a priority basis.

5. *The respiratory rate increases.* When oxygen demands are increased, the respiratory rate and depth increase.

The blood pressure may not be elevated. Epinephrine increases cardiac output and adjusts the tone of the blood vessels to permit maximum flow to the areas in need. This entails selective vasoconstriction (narrowing of vessels) and vasodilation (widening of vessels) called *redistribution* (flow is restricted to some organs while preserved or increased to other organs). For example, the vessels to the skin and GI tract constrict, and vessels to the brain, heart, and skeletal muscles dilate. Redistribution resulting from epinephrine preferentially feeds the organs and tissues needed to fight, or flee from, danger.

During the disease process or after trauma, signs of epinephrine release should be sought. Signs of epinephrine release are often considered as part of a compensatory mechanism that the body uses to survive. The importance of this mechanism is stressed in the assessment of the compensatory response to hypovolemia. In shock, the body selectively redistributes blood flow to the organs most essential for survival, especially the brain and the heart, so that the patient remains awake and maintains blood pressure. Other body organs are underperfused and starved for oxygen (in shock). Individuals with massive injuries and bleeding may be alert and have a normal blood pressure. In these patients, as an EMT, you must look for signs that indicate shock other than mental status and blood pressure. It is not appropriate to wait until a patient is unresponsive or hypotensive to consider shock because these are relatively late events.

REAL*World*

Some people take medications that may alter their body's ability to compensate for shock. Usually these medications are taken to control high blood pressure, keeping the heart rate slow or the blood vessels from constricting. If a patient is taking this type of medication, the progression to shock may be hidden until it is too late to stop. A good history and high index of suspicion can be the EMT's best tool.

External Bleeding

Personal Precautions

While controlling external bleeding, standard precautions related to blood and body fluids must be observed. Some diseases are transmitted through blood-to-blood contact, but simple precautions can reduce the chances of disease transmission. These precautions include the use of gloves, goggles, masks, and gowns to prevent the patient's blood from coming in contact with open sores or mucous membranes. Standard precautions are used during airway management, bleeding control, and wound management according to the potential for splashing of the patient's blood and body fluids.

Severity of Blood Loss

Blood is important for its oxygen-carrying ability, volume, and various cellular components. Severe bleeding results in a loss of all these elements. Blood loss leaves a person depleted of RBCs and hemoglobin (necessary to carry oxygen), blood volume (necessary to fill the vascular space), and platelets and clotting factors (necessary to stop bleeding).

The sudden loss of 1 L (1000 mL) of blood in an adult, ½ L (500 mL) in a child, or 100 to 200 mL in an infant is considered serious. The severity of blood loss must be based on the patient's signs and symptoms and the general impression of the amount of blood loss.

If left untreated, individuals who lose about half their blood volume experience circulatory arrest and die. The sudden loss of blood volume is the earliest cause of shock and death in the bleeding patient.

Case in Point

A 15-year-old boy has fallen from a bicycle and sustained a severe laceration to his midthigh region. He has bright-red blood flowing from the wound. The first EMT, who donned gloves while leaving the ambulance, applies direct pressure to the wound using several dressings. He sees active bleeding through the dressing and applies additional dressing to facilitate the clotting process, maintaining direct pressure. The wound continues to bleed. The EMT then applies a pressure point in the crease of the thigh, halfway between the crest of the pelvis on the hip and the pubic area, while his partner attaches a pressure dressing. The bleeding is controlled within a few minutes.

Loss of Blood Cells

Normally a person has three or four times the amount of RBCs and hemoglobin necessary to sustain life. Many patients with chronic diseases live with about half-normal levels of hemoglobin. Patients with a low supply of hemoglobin are said to be *anemic.*

The lower number of RBCs in an anemic patient causes a change in the normal skin color (**Figure 20-2**). With a diminished amount of hemoglobin, the pink color of oxygenated hemoglobin visible in superficial body areas (skin, nail beds, palm creases, conjunctivae) is less intense, leading to pallor (paleness). The temperature and moisture of the skin are not affected as they would be with epinephrine-induced vasoconstriction; rather, they appropriately reflect environmental temperatures and other conditions. The anemic person may complain of weakness and drowsiness.

Loss of Blood Volume

Hemorrhage results in equal loss of blood volume and hemoglobin. Although the body can adjust to the loss of half its hemoglobin (resulting in anemia) over time, a sudden loss of half the blood volume causes circulatory arrest. Even though the body can limit the areas perfused when blood loss occurs, with the loss of half the normal blood volume, insufficient blood is available to fill the smallest possible vascular space, and circulation ceases. Patients in cardiac arrest caused by hemorrhage cannot be resuscitated until their blood volume is restored.

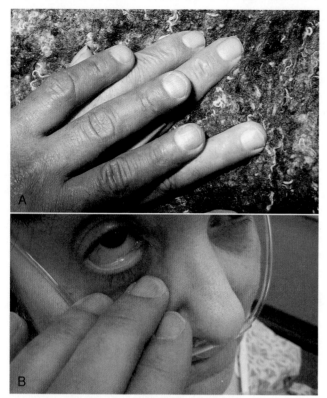

Figure 20-2 Anemia. Check the nail beds and conjunctivae for pallor. Pale coloring of the nail beds and conjunctivae can indicate a deficiency of red blood cells and their pigment, hemoglobin. **A,** The patient *(bottom hand)* has half the normal amount of red blood cells. Note contrast of patient's nail beds with the examiner's hand *(on top).* Regardless of skin pigment, the nail beds provide a quick check during the respiratory and circulatory assessment. **B,** Note pallor of conjunctiva in the same patient with severe anemia (low blood hemoglobin).

LEARNING OBJECTIVES
- Differentiate among arterial, venous, and capillary bleeding.
- Describe methods of emergency medical care for external bleeding.
- Establish the relationship between body substance isolation and bleeding.
- Establish the relationship between airway management and the trauma patient.

Types of Bleeding

By noting several important details about a patient who is losing blood, the EMT is better able to evaluate and treat the patient. **Table 20-1** summarizes the three types of external bleeding.

Type of Vessel Injury

When arterial vessels sustain trauma (where there is a significant muscular layer), the type of injury may influence the amount of bleeding. When smaller arteries are completely severed, the circular muscle within the arterial wall tends to constrict and prevent further blood loss. Small veins also tend

Table 20-1	Types of External Bleeding		
Vessel	**Flow**	**Color**	**Location**
Artery	Pulsatile or spurting	Red	Deeper vessels, except at joints
Capillary	Continuous oozing	Dark red	Superficial
Vein	Continuous	Dark red or purple	Superficial flow compared with arteries

to collapse if they are completely severed. The worst type of injury to an artery is one that severs only part of the wall. In this case, the muscle cannot fully constrict to prevent blood loss because the continuous surface of part of the artery holds it open.

Quality of Blood Flow

If the blood vessel walls are severed, bleeding results. The rate of bleeding depends on the size and type of vessel injured. Because they are high-pressure vessels, the arteries bleed the fastest, and blood spurts or pulsates from the wound. The veins exhibit continuous blood flow. Although the capillaries also show a continuous flow, because of their small size the blood seems to ooze. The larger the vessel severed, the faster is the rate of blood loss. In fact, when the largest vessels (e.g., aorta) are severed, death can occur in seconds.

Color

Recognizing the types of external bleeding is also aided by the color of the blood flowing from a wound. Arterial blood is bright red because its hemoglobin is rich in oxygen. Venous blood is a darker red because it contains less oxygen. The color of capillary blood is between the two.

Location

External veins tend to be more *superficial* (close to the body's surface) than arteries. Arteries tend to run deeper in the body and along bony surfaces, making them vulnerable to injury caused by fractures. The arteries are forced to come toward the surface at the joints of long bones.

Clotting

Clotting normally begins soon after an injury occurs, generally within 4 to 6 minutes. Capillaries tend to clot faster than other vessels. A partially severed artery is least likely to clot because of the high pressure of the blood flowing through it. Clotting may not occur if very large vessels are injured because the continuous flow of blood displaces the clotting elements.

Control of Bleeding

As previously noted, standard precautions should be routine with severe bleeding and the risk of splashing blood. Loss of blood volume and hemoglobin is a critical event. Thus, recognition and control of external bleeding are part of the initial (primary) assessment. Obvious external bleeding

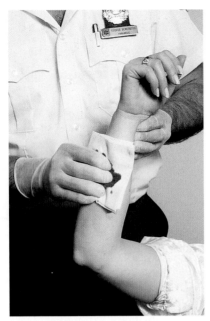

Figure 20-3 Direct pressure is applied over the wound site (with elevation) with sufficient pressure to control bleeding but not obstruct distal arterial blood flow.

requires immediate attention and is treated in conjunction with *a*irway control and *b*reathing as part of the ABCs (*c*irculation).

The primary method to control bleeding is applying pressure directly over the wound. In severe cases, pressure applied over a major artery (pressure point) may be needed to assist in bleeding control; as a last resort, application of a tourniquet (constricting device) may be necessary. If the site of bleeding is an extremity, elevating and, if indicated, splinting the affected part may further control blood loss (**Box 20-1**).

Direct Pressure

The best and first measure used to control bleeding is the immediate application of direct pressure. Ideally, a sterile dressing should be applied to any open wound to minimize the possibility of infection. Control of bleeding is of such high priority, however, that any clean cloth (e.g., scarf, shirt, gloved hand) should be used if a sterile dressing is not immediately available (**Figure 20-3**).

Direct pressure compresses bleeding vessels so that they collapse and obstruct further loss of blood. The amount of pressure required to control the bleeding depends on the type of bleeding. Although minimal pressure controls capillary bleeding, more force is necessary to control bleeding from an artery. For large, gaping wounds, packing the wound with sterile gauze

Box 20-1	Methods of Bleeding Control*

1. Direct pressure
2. Elevation
3. Pressure points
4. Tourniquet

*In order of application.

and using your hand to apply direct pressure may be necessary if "fingertip" pressure does not control bleeding.

Once in place, the dressing generally should not be removed. Its removal might disrupt blood clots and cause bleeding to recur. If the dressing becomes soaked with blood and bleeding appears to be uncontrolled, you must assess whether you have directed pressure over the point of hemorrhage. The general rule is to apply additional dressings over the blood-soaked dressings and then reapply direct pressure. Some EMTs favor placing a roll of gauze over the original dressing and then applying direct pressure, believing it helps focus pressure more directly over the bleeding point (**Figure 20-4**).

A few exceptions exist to the general rule not to remove a dressing once it is applied. If continued bleeding through a dressing is evident, and you clearly have not accomplished

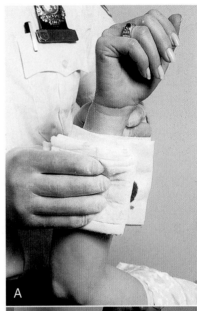

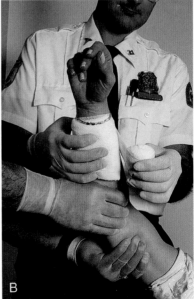

Figure 20-4 **A,** The dressing can be reinforced. **B,** A pressure bandage can be applied to provide continued direct pressure.

bleeding control through traditional means, you may need to quickly inspect the wound. Look to determine if a particular part of the wound is bleeding the most severely (as from an arterial "pumper") and where direct pressure must be focused to accomplish bleeding control. This may be particularly important if the first dressing has not controlled bleeding and was applied before your arrival by the patient or a bystander. The Case in Point provides an example of this exception to the rule.

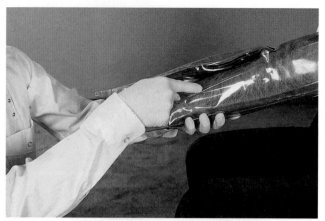

Figure 20-5 An air splint might be used for continued direct pressure to control bleeding on a large area on an extremity.

Case in Point

A patient with a head wound has had a dressing applied on the skull above the ear with a pressure bandage wrapped around the head. The bandage and dressing are soaked with blood. On arrival at the hospital, the patient states, "I am going to pass out," an ominous statement in a patient with blood loss. His systolic blood pressure is 60 mm Hg by palpation. The dressing is removed and reveals spurting blood from the temporal artery, which is quickly and completely controlled with *focused direct pressure.* After subsequent repair of the wound and restoration of blood volume, the patient makes a full recovery from what otherwise might have been a fatal scalp wound.

Pressure Bandage

To allow attention to other tasks, once bleeding has been controlled with direct pressure, you should apply a bandage circumferentially to form a pressure dressing (except around the neck). Sufficient sterile gauze pads are used to cover the wound, and additional dressings are placed on top of the sterile pads. Additional gauze pads can be used to build up the dressing. Adding bulk over the dressing focuses the bandage's pressure more directly over the wound.

A roll bandage 3 to 4 inches (7.5-10 cm) wide can be rolled over the dressing three or four times and then secured by tying it or affixing tape. If the pressure dressing is inadequate to maintain bleeding control, or if the site of injury does not permit application of a circumferential dressing, continuous application of manual direct pressure is required. Caution is necessary when applying direct pressure to the skull. In general, the pressure should be distributed over a larger surface area to avoid the risk of depressing bone fragments if the skull is fractured beneath the wound.

The ideal pressure dressing should be tight enough to control all bleeding yet still permit some blood flow to the structures beyond. When circumferential pressure dressings are applied around a limb, a careful check of distal pulses and evidence of distal blood flow is required. If the bandage covers the distal pulse site, the capillary refilling time test can be used to gauge blood flow to the distal extremity. If no distal pulses are felt, the dressing is acting as a tourniquet, which is the method of last resort in bleeding control. The application of dressings and bandages is discussed in detail in Chapter 21.

An air splint also can be used to apply direct pressure over an extremity (**Figure 20-5**). It might be useful for a large wound (e.g., abrasion) that is oozing blood. Because the air splint is clear, the dressing (and bandage) can be observed under the splint and reassessed periodically.

The **pneumatic antishock garment (PASG)** can apply direct pressure over a lower extremity. Some experts have recommended use of the PASG for extensive lacerations or extensive soft tissue injury to the lower extremities, as a means to apply direct pressure, especially in situations with limited numbers of EMTs who must tend to other critical tasks. However, other experts express concern that a PASG would obscure the wound and that direct pressure with circumferential bandaging is more effective. The PASG is described later in this chapter.

Elevation

To control bleeding from the extremities, elevation is used in conjunction with direct pressure. This is recommended unless contraindicated by certain fractures (e.g., humerus). The limb should be elevated with a sling, pillow, or rolled blanket so that the wound is above the level of the heart.

Splinting

Broken bone fragments may continue to grate on blood vessels and increase bleeding if they are not immobilized. Muscular activity can also increase the rate of blood flow, and thus the bleeding, in an extremity. Therefore, splinting an extremity is useful as part of the approach to bleeding control when fractures are suspected or when the injury is deep into the muscular tissues. Apply a pressure bandage to control external bleeding, then splint the extremity.

Pressure Points

Bleeding is sometimes difficult to control with direct pressure alone. Depending on the wound's location, application of pressure directly over a major artery (or on a pressure point) that feeds that body area may be helpful. Pressure can be applied at the common pulse points, where arteries can be palpated. For bleeding from the extremities, pressure over the brachial or femoral artery may be useful. Compress the brachial artery against the humerus with the fingers (**Figure 20-6**). Use the heel of the hand over the femoral artery to compress it against the pelvis and help control bleeding in a lower extremity.

The pressure applied collapses the arteries and reduces or stops the blood flow. Pressure points are an adjunct to direct

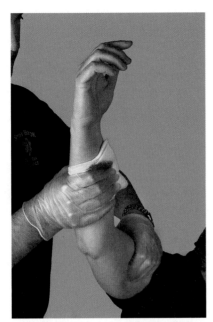

Figure 20-6 The pressure point for the upper extremity is located on the medial aspect of the upper arm.

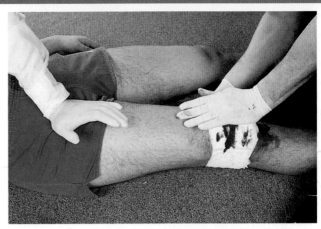

Figure 20-7 The pressure point for the lower extremity is located halfway between the pubic bone and the iliac crest. Place the heel of your hand in that location while your partner maintains direct pressure.

pressure in the control of bleeding. For example, while one EMT holds a pressure point, another EMT should try to apply or reinforce a direct-pressure dressing (**Figure 20-7**).

Tourniquets

A tourniquet might be required as a last resort for uncontrolled bleeding. The tourniquet is a constricting band applied over an extremity with enough pressure to stop blood flow beyond the site of application. The lumen of the arteries is obliterated because the external pressure is greater than the internal pressure. No blood can flow beyond the tourniquet. In fact, a blood pressure cuff, inflated above the systolic blood pressure, could be used as an effective tourniquet. A tourniquet should be placed just proximal to the wound, and it should not be applied directly over any joint (**Skill 20-1**).

Because a tourniquet completely stops blood flow, thereby starving the distal tissues of oxygen, a possible complication from prolonged use of a tourniquet is loss of the extremity. The pressure of the tourniquet is transmitted to the nerves as well. Nerves can tolerate pressure for only a short time before permanent damage ensues. Furthermore, the nerves are more susceptible to injury at some sites, such as the elbow or knee, where they must surface to cross the joint. No material that will cut into skin or tissue, such as wire or rope, should be used.

If a tourniquet is not applied tightly enough, it will obstruct venous return from the extremity but permit arterial flow to the limb and exacerbate rather than control bleeding. When the decision to apply a tourniquet is made, it must be placed properly. The indication for tourniquet placement is control of blood loss when other methods fail. Although few cases require tourniquet use, they do exist; for these patients the use of a tourniquet is lifesaving. Learn how to apply a tourniquet properly so that you can apply one to save a patient's life if severe blood loss cannot be controlled by other means.

Special Areas of Bleeding

Bleeding from the nose and mouth deserves special consideration to ensure that blood stays out of the airway. Nosebleeds (**epistaxis**) are common and can result from the following:

- Trauma to the skull
- Digital trauma (e.g., nose picking)
- Medical conditions (e.g., high blood pressure, sinusitis, other respiratory infection)
- Coagulation or clotting disorders

Nosebleeds can be serious enough to cause severe blood loss. Most nosebleeds arise from the anterior section of the nose (**Figure 20-8**). Control of bleeding is best accomplished with direct pressure to both sides of the nostrils, held in place for at least 5 minutes so clotting can occur, with the patient sitting and leaning forward to reduce the chance of aspiration of blood in the airway (**Figure 20-9**).

REAL*World*

Geriatric patients typically have conditions that make them prone to nosebleeds. Dehydration is common, as well as medical conditions such as high blood pressure. They may be taking medications to help prevent blood clots, which will increase bleeding time. Occasionally an elderly patient will present to EMS with posterior epistaxis (nosebleed at back of nasal passages). This type of nosebleed in a geriatric patient should be considered a life-threatening condition. In addition to the airway being at risk, none of the standard methods of bleeding control can be used with a posterior nosebleed. The EMT should have the patient sit upright and lean forward so that the blood can flow from the nose and mouth. Rapid transport is required to have the nosebleed controlled in the emergency department (ED).

Skull fractures sometimes are accompanied by bleeding from ears or nose. The discharge may be blood mixed with cerebrospinal fluid (CSF). In these cases, no attempt should be made to stop bleeding because disruption of the covering of the brain may have occurred and risk of infection exists. Instead, a loose sterile dressing is used to prevent entry of outside debris.

Bleeding from the mouth is of concern because it may contribute to aspiration and related airway obstruction. Suction should be available; if needed, you should position the patient to allow for drainage of blood or other fluids. When spinal injury is suspected, log-roll the patient while maintaining spinal immobilization.

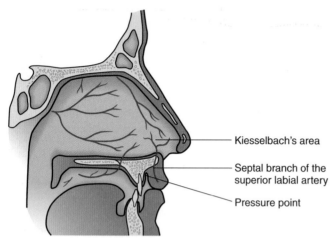

Figure 20-8 Blood supply to the nose. Key areas where bleeding control can be applied include Kiesselbach's area and the vessels in the upper lip (anterior nosebleeds). Pinching the nostrils controls most anterior nosebleeds. Some experts also recommend placing roll gauze under the upper lip. Deeper vessels that can cause posterior bleeding in the nose may need hospital intervention and nasal packing for control of bleeding. *From Kulig K: Epistaxis. In Rosen P et al, editors:* Emergency medicine: concepts and clinical practice, *St Louis, 1983, Mosby.*

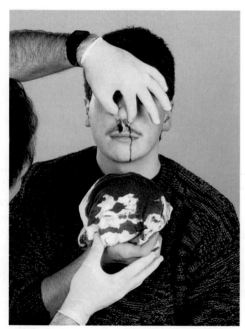

Figure 20-9 To control anterior nosebleeds, apply pressure by pinching the nose closed on either side and holding for 5 minutes.

> **LEARNING OBJECTIVES**
> - Establish the relationship between the mechanism of injury and internal bleeding.
> - List the signs of internal bleeding.
> - List the steps in the emergency medical care of the patient with signs and symptoms of internal bleeding.

Internal Bleeding

Signs of internal bleeding are obvious when a patient is vomiting blood or has heavy vaginal or rectal bleeding. Other obvious evidence of GI bleeding is "coffee grounds" vomitus or dark, tarry stools. After injury, bleeding in the subcutaneous tissues is indicated by large contusions on the skin that are swollen and discolored (black and blue). Internal bleeding should be suspected in patients with painful swelling of a limb, such as with a fracture of the femur.

As an EMT, you must also be aware of the possibility of internal bleeding from either the mechanism of injury or the typical complaints associated with diseases that can result in rapid blood loss.

Major trauma, blunt or penetrating, should always dictate a careful search for signs of bleeding. Common mechanisms include falls, motorcycle or motor vehicle crashes, striking of a pedestrian, blast injuries, and knife and gunshot wounds. Fractures may result in large amounts of blood loss, especially when they involve the femur or pelvis. Skull fractures rarely result in significant bleeding within the skull because the cranium is a nonexpandable space. The exception to this is open wounds or skull fractures in an infant. The bones of the skull in an infant have not fused, and the size of the skull can expand if there is bleeding within the cranium, allowing a critical amount of blood loss to occur.

Medical conditions, such as ulcers of the stomach and duodenum or a history of an abdominal aneurysm, should prompt consideration of internal bleeding as the reason for a patient's complaint of weakness. In women of childbearing age, a ruptured ectopic pregnancy should always be considered. Sometimes the abdomen is distended, tender, or rigid. **Table 20-2** lists some sites of internal bleeding with hidden blood loss.

Regardless of whether bleeding is internal or external, as an EMT you must be familiar with the early signs of hypovolemia,

> ### Case in Point
>
> Two EMTs respond to a 47-year-old woman complaining of abdominal pain, vomiting, and dizziness. During the initial (primary) assessment and the focused (secondary) assessment, the EMTs note pain and tenderness in the epigastric region of the abdomen. The patient states she has vomited several times during the last hour. One EMT looks in the bathroom and notes bright-red blood in the toilet bowl. The patient is lethargic and has a weak pulse of 130 beats/min. Her skin is pale, cool, and clammy. The blood pressure is 90/70 mm Hg. Respirations are 24 breaths/min and shallow. The EMTs administer high-concentration oxygen and initiate rapid transport with the patient's legs elevated, covering the patient to maintain body temperature. En route they reassess the patient and notify the trauma center of the impending arrival of a victim of an apparent episode of gastrointestinal bleeding and related hypovolemic shock.

Table 20-2	Potential Sites of Hidden Blood Loss*	
Site	**Amount†**	**Percentage of Total Blood Volume**
Hemithorax	2 L	40%
Abdomen	≥3 L	≥50%
Femur	≥1 L	20%
Pelvis	0.5 L per fracture	10% per fracture‡
Skull	Not significant unless an infant	

*Calculated for a 70-kg man with a total blood volume of 5 L. Large amounts of blood may fill various body cavities without external signs.
†Amount of blood that can accumulate in a body area with heavy bleeding.
‡Because the pelvis is a ring, an "unstable" pelvic fracture detected by movement with compression of the iliac crests has at least two fractures and potential 1 L of blood loss.

or abnormally decreased blood volume. The body compensates for blood loss so effectively that the initial loss of blood may not be appreciated on first assessment without a high level of suspicion and knowledge of the compensatory mechanism. Continued bleeding at the same rate may lead to rapid deterioration of the patient's condition and to shock.

The prehospital management of internal bleeding includes recognizing its existence, maintaining the patient's oxygenation and ventilation, controlling any external bleeding, and providing rapid transport. The patient with suspected internal bleeding should be watched for any signs and symptoms of shock.

> **LEARNING OBJECTIVES**
> - List the signs and symptoms of shock.
> - Outline the steps in the emergency medical care of the patient with signs and symptoms of shock (hypoperfusion).
> - Explain the sense of urgency to transport patients who are bleeding and who show signs of shock (hypoperfusion).

Shock

Shock is the failure of the circulatory system to adequately perfuse and oxygenate the tissues of the body. Shock has many causes, but ultimately all result in inadequate tissue perfusion and oxygenation. Shock is caused by a disruption of any of the components of the circulatory system and may be present in varying degrees. In some cases, it may be slight, transient, and self-correcting. In other cases, shock may be severe enough to result in death. The onset of shock may be immediate or delayed. Because early recognition of shock is important in ensuring prompt treatment, the EMT must be familiar with the signs and symptoms of this life-threatening condition.

The ability to assess shock is aided by knowledge of the compensatory mechanisms that the body uses to survive. These compensatory mechanisms work to keep the mind alert and the blood pressure normal until the last moments. When you are aware of the ways the body tries to compensate for bleeding, you can recognize signs of shock and treat patients in the early stages, when they have the greatest chance of survival.

Classification of Shock

Although many different conditions can lead to circulatory failure, they are usually classified as problems of one of the following:
- Heart
- Blood volume
- Vascular system

Heart failure results in a direct decrease in cardiac output because the heart itself is damaged. Loss of blood volume or dilation of the vascular system can also cause decreased perfusion.

Cardiogenic Shock

With severe heart failure, cardiac output is inadequate to meet the body's needs at rest, and the patient is in shock. This shock is termed cardiogenic because it stems from heart failure or pump failure. The most common cause of cardiogenic shock is myocardial infarction, in which the blood supply to the heart muscle itself is obstructed and part of the heart muscle starts to die. A decrease in cardiac output can also be caused by abnormal heart rhythms.

The effects of pump failure are seen on both the arterial and the venous side of the circulation. On the arterial side, less blood flows to tissues and organs, resulting in decreased perfusion to the affected part. This may occur with or without hypotension. At the same time, because the ventricles cannot pump effectively, blood returning to the heart backs up in the venous system. This backup forces fluid from the blood into the alveoli and tissues, causing edema.

Distended neck veins result from backup on the systemic side of the circulation. Backup on the pulmonary side is evidenced by signs of fluid in the lungs, such as shortness of breath, noisy breath sounds, and an increased work of breathing.

The mortality rate from cardiogenic shock is high. Early hospital treatment is mandatory. Prehospital therapy is supportive and limited, with recognition the key to early hospital care. Patients may have both hypotension and pulmonary edema. The decision to position the patient in the supine rather than the sitting position on the stretcher should be dictated by the patient's comfort. If the patient can tolerate it, the sitting position is preferred because it aids breathing. If the patient is weak and has an altered mental status, the supine position may improve brain perfusion. Once the patient is in the supine position, however, the need for positive-pressure ventilation should be evaluated. High-concentration supplemental oxygen should be administered to the patient. The patient's airway and ventilations should be constantly monitored. Suction and positive-pressure ventilation devices should be readily available. Patients with cardiogenic shock are at high risk for cardiopulmonary arrest.

Hypovolemic Shock

With a decrease in blood volume, the amount of blood returning to the heart decreases along with cardiac output. The most life-threatening cause of low blood volume is severe and rapid bleeding, or hemorrhage. Hypovolemic shock is shock caused by low blood volume.

Other causes of decreased volume of circulating fluid or plasma (hypovolemia) in the body include the following:

- Gastrointestinal illnesses
- Fever
- High environmental temperatures
- Prolonged exercise
- Metabolic problems, such as diabetes

Any condition resulting in water loss that exceeds the amount of water taken in causes the body to become dehydrated. Signs and symptoms of dehydration include the following:

- Thirst
- Absence of tearing and sweating
- Dry tongue and mucous membranes
- "Tenting" of the skin (pinching the skin leaves it "tented" rather than rapidly returning to normal)

You may frequently encounter patients who are dehydrated as a result of not being able to care for themselves because of an illness, some underlying condition, or extremes of age (infants and elderly people). Often these patients are individuals who require the assistance of a caregiver.

Signs and Symptoms of Blood Loss. The loss of blood results in dynamic changes in the circulatory system as the heart and vessels attempt to compensate for the diminishing blood volume. Many compensatory mechanisms are available. The degree of blood loss determines the type of compensatory mechanisms the body uses to maintain blood flow, which include the following:

- Constriction of veins
- Constriction of the arteries
- Increased heart rate
- Increased rate of breathing

In turn, these mechanisms alter the clinical presentation of the patient. By learning the signs of early shock, the EMT often can provide appropriate treatment at the scene and rapid transport to the hospital before irreversible shock occurs.

Stages of Hypovolemic Shock. The body compensates for acute bleeding in different ways, depending on the amount of blood loss.

Blood Loss of 10% to 15%. The first response to blood loss is constriction of the circular muscles in the venous system. The venous system contains more than half the total blood volume. Constricting the veins reduces the size of the total vascular space that must be filled by the remaining blood volume.

The veins can change the space that blood must occupy to compensate for the loss of 15% of the total blood volume. Thus, no signs or symptoms of blood loss may be present with this amount of blood loss.

With few or no accompanying signs or symptoms, a blood loss of less than 15% (or the first 700 mL of blood) is the most difficult amount to evaluate. You should look for blood in the surrounding area as a result of external bleeding; for signs of internal bleeding, such as vomiting blood; and for the mechanism of injury, because a patient with blood loss of less than 15% may show no other signs or symptoms.

Blood Loss of Up to 30%. When bleeding surpasses 15% of blood volume, constriction of the veins is insufficient to compensate and maintain perfusion. Less blood returns to the heart, cardiac output decreases, and less blood is pumped out with

Table 20-3	Capillary Refilling Time Test*
Result	**Total Blood Loss**
Normal (capillary return within 2 seconds)	Minimal
Delayed (>2 seconds)	Moderate
Prolonged, absent	Severe

*Correlation of capillary refilling time testing and blood loss.

each beat. The body senses an imminent fall in blood pressure, and the sympathetic nervous system and epinephrine cause a compensatory increase in heart rate and constriction of arterial vessels. The constriction of arteries is selective. Arteries are closed in less important areas, redistributing the remaining blood to the brain, head, and lungs at the expense of the skin, muscles, and digestive tract.

The blood pressure is maintained by these mechanisms within normal ranges. However, signs of epinephrine release are evident. The patient has a rapid and thready pulse. Because of the redistribution of blood away from the skin, the skin is cool, pale, and clammy. The patient is alert (and apprehensive) because blood is sent preferentially to the brain. The pupils dilate. The patient may have a "funny" feeling in the stomach or may feel like vomiting.

If the patient is further stressed by attempting to sit or stand from the lying position, he or she feels weaker, faint, or dizzy and must lie back down. The heart is unable to maintain the blood pressure against this added force of gravity, or it may be able to maintain the blood pressure only with a still greater increase in heart rate.

Capillary refilling time may be a useful test to help gauge blood loss. This test is more reliable in children than adults and is used for patients younger than 6 years. Gentle finger pressure is placed on a nail bed and then released. Normally, when the nail is compressed, blood is squeezed from the capillaries under the nail, and the nail bed becomes pale. When pressure is released, the capillaries immediately refill with blood, and a pink color returns. After significant blood loss, the time required for the capillaries to refill with blood increases (**Table 20-3**). With blood loss less than 15%, the capillaries refill immediately or within 2 seconds. However, after about 20% to 25% blood loss, the capillaries refill more slowly. If the time for refilling is more than 2 seconds, a person is said to have "delayed" capillary refilling time. Two seconds is about the time it takes to say "capillary return." With still greater blood loss, the time for refilling may be prolonged to the point that capillary refill seems absent. However, delayed capillary refilling is not always a reliable indicator of hypovolemia. Capillary refilling time may also be prolonged without blood loss in patients exposed to cold environments and in some older patients.

The body attempts to pull additional fluid into the capillaries to restore blood volume. Although this is a slow process, the cells are sensitive to water loss, and the patient may be thirsty. If the patient may need surgery under general anesthesia, the patient should not be allowed to drink fluids because it increases the danger of vomiting during intubation.

A normal blood pressure when the patient is supine may be misleading; all the compensatory efforts are working to maintain a sufficient perfusion pressure for the vital organs.

Blood Loss of 30% to 45%. With still greater blood loss, the compensatory mechanisms are all working to their maximum capacity, but blood return to the heart has fallen even further. The cardiac output is half of normal, and blood pressure falls. Hypotension is a relatively late event in blood loss, occurring only after all the body's compensatory mechanisms are exhausted.

The patient's mental status starts to deteriorate, and the patient may gasp for air. With further blood loss, the next most oxygen-dependent organ, the heart, starts to fail. The heart has been beating faster and stronger in its attempt to maintain the cardiac output. This increased activity requires an increased supply of oxygen to the heart muscle. At this point, however, the blood pressure is falling despite the heart's efforts. Because the blood pressure is the driving force for the coronary circulation, the heart itself is inadequately perfused and loses its ability to continue both rapid and powerful contractions. In fact, the heart rate may slow as shock progresses.

The patient initially had hypovolemic shock; the ability of the body to compensate has now been severely hampered by the inadequate perfusion of the heart muscle, and now the patient is in great jeopardy. The patient still has more than half the normal hemoglobin. The sudden loss of volume is the critical factor in acute hemorrhage.

Blood Loss of Greater than 45%. With still greater blood loss, circulatory collapse follows. The constriction of the venous and arterial vessels, which reduces the size of the vascular space, requires muscular contraction. As the patient becomes hypotensive, the constricting muscles in the vascular tree are less perfused. These muscles become exhausted, and the vessels begin to dilate. A decrease in blood pressure results in total circulatory collapse and then cardiac arrest. The patient must receive hospital intervention within minutes or death is certain.

Table 20-4 summarizes the signs and symptoms of severe bleeding in relation to the percentage of blood loss.

Infants and Children. Infants and children may maintain their blood pressure until their blood volume is depleted by more than half. With young and healthy hearts, these patients can compensate even after extensive bleeding. When blood pressure does decrease, however, infants and children may decompensate rapidly.

Vasodilatory Shock

The circulatory system also fails when the vascular system loses its ability to constrict and blood pressure falls.

Anaphylaxis and Spinal Injury. Two serious conditions that can cause vasodilatory shock are anaphylaxis and spinal cord injuries. In anaphylaxis, as a result of a severe allergic reaction, the body releases chemicals that directly cause vasodilation. In shock caused by spinal cord injuries, damage to the upper spinal cord can result in loss of the sympathetic nervous system's ability to constrict the blood vessels (resulting in vasodilation) and to increase the heart's rate (to allow a compensatory increase in cardiac output). (See chapters 14 and 24.)

Table 20-4	Correlation of Signs and Symptoms with Degree of Blood Loss	
Blood Loss*	**Compensatory Effect**	**Signs and Symptoms**
<15%	Veins contract	None or transient
15%-30%	Epinephrine response Arteries constrict to maintain blood pressure, reducing flow to skin, gut, and muscle Increased heart rate	Rapid and thready pulse Cool, pale, clammy skin Thirst Weakness Faintness or dizziness; anxiety; rapid, shallow breathing Delayed capillary refilling time† Blood pressure may be normal
30%-45%	Decompensation; cardiac output falls to half of normal	Hypotension Deteriorated mental status Combativeness, restlessness Rapid, shallow, "air-hungry" respirations

*As percentage of total blood volume.
†More reliable in infants and children.

Psychogenic Shock. Another cause of vasodilatory shock is an emotional reaction that stimulates the parasympathetic nervous system, such as hearing distressing news (e.g., sudden death of loved one) or fright. The result is dilation of the blood vessels and a slowing of the heart rate, the combination of which is sufficient to result in fainting. If the patient is placed in a horizontal position with the legs elevated, the problem usually is corrected because the effect of gravity on blood pooling in the lower extremities is reduced and the initial nervous reaction is brief. Because of the emotional origin of this condition, this type of shock is often referred to as *psychogenic* (originating in the mind).

Patients in psychogenic shock do not usually require additional prehospital treatment. When they faint, they may fall to the ground; the change in posture helps restore brain perfusion by changing the gravitational forces on venous pooling.

Septic Shock. Shock resulting from massive infection is caused mainly by vasodilation. Vessels throughout the body dilate, particularly in the infected areas. Septic shock can be further complicated by the leakage of fluid through the blood vessel walls, resulting in hypovolemia. Thus, septic shock can have both vasodilatory and hypovolemic components. A further complication can result from the release of chemicals that depress the pumping ability of the heart.

Time Constraints

Shock must be diagnosed and treated rapidly to prevent permanent damage to the tissues and death. For example, in patients with hypovolemic shock caused by hemorrhage, delaying diagnosis and treatment until the patient is hypotensive (blood pressure <80 mm Hg) with a deteriorating mental status greatly increases the mortality risk.

Therefore a goal of an emergency medical services (EMS) system is to recognize, treat, and transport patients in shock before they become hypotensive, when they have the best chance for survival. To accomplish this, you will need assessment skills that recognize the early signs of shock.

EXTENDED_Transport_

The best chance of survival in a patient with hemorrhagic shock is emergency surgery. When treating this patient, the EMT is racing the clock. The EMT must consider the fastest way to transport the patient to surgery. Alternative modes of transportation such as helicopter should be considered. While transporting for long periods or waiting for alternate transportation, basic skills are most beneficial. Monitor the patient's airway and provide oxygen; stop external bleeding; and keep the patient warm.

Management

After attention to airway, breathing, and bleeding control, treatment for shock is initiated. In cases of shock from blood loss, bleeding control is the fundamental and most important step in treatment. The following measures should be taken:

1. Give high-concentration supplemental oxygen to patients in shock to ensure that the circulating hemoglobin is completely saturated with oxygen.
2. If the patient's condition permits, elevate the legs 8 to 12 inches (20-30 cm).
3. If the patient's condition permits, splint bone or joint injuries. If rapid transport is indicated, immobilize the patient to the long spine board.
4. Maintain the patient's body temperature with blankets. The patient in shock has trouble regulating body temperature and cannot afford additional heat loss. When environmental temperatures exceed body temperature, leave the patient uncovered.

Many patients with hypovolemic shock can be resuscitated if they receive timely treatment. They are often transported to trauma centers because definitive care for many of these patients can be given only in the operating room. The ultimate therapy for a patient with hypovolemic shock is outside the bounds of the prehospital sphere.

Again, a goal of EMS systems is to bring patients to definitive therapy as quickly as possible. The transport decision, or the point during the prehospital assessment when transport should begin, is one of the most important decisions that an EMT makes. The advantage you bring to the patient is recognizing shock, making an early transport decision to the appropriate hospital, and communicating with the hospital before arrival so staff can expedite care. The only acceptable delays at the scene are for lifesaving treatments. The EMT must consider the risks and benefits of time spent on the scene.

Pneumatic Antishock Garment

Your EMS system may use the PASG. In the past, use of the PASG was mandatory training for all EMTs. Studies over the years, however, have reappraised its use, and indications for the PASG have now changed in most EMS systems (see References).

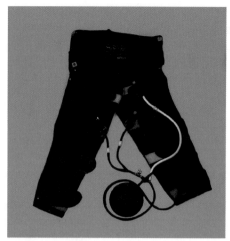

Figure 20-10 Pneumatic antishock garment (PASG) with a foot pump and a pressure gauge.

Description. The PASG is an air-filled pair of pants that surrounds the legs and the abdomen (**Figure 20-10**). The leg and abdominal sections (bladders) can be inflated to pressures up to 100 mm Hg. By their application and inflation, the bladders transmit their inflated pressure circumferentially to structures within the legs and abdomen. This increased pressure reduces the size of the vascular space and increases the vascular resistance, thereby increasing blood pressure. A small amount of blood is "autotransfused" from the compressed vessels to the thorax. The PASG may help control bleeding beneath the garment when the pressure of the PASG exceeds the pressure of the vessels underneath and causes their collapse. The PASG may also help tamponade bleeding within the abdomen and pelvis.

Skill 20-2 illustrates the application of the PASG.

Indications. Although the PASG was once used widely in EMS throughout the United States, its use is currently controversial. PASG may be used to treat shock, and suspected pelvic fractures specifically, if signs of shock are present and the lower abdomen is tender and pelvic injury is suspected, with no evidence of chest injury. Other experts would limit PASG use to patients with pelvic fractures and shock when transport times are prolonged and the pelvis is grossly unstable when tested with pressure on the iliac crests.

The PASG might be useful as a pressure splint to help control bleeding in massive soft tissue injuries to the lower extremity. In patients with fractures or extensive crush injury in the lower leg, the PASG might cause compartment syndrome or ischemia of muscle and other tissues from arterial compression. As a result, many experts limit PASG use for bleeding control in the lower extremity to patients whose bleeding is otherwise uncontrollable.

Some EMS systems advocate use of the PASG for patients with severe hypovolemic shock (systolic blood pressure <50 mm Hg) or a palpable pulse but no measurable blood pressure. The PASG was shown to benefit survival of patients with systolic blood pressure less than 50 mm Hg, but not those with blood pressure greater than 50 mm Hg.

Because the PASG compresses all tissues beneath, some physicians advocate its use if the source of bleeding is in the pelvis or abdomen, arguing that the *tamponade* effect (compression of blood vessels) should limit bleeding. Some experts believe it is a benefit to some medical causes of abdominal hemorrhage, such as bleeding from abdominal aortic aneurysm.

Removal. In general, once the PASG is applied, it should not be deflated in the field unless the EMT is instructed to do so by a physician. If so directed, the device is deflated in stages, starting with the abdominal section, monitoring vital signs carefully.

Contraindications. Penetrating chest injuries are a clear contraindication to use of the PASG. Other conditions that can be made worse with the PASG include rupture of the diaphragm, in which the abdominal contents are pushed upward through a hole in the diaphragm and enter the thoracic cavity. Cardiac tamponade, caused by buildup of fluid or blood in the pericardium, may also be worsened by the PASG because it increases systemic vascular resistance (SVR), and the heart must pump harder to deliver the same stroke volume. Because it is difficult to detect these conditions with certainty in the field, signs of significant chest injury or abnormal breath sounds might be contraindications to use of the PASG.

Because the PASG raises SVR, it increases the work placed on the heart as it tries to pump blood out through the arteries. Therefore, its use is contraindicated in cardiogenic shock, acute myocardial infarction, and pulmonary edema. Such patients might experience difficult and noisy breathing, low blood pressure, and complaints of chest pain.

Use of the PASG is contraindicated in conditions involving the abdomen, such as pregnancy and exposed abdominal organs. In a patient with these conditions, direct pressure from the PASG may compromise the viability of the fetus or the exposed bowel. An impaled object in the abdomen would be an obvious contraindication to inflating the abdominal portion of the PASG.

The EMT should always be aware of indications and contraindications for the PASG according to local protocols. For many situations, when few or conflicting data exist, the risk/benefit determination is a medical decision made by local medical direction.

Traumatic Cardiopulmonary Resuscitation

Patients in cardiopulmonary arrest from trauma or internal bleeding are so rarely resuscitated by measures used in the field that most EMS systems have policies to address this situation. Often the policy recognizes that for *pulseless* patients, the only chance for survival may be rapid surgical intervention and blood and fluid therapy in an ED and operating room. This would apply primarily to patients who do not have a documented pulse in the field when EMS arrives or who lose the pulse during transport. In such patients, especially those with penetrating heart wounds, lives have been saved as a result of rapid transport.

However, for most patients in the field who are found pulseless because of trauma, particularly blunt trauma, the chance for survival is so remote that the patient is often treated as *expectant*. They may be left at the scene and transported by the medical examiner, or they may be transported to the hospital for formal pronouncement of death, depending on circumstances and local policy. However, transporting these patients with lights and sirens or air transport makes no sense in such situations, because the risk of a crash and injury to others exceeds any chance of benefit to the patient. You should consult local protocols to best handle these situations.

Scenario Follow-up

This scenario illustrates the importance of (1) direct pressure for controlling external bleeding and (2) effective patient assessment to identify potentially life-threatening internal bleeding. This patient's vital signs are highly suggestive of internal bleeding and the early stages of shock. The increasing pulse rate indicates the body's attempt to improve circulation with the available blood volume. The pale skin is caused by the redistribution of blood from the skin to vital organs. These actions largely result from the release of epinephrine (adrenaline). The patient is beginning to show signs of *decompensation* with a slight drop in blood pressure.

An awareness of these signs is critical to good decision making in prehospital care. The early decision to transport to the local trauma center gave this patient the best chance for survival. The only definitive treatment of uncontrolled internal bleeding is surgery.

Summary

Evidence of bleeding and shock is elicited during the initial (primary) assessment and focused (secondary) assessment (patient history, physical examination). Control of external bleeding is an essential skill and part of the ABCs. Bleeding control is accomplished by direct pressure, elevation, pressure points, and as a last resort, a tourniquet. Internal bleeding is controlled at the hospital. Because patients with significant blood loss may be alert and have "normal" blood pressure, it is important to look for other signs and symptoms to recognize shock and internal bleeding before the patient's condition deteriorates. Rapid transport to the hospital for definitive care is the primary part of the treatment plan for all patients with serious bleeding or signs of shock.

Skills

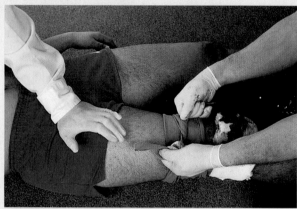

1. Place a piece of soft material (4 inches wide, six to eight layers deep), such as a folded triangular bandage or a commercial tourniquet, proximal to the wound (but as distal as possible). Wrap the material around the extremity twice, then secure with a half-knot.

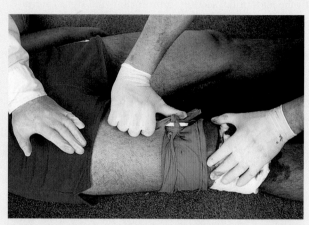

2. Place a stick or pencil in the half-knot and secure with a square knot.

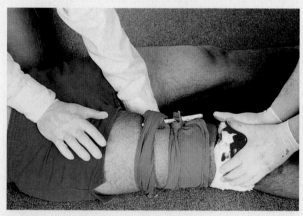

3. Twist the stick until bleeding stops, and then securely attach it next to the extremity.

Clearly note on the prehospital record that a tourniquet has been applied and the time of application so that hospital personnel do not overlook it during resuscitation efforts.

Note: Once a tourniquet is applied, only hospital personnel should remove it. Leave the tourniquet exposed in clear view, and directly inform hospital personnel that a tourniquet has been applied. You may write "TK" across the patient's forehead (or on tape that is applied to the forehead) as another reminder.

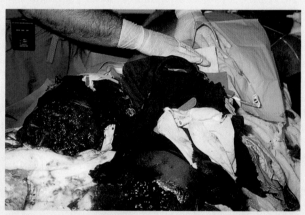

4. An example of the type of patient for whom tourniquets may be needed would be this patient with bilateral leg amputations caused by a train accident and severe blood loss (systolic blood pressure 60 mm Hg by palpation). Tourniquets were placed by EMS personnel in the field, and the patient survived.

Skill | 20-2   *Applying the Pneumatic Antishock Garment (PASG)*

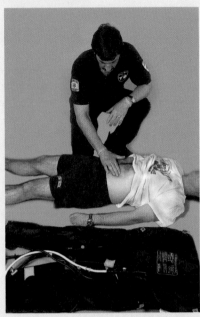

1. Examine the patient's abdomen and legs to determine the extent of injuries; once the PASG is applied, these areas will not be accessible. If possible, remove the patient's trousers, socks, and other clothing. If this is impossible, remove bulky objects, such as a wallet, belt buckle, or keys.

2. Lay the PASG open on the stretcher, then lay the patient on the garment with a log-roll procedure. If spinal injuries are suspected, take the appropriate precautions.

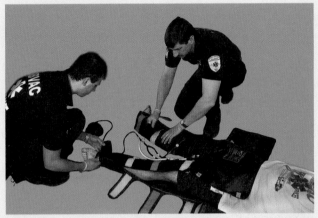

3. The top of the abdominal section of the PASG should lie below the lowest rib.

4. Fasten the Velcro straps. Try to ensure that at least three fourths of the Velcro surface area is covered; otherwise, the Velcro straps may loosen with increasing pressure.

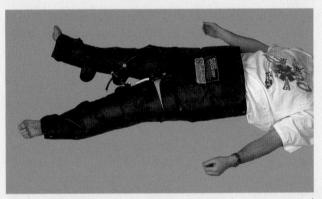

5. If the foot pump is not already connected, connect it and open the stopcock valves.

6. Inflate the legs and (if not contraindicated) abdominal sections. Check for evidence of clinical response: improvement in vital signs, capillary refilling time, skin color, and mental status.

The Bottom Line

Learning Checklist

✓ The circulatory system is the transport system of the body. It delivers oxygen and nutrients to the tissues and returns the waste products of metabolism (carbon dioxide and cellular wastes) to the lungs and kidneys for excretion.

✓ The circulatory system consists of the heart, blood, and blood vessels. The blood consists of plasma and white blood cells (combat infection), red blood cells (transport oxygen and carbon dioxide attached to hemoglobin), and platelets (for clotting).

✓ Blood pressure consists of two components; systolic pressure is exerted on the walls of the artery when the ventricle contracts; diastolic pressure is exerted on the walls of the artery when the ventricle relaxes.

✓ External bleeding is controlled by direct pressure, elevation, pressure points, and as a last resort, a tourniquet.

✓ A pressure bandage can be applied for continuous control of bleeding.

✓ Anterior nosebleeds (epistaxis) can be controlled by pinching the nose while the patient leans forward to avoid aspiration and swallowing of blood.

✓ Internal bleeding can be recognized when a patient vomits or coughs up blood or when there is bleeding from other body openings.

✓ Blood loss of 10% to 15% results in constriction of the venous system and may not present with any signs or symptoms.

✓ Blood loss of 15% to 30% may result in weakness; anxiety; rapid and thready pulse; pale, cool, and clammy skin; delayed capillary refilling time (children); and thirst. These patients may have a normal blood pressure.

✓ Blood loss of 30% to 45% may result in hypotension, altered mental state, combativeness, restlessness, and rapid and shallow breathing.

✓ Shock is the failure of the circulatory system to adequately perfuse the body's tissues.

✓ Shock can be caused by the loss of blood volume, failure of the heart, or dilation of the blood vessels.

✓ General emergency care for shock can include oxygen administration, leg elevation (8-12 inches), prevention of heat loss, and rapid transport to the hospital.

✓ The pneumatic antishock garment (PASG) can increase the blood pressure by increasing systemic vascular resistance.

✓ The PASG can exacerbate bleeding from penetrating thoracic injuries by raising blood pressure before bleeding is controlled.

Key Terms

Blood pressure Force exerted by the blood volume on the walls of the vessels.

Direct pressure First step in controlling bleeding. This pressure is applied over the site of the wound. Use a gloved hand or absorbent material, such as gauze.

Epistaxis Nosebleed; hemorrhage from the nose.

Hemorrhage Profuse bleeding.

Hypoperfusion Decreased blood flow through an organ; if prolonged, can result in cellular dysfunction and death; also called *shock*.

Hypovolemic shock Shock resulting from low blood volume caused by excessive bleeding, burns, metabolic disorders, or other causes of body fluid loss.

Pneumatic antishock garment (PASG) Air-filled pants that surround the legs and abdomen; when inflated, can be used to treat shock, immobilize fractures, and control bleeding.

Pressure point Common pulse location where pressure can be applied to collapse an artery and thereby reduce or stop blood flow to a wound.

Shock Failure of the circulatory system to adequately perfuse and oxygenate the vital organs of the body; also called *hypoperfusion*.

Tourniquet Constricting band applied over an extremity with enough pressure to completely stop blood flow beyond the site of application.

Review Questions

1. A 55-year-old man is walking and suddenly feels dizzy. EMTs arrive and note that his blood pressure is very low. Which of the following physiologic parameters *directly* affects the blood pressure?
   a. Cardiac output
   b. Diameter of the blood vessels
   c. Tidal volume
   d. Vital capacity

2. A 25-year-old male has sustained a slash injury to his neck. Dark blood is flowing in a steady stream from the wound. Which type of bleeding is the patient experiencing?
   a. Capillary
   b. Venous
   c. Arterial
   d. Arteriole

3. What is the correct order of the following actions for controlling bleeding?
   a. Tourniquet, pressure point, direct pressure
   b. Direct pressure, tourniquet, pressure point
   c. Direct pressure, pressure point, tourniquet
   d. Pressure point, direct pressure, tourniquet

4. You note that a patient has head and facial wounds with spurting blood. The appropriate personal precautions would include:

   a. Gloves only

   b. Gloves and goggles

   c. Gloves, goggles, and mask

   d. Gloves, goggles, mask, and gown

5. You respond to a man struck by a car. He has contusions to his head, abdomen, arm, and leg. Which mechanism of injury would you expect to cause severe internal bleeding?

   a. Head

   b. Abdomen

   c. Arm

   d. Leg

6. Which of the following is a late sign of hypovolemic shock?

   a. Pale skin

   b. Tachycardia

   c. Hypotension

   d. Increased respiration

7. The pneumatic antishock garment (PASG) has been recommended in the treatment of:

   a. Cardiogenic shock

   b. Bleeding in the chest

   c. Head injury associated with shock

   d. Pelvic injuries with associated shock

8. Which of the following is a recommended treatment for patients in hypovolemic shock (hypoperfusion) without evidence of serious injuries?

   a. Elevate the lower extremities 8 to 12 inches.

   b. Seat the patient in the upright position.

   c. Place the patient in the prone position.

   d. Position the patient in the semireclining position.

For Further Review

In the Student Workbook

- Multiple-choice questions
- Fill-in-the-blank questions
- True-false questions
- Case scenario questions

On Evolve

- Chapter challenge
- Weblinks
- Lecture notes
- Exercises

Learning Objectives

Cognitive Objectives

- Describe the structure and function of the circulatory system.
- Differentiate among arterial, venous, and capillary bleeding.
- Describe methods of emergency medical care for external bleeding.
- Establish the relationship between body substance isolation and bleeding.
- Establish the relationship between airway management and the trauma patient.
- Establish the relationship between mechanism of injury and internal bleeding.
- List the signs of internal bleeding.
- List the steps in the emergency medical care of the patient with signs and symptoms of internal bleeding.
- List signs and symptoms of shock (hypoperfusion).
- Outline the steps in the emergency medical care of the patient with signs and symptoms of shock (hypoperfusion).

Affective Objectives

- Explain the sense of urgency to transport patients who are bleeding and show signs of shock (hypoperfusion).

Psychomotor Objectives

- Demonstrate direct pressure as a method of emergency medical care of external bleeding.
- Demonstrate the use of diffuse pressure as a method of emergency medical care of external bleeding.
- Demonstrate the use of pressure points and tourniquets as a method of emergency medical care of external bleeding.
- Demonstrate the care of the patient exhibiting signs and symptoms of internal bleeding.
- Demonstrate the care of the patient exhibiting signs and symptoms of shock (hypoperfusion).
- Demonstrate completing a prehospital care report for the patient with bleeding and/or shock (hypoperfusion).

References

O'Connor RE, Domeier RM: An evaluation of the pneumatic antishock garment (PASG), *Prehosp Emerg Care* 1:36, 1997.

Pepe PE: The pneumatic anti-shock garment. In Kuehl AE, editor: *Prehospital systems and medical oversight,* Dubuque, Iowa, 2002, Kendall/Hunt.

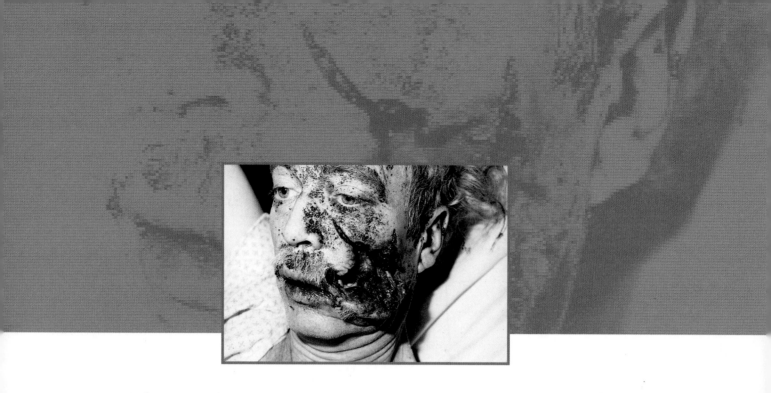

21 Soft Tissue Injuries

CHAPTER OUTLINE

Anatomy and Physiology

Wounds

Dressings and Bandages

Facial Injuries

Burns

Skills

Scenario

You respond to the scene of a stabbing. Police are there, and it is safe to begin patient care. A young man in his 20s is lying on the street, bleeding from both arms, with a knife protruding from the center of his chest. He is breathing adequately, and his pulse is 100 beats/min and blood pressure 120/86 mm Hg. You note lacerations on both forearms and across the left palm. The lacerations on the forearms of this patient could be a source of significant bleeding and were most likely the result of defensive maneuvers during the knife attack. You control bleeding with direct pressure using dressings, then you bandage the dressings in place. You treat the knife in the chest as an impaled object, securing it with bulky dressings to minimize movement or inadvertent dislodgement.

Almost all trauma patients injure the skin and soft tissues at the point of impact. The soft tissues include the skin, the subcutaneous layer of fat and connective tissue beneath the skin, and the skeletal muscles, tendons, and ligaments. Injuries to the soft tissue are classified as open or closed. With *open* injuries the skin is broken; with *closed* injuries the skin remains intact.

This chapter focuses on the general care of open and closed wounds to the skin and soft tissues and on techniques of wound management, including basic dressing and bandaging. The management of soft tissue injuries to specific body areas is included in the respective chapters of this text.

To appreciate the consequences of damage to the skin and the layers of tissue underneath, you must understand the anatomy of the skin. Soft tissue injuries themselves are usually not life threatening; however, they may suggest the existence of more serious injuries to underlying organs or major blood vessels. Therefore you should look at the skin in conjunction with the mechanism of injury for clues to the type of trauma sustained and possible underlying injuries.

> **LEARNING OBJECTIVES**
> * State the major functions of the skin.
> * List the layers of the skin.

Anatomy and Physiology

The skin is the largest organ of the body, providing a protective covering and insulation. It separates the internal environment from the external environment. It is a barrier to infection and loss of body fluids and is important for regulation of body temperature.

The skin has two major layers, the epidermis and the dermis, that rest on the subcutaneous tissue (**Figure 21-1**).

Epidermis

The surface, or outermost, layer of the skin is called the **epidermis.** The epidermis is *avascular* (no blood supply) and consists of four separate sublayers. When intact, the epidermis is impermeable and cannot be penetrated by microorganisms. It is also responsible for preventing water loss from the cells underneath. The most superficial layer of the epidermis is dead tissue that is constantly rubbed or flaked away and replaced by the living cells underneath, which migrate upward. The layers of the epidermis become filled with a protein called *keratin* as the new cells move toward the skin surface. This protein is partly responsible for the skin's impermeable barrier.

The epidermis is also responsible for the color of the skin. It contains a special pigment called *melanin,* which helps protect the body from the sun's radiation. This pigment is produced deep within the layers of the epidermis.

Skin color is also influenced by the blood flow in the skin capillaries contained within the dermis. Increased blood flow, as occurs in a hot environment, gives the skin a pink appearance. When blood flow to the skin is reduced as a result of vasoconstriction (e.g., hypovolemic shock, cold temperatures), the skin may appear pale.

Dermis

The **dermis** is composed of dense connective tissue that contains the nerves, blood vessels, sweat glands, sebaceous glands, and hair follicles. The connective tissue gives strength to the skin and serves to anchor and support the other structures.

The *nerves* in the dermis have various specialized endings that can perceive different sensations, such as pressure, vibration, pain, warmth, and cold. If this layer of skin is completely damaged, such as in third-degree burns, there is no sensory perception.

The *blood vessels* within the dermis play an important role in temperature regulation. They can constrict to prevent heat loss to the environment and dilate when the body needs to radiate heat.

The *sweat glands* are also important in the regulation of body temperature. Evaporation is an important means of cooling, particularly in extremely hot environments or when there is a rapid buildup in internal heat production, as in exercise.

The *sebaceous glands* secrete an oily substance called **sebum,** which helps moisturize the skin. The sebaceous glands are located near the hair follicles, which guide the sebum out to the surface of the skin, where the oily substance spreads out.

Hairs grow from the *hair follicles,* which are located within the dermis. Injuries that spare part of the dermis may allow for regrowth of new skin from cells that make up the hair follicles and sweat glands.

Injuries that destroy all the structures within the dermis require skin grafting.

Subcutaneous Tissue

Beneath the skin is a layer of fat and connective tissue called the subcutaneous tissue. It serves as a body insulator, and the fat can be used for energy as needed. Beneath the subcutaneous tissue is the fascia. The **fascia** is a fibrous membrane covering that separates the subcutaneous tissue from the skeletal muscles. Knowledge of the skin and its subcutaneous layers is important in understanding the severity and complications of burns.

Table 21-1 summarizes the layers and functions of the skin.

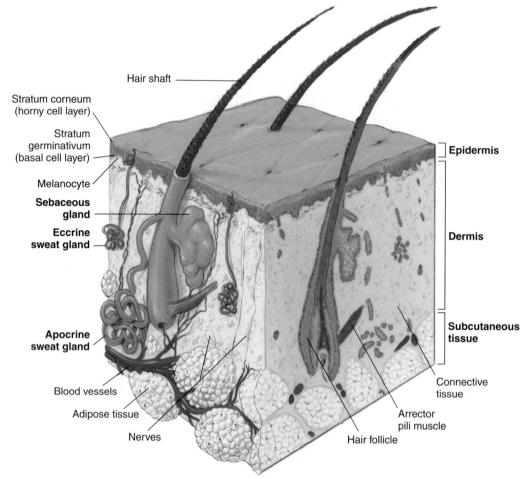

Figure 21-1 Layers and structures of the skin. *From Jarvis C: Physical examination and health assessment, ed 5, Philadelphia, 2008, Saunders.*

Table 21-1	Anatomy and Physiology of the Skin
Layer	**Function**
Epidermis	
Outer layer (keratin)	Protective barrier to infection; prevents water loss
Melanin	Protects from sun's radiation
Dermis	
Blood vessels	Body temperature regulation; constrict to conserve heat, dilate to remove heat
Nerve endings	Sensation
Sebaceous glands (sebum)	Moisturize
Sweat glands	Temperature regulation; cool by evaporation
Hair follicles	Guide sweat and sebum to the skin surface
Subcutaneous Layer	
Connective tissue and fat	Insulation; stores energy (fat)

Mucous Membranes

As skin continues into a body orifice, it changes its character. The layer of the epidermis containing keratin is absent and is replaced by mucous membranes. Mucous membranes line the internal surface of the body, such as the oropharynx, nasopharynx, ureters, bladder, lungs, intestines, and vagina. This membrane is rich in mucous glands, which secrete a lubricating fluid (mucus) to protect the body from invading organisms.

> **LEARNING OBJECTIVES**
> • List the types of closed soft tissue injuries.
> • State the types of open soft tissue injuries.

Wounds

Wounds are considered either open or closed. *Closed wounds* are the result of blunt forces that do not break the integrity of the skin. *Open wounds,* by definition, are those in which the skin surface is broken. The mnemonic *DCAP-BTLS* serves as a reminder of the types and signs of injury encountered during your assessment: *d*eformities, *c*ontusions, *a*brasions, *p*unctures, *b*urns, *t*enderness, *l*acerations, and *s*welling.

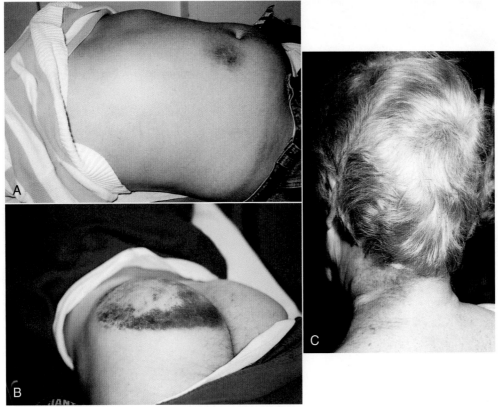

Figure 21-2 **A,** Ecchymosis caused by a kick to the abdomen 1 day earlier. **B,** Contusion to buttock after striking a tree while sledding. **C,** Severe hematoma, visible on occipital area of the scalp, was caused by a fall from fainting 3 days earlier. Blood under the scalp has gravitated down to the neck, causing ecchymoses along its path.

Closed Wounds

When blunt or compression forces are applied to the skin, the blood vessels may leak or rupture. This may be accompanied by swelling from leakage of plasma (edema) into the injured area. There may be tenderness or pain at the site of injury. This type of injury is commonly referred to as a "bruise," or **contusion.**

Contusions can be accompanied by leakage of blood from injured vessels. This bleeding may be visible just under the skin as a black-and-blue area and is called **ecchymosis.** Over time the color changes to greenish brown and then to yellow as the blood products break down and are absorbed. When blood collects in a pocket beneath the skin, a **hematoma** (tumor or swelling containing blood) may form (**Figure 21-2**).

Open Wounds

Any wound that results in a break in the skin is referred to as an open wound. Types of open wounds range from a scraping of the outermost layers of the skin to complete amputation of an extremity.

Abrasions

An **abrasion** is a scraping of the surface of the skin or mucous membrane. It may damage superficial capillaries, causing an oozing of blood at the skin's surface. Although often painful, abrasions themselves do not usually result in significant blood loss, but as with other open wounds, they are subject to infection (**Figure 21-3**).

Lacerations

A **laceration** is a tearing of the skin or other soft tissues. It may result from a blunt tearing force or a sharp object. The extent of surrounding tissue damage is a function of the mechanism of injury. Blunt forces that tear the skin may cause significant damage to tissues. A sharp object is more likely to cause an incision-type wound and minimal damage to the surrounding tissue (**Figure 21-4**). Bleeding from lacerations can be severe.

Avulsions

An **avulsion** is a tearing away of the skin's surface. A *complete* avulsion injury may tear away a complete segment of skin. An *incomplete* avulsion occurs when the skin is torn back and a characteristic flap forms. This flap may be attached by a *pedicle,* or small piece of skin. This pedicle represents the remaining source of blood and nerve supply to the avulsed flap and should be handled carefully (**Figure 21-5**).

Punctures and Penetrations

A **puncture** occurs when a sharp instrument is driven through the skin's outer layer. Punctures can be deceiving. A small puncture wound may be caused by an object (e.g., ice pick) that has penetrated to a significant depth, causing damage to underlying structures (**Figure 21-6**). There may be little external bleeding but severe internal bleeding. At times an exit wound may be evident, as with a gunshot wound.

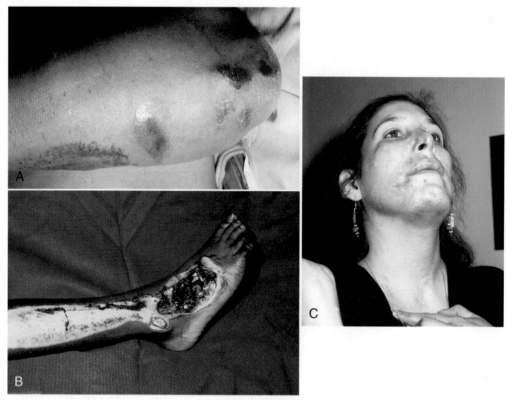

Figure 21-3 **A,** Abrasions sustained in a fall to the pavement after the patient was struck by a car. **B,** Deep abrasion through all levels of the skin after the patient was dragged by a vehicle on the road. **C,** Abrasions of the face caused by airbag deployment.

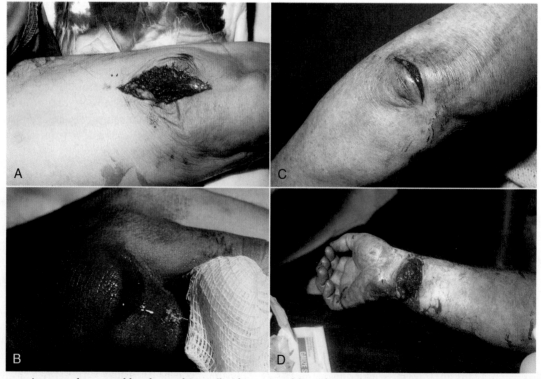

Figure 21-4 Lacerations can be caused by sharp objects (knife, saw) or blunt force (fall). **A,** Deep laceration to the thigh caused by a circular saw. **B,** Laceration over knuckle on lateral aspect of the hand was caused when the patient struck another person in the teeth. Lacerations in this area suggest contamination from human bite wounds. **C,** Laceration of the elbow caused by a fall on the street. **D,** Laceration to the wrist.

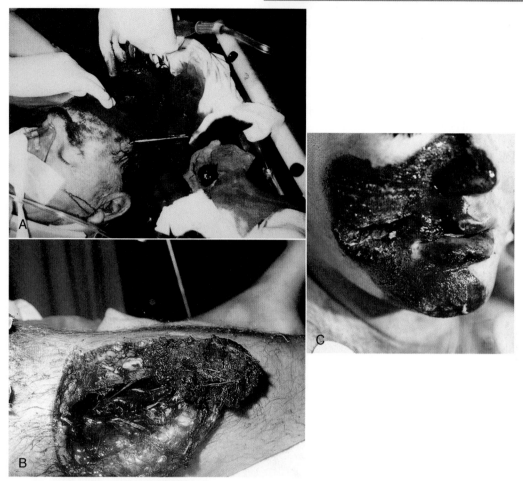

Figure 21-5 A, Severe avulsion of the scalp caused by blunt trauma. **B,** Deep avulsion of the leg after the patient was thrown off a motorcycle in a crash. This wound is grossly contaminated from contact with the ground. **C,** Avulsions and severe abrasions of the face after ejection from an automobile.

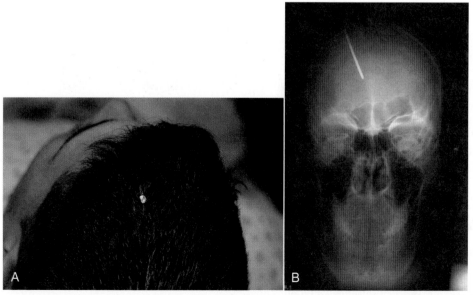

Figure 21-6 A, Puncture wound of the head shows head of the nail from a nail gun. **B,** X-ray film of the skull of the same patient showing penetration of the nail into the brain.

Amputations

An **amputation** involves the cutting away from the body of a limb or protruding structure. Sharp or crushing forces may result in amputation (**Figure 21-7**). Because the amputated part has no blood supply, time to surgical intervention and care of the amputated part are important factors in successful replantation. Bleeding can be massive or limited.

Crush Injury

Crush injuries may result in both open and closed wounds. A **crush injury** is the result of the severe compressing force that damages and sometimes tears the soft tissues and underlying structures. Examples include a car tire rolling over a leg, a finger crushed under heavy furniture, or an extremity caught in a meat grinder (**Figure 21-8**). Crush injuries can cause significant damage to underlying structures with minimal or no external bleeding.

Severity and Complications

The *severity* of a wound depends on the following:
- Mechanism of injury
- Site of injury
- Extent of the injury
- Introduction of foreign bodies or contamination into the wound

It is important to consider damage to underlying structures, including blood vessels, nerves, ligaments, bones, joints, and organs within the body cavities. Common *complications* of wounds include the following:
- Bleeding
- Infection
- Damage to underlying structures

Nerve damage, fractures, and injury to muscles, tendons, and ligaments may result in loss of function. Wounds over the major body cavities—the head, chest, and abdomen—carry the risk of damage to internal organs.

> **LEARNING OBJECTIVES**
> - Establish the relationship between body substance isolation and soft tissue injuries.
> - Describe the emergency medical care of the patient with a closed soft tissue injury.
> - Describe the emergency medical care of the patient with an open soft tissue injury.
> - Establish the relationship between airway management and the patient with chest injury, burns, blunt injury, or penetrating injury.

Wound Management

As an emergency medical technician (EMT), protect yourself with appropriate personal precautions. For closed injuries or minor open injuries, only gloves may be necessary. For spurting wounds or massive bleeding, or when splashing of blood is possible, you may need eyewear, mask, and gown. Routine handwashing should precede and follow every call.

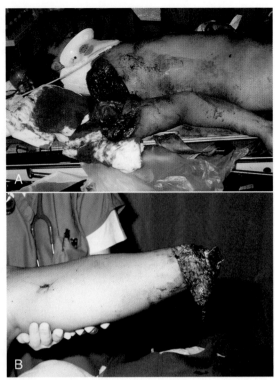

Figure 21-7 A, Near-complete amputation of the arm at the shoulder. **B,** Amputation of the foot after a motor vehicle crash.

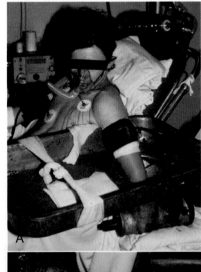

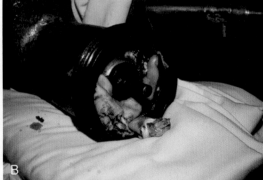

Figure 21-8 Crush injury. A man with his arm caught in a meat grinder is brought to the hospital along with part of the grinder.

You should obtain a history of the mechanism of injury. Life-threatening conditions to the airway, breathing, and circulation (ABCs) take priority. Wounds that involve the airway or result in external hemorrhage should be recognized and treated during the initial assessment. Consideration of the location of the wound may suggest underlying organ damage or internal bleeding. In the case of a projectile injury, look for an exit wound. If there is loss of function, consider damage to bones and muscles as well as to nerves and vessels. Check for neurovascular function distal to the injury, and record your findings.

Procedures used in wound management include the following:
- Control of bleeding
- Prevention of further contamination
- Immobilization of the affected part
- Preservation of avulsed or amputated parts
- Stabilization of all impaled objects (except those lodged in the cheek)

Bleeding Control

To manage a wound, you must first expose the wound and then control any bleeding by direct pressure, elevation, use of pressure points, and, if necessary, application of a tourniquet (see Chapter 20). The extent of blood loss (both internal and external) should be assessed, and you should search for any signs of hypovolemic shock.

Do not underestimate the significance of external blood loss in infants and small children. What would be a minor blood loss for an adult could be lethal for a small child. With a pediatric patient, you should estimate the significance of any external blood loss in consideration of the child's size. For example, infants have a blood volume of 80 to 100 mL/kg of body weight. Therefore an 11-pound (5-kg) baby has a total blood volume of 500 mL, and a small-volume blood loss can be lethal.

With closed wounds, minimal care may be necessary for minor bruises. However, with larger contusions accompanied by swelling or hematomas, counterpressure with a pressure dressing may be used to prevent further bleeding beneath the skin. Application of ice or cold packs may reduce further swelling by vasoconstriction of the underlying vessels. Elevation of the extremity may provide some pain relief and may minimize further swelling by the gravitational effect on blood flow. If a patient complains of pain on movement or has swelling and deformity of the affected part, splinting of the extremity may be appropriate. Patients should minimize their activity and movement.

Open wounds must be covered with a sterile dressing to control bleeding and prevent further contamination. When needed, a bulky dressing may be applied to help focus the direct pressure over the wound. Always think about the underlying organs and the mechanism of injury. As mentioned earlier, a patient is usually at greatest risk from the associated injuries, not those to the soft tissues themselves (see Chapter 20).

Infection

All open wounds are subject to infection. Sterile dressings should be applied when possible. Superficial abrasions that are particularly dirty may be washed gently with sterile saline solution or sterile water before the dressing is applied, if there are no associated critical injuries and if circumstances permit. Likewise, gross contamination and debris on avulsed flaps or amputations may be rinsed before the dressing is applied.

Special Considerations

Some wounds require special treatment. These include chest injuries and abdominal injuries with exposed organs, amputations, impalement injuries, and open neck wounds.

Chest and Abdominal Injuries.
Chest and abdominal wounds may require special attention because of the major organs and organ systems that lie within these two major body cavities. The chest contains the airway and the lungs. The nature of the cavity is unique because it contains the pleural space, which maintains a negative pressure and keeps the lungs in a state of expansion. When this space is penetrated, air can enter the pleural space and collapse the lung. Wounds through the chest wall require special attention, including the application of an airtight, occlusive dressing. An *occlusive* dressing seals off and prevents air from entering the wound.

Abdominal wounds with exposed organs also require special attention because the organs can dry out and can be damaged when exposed to air for an extended period. This type of injury, called an *evisceration,* should be covered with a moist, sterile dressing.

Management of chest and abdominal injuries is discussed in detail in Chapter 22.

LEARNING OBJECTIVES
- Describe the emergency medical care of a patient with an amputation.
- Describe the emergency medical care of a patient with an impaled object.

Amputations and Avulsions.
In certain cases an avulsed portion of skin may be reattached to cover an open wound, or an amputated part may be reattached in the hospital. Retrieval and proper handling in the field of any separated body part increase the chances for successful reattachment. Avulsed flaps of skin must be handled gently to preserve the remaining blood supply to the flap. They may be returned to their normal anatomic position after irrigation of gross debris.

Parts detached from the body remain viable for a few hours when left at room temperature. If the part can be cooled, it can remain viable for up to 18 hours. As with any body tissue, however, amputated or avulsed parts can incur frostbite; to cool without causing cold injury to the part itself, never place the severed tissue directly on ice. Rinse off gross contamination of the detached part with sterile saline solution or sterile water, then cover the part with a sterile dressing and place in a watertight plastic bag. Place the bag in another container with ice or ice and water, label it, and transport it with the patient to the hospital (**Figure 21-9**).

Impalement Injury.
When you encounter an object that has impaled the patient's tissue, you must act to avoid any complication to underlying structures. A knife or other object may be implanted in such a way that it actually stops blood flow from a severed blood vessel and controls bleeding (**Figure 21-10**). Removal of such an object may cause active bleeding. Any impaled object should be stabilized in place with bulky dressings,

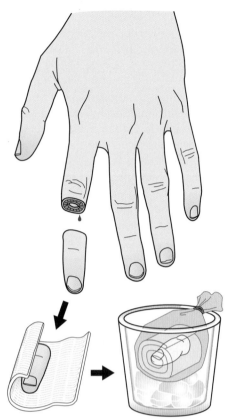

Figure 21-9 Amputated parts should be carefully rinsed with sterile saline or water, wrapped in sterile gauze and placed in a plastic bag, and transported on ice.

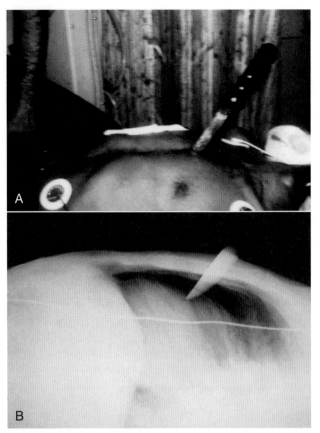

Figure 21-10 **A,** Knife has impaled the anterior chest. In the field, impaled objects are stabilized in place with a bulky dressing. **B,** On the x-ray film, the tip of the knife lies just short of the cardiac shadow.

---

unless it is in the cheek or otherwise obstructing the airway. If the object is too large to be stabilized, or it will not allow patient movement, it may be cut or shortened to facilitate management and transport (e.g., if a patient is impaled on a fence post). Impaled objects should also be removed if they interfere with the performance of cardiopulmonary resuscitation (CPR).

When a patient is impaled on a large structure such as a fence, special rescue techniques may be needed to cut the object and transport it with the patient to the hospital. Consult your local emergency medical services (EMS) system to identify available resources when special rescue techniques may be needed.

Neck Wounds. Neck and upper chest wounds may lead to an **air embolism** when the large veins are torn. Because changes in air pressure within the chest occur during breathing, air may be sucked into the veins and travel through the blood vessels. An air embolism can become trapped within the blood vessels or heart and obstruct blood flow. An air embolism is more likely to develop if the patient is sitting and if the wound is above the level of the heart. Such a wound should be covered with an occlusive, airtight dressing, and the patient should be transported in a supine or head-down position to reduce the chances of an air embolism **(Figure 21-11).**

When the neck is torn or lacerated, bleeding is likely to be severe because the neck is highly vascular. Use direct pressure to control bleeding, but take care to compress the carotid artery only as a last resort. Continuous compression of the carotid artery may obstruct blood flow to the brain.

LEARNING OBJECTIVES
- List the functions of dressing and bandaging.
- Describe the purpose of a bandage.
- Describe the steps in applying a pressure dressing.
- Describe the effects of improperly applied dressings, splints, and tourniquets.

Dressings and Bandages

A **dressing** is any material that covers a wound. It prevents introduction of further contamination into the wound and aids in bleeding control. The dressing should be sterile, but if a sterile dressing is not immediately available, any clean material, or even your gloved hand, should be used for initial control of blood loss.

A **bandage** is material used to secure a dressing in place and provide pressure over the dressing to aid in the continuous control of bleeding.

Dressings

Suitable dressings include any sterile material used to cover a wound. Many types of dressings are available. A basic dressing is sterile gauze or other absorbent material that is applied directly to the wound. The dressing may vary in size and thickness according to the wound. Wounds that cover a large surface area

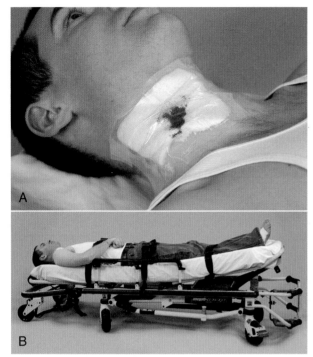

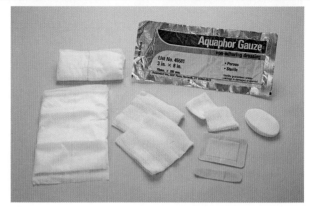

Figure 21-12 Common dressings used in prehospital care.

Figure 21-11 **A,** Airtight dressing to the neck. **B,** Head-down position helps to decrease the risk of air embolism.

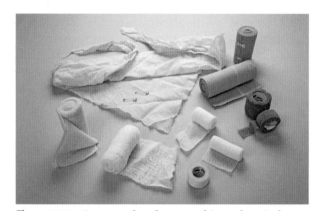

Figure 21-13 Common bandages used in prehospital care.

(e.g., extensive abrasions, burns) may require a *multitrauma* or *universal dressing,* made of thick, absorbent material 9 × 36 inches in size. It is folded on itself and packed within a sterile cover. This dressing can also be used as a pressure dressing over long, open wounds or as padding for splints.

Most punctures or lacerations can be effectively covered with a 4 × 4–inch gauze dressing. If an occlusive or airtight dressing is needed, sterile plastic wrap or sterile aluminum foil may be used. Some dressings, similar to adhesive bandages, come pre-packed with adhesive and are ideal for small and minor wounds (**Figure 21-12**).

Bandages

A bandage holds a dressing in place and allows the EMT to attend to other tasks. A bandage must be tight enough to control bleeding but must not cut off circulation to the limb. The various types include self-sticking or self-adherent, gauze roller, and triangular bandages (**Figure 21-13**).

Self-Adherent Bandages

Self-adherent bandages are supplied as rolls of slightly elastic, gauzelike material that can be wrapped around the dressing on the affected part or extremity. The self-adherent quality makes it easy to work with and allows for rapid application. The elastic quality of this bandage helps in applying pressure to control bleeding.

Elastic (Ace) bandages, which are used to support joints, should not be confused with self-adherent bandages. Elastic bandages are stretchy; if not properly applied, they result in uneven pressure to the limb and may cause possible complications from obstruction of distal blood flow and pressure on local nerves (e.g., they can act as a tourniquet).

Gauze Roller Bandages

The gauze roller bandage is a cotton and relatively nonelastic roller bandage that comes in various widths. It is most often used for extremity and head dressing applications.

Triangular Bandages

Triangular bandages are probably the most versatile of all bandages. Formed by cutting a 36- to 42-inch square of cloth (usually muslin) diagonally, the resulting triangle can be folded as necessary for multiple uses. This versatility allows for rapid application of direct pressure or support to almost any portion of the body. These bandages may be used as slings in the triangular form, or they may be folded and used as cravat-type bandages. A *cravat bandage* is simply a triangular bandage folded to form a band around an injured part. Triangular bandages are also used in the application of tourniquets.

Related Materials

Adhesive Tape. Adhesive tape is used to secure self-adherent or roller bandages, occlusive dressings, or 4 × 4–inch squares of gauze. For small abrasions or less serious wounds, adhesive tape may be used to attach a dressing in place.

Pneumatic Antishock Garment. For wounds to the extremities with associated fractures, or when immobilization is indicated, a pneumatic antishock garment (PASG) may be applied over a dressing and bandage. The PASG is particularly useful when there are multiple extremity wounds in association with shock.

Blood Pressure Cuffs. When added pressure is needed to control hemorrhage, a blood pressure cuff may be used as a bandage. The pressure of the cuff can be inflated until arterial bleeding is controlled.

When using a blood pressure cuff or other tightly applied bandage, pay careful attention to distal blood flow. Evaluate distal blood flow by checking for the presence of a distal pulse and movement and sensation. In some cases the amount of pressure needed to control bleeding in a large artery may require total occlusion of arterial blood flow.

Bandage Application

Dressings may be attached in many ways to various parts of the body: the extremities, head, and trunk.

The roller bandage is the most common type of bandage used in prehospital emergency care. It comes in either self-adherent or gauze material and in various widths for different areas to be bandaged. **Skill 21-1** illustrates the use of a roller bandage as a pressure dressing to control bleeding. **Skill 21-2** illustrates the application of a head bandage.

Bandages for the extremities are probably the simplest to apply. The cylindrical shape of the arm or leg lends itself to easy bandage attachment. A figure-eight bandage secures a dressing over a joint and also allows for mobility (**Skill 21-3**).

If an object is impaled in the patient, it should be stabilized to limit movement (**Skill 21-4**). You should never remove an impaled object unless it is penetrating the cheek or is interfering with CPR. Gently remove objects in the cheek because these may interfere with airway and respiration. If significant bleeding occurs in the cheek after removal, apply a dressing from within the mouth, with finger pressure applied to control bleeding (**Skill 21-5**).

Most dressing applications to the chest and back can be done with tape across the skin's surface. At times the skin surface may be sweaty or wet, and you may have difficulty attaching tape. In these cases a triangular bandage can be used to hold dressings in place over abrasions or superficial wounds. When securing the bandage around the circumference of the chest, be careful not to exert excessive pressure that may restrict chest movement. Penetrating wounds require an occlusive dressing, and wounds with active bleeding require direct pressure.

Facial Injuries

When encountering a patient with injuries to the face and neck, your first concern is the airway. The facial bones give structural support to the airway, and loss of their integrity can compromise airway patency. Bleeding, foreign bodies, broken teeth and dentures, and vomitus can obstruct the air passage. Maintaining a clear airway in the presence of bleeding and foreign bodies is often difficult, and many techniques may need to be used. These techniques include manual extraction of foreign bodies, control of bleeding, suctioning, use of appropriate airway techniques, and positioning of the patient to permit drainage.

> **EXTENDED***Transport*
>
> When transporting a patient with an injury to the face or neck for an extended time, frequent reassessment is crucial. Scene assessment may reveal a patent airway with no signs of respiratory difficulty. During transport, however, injured tissue can swell, resulting in airway compromise. If the patient develops a cough, has difficulty clearing the airway, or has a change in the sound of the voice, the EMT should consider a developing airway obstruction.

The face has a rich blood vessel supply, and injuries can cause extensive bleeding. Because the facial bones are part of the skull and offer protection to the brain, trauma to the face should lead the EMT to search for signs of injury to the brain and cervical spine. The facial bones also offer protection to the eye and the middle and inner ear; the EMT must be able to institute special handling techniques for these sensitive organs.

Bleeding after injuries to the face is of great concern when the blood enters the airway and interferes with ventilation. Remove blood, blood clots, loose teeth, or other foreign bodies from the airway with a finger sweep or suction. If no injury to the cervical spine is suspected, a conscious patient may be allowed to sit and should be encouraged to clear the airway by coughing. Unconscious patients may be placed in the lateral recumbent position with the head down to facilitate drainage. If there is the possibility of cervical spine injury, try to maintain cervical alignment while providing for airway clearance and drainage as the situation dictates. Swelling and hematomas may form within the oral cavity and under the tongue, compromising the airway, and may require advanced airway maneuvers. Partial compromise may evolve to severe compromise as airway swelling progresses.

Bleeding from the face should be controlled with direct pressure. Bleeding within the oral cavity may also be controlled with direct pressure if it is within reach of your fingers. A rolled 4 × 4–inch gauze bandage can be pressed with the finger against oral lacerations, with counterpressure supplied by other fingers on the outside of the cheek. A rolled 4 × 4–inch gauze bandage, similar to that used in a dentist's office, can be placed between the cheek and gums of a conscious patient to control bleeding in that area.

Impaled objects in the cheek should be removed, if possible, because they may interfere with breathing. Gently try to pull the object back through the wound, and control bleeding (see Skill 21-5). Do not use excessive force if resistance is encountered. Rather, control bleeding with the object in place, stabilize the object, and position the patient to allow for drainage if necessary.

Eye Injuries

Anatomy and Physiology

The eye is a delicate organ whose unique structure demands special handling. An appreciation of the structure and function of the eye and the structures that protect and surround it will help you understand the proper steps in care. Proper treatment in the field can preserve eye function after potentially blinding injuries. Conversely, improper handling of an injured eye may result in further damage and loss of vision.

The eye is a globular structure filled with a gel-like fluid called *vitreous humor* (**Figure 21-14**). It rotates within the bony orbit through the action of the orbital muscles.

The outer layer of the eye, called the **sclera,** is composed of a tough, fibrous, and *opaque* (not transparent to light) protective membrane, except for the portion over the iris and pupils. Here the outer layer is called the *cornea.* The cornea is transparent to light so that light rays can enter the opening of the eye, the *pupil.*

Surrounding the pupil is the pigmented or colored portion of the eye, called the *iris.* The iris is a circular muscular structure that controls the amount of light that enters the eye through the pupil. The iris is made of constricting and dilating muscles. Depending on the tone of these two types of muscles, the pupil changes in size. The pupil constricts in response to bright light and dilates in dim light, permitting more light to enter. It also changes in size (to a lesser degree) when focusing on near or far objects, dilating to improve far vision and constricting when focusing on close objects. Because the muscles of the iris are directed by cranial nerves, pupillary size is often used to evaluate brain function and the effects of drugs and other factors on the central nervous system.

As light passes through the pupil, the lens focuses it onto the posterior wall of the eye or the retina. Ciliary muscles are attached to the lens to change its shape so that light can be focused. The retina is composed of millions of sensory receptors that convert light into nerve impulses, which are then transmitted by the optic nerve to the brain for interpretation as a visual image.

Chambers of the Eye. Anatomically, the eye can be divided into anterior and posterior chambers by the lens. The anterior chamber is filled with a circulating watery fluid called the *aqueous humor.* The posterior chamber is filled with the firmer, gel-like vitreous humor. The aqueous and vitreous humors are under slight pressure and give shape and firmness to the eye.

Aqueous Humor. Specialized capillaries continuously form the aqueous humor. This substance circulates within the anterior chamber and is then drained and reabsorbed back into other capillaries. When drainage of the aqueous humor is obstructed, pressure builds up and causes a condition known as *glaucoma.* If the blockage is not corrected, the increased pressure can damage the nerves and result in loss of vision.

Vitreous Humor. The vitreous humor is not formed or drained continuously. This gel-like substance cannot be lost without permanent damage. Loss of the vitreous humor from a penetrating wound to the eye can result in permanent loss of eye shape and function. Therefore, direct pressure must never be applied to an injured eyeball.

Protection. The eye is set deep within orbits, or sockets, formed by many bones (**Figure 21-15**). The outer palpable ridges are composed of parts of the frontal and zygomatic bones and the maxilla. The eye is protected in front by the eyelids. The eyelids can blink quickly to protect the eye from oncoming objects. The eyelashes act as filters to help prevent small particles from entering the eye. The *conjunctiva,* a mucous membrane, lines the interior surface of the eyelids and covers the anterior surface of the eye. It changes its composition as it extends over the sclera and again over the cornea. When the conjunctiva is irritated by a foreign body or inflamed (from an infection or allergy), the capillary vessels become prominent, and *conjunctivitis* ("pinkeye") results (**Figure 21-16**).

The *lacrimal glands,* located at the superior lateral surface of each eyeball, secrete tears. Tears are secreted continuously, moistening and cleaning the eyeball and providing lubrication for smooth passage of the eyelids over the eyeball. Tears are drained through the lacrimal canals located at the medial portion of each eyeball.

A layer of fat behind the eye serves as an additional cushion between the eyeball and the bony orbit. This explains why eyes may appear sunken with malnutrition.

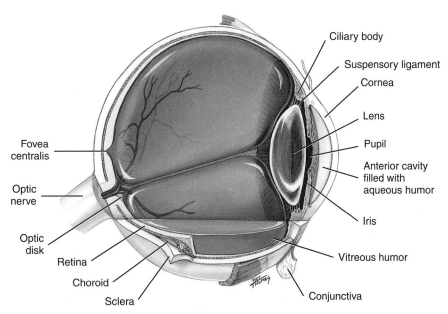

Figure 21-14 Anatomy of the eye. *From Applegate EJ:* The anatomy and physiology learning system, *ed 3, Philadelphia, 2006, Saunders.*

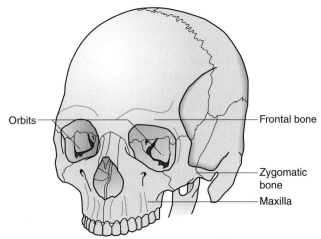

Figure 21-15 Major bones that make up the orbits, or sockets, of the eye.

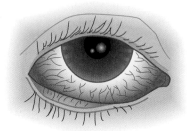

Figure 21-16 Conjunctivitis.

Management of Eye Injuries

The following three principles are important to remember when caring for eye injuries:

1. *Avoid pressure.* Do not apply any pressure onto an eye that may have had a penetrating injury.
2. *Cover both eyes to limit movement.* Cover both eyes to limit movement of one eye.
3. *The patient's cooperation is needed.* Patient cooperation is important, especially during eye irrigation or during treatment for foreign bodies. The eye is extremely sensitive, especially after irritating injuries. Explain your actions to gain the patient's cooperation. Have the patient lie supine.

Foreign Bodies. Foreign bodies are extremely irritating and can cause considerable pain. They may be noticed on the eyeball itself, on the lower eyelid, or under the upper eyelid. The patient may feel a foreign object under the upper lid when blinking. Some foreign bodies may be superficial and easily removed. For example, if dust or dirt falls or is blown into the eye, the tearing mechanism may be adequate to remove it. Other foreign bodies may be deeply embedded, and eye surgery may be necessary. For example, if a person is hammering and a piece of metal ricochets into the eye, it can enter with considerable force and may have to be removed by a physician.

On inspection, the lower lid and most of the eyeball are easily visualized. Have the patient look to either side and up and down

so that you can inspect most of the anterior surface. Objects may become trapped under the upper lid. To inspect this area fully, ask the patient to look downward while you invert the upper lid with a cotton-tipped applicator. Grasp the eyelashes with your thumb and finger (make sure your hands are clean, and preferably use gloves). With the cotton-tipped applicator, place the end of the applicator in the middle of the upper lid (**Figure 21-17**). Using the applicator as a lever, pull the lid forward and upward, causing it to fold back over the applicator, thus exposing the inside surface of the lid. While maintaining the lid, have your partner rinse any foreign body away with irrigating solution (**Skill 21-6**).

Corneal Abrasions. The cornea is particularly sensitive. Scratches on the cornea from brushing against a tree branch or from foreign bodies are painful. The feeling may persist even after the foreign body is removed from the cornea by irrigation. You might notice a small defect on the normally smooth corneal surface. This may be more apparent if you shine a light on the eye from the side. There may be accompanying inflammation of the conjunctiva over the nearby sclera, noticeable as pinkness from the dilating capillaries. Patching an eye with corneal abrasions is recommended and may provide some pain relief.

Impaled Objects. If an object is protruding from the eyeball, *never remove it.* Doing so risks loss of the vitreous humor and permanent damage to the eye. Instead, stabilize the object with a dressing of several 4 × 4–inch gauze squares built up around the object. Cover the dressing with a paper cup or piece of cardboard folded into a cone shape. The cone-shaped dressing

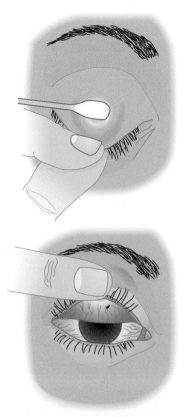

Figure 21-17 Inverting the upper lid to examine for a foreign body.

(1) prevents the object from becoming more deeply embedded in the eye and (2) prevents any pressure from being transmitted to the eyeball itself. Have the patient close the other eye, and tell the patient not to move the eyes. Secure the cone in place with a self-adherent bandage. Cover the other eye, keeping the patient calm. Transport the patient in the supine position.

Lacerations. Lacerations to the eyelids can cause brisk bleeding because of the rich blood supply. Check to see whether there is accompanying damage to the eye itself. Use gentle and direct pressure to control bleeding from the eyelid, but avoid transmitting pressure to the eye itself. Possible associated injury to the eyeball may not be obvious on initial inspection in the field (**Figure 21-18**). Loss of the internal contents of the eye by direct pressure on the eyeball can result in loss of sight. For lacerations to the eye itself, cover the eye with a plastic eye shield or cup to protect it from external pressure.

Extruded Eyeball. If the eyeball is extruding from the socket, do not attempt to replace it (**Figure 21-19**). Rather, place several layers of 4 × 4–inch gauze squares with a hole cut in the center and moistened with sterile saline solution around the extruding eyeball. Attach a cup or cone-shaped cardboard over the dressing with bandages, then cover the opposite eye and transport the patient to the hospital (**Figure 21-20**).

Fracture of the Orbit. Significant blows to the orbit of the eye can result in fractures. There may be tenderness and signs of soft tissue trauma along the orbital ridge. At times, orbital fractures are complicated by impaired eye movement and visual disturbance. The muscles that move the eye occasionally become entrapped in the fracture. The patient may not be able to move both eyes symmetrically in all directions. As a result, the patient may complain of double or impaired vision.

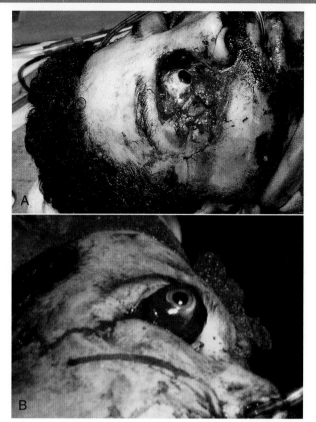

Figure 21-19 **A,** Trauma with an exposed and extruding eyeball. **B,** Trauma with an exposed and extruding eyeball and large hemorrhage below the conjunctiva.

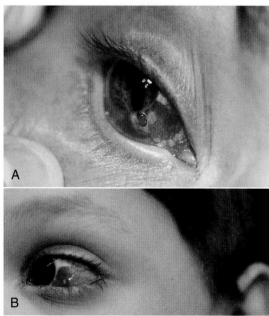

Figure 21-18 **A,** Laceration to the eyeball, with deformity of pupil and contents of eyeball (vitreous humor) extruding. **B,** Laceration to the eyeball with exposure of vitreous humor.

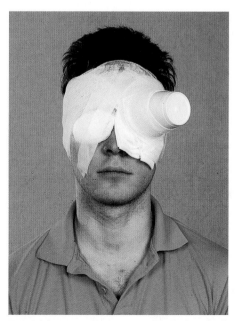

Figure 21-20 Use a cup to protect an extruded eyeball. Preformed plastic eye cups are available, you can improvise with a paper cup or other suitable container as shown in the figure.

Ear Injuries

Anatomy and Physiology

The functions of the ear include hearing, establishing positional sense, and providing balance. Sound waves are transmitted into fluid waves and finally into nerve impulses, which enable the brain to "hear." Movement of the head and changes in body position cause changes in fluid-filled structures of the ear, which are relayed as nerve impulses to different parts of the brain.

Because much of the ear is enclosed within the skull, blood extruding from the ear after trauma is a sign of possible skull fracture. Also, because of the location of the middle and inner ear, infections of the ear are a potential cause of meningitis.

Each ear is composed of three sections called the external, the middle, and the inner ear (**Figure 21-21**).

External Ear. The external ear is composed of the *auricle,* or pinna, which is the outer visible earflap, and the *external auditory canal,* a curving tube leading inward through the temporal bone to the tympanic membrane. The auricle, made up of skin and cartilage, provides protection to the opening and directs sound waves into the auditory canal. The auditory canal is lined with modified sweat glands, which secrete earwax to trap particles and bacteria that may enter the ear.

Middle Ear. The middle ear is an air-filled cavity that transmits sound waves from the external to the inner ear. It begins at the *tympanic membrane,* or "eardrum," and ends at the *oval window* of the inner ear. Communicating across from the eardrum are three tiny bones called, in order, the *malleus* (hammer), the *incus* (anvil), and the *stapes* (or stirrup). These three small bones, known as the **auditory ossicles,** are attached to each other and act as a series of levers to transmit sound waves collected at the eardrum to the inner ear.

The middle ear communicates with the nasopharynx by the *eustachian tube,* which allows the equalization of air pressure between the middle ear and the outside or atmospheric pressure. Because of this communication, infections of the pharynx can travel up the eustachian tube and cause infections of the middle ear.

Inner Ear. The inner ear is encased within the skull. It contains coiled and looped tubes that are filled with fluid and lined with special sensory cells.

Management of Ear Injuries

Blunt trauma can cause contusions and hematoma formation in the auricle. Severe blows can also damage the eardrum, with resulting pain or bleeding from the middle ear, which may be visible in the auditory canal. After significant trauma, blood or clear fluid draining from the ear should always be considered a possible sign of skull fracture. In such cases, apply a loose, sterile dressing.

Because the auricle projects outward, it is susceptible to laceration, avulsion, and complete amputation (**Figure 21-22**). If possible, remove gross contamination and apply a sterile dressing; then apply a bulky dressing around the auricle before bandaging. Treat incompletely avulsed parts of the auricle by approximating their anatomic position and then holding them in place with a bulky dressing until a bandage can be applied. Treat completely avulsed or amputated parts as you would any other, by removing gross contamination, wrapping the amputated part in gauze moistened with sterile saline solution,

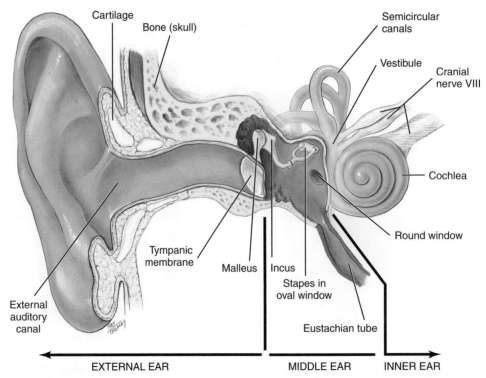

Figure 21-21 Anatomy of the ear. *From Jarvis C: Physical examination and health assessment, ed 5, Philadelphia, 2008, Saunders-Elsevier.*

and then placing the part in a plastic bag. Keep the part cool by placing it over ice or in water with ice added.

Foreign Bodies. Foreign bodies that are lodged in the ear canal should be removed in the emergency department unless you are otherwise directed by local protocol. The eardrum is extremely sensitive, and objects that have penetrated the eardrum may cause pain and bleeding. Be careful not to obstruct blood flow from the ear canal.

Barotrauma (Pressure-Related Injuries). During exposure to changing environmental pressures, as in flying or underwater diving, the middle ear maintains equal pressure on each side of the tympanic membrane by air movement through the eustachian tubes (**Figure 21-23**).

If pressures change before equalization can occur, unequal pressures on the tympanic membrane may cause distortion and rupture (**Figure 21-24**). This condition, called *barotrauma*, can occur when divers or airplane passengers change depth or altitude too quickly, without time for equalization to occur.

Patients with barotrauma of the ear are likely to have pain or hearing loss. Upper respiratory tract infections may predispose patients to barotrauma during airplane trips because of clogging of the eustachian tubes, which prevents equalization. For the same reason, divers should not dive when they have a cold.

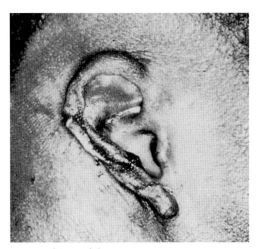

Figure 21-22 Avulsion of the ear. *From Zuidema GS, Rutherford RB, Ballinger WF: The management of trauma, ed 4, Philadelphia, 1985, Saunders.*

> **LEARNING OBJECTIVES**
> - List the categories of burn injuries.
> - Define superficial burn.
> - List the characteristics of a superficial burn.
> - Define partial-thickness burn.
> - List the characteristics of a partial-thickness burn.
> - Define full-thickness burn.
> - List the characteristics of a full-thickness burn.

Burns

Burns can be caused by thermal (heat), chemical, or electrical injury. The organ most often injured by burns is the skin, which accounts for about 15% of body weight in the adult. As previously stated, the skin serves as a protective barrier against

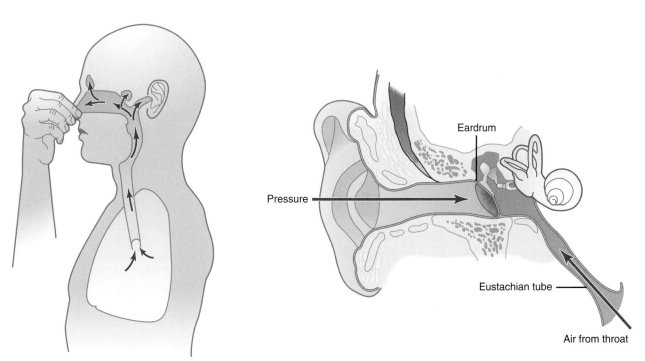

Figure 21-23 Unequal pressure on both sides of the eardrum may cause distortion or injury. This is felt when descending from high altitudes, especially when the person has a cold. In this circumstance, the person attempts to exhale while closing the nose and mouth, increasing the pressure in the internal air spaces, such as the eustachian tubes. *Modified from Neuman TS: Unusual forms of trauma. In Baxt WB, editor: Trauma: the first hour, Norwalk, Conn, 1985, Appleton-Century-Crofts.*

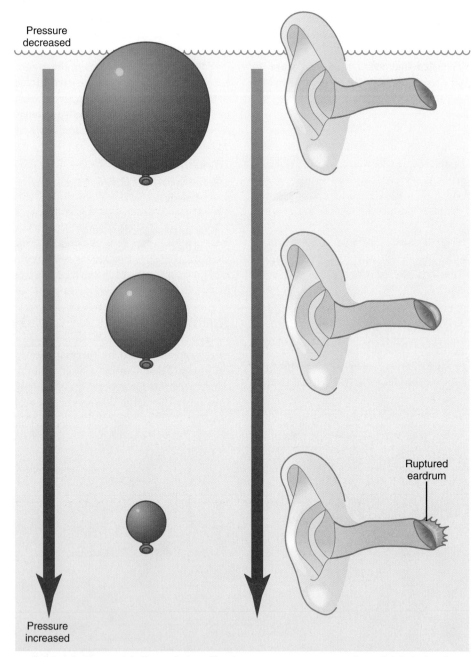

Figure 21-24 Barotrauma to the eardrum. A balloon descending in water serves as a good model for what happens in the ear of a diver submerging. As a balloon descends, the effective atmospheric pressure increases relative to the depth of the water. Air that fills a balloon at the surface is compressed as it descends as a result of the increased pressure from the water on all sides. The tympanic membrane is also subject to these pressures. Pressure on the inside of the tympanic membrane normally increases to match the atmospheric pressure. If a diver cannot equalize pressure on both sides of the tympanic membrane because of blockage of the eustachian tube, rupture of the eardrum can result. *Modified from Neuman TS: Unusual forms of trauma. In Baxt WB, editor:* Trauma: the first hour, *Norwalk, Conn, 1985, Appleton-Century-Crofts.*

infection, as a barrier to water loss, as a major thermoregulatory organ, and as a sensory organ for touch, pain, temperature, and pressure perception.

The different layers of the skin contribute to these functions. The outer epidermis is relatively impermeable to water and bacteria. The dermis contains the blood vessels, nerves, and other structures (e.g., hair follicles, sweat glands, sebaceous glands), which extend by ducts to the epidermis. Underneath the dermis is a layer of subcutaneous tissue that protects and insulates.

Burns result in a loss of temperature control, loss of body fluids and water, and susceptibility to infection.

Thermal Burns

Thermal burns affect about 2 million individuals annually, and 3% to 5% of these burns are life threatening. Most thermal burns occur in the home as a result of flames or scalding water. For children younger than 3 years, hot liquids are the most common source of burns. Small children can sustain burns when they reach for pots on a stove, spill hot liquids such as coffee or tea, or place their hands under hot-water taps. From ages 3 to 14 years, burning clothing is the most common source of burns. Over age 60 years, complicating factors such as momentary blackouts or general debilitation may contribute to household incidents or may impede the ability to escape.

The smoke produced by burning materials can contain a number of toxins, the most common being carbon monoxide (CO), a colorless, tasteless, odorless gas that impairs oxygen transport and contributes to more than half of all deaths from fires. In fact, many deaths from fires are the result of smoke inhalation alone, without thermal burns. Because the inhalation of smoke has rapid and lethal effects, all victims must be promptly removed from the toxic environment, and high-concentration oxygen must be given to facilitate CO removal.

Assessment of Burn Injuries

Burn injuries can be classified by widely accepted criteria used to assess their severity. These criteria include the depth, extent, and location of the burn, as well as complicating factors such as age, respiratory involvement, and associated medical or traumatic conditions.

Depth of Burns. The classification of burn depth is based on skin anatomy and referred to in terms of degree (**Figure 21-25**).

Superficial (First-Degree) Burns. **Superficial burns** involve the epidermis only and spare the deeper layers. Sunburn is a common example of a first-degree burn. These burns can also result from minor flash injury or occur at the periphery of more severe burns. The skin appears reddened (erythema) and is dry and warm to the touch. First-degree burns are generally painful because the nerves in the deeper layers are left intact. The pain may not occur for several hours, as with sunburn. There may be slight edema resulting from congestion and dilation of the intradermal vessels.

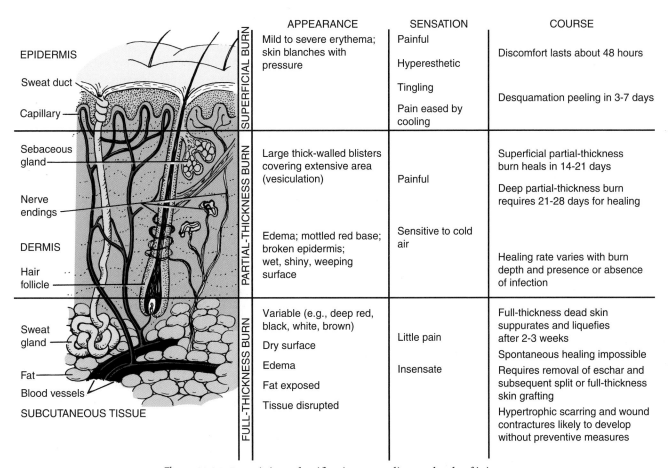

		APPEARANCE	SENSATION	COURSE
EPIDERMIS / Sweat duct / Capillary	SUPERFICIAL BURN	Mild to severe erythema; skin blanches with pressure	Painful / Hyperesthetic / Tingling / Pain eased by cooling	Discomfort lasts about 48 hours / Desquamation peeling in 3-7 days
Sebaceous gland / Nerve endings / DERMIS / Hair follicle	PARTIAL-THICKNESS BURN	Large thick-walled blisters covering extensive area (vesiculation) / Edema; mottled red base; broken epidermis; wet, shiny, weeping surface	Painful / Sensitive to cold air	Superficial partial-thickness burn heals in 14-21 days / Deep partial-thickness burn requires 21-28 days for healing / Healing rate varies with burn depth and presence or absence of infection
Sweat gland / Fat / Blood vessels / SUBCUTANEOUS TISSUE	FULL-THICKNESS BURN	Variable (e.g., deep red, black, white, brown) / Dry surface / Edema / Fat exposed / Tissue disrupted	Little pain / Insensate	Full-thickness dead skin suppurates and liquefies after 2-3 weeks / Spontaneous healing impossible / Requires removal of eschar and subsequent split or full-thickness skin grafting / Hypertrophic scarring and wound contractures likely to develop without preventive measures

Figure 21-25 Burn injury classification according to depth of injury.

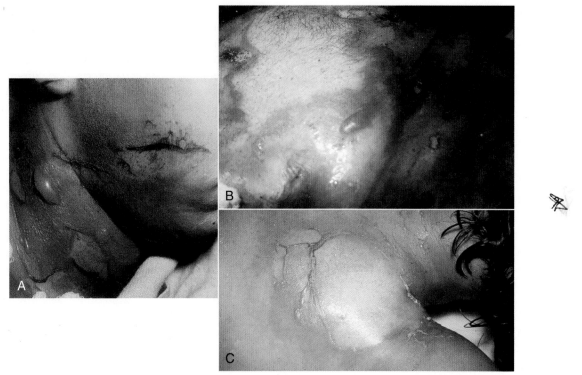

Figure 21-26 A, Partial-thickness burns from brief exposure to flame. **B,** Deep partial-thickness burn with blistering surrounded by a full-thickness burn. **C,** Partial-thickness burn on the shoulder resulting from a scald injury.

Superficial burns heal spontaneously after small scales of the epidermis peel off. Because there is no loss of skin function, first-degree burns are not included in estimating the extent of burn injury, even though some individuals with extensive sunburn feel ill and may have a slightly elevated body temperature.

Partial-Thickness (Second-Degree) Burns. **Partial-thickness burns** involve the epidermis and extend into, but not through, the entire dermis. They are typically caused by flash injuries or hot-liquid scalds.

Partial-thickness burns can have different appearances depending on the extent of dermal injury. A common characteristic is edema and blister formation caused by tissue damage and accumulation of plasma from injured capillaries **(Figure 21-26).** The blisters and wound surface may be moist or weeping. Blisters should generally be left intact because they provide a barrier to infection. The edema may restrict blood flow, particularly if it completely circles an extremity.

The color may vary, depending on the depth of the burn. The burn may appear pink or red and blotchy; deeper burns may be darker or pale and colorless.

Partial-thickness burns vary in their sensitivity, depending on the depth. More superficial partial-thickness burns can be extremely painful and sensitive to touch and air movements. Deeper partial-thickness burns may have normal or decreased sensation to touch. Very deep partial-thickness burns may have no sensation, and it is difficult to distinguish these from full-thickness (third-degree) burns.

Skin functions are lost with partial-thickness burns, leading to fluid loss, body heat loss, and susceptibility to infection.

However, partial-thickness burns can heal spontaneously because some skin tissue and structures, such as hair follicles or sweat glands, which can regenerate skin, are spared.

Full-Thickness (Third-Degree) Burns. **Full-thickness burns** involve the entire thickness of the epidermis and dermis. They can be caused by extreme heat, prolonged exposure to flames, or immersion scalds. The skin can appear charred, yellow-brown, dark red, or white and translucent **(Figure 21-27).**

In contrast to superficial and partial-thickness burns, there is no pain or sensation because the nerves in the deeper layers of the dermis are destroyed.

The texture of the skin in full-thickness burns is leathery. Having lost its normal resilience, such skin can restrict movement and the expansion of underlying structures. This is particularly true if the burn extends over a large surface or circles a limb or the torso. For example, full-thickness burns of a large portion of the chest wall can limit lung expansion. Circumferential burns of the extremities can constrict blood flow. The constriction can progress over time, and in the hospital setting, incisions are sometimes made through the leathery skin to allow chest wall expansion or distal blood flow to an extremity.

Full-thickness burns heal only from the margins of the wound because there are no cells left in the destroyed dermis capable of generating new skin tissue. Therefore these burns require skin grafting, which involves transplantation of skin from an unaffected body area to the burn site.

Other Burns. Burns can involve tissues beneath the skin as well, including subcutaneous tissue, muscle, and even bone; this is sometimes called a "fourth-degree burn." Electrical burns

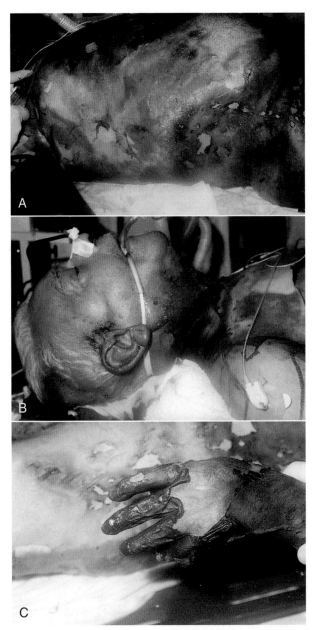

Figure 21-27 **A,** Full-thickness burns covering most of the torso. Red and charred areas have a leathery feel. **B,** Full-thickness burns around the neck. Circumferential burns can impair circulation and breathing. **C,** Full-thickness burns to the hand. Note charring of the fingers with sloughing of the nails and skin.

can cause damage to deeper underlying structures as the current travels through the body.

It is important to note that many burns are a combination of superficial, partial-thickness, and full-thickness burns.

Extent of Burns. The amount of skin burned plays a large role in the severity of a burn injury. Calculations of the extent are made according to the "rule of nines" (**Figure 21-28**). For adults, the body is divided into surface areas of 9% and 18% to help estimate the extent of a burn. The head and neck and each arm are each considered 9% of the body surface area (BSA). The front of the torso, back of the torso, right leg, and left leg are each considered 18% of BSA. The genitalia

are considered 1% of BSA. The palm represents about 1% as well and might be used to estimate and describe smaller areas of burn.

An adjustment is made in the calculations for infants, who have a greater surface area on the head in comparison with the rest of the body. The head in children accounts for 18% of BSA and each lower limb, 13.5%. The trunk and arms remain the same (18% and 9%).

Always describe the depth and extent of areas burned in reports and communications, such as "partial- and full-thickness burns to the entire right arm (9%) and anterior trunk (18%)." For reports you may want to distinguish partial-thickness and full-thickness areas on a patient diagram by using different marking techniques. The exact determination of degree and extent of burn are not as important as recognizing a critically burned patient and transporting quickly to the nearest, most appropriate hospital (burn center if available). Do not delay transport to calculate burn severity.

> ### Case in Point
>
> Two patients have sustained burns over their head and neck. One is 36 years old, and the other is 1 year old. Which of these patients has a burn involving 18% of their body surface?

Location of Burns. Body areas where burns are more critical because of the tendency to result in infection, loss of function, or respiratory involvement include the face, perineum and genitalia, and feet and hands.

Burns to the perineum and genital area are prone to infection as a result of contamination from fecal bacteria. Significant burns to the hands and feet require special handling to avoid permanent damage. Facial burns are more severe because they can involve special structures and may be accompanied by respiratory tract involvement. If burns are circumferential, they are considered severe because the loss of elasticity or edema around an entire extremity or body cavity can compromise blood flow or breathing. Circumferential burns can involve the extremities, neck, or torso.

Complicating Factors. Certain historical or physical factors (e.g., age) make recovery from a burn more difficult or even increase the likelihood of death. Other factors include the presence of inhalation injuries, associated injuries or medical conditions, and certain preexisting conditions.

Age. The severity of a given burn is increased if the patient is at an extreme of life. Adults older than 55 years and children younger than 5 years are generally considered at increased risk.

Inhalation Injuries. Inhalation injury is the most common cause of death in fires. Inhaled steam or extremely hot air, smoke particles, and toxic gases can cause direct damage to the respiratory tract. This can result in airway compromise or damage to the lungs themselves. Steam carries more heat than air and can overwhelm the ability of the upper respiratory tract to cool air to body temperature before it reaches the alveoli. Particles of smoke carry heat as well as toxic chemicals deep into the respiratory tract.

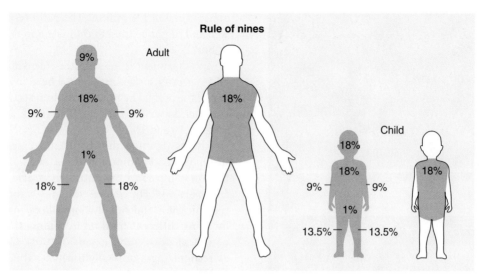

Figure 21-28 The "rule of nines" is a fairly accurate and simple approach for estimating the extent of a burn. _From NAEMT: Prehospital trauma life support, ed 6, St Louis, 2007, Mosby-Elsevier._

Smoke is hot air containing noxious gases as well as small particles of various sizes to which toxic chemicals are attached. The type of gases given off during fires depends on the substance burned and varies with the heat of the fire. Specific toxic gases are covered in Chapter 15.

Death from smoke inhalation results from lack of oxygen. Smoke interferes with oxygen delivery and use in the following four ways:

1. Fires consume oxygen, lowering the percentage of oxygen in the air. This is a particular problem if the fire is in a closed space.
2. Carbon monoxide, the most common toxic gas, is a by-product of combustion. CO binds with hemoglobin and interferes with oxygen transport to the tissues. Small concentrations of this odorless, colorless, tasteless gas in the air breathed can result in lethal levels in the blood because CO has a 200 times greater affinity for hemoglobin than does oxygen. All victims of smoke inhalation should be considered to have inhaled CO and should be treated with oxygen.
3. Smoke may impair the tissues' ability to use oxygen. For example, cyanide gas is produced in some fires. Cyanide poisons the tissues and interferes with oxygen metabolism at the tissue level. Sources of cyanide include burning polyurethane, polyacrylonitrile, wool, and silk.
4. Heat and irritant gases in smoke can lead to swelling of the airway, bronchospasm, and damage to the delicate alveoli. Irritant gases, such as hydrochloric acid, chlorine, and phosgene, produce an inflammatory reaction and can damage capillaries and cause edema in the airways or alveoli. These irritant gases can form from burning plastics or industrial fires.

Physical signs that should raise suspicion of inhalation injury include the following (**Figure 21-29**):

- Singed nasal hairs
- Sputum with black particles (_carbonaceous_ sputum)
- Burns around the mouth and nose
- Hoarseness of the voice
- Respiratory distress

**Associated Conditions.** Associated traumatic injuries may take precedence over the burn injury as the greatest immediate threat to life and may complicate the treatment of the burns. Preexisting medical conditions that may hamper recovery may also raise the severity of a burn injury. Such conditions include lung and heart disease, diabetes, or other severe injury or illness.

Burn Severity. Burns are classified by severity for patient triage and transport decisions. Local protocols often use burn severity as the criterion for determining which facility (e.g., burn center) should be selected. This decision is often made in the field. Nationally accepted criteria may be adjusted to reflect local resources. **Box 21-1** summarizes the criteria for a critically burned patient who should go to a burn center for specialized care.

The depth and extent of burns are the major determinants in classifying the severity of a burn. Only partial-thickness and full-thickness burns are counted in assessing extent of the burn, because superficial burns do not result in loss of skin function. Other factors, as discussed, are also used in determining whether a patient should be considered as having sustained a minor, moderate, or major burn injury.

EXTENDED_Transport_

Burns are a dynamic injury. The tissues changes associated with a burn continue several hours after the initial injury. During extended transport, the burn patient may develop airway obstruction secondary to swelling the facial and neck structures. Pulmonary edema may develop, and if bandages or splints have been placed, frequent evaluation of distal pulses and sensation is important to ensure that tissue swelling has not made the bandages or splints too tight, compromising circulation. If distal circulation has been occluded, the device should be loosened to allow for return of circulation.

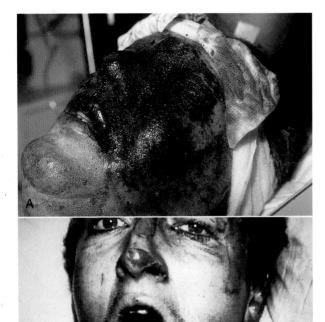

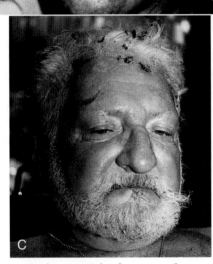

Figure 21-29 **A,** Carbon particles from a gas-burner explosion account for a blackened appearance. **B,** Burns on the face and carbonaceous sputum. **C,** Signs of inhalation injury include burns around the mouth and nose and singed nasal hairs.

Box 21-1	Critical Burns Requiring Transport to a Burn Center

Full-thickness burns in any age group
Partial-thickness burns in greater than 10% of the body's total surface area
Any burn associated with inhalation injury
Any burn that involves the face, hands, feet, genitalia, perineum, or major joints
Electrical burns (including lightning)
Chemical burns
Any burn complicated by another trauma (such as a fracture)

LEARNING OBJECTIVES
• Describe the emergency medical care of the patient with a superficial burn.
• Describe the emergency medical care of the patient with a partial-thickness burn.
• Describe the emergency medical care of the patient with a full-thickness burn.

Management of Burns

The management of burns includes the following steps:
1. Stop the burning process.
2. Remove the patient from the smoky environment.
3. Provide high-concentration supplemental oxygen to reverse the effects of carbon monoxide.
4. Treat the patient for shock.
5. Prevent infection.
6. Transport the patient to the appropriate facility.

The major emphasis must be given to assessing and treating life-threatening complications, such as smoke inhalation, airway obstruction, and associated injuries or complicating medical conditions. Once the burning process has been stopped, the prehospital treatment of burns concentrates on preventing infection, maintaining body temperature, and minimizing pain.

Stop the Burning. Remove the patient from the burning or smoky environment and extinguish the flames with blankets or water. The patient whose clothing is burning should be covered with a blanket, placed on the ground, and rolled slowly to extinguish the flames. Running in panic allows flames to spread and rise upward toward the face. Remove smoldering clothing and jewelry if it is not adhered to the skin. Pour cool, sterile water over smoldering articles of clothing that are adhered to the skin to stop the burning process. Cool, sterile water, applied with a face cloth, may help limit the severity of certain burns, such as scalds.

Use caution in applying cool, wet compresses to extensive areas of burned skin because of the chance of inducing hypothermia. Generally, once smoldering has been stopped, do not leave cool, wet compresses on more than 20% of BSA. Cool, wet compresses should be left on for only a few minutes, until the burned skin returns to normal body temperature.

Treat Life-Threatening Conditions First. Patients should be assessed carefully for the presence of airway compromise and respiratory distress. Look for the following signs:
• Stridor
• Hoarseness
• Use of accessory muscles
• Cyanosis
• Other signs of respiratory distress
• Signs of inhalation injury

If there is evidence of inhalation injury, shock, or extensive burns, administer high-concentration supplemental oxygen to the patient. You should assume that patients with inhalation injury have inhaled CO, for which high-concentration oxygen is the main treatment.

Assess the patient for associated trauma and shock caused by other injuries. Shock can result from hypovolemia caused by blood loss from other injuries, fluid loss from the burns, and sometimes from vasodilation caused by pain. The shock from burns is typically not severe within the first hour, and fluid replacement for burn fluid loss can be done in the hospital setting.

Obtain a history that includes the circumstances surrounding the burn and the source and duration of the thermal injury or smoke inhalation. For example, was the patient in a closed space or unconscious? Inquire about preexisting medical conditions that may complicate therapy.

Cover the Wound. The burn wound should be covered with sterile or clean dressings or sheets. Remove rings or bracelets that may become constricting. Jewelry retains heat, and fingers and extremities may swell later. Never apply ointments or any other substance on the burn because the ointment will have to be removed in the hospital to allow for proper assessment, cleansing, and more definitive care. Leave blisters intact. Covering the wound often gives the patient some pain relief.

In cool environments, use blankets to insulate and maintain body temperature because burn patients are susceptible to hypothermia. Transport the patient according to local protocols.

LEARNING OBJECTIVES
- Describe emergency care for the patient with a chemical burn.
- Describe emergency care for the patient with an electrical burn.

Chemical Burns

Chemicals cause burns similar to thermal burns. The type and concentration of the product and the duration of exposure are important variables in determining the severity. The key difference between chemical and thermal burns is that chemicals continue to burn until they are removed. Therefore the general principle to follow in managing chemical burns is to initiate *immediate and thorough irrigation* of the affected areas. Large amounts of water (gallons) should be used, and irrigation should continue for 20 to 30 minutes.

You should take care to position the patient and yourself to avoid runoff and splashes because these contaminate unaffected areas as well as the rescuer. Take the necessary safety precautions to protect yourself from exposure to hazardous materials. Wear gloves, eye protection, gown, and mask if splashes are likely. Garden hoses or showers are ideal for irrigation because they provide a continuous stream that dilutes and washes away the caustic elements. The pressure from a hose should be adjusted to avoid high-pressure streams and resultant traumatic injury to injured tissues. The EMT may be prone to "run to the hospital" for treatment of a chemical burn. In the absence of life-threatening conditions, however, it is best to provide vigorous irrigation on the scene, where there is a good source of water, rather than in the ambulance. This is particularly true when faced with long transport times. Failure to irrigate the affected area on the scene can result in continuation of the burning process during transport and further damage to the soft tissues.

Acids and *alkalis* are the most common chemicals that produce burns. Alkalis tend to take longer to remove. In general, you should irrigate as soon as possible after exposure; there is a difference in severity with a delay as short as 2 minutes.

If powders or dried chemicals are involved, these should be brushed off and contaminated clothing and shoes removed before irrigation. Dried chemicals may collect in pant cuffs and shoes. *Lime* is a good example of such a chemical. Lime *(calcium oxide)* is converted to a very caustic chemical, *calcium hydroxide,* with the addition of water. Large amounts of water, sufficient to provide a continuous and thorough irrigation, must be available because small amounts can activate the chemical but not remove it.

Yellow phosphorus or *white phosphorus* is a chemical used in munitions and industries that make insecticides, poisons, and fertilizers. Because phosphorus combusts spontaneously when exposed to air, affected parts should be kept submerged in water or covered with soaked dressings.

Sodium and *potassium* metals also ignite spontaneously in air, but react with water to form more caustic products. Therefore, smoldering fragments of sodium or potassium that are embedded in the skin should be extinguished with a fire extinguisher, smothered with sand, or covered with petroleum jelly.

Hydrofluoric acid is used in industry and is present in grout cleaners. It is caustic to the skin and also readily penetrates into the dermis, where it dissociates and continues to cause injury until it is deactivated. As with other acid burns, water is used for irrigation. However, deactivation of hydrofluoric acid that has penetrated the skin may require the application of dressings soaked in calcium chloride, calcium gluconate, or magnesium oxide paste. In the hospital, calcium salts can be injected into the skin to accomplish this purpose.

Water irrigation usually remains the treatment of choice and should be used immediately unless dealing with metallic sodium or potassium.

Once irrigation techniques are initiated, call the regional poison control center for further instructions when appropriate. Caustic substances in the eye require continuous irrigation, with the eye held open by force if necessary, for at least 20 minutes or until the procedure is discontinued by hospital staff.

Burns to the Eyes

Chemical damage depends on the nature of the chemical and the duration of contact with the eye. Alkaline and acid materials are particularly harmful. Other toxic chemicals can have variable effects. For example, the methylisocyanate gas leak in Bhopal, India, that killed thousands of people also caused blindness in many of the survivors. Because it is often difficult to predict what effects a particular chemical may have, the rule is to flush the eye immediately with clean water or other irrigating solution (e.g., sterile saline). Irrigate in the same manner as you would to remove a foreign body—that is, from the middle of the eye out toward the side. Hold the eyelids open with your fingers. Continue irrigating for at least 20 minutes, and longer if the chemical agent is alkaline.

If an irrigating solution is not readily available, use tap water and irrigate with any of several methods, such as having the patient's eyes held open under a gently flowing faucet, pouring

Case in Point

You are called to the site of an industrial accident. A worker has been splashed in her right eye with a sodium hydroxide solution. She has initiated irrigation at the scene, but the nearest hospital with an ophthalmologist is 30 minutes away. The nurse at the worksite has placed anesthetic drops in the patient's eye to allow her to tolerate irrigation better. You are given 4 liters of sterile saline to take during your transport to the hospital so you can continue continuous irrigation en route. You buckle yourself in the captain's chair and assemble the irrigating materials so you can continue this emergency decontamination safely as you transport the patient.

water from a glass or other container onto the eyes, or placing the patient's face in a large pan of water and having the patient blink. The patient's face can be placed in a pan of sterile or clean water for short periods, with the patient taking a breath before resubmerging. The water should be changed every few minutes. Remember, the longer the chemical is in contact with the eye, the greater the risk of injury.

Exposure to too much infrared light from the sun or to ultraviolet light from arc welding without protective goggles can result in painful burns to the cornea. The pain usually occurs a few hours after exposure. Cover the eyes with moist patches, and transport the patient to the hospital.

Burns to the eyelids may occur after exposure to fire and intense heat. Cover the eyelids with a moist, sterile dressing, and transport the patient to the hospital.

Electrical Burns

In the United States, about 1000 people die each year from electrical injuries. At high risk are industrial workers and children. Electrical incidents result from downed power lines, malfunctioning home appliances, children chewing through electrical cords, and contact with high-tension power lines.

When electricity traverses the body, it is converted to heat that burns the tissues in its path. High-voltage arcs generate intense amounts of heat and can burn a person nearby. Death can result from the passage of current through vital organs, which causes respiratory or cardiac arrest.

Emergency medical technicians must take precautions to protect themselves and the patient from further injury. Knowing basic properties of electricity can help guide you to take correct actions.

Electricity Basics

Electricity is the movement of electrons from a point of higher concentration to a point of lower concentration. Electricity is often described in terms of the following three variables:

- *Amperage* is the number or volume of electrons flowing.
- *Voltage* is the force with which movement occurs.
- *Resistance* is the degree of hindrance to electron flow

These three concepts are interrelated by the following formula:

$$A\,(\text{amperage}) = \frac{V\,(\text{voltage})}{R\,(\text{resistance})}$$

Current can be direct or unidirectional in flow, or it can alternate or switch the direction of electron flow at a given number of cycles per second (hertz, Hz). Flow from a battery is an example of direct current (DC); household electrical flow is usually a form of alternating current (AC).

Generally, exposure to low voltage is less serious than exposure to high voltage. However, fatalities have occurred with voltage as low as 45 to 60 Hz. Household current is capable of causing a sustained muscular contraction, preventing release of the electrified object by the patient. Amperage, which is not usually known, also does more damage as the number of milliamperes increases. Symptoms can range from tingling to sustained muscular contraction to fatal organ damage. If current passes through the brain, it may cause respiratory arrest. If it passes through the heart, it may cause cardiac arrest.

Resistance is defined as a measure of the hindrance to electron flow through a given material. Materials vary tremendously in their resistance. For example, copper wires offer relatively low resistance and conduct electricity readily; they serve as *good conductors*. Rubber has a very high resistance to electrical flow; it serves as an *insulator*. Good conductors offer low resistance. Poor conductors offer high resistance. Lightning rods, for example, are made of metal, which is a good conductor, and are used to direct electricity from the roof of a house along insulated wires to the ground. Because electricity seeks to flow along the path of least resistance from a higher to a lower potential, lightning rods prevent electricity from traveling through a highly resistant wooden roof, which would generate heat and fire. Instead, the electricity is directed to the earth, which can absorb the current.

Vehicles are insulated from the ground by their rubber tires. Thus a downed power line in contact with a vehicle may leave the occupants unharmed as long as they avoid direct contact with the ground. However, if they step out of the vehicle while holding onto the door, they will be part of the *circuit* consisting of the wire, the vehicle, their bodies, and the ground, and they will sustain electrical injury.

Electrical Effects on the Body

When electrical current passes through the body as part of its circuit (usually to the ground), it follows an internal path of least resistance. Skin and bone offer high resistance to electrical current, muscle offers less, and the vessels and nerves offer the least resistance to electrical flow **(Figure 21-30)**. Therefore, current passing from arm to arm tends to pass along the vessels and nerves in the arms and thorax. Even high current can enter and exit at relatively small surface areas; you therefore cannot gauge the extent of internal injury from the external appearance.

Wet skin, offering less resistance, is more easily penetrated by electricity than dry skin. Even household current that penetrates wet skin can cause cardiac arrest.

Burns to the soft tissues, because of the heat generated from electrical current, can extend from superficial to full-thickness burns. Full-thickness burns can vary from those that look gray-white to those that appear charred. Thermal burns can also be caused by the intense heat generated by

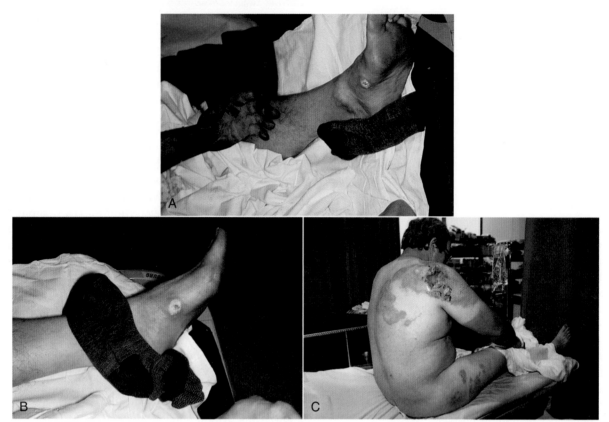

Figure 21-30 A, Electrical burns. High-voltage entrance wound in the hand, with exit wound in the foot. **B,** Close-up view of exit wound in the foot in *A.* The current burned a hole in the patient's sock. **C,** This patient's shoulder was touched by a high-voltage wire. The entrance wound was in the shoulder, with exit in the hip.

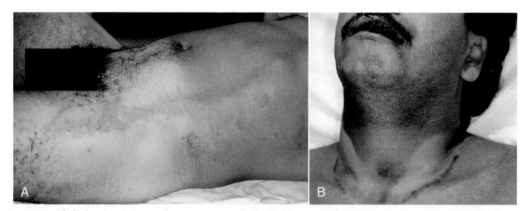

Figure 21-31 A, Patient with lightning injury where current splashed skin. **B,** Lightning burst a metal necklace chain off the patient, leaving a burn mark. The patient went into cardiac arrest and was resuscitated by bystanders administering CPR.

electrical arcs that are nearby but not in direct contact with the body. In general, the longer the duration of contact, the greater is the severity of the burn. Electrical burns tend to be more extensive than they appear, as judged from their external marks.

The most immediate life-threatening effects of electrical injuries are respiratory and cardiac arrest. Early resuscitation can improve patient outcome. For example, respiratory arrest after a lightning injury can be prolonged, but patients who have received early respiratory support have recovered. Associated falls

may cause fractures and other injuries. Lightning injuries also burn the skin and soft tissue (**Figure 21-31**).

Assessment and Management

The first priority is to assess whether hazards continue to exist. Are there fallen wires? Any downed wire should be considered as charged until the appropriate authorities, such as power company personnel, confirm that the power is off. Rescuers should not attempt to secure power lines with a stick or rope or other nonconductive material because the risk of injury to the rescuer is high.

When encountering patients trapped in a vehicle in contact with a downed wire, have them remain in the vehicle. Do not touch the vehicle or patient yourself, because this will place you in a circuit from the vehicle to the ground. After ensuring rescuer safety, assess and manage any life-threatening conditions with appropriate concern for the cervical spine if falls or violent contractions have occurred. Look closely for any fractures, and splint appropriately. When assessing the skin, look for both entrance and exit wounds. Cover the wounds with sterile dressings, and transport the patient to the hospital.

Scenario Follow-up

At the Trauma Center it was determined the knife did not hit the heart, but it did hit a lung resulting in a pneumothorax. The Trauma surgeon complimented you and your partner on how well you immobilized the knife. Showing you the x-ray she pointed out that any movement would have lacerated the heart. The patient was taken to surgery and was expected to make a full recovery.

Summary

The management principles for soft tissue injuries are to ensure a patent airway, control bleeding, prevent infection, immobilize the affected part, and preserve avulsed or amputated parts. When wounds to the face threaten the patency of the airway, be prepared to control bleeding, suction, and, if necessary, remove embedded objects that obstruct the airway. Use direct pressure, elevate the affected part, and occasionally use pressure points to control bleeding. A tourniquet is rarely needed, but once applied, it should remain in place until the patient reaches the hospital. Cold packs can be used to reduce internal bleeding or swelling. Treat open wounds with the application of a sterile dressing to prevent infection.

Skills

Skill | 21-1   *Applying a Pressure Dressing with a Roller Bandage*

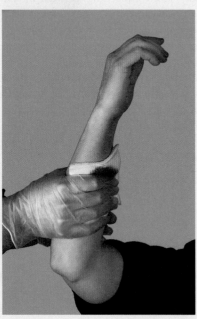

1. Cover the wound with the appropriate sterile dressing while applying firm pressure with your hand until the bleeding stops.

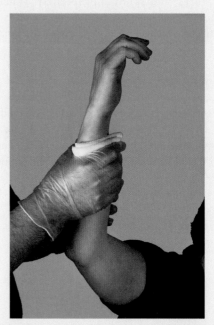

2. If the bleeding continues, reinforce the dressing with more absorbent material and apply more direct pressure.

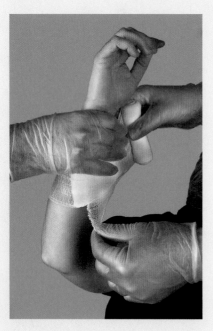

3. Once bleeding is controlled, continue to apply pressure, and attach a self-adherent or roller bandage around the affected part. Apply just enough pressure to control bleeding. Working at a steady pace, roll the bandage evenly over the body surface. Maintain uniform pressure during the application, and avoid clumping of the bandage material. Hold one corner end of the start of the bandage to use as an anchor.

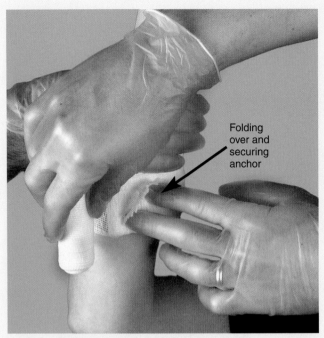

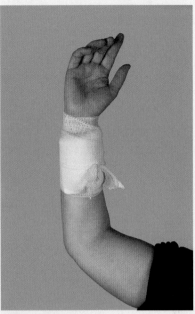

4. After encircling the body part once, anchor the bandage in place by folding a corner end over the second layer of the bandage. Cover the fold to prevent slippage with the next layer. Overlap the subsequent layers approximately halfway over the previous layer. The bandage should be tight enough to control bleeding but loose enough to allow distal blood flow.

5. Once the bandage is in place, attach the end with adhesive tape, or tie off the end.
Note: The EMT should be especially cautious when using self-adherent bandages, which can become extremely tight because of their elastic quality.

Skill | 21-2   *Applying a Head Bandage*

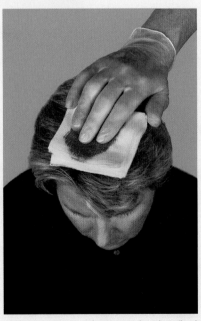

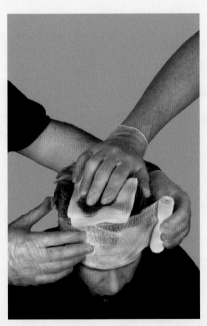

1. Apply gentle pressure to the wound with a flat hand.

2. Begin the head bandage by anchoring the bandage below the occipital protuberance. Circle the head completely once or twice.

Continued

Skill | 21-2   *Applying a Head Bandage–cont'd*

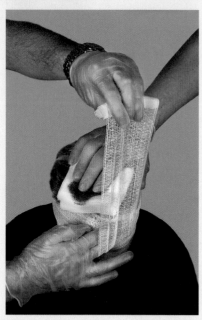

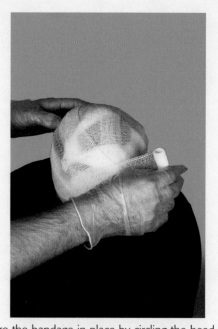

3. Begin to traverse the bandage back and forth across the top of the head until the area with the dressing is completely covered. Once the dressing is traversed, your assistant can help by holding the bandage in back of the head until it is secured.

4. Secure the bandage in place by circling the head once or twice and taping the bandage in place.
Note: Application of this type of bandage takes two persons. The bandage is useful for isolated scalp lacerations if spinal injury is not suspected. If rapid transport is indicated, a delay at the scene to apply this type of bandage is not warranted.

Skill | 21-3   *Applying a Bandage to the Knee or Elbow*

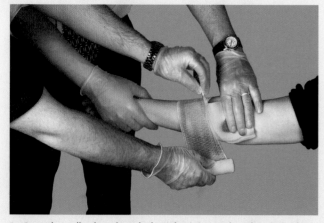

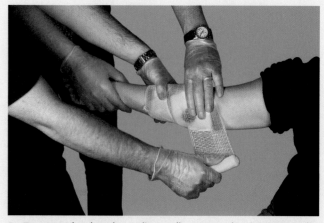

1. Start the roller bandage below the joint and anchor it in place.

2. Traverse the bandage diagonally across the joint over the dressing.

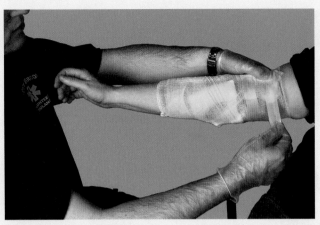

3. Circle the bandage above the joint. After circling the proximal portion, traverse downward to form an X over the dressing on the joint. Continue this pattern until the bandage is complete.

Skill | 21-4   *Stabilizing an Impaled Object*

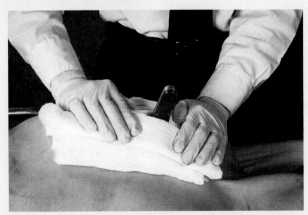

1. Stabilize the impaled object by placing surgical pads or a multitrauma dressing on both sides of it. The bulk should be sufficient to limit any movement of the object.

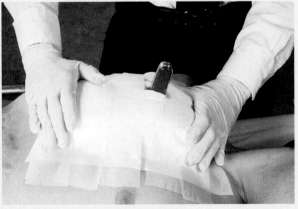

2. Tape the dressing on all four sides.

Skill | 21-5   *Management of an Impaled Object in the Cheek*

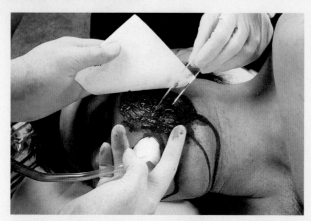

1. As the object is withdrawn, be prepared to control bleeding from the inside.

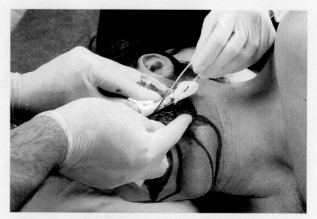

2. Manual control of bleeding outside the cheek may also be required.

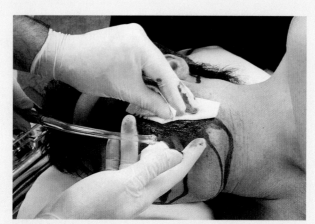

3. Keep suction ready to remove blood and secretions from the airway as needed. Position the patient to permit drainage of blood collecting in the mouth to prevent aspiration.

Skill | 21-6 *Removing Foreign Bodies from the Eye*

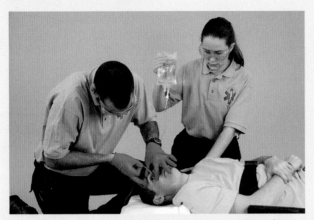

1. Use sterile water or saline or an intravenous (IV) administration set or specially packaged eye-irrigating solution. Explain your actions to gain the patient's confidence and cooperation. This is especially important with children, who may be frightened by having both eyes covered.

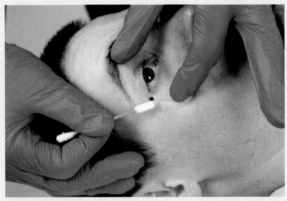

3. If removal by irrigation is not successful, gently whisk the foreign body off the eye with a clean, moistened, cotton-tipped applicator.

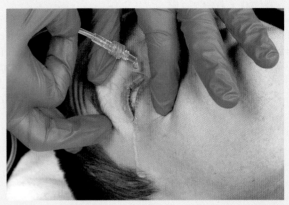

2. Allow a gentle stream of water to pass from the medial portion of the sclera over the rest of the eyeball as you attempt to flush away the foreign body. Respect the delicacy of the eyeball. Do not use a high-pressure stream. Rinse the affected portion of the eyelid if necessary.

CAUTION: Do not use an applicator to remove foreign bodies from the cornea. Scratches to the cornea may result, causing scar formation and impaired vision. The only method advised for removal of foreign bodies on the cornea is *irrigation.*
Once foreign bodies are removed, patch the eye if the patient complains of pain or foreign body sensation. Use a specially prepared eye patch, and tape it with plain cellophane tape or adhesive tape. A 4 × 4–inch gauze can be folded to serve the same purpose.
Note: At times, foreign bodies cannot be removed in the field by the above measures. In this case, you may cover both eyes to limit eye movement because both eyes move symmetrically. It is desirable to limit eye movement because a foreign body embedded under the upper lid may continue to scratch the eyeball that is moving underneath. Have the patient lie supine on the stretcher, and keep the patient calm.

The Bottom Line

Learning Checklist

✓ The skin has two major layers; the epidermis is the outer layer and provides protection from the sun's radiation, prevents water loss, and provides protection against infection. The dermis is the inner layer that contains hair follicles, sweat glands, sebaceous glands, nerves, and blood vessels.

✓ Subcutaneous tissue lies beneath the skin and consists of fat and connective tissue.

✓ Closed wounds, such as contusions, ecchymoses, or hematomas, are caused by blunt trauma.

✓ Open wounds are caused by blunt or penetrating trauma and include lacerations, abrasions, avulsions, amputations, punctures, and penetrations.

✓ Crush injuries may result in closed or open wounds.

✓ Severity or complications of wounds are determined by the mechanism of injury, site of the injury, extent of the injury, and introduction of foreign bodies or contaminants into the wound.

✓ Common complications of wounds include bleeding, infection, and damage to underlying structures.

✓ Wound management may include control of bleeding, immobilization of the affected part, prevention of contamination, preservation of avulsed or amputated parts, and stabilization of impaled objects (except those in the cheek, which can be removed).

✓ Partially avulsed body parts should be rinsed of gross debris, dressed, and bandaged in their original anatomic position.

✓ Amputated parts should be rinsed of gross debris, wrapped in sterile gauze, and placed in a plastic bag that is placed on ice.

✓ A dressing is any material used to cover a wound. A bandage is any material used to secure a dressing in place or provide pressure over the wound.

✓ Foreign bodies in the eye should be irrigated out of the eye or removed with a cotton swab. (Invert the eyelid if the object is beneath the lid.)

✓ Impaled objects should never be removed from the body, except from the cheek to ensure control of the airway.

✓ Cover extruded eyeballs with a moistened dressing and a cup and bandage. Cover the good eye to avoid sympathetic eye movement.

✓ Burns may be caused by thermal, electrical, or chemical mechanisms.

✓ General burn management includes stopping the burning process, removing the patient from the burning environment, providing supplemental oxygen, treating for shock, preventing shock, and transporting the patient to the appropriate facility.

✓ There are three major categories of burn injuries: superficial (first-degree), partial-thickness (second-degree), and full-thickness (third-degree) burns.

✓ Superficial burns are painful and cause reddened and dry skin that is warm to the touch (e.g., sunburn).

✓ Partial-thickness burns are very painful and are characterized by a pink, red, or blotchy appearance (deeper partial-thickness burns may be pale) and a wet, weepy surface with edema and blisters.

✓ Full-thickness burns are not painful and are characterized by a deep-red, black, or brown appearance; edema; and disrupted skin; and may have no sensation to touch (although the surrounding partial-thickness areas will be painful).

✓ The extent of burns is evaluated with the "rule of nines"; 9% for each arm, 9% for head (except for children [18%]), 18% for anterior or posterior trunk or torso, 18% for each leg (except for children [13.5%]), and 1% for the groin.

✓ Factors that complicate or affect the severity of burns include inhalation injuries, age (older than 55 years or younger than 5 years), associated conditions (heart or lung disease, diabetes, severe illness), and location of the burn (face, perineum, feet and hands).

✓ Irrigate chemical burns for at least 20 to 30 minutes before or during transport to the hospital.

✓ Brush dry chemicals from the skin before irrigation.

✓ Electrical burns have entrance and exit wounds and may be more extensive than they appear on the surface.

✓ Electrical injuries may cause fractures or lead to respiratory or cardiac arrest.

Key Terms

Abrasion A scrape on the surface of the skin or mucous membrane.

Air embolism An air bubble introduced into the circulatory system (as through an open wound) that can result in obstruction of blood flow.

Amputation Cutting away of a limb or protruding structure from a person's body.

Auditory ossicles Consisting of the malleus, incus, and stapes, these bones transmit sound waves to the inner ear.

Avulsion Tearing away of a body part or structure; the part is often still attached to the body by a small flap of skin.

Bandage Material used to secure a dressing in place and provide pressure over the dressing to aid in control of bleeding.

Contusion Bruise caused by external violence and characterized by leakage of blood and swelling under the skin.

Crush injury Injury resulting from the severe compressing force that damages and sometimes tears soft tissues and underlying structures.

Dermis Skin layer below epidermis composed of dense connective tissue that contains the nerves, blood vessels, sweat and sebaceous glands, and hair follicles.

Dressing Any material that covers a wound, prevents introduction of further contamination into the wound, and aids in bleeding control.

Ecchymosis Black-and-blue marks caused by bleeding beneath or within layers of the skin.

Epidermis Outermost layer of skin.

Fascia Fibrous membrane covering that separates tissue from bone.

Full-thickness burns Burns that involve the entire thickness of the epidermis and dermis; also called *third-degree burns.*

Hematoma Collection of blood beneath the skin.

Laceration Tear or cut in the skin or other soft tissues.

Partial-thickness burns Burns that involve the epidermis and extend into, but not through, the dermis; also called *second-degree burns.*

Puncture Penetrating injury caused by a sharp, pointed object.

Sclera Outer layer of eye.

Sebum Oily substance secreted by the sebaceous glands that helps moisturize the skin.

Superficial burns Burns that involve the epidermis, the superficial layer, of the skin; also called *first-degree burns.*

Review Questions

1. The outermost layer of the skin is called the:
   a. Superficial
   b. Fascia
   c. Epidermis
   d. Dermis

2. A third-degree burn implies that the burn has damaged which layer of the skin, composed of dense connective tissue that contains the nerves, blood vessels, sweat and sebaceous glands, and hair follicles?
   a. Subcutaneous layer
   b. Fascia
   c. Epidermis
   d. Dermis

3. If the dermis is completely damaged, as in full-thickness burns, there will be _____ sensory perception.
   a. increased
   b. extremely painful
   c. no
   d. tingling

Questions 4-8. Match the description in column B with the type of wound in column A.

Column A	Column B
4. Contusion	a. Tearing away of body part or structure, but still attached by pedicle.
5. Abrasion	b. Penetrating injury caused by sharp, pointed object.
6. Laceration	c. Scraping of skin surface or mucous membrane.
7. Avulsion	d. Tearing of the skin or other soft tissues.
8. Puncture	e. Bruise.

9. In general, embedded objects that have impaled the body should be:
   a. Stabilized in place.
   b. Carefully removed.
   c. Pushed through.
   d. Left alone.

10. Objects that have impaled the cheek should be:
    a. Stabilized in place.
    b. Carefully removed.
    c. Pushed through.
    d. Left alone.

11. Which vessels are likely to allow an air embolism to form if they are cut?
    a. Arteries in the neck
    b. Veins in the neck and upper chest
    c. Capillaries in the chest
    d. Arteries in the chest

12. The first concern for a patient with injuries to cheek and teeth is the:
    a. Cervical spine
    b. Airway
    c. Eye
    d. Brain

13. Complete and deep avulsions of the facial skin should be treated by placing a(n) _____ dressing directly over the wound.
    a. petroleum jelly
    b. aluminum foil
    c. moistened
    d. Surgi-Pad

14. A general principle for treating eye injuries is:
    a. Always irrigate and apply firm pressure.
    b. Avoid pressure to the eyeball.
    c. Never treat in the field.
    d. Use petroleum gauze, and never cover both eyes.

15. A preferred method for removing foreign bodies of the eye in the field is:
    a. Blow-by oxygen
    b. Irrigation
    c. A cotton-tipped applicator
    d. None of the above

16. Chemical burns to the eye are treated by:
    a. Bandaging the affected eye.
    b. Irrigating with water or sterile saline.
    c. Irrigating with a neutralizing solution.
    d. Rapid transport without field treatment.

17. The most common cause of a burn in a child younger than 3 years is:
  a. Sunburn
  b. Scalding injury
  c. Electrical injury
  d. Chemical injury

18. Skin that appears charred, yellow-brown, dark red, or white and translucent is probably related to a _____ burn.
  a. superficial
  b. partial-thickness
  c. full-thickness
  d. Both a and b

19. Two patients are removed from a burning hotel. One man is 65 years old and has partial-thickness burns over his left arm and anterior chest and singed nasal hair. The other patient is 35 years old and has third-degree burns over his right hand and a history of recent surgery for hernia repair. The fire chief asks if either patient needs to go to the burn center. What criteria would dictate burn center transport, if indicated, for these patients?
  a. Partial-thickness burns greater than 5%, facial involvement, extremes of age, recent hospitalization
  b. Partial-thickness burns greater than 10%, any burn associated with inhalation injury, age over 55 or under 5, full-thickness burn
  c. Partial-thickness burns greater than 15%, nasal burn, age over 65 or under 5, full-thickness burn over 5%
  d. Partial-thickness burns greater than 10% in adult and 5% in children, singed nasal hair, burns to hand

20. A 3-year-old child has burns from a spilled pot of boiling water, with redness and blistering over the entire left arm, anterior chest, and anterior surface of both legs. What is the approximate body surface area involved?
  a. 10%
  b. 20%
  c. 30%
  d. 40%

For Further Review

In the Student Workbook

- Multiple-choice questions
- Matching questions
- Short-answer questions
- Case scenario questions
- Skill check questions

On Evolve

- Anatomy challenge
- Weblinks
- Lecture notes
- Exercises

Learning Objectives

Cognitive Objectives

- State the major functions of the skin.
- List the layers of the skin.
- List the types of closed soft tissue injuries.
- State the types of open soft tissue injuries.
- Establish the relationship between body substance isolation and soft tissue injuries.
- Describe the emergency medical care of the patient with a closed soft tissue injury.
- Describe the emergency medical care of the patient with an open soft tissue injury.
- Establish the relationship between airway management and the patient with chest injury, burns, blunt injury, or penetrating injury.
- Describe the emergency medical care of a patient with an amputation.
- Describe the emergency medical care of a patient with an impaled object.
- List the functions of dressing and bandaging.
- Describe the purpose of a bandage.
- Describe the steps in applying a pressure dressing.
- Describe the effects of improperly applied dressings, splints, and tourniquets.
- List the categories of burn injuries.
- Define superficial burn.
- List the characteristics of a superficial burn.
- Define partial-thickness burn.
- List the characteristics of a partial-thickness burn.
- Define full-thickness burn.
- List the characteristics of a full-thickness burn.
- Describe the emergency medical care of the patient with a superficial burn.
- Describe the emergency medical care of the patient with a partial-thickness burn.
- Describe the emergency medical care of the patient with a full-thickness burn.
- Describe emergency care for the patient with a chemical burn.
- Describe emergency care for the patient with an electrical burn.

Psychomotor Objectives

- Demonstrate the steps in the emergency medical care of patients with each of the following:
  - Closed soft tissue injuries
  - Open soft tissue injuries
  - Open chest wounds
  - Open abdominal wounds

- An impaled object
- An amputation
- Superficial burns
- Partial-thickness burns
- Full-thickness burns
- An electrical burn
- A chemical burn

- Demonstrate the steps in the emergency medical care of an amputated part.
- Demonstrate completing a prehospital care report for patients with soft tissue injuries.

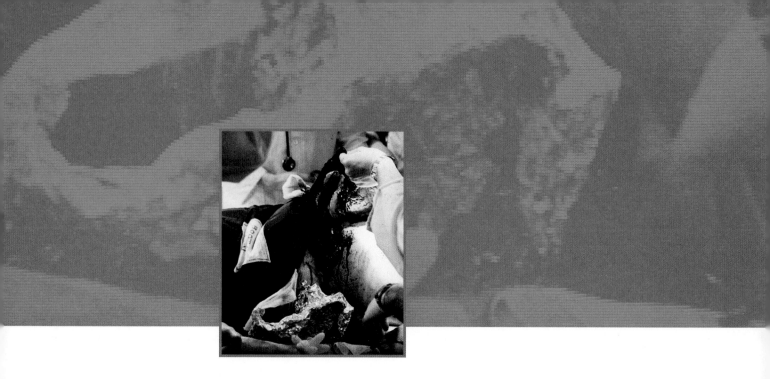

22 Chest and Abdominal Emergencies

CHAPTER OUTLINE

Scenario

You respond to a call for a "stabbing." On arrival you find a 23-year-old man who has been stabbed in the chest and has a large slash wound across his anterior abdomen. The chest wound is bubbling with each breath and making a "sucking" sound. The patient's bowel is protruding from the abdominal wound. The patient is alert, pale, and sweaty. His respirations are 22 breaths/min and shallow, pulse 120 beats/min and thready, and blood pressure 90/60 mm Hg. While your partner prepares the patient for rapid transport, you seal the chest wound with an occlusive three-sided dressing and administer high-concentration oxygen by nonrebreather mask. You also place a sterile dressing around the protruded bowel, moisten it with sterile water, cover it with a dry sterile dressing, and tape it in place.

The thoracic and abdominal cavities are highly vascular and contain vital organs; injury can result in hemorrhage, damage to organs, and death. Both cavities are large enough to contain the body's entire blood volume, concealing internal bleeding. Damage to vital organs in the chest can result in respiratory compromise or cardiac failure. Injury to organs in the abdomen can result in bleeding and leakage of contents of the hollow organs within the abdominal cavity.

Early recognition of thoracic and abdominal injury is aided by a working knowledge of anatomy and physiology. Based on the mechanism of injury, you can anticipate certain organ injuries and search for related signs. For example, blunt trauma to the anterior chest wall can result in fractures of the ribs and flail chest, which make breathing ineffective. Knowing the meaning of key signs such as paradoxical movement of the chest wall will alert you to the need for special treatment considerations. Management of thoracic injuries may require application of airtight or occlusive dressings, stabilization of multiple rib fractures, and ventilation and oxygenation. With open abdominal wounds, organs may extrude (evisceration), requiring special handling. By understanding the importance of injuries to the chest and abdomen, learning signs of injury requiring emergency care at the scene and early transport, and learning how to handle special situations unique to injuries of the chest and abdomen, you will provide optimal care for your patients.

Chest

Anatomy and Physiology

The thoracic cavity begins just below the neck and extends down to the diaphragm (respiratory muscle that separates thorax and abdomen). The rib cage surrounds the thoracic cavity on both sides and provides structure for ventilation and protection of the vital organs. The upper 10 pairs of ribs are attached to the sternum on the anterior side and to the thoracic spine on the posterior side. These ribs are attached to the sternum by soft cartilage that allows for chest wall movement during ventilation. The eleventh and twelfth pairs of ribs are not attached to the sternum. They are attached only to the eleventh and twelfth thoracic vertebrae and are referred to as "floating" ribs. The sternum

is composed of three separate bones: upper manubrium, middle body, and lower xiphoid process (**Figure 22-1**).

The clavicles, or collarbones, lie over the anterior upper ribs and extend from the sternum to the shoulders. The scapulae, or shoulder blades, lie over the upper posterior ribs and attach to the clavicles and humerus to form the shoulder. The bony tip of the shoulder is the acromion (acromial process).

The diaphragm is a dome-shaped muscle that forms the base of the thoracic cavity. It contracts and pushes down into the abdomen, expanding the size of the thoracic cavity and allowing air to enter the lungs during inspiration. The diaphragm relaxes and rises within the thoracic cavity during expiration. As mentioned, the diaphragm forms the division between the thoracic and abdominal cavities. Because it moves with breathing, the boundary between these two cavities may move as well, which is a consideration when evaluating penetrating injuries. With forced exhalation, for example, the upper portion of the right side of the diaphragm can extend as high as the fourth costal cartilage anteriorly and to the eighth rib posteriorly, with the left diaphragm being slightly lower.

The attachments of the diaphragm are the xiphoid process of the sternum, the lower six ribs, and the upper lumbar vertebrae. There are openings in the diaphragm for the aorta, venae cavae, and esophagus.

Contained within the thoracic cavity are the heart, lungs, and great vessels. The esophagus travels through the middle of the thoracic cavity posterior to the trachea.

The thoracic cavity is subdivided into two smaller spaces: the *mediastinum* in the center and the *pleural spaces* on either side. The mediastinum is occupied by the heart, great vessels (venae cavae, aorta), esophagus, trachea, and main stem bronchi. The lungs occupy the pleural spaces.

> **LEARNING OBJECTIVES**
> - Discuss the emergency medical care considerations for a patient with a penetrating chest injury.
> - Differentiate the care of an open wound to the chest from an open wound to the abdomen.
> - Establish the relationship between airway management and the patient with chest injuries.

Chest Injuries

Mechanism of Injury

Motor vehicle crashes are the major cause of severe blunt injury to the chest. Although unrestrained individuals are at greatest risk, even restrained drivers and passengers can sustain severe blows to the chest wall if there is intrusion into the passenger compartment. *Deceleration injuries* can cause tears of major vessels, especially the aorta. Deceleration injuries usually occur to structures that have both mobile and fixed portions. Although the victim may stop on impact, mobile portions of an organ continue to move within the body cavity, tearing from the fixed portion of the same organ at the point of attachment.

Penetrating injuries from knives and guns can strike vital structures. Knife wounds that enter the neck are often directed from above in a downward direction. As an emergency medical

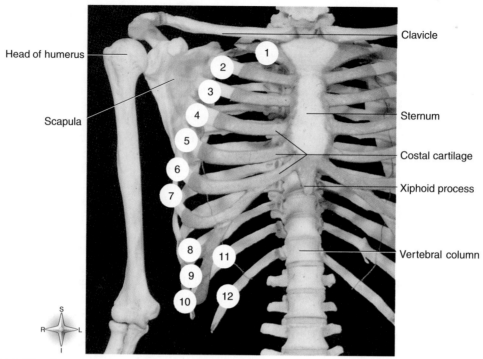

Figure 22-1 The thoracic cavity. *From Thibodeau G:* Structure and function of the body, *ed 11, St Louis, 2003, Mosby.*

technician (EMT), you should be alert to the possibility that such wounds can enter the thoracic cavity, particularly if the entry wound is to the lower neck. Missile wounds are notorious for changing their path after entry (e.g., bullets may bounce off bones or break into fragments). You should maintain a high suspicion in these cases and look for signs of **pneumothorax** (air in pleural space), **hemothorax** (bleeding in pleural space), injury to the great vessels, and **pericardial tamponade,** or **cardiac tamponade** (blood or fluid collecting between layers in covering of heart, causing cardiac compromise).

Rib Fractures

In general, an isolated rib fracture usually is not a serious emergency. However, broken ribs can puncture a lung or a blood vessel, resulting in pneumothorax (collapse of a lung from air in pleural space), hemothorax (bleeding within thoracic cavity), or a **flail chest** resulting from fractured ribs. Fracture of lower ribs may signal injury to the abdominal organs underneath, specifically the liver, spleen, and kidneys, with signs of internal bleeding. Rib fractures are most often the result of blunt trauma (steering wheel injuries, falls, assault involving blows to chest).

Often a patient with a broken or bruised rib will complain of increased pain with breathing when the injured area is moved. To avoid pain, the patient tends to reduce movement of the injured area of the chest wall, called "splinting." Patients with splinting may display unequal chest wall movements, noticeable on inspection of the thorax. Local tenderness is present over the injured part, and *crepitus* can be felt.

Flail Chest

Flail chest is defined as two or more ribs fractured in two or more places (**Figure 22-2**). This results in a portion of the chest wall being unstable, which alters the mechanics of breathing. With

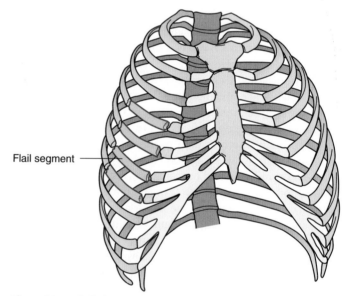

Figure 22-2 Flail chest occurs when two or more ribs are fractured in two or more places; the affected rib segment becomes dissociated from the remaining chest wall.

normal breathing, the chest cavity expands during inspiration, causing a relative negative pressure inside compared with atmospheric pressure. No longer fixed to the thorax, the unstable or flail portion of the chest wall is pulled inward by this "negative" pressure. Conversely, with exhalation, when the pressure within the chest cavity increases the flail segment is pushed out. In essence, the flail segment is moving in the direction opposite the remaining chest wall (**Figure 22-3**). This is called *paradoxical breathing,* or **paradoxical motion** during breathing, and is a key sign of flail chest. Mechanisms of injury causing flail chest include driver impact from the steering wheel in motor vehicle

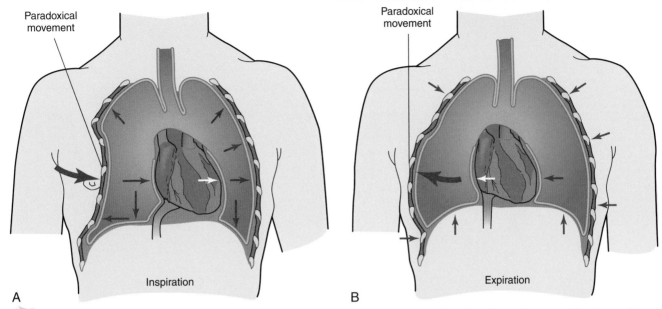

Figure 22-3 Paradoxical motion of breathing. The flail segment moves in the opposite direction from the rest of the intact chest wall. This opposite movement compromises the normal bellow effect of ventilation.

crashes, pedestrian impact from an automobile, and falls (particularly in elderly persons).

Alerted by the mechanism of injury, you may observe paradoxical motion during breathing. The flail segment will be tender and may feel mobile during palpation. You should look for any signs of underlying injury, such as pneumothorax. Breath sounds in the affected area may be diminished. Flail segments can range from relatively small areas of the chest to separation of the entire sternum from the anterior thorax.

Management of a flail chest includes the administration of supplemental oxygen and methods to restore the normal mechanics of breathing. If paradoxical motion is noticeable, you can splint the flail segment to the remaining thoracic cage by using manual pressure on the flail segment. You can also place the patient with the injured side down or place a padded splint board over the flail segment and tape it to the adjacent ribs. All these measures will help prevent outward movement of the flail segment during expiration. If the patient still has inadequate breathing, positive-pressure ventilation is needed. Positive-pressure ventilation does not rely on the patient's chest wall expansion to "pull in" air. Rather, air is forced into the lungs, resulting in uniform expansion. When a patient is breathing spontaneously, coordinate or synchronize your efforts with the patient's attempts to breathe. As the patient begins a breath, provide an assisted ventilation to supplement the patient's own effort to provide an adequate tidal volume.

Traumatic Asphyxia

Traumatic asphyxia is a condition resulting from severe compression of the thorax, such as from high-speed injuries, steering wheel injuries, or heavy weights falling across the chest (e.g., vehicle falling off a jack onto person below). When these types of injuries occur, the heart is compressed, and the blood within the veins is driven into the upper thorax, neck, and brain, causing severe swelling and ecchymosis of the neck and face (**Figure 22-4**).

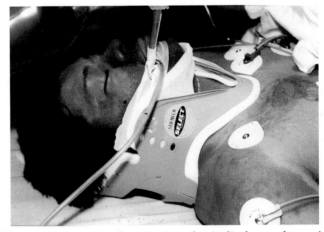

Figure 22-4 A victim of traumatic asphyxia displays ecchymosis and swelling above the level of the heart. A truck with a rear tire removed had slipped off the jack, trapping the patient underneath. At rescue he was in cardiac arrest. Prompt cardiopulmonary resuscitation by bystanders and early EMS response restored his circulation. He survived the injury.

Although the discoloring and swelling are most noticeable, the associated injuries to the heart, lungs, and chest wall, with or without inability to breathe because of weight on the chest, are all life-threatening factors. Therefore the assessment of the patient with suspected traumatic asphyxia should include looking for associated injuries to the lungs and chest wall.

Management of the patient with suspected traumatic asphyxia includes high-concentration supplemental oxygen and positive-pressure ventilation as needed.

Pneumothorax

A pneumothorax is a collection of air in the pleural space that results in collapse of the lung. It occurs when air enters the normally closed space between the linings of the chest wall and the

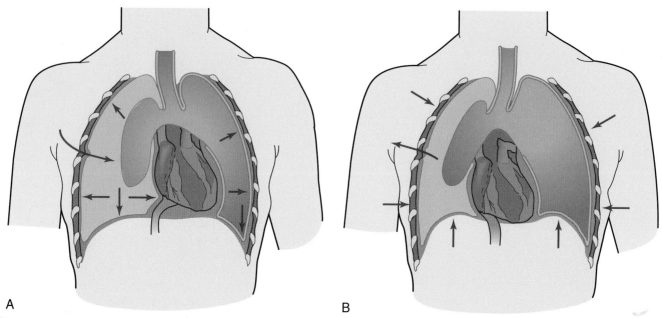

Figure 22-5 Decreased respiratory function in open pneumothorax. **A,** When the chest cavity is penetrated, air may enter the pleural space, causing the lung to collapse. A hole in the chest wall can interfere with the normal air movement of breathing. When the chest cavity expands, air rushes through the hole in the chest wall as well as the trachea. If the hole in the chest wall is extremely large, air preferentially enters through the hole rather than through the airway, resulting in severe hypoventilation and hypoxia. Note the tracheal shift away from the injured side. **B,** During exhalation, as air leaves the hole in the chest cavity, the structures in the mediastinum shift toward the affected side.

lungs (visceral and parietal pleurae). Normally the visceral and parietal pleurae slide against each other during movement of breathing and act as if tightly adhered to one another. When air enters this space, it can dissect along the two pleurae, resulting in loss of adherence and lung collapse. When a lung or part of a lung collapses, less alveolar space is available for diffusion of oxygen, and hypoxia can result.

The following two mechanisms may cause pneumothorax, resulting in air entering the pleural space:

1. Blunt or penetrating trauma may puncture or damage the chest wall or the lung. A pneumothorax can occur when a missile (e.g., bullet, piece of shrapnel), sharp object, or a broken rib penetrates the chest wall or lung. When blunt force is applied to the thoracic cavity, it may cause the lung to rupture or tear. This may occur when a person takes a deep breath and holds it just before an automobile collision. As the person's chest cavity strikes the steering wheel, the trapped air causes the lungs to rupture. This is commonly called the "paper bag effect."

2. The lung wall may spontaneously rupture as a result of a *bleb,* or blisterlike defect, in the lung tissue (see Chapter 11).

You will encounter various presentations of pneumothorax, including open and closed pneumothorax, tension pneumothorax, and hemothorax (when accompanied by bleeding).

Open Pneumothorax. When the chest wall is punctured, the hole in the chest wall may stay open. Air may then be drawn into the pleural space during inspiration. This can create a "sucking" sound, and this type of injury is frequently referred to as a *sucking chest wound* or an **open pneumothorax.**

The larger the hole in the chest wall, the more serious is the effect of the open pneumothorax on breathing. The mechanics

of breathing create a negative pressure relative to air within the thoracic cavity during inhalation. Air then moves into the lungs through the trachea until the pressure equalizes with the atmosphere. However, air will also enter the thoracic cavity from a hole in the chest wall. The larger the hole, the more air will enter. When the size of the hole in the chest wall is larger than the diameter of the trachea, more air will enter through the hole in the chest wall than will enter the lungs through the airway **(Figure 22-5).** The result is an inadequate tidal volume because insufficient air is entering through the trachea, and the lung is being collapsed by the air entering into the plural space through the hole in the chest.

Fortunately, as an EMT you can take immediate action to restore the mechanics of breathing by recognizing and sealing an open chest wound. This action converts the potentially life-threatening open pneumothorax into a closed pneumothorax.

If the chest wall has been penetrated, an open chest wound may be audible and visible. The patient with a pneumothorax may complain of difficulty breathing and chest pain that is worse with breathing. Breath sounds on the affected side may be diminished or absent. Subcutaneous emphysema may be present as well as chest wall tenderness **(Figure 22-6).** Management is directed at ensuring an adequate airway, preventing further air from entering the pleural space, giving supplemental oxygen, and rapidly transporting to a hospital.

When a penetrating wound is discovered on the chest wall, you should immediately apply manual pressure with your gloved hand. An occlusive or airtight dressing consisting of aluminum foil or plastic wrap should then be taped securely to the chest wall. Overlap the tape around three sides of the dressing to act as a flutter valve to prevent any further air from entering

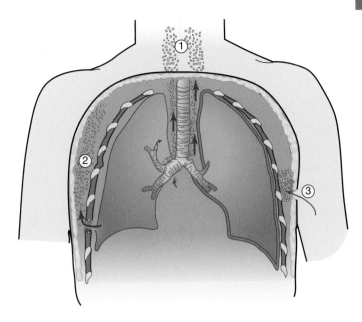

Figure 22-6 Subcutaneous emphysema, or air under the skin, may feel like crepitus (or "crackling"), and there may be obvious swelling. *1,* In the neck, air dissects along deep tissue planes from tears in the esophagus, bronchus, or mediastinal surface of a lung. *2,* Air may be felt along the chest wall over a tear in the pleura and intercostal muscles or from a pneumothorax with rib fractures. *3,* In the area of an external wound, air may accumulate at the sight of injury. *From Zuidema GD, Rutherford RB, Ballinger WF: The management of trauma, ed 4, Philadelphia, 1985, Saunders.*

the chest wall while still allowing air to escape when or if the pressure rises within the chest cavity. **Skill 22-1** illustrates the management of an open chest wound.

The patient should then be placed in the position of comfort (unless spinal injury is suspected). High-concentration oxygen should be administered through a nonrebreather mask. If the patient is hypoventilating or is in respiratory arrest, you should take care during positive-pressure breathing to reduce the probability of more air entering the pleural space. To avoid unnecessarily high pressure during positive-pressure ventilation, use the lowest effective pressure by giving breaths slowly over 1 to 2 seconds while observing chest rise.

Closed Pneumothorax. A pneumothorax without an open wound to the chest is a closed, or simple, pneumothorax. This injury can occur when a broken rib pierces the lung and causes air to flow into the pleural space. The patient with a closed pneumothorax may complain of difficulty breathing and chest pain associated with breathing. Breath sounds on the affected side may be decreased or absent.

Management of the patient with a closed pneumothorax includes administration of high-concentration supplemental oxygen and assisted positive-pressure ventilation as needed. The patient should be rapidly transported to the hospital and watched carefully for any signs of a developing tension pneumothorax.

Tension Pneumothorax. A closed pneumothorax can occasionally develop into a **tension pneumothorax,** a condition in which

air entering the chest cavity becomes trapped within the pleural space. This causes a buildup of pressure and can cause collapse and shifting of the chest contents. When air enters the pleural space during inspiration but cannot exit when the patient exhales, more and more air becomes trapped in the pleural space with every breath, and the pressure increases. This pressure is exerted on all the structures within the chest cavity. The lung collapses, and the structures of the mediastinum are compressed and pushed to the opposite side. The increased pressure can collapse the superior and inferior venae cavae, reducing blood return to the heart and causing profound shock **(Figure 22-7).**

Open chest wounds may also function as one-way valves, causing tension pneumothorax. Air enters the pleural space during inhalation but closes the flap of tissue during exhalation, trapping the air within. Closing an open chest wound prevents outside air from entering the chest cavity.

Signs of a tension pneumothorax include the following:
- Breath sounds noticeably absent on the affected side
- Distended neck veins (caused by obstruction of blood returning through large veins)
- Signs of shock, such as tachycardia and hypotension
- Shifting of the trachea away from the affected side (late sign)

If these signs develop after the application of an airtight dressing to an open chest wound, the dressing should be removed immediately. This may permit trapped air to escape from the chest cavity and release the tension. You should immediately reseal the dressing after the release of air and observe the patient closely for indications of further tension.

If signs of tension pneumothorax develop after blunt trauma or with a spontaneous pneumothorax (collapse of part of lung in a medical patient), transport the patient immediately to the hospital. A needle must be placed into the chest cavity to relieve the tension as soon as possible **(Figure 22-8).** Some emergency medical services (EMS) systems permit paramedics to perform this procedure. If this is the case in your region, you may be directed to request an advanced life support (paramedic) intercept.

Hemothorax

A hemothorax occurs when a blood vessel in the chest cavity is injured and blood begins to accumulate in the pleural space. A hemothorax can be the result of penetrating or blunt trauma, and bleeding can be severe enough to cause shock. Both hemothorax and pneumothorax can occur independently or in combination.

Management of the patient with a hemothorax includes administration of high-concentration supplemental oxygen and positive-pressure ventilation if needed. The patient should also be observed closely for any developing signs and symptoms of shock as a result of the blood loss.

Pulmonary Contusion

Severe blows to the chest wall can result in bruising of the lungs, or pulmonary contusion. The swelling and fluid buildup that result within the lung tissue decrease the diffusion of oxygen into the capillaries. Although a pulmonary contusion may not be initially evident, it can progress during the first hours after injury.

Management of the patient with a pulmonary contusion includes high-concentration supplemental oxygen.

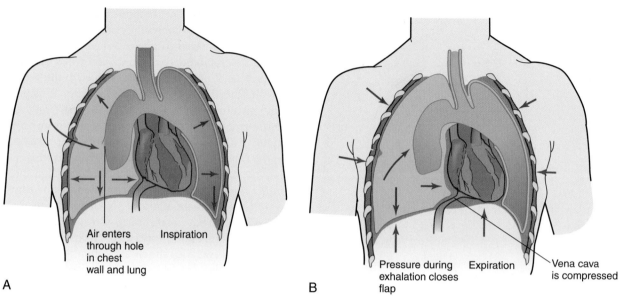

Figure 22-7 Decreased respiratory and cardiovascular function in tension pneumothorax. **A,** Flap of tissue on the lung or chest wall acts as a one-way valve. Air enters the chest cavity during inspiration as the flap opens. **B,** During expiration, pressure within the thorax closes the flap, preventing air in the pleural space from exiting. Air begins to collect in the pleural space, gradually increasing in pressure. Because of the increased pressure, the diaphragm is pushed downward, the mediastinum is pushed away from the affected side (tracheal shift), and the vessels collapse within the mediastinum, obstructing venous return to the heart. The obstructed venous return might be suspected by observing distended neck veins.

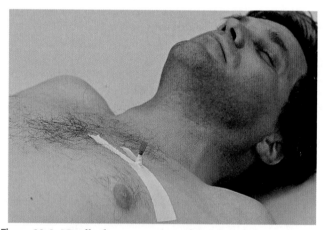

Figure 22-8 Needle decompression of the chest is a simple procedure that can relieve a tension pneumothorax. This technique is used by paramedics in some EMS systems. By placing a small needle in the chest, air under pressure rushes out, relieving the tension. *From NAEMT: Prehospital trauma life support, ed 6, St Louis, 2007, Mosby-Elsevier.*

entry of the returning venous blood. With less blood in the ventricles, less blood volume is ejected with each heartbeat, and blood pressure falls. The blood backs up in the veins and may be evident as distended neck veins.

The patient with cardiac tamponade needs rapid hospital intervention.

Aortic Tear

The aorta can be torn by deceleration forces as the unattached or mobile portion of the aorta continues to move forward after impact while the portion of the aorta attached to body structures suddenly stops. Shearing forces can tear the aorta at this point, where mobile and attached portions meet. The blood loss from this type of injury is so severe and immediate that 80% of such patients die at the scene. Some patients may complain of chest pain or shortness of breath; others show signs of inadequate blood flow to the extremities.

As an EMT, you will not be expected to detect aortic tear in the field, but you should remember that severe injury can result from deceleration forces with few outward signs of direct impact.

Pericardial Tamponade

Pericardial tamponade is the mechanical compression of the heart by large amounts of fluid or blood within the pericardial space. This compression limits the normal range of motion and function of the heart. A penetrating wound to the heart can cause bleeding in the space between the heart and its covering (pericardium). If this occurs rapidly, the blood within the pericardium will compress the chambers of the heart and restrict

---

LEARNING OBJECTIVES

- State the emergency medical care considerations for a patient with an open wound to the abdomen.
- Relate anatomy to the mechanism of injury to determine potential organ damage.
- State the emergency medical care considerations for a patient with nontraumatic, acute abdominal distress.

Abdomen

Anatomy and Physiology

The abdominal cavity is bounded by the diaphragm superiorly and the bony pelvic cavity inferiorly. Posteriorly it is protected by the spine. The sides and anterior portions are protected by layers of muscle. It is important to remember that the superior abdominal border is the diaphragm, and that some of the upper abdominal organs are under the lower ribs. Because the diaphragm is mobile, penetrating wounds to the lower chest may enter the abdominal cavity. With forced expiration, for example, the upper portion of the right side of the diaphragm can extend as high as the fourth costal cartridge anteriorly to the eighth rib posteriorly, with the left part of the right side of the diaphragm being slightly lower than the right part.

The abdominal cavity contains several organs of digestion and excretion, including the stomach, small and large intestines, liver, gallbladder, pancreas, kidneys, and ureters. The spleen is also contained within the abdominal cavity. Many organs in the abdomen are hollow or tubular, containing and promoting flow of contents such as food, bile, and urine. Other organs are solid; some, such as the liver, spleen, and kidneys, are rich with blood vessels and can bleed extensively if ruptured.

The pelvic cavity is the lowermost portion of the abdominal cavity. The "pelvic girdle" is a ring of bones formed by the sacrum, left and right ilium, left and right ischium, and left and right pubis. They provide protection to the pelvic organs within, including parts of the lower intestine, rectum, and urinary bladder, as well as the reproductive organs in females. The top of the ilium bone is called the *iliac crest.* The point where the pubic bones meet anteriorly is called the *pubic symphysis.* The pelvic bone can bleed heavily and cause injury to pelvic organs when fractured (**Figure 22-9**).

The lining of the inner abdominal cavity is called the *peritoneum;* this smooth membrane lines the abdominal wall and

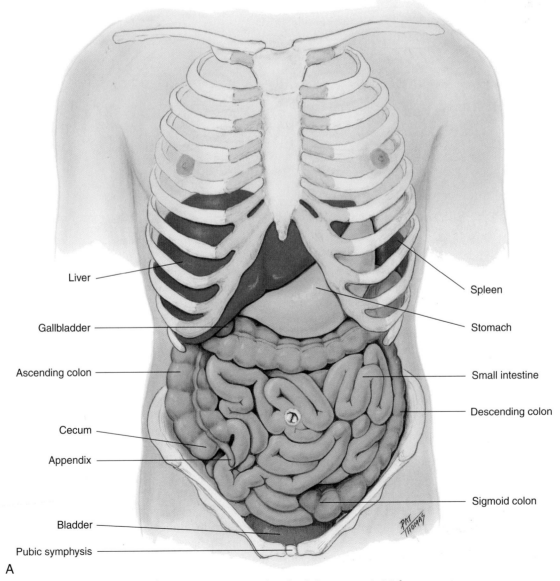

A

Figure 22-9 Abdominal and pelvic organs. **A,** Male.   *Continued*

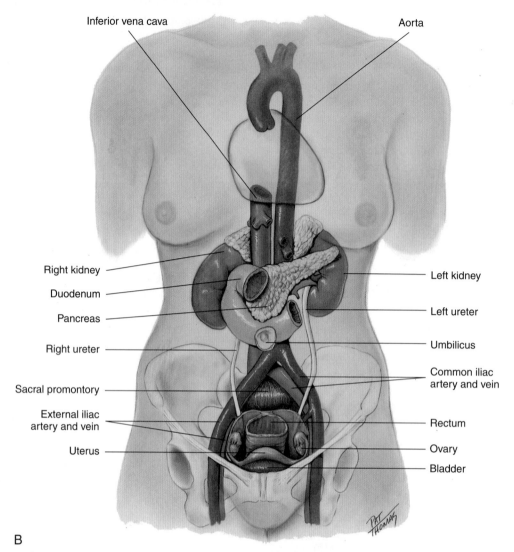

Inferior vena cava

Aorta

Right kidney

Duodenum

Pancreas

Right ureter

Sacral promontory

External iliac artery and vein

Uterus

Left kidney

Left ureter

Umbilicus

Common iliac artery and vein

Rectum

Ovary

Bladder

B

Figure 22-9, cont'd B, Female. *From Jarvis C:* Physical examination and health assessment, *ed 5, Philadelphia, 2008, Saunders-Elsevier.*

the contents of the abdomen. It has two parts, the *parietal* peritoneum, which lines the abdominal and pelvic walls, and the *visceral* peritoneum (internal layer), which covers most of the intraabdominal organs. The space between the visceral and the parietal peritoneum is called the *peritoneal cavity.* **Peritonitis** (inflammation of the peritoneum) can affect the entire abdomen and cause diffuse abdominal pain, tenderness, and involuntary "guarding" (contraction of abdominal musculature). The kidneys and other major structures are located behind the peritoneum (retroperitoneum).

Abdominal Quadrants

The abdominal-pelvic cavity can be divided in various ways to describe the location of pain, tenderness, or other physical findings. A common system is to divide the abdomen into quadrants by two imaginary lines that intersect at the umbilicus, or navel. Horizontal and vertical lines through the umbilicus form right and left upper quadrants and right and left lower quadrants (**Figure 22-10**). Some organs are contained within a single quadrant, and others lie in more than one quadrant. Knowing the location of organs within the different quadrants is helpful

in assessing patients and communicating findings at the hospital or on the prehospital care report. For example, bleeding from the liver would be suspected after a stab wound to the right upper quadrant. Bleeding from the spleen is a concern with fractures of the lower left ribs.

Abdominal Pain

One reason that patients may have difficulty describing their abdominal complaint is because abdominal pain is transmitted by two distinct pain pathways. One pathway, the *visceral pathway,* gives perceptions that are imprecise regarding both the quality and the actual location of the pain. The second pathway, the *somatic pathway,* is perceived more clearly, with the pain having a sharp (even knifelike) quality, and is localized anatomically near the affected organ.

Visceral pain is diffuse, cramping, and aching. Patients may have difficulty finding adjectives to describe this pain. Visceral pain may be accompanied by symptoms such as nausea, vomiting, sweating, and contractions of the abdominal wall muscles.

Somatic pain fibers innervate the parietal (outer layer) peritoneum and abdominal wall and travel through spinal nerves.

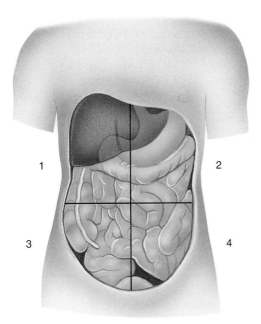

Figure 22-10 The abdomen can be roughly divided into quadrants—upper, lower, left, and right—intersecting at the umbilicus. Knowing the location of organs in different parts of the quadrants can alert you to injuries sustained from trauma.

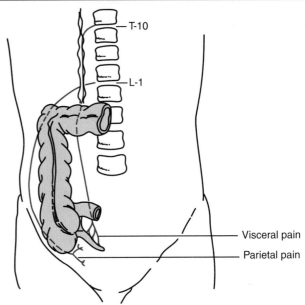

Figure 22-11 Pain pathways in appendicitis. The visceral pain is perceived as coming from the umbilical area. The somatic pain, felt later in the illness, is perceived as coming from the right lower quadrant, where the appendix usually lies. Early in the illness the patient may describe a dull, continuous pain in the midabdomen, which may be accompanied by nausea and vomiting and loss of appetite. As the appendix becomes more inflamed, it can irritate the parietal peritoneum on the adjacent abdominal wall. At this stage the pain is perceived as sharp and in the right lower quadrant. It may be accompanied by guarding. *From Guyton A, Hall J:* Textbook of medical physiology, *ed 11, Philadelphia, 2006, Saunders.*

The brain perceives a sharp pain localized to the abdominal wall overlying the inflamed abdominal organ and may initiate a reflex contraction (guarding) of the overlying musculature. **Figure 22-11** illustrates how these two pathways influence pain perception in a case of appendicitis.

Rather than being attributed to the organ itself, a patient may feel the pain in an area distant from the anatomic source. The location of this "referred" pain corresponds to the segment of the body from which an organ originally developed in the embryo. Although the organ moved to a different location as the embryo and fetus developed, it continued to share nervous innervations with structures from its point of origin. The brain can confuse the pain as arising from its origin. For example, the diaphragm originated from the cervical plexus (groups of nerves arising from cervical region of spine), and pain can be referred from the diaphragm to the shoulder. Likewise, pain from the heart can be referred to the neck, jaw, and arm, shared points from its developmental origin.

Case in Point

An ambulance has been called to the home of a 42-year-old woman complaining of left shoulder pain. As the EMTs complete their focused (secondary) assessment, they inspect the shoulder and see no abnormal findings. They then palpate the shoulder and feel nothing abnormal, and they cannot reproduce the pain while touching. During their detailed physical examination, the EMTs determine that the patient has abdominal pain and increased shoulder pain when her upper abdomen is palpated. They later discover the patient has an inflamed spleen, causing pain being referred to her shoulder. This specific referred-pain presentation is known as *Kehr's sign.*

Abdominal Injuries

Because of the large vessels and highly vascular organs within the abdomen, injuries can result in rapid blood loss and death. Because the abdomen is such a large cavity, *distention* (bulging or protrusion) of the abdomen may not be apparent, even after significant abdominal bleeding. You must therefore maintain a high level of suspicion when encountering a patient with abdominal trauma to provide the patient with the best chance for survival.

Abdominal trauma may result from blunt or penetrating forces. Persons in motor vehicle crashes and pedestrians struck by a vehicle account for most cases of blunt trauma to the abdomen. Other causes include blows to the abdomen and falls.

Penetrating injuries may result from stab wounds or missile injuries. Stab wounds are caused by assault with knives or other sharp objects, self-inflicted injuries, or impalement by objects after a collision or fall. Missile injuries can result from gunshot wounds or explosive fragmentation devices.

The primary goal of prehospital care for patients with abdominal injuries is to recognize life-threatening injuries quickly and provide rapid transport while administering essential life support treatments en route. Most serious abdominal injuries require surgical intervention and cannot be managed in the field. In most regional emergency medical services (EMS) systems, a patient with a penetrating injury to the abdomen is a trauma center candidate.

A special circumstance requiring careful prehospital handling and dressing is **evisceration,** or the extrusion of abdominal contents (e.g., bowel) through a penetration in the abdominal wall.

Mechanism of Injury

The mechanism of injury is an important means of suspecting the presence of intraabdominal injuries. Internal bleeding may not be obvious, and you must remain alert for early signs of shock. Tears or perforations of hollow organs can cause spillage of contents into the peritoneum, and signs of peritonitis may be present.

Blunt Abdominal Trauma. Blunt trauma may result in injuries from compression or deceleration type of forces.

Compression Injuries. Compression injuries occur when two opposing forces compress intraabdominal organs, resulting in contusions, tears, or rupture. In motor vehicle crashes the unbelted driver may be thrown against the steering wheel, suddenly stopping the forward motion of the anterior wall of the chest and abdomen. As the rest of the body moves forward, the posterior abdominal wall and spine compress the intraabdominal organs within. Solid organs such as the spleen, liver, and kidneys are fragile and highly vascular. When torn or ruptured, they can bleed profusely, causing hypovolemic shock. The pancreas, extending across both upper quadrants, can be compressed by the vertebral bodies. When hollow organs such as the stomach or intestines burst or are torn or ruptured, their contents may be spilled into the peritoneal cavity, resulting in severe inflammation and infection. Compression of the abdominal contents can exert such pressure that the abdominal cavity itself is violated. One such example is rupture of the diaphragm with the abdominal contents squeezed upward into the thorax.

Deceleration Injuries. Deceleration injuries result when organs or vessels tear at a point of attachment during a sudden stop. After a vehicle hits a wall and the occupant strikes the steering wheel or dashboard, the mobile organs within the body will continue to move. Initially, they all move at the same speed. The rate of deceleration and the distance the organs move depend on their relative mobility within the body, and these differences create shearing forces that can tear and rupture organs. For example, the liver, a relatively mobile organ, is attached to the abdominal wall by a large, fixed ligament. During deceleration, the liver continues to move beyond its supporting ligament and literally splits over the structure.

The kidneys are attached to the ureters by a group of major vessels off the aorta and venae cavae. With deceleration, shearing forces can cause tears in the renal artery. The intestines and spleen can also be affected by this type of injury.

Deceleration injuries can be deceiving because there may be no external evidence of trauma to the abdominal wall.

Seat Belt Injuries. A properly worn seat belt is applied across the pelvis between the anterior-superior iliac spine and the femur at a 45-degree angle with the floor, tight enough to remain in that position. This approach helps the bony pelvis to protect the soft organs within. If the seat belt is improperly positioned, forces can be transmitted to the abdominal wall and compress the abdominal organs. Abrasions, contusions, and ecchymosis in a band across the abdominal wall are indications of the point of compression of a seat belt. Even if the seat belt is properly worn, you should be concerned about deceleration forces on internal organs.

REAL*World*

Seat belts in vehicles are designed to fit adults. When small children are strapped into a vehicle with only the seat belts instead of also using a car seat, the seat belts will sit high across the abdomen and high across the chest and neck. In a collision, a child could sustain severe thoracic and abdominal injuries secondary to the seat belt. The EMT's duties on an accident scene include determining if the occupants were restrained and, if so, how were they restrained. Children improperly restrained should be evaluated and treated with a high index of suspicion by the EMT.

Penetrating Trauma. Penetrating wounds can range in severity from simple superficial punctures and lacerations of the skin to penetration of major organs and vessels. The structures that are punctured or lacerated are determined by *location* of the wound, *size* of the object, and *direction* at which the object entered the abdominal cavity. Objects that puncture major vessels such as the aorta or vena cava are more likely to result in massive blood loss and death. It is important to know what instrument caused the penetration. You should always be highly suspicious that there is internal bleeding. A small puncture may appear benign and lull the EMT into underestimating the extent of the injury.

Missile injuries are generally more severe than stab wounds. In gunshot wounds the speed at which the bullet travels is a major factor in determining the severity of injury and an important part of the history of the event. The greater the speed of the missile, the higher is the level of energy and the larger the zone of injury.

Finally, the location of the wound and trajectory of the bullet also affect the severity of the injury. However, it is extremely difficult to determine the path of a bullet or other missile because it may ricochet off the bone and travel from the abdomen to the chest. You should carefully check for entrance and exit wounds when evaluating gunshot or other missile wounds.

Assessment and Management

Because injury is often hidden within the abdominal cavity, you must rely on two major factors to identify life-threatening problems: the mechanism of injury and early signs of hypovolemic shock.

Scene Size-up

Obtaining the mechanism of injury must be included as part of your scene size-up. A patient who has fallen from a height of 20 feet or who has been shot in the abdomen does not need to exhibit signs of shock to be treated as having a severe injury. Rather, you would initiate rapid transport for such a patient because of the mechanism of injury alone. Transporting a patient to the emergency department or operating room before shock occurs improves the patient's chance for survival.

You should document the mechanism of injury with sufficient detail to allow hospital personnel to reconstruct your observations from the scene. Documentation should include time of injury and particular circumstances as warranted.

Initial (Primary) Assessment

You should begin your search for hypovolemia during the initial (primary) assessment. Signs of poor skin perfusion, including rapid and thready pulse, rapid breathing, and sweaty skin, are early signs of shock. Hypotension and altered mental status are late signs of shock.

Focused (Secondary) Assessment

With blunt trauma, look for bruises, tire marks, and seat belt marks on the abdominal wall. Is the abdomen distended? Remember the mnemonic DCAP/BTLS? Broken bones raise the suspicion of significant internal injury. Evaluate the ribs, especially noting tenderness of the ribs over the liver or spleen. Palpate the abdomen, noting any tenderness and guarding in the four quadrants. Ask the patient where the pain is located before you examine the abdomen, and begin your examination away from that area, examining it last. With gentle pressure, compress the iliac crests medially and then posteriorly, looking for pain or any instability. Stop if you feel movement of the pelvic bones, because movement is evidence of a pelvic fracture. Pelvic fractures can cause significant blood loss as well as injury to pelvic organs.

Remember that many factors can mask signs of severe injury. Alcohol or other drugs may mask an injury. Associated head injuries or spinal injuries may be present, with loss of pain perception and the normal sympathetic nervous system response to hypovolemia. Is the patient elderly, or taking medications such as beta blockers that may slow the heart rate? Age and certain drugs can decrease heart rate. All these factors are important to ascertain when evaluating the patient.

You should take a SAMPLE history, noting signs and symptoms, allergies, medications, pertinent past medical history, last oral intake, and events leading up to the trauma.

REALWorld

Geriatric and pediatric patients present different challenges to the EMT. When hurt or traumatically injured, the geriatric or pediatric patient may have a difficult time identifying or describing the pain. Children may be frightened by the pain and may have an exaggerated response to a minor injury. Geriatric patients have decreased pain sensation and thus may not have the typical presentation with a serious injury. Pediatric patients can compensate for injuries and illnesses with minimal changes in vital signs until they deteriorate suddenly, possibly catching the EMT off guard. Geriatric patients can no longer compensate rapidly and may not show some of the initial signs of shock, such as tachycardia, again possibly catching the EMT off guard. The EMT must evaluate mechanism of injury, evaluate the patient thoroughly, and maintain a high index of suspicion monitoring for changes in the patient's presentation.

Management

Definitive management of major traumatic abdominal emergencies should be done within the hospital. Some patients may require rapid transport and treatment for shock. Other factors to consider are listed in **Box 22-1**.

Box 22-1 Protocol for Treating Traumatic Abdominal Emergencies

1. Treat the whole patient. In the setting of multiple blunt trauma, immobilize the spine as indicated and treat life-threatening injuries.
2. Maintain the airway, especially with vomiting. Patients with altered mental status and vomiting should be placed in the lateral recumbent position, with suction on standby to aid in keeping the airway clear during transport. For patients immobilized on a long spine board, be aware that the patient may have to be turned as a unit if vomiting occurs. Suction must be available.
3. Give high-concentration oxygen.
4. Control external bleeding, secure penetrating objects in place, and dress open wounds. If there is evisceration of bowel, cover with a moistened sterile dressing and then a dry multitrauma dressing, and secure in place.
5. Treat for shock if present. Maintain body temperature, elevate legs, and consider the pneumatic antishock garment if bleeding from a broken pelvis is suspected.
6. Position the patient according to the need for spinal immobilization, airway maintenance, positive-pressure ventilation, shock treatment, and comfort. Patients with abdominal injuries may find the most comfort from being transported supine with hips and knees flexed. A pillow may be placed under the knees.
7. Give nothing by mouth. The patient with an abdominal emergency may require surgery.
8. Complete the examination en route to the hospital. Repeat vital signs as indicated. Record your findings.
9. Select the hospital by local protocols for trauma center candidates. Notify the hospital of the impending arrival.

Special Considerations

Evisceration. Evisceration is the presence of abdominal contents, usually intestines, protruding through the abdominal wall. It occurs after slash injuries in which a large opening is created in the abdomen. You should not attempt to put the organs back into the abdominal cavity. Instead, cover the exposed organs with a moist, sterile dressing or an airtight dressing to prevent the exposed bowel from drying out (**Figure 22-12**).

To make a moist dressing, apply a large, sterile multitrauma dressing moistened with sterile saline around the exposed organs, then cover the moist dressing with a dry multitrauma dressing and tape it in place. To secure an airtight dressing, wrap the exposed bowel loosely with sterilized aluminum foil or plastic wrap, and secure all edges with tape to prevent air from entering the dressing. **Skill 22-2** illustrates the management of an evisceration. The patient should be transported in the supine position with the hips and legs flexed, with a pillow placed under the knees to help maintain this position.

Urinary Tract Injuries. Urinary tract injuries can have various presentations. Kidney injuries are suspected with bruises over the flank. Injuries to the pelvis can cause bladder or urethral tears. There may be blood at the tip of the penis or a hematoma of the scrotum, evidenced by black or bluish discoloration of

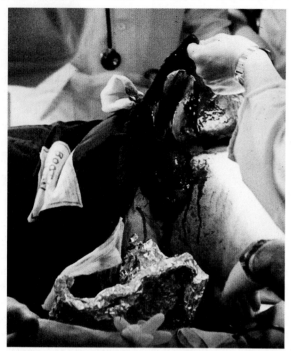

Figure 22-12 Evisceration caused by a self-inflicted slash wound across the abdomen.

the scrotum caused by blood extending downward through the tissues.

Direct injuries to the male genitalia can result in laceration, bruising, avulsion, or even amputation. Use direct pressure (moisten dressings applied to denuded or "skinned" areas) to control bleeding. Bring avulsed or amputated parts to the hospital, wrapping them in a moist sterile dressing and putting them into a plastic bag placed over ice.

Injuries to the female genitalia may occur from direct trauma or straddle injuries, which involve falling onto an object with the main force applied to the perineum. External bleeding may be present and should be controlled with direct pressure. Do not place dressings within the vagina. If necessary, hold dressings in place with a triangular bandage. For blunt trauma in pregnancy, see Chapter 19. Leave foreign bodies in the genitalia or urethra in place for removal at the hospital.

> **REAL***World*
>
> Traumatic injuries to the genitalia in men and women can be the result of a sexual assault or rape. The EMT must remember to consider the emotional state of their patient as well as the legal implications and responsibilities of the EMT. (See Chapter 18 for further discussion.)

Penetrating objects in the abdomen should be left in place and removed at the hospital. You should stabilize the penetrating object with a bulky dressing on all sides of the object secured by tape (see Chapter 21): If the patient is impaled on a fence post or other large object, it may be necessary to cut the object so that the patient can be moved with the impaled object stabilized in place.

LEARNING OBJECTIVES
- Recognize a patient with an acute abdomen.
- Discuss the emergency medical care considerations for a patient with acute abdomen.

Acute Abdomen

"Acute abdomen" is a general term commonly used to identify abdominal pain of recent onset. The pain is not traumatically induced, but rather has other causes, such as, infection, obstruction or occlusion, perforation, nontruamatic bleeding (as from gastric ulcer), and chronic organ failure. For many patients with acute abdominal pain, their outcome depends on early diagnosis and surgical intervention.

Digestive System

The function of the digestive system is to break down foods, absorb them into the bloodstream, and process them into useful forms for energy, growth, and other body functions. Food is broken down both mechanically and chemically. It is mechanically made smaller by chewing in the mouth and churning in the stomach and intestines. Food is chemically broken down by acids and enzymes that are secreted into the mouth, stomach, and intestines. As food travels through the digestive tract, it becomes smaller and smaller until it is either absorbed or excreted as feces.

Esophagus

The esophagus travels through the chest cavity just posterior to the trachea. It enters the abdominal cavity through the diaphragm. The esophagus is a muscular tube that propels food from the mouth to the stomach through the process of peristalsis. *Peristalsis* is muscular action that moves food in a coordinated manner through the entire digestive system.

Esophageal disorders may cause complaints such as indigestion or heartburn. Gastric acid may reflux (flow back) into the esophagus (gastroesophageal reflux), causing irritation of the esophageal wall, resulting in a burning sensation or chest pain. Esophageal disorders can be confused with myocardial infarction. It is important to collect the history carefully as related to the character of the chest pain and the past medical history. The patient may have taken antacids; inquire whether or not this relieved the pain. Pain related to this disorder may also be reduced or relieved while sitting. When in doubt, treat for myocardial infarction. Remember that patients with ischemic chest pain may attribute their discomfort to "indigestion."

Hemorrhage. The esophagus may also be the site of hemorrhage. Patients with severe liver disease, often related to heavy alcohol use, may have *esophageal varices,* balloonlike blood vessels that can protrude through the lower esophageal wall, where they can be subject to erosion from gastric acids. A varix may rupture and result in massive bleeding. Signs of esophageal bleeding include *hematemesis* (vomiting blood) and possibly *melena* (blood in stool that appears black, with tarry consistency and distinct foul odor).

Esophageal Perforation. The esophagus can also perforate from a variety of mechanisms. Forceful vomiting or retching may cause tears in the esophagus, causing profuse bleeding. Ingestion of caustic or corrosive substances can cause perforation. Esophageal perforation is life threatening and requires immediate surgical intervention.

Stomach

The stomach is a J-shaped organ located in the left upper quadrant (LUQ). It has two openings, one connecting with the esophagus and the other leading to the duodenum, the first phase of the small intestine. The volume of the stomach varies tremendously; it can expand to 10 times its empty size. The stomach stores food and breaks it down mechanically through contraction and relaxation of muscles and chemically by strong acids and enzymes.

Ulcers and Gastritis. Peptic ulcer disease and gastritis are common disorders in which the digestive action of the gastric juices begins to work on the organ's own lining. Under a variety of conditions, the acidic gastric juice bores a hole in the wall of the stomach or duodenum. This hole causes pain in the epigastric region or in the back, depending on the location of the crater. The pain may be relieved by the administration of antacids or milk. Aspirin ingestion or coffee may aggravate or precipitate the pain. The pain may be described as burning or indigestion. The patient often has a past medical history of ulcers or gastritis. Common medications that the patient may be taking include Tagamet (cimetidine), Zantac (ranitidine), Pepcid (famotidine), and antacids.

Ulcer disease can cause several complications, with bleeding the greatest concern. The ulcer may bore through a blood vessel and cause massive bleeding. Abdominal pain associated with hematemesis, melena, or signs of hypovolemic shock suggests bleeding ulcers.

Small Intestine

Food travels from the stomach into the small intestine. The small intestine is located in the central part of the abdominal cavity throughout all four quadrants. The small intestine ranges from 10 to 20 feet (3-6 m) in length and provides the large surface area through which nutrients are absorbed. The mall intestine is divided into three segments. The first part is the *duodenum*, which extends from the stomach. It is U shaped, leaving the stomach to the right and hooking back to the left, where it connects to the second segment of the small intestine, the *jejunum*. Attached to the duodenum is the drainage tube from the liver, pancreas, and gallbladder. The jejunum connects with the *ileum*, the third part of the small intestine. The ileum ends at the ileocecal junction, where the large and small intestines meet.

The most common emergency arising from the small intestine is *duodenal ulcers.* The second most common is *obstruction.* Obstruction can result from external compression or internal blockage and from twisting or kinking of the intestine. External compression includes the condition of "incarcerated hernia."

Hernia. Hernias are outpocketings (protrusions) of the peritoneum into abnormal openings in the abdominal wall. The most common is an *inguinal hernia,* and patients may complain of pain or a swelling in the groin. With inguinal hernia, the bowel enters the inguinal canal and can present as swelling anywhere along the entire path of the canal and even into the scrotum in males. This is a common condition and does not by itself constitute an emergency as long as the bowel can easily slide back into the peritoneal cavity. If the small intestine becomes trapped or incarcerated, however, a blockage of flow through the small intestine occurs, and the blood flow to the trapped segment of bowel can be compromised.

Intestinal Obstruction. Intestines can also twist around scars from previous abdominal surgery, and this is a common cause of intestinal obstruction. Internal obstruction can occur anywhere in the small intestine when a foreign body becomes lodged in the lumen.

The initial symptom of obstruction is crampy, intermittent abdominal pain. The pain is diffuse and cannot be described as arising from a particular area but may be centered in the area of obstruction. As the buildup continues, the pain becomes more steady and severe, with marked abdominal distention and vomiting as intestinal contents back up.

If you suspect intestinal obstruction, you should inquire about the last bowel movement or the passage of gas. Patients with obstruction have a history of no recent bowel movements or gas.

Pancreas

The pancreas has two general functions: (1) secreting digestive enzymes into the digestive tract to aid in the breakdown of food and (2) secreting the hormone insulin into the blood to regulate glucose use by the body's cells. The pancreas extends across the upper abdomen behind the stomach and in front of the spine, in the retroperitoneal space.

In its role as an endocrine organ, the pancreas secretes insulin, which regulates glucose metabolism. The most common medical problems related to the pancreas are diabetic states and pancreatitis. Diabetes results from failure of the pancreas to produce sufficient insulin (see Chapter 13).

Pancreatitis. Pancreatitis exists in two forms, *acute* and *chronic,* and can be life threatening. The basic abnormality is the inflammation of pancreatic tissues. The most common causes are heavy alcohol consumption and gallstones that block pancreatic duct outflow.

The attack of pancreatitis can begin with sudden, severe epigastric pain that may radiate to the back. Some patients perceive it as right upper quadrant (RUQ) or LUQ pain. The character of the pain varies but is often described as "knifelike." The pain may be aggravated by lying down and somewhat relieved by sitting up. Eating or drinking may worsen the symptoms. Vomiting, fever, and tachycardia are other common signs of pancreatitis. Ecchymosis may be seen in severe cases in the periumbilical region or over the flank. Ultimately, the patient may develop hypovolemic shock.

Liver

The liver is a large, solid, soft organ located in RUQ of abdomen, just below the diaphragm and partially protected by the lower ribs. One of the main functions of the liver is to filter out toxins from the blood. It detoxifies drugs, alcohol, and other potentially poisonous substances. When the liver is overwhelmed by toxins, liver failure may occur, as with chronic alcohol ingestion or an overdose of certain drugs, such as acetaminophen. Patients who have reduced liver function may need adjustments during drug therapy because of their decreased ability to detoxify the substance. The liver also produces proteins that play an important role in fluid balance and blood clotting. Patients with severe liver disease are at increased risk for bleeding.

Liver Disease. As with pancreatitis, alcohol consumption is a major cause of liver disease, leading to **hepatitis** (inflammation) or **cirrhosis** (scarring). Other causes of liver disease are infections and drug reactions. Infectious hepatitis is a special concern to EMTs and all healthcare workers.

Liver disease may be accompanied by jaundiced (yellow) skin or mucous membranes. The earliest jaundice tends to appear in the sclera (white portion of eye) or mucous membranes. Jaundice is caused when liver damage has blocked the bile ducts, resulting in a buildup of bilirubin (breakdown product of red cells) in the blood. Other signs and symptoms of liver failure include vomiting, lethargy, and anorexia. End-stage liver failure can result in hepatic coma from a buildup of toxins in the blood, which alters brain function.

Gallbladder

The gallbladder stores and concentrates bile produced by the liver. It is located under the liver in the RUQ of the abdomen. The presence of fatty food in the duodenum stimulates the gallbladder to secrete bile into the small intestine. Depending on the site of obstruction in the duct system, the patient may develop problems related to the gallbladder, liver, or pancreas.

Cholecystitis. The major medical emergency related to the gallbladder is **cholecystitis** (inflammation or low-grade, chronic infection). This usually occurs when *gallstones,* or rock-like concretions of cholesterol, bile pigment, and calcium, block the bile exit from the gallbladder. The gallbladder can become distended and inflamed.

Initially, the patient with gallbladder disease may complain of RUQ pain, which is aggravated by the ingestion of fatty foods. The pain may be located in the RUQ or referred to the right subscapular region posteriorly and may be confused with pancreatitis or ulcer disease. The patient with acute cholecystitis may also exhibit vomiting, fever, and jaundice from blockage of the bile duct by gallstones. On palpation, the RUQ may be tender; the pain may be aggravated on inspiration. Some patients may describe pain similar to that of myocardial infarction. Finding tenderness on palpation of the abdomen in the RUQ would favor gallbladder disease.

Large Intestine

The large intestine begins in the right lower quadrant (RLQ), continuing the flow of digestive contents from the ileum. It begins with the cecum and appendix, then the ascending colon, transverse colon, descending colon, and sigmoid colon. The *cecum* is the junction between the ileum and the ascending colon. The *appendix* is a wormlike outpocketing of the cecum with an extremely narrow lumen and no known function. The colon wraps around the boundary of the peritoneal cavity, first up the right side *(ascending colon)* and then across the upper portion of the abdomen *(transverse colon)* anterior to the duodenum,

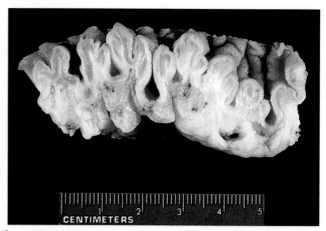

Figure 22-13 Diverticulosis. Section through the sigmoid colon showing multiple saclike diverticula protruding through the muscle wall into the mesentery. *From Kumar V et al: Robbins and Cotran pathologic basis of disease, ed 7, Philadelphia, 2005, Saunders.*

pancreas, ileum, and jejunum. It then travels down the left side *(descending colon)* of the abdomen to meet the sigmoid colon. The *sigmoid colon* travels into the pelvis, is relatively mobile, and leads into the rectum.

The functions of the large intestine are (1) absorption of water and electrolytes from contents delivered by the small intestine and (2) formation of feces. With constipation, the colon contains feces for a longer time and absorbs excess water, resulting in hard stools. With diarrhea, the colon absorbs little water and may have increased secretions (at times with blood). The colon normally contains bacteria, a major constituent of the feces. Many diseases that you may encounter as an EMT arise from the large intestine.

Diverticula. Diverticula of the bowel are common and usually asymptomatic. A bowel **diverticulum** is an outpouching of the inner wall of bowel tissue into the muscle layer of the bowel **(Figure 22-13)**. Diverticula most often occur on the left side of the large intestine. Diverticula that occur near arteries may cause painless bleeding. This bleeding may become severe and is responsible for most massive lower gastrointestinal (GI) "bleeds." Bleeding can have a sudden onset.

The diverticula may become clogged with feces and pus and lead to infection of the large intestine, called *diverticulitis.* This causes mild to moderate pain, usually in the left lower quadrant (LLQ). The character of the pain is dull or aching and may be associated with anorexia and nausea. Fever is also common. The patient may have LLQ tenderness and other signs of peritoneal inflammation. Complications of diverticulitis include obstruction secondary to massive swelling, perforation of the bowel, peritonitis, and bleeding. The patient may have developed hypovolemic or septic shock, depending on the duration and extent of the problem.

Intestinal Obstruction. Obstruction of the large intestine occurs for a variety of reasons. The bowel may twist on itself in areas where it is mobile, such as the sigmoid colon. A cancerous tumor can encroach on the lumen, and the patient may note narrow stools for a time before complete obstruction. Patients with large-bowel obstruction fail to pass gas and stool and have pain and abdominal distention. In contrast to small-bowel obstruction, vomiting does not usually occur because of the distance from the upper GI tract, and because the ileocecal junction acts as a valve, which prevents backflow of material.

Appendicitis. Appendicitis is the most common surgical emergency. It is thought that appendicitis occurs when bowel contents become clogged in the lumen of the appendix. As the normal mucosal secretions continue to collect within the blocked appendix, it distends. Nerve fibers produce a mild, vague pain that the patient usually interprets as being in the umbilical region. As time passes and further distention develops, there is more severe pain and an associated loss of appetite, with nausea and vomiting. As the intestinal wall is compromised from the swelling and bacteria begin to invade the tissue, signs of infection develop (e.g., fever). As the parietal peritoneum is stimulated, pain localizes in the RLQ. The combination of RLQ pain, fever, nausea, and vomiting is highly suggestive of appendicitis. If untreated, the appendix can become gangrenous and rupture, spilling its contents into the peritoneum.

On physical examination the patient may complain of RLQ tenderness, and there is voluntary guarding of the abdomen. As the disease progresses, peritonitis may develop, and the patient may present with acute pain and flexion of the lower extremities. At this point, the disease becomes life threatening.

The definitive therapy for appendicitis is surgery. The main complication is perforation, which spills pus into the peritoneal cavity. At first the pus irritates the RLQ and the pain is local, but ultimately pus spreads to a larger area of the abdomen. As the infection progresses, septic shock may develop. Once the infection spreads, the pain and fever increase. The physical examination shows peritoneal signs, including diffuse tenderness localized to the right side, involuntary guarding, rebound tenderness, and distention.

Urinary System

The urinary system is composed of two kidneys, two ureters, the urinary bladder, urethra, and external genitalia. The functions of the urinary system are (1) to regulate fluid volume and blood salt concentration and (2) to filter the blood of toxins.

Kidneys and Ureters

The kidneys are located in the retroperitoneum, high up on the posterior abdominal wall just under the diaphragm. A large portion of the kidneys is protected by the posterior rib cage. They are connected to the urinary bladder by tubes called *ureters*. The kidneys are slightly mobile and can move with respiration. These highly vascular organs play a major role in regulating fluid levels in the body. When the body is overhydrated, as occurs during excessive fluid intake, the kidneys excrete larger volumes of water, a process known as *diuresis*. When the body is dehydrated, the kidneys conserve water, and urine output is restricted. In severe hypovolemic states caused by bleeding, diarrhea, or other problems, the kidneys may shut down completely, resulting in no urine output.

The kidneys also act as filters of toxins in the blood. They filter poisons, medications, and a byproduct of metabolism called *urea*.

Renal Failure. Kidney failure, or renal failure, can be acute or chronic, with numerous causes. *Acute renal failure* (ARF) may be caused by decreased blood flow resulting in a shocklike state, by intrinsic renal disease from infection, by drug reactions (adverse reactions to antibiotics), or by uncommon systemic disease. ARF may also result from obstruction to urine outflow, either at the ureter (e.g., stone, tumor) or at the urethra (e.g., enlargement of prostate gland). *Chronic renal failure* (CRF) may be caused by diabetes, hypertension, and as with ARF, intrinsic renal disease and uncommon systemic disease.

Patients in renal failure require *dialysis*, which artificially filters the blood.

Pyelonephritis. The most common emergency related to the kidney is **pyelonephritis.** This severe infection of the kidney affects women more often than men. Pregnancy, neurologic conditions that affect the bladder (as in quadriplegic patients), and diabetes are risk factors. Patients with pyelonephritis may present with high fever, shaking chills, abdominal and back pain, nausea, vomiting, diarrhea, and dysuria. They often have pain in the flanks, below the ribs and above the ilium. The urine usually contains pus or blood, and septic shock may occur.

Kidney Stones. Kidney stones form when excess amounts of certain products accumulate in the urine. *Renal colic* is caused by passage of a stone from the kidney into the ureters, causing partial or total obstruction of urine flow. With peristaltic waves of the ureter come spasms of intermittent pain, causing the patient to roll and move around in an attempt to find a position of comfort. The pain is felt in the back or along the path of the urinary system, sometimes radiating into the groin or testicles. The condition may be accompanied by blood in the urine. Men are affected more often than women (3:1 ratio), with most cases occurring between ages 20 and 50. The backup of urine can cause kidney damage.

Urinary Bladder and Urethra

The bladder is located anteriorly, low in the pelvis. When distended with urine, the bladder can be felt in the lower abdomen. Ureters bring urine to the bladder from the kidneys. The function of the bladder is to store urine. It releases urine under voluntary control by relaxation of sphincter muscles at its junction with the urethra.

Bladder emergencies may result from infections. They occur more often in women and rarely are serious enough to require the assistance of an EMT. If left untreated, however, bladder infections can ascend and involve the kidneys. Patients with pelvic pain, difficult or painful urination, and blood in the urine, along with fever, suprapubic tenderness, and voluntary guarding, should be suspected of having a bladder infection.

Reproductive System

Male Reproductive System

The male reproductive system includes the testicles (testes) and epididymis, seminal vesicles, prostate gland, penis, urethra, vas deferens, and scrotum (pouch with testes and epididymis). The testes are suspended in the scrotum by the spermatic cord, which passes down from the abdomen through the inguinal canal. The left testicle usually lies slightly lower in the scrotum than the right testicle. The testes produce the male hormone *testosterone*, as well as spermatozoa and semen (seminal fluid). The sperm are transported via the vas deferens up through the spermatic cord to the base of the bladder. Here the vas deferens joins the seminal vesicles (which store semen) to form the ejaculatory duct, which travels through the prostate, where it opens into the prostatic portion of the urethra, a tube through which both urine and semen pass. The prostate gland secretes fluid that mixes with the semen.

Medical complaints involving the male urinary/reproductive system encountered by EMTs may include acute urinary retention, testicular torsion, and infections.

Testicular Torsion. Torsion of the testes is most common in younger men and adolescents. A testicle can twist within the scrotum about the spermatic cord, which not only supports but also carries the vas deferens, arteries, and veins to the testicle. The blood supply to the testicle can be shut off with torsion. This is a surgical emergency. If the torsion is not relieved within hours, gangrene of the testicle can result. There may be swelling in the scrotal area and marked pain, which is referred to the testicle; in some cases, however, only abdominal pain accompanied by nausea or vomiting may be present.

Infection. Infections can cause pain and burning on urination and pain and swelling of the testes and epididymis. Infections can involve the prostate, urethra, bladder, and testes and epididymis. Patients with urinary tract infections complain of *dysuria* (painful urination), *hematuria* (blood in the urine), frequency of urination, and discharge of pus from the urethral opening.

Female Reproductive System

The female reproductive system has the potential to cause an acute abdomen as well. These conditions as well as anatomy and physiology are discussed in Chapter 19.

Assessment

Because it is extremely difficult to diagnose the cause of abdominal pain in the field, and because many patients may need timely hospital interventions, you should focus on identifying life-threatening conditions and bring these patients to the hospital as quickly as possible. Life-threatening conditions include bleeding and signs of an acute abdomen. The bleeding patient may present with signs of shock, with or without obvious evidence of blood loss. An acute abdomen may require rapid surgical intervention, administration of antibiotics, and restoration of fluids and blood.

In the prehospital setting the following findings are indicative of acute abdomen:

- Patient positioned to avoid any movement of the abdomen (supine or on the side with knees raised and shallow breathing) (**Figure 22-14**)
- A distended and tense abdomen
- Abdominal tenderness
- Abdominal guarding (voluntary or involuntary)

Although additional historical and physical information may be helpful to the physician in making a diagnosis, accumulation of such data should not delay hospital transport. Data can be gathered en route to the hospital or at the hospital.

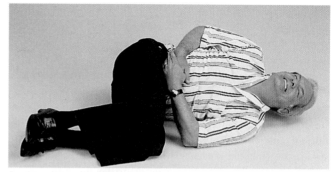

Figure 22-14 Often the most comfortable position for a patient experiencing acute abdominal pain is flat on the back (or side) with the knees drawn up to the chest. *From Shade B et al:* Mosby's EMT-Intermediate textbook for the 1999 National Standard Curriculum, *ed 3, St Louis, 2007, Mosby-Elsevier.*

Initial (Primary) Assessment

If signs of shock are present, rapid transport is indicated. Establishing an airway and administration of supplemental oxygen should be early steps. The position of choice during transport is determined by the mental status of the patient, the position of comfort, and the need to maintain the airway to prevent aspiration, particularly if the patient is vomiting.

Patient History

Pain and bleeding are common chief complaints. Associated complaints may include weakness, vomiting, change in bowel habits, and inability to urinate. You should gather a SAMPLE history with the OPQRST approach (**Box 22-2**).

Focused (Secondary) Assessment

After the initial (primary) assessment and vital signs are taken, look for findings associated with abdominal complaints during the focused physical examination. Is there jaundice in the sclera or skin? Are there signs of dehydration such as dry lips and skin?

From your first approach to the patient, note whether the patient is lying still or is moving about in an unsuccessful attempt to find a position of comfort. You should inspect the abdomen, looking for obvious distention and scars from previous surgery. Lightly touch the abdomen and feel whether it is tense or soft. If the muscles are rigid, ask the patient to try and relax them.

Ask the patient to point to any area of pain, and begin palpation away from that quadrant, examining the painful area last. Gently palpate the abdomen with the pads of your fingertips in each quadrant. Note areas of tenderness. Is there any firmness or rigidity of the abdominal wall muscles? If so, is it generalized, or localized to one quadrant? Note the presence of any masses.

Management

Management for an acute abdomen is essentially the same as for an injured abdomen (see Box 22-1). Treatment for major abdominal emergencies takes place in the hospital. Rapid transport and shock treatment may be required for some patients.

| Box 22-2 | Collecting a SAMPLE History for Patients with Abdominal Complaints |

Signs and Symptoms

Why did the patient call for the ambulance?

Abdominal pain and bleeding are common chief complaints. Associated complaints may include weakness, vomiting, change in bowel habits, and inability to urinate. If there are associated complaints, establish the sequence of events, then develop the chief complaint and history of the present illness more fully using the *OPQRST* approach, as follows:

Onset: When did the pain begin? Was it gradual in onset or sudden and acute? Were there other symptoms associated with the onset of pain, such as syncope or faintness, nausea and vomiting, or an urge to move the bowels? Is the pattern of pain continuous and steady or intermittent and crampy?

Provocation: Does anything make the pain better or worse? Are there relieving or aggravating factors? Has the patient taken medications such as antacids? Does eating aggravate or relieve the pain? Look at the position of the patient. Is the patient lying in one position, trying to avoid any movement? Or is the patient moving about, trying without success to find a position of comfort?

Quality: Use the patient's own words to describe the quality of the pain. What adjectives does the patient use to describe it: knifelike, tearing, dull, or crampy? Is the pain diffuse and poorly localized, or can the patient point to an area of the abdomen?

Radiation: Does the pain radiate? Remember that a patient's pain may be referred to another area, even outside the abdomen; for example, pain from the spleen is often referred to the left shoulder. Pain from a gallbladder attack, kidney stone, or aortic aneurysm can be referred to the back.

Severity: How does the patient rate the severity? Use a 1 to 10 scale, with 1 being barely perceptible and 10 being the worst pain ever experienced.

Time: How long has the pain been present? Did it change in quality or location? If so, when?

When taking a SAMPLE history from patients with abdominal pain, you may note associated complaints that include the following:

Bleeding: Bleeding from the mouth, rectum, urinary tract, or vagina may be present. What are the characteristics of the bleeding? Vomiting resulting from upper gastrointestinal (GI) bleeding may be manifested by bright-red or dark-red blood alone. There may be blood mixed with vomitus, or the vomit may resemble coffee grounds, a sign of upper GI bleeding. A sample of the latter may be brought to the hospital to be tested for the presence of blood. Blood from the rectum may appear as melena, bright-red blood, or blood mixed with stool. Are there complaints of vaginal bleeding? Are they associated with abnormal pain? Is vaginal bleeding occurring during the menstrual period, or outside the normal cycle? Does the patient think she may be pregnant?

Jaundice: Color can range from a faint yellowish tinge to the sclera to a marked orange color to the skin. Jaundice often indicates liver or gallbladder disease. Did the patient notice jaundice? If so, when?

Nausea and vomiting: Ask the patient if there was any nausea or vomiting. When did vomiting begin? Is it associated with pain? What was present in the vomitus: undigested food, mucus, bile, coffee-grounds material, blood? Was there a fecal smell to the vomitus, signifying a lower GI obstruction?

Distention: Does the patient complain of fullness in the abdomen and an increase in girth? On inspection, is there noticeable distention? Distention can occur from buildup of fluid and from obstruction of the GI tract **(Figure 22-15).**

Chills and fever: The patient may complain about fever or chills, which could signify an infectious process.

Urinary symptoms: Are there problems related to the urinary tract, such as dysuria (burning on urination), hematuria (blood mixed with urine), frequency (urge to urinate more often than usual), polyuria (frequent urination with large amounts of urine)? (Note that diabetic ketoacidosis can present as abdominal pain.) Does the patient complain of a discharge from the penis or vagina?

Cardiopulmonary symptoms: Does the patient have complaints that may be associated with the cardiopulmonary system, especially in the face of upper abdominal pain? Remember that pneumonia can cause abdominal pain, particularly in children. Also remember that myocardial infarction can present with abdominal pain and vomiting.

Allergies and Medications

Is there a history of allergies? Is the patient taking medications for abdominal problems? What other medications is the patient taking?

Pertinent Past Medical History

The past medical history may be informative. In addition to the usual questions about heart disease, chronic obstructive pulmonary disease, hypertension, and diabetes, does the patient have a history of abdominal disease, such as liver disease, ulcers, or urinary tract infection? Has the patient ever had abdominal surgery? Does the patient have a history of abdominal aneurysm?

Has the patient had similar episodes in the past? If so, what was the diagnosis?

Last Oral Intake

When was the last time the patient ate or drank something?

Events Leading up to Present Illness

If the patient has multiple complaints or associated complaints, establish a brief chronology of events and further develop additional complaints with the OPQRST approach outlined above.

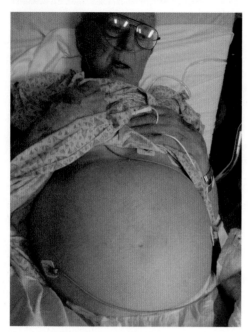

Figure 22-15 An example of abdominal distension.

Scenario Follow-up

Quick thinking and rapid occlusion of the sucking chest wound stopped the development of a tension pneumothorax. The patient was transferred to a Level I trauma center, where he was immediately taken to surgery. The patient is expected to make a full recovery.

Summary

The assessment and management of chest and abdominal emergencies represent a unique challenge to the EMT. Because both the thoracic and the abdominal cavity have the ability to store great quantities of blood, you must maintain a high index of suspicion about internal bleeding. Monitor vital signs frequently; initiate rapid transport when early signs of hypovolemic shock appear, and consider the mechanism to predict injury.

Serious injuries may be present within the thoracic cavity that require interpretation of signs elicited during the focused (secondary) assessment. Special findings include a sucking chest wound, paradoxical motion during breathing, deviation of the trachea, distended neck veins, and decreased or absent breath sounds. Seal an open pneumothorax with an occlusive dressing sealed on three sides. A flail chest may require splinting and positioning to reduce paradoxical movement during exhalation. Findings indicating tension pneumothorax or pericardial tamponade require rapid transport to hospital intervention. Supplemental oxygen, careful assisted ventilations, and repeated monitoring of any changes are basic and fundamental aspects of care.

For patients with abdominal emergencies, the EMT should look for signs of internal bleeding. The focused (secondary) assessment should determine any tenderness, rigidity, or firmness of the abdomen as well as any abdominal distention. Eviscerated bowel is covered with a moistened sterile dressing and then covered to prevent drying and further exposure to the environment. With medical patients, abdominal emergencies can involve serious bleeding as well as signs of an acute abdomen, including tenderness, guarding, and positioning to avoid movement of the abdomen.

Skills

Skill | 22-1   *Management of an Open Chest Wound*

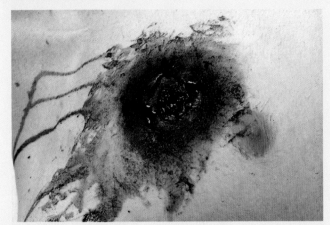

1. Assess the open wound on the chest wall.

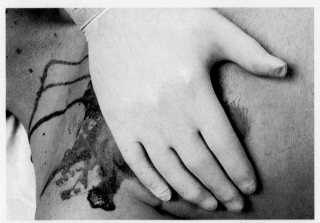

2. If an airtight dressing is not immediately available, cover the hole with a gloved hand.

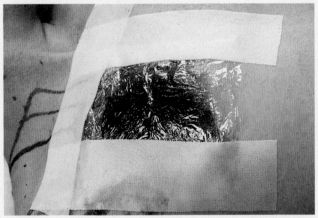

3. Apply an airtight dressing of plastic wrap. Ask the patient to exhale forcefully; place an occlusive dressing over the wound. Tape the dressing on three sides. This prevents air from entering the wound during inspiration (dressing is sucked against wound) but allows air to exit during expiration.

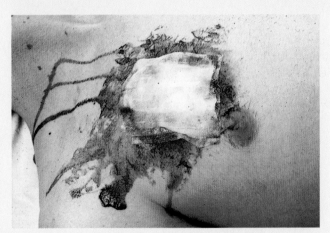

4. Apply an airtight dressing of gauze. Place gauze so that it extends at least 2 inches (5 cm) in each direction over the wound. Place the sterile side of the aluminum foil over the gauze, and tape on three sides. Some protocols advocate taping all four sides. In either case, the patient with a "sealed" open pneumothorax must be watched carefully for signs of a tension pneumothorax. If such signs occur, loosen the seal during expiration to allow release of built-up air pressure.

Skill | 22-2   *Management of an Evisceration*

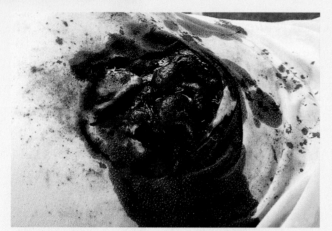

1. Assess the evisceration.

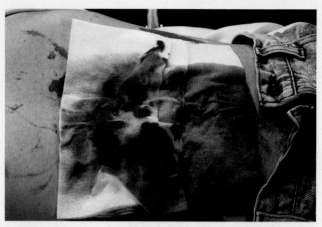

2. Place a moistened multitrauma dressing around the exposed viscera.

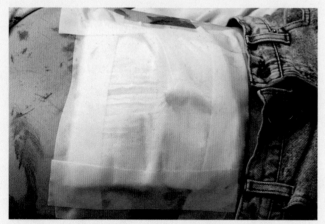

3. Cover with a dry, sterile dressing and tape in place.

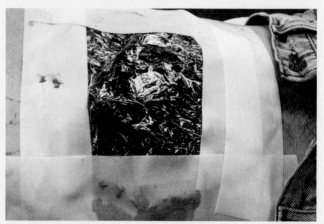

4. Cover the exposed viscera with plastic wrap, and tape completely around the border of the dressing to ensure an airtight seal.

The Bottom Line

Learning Checklist

✓ The chest and abdomen are large cavities that can hold the entire blood volume and mask severe internal bleeding.

✓ Signs of rib fractures include pleuritic chest pain, splinting of the chest wall, and bruising on the chest wall.

✓ A flail chest is defined as two or more ribs fractured in two or more places.

✓ Flail chest is treated by splinting the chest and providing positive-pressure ventilation.

✓ Pneumothorax (air in the pleural space) may be traumatic or spontaneous and open or closed.

✓ Signs of pneumothorax include open chest wound, pleuritic chest pain (pain during breathing), subcutaneous emphysema, dyspnea, absent or diminished breath sounds on the affected side, and signs of inadequate breathing.

✓ Open chest wounds are treated by applying a three-sided occlusive dressing to the wound to prevent air from entering the pleural space, while allowing air to escape, and preventing tension pneumothorax.

✓ Tension pneumothorax is caused by air trapped in the pleural space. Tension can be exerted on the diaphragm, heart, and great vessels, which can obstruct venous return and result in shock.

✓ Signs of tension pneumothorax include dyspnea, absent or diminished breath sounds on the affected side, distended neck veins, tracheal shift, and other signs of shock.

✓ If an occlusive dressing is applied and a tension pneumothorax develops, remove the dressing until signs of tension are alleviated.

✓ Pericardial tamponade is caused by a buildup of blood or fluid in the space between the heart and the sac around the heart, causing pressure and obstruction of venous return.

✓ Signs of pericardial tamponade include distended neck veins, narrow pulse pressure (minimal difference between the systolic and diastolic pressures), and signs of shock.

✓ Eviscerations are treated by placing a dressing moistened with sterile water around the bowel and covering with a dry dressing.

✓ The position of transport for patients with abdominal injuries is dictated by the need for airway management, spinal immobilization, and the position of comfort. Patients with abdominal pain often prefer to be placed supine with legs flexed.

✓ An acute abdomen is nontraumatically induced abdominal pain of recent onset.

✓ Acute abdomen can be caused by the following:
  ✓ Intestinal obstruction
  ✓ Infection
  ✓ Hemorrhage
  ✓ Perforation
  ✓ Renal failure

Key Terms

Cardiac tamponade See *pericardial tamponade.*

Cholecystitis Inflammation or low-grade chronic infection of the gallbladder.

Cirrhosis Scarring of the liver.

Diverticulum Outpouching of the inner wall of bowel tissue into the muscular layer of the bowel; plural *diverticula.*

Evisceration Spilling of the abdominal contents through a wound in the abdominal wall.

Flail chest Condition in which two or more ribs are fractured in two or more places, resulting in dissociation of part of the chest wall structure.

Hemothorax Bleeding within the pleural cavity.

Hepatitis Inflammation of the liver.

Open pneumothorax A pneumothorax in which the chest wall is punctured; also called a *sucking chest wound.*

Paradoxical motion Type of breathing in which the chest wall moves opposite to normal chest movement; also called *paradoxical breathing.*

Pericardial tamponade Mechanical compression of the heart by large amounts of fluid or blood within the pericardial space; also called *cardiac tamponade.*

Peritonitis Inflammation of the peritoneum.

Pneumothorax Air within the pleural space.

Pyelonephritis Severe infection of the kidney.

Tension pneumothorax Air trapped in the pleural space caused by a one-way valve effect created on the chest wall or lung wall; results in increased intrathoracic pressure, respiratory failure, and shock.

Review Questions

1. Which of the following is the most common breath sound associated with a tension pneumothorax?
   a. Diminished or absent on one side
   b. Wheezes on one side
   c. Rhonchi on one side
   d. Friction rub on one side

2. A patient with a penetrating wound to the chest who becomes increasingly short of breath, cyanotic, and unresponsive after application of an airtight dressing, and also exhibits distended neck veins, most likely has which of the following?
   a. Pericardial tamponade
   b. Flail chest
   c. Traumatic asphyxia
   d. Tension pneumothorax

3. What is the primary sign of a flail chest?
   a. Absent breath sounds on both sides
   b. Paradoxical movement of the chest wall
   c. Bleeding from the airway
   d. Hematoma over the floating ribs

4. Which of the following is the best treatment for a flail chest?
   a. Splinting the chest wall
   b. Positive-pressure ventilation
   c. Oxygen by nasal cannula
   d. Both a and b

5. Which of the following would be the best treatment for an evisceration?
   a. Inserting the bowel back into the abdominal cavity.
   b. Applying a moistened dressing, covered with a dry dressing.
   c. Applying a petroleum jelly dressing over the exposed bowel.
   d. Taping the exposed bowel to the abdominal wall.

6. During the focused (secondary) assessment, you note a wound at the lower margin of the rib cage that is bubbling and creating a sucking sound. Which body cavity do you believe is penetrated?
   a. Abdominal cavity
   b. Chest cavity
   c. Pelvic cavity
   d. Retroperitoneal cavity

7. Your patient complains of abdominal pain and denies trauma. The pain is knifelike in the upper abdomen and radiates to the back. The patient is a known alcoholic. Which of the following would most likely explain these symptoms?
   a. Pancreatitis
   b. Appendicitis
   c. Epididymitis
   d. Diverticulitis

For Further Review

In the Student Workbook

- Multiple-choice questions
- Fill-in-the-blank questions
- Short-answer questions
- True/false questions
- Case scenario questions

On Evolve

- Anatomy challenge
- Weblinks
- Lecture notes
- Exercises

Learning Objectives

Cognitive Objectives

- Discuss the emergency medical care considerations for a patient with a penetrating chest injury.
- Differentiate the care of an open wound to the chest from an open wound to the abdomen.
- Establish the relationship between airway management and the patient with chest injuries.
- State the emergency medical care considerations for a patient with an open wound to the abdomen.
- Relate anatomy to the mechanism of injury to determine potential organ damage.
- State the emergency medical care considerations for a patient with nontraumatic, acute abdominal distress.
- Recognize a patient with an acute abdomen.
- Discuss the emergency medical care considerations for a patient with acute abdomen.

Psychomotor Objectives

- Demonstrate the steps in the emergency medical care of a patient with an open chest wound.
- Demonstrate the steps in the emergency medical care of a patient with open abdominal wounds.
- Demonstrate the steps in the emergency medical care of a patient with acute abdomen.

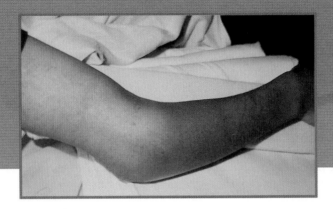

23 Musculoskeletal Care

CHAPTER OUTLINE

Anatomy and Physiology
Musculoskeletal Injuries
Skills

Scenario

You respond to the scene of a motorcycle crash. The rider, a 30-year-old woman, has been thrown over the handlebars. She is lying on her back, moaning in pain. Primary (initial) assessment reveals that the patient is alert and has rapid, deep breathing; a rapid, thready pulse; and pale, cool, clammy skin. There are abrasions on both forearms and the forehead and tenderness across the left lower lateral chest wall. On palpation of the pelvis, you note movement as you gently palpate the iliac bones. The patient's blood pressure is 90/70 mm Hg. You immobilize the neck, place the patient on a long spine board, and initiate transport to the trauma center.

Injuries to bones, ligaments, tendons, and muscles account for a significant number of all traumas. Motor vehicle crashes, falls, and sports injuries are common causes. Elderly persons are particularly susceptible to fractures from weakening of the bones with age. Musculoskeletal injuries are usually very painful and can result in swelling and deformity, temporary or permanent loss of function, and even death from the complications associated with fractures.

Bones provide support and protection for the body. The forces required to break or fracture a bone are usually more than sufficient to result in damage to nearby or underlying soft tissues and organs. Complications of musculoskeletal injuries include hemorrhage and damage to nearby vessels and nerves.

A working knowledge of anatomy aids recognition of injuries and their complications. Establishing the mechanism of injury and relating it to anatomic structures provide the first clues to evaluation and treatment. Musculoskeletal injuries often occur in patterns, and recognition of injury to one part of the body often raises suspicion that an associated injury in another part of the body has also occurred. For example, an injury of the heel after a fall alerts the emergency medical technician (EMT) to the possibility of an associated injury to the vertebral column. A search for complications of musculoskeletal trauma, such as neurologic and vascular injury and serious hemorrhage, is also part of the assessment.

Obvious deformities may distract the EMT, causing more serious or associated injuries to be overlooked. As an EMT, you should remember that life-threatening conditions take priority. Treatment of musculoskeletal injuries is directed toward immobilizing the injured part to prevent pain and further injury. Techniques used to immobilize and support injured extremities include rigid splinting, traction splinting, use of sling and swathe, and use of the long spine board and other materials.

LEARNING OBJECTIVES
- Describe the function of the muscular system.
- Describe the function of the skeletal system.
- List the major bones or bone groupings of the spinal column, the thorax, the upper extremities, and the lower extremities.

Anatomy and Physiology

Skeletal System

The skeletal system provides a framework for support and protection of the body. Muscles are attached to the skeletal system to allow movement of one part relative to another. The size and functions of bones vary widely, ranging from the tiny bones of the middle ear, which transmit sound waves for hearing, to large bones such as the femur, which must support the body's weight during walking and running. There are 206 bones that make up the skeleton. Many of these bones are discussed in earlier chapters; see Chapter 4 for review of the skull, face, spinal column, and thoracic cage.

The skull and face, the spinal column, and the thoracic cavity are collectively referred to as the *axial skeleton*. The axial skeleton is designed primarily for support and protection of the internal organs. Some movement occurs within the vertebral column. The upper and lower extremities, the shoulder, and the pelvis make up the *appendicular skeleton* which is primarily concerned with movement and support of the body in the erect position. The appendicular skeleton also protects the internal organs within the pelvis.

The skeletal system is composed of connective tissue. The major connective tissues include bone, bone marrow, cartilage, ligaments, and tendons (**Figure 23-1**).

Bone is a calcified connective tissue that gives strength to the skeleton. *Bone marrow,* inside the bone, is the source of blood cells. *Cartilage* is the softer precursor to the bony skeleton in the fetal stage, when formation and calcification of bone begin. Cartilage persists at the sites of bone growth (growth plates, or *epiphyses*) and within the bones during childhood. At the end of adolescence, after growth of the bones is essentially complete, the cartilage within the growth centers becomes calcified as well. Cartilage persists in adult life, until old age, as the costal cartilage along the anterior ends of the ribs. Cartilage is present throughout life at the joints of two or more bones, where it serves as a cushion and provides a friction-free surface. The special cartilage found at joints or articulations of bones is called *articular cartilage*. Cartilage is also found within the respiratory tract and in the ears, where it gives support to such structures as the larynx, trachea, bronchi, nose, and pinna (outer ear).

Ligaments are tough connective tissue bands that bind one bone to another at joints. Many extremity injuries involve the tearing or stretching of ligaments, resulting in instability of the joints. Injuries to ligaments are called *sprains*.

Tendons are tough connective tissue bands that connect muscle to bone and serve to pull or move bones as muscles contract. Tendons can be overstretched or torn after trauma or violent contractions of muscles. Injuries to the muscles or tendons are called *strains*.

Muscular System

The *muscles* are tissues capable of contraction or shortening. They are attached and designed in such a way that the power of their contraction results in movement. The three types of muscle include voluntary (skeletal), involuntary (smooth), and cardiac.

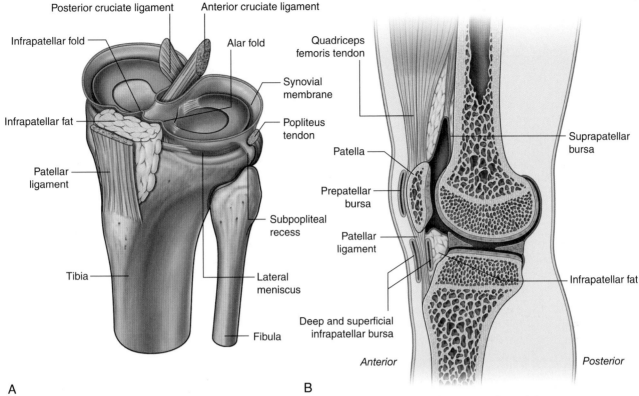

Figure 23-1 Synovial membrane of the knee joint and associated bursae. **A,** Superolateral view; patella and femur not shown. **B,** Paramedial sagittal section through the knee. *From Drake RL et al:* Gray's anatomy for students, *2005, Oxford, Churchill Livingstone.*

Contraction of the *voluntary muscles* results in movement of the skeleton. Voluntary muscles are under the individual's conscious control. They are attached to bone directly or by tendons in such a way as to allow movement of one bone relative to another.

Contraction of the *smooth muscles* results in automatic functions such as peristalsis, which causes movement of food through the digestive tract. Involuntary or smooth muscles are not under an individual's conscious control. They are found within the internal organs such as blood vessels, the digestive and urinary systems, and the respiratory system.

Cardiac muscle is similar in structure to skeletal muscle. However, it functions automatically to pump blood with each heartbeat. It is also not under an individual's conscious control. Instead, cardiac muscle functions under control of its own pacemaker and is directed by the involuntary nervous system.

Extremities

A working knowledge of major bones and joints is useful. By palpating the major bones and joints and thinking about their normal alignment and movement, it will be easier to detect deformity and abnormal function when you assess patients. Although you are not expected to memorize the name of every bone, acquiring a growing vocabulary of the major bones and their *articulation* (joining one with another) will improve your ability to assess and communicate.

Upper Extremities

The upper extremities consist of the shoulder, arm, elbow, forearm, wrist, and hand. The shoulder is formed by the articulation (joining) of the humerus with the scapula and receives support from attachments between the scapula and the clavicle.

Shoulder and Humerus. The shoulder is formed by three bones and the muscles that are attached. The *scapula* (shoulder blade) is an irregularly shaped bone that lies on the upper part of the back. Its acromial process can be felt at the lateral edge of the shoulder. Just below the acromion is the glenoid fossa (cavity), which serves as a shallow socket for articulation with the head of the humerus (**Figure 23-2, A**). The triangular, lower portion of the scapula lies over the posterior ribs, where it is covered by thick muscles, but the medial border is readily seen and felt.

The *clavicle* (collarbone) can be palpated from its attachment to the sternum to its attachment with the acromion. The clavicle serves as the attachment of the upper extremity to the axial skeleton. It is often fractured when forces that exceed the strength of the bone are transmitted from falls on the arm or shoulder.

The *humerus* is the bone of the upper arm (**Figure 23-2, B**). It is a long bone extending from the glenoid process of the scapula, where the rounded head of the humerus forms a ball-and-socket joint. Ball-and-socket joints permit a wide range of motion in all planes. The main portion of the humerus is referred to as the *shaft*. The shaft widens as it nears the elbow to form the surface for articulation with the bones of the forearm.

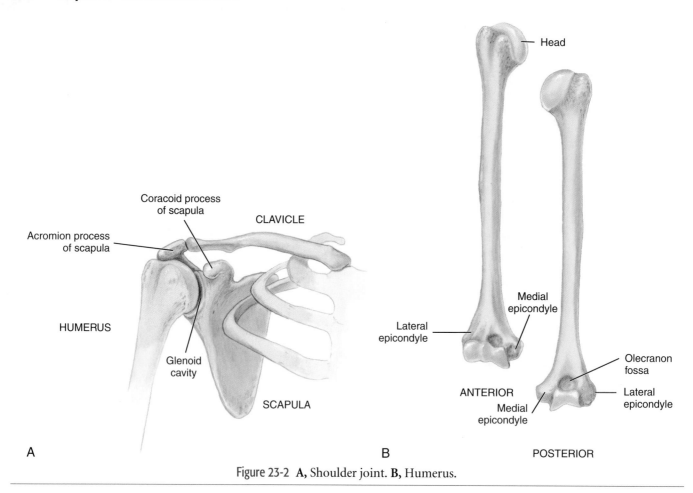

Figure 23-2 **A,** Shoulder joint. **B,** Humerus.

The outer palpable projections of the lower humerus are called the medial and lateral *epicondyles,* which serve as the points of attachment of the muscles of the forearm. Major muscles of the shoulder include the deltoid, pectoralis major, trapezius, and latissimus dorsi.

Elbow and Forearm. The elbow is made up of the articulation of the lower humerus and the proximal ends of the radius and ulna **(Figure 23-3).** The *ulna* is located medially along the length of the forearm. It is a superficial bone and can be palpated along its entire length from the *olecranon,* or posterior point of the elbow, to the wrist. The *radius* lies parallel to the ulna on the lateral aspect or thumb side of the arm. The radius and ulna are joined by ligaments that allow rotation of the radius about the ulnar bone. Just distal to the lateral epicondyle of the humerus, the radial head can be palpated and felt to rotate during rotation of the arm. The *elbow* is a complex joint because the three bones articulate with each other in different ways. The hinge properties of the joint allow for flexion and extension, whereas the other articulations allow for rotation of the forearm.

The muscles moving the forearm cause flexion, extension, and rotation. The principal muscle that flexes the arm is the biceps. The major muscle extending the arm is the triceps.

Wrist and Hand. The wrist is composed of eight small bones, called *carpal bones,* in two rows of four **(Figure 23-4).** These bones articulate with the radius and the ulna proximally and with the metacarpals distally. The *metacarpals* consist of five bones that extend from the wrist to the knuckles, where they articulate with the first row of finger bones *(phalanges).* The wrist is a complex joint that allows for flexion, extension, abduction, adduction, and circumduction (a circular motion).

Lower Extremities

Pelvis and Femur. The *pelvis* is a ringlike structure consisting of the sacrum and the coccyx posteriorly, the pubic symphysis anteriorly, and three fused bones (ilium, ischium, and pubis) making up each side **(Figure 23-5).** The *ilium* is a winglike bone forming the superior lateral aspect of the pelvis; its uppermost portion is known as the *iliac crest.*

The *ischium* forms the posterior portion, and the *ischial tuberosity* (protuberance) bears the weight of the body in the sitting position. It is palpable with the thigh flexed and buttock relaxed. It is the site of placement for the proximal portion of the traction splint.

The *pubis* is composed of a body and superior and inferior pubis rami.

The ilium, ischium, and pubis join together at the *acetabulum,* which is the socket for the hip joint. The pelvis protects the internal organs in the pelvic cavity and supports the weight of the body. The body's weight is transmitted to each femur when a person is standing or to the ischial tuberosities when one is sitting.

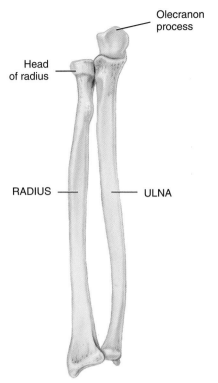

Figure 23-3 Radius and ulna.

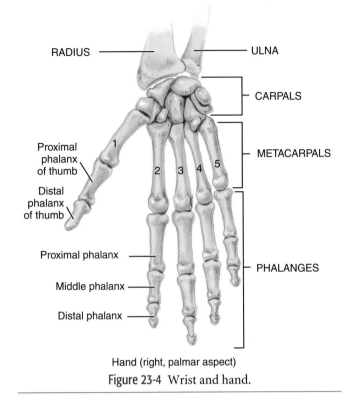

Hand (right, palmar aspect)

Figure 23-4 Wrist and hand.

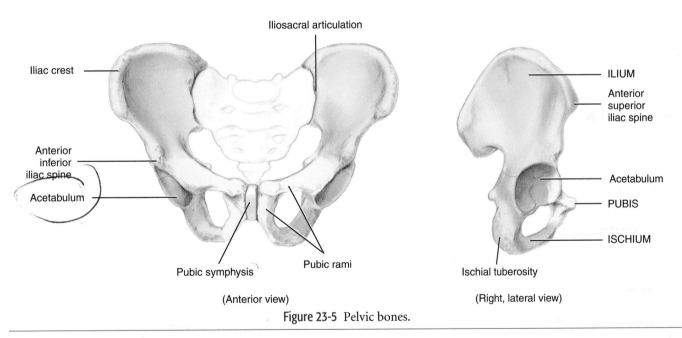

(Anterior view)

(Right, lateral view)

Figure 23-5 Pelvic bones.

The *femur* is the longest and strongest bone in the body (**Figure 23-6**). It has a rounded head, which articulates with the acetabulum to form the hip joint, a ball-and-socket joint. The femoral neck extends for about 2 inches (5 cm) and attaches the head of the shaft of the femur at the greater and lesser *trochanters,* which are projections of bone serving as attachments for muscles. The shaft of the femur widens distally before articulation at the knee joint, where you can palpate the medial and lateral *condyles,* which are prominent surfaces whose surface meets the condyles of the tibia to form the knee joint.

Knee and Lower Leg. The *tibia* is the major weight-bearing bone of the lower leg. It is widened both proximally and distally for articulation at the knee and ankle joints (**Figure 23-7**). The tibia runs anteriorly and superficially along the entire lower leg. Proximally, the medial and lateral tibial condyles form a surface for articulation with the femoral condyles. Strong ligaments hold the joint together. At the knee, the *patella* (kneecap), a small flat bone, is easily palpable anteriorly. It is contained within the tendon on the quadriceps muscle. The knee joint is a hinge joint permitting flexion and extension and some rotation when the knee is in the flexed position (see Figure 23-1).

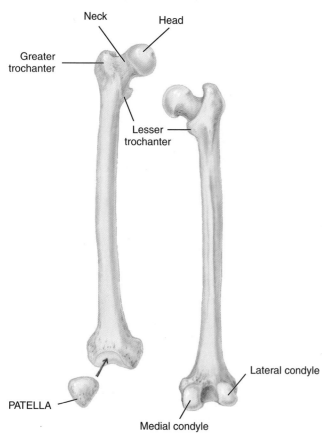

FEMUR and PATELLA (right)

Figure 23-6 Femur.

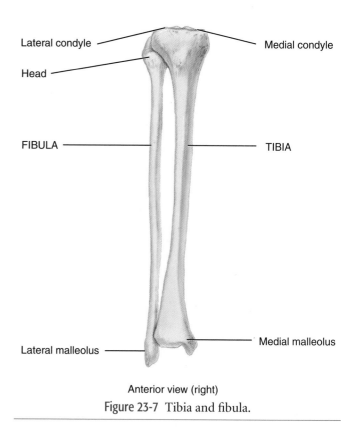

Anterior view (right)

Figure 23-7 Tibia and fibula.

The *fibula* is a smaller long bone running parallel, lateral, and posterior to the tibia (see Figure 23-7). The proximal head of the fibula articulates with the tibia and can be palpated on the lateral and posterior aspect of the lower leg just below the knee. It is not a weight-bearing bone but serves as a point of attachment for muscle and forms part of the ankle joint.

Ankle and Foot. The bones of the foot include seven tarsal bones, five metatarsal bones, and 14 phalanges (**Figure 23-8**). The ankle joint is formed by articulation of the tibia and fibula and the talus bone (one of the tarsals). The *talus* rests on the *calcaneus,* or heel bone, and is attached to the rest of the foot through the other five tarsal bones, transmitting the weight of the body to the foot. Ligaments attach the palpable lateral and medial malleoli to the talus and calcaneus. The primary movement at the ankle is flexion and extension. The articulation with the talus bone permits other complex motions of the ankle and foot.

Extending from the tarsal bones are the metatarsal bones and phalanges. The foot functions as a support for the body's weight during standing and acts as a springboard during walking and running.

Major Muscles. Major muscles of the lower limb include the gluteus maximus, quadriceps, hamstrings, gastrocnemius, and tibialis anterior. The *gluteus maximus* extends from the pelvis to the femur. It extends and abducts the thigh and rotates it laterally. Flexion and adduction of the thigh are functions of adductor muscles extending from the pubis, ilium, and lower vertebrae to the femur. Extension of the leg is accomplished by

the *quadriceps,* four muscles inserted by a common tendon on the tibia. The quadriceps, with its muscular thickness that extends from the ilium to the tibia, also helps protect the thigh. Flexion of the lower leg is accomplished by the hamstrings, extending from the ischium and femur to the tibia. Dorsiflexion (upward flexion) of the foot is accomplished by the tibialis anterior extending from the tibia to the foot. Plantar flexion (downward movement) of the foot is accomplished by the gastrocnemius and the soleus extending from the condyles of the femur and proximal tibia and fibula to the calcaneus. (See Figure 4-16.)

LEARNING OBJECTIVE
- Differentiate between an open and a closed painful, swollen, deformed extremity.

Musculoskeletal Injuries

Injuries to the musculoskeletal system include fractures, sprains, strains, and dislocations. A **fracture** is defined as a break in the continuity of bone. This break may be *complete,* with the two ends widely separated, or *incomplete,* with a hairline crack along a portion of the bone. Fractures can be classified as closed or open. A *closed fracture* has no break in the skin over the fracture site, and the fracture is not open to the external environment. *Open fractures* are exposed to the external environment because the skin above the site has been broken. Open fractures carry the risk of infection and should be covered with a sterile dressing. Open fractures can result from penetrating wounds, lacerations from crush injuries to a limb, or sharp bone fragments tearing through the surrounding soft tissue and skin (**Figure 23-9**).

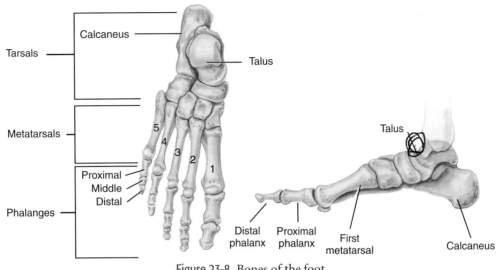

Figure 23-8 Bones of the foot.

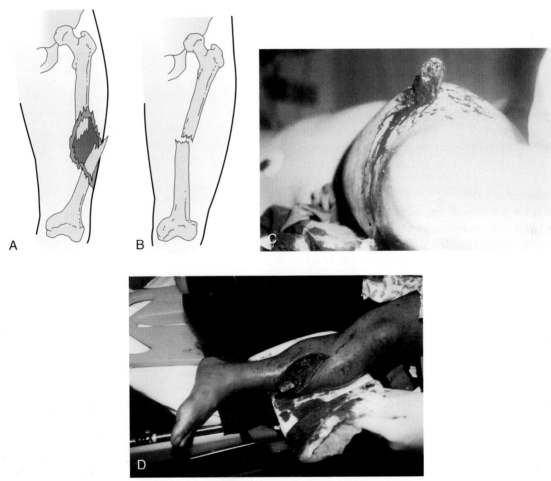

Figure 23-9 **A,** Open fracture. **B,** Closed fracture. **C,** Motorcycle rider with open fracture of femur. **D,** Open fracture of lower leg.

Sprains are injuries to ligaments, usually resulting from stretching forces. **Strains** are injuries to muscles or their tendons, again usually from overstretching or violent contractions. Sprains and strains may be minor, with only overstretching of some of the fibers, or major, resulting in complete disruption of the ligament or tendon. A **dislocation** is a displacement of the bones in a joint from their normal anatomic position. For a dislocation to occur, stretching or tearing of the joint ligaments must take place as well. Dislocations can be associated with fractures, sprains, and strains. The forces causing these injuries are similar in many cases, as are many of the signs and symptoms.

In prehospital care, a painful, swollen, deformed extremity is treated as if a significant bony or soft tissue injury exists.

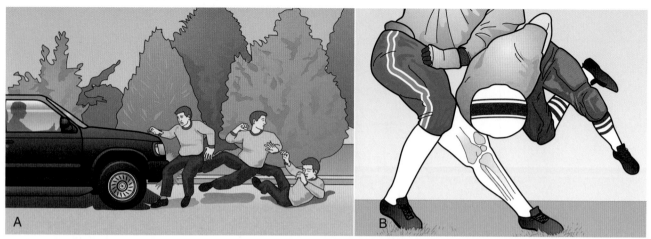

Figure 23-10 A, Direct force. A bumper striking a pedestrian is an example of a common mechanism causing direct injury to the tibia and other body parts. **B,** Direct force from sports injury. Ligaments of the knee may be injured when the leg in a normally immovable position (front foot fixed in ground) has an overpowering force (in this case a blocker) applied against it.

Mechanism of Injury

The mechanism of injury can help you predict the location and type of musculoskeletal injury. Reconstructing the mechanism of injury is an important step in assessing any trauma patient. The mechanism of injury may generate a high level of suspicion of certain types and patterns of injuries. For example, you would suspect that the unrestrained passenger in a front-end collision would have injuries to the head, neck, and chest because the head and thorax are thrown against the windshield and dashboard. Furthermore, as a knee hits the dashboard, force is transmitted from the knee along the femur to the hip and pelvis, and a search for injury along the line of transmitted force is indicated. Always include the mechanism of injury in the prehospital care record and communicate it to the hospital staff. This information helps the staff in their search for and treatment of both direct and associated injuries.

Forces that cause fractures can be direct or indirect. Examples of *direct forces* applied to a bone include a vehicle bumper striking the tibia of a pedestrian, a gunshot wound shattering a bone, a falling person landing on both feet and breaking the heel bones, or sports injuries (**Figure 23-10**).

Indirect forces are usually forces that are transmitted along the axes of bones, resulting in an injury at a location other than the point of impact (**Figure 23-11**). For example, a person falling on an outstretched hand may have a fracture of any of the bones of the upper extremity because different transmitted forces are generated according to the exact position of the hand and arm at the time of impact (**Figure 23-12**). Another example of indirect force is a twisting force. Such an injury can occur, for example, when a skater catches one of the blades in the ice while doing a spin. The planted blade acts as a fixation point while the leg continues to rotate, transmitting a twisting force along the axis of the bones (**Figure 23-13**). Another indirect force that can cause fractures is the violent contraction of muscles, which tears off the bony attachment.

Case in Point

A 10-year-old boy is crying on the sidewalk and holding his right arm. He fell backward off his skateboard and tried to break the fall with his right hand. He has abrasions over the palm of the right hand and a deformity of the right elbow with tenderness and swelling.

Fractures of the upper extremity because of falls on the outstretched hand are common in children. The location of the fracture varies with the position of the body and extremity at the time of impact. Obtaining an accurate description of the mechanism of injury is useful in understanding the physical findings and making an accurate diagnosis.

Assessment

As with any assessment, be sure to use appropriate personal precautions with musculoskeletal injuries. During the scene size-up, determine the potential mechanism of injury by observing the immediate environment and briefly questioning the patient and bystanders. As always, undertake the initial (primary) assessment while considering the possible presence of spinal injuries. Assessment of the airway, breathing, circulation (ABCs), control of bleeding, and identification of other life-threatening conditions, such as open chest wounds and shock, take priority over fractures. Do not become distracted by a grotesquely angulated or deformed extremity. Life-threatening conditions always come first and in some cases may indicate rapid transport, with the patient immobilized to a long spine board, along with primary life support measures.

Begin the focused (secondary) assessment (patient history and physical examination) by obtaining more information about the mechanism of injury and the conditions immediately surrounding the injury. It is helpful to determine the position of an injured automobile passenger, whether a seat belt was worn or an airbag was inflated, the speed of impact, the height from which a patient fell, and the position of the body on impact. A history of events immediately preceding an injury may point to medical conditions that might have caused the incident. For

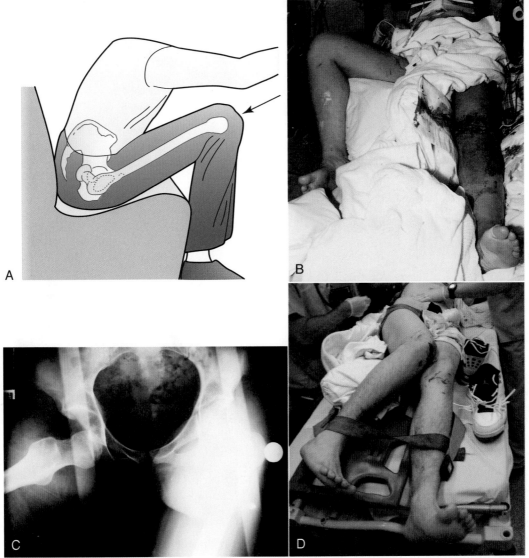

Figure 23-11 A, Indirect force. The knees strike the dashboard, and the force from the dashboard is transmitted along the axis of the bone. The bone can fracture, or in this case, dislocate at the hip. **B,** Patient with dislocation of right hip and laceration to the left leg from striking the dashboard (unrestrained driver and front-end collision). **C,** Radiograph of the patient in C. **D,** Posterior dislocation of hip with internal rotation.

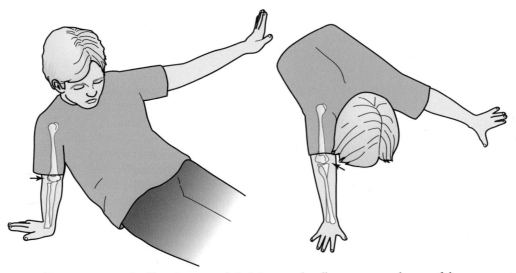

Figure 23-12 Fall on an outstretched hand can result in injury to the elbow or to any bones of the upper extremity.

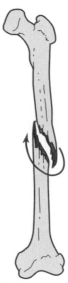

Figure 23-13 Twisting force transmitted along axis of a bone resulting in a spiral fracture.

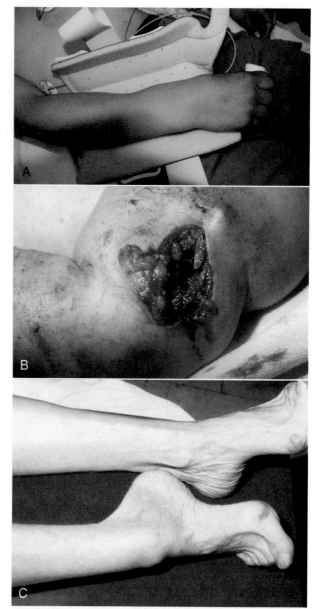

Figure 23-14 A, Deformity of wrist. **B,** Deformity and protuberance of bone end against soft tissue. **C,** Deformity in an elderly woman resulting from ankle fracture dislocation caused by a fall off the curb.

example, did a patient trip and fall, or become dizzy, lose consciousness, and then fall? Following a head-to-toe survey approach ensures that adequate attention is paid to the thorax, abdomen, and spine. You should open or cut away clothing, if necessary, to visualize the soft tissues and inspect the patient for abrasions, bruises, deformities, and other signs of injury (DCAP/BTLS: *d*eformities, *c*ontusions, *a*brasions, *p*unctures or *p*enetrations, *b*urns, *t*enderness, *l*acerations, and *s*welling). Patterns of skin wounds and the nature of the injury may help you visualize the forces experienced by the patient during the trauma.

Some types of injuries can be anticipated by the mechanism of injury. For example, you can suspect that patients with lap belt injuries may have a compression injury to the abdominal organs, bruising of the abdominal wall, and a spinal injury from hyperflexion of the lower spine.

Signs and Symptoms

Pain and Tenderness. Pain is probably the most common symptom of a bone or joint injury. Sometimes the pain is referred distal or proximal to the site of the injury, so examination of the entire extremity is essential. For example, problems with the hip sometime present with a complaint of pain in the knee.

Deformity or Angulation. The angulation of long bones, protuberance of the bone end against the soft tissues, and overriding or separation of bone fragments by opposing muscles can result in visible and palpable deformities (**Figure 23-14**).

Swelling and Discoloration. Fluid or blood loss at the site of injury can result in swelling or discoloration of the affected part. This can be an early sign or it may not be apparent for some time after injury. By comparing extremities, you can gauge the extent of swelling (**Figure 23-15**).

Loss of Use. Loss of function of a skeletal part occurs with injury. This can result from pain on attempted movement or gross disruption of bones, ligaments, or tendons. Therefore, you should never attempt to force movement when a patient does

not voluntarily move a limb. Other reasons for loss of function include nerve or vascular injury, making assessment of nerve and vascular function distal to an injury essential.

Grating or Crepitus. During palpation, you may note a grating sensation or sound (**crepitus**) indicating bone fragments rubbing against one another. You should not deliberately attempt to elicit this finding but should recognize its significance if you encounter it during the initial palpation.

Exposed Bone. Bone ends protruding through the skin are an obvious sign of an open fracture (**Figure 23-16**). However, pain and tenderness are often the only signs of a fracture.

Joint Locked into Position or Dislocation. A *dislocation* is a complete or partial separation of the bones in a joint, resulting in

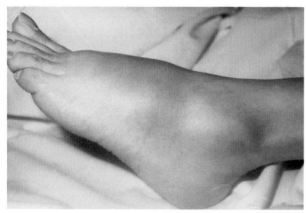

Figure 23-15 Swelling and discoloration of foot and distal fibula.

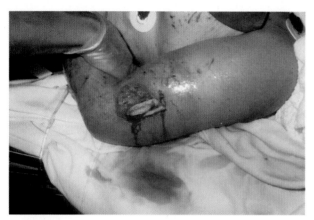

Figure 23-16 Open fracture with exposed bone ends.

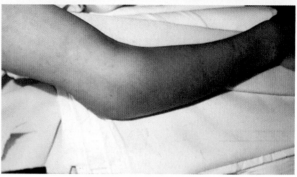

Figure 23-17 Dislocation of elbow with resulting deformity.

Table 23-1	Average Blood Loss with a Closed Fracture	
Fracture Site	**Amount of Blood Loss (mL)**	
Radius or ulna	250-500	
Humerus	500-750	
Pelvis	1500-3000	
Femur	1000-2000	
Tibia and fibula	500-1000	

Associated Injuries

Many associated injuries and complications can occur with musculoskeletal injuries.

Bleeding. *Bleeding can be a life-threatening complication of fractures,* especially if there are multiple or open fractures. Fractures of the pelvis and femur are particularly serious in terms of associated blood loss. **Table 23-1** shows the range of blood loss from certain closed fractures.

Case in Point

A 40-year-old motorcycle rider was thrown forward against the handlebars after a collision. You find the patient moaning in pain with a rapid pulse and blood pressure of 86/60 mm Hg. His airway is open, and breathing is adequate and rapid. On inspection you note deformity of the left wrist, and on gentle compression of the lateral aspect of the pelvis you note movement as the patient moans in pain. You are 30 minutes from the nearest hospital, and there is no medevac available. You apply the pneumatic antishock garment (PASG) as an air splint for the pelvis and initiate transport.

Movement of the pelvis means the pelvic ring is broken. These fractures are unstable and can result in significant blood loss. Limiting movement of the pelvis during transport may minimize further bleeding.

---

loss of the normal anatomic alignment (**Figure 23-17**). A dislocation can result from both direct and indirect injuries. Some patients have recurrent dislocations of the shoulder caused by previous injuries that overstretch the joint structures or from voluntary muscle contraction without any trauma.

Case in Point

An 80-year-old woman is found on the sidewalk, unable to stand. She was walking across the street when she slipped on the edge of a curb and fell. Her right ankle has an obvious deformity.

Elderly patients are more susceptible to fractures from low falls because of *osteoporosis,* which leads to weakening of the bones (see **Figure 23-14,** *C*).

A dislocation may be associated with a fracture, and signs and symptoms of a fracture may be present. The following signs are more specific for dislocation:

- Loss of movement and deformity at a joint, with the joint possibly locked in a deformed position
- Pain and swelling over the joint

Dislocations can occur at any joint, and common sites include the shoulder, elbow, fingers, hip, knee, and ankle.

Vascular Injuries. Vessels can be pinched or torn by bone fragments. Vessels can also be damaged directly by the same force that caused the fracture (especially with such penetrating injuries as gunshot wounds). Vessels can also go into spasm, can be compressed by soft swelling, or can be occluded by clots. Common sites in which fractures or dislocations are associated with vascular injury include the shoulder, elbow, knee, bones of the foot, and temporoparietal region of the skull (middle meningeal artery).

Vascular injuries can result in loss of blood flow to distal tissues as well as blood loss if the vessel is torn. Without early restoration of the blood supply, the limb may be lost. The presence of vascular compromise is determined by assessing the following factors:

- Distal pulses
- Skin color and temperature
- Capillary refilling time
- Pain
- Numbness
- Tingling
- Prickling
- Sensory loss
- Paralysis distal to the injury

One way to remember the signs of ischemia of a limb is to keep in mind the five "P"s: pain, pulselessness, pallor, paresthesia (numbness or tingling, prickling), and paralysis. Always check for vascular compromise before and after applying splints.

Peripheral Nerve Injury. In cases of trauma to an extremity, nerves are injured more often than arteries. Mechanisms similar to those that injure arteries can also cause nerve contusion or complete disruption of a nerve. For example, torn bone ends can tear or pinch the nerve; displaced joints can stretch or compress a nerve; and violent forces, such as gunshot wounds, can cause direct damage (**Figure 23-18**).

Common sites where fractures or dislocations cause disruption of nerves include the clavicle, shoulder, humerus, elbow, wrist, hip and femur, knee, and spinal cord. The signs and symptoms of nerve injury are as follows:

- Numbness
- Pain
- Abnormal sensation (different from that in the other limb)
- Loss of motor ability

Although most fractures are not complicated by nerve or vessel injury, nerve and vascular function must be evaluated in every case. Check for signs of circulation (pulse, temperature, color, and possibly capillary refilling time) and nerve function (sensation and movement) distal to the injury. Continued swelling after an injury or constriction caused by tightly applied splints can cause nerve and vascular problems after the event, so reevaluate the nerve function and vascular status periodically during transport.

Injuries to Internal Organs. Force can be transmitted to underlying organs. For example, fractures of the pelvis may injure organs within the pelvic cavity, such as the bladder, urethra, rectum, lower intestine, and reproductive organs. Injuries to the thorax may cause hemothorax, pneumothorax, or rupture of the spleen and liver.

Management

As mentioned, life-threatening conditions should be managed first. Administer oxygen to a patient with musculoskeletal injury if indicated. You can splint injuries in preparation for transport if appropriate, or you can splint them en route. You can apply cold packs to areas of painful, swollen, deformed extremities to reduce swelling. If applicable, elevate the injured and splinted extremity.

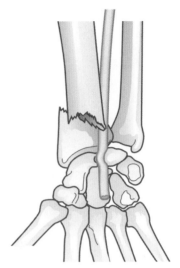

Figure 23-18 Nerve injury caused by fracture and dislocation of a bone.

LEARNING OBJECTIVES
- State the reasons for splinting.
- Explain the rationale for splinting at the scene versus "load and go."
- Explain the rationale for immobilization of a painful, swollen, deformed extremity.
- List the general rules of splinting.
- List the complications of splinting.
- List the emergency medical care for a patient with a painful, swollen, deformed extremity.

Splinting

The goals of management for patients with musculoskeletal injuries are to reduce pain and prevent further injury by immobilizing or splinting the injured part. Minimizing any complications from fractures speeds healing. Splinting prevents the further motion of bone fragments or dislocated joints and thereby minimizes pain and further damage to the surrounding soft tissues. Splinting may also reduce blood loss. Without proper immobilization, broken bone fragments can cause further damage by tearing or pinching surrounding vessels, nerves, muscles, and other soft tissues. In extreme cases, a closed fracture might even be converted to an open fracture if sharp bone fragments move about and tear through overlying skin.

Splinting Principles. Many methods of immobilization and different types of splints are available. Certain principles of management should be adhered to regardless of the specific technique used.

Use a Long Spine Board to Immobilize Patients in Critical Condition. Saving the patient's life is the first priority. Assess and address life-threatening conditions before caring for extremity fractures. In some cases the need for rapid transport may preclude splinting in the field because the time to apply splints may delay treatment for life-threatening conditions. The long spine board should be used for these patients.

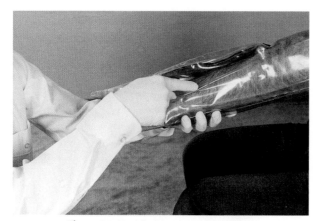

Figure 23-19 Air (pneumatic) splint.

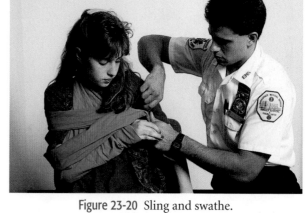

Figure 23-20 Sling and swathe.

When in Doubt, Splint the Injury. Some bony injuries may still allow function and normal motion of the extremity. However, if pain, tenderness, or the mechanism of injury suggests that a bony injury is possible, treat it as such. Do not be misled by the absence of more obvious signs, such as deformity, disability, and crepitus.

Splint before Moving. Whenever possible, patients should be immobilized before moving them. You should attempt to eliminate all unnecessary movement of the patient's injured part. However, hazardous or life-threatening conditions may preclude splinting before movement.

Pad Splints and Remove Clothing. The surface of the splint in contact with the patient should be well padded to avoid pressure points against soft tissues. You should remove or cut away clothing to expose the injured part so that folds of clothing do not act as pressure points beneath a splint. When applying a rigid splint, you should pad all "voids," such as joints, to avoid pressure points.

Immobilize Joints or Bones above and below the Injury. To immobilize a bone effectively, immobilize the joints above and below the injury site. For example, when splinting fractures of the midforearm, immobilize the elbow and wrist. Similarly, to immobilize an injured joint, splint the bones above and below. For example, when splinting a fractured or dislocated elbow, include the humerus and the forearm.

Check and Recheck Nerve and Vascular Function. Check distal pulses, capillary refilling time, skin color and temperature, sensation, and motor function before and after splinting, and record your findings.

Straighten Extremity in Severe Injuries. As a rule, joint injuries are splinted in the position in which they are found. However, if the extremity is cyanotic or lacks a distal pulse, some protocols will allow you to attempt to straighten the extremity. At times, straightening an extremity may restore blood flow by releasing entrapped vessels. If resistance is encountered or if the patient complains of increased pain, however, splint the extremity in the position in which it is found.

Cover Open Wounds. Dress and bandage all open wounds over suspected fractures before splinting.

Treat Protruding Bones. If bone ends are protruding, do not attempt to reintroduce them back in through the wound by traction. Cover protruding bone fragments with a sterile, moistened dressing covered by a dry dressing.

Types of Splints. Several varieties of splints are used to immobilize bony injuries. As an EMT, you should be familiar with the advantages and disadvantages of each type.

Rigid splints are made of a rigid material, such as cardboard, wood, metal, or plastic, and should be well padded. These splints come in lengths of a few inches for fingers to 5 feet for fractures of the lower extremity not requiring traction. They are applied on either side of a fractured extremity and secured with roller bandages or cravats. Rigid splints can be made from readily available materials and also are commercially available both as preformed and ready to apply and as rolls of padded aluminum that can be cut and shaped for application. They are versatile and can be adapted as needed to immobilize angulated fractures.

Pneumatic (air) splints are plastic splints that are filled with air to provide circumferential support to an injured extremity. They come in various lengths and configurations for use on distal upper and lower extremity fractures (**Figure 23-19**). The pneumatic antishock garment (PASG) can serve as an air splint for patients with lower extremity or pelvic fractures in the presence of shock. The air pressure within an air splint must be reevaluated with changes in environmental temperature.

A **sling** is a triangle-shaped bandage that is used to support the weight of the arm, and a **swathe** is a folded triangular bandage or roller bandage used to bind the upper arm to the chest wall. The sling and swathe combination is used in the treatment of most upper extremity injuries as a primary method of immobilization or as an adjunct to splints. A sling and swathe combination can be bought commercially or improvised (**Figure 23-20**).

Traction splints are devices consisting of a metal frame and a pulley system to apply traction to the lower extremity. They range from a simple metal frame used with bandage materials to apply traction to sophisticated commercial devices with self-grip fasteners and mechanical pulleys. Traction splints are used to immobilize fractures of the midthigh (femur) (**Figure 23-21**). The Sager splint can also be used to immobilize fractures of the proximal thigh (check local protocols).

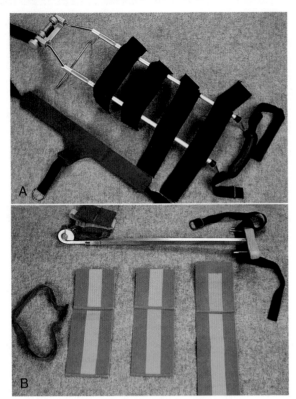

Figure 23-21 **A,** Hare traction splint. **B,** Sager traction splint with ankle hitch and straps.

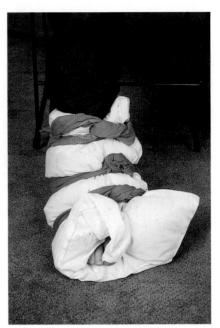

Figure 23-22 Pillow splint.

Case in Point

A young man was thrown off his motorcycle at a high rate of speed. He is alert, is breathing rapidly, and has blood pressure of 100/70 mm Hg and pulse of 120 beats/min. His skin is cool, pale, and diaphoretic. He has multiple abrasions over his left side, and his left midthigh is swollen and tender with angulation. You are 30 minutes from the nearest hospital. You apply a traction splint, which supports and realigns the extremity before loading the patient onto the backboard and beginning transport. The patient maintains his blood pressure during transport.

The traction splint was first developed by Hugh Owen Thomas in the mid-1800s for "enforced, uninterrupted, and prolonged" immobilization to allow fractures of the lower extremity time to heal. The Thomas splint found widespread use in World War I, and mortality from compound fractures of the femur fell from 80% in 1916 to less than 8% in 1918.

With fractures of the femur, traction helps to realign the bone and prevent unwanted motion during transport, and it returns the shape of the thigh to a cylinder, which helps control bleeding. Femoral fracture can result in severe, even fatal, blood loss.

Development of the precursor for the midline traction splint was in response to EMS concerns about patients with femoral fracture requiring prolonged transport in rural Canada. A physician in an outlying rural hospital developed the prototype—a crutch and fishing scale—to maintain immobilization over the long journey to Vancouver. This device currently is known as the Sager traction splint.

Blankets, magazines, cardboard, and other material can be used as an improvised splint to accomplish the objectives of immobilization. The device is less important than the principles of management. A pillow can be used as a splint for an ankle or as an adjunct in the immobilization of dislocations. It can be attached with safety pins, bandages, or cravats (**Figure 23-22**).

Precautions. It is important to learn when and how to apply splints properly and monitor their effectiveness during patient transport. The first consideration is when and where to apply a splint. Again, life-threatening conditions must be treated first. Never delay care for life-threatening injuries to splint an extremity. Rather, immobilize the patient on a long spine board, and provide subsequent care to the limb en route if conditions permit.

An improperly applied splint can aggravate bone or joint injury and compress nerves, tissues, and blood vessels. For example, if the splint is applied too tightly, it can reduce distal circulation. If it is too loose or improperly applied, the bones may not be immobilized and can cause or aggravate tissue, nerve, vessel, or muscle damage from excessive movement.

Techniques. As an EMT, you should be familiar and adept with various splinting techniques to allow treatment of the different types of musculoskeletal injuries encountered in the field (**Table 23-2**). This section describes methods to splint long bones and joints and to apply traction.

Splinting of a long bone can be achieved by applying a rigid splint, air splint, or sling and swathe. The long board splint can be used to immobilize fractures of the knee, tibia, and fibula in the straightened position (**Figure 23-23**). **Skill 23-1** illustrates the application of a rigid splint to the lower extremity.

To immobilize fractures of the midforearm, use a rigid splint extending from the palm of the hand past the medial aspect of the elbow. When the arm is found in a straightened position and a fracture of the forearm or elbow is suspected, the arm can be splinted in the extended position with a rigid splint. **Skill 23-2** illustrates the application of a rigid splint to the forearm in a straightened position.

Fingers are splinted with a flexible aluminum splint or a tongue blade (**Figure 23-24**). The splint can be attached with ½-inch tape or 2-inch roller gauze, taking care not to constrict distal blood flow. Multiple finger fractures may be immobilized with a rigid board splint or air splint.

Table 23-2	Specific Musculoskeletal Injuries*

Bone	Common Mechanisms of Injury	Possible Signs and Symptoms	Treatment
Clavicle	Fall on outstretched arm	Obvious deformity Dropped shoulder Arm held against chest	Sling and swathe
Shoulder injuries	Fall on outstretched hand or direct blow to shoulder	Loss of rounded contour to shoulder Obvious deformity Limited motion	Sling and swathe
Upper arm (humerus)	Fall on outstretched hand	Obvious swelling and deformity	Sling and swathe with rigid splint to medial portion of humerus
Elbow	Fall on outstretched hand	Obvious swelling and deformity	Rigid splint and sling
Forearm and wrist	Fall on outstretched hand; "defensive" protection injury	Deformity	Rigid splint and sling and swathe
Hand	Punch, crush, fall	Deformity, loss of function	Position of function, rigid splint (tongue blade for fingers), sling and swathe
Pelvis	Crush, fall, direct compression	Pain, shock, mobility of pelvic ring on compression	Spine board, PASG if signs of shock present
Dislocated hip	Dashboard injury, direct blow to thigh or hip	Pain and locked joint	Immobilization of one leg to the other with support with pillows and blankets and transport on spine board
Hip injury	Fall	Shortened and externally rotated extremity	Immobilization of one leg to the other with support and transport on spine board
Thigh (femur)	Direct blow, torsion, or indirect forces (e.g., knee to dashboard)	Swelling, deformity, signs of shock	If isolated midthigh, traction; if associated with shock, PASG Check local protocols; note Sager-type splint may be used for proximal thigh fractures in some EMS systems.
Knee	Dashboard, direct blow, fall, sports injury	Deformity, locked, unstable	If straight, rigid splint; if angulated and compromised circulation, attempt to straighten; if locked, splint in the position in which found.
Lower leg	Direct blow (e.g., bumper injury) or twisting force	Deformity	Rigid splint
Ankle and foot	Fall, twisting	Pain, deformity	Pillow splint

*All musculoskeletal injuries can present with painful, swollen, and deformed extremities. The mechanism of injury, signs and symptoms, and treatments are related to the location of the injured part.
PASG, Pneumatic antishock garment.

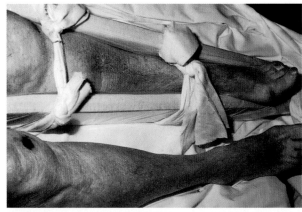

Figure 23-23 Fracture of lower leg immobilized with long board splint.

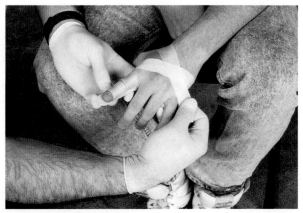

Figure 23-24 Applying a finger splint. Extend a tongue blade or commercial finger splint from the tip of the finger to the heel of the hand, and tape in place.

Joint injuries can be immobilized in the straightened or angulated position. If the extremity is cyanotic or lacks pulses, you should attempt to straighten the extremity. If you encounter resistance, you should splint the extremity in the angulated position.

EXTENDED *Transport*

A musculoskeletal injury may swell as the body begins the healing process. If an EMT places a splint on an injured extremity and has an extended transport time, the injured extremity must be evaluated frequently. As the extremity swells, the splint can act as a tourniquet, limiting blood supply to the distal extremity. If ongoing assessment (reassessment) shows that the extremity has lost distal pulses or that capillary refill has slowed, the EMT should loosen the splint to allow for distal perfusion.

The wrist and hand region is immobilized by attachment of a rigid splint that extends from the proximal joint of the phalanges to the midforearm. The forearm is then placed in a sling. **Skill 23-3** illustrates the application of a rigid splint to the forearm and wrist.

If the injury is proximal to the wrist, check radial and ulnar pulses, as for all upper extremity injuries. If the injury is to the wrist and hand, use skin color and temperature and capillary refilling time to gauge distal vascular function.

If an elbow is angulated and locked because of a dislocation, it may be immobilized in the position found. A rigid splint can be bridged from the humerus to the distal forearm to prevent movement of the elbow **(Skill 23-4)**. **Figure 23-25** illustrates the deformity of a splinted elbow injury and a related radiograph.

The sling and swathe combination is the primary immobilization technique for fractures to the clavicle, scapula, shoulder, and humerus. It is also useful for fractures of the elbow and forearm. When applying the sling and swathe, take care not to apply excessive pressure over the axillary region on the opposite side. The sling supports the weight of the arm and keeps the forearm elevated. The swathe serves to bind the upper extremity to the chest wall to prevent movement. Place the knot made in the sling on the side of the patient's neck to avoid pressure and discomfort **(Skill 23-5)**.

Traction splints are used to immobilize isolated painful, swollen, deformed midthigh injuries with no joint or lower leg injury. Contraindications to the use of a traction splint include the following:
- Injury close to the knee
- Injury to the knee
- Injury to the hip
- Injured pelvis
- Partial amputation or avulsion with bone separation; distal limb is connected only by marginal tissue (traction would risk separation).
- Lower leg or ankle injury

The *Hare traction splint* is an adjustable leg splint with a mechanical pulley to establish traction for midshaft fractures of the femur. The splint comes with padded ankle hitches, self-grip leg bands, and a self-grip groin strap to prevent the splint from slipping upward when traction is applied. If needed, an ankle hitch can also be improvised with a cravat bandage. Traction is achieved by fixing the splint against the ischial tuberosity of the pelvic bone, located at the base of each buttock **(Skill 23-6)**.

The *Sager traction splint* is an adjustable leg splint with a mechanical pulley to establish traction. The Sager traction splint has a single adjustable bar that can be placed on the medial or lateral aspect of the leg. Traction is achieved by fixing the splint against the perineum **(Skill 23-7)**. The Sager traction splint can also be used for fractures of the proximal thigh (check local protocols).

For certain types of extremity injuries, special approaches are needed for immobilization because of the urgent nature of the patient's condition or the unusual position of the extremity. An *air splint* can be used in place of a rigid splint for fractures of the upper extremity. Air splints are available in full arm and leg and partial arm and leg lengths **(Skill 23-8)**. Be sure to monitor splint pressure when you move from one environment to another because temperature changes can increase or decrease pad pressure.

Dislocations of the hip are often locked and resist straightening. You should place the patient on a long spine board, with pillows between the knee area and the board to provide support. The legs can then be tied together for additional support. Traction splints are contraindicated for immobilization of hip dislocations because of the angulation and locking of the extremity.

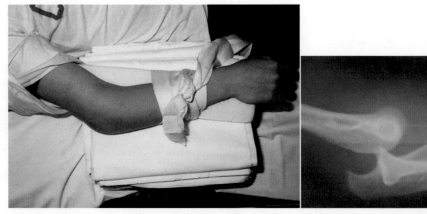

Figure 23-25 Type of injury for which an elbow splint in the angulated position is indicated, with associated radiograph illustrating the bone position and deformity of an elbow dislocation.

Patients who are in shock or who have a critical injury or an injury to the pelvis are best immobilized with a long spine board. PASG can be considered if indicated by local protocols. A long spine board is used for all pelvic fractures. The patient should be securely attached with straps. The legs of the patient can be tied together after padding is placed between the legs to offer further immobilization.

Scenario Follow-up

The motorcyclist thrown from her bike sustained direct compression of her pelvis with force sufficient to break the ring of the pelvis, making it unstable. These fractures can be associated with significant blood loss. Avoiding further movement of the fracture site during transport can be aided by using a device such as the PASG to support the bony structure and provide some compression to help control bleeding.

Summary

Musculoskeletal injuries are often encountered by EMTs. Proper immobilization is important to minimize pain and damage to vessels, nerves, soft tissue, organs, and muscles. Immobilization also reduces the chance of permanent damage or disability and prevents conversion of a closed injury to an open injury. Cool compresses and elevation may be applied to decrease swelling.

Splinting is usually done before the patient is moved. However, if life-threatening injuries are encountered, the patient may be immobilized to a long spine board so that transport to hospital care can begin immediately. Further care to injured extremities can be conducted en route.

Assessment for musculoskeletal injuries is aided by an understanding of the mechanism of injury and examination for deformity and angulation, pain and tenderness, grating, swelling, bruising, exposed bone ends, and joints locked into position. General rules for splinting call for assessment of pulse, motor, and sensory functions distal to the injury before and after splinting, with documentation of the findings. Immobilize the joint above and below the injury. Remove or cut away clothing, cover open wounds with a sterile dressing, and pad splints to prevent pressure and discomfort to the patient. If there is a severe deformity or if the distal extremity is cyanotic or lacks pulses, align with gentle traction before splinting. Do not intentionally replace the protruding bone ends in an open fracture.

Immobilization devices include rigid splints, traction splints, air splints, improvised splints (pillow), and PASG. The EMT uses the procedures for long-bone splinting, splinting joint injuries, and traction splinting to care for most types of musculoskeletal injuries.

Skills

Skill │ 23-1   *Applying a Rigid Splint to the Lower Extremity*

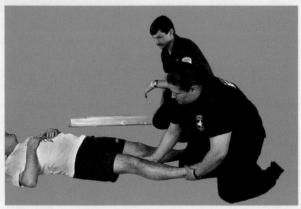

1. Using appropriate personal precautions, apply manual stabilization.

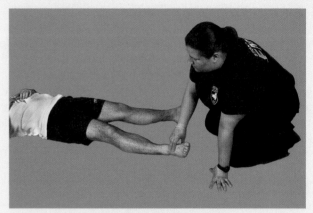

2. Assess pulse, motor, and sensory function.

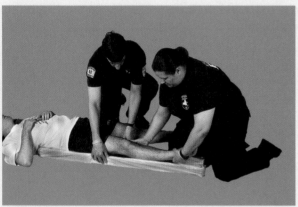

3. If there is a severe deformity or if the distal extremity is cyanotic or lacks pulses, align with gentle traction (as protocols allow) before splinting. Measure the splint.

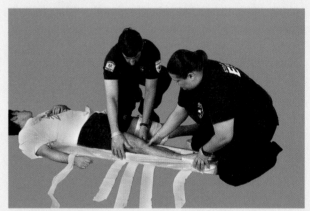

4. Apply the splint, immobilizing the bone and joint above and below the injury. Immobilize the foot in a position of function.

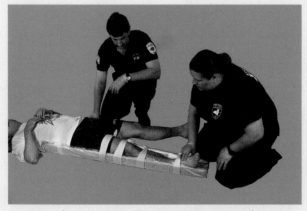

5. Secure the entire injured extremity. Reassess pulse, motor, and sensory function after application of the splint, and record your findings.

Skill | 23-2   *Applying a Rigid Splint to the Forearm in the Straightened Position*

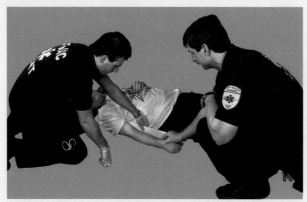

1. For patients transported in the supine position, the arm may be splinted in the straightened position with the elbow extended. Maintain the arm in alignment. Check distal circulation and nerve function prior to splinting.

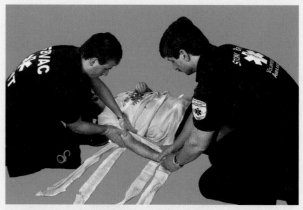

2. Place a padded rigid splint along the medial surface from the armpit to the hand. You can place a roller bandage between the hand and splint to keep the hand in the position of function, as if holding a can.

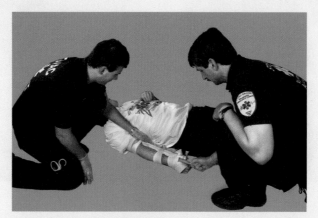

3. Attach with cravats or bandage and secure to torso; assess distal circulation and nerve function.

Skill | 23-3   *Applying a Rigid Splint to the Forearm and Wrist*

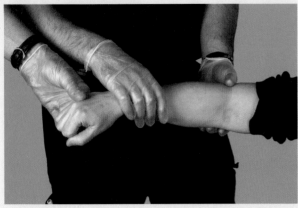

1. Using appropriate personal precautions, apply manual stabilization.

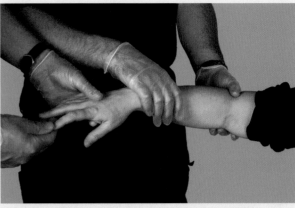

2. Assess pulse, motor, and sensory function. Reassess distal circulation and nerve function prior to splinting.

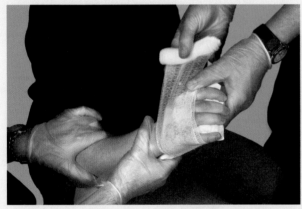

3. Align with gentle traction (as protocols allow) if the distal extremity is cyanotic or lacks pulses and no resistance is met. Immobilize the site of injury with a padded rigid splint.

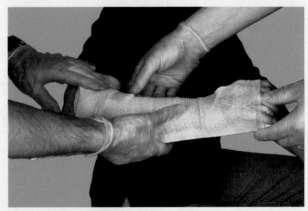

4. Immobilize the bone above and below the site of injury.

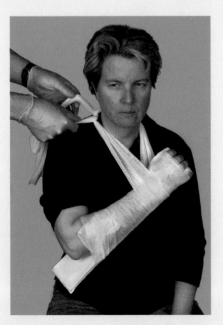

5. Reassess pulse or circulation and motor and sensory function after application of splint, and record findings. Use the sling and swathe combination to support and elevate the arm and to limit movement.

Skill | 23-4   *Applying a Rigid Splint to the Elbow in the Flexed Position*

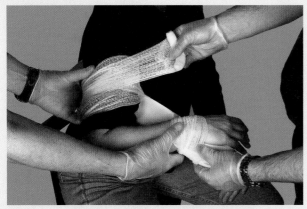

1. Apply a padded rigid splint from the armpit area to the wrist, and secure in place with a cravat or bandage.

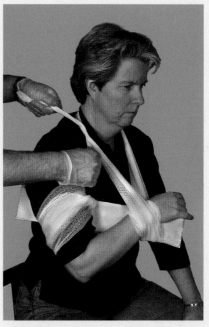

2. Use a cravat bandage to form a sling to support the weight of the arm.

Skill | 23-5   *Applying a Sling and Swathe*

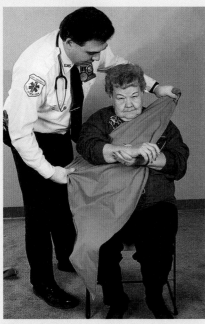

1. Place the sling with the long end over the opposite shoulder and the apex toward the injured side. Check distal circulation and nerve function prior to splinting.

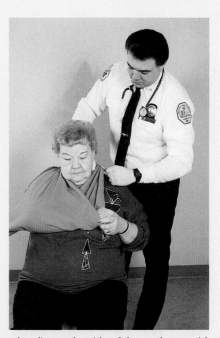

2. Secure the sling at the side of the neck to avoid pressure.

Continued

Skill | 23-5   *Applying a Sling and Swathe—cont'd*

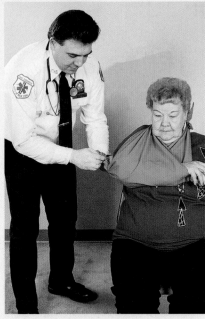

3. Secure the end of the sling with a knot or twist.

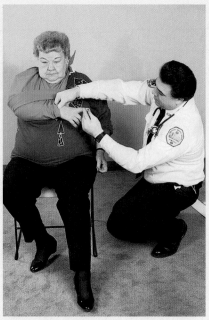

4. Attach the swathe, and check distal circulation.

Skill | 23-6   *Applying a Hare Traction Splint*

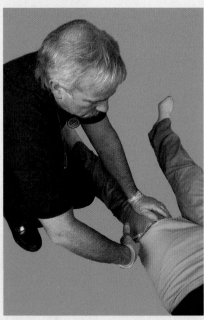

1. Using appropriate personal precautions, cut away clothing.

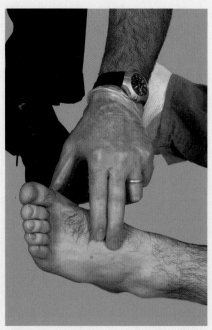

2. Assess pulse, motor, and sensory function distal to the injury and record findings.

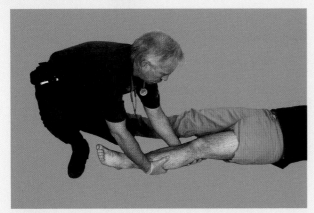

3. Perform manual stabilization of the injured leg.

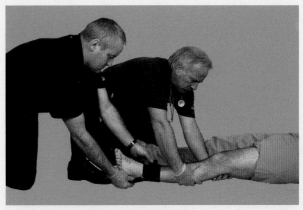

4. Apply distal securing device.

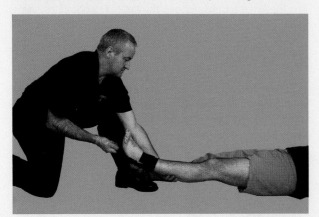

5. Apply manual traction (required when using a bipolar traction splint).

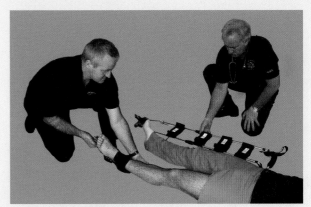

6. Prepare and adjust splint to the proper length.

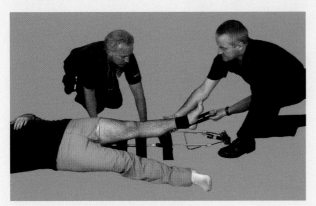

7. Position splint under the injured leg.

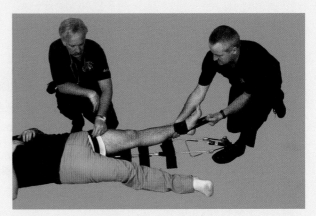

8. Apply proximal securing device (ischial strap).

Continued

Skill |23-6   *Applying a Hare Traction Splint–cont'd*

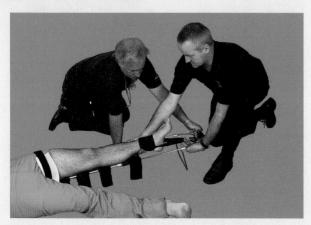

9. Apply mechanical traction.

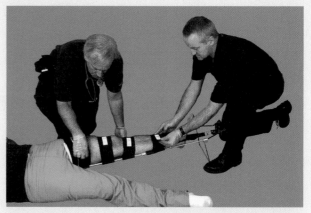

10. Position and secure support straps. Place two straps below the knee and two above the knee. Do not place straps directly over the site of the injury.

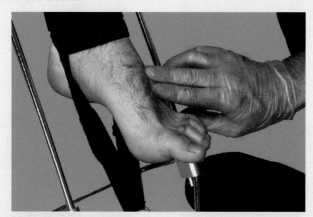

11. Reevaluate the proximal and distal securing devices, and reassess pulse, motor, and sensory function. Secure the torso to the long board to immobilize the hip, and secure the splint to the long board to prevent movement of the splint.

Skill | 23-7   *Applying a Sager Traction Splint*

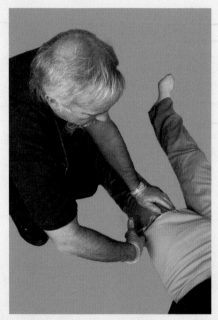

1. Using appropriate personal precautions, remove or cut away clothing.

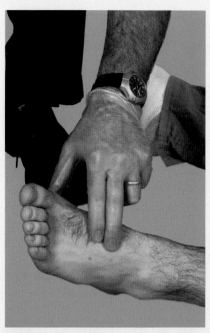

2. Assess pulse, motor, and sensation distal to the injury and record findings.

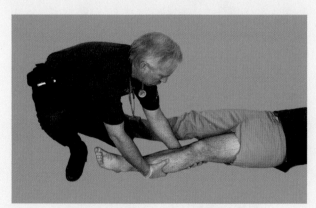

3. Perform manual stabilization of the injured leg.

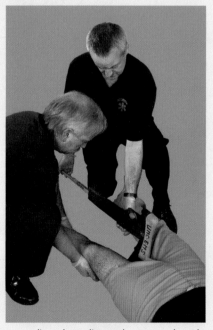

4. Prepare or adjust the splint to the proper length.

Continued

Skill | 23-7   *Applying a Sager Traction Splint—cont'd*

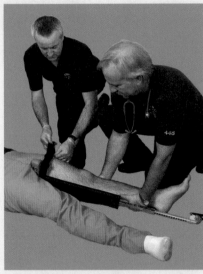

5. Apply a proximal securing device (ischial strap).

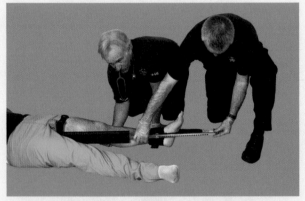

7. Apply mechanical traction. As a rule, traction should not exceed 10% of the patient's body weight, or approximately 15 pounds of traction in this case.

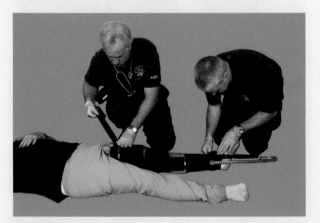

9. Reevaluate proximal and distal securing devices.

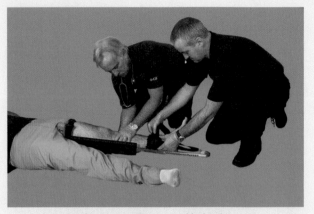

6. Apply a distal securing device (ankle hitch).

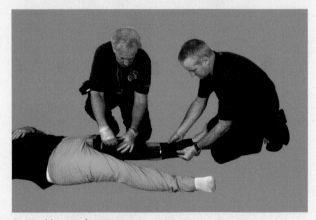

8. Position and secure support straps.

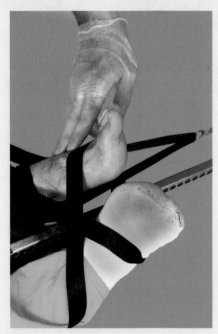

10. Reassess pulse, motor, and sensory function distal to the injury after application of the splint, and record findings. Secure the torso to the long spine board to immobilize the hip. Secure the splint to the long spine board to prevent movement of the splint.

Skill | 23-8   *Applying an Air Splint*

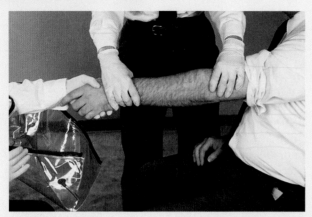

1. Using appropriate personal precautions, apply manual stabilization.

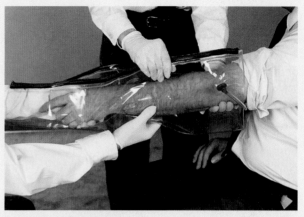

2. Assess pulse, motor, and sensory function. Apply splint, immobilizing the bone and joint above and below the injury.

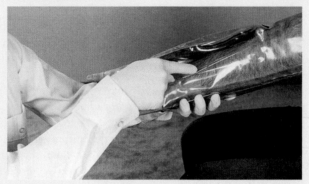

3. Check pressure in the splint, noting a slight dent with finger pressure. Reassess pulse, motor, and sensory function after application of the splint, and record findings.

The Bottom Line

Learning Checklist

✓ A fracture is a break in the continuity of bone.

✓ Sprains are injuries to ligaments, usually resulting from stretching forces.

✓ Strains are injuries to muscles or their tendons, usually from overstretching or violent contractions.

✓ A dislocation is a displacement of bones in a joint from the normal anatomic position.

✓ A painful, swollen, deformed extremity is treated as if a significant bony or soft tissue injury exists.

✓ Forces that cause fractures may be direct or indirect.

✓ Examples of direct forces applied to a bone include a vehicle bumper striking the tibia of a pedestrian, a gunshot wound shattering a bone, or a falling person landing on both feet and breaking the heel bones.

✓ Indirect forces are forces that are transmitted along the axis of bones, resulting in an injury at a location other than the point of impact. A person falling on an outstretched hand and fracturing the shoulder is an example of an indirect force.

✓ Fractures can be classified as closed or open.

✓ A closed fracture has no break in the skin over the fracture site, and the fracture is not exposed to the external environment.

✓ An open fracture is exposed to the external environment because the skin above the site has been broken.

✓ Pain is the most common symptom of a bone or joint injury. Pain may be referred distal or proximal to the site of the injury, so examination of the entire extremity is essential.

✓ Angulation of long bones, protuberance of the bone end against the soft tissues, and overriding or separation of bone fragments by opposing muscles can result in visible and palpable deformities.

✓ Fluid or blood loss at the site of injury can result in swelling or discoloration of the affected part.

✓ Loss of function of a skeletal part occurs with injury.

✓ Never attempt to force movement when a patient does not voluntarily move a limb.

✓ Crepitus is a grating sensation or sound indicating that bone fragments are rubbing against one another. Do not deliberately attempt to elicit this finding.

✓ Bone ends protruding through the skin are an obvious sign of an open fracture.

✓ Signs specific for dislocation include loss of movement and deformity at a joint, joint locked in a deformed position, and pain and swelling over the joint.

✓ Common sites of dislocations include the shoulder, elbow, fingers, hip, knee, and ankle.

✓ Vascular injuries can result in loss of blood flow to distal tissues as well as blood loss at the site of injury.

✓ The presence of vascular compromise is determined by assessing distal pulses, skin color and temperature, capillary refilling time, pain, numbness, tingling, prickling, sensory loss, and paralysis distal to the injury.

✓ Common sites where fractures or dislocations cause disruption of nerves include the clavicle, shoulder, humerus, elbow, wrist, hip, femur, knee, and spinal cord.

✓ Signs and symptoms of nerve injury include pain, abnormal sensation, and loss of motor ability.

✓ General rules of splinting include immobilize critical patients with a spine board; when in doubt, splint the injury; splint before moving; pad splints and remove clothing; immobilize the joint/bone above and below the injury; check and recheck neurovascular function; and cover open wounds.

✓ Long board splints can be used to immobilize fractures of the knee, tibia, and fibula in the straightened position.

✓ Immobilize fractures of the midforearm with a rigid splint extending from the palm of the hand past the medial aspect of the elbow.

✓ Suspected fractures of the forearm or elbow can be splinted in the extended position with a rigid splint.

✓ Fingers are splinted with a flexible aluminum splint or a tongue blade.

✓ Joint injuries can be immobilized in the straightened or angulated position.

✓ If the extremity is cyanotic or lacks pulses, try to straighten the extremity as allowed by local protocols. If you encounter resistance, splint the extremity in the angulated position.

✓ The wrist and hand region is immobilized by attachment of a rigid splint that extends from the proximal joint of the phalanges to the midforearm. The forearm is then placed in a sling.

✓ An elbow that is angulated and locked because of a dislocation may be immobilized in the position found. A rigid splint can be bridged from the humerus to the distal forearm to prevent movement of the elbow.

✓ The sling and swathe combination is the primary immobilization technique for fractures of the clavicle, scapula, shoulder, and humerus.

✓ Traction splints are used to immobilize painful, swollen, and deformed midthigh injuries with no joint or lower leg injury. In some systems, the Sager-type splint is also used for proximal thigh injury.

✓ Contraindications to the use of a traction splint include injury close to or at the knee, hip, or pelvis; partial amputation or bone separation; and lower leg or ankle injuries.

Key Terms

Crepitus Sensation felt during palpation caused by air beneath the skin or broken bone ends rubbing together.

Dislocation Displacement of the bones in a joint from their normal anatomic position.

Fracture A break in the continuity of bone.

Pneumatic (air) splint Plastic splints filled with air to provide circumferential support to an injured extremity.

Rigid splint Splint made of rigid material such as cardboard, wood, metal, or plastic; should be well padded.

Sling A triangle-shaped bandage used to support the weight of the arm.

Sprain Injury to ligaments, usually resulting from stretching forces.

Strain Injury to muscles or their tendons, usually from overstretching or violent contractions.

Swathe Folded triangular bandage or roller bandage used to bind the upper arm to the chest wall.

Traction splint Device consisting of a metal frame and a pulley system to apply traction to the lower extremity.

Review Questions

1. Which of the following best defines a strain?
   a. Tearing of a ligament
   b. Dislocation of a joint
   c. Type of fracture to the flat bones
   d. Tear to the muscle and/or tendon

2. Forces transmitted along the axis of bones that cause fractures in locations other than the point of impact are called:
   a. Direct forces
   b. Indirect forces
   c. Displaced forces
   d. Tangential forces

3. An injury to bony structures that does not cause a related break in the skin is called a(n):
   a. Open injury
   b. Closed injury
   c. Complex injury
   d. Compound injury

4. In the pneumonic DCAP BTLS, what does the "D" stand for?
   a. Debilitating
   b. Distinctive
   c. Discoloration
   d. Deformity

5. Which of the following is a general rule of splinting?
   a. Immobilize the joint above and below the injury.
   b. Apply traction to all injured extremities.
   c. Place the hand and foot in the straightened position.
   d. Splints should be firm and nonpadded.

6. What should be routinely done before and after applying any splint?
   a. Check for patient orientation.
   b. Check blood pressure in the affected limb.
   c. Assess pulse, motor, and sensory function.
   d. Put gentle traction on the affected extremity.

7. Traction splints are indicated for:
   a. Knee injuries
   b. Lower leg injuries
   c. Midthigh injuries
   d. Pelvic injuries

8. Which of the following fractures is associated with bleeding sufficient to cause a 40% or greater blood loss in a man with an estimated total blood volume of 5000 mL?
   a. Both humeri
   b. Pelvis
   c. Tibia
   d. Ankle and humerus

9. Which of the following side effects of splinting an extremity is of *least* concern?
   a. Compression of nerves, tissues, and blood vessels from the splint.
   b. Inability to assess distal nerve and vascular function.
   c. Aggravation of the bone or joint injury.
   d. Slowing of the pulse from stimulation of the autonomic nervous system.

10. Which of the following is the most important reason for splinting?
    a. Splinting takes away all the pain.
    b. Takes the patient's mind off the injury.
    c. Minimizes damage to muscles, nerves, or blood vessels by broken bone ends.
    d. Converts an open injury to a closed injury by retracting the protruding bone end.

For Further Review

In the Student Workbook

- Multiple-choice questions
- Matching questions
- Fill-in-the-blank questions
- Short-answer questions
- Case scenario questions
- Crossword puzzle

On Evolve

- Anatomy challenge
- Weblinks
- Lecture notes
- Exercises

Learning Objectives

Cognitive Objectives

- Describe the function of the muscular system.
- Describe the function of the skeletal system.

- List the major bones or bone groupings of the spinal column, the thorax, the upper extremities, and the lower extremities.
- Differentiate between an open and a closed painful, swollen, deformed extremity.
- State the reasons for splinting.
- List the general rules of splinting.
- List the complications of splinting.
- List the emergency medical care for a patient with a painful, swollen, deformed extremity.

Affective Objectives

- Explain the rationale for splinting at the scene versus "load and go."
- Explain the rationale for immobilization of the painful, swollen, deformed extremity.

Psychomotor Objectives

- Demonstrate the emergency medical care of a patient with a painful, swollen, deformed extremity.
- Demonstrate completing a prehospital care report for patients with musculoskeletal injuries.

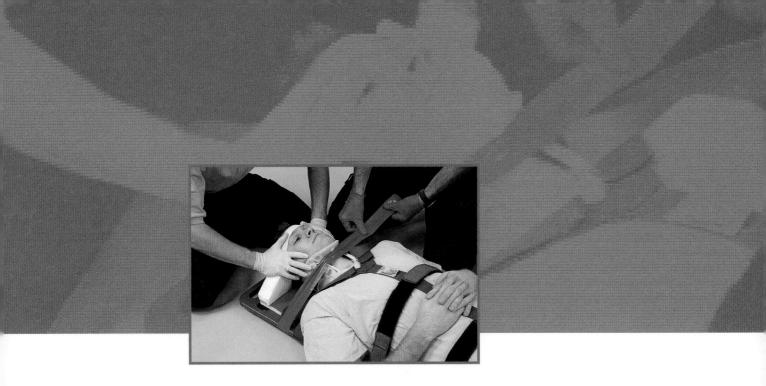

24 Injuries to the Head and Spine

CHAPTER OUTLINE

Scenario

You respond to a call for a 14-year-old boy who fell approximately 7 feet from a swing and struck the left side of his forehead on a soft rubber mat, knocking him unconscious. After 30 seconds, he awoke and said he felt "all right." You find the patient alert and breathing with his abdominal muscles at a rate of 24 breaths/min. His pulse is 68 beats/min and regular, and his blood pressure is 90/60 mm Hg. The patient cannot move his arms and legs and has sensation above the clavicle but none at the nipple line. You also note the presence of priapism.

You immediately begin delivery of high-concentration oxygen by nonrebreather mask as you provide manual inline stabilization of the cervical spine, then log-roll him onto a long spine board. En route to the hospital, the patient's mental status changes to unresponsive, his respiratory rate drops to 8 breaths/min, and he becomes cyanotic. You begin positive-pressure ventilation with a bag-mask device. On arrival at the trauma center, the patient's color has improved, and he is responsive to verbal stimuli.

One of the major goals of emergency care is to ensure brain viability. The majority of deaths from trauma result from direct injury to the nervous system. In addition, because the brain is the controlling center for other vital organ systems, such as respiration and circulation, brain dysfunction may result in cardiopulmonary failure and death. Because of the interdependence of the heart, lungs, and brain, signs of brain function are used to assess the status of other vital organs.

The nervous system is the center of consciousness and the intellectual, emotional, and behavioral functions that make up many characteristics of personality and human behavior. It receives and interprets stimuli from the internal and external environment, and it directs and regulates other organs and tissues. Some of its activity is conscious or willful, but much of the brain's activity is unconscious or involuntary in response to the environment.

This chapter reviews the anatomy and physiology of the nervous system and discusses the assessment and management of head and spinal injuries.

> **LEARNING OBJECTIVES**
> - State the components of the nervous system.
> - List the functions of the central nervous system.
> - Define the structure of the skeletal system as it relates to the nervous system.

Anatomy and Physiology

The nervous system is composed of the *central nervous system* (CNS) and the *peripheral nervous system* (PNS). The CNS is the "computer," and the PNS is the "communicator." The CNS is made up of the brain, the brainstem, and the spinal cord.

The CNS receives information about the outside environment and about functions within the body itself. In turn, it organizes and analyzes this information and directs the activities of the organs, muscles, and other tissues. The CNS receives and transmits information by nerves or special tracts of nerve tissue that extend through the CNS and extend into the PNS.

The PNS is composed of the nerves outside the CNS, which extend from the brainstem and spinal cord. The PNS has *sensory nerves* that carry messages to the spinal cord and brain and *motor nerves* that carry messages back to the muscles and various organs.

Central Nervous System

The CNS is composed of the brain and the spinal cord (**Figure 24-1**). The brain is the central computer. It processes sensory input from sensory nerves and organizes responses, which are then transmitted to the body by outgoing motor nerves.

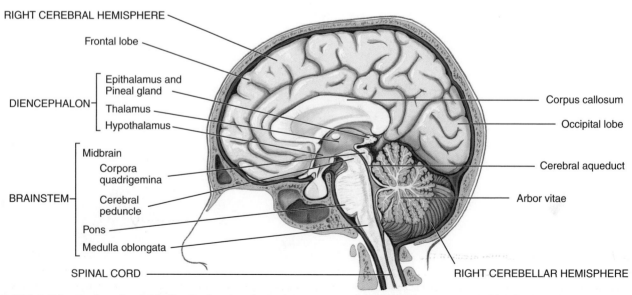

Figure 24-1 Midsagittal section of the brain showing the major portions of the brain, brainstem, and beginning of the spinal cord. *From Applegate EJ:* The anatomy and physiology learning system, *ed 3, St Louis, 2006, Saunders.*

Brain

The largest and most superior portion of the brain is called the **cerebrum.** The cerebrum is divided into right and left halves called *hemispheres.* Generally, the right hemisphere controls the left side of the body, and the left hemisphere controls the right side of the body. The convoluted hemispheres are further subdivided into different *lobes,* or sections, that have specific and distinct functions (**Figure 24-2**). The lobes are generally named according to their location with respect to the overlying skull bones: *frontal lobe* (area responsible for intellectual functions and motor control of skeletal muscles), *parietal lobe* (center for sensory perception), *occipital lobe* (center for receiving and processing visual stimuli), and *temporal lobe* (receives olfactory and auditory signals). Loss of brain tissue in a specific area can result in distinct and limited losses of function, which point to the subdivision of labor within the brain itself.

The **brainstem** is the lower part of the brain. It is made up of bundles and tracts of nerves traveling down to the spinal cord from the cerebrum. The brainstem has distinct nerve cell centers of its own. Some nerve centers located in the brainstem control muscles of the eyes and iris. They communicate by peripheral nerves called *cranial nerves,* which originate in the brainstem and travel through the skull. Other nerve centers in the brainstem monitor and direct respiratory and circulatory functions of the body. Because these areas are so close together, loss of function in some structures (e.g., control of pupillary size or eye movement) means that the neighboring centers that control respiration and much of circulation may also be damaged, leading to loss of vital function. Checking the pupils is part of the assessment for patients with a head injury, an altered mental status, or loss of nerve function. Damage to certain parts of the brainstem (pons and medulla) can result in abnormal breathing patterns.

The **cerebellum** is an outpocketing of the brain located posterior to the brainstem. It is primarily concerned with coordination of movement and balance.

Spinal Cord

The spinal cord emerges from the brainstem and is a continuation of nerve tracts from all parts of the brain. It also has its own processing centers, such as reflex action. For example, touching a hot iron causes an immediate reaction to remove your hand even before the brain receives the message that damage has occurred. This type of action can occur through the reflex arcs along each segment of the spinal cord (see Chapter 4).

Protection of Brain and Spinal Cord

Because the brain and spinal cord are of such central importance and so sensitive to pressure, they are protected and encased within strong bones that make up the skull and vertebral column. Three layers of membranes under the bones separate bone from the brain and spinal cord and offer further protection. In addition, between the two innermost membranes lies the *cerebrospinal fluid* (CSF), which can absorb shocks from sudden blows and adds still another layer of protection. The clear, colorless CSF also provides some nutrition to the nerve cells.

Skull. The skull is made up of several bones that compose the cranium, the face, and the lower jaw, or mandible (**Figure 24-3**).

The bones making up the cranium are flat and irregularly shaped. These bones are separate at birth to allow for passage of the skull through the birth canal. Over time, they fuse together at suture lines. The bones making up the outer surface of the cranium include the *frontal bone* anteriorly (the forehead), the *occipital bone* posteriorly, and the *parietal and temporal bones,* which form the lateral surfaces of the cranium.

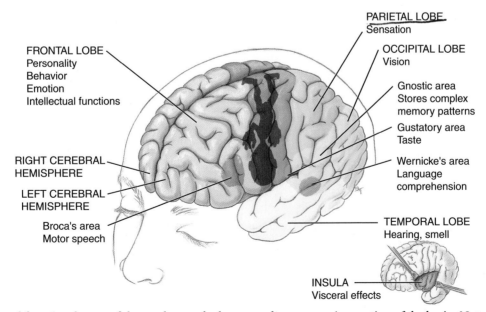

FRONTAL LOBE
Personality
Behavior
Emotion
Intellectual functions

RIGHT CEREBRAL HEMISPHERE

LEFT CEREBRAL HEMISPHERE

Broca's area
Motor speech

PARIETAL LOBE
Sensation

OCCIPITAL LOBE
Vision

Gnostic area
Stores complex memory patterns

Gustatory area
Taste

Wernicke's area
Language comprehension

TEMPORAL LOBE
Hearing, smell

INSULA
Visceral effects

Figure 24-2 Lobes and functional areas of the cerebrum, the largest and most superior portion of the brain. Note the body drawing overlying the junction of the frontal and parietal lobes. The distorted appearance of the figure is in proportion to the amount of brain surface area devoted to a particular body function. Use of the hands, eating, swallowing, and speech are complex tasks; therefore more brain cells are delegated for these functions than for tasks such as bending at the waist. *From Applegate EJ:* The anatomy and physiology learning system, *ed 3, St Louis, 2006, Saunders.*

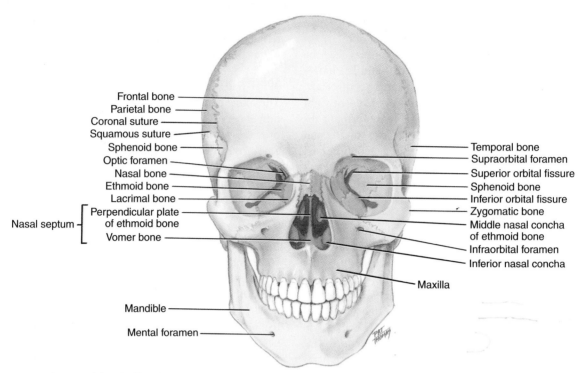

Figure 24-3 Frontal view of the skull with bones composing the cranium, face, and lower jaw. *From Applegate EJ: The anatomy and physiology learning system, ed 3, St Louis, 2006, Saunders.*

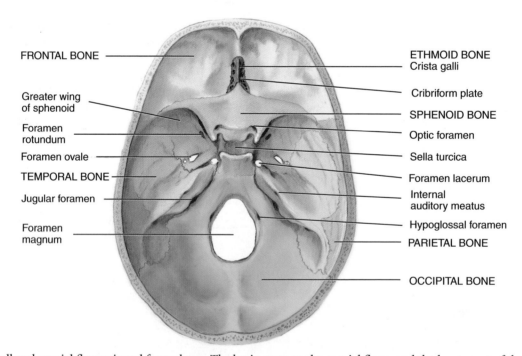

Figure 24-4 Skull and cranial floor, viewed from above. The brain rests on the cranial floor, and the lower part of the brain, the brainstem, travels through the foramen magnum to join with the spinal cord. Other foramen in the figure allow for passage of nerves and blood vessels through the base of the skull. *From Applegate EJ: The anatomy and physiology learning system, ed 3, St Louis, 2006, Saunders.*

After birth and during infancy, the bones do not meet at all points, and soft spots are present at two sites. These are the anterior and posterior *fontanels,* located in the midline of the top of the skull at the ends of both parietal bones.

The largest part of the brain, the cerebrum, sits within the cranium and rests on numerous bones that are fused together, forming the base of the skull. In the midline of the base of the skull is an opening called the *foramen magnum.* The lower part of the brain, the brainstem, travels through the foramen magnum as it leaves the cranium to connect with the spinal cord **(Figure 24-4).**

The space within the cranium holds approximately 1 L of fluid. After infancy, when the cranial bones are fused, the

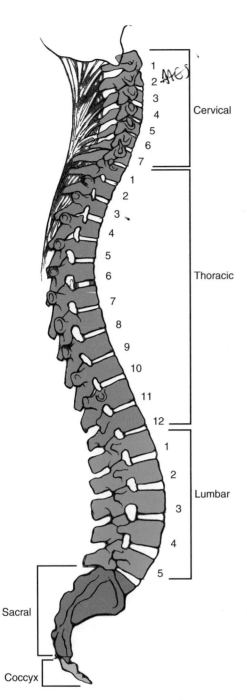

Figure 24-5 The spinal column has a central opening that protects the spinal cord.

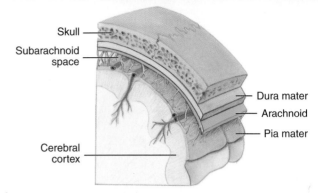

Figure 24-6 Meninges of the central nervous system. *From Applegate EJ:* The anatomy and physiology learning system, *ed 3, St Louis, 2006, Saunders.*

cranial space is nonexpandable. This space is filled almost entirely with brain tissue, with spinal fluid and circulating blood the remaining contents. If bleeding occurs within this nonexpandable space, pressure is transmitted to brain tissue itself. Because brain tissue is very susceptible to pressure, this causes loss of brain function. If pressure is severe, the brain may *herniate* (protrude, rupture) through the only opening in the cranium, the foramen magnum. This dire emergency calls for prompt neurosurgical evaluation.

Spinal Column. The spinal column consists of 33 vertebrae extending from the base of the skull to the *coccyx* (tailbone). Most vertebrae are held together by ligaments and separated by cartilaginous disks that serve as cushions. The ligaments allow for movement such as bending and rotation while maintaining proper alignment of the vertebral column. Proper alignment is essential because the spinal cord passes through the vertebral column.

The spinal vertebrae are named according to their location and structure. Starting from the head, the first seven vertebrae are called the *cervical* vertebrae (C1 to C7). The next 12 vertebrae are the *thoracic* vertebrae (T1 to T12), which provide the main support for the rib cage, with each pair of ribs joining the corresponding vertebrae. The next five vertebrae are *lumbar* (L1 to L5). The lumbar vertebrae extend to the *sacrum,* which consists of five vertebrae fused together. Extending from the sacrum are four fused vertebrae that make up the coccyx **(Figure 24-5).**

The vertebrae have an anterior body and a posterior spinous process that allow for attachment of ligaments. Arcs of bone connect the body and spinous process of each vertebra, leaving a central opening through which the spinal cord travels. At the level of each vertebra are openings through which the peripheral nerves leave the spinal column and travel to the various parts of the body.

Membranous Coverings. The *meninges,* or membranous coverings of the brain and cord, have three layers. The outer layer closest to the skull and vertebral column is a tough, leathery layer called the *dura.* The middle layer is called the *arachnoid.* Between the dura and the arachnoid layer are many veins and venous sinuses. The innermost layer is called the *pia mater,* which is adherent to the brain tissue itself. It is between the arachnoid and the pia mater that CSF circulates **(Figure 24-6).** Bleeding from torn arteries or veins can occur between these layers and can put pressure on the brain.

Cerebrospinal Fluid. The CSF helps protect and cushion the brain and acts like a liquid shock absorber. It is continually being formed and absorbed from blood-rich plexuses. CSF serves a nutritional role as it circulates around the brain and spinal cord, within ventricles (hollow cavities) within the brain, and within the innermost center of the spinal cord itself.

Peripheral Nervous System

Each spinal nerve has both sensory and motor components. One spinal nerve leaves from each side of the vertebral column. There are 31 pairs of spinal nerves. Together with the 12 cranial

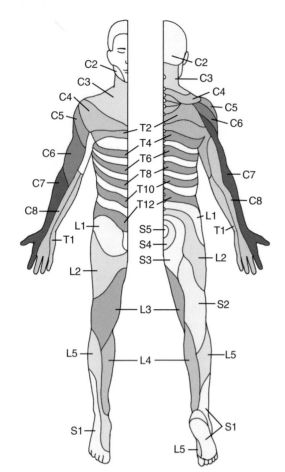

Figure 24-7 Map of the dermatomes. *From Aehlert, B:* paramedic practice today, above and beyond, *St. Louis, 2010, Mosby.*

nerves leaving the brainstem, they compose the PNS. These peripheral nerves continue to subdivide until they form an extensive network that innervates (supplies with nerves), or connects with, the various tissues, organs, and muscles.

The *sensory* branches bring information to the spinal cord and brain. The *motor* nerves transmit information from the brain and spinal cord to organs, muscles, and tissues, regulating their activity. As an emergency medical technician (EMT), you are expected to test for motor function and muscle strength of both the lower and the upper extremities. This is helpful in identifying spinal injury and one-sided signs that may indicate structural brain injury. Because the spinal nerves are the communicating wiring to and from the brain, any disruption along the nerve pathways can result in loss of sensory and motor function. This loss always occurs distal to the site of injury.

Dermatomes

Knowledge of the anatomy of the spinal cord and peripheral nerves can help determine the level of injury. If you follow the wiring diagram of the nervous system, you will find that nerves exiting from nearby segments of the vertebral column innervate particular segments of skin, or *dermatomes.* The sensory components of the nerves follow dermatome patterns (**Figure 24-7**). The same is true for skeletal muscles.

As shown in the diagram, sensation from the skin over the collarbone anteriorly is transmitted through the nerve entering the vertebral column at the fourth cervical vertebra (C4). Sensation from skin around the nipple is transmitted through the spinal nerve entering the vertebral column at the fourth thoracic vertebra (T4). If the vertebral column is damaged, crushing the spinal cord at the first thoracic vertebra (T1), function below or distal to the injury is lost. Such a patient could still feel sensation over the collarbone (C4) but would not have sensation in the nipple dermatome (T4).

You are not expected to memorize the dermatome chart. However, you should know that patients can present with no sensation below the level of injury.

Function of the Nervous System

The nervous system can also be divided by function. The *voluntary* (or somatic) nervous system connects the CNS with sensory and motor nerves that direct conscious activities, such as the control of skeletal muscles.

The *involuntary* (or autonomic) nervous system controls vital body functions such as heart rate, contraction and relaxation of smooth muscle, and body temperature. The involuntary nervous system is further divided into *parasympathetic* and *sympathetic* divisions. In general, these divisions have opposite effects on a given organ or tissue. For example, the parasympathetic division slows down the heart rate, whereas the sympathetic division speeds it up. These two divisions, with their opposite effects, tend to counterbalance each other and allow the brain to meet the body's changing needs at any given time.

Oxygen and Glucose: Essential Nutrients of the Central Nervous System

The nervous system depends on an adequate supply of oxygen and glucose. If complete cessation of oxygen delivery occurs, as in cardiac arrest, CNS activity ceases in about 5 seconds, and the patient becomes unconscious. If some oxygen is not delivered to the brain within about 4 to 6 minutes, irreversible brain damage occurs. This explains why early application of cardiopulmonary resuscitation (CPR) is so important. Other conditions that result in inadequate delivery of oxygen to the brain (e.g., hypoxia, hypotension) can cause various degrees of cell damage.

Patients who are hypoxic have altered brain function. The most sensitive areas are those concerned with intellect, behavior, and consciousness. Changes in behavior, ability to reason, judgment, and level of consciousness are often referred to as "alterations in mental status." In fact, altered mental status is the most sensitive indication of inadequate oxygen and explains why the check for responsiveness is the first step in the initial (primary) assessment. One form of altered mental status is agitated or even combative behavior, which can be confused with intoxication or a behavioral disorder. The finding of unresponsiveness or altered mental status leads the EMT to question whether adequate oxygen is being delivered to the brain.

Glucose is another essential nutrient of the CNS. When glucose levels in the blood are too low, the patient may have altered brain function, ranging from agitation to coma.

Nerve Cells and Pressure

Nerve cells are very sensitive to pressure. If an outside force is applied to the nerves, nerve function becomes compromised. Both the amount of pressure transmitted to the nerve cells and the time during which it is applied affect the amount of nerve damage that occurs. A sudden force, applied over a few milliseconds, may disrupt nerve or brain function temporarily or permanently, depending on the amount of force applied. Lesser forces sustained over long periods result in damage in proportion to the time over which the force is applied.

Case in Point

Two EMTs respond to a 15-year-old boy who fell off a bridge into 1 foot of water. Bystanders indicate that he fell directly on his head and was unresponsive for about 3 minutes. They dragged him from the water and placed him on his back. The EMTs' examination reveals that the patient is lethargic, complaining of pain in his neck, and experiencing shortness of breath. His vital signs are pulse 70 beats/min and regular, respirations shallow at 28 breaths/min with abdominal movement only, and blood pressure 86/70 mm Hg. He is talking in short sentences to catch his breath. The neurologic examination reveals no sensation or movement below the collarbone. During the head-to-toe survey the EMTs note a large contusion on the upper left quadrant of the boy's abdomen and priapism. They administer high-concentration oxygen by nonrebreather mask and immobilize the boy on a long spine board. The EMTs notify the hospital of the patient's imminent arrival and closely monitor his vital signs en route.

LEARNING OBJECTIVES
- Relate mechanism of injury to potential injuries of the spine.
- Describe the implications of not properly caring for patients with potential spinal injuries.
- State the signs and symptoms of potential spinal injury.
- Describe the method of determining if a responsive patient may have a spinal injury.

Injuries to the Spine

Injuries to the head are often associated with spinal injuries, so assessment of head and spinal injuries is integrated in the EMT's approach to the patient.

Mechanism of Injury

Most injuries to the spinal cord occur because of damage to the spinal column that protects the cord. The spinal cord is a soft tube that can be torn, crushed, or contused when the bony vertebrae are broken or displaced from their normal alignment. Motor vehicle crashes are the most common cause (>50%) of spinal cord injury, followed by falls and sports-related injuries. Diving is a common cause of sports-related injuries.

The spinal column can be crushed, displaced in any direction, or broken. Although injuries can occur at any site along the spinal column, certain sections of the column are more vulnerable than others. The most common sites of vertebral injury are where vertebrae that allow motion meet vertebrae that are fixed.

The thoracic vertebrae are fixed by the ribs and allow little motion. The cervical vertebrae are highly mobile, allowing a greater range of motion of the head and neck. It is easy to visualize the results of a sudden deceleration injury, such as a motor vehicle crash. A driver wearing a seat and shoulder belt experiences little movement of the thorax. However, the head continues to move forward after the chest has stopped. The junction of lower cervical vertebrae and upper thoracic vertebrae is the site of both bony fracture and tearing of the supporting ligaments.

With this concept in mind, the same potential exists at the other end of the thoracic vertebrae. Here, the fixed thoracic vertebrae T1 through T10 meet the more mobile lower two thoracic vertebrae, T11 and T12. Again, mobile and fused vertebrae meet because the eleventh and twelfth ribs are "floating" ribs that are not attached to the sternum anteriorly. A common site of injury is from T10 to the first lumbar vertebra (L1).

Because the sacrum is composed of vertebrae that are fused together, a similar site exists where the lower lumbar vertebrae meet the sacrum. Many patients with back injuries experience problems at the level of L4 and L5.

Specific Mechanisms of Injury

There are many different mechanisms of spinal injury. In addition to recognizing direct blows, you must understand the dynamic forces that are set in motion after impact. By appreciating these potential mechanisms, you can maintain the appropriate level of suspicion when approaching injured patients. Because most spinal cord injuries are closed injuries, there may be little gross evidence of damage to the spinal column. The mechanism of injury should be documented and relayed to hospital personnel so that they can continue to check for related complications while further evaluation (e.g., physical examination, with or without radiographic studies) proceeds.

Compression Injuries. Compression forces occur when one spinal vertebra is driven onto another. The force may be transmitted from above (the head) or below. Examples include incidents in which a person dives into shallow water with the head and neck in normal alignment (not flexed) or falls from a height and lands on the feet or buttocks. These forces often compress vertebrae to the point in which the bones are crushed. Damage to the spinal cord follows if the resulting bone fragments are driven into the spinal canal and impinge on the soft, vulnerable cord (**Figure 24-8**).

Flexion Injuries. Flexion forces usually involve fixed and mobile vertebrae. In these situations the head is driven forward by sudden deceleration (as described previously) or when force is applied to the back of the skull. The bodies of the adjacent vertebrae are wedged together anteriorly, with resulting fracture to the body of the vertebra. In some cases a flexion injury can tear the posterior ligament that supports the spine, allowing one vertebra to slide forward onto another, compressing the cord between them.

Flexion forces occur when the head is jolted forward in a head-on collision from deceleration forces or when the top of the head strikes the windshield with the neck in a flexed position. Flexion injuries also can result from falls when the spine is sharply flexed and jackknifes at the waist. A final example includes lap belt injuries, when the pelvis is held stationary and

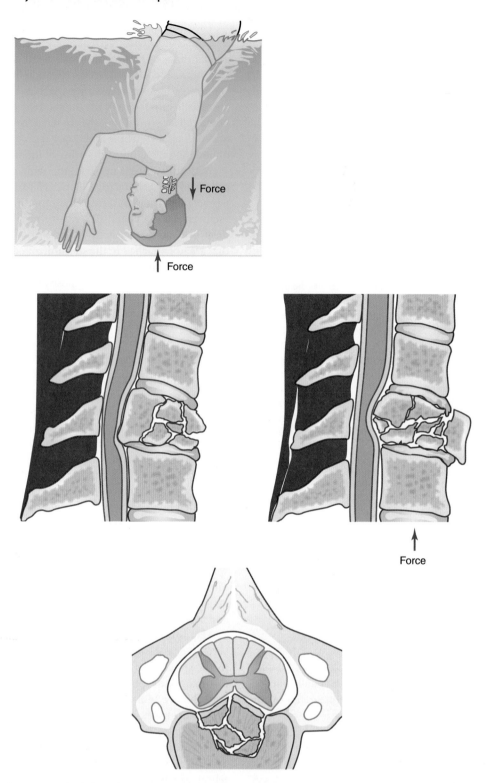

Figure 24-8 When a force is applied directly along the path of the vertebral column, the vertebrae are compressed onto one another, compressing the bone and causing fractures of the vertebral body. When bone fragments extrude into the vertebral canal, they may injure the spinal cord.

the deceleration forces place maximal stress on the thoracic and lumbar vertebrae (**Figure 24-9**).

Extension Injuries. Hyperextension injuries can occur when the head is suddenly jolted backward. An example would be striking the windshield of a vehicle with the face. The anterior ligaments supporting the spine can tear, with consequent swelling and possible instability resulting in dislocation (**Figure 24-10**).

"Whiplash injury" is a common term used to describe hyperextension of the neck resulting from motor vehicle crashes.

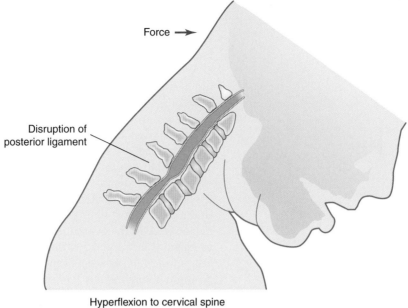

Force →

Disruption of
posterior ligament

Hyperflexion to cervical spine

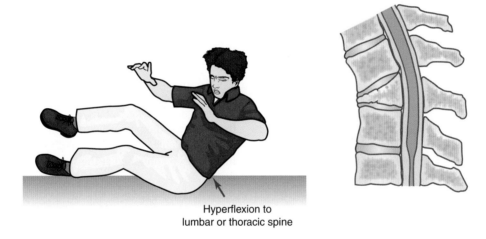

Hyperflexion to
lumbar or thoracic spine

Figure 24-9 When the spine is exposed to extreme flexion forces, the supporting posterior ligaments can tear, allowing the vertebrae to slide forward over one another and compressing the cord. In other cases, compression of the bone results in fracture.

Whiplash injury occurs when the head is suddenly jolted backward when a vehicle is struck from behind. The muscles in the anterior of the neck try to overcome this violent change in head position and can tear if sufficient force is exerted. A whiplash injury usually causes more muscle soreness and stiffness than a column or cord injury. However, reliably establishing the severity is impossible at the scene, and cervical immobilization should be applied. Other forces may cause excessive rotation or lateral bending of the spine. Distraction forces, such as hanging, can cause disruption of ligaments holding the vertebrae together and damage to the spinal cord.

Gunshot wounds may damage the spinal cord directly or drive bone fragments into the spinal canal. The course of a bullet within the body is unpredictable. It may ricochet off other bones and change course. Knife wounds may enter the spinal canal between vertebrae and damage the cord. Fortunately, these injuries are less common than those previously described.

When spinal injury is suspected, the patient should be appropriately immobilized.

It is important to reconstruct the mechanism of injury during the scene size-up and conceptualize the forces that may have caused spinal injury. In some patients with no external evidence of injury, the mechanism of injury itself provides the rationale for immobilization and treatment.

Assessment

One of the goals of every patient assessment is to determine whether the possibility of spinal injury exists and, if it does, to determine and document the level of injury. Understanding the possibility of spinal injury leads to proper care and handling at the scene and immobilization before and during transport to prevent further injury. Knowledge of the presence and level of spinal injury helps to identify and anticipate the complications requiring respiratory and circulatory support.

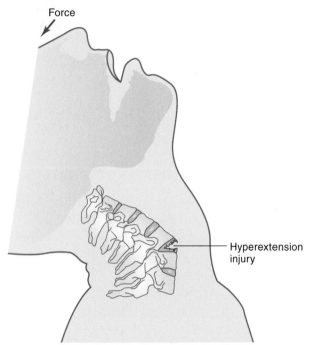

Figure 24-10 When forces are applied to the forehead or face, hyperextension injuries can occur. This figure illustrates an example of a hyperextension force and the tearing of supporting ligaments and the related displacement of vertebrae.

Scene Size-up

During the scene size-up, you should try to determine the mechanism of injury and conceptualize what types of forces occurred during the event. You should assume that all unconscious patients have a possible spinal injury. If the patient was a victim of a motor vehicle crash, a significant fall, or other significant injury, approach the patient with a high level of suspicion. This is important to prevent aggravating a possible spinal injury during the assessment phase. Bruising or lacerations about the head, face, and forehead should raise your suspicion, as should signs of trauma to the shoulders or pelvis, because forces causing these injuries may be transmitted to the spine. Patients may also have another injury as their major complaint, such as a fractured extremity, that is more painful than the spinal injury. Such associated injuries may distract their attention from their spinal injury.

Patients may deny or minimize their injuries. A primary goal is to prevent further spinal injury from occurring.

Initial (Primary) Assessment

Most patients sustain spinal injury as a result of motor vehicle crashes. Some patients may still be trapped in the vehicle when help arrives. Therefore, gaining access and initiating essential treatment are often the initial steps in the rescue process.

Patients still in a vehicle should be evaluated with a focus on the cervical spine. Either you or your partner must maintain the head and neck in the neutral position while supporting the weight of the head. This is true for both conscious and unconscious patients. If the initial (primary) assessment shows no immediate danger to life, the ideal means of extrication is to apply a cervical collar and immobilize the patient on a short spine board before removal. Once removed, the patient should be placed on a long spine board in anticipation that injuries to the thoracic or lumbar spine may also have occurred.

When the initial assessment shows that CPR or other lifesaving measures are needed, or that another hazard exists, there is no time to use the short spine board, and rapid extrication should be done instead (see Chapter 5).

When spinal injury is suspected, the primary assessment includes immediate inline immobilization of the cervical spine. You should open the airway with the modified jaw thrust to prevent hyperextension of the neck. If a patient is found with the head flexed, you should return the head to the neutral position and support it. If you encounter resistance in returning the neck to the neutral position, evaluate the adequacy of ventilations in the position found. In certain types of dislocation injuries, the vertebrae can become locked in a dislocated position. If the patient is hypoventilating or apneic, you should provide positive-pressure ventilation, again avoiding extension of the neck if possible by using a jaw thrust to open the airway. With possible spinal injuries, spend extra time immobilizing the patient securely before transport, unless signs of inadequate ventilation and circulation or other life-threatening conditions exist that require rapid transport to the hospital.

Focused (Secondary) Assessment

During the patient history you should attempt to reconstruct the mechanism of injury and the events leading up to the injury. You may need the help of bystanders or witnesses to reconstruct the events. If the patient is unconscious, this may be the only means available. The condition of the patient may dictate that the history be obtained at the same time that treatment is rendered.

Important questions and observations include the following:

- When did the injury occur?
- What was the position of the patient at the time of injury? Was the patient thrown by the impact (e.g., unrestrained passenger ejected from vehicle)?
- In motor vehicle crashes, what damage occurred to the vehicle? Estimate the speed of impact, and determine the position of the patient in the vehicle. Was the patient wearing a seat belt? Has the patient been moved? Did he or she move initially?
- Did the patient lose consciousness before the injury?
- Did the patient experience a period of cyanosis or apnea?
- In falls, what is the estimated height of the fall, and what surface did the patient strike on landing?
- Do you suspect alcohol or drug use?
- What is the patient's previous medical history? Is it related to the cause of the injury (e.g., a diabetic patient with hypoglycemia or fainting)?

Box 24-1 lists signs and symptoms of a spinal injury.

Rapid Trauma Assessment

You should pay special attention to the spine during the rapid trauma assessment. Using a log roll (see Chapter 7), assess the cervical, thoracic, and lumbar spine for tenderness or deformities and

| **Box 24-1** | Signs and Symptoms of Spinal Injuries* |

Tenderness in the area of injury (especially tenderness of the spine)
Pain associated with moving
Pain independent of movement or palpation
Obvious deformity of the spine on palpation
Soft tissue injuries associated with trauma:
    Head and neck to cervical spine
    Shoulders, back, or abdomen—thoracolumbar spine
    Lower extremities—lumbosacral spine
Numbness, weakness, or tingling in the extremities
Loss of sensation or paralysis below the suspected level of injury
Loss of sensation or paralysis in the upper or lower extremities
Incontinence

*Lack of pain or the ability to walk, move extremities, or feel sensation does not rule out the possibility of spinal column or cord damage. You should tell the patient not to move while asking questions.

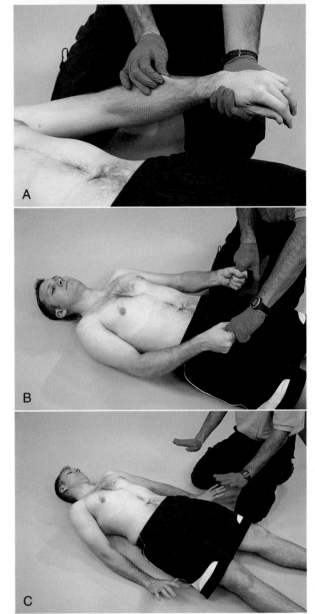

look for other signs of injury (DCAP/BTLS). Important questions to ask the patient include the following:

- "What happened?"
- "Does your neck or back hurt?"
- "Where does it hurt?"
- "Can you move your hands and feet?"
- "Can you feel me touching your fingers and toes?"

A brief examination of the sensory and motor functions should be performed before transport. Check both hands and feet for the ability to feel touch and pain and for motor function.

A systematic examination is important to identify the level of injury and to compare one side with the other. You should proceed to check the arms, starting at the hands and checking first for sensation and then for movement. Have the patient grasp your fingers in the palm of one hand and squeeze to check for strength. Again, compare the two sides and document your findings (**Figure 24-11**).

You should then check sensation in the lower extremities (**Figure 24-12**). To assess motor function of the lower extremities, ask the patient to move the toes up and down. Then place your hands against the soles of both feet. Have the patient try to push your hands away, using only the toes, to gauge the patient's strength. The muscle strength should be noted as absent, weak, or present (**Figure 24-13**).

Special Assessment Considerations

Respirations. Look closely at the rate and depth of respirations. Shallow breathing may indicate that the muscles of respiration are impaired. Look at the type of breathing. Is it abdominal breathing only? Ask the patient to take a deep breath to check for the effectiveness of the intercostal muscles. Does the chest rise and expand equally? You can also ask the patient to exhale vigorously or cough to check abdominal muscle function.

A major concern with spinal cord injury is respiratory function. All the nerves that innervate the respiratory muscles pass through the cervical and thoracic portions of the spinal

Figure 24-11 **A,** Sensory examination. Have the patient close the eyes, and provide stimuli on both surfaces of the upper extremities with a pinch or touch with a blunt object. Have the patient indicate when the stimuli are felt. If the patient is unable to speak, observe for responsiveness while you are applying the stimuli. **B,** Motor examination. Have the patient hold both your hands at the same time and squeeze with equal pressure. **C,** Motor examination. Have the patient extend his or her hands.

column. Injuries to the cervical and thoracic spine may affect a patient's ability to breathe. The main muscle of respiration, the diaphragm, is innervated by the phrenic nerve, which arises from branches off the third, fourth, and fifth cervical vertebrae (C3 to C5). Nerves from the second through eighth thoracic vertebrae (T2 to T8) innervate the intercostal muscles. Nerves from T8 to T12 innervate the abdominal muscles.

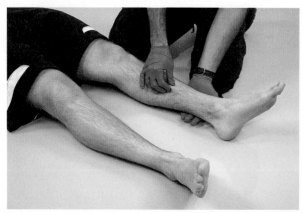

Figure 24-12 Sensory examination. Have the patient close the eyes, and provide stimuli to the lower extremities with a pinch or touch with a blunt object. Have the patient indicate when the stimuli are felt. If the patient is unable to speak, observe for responsiveness while you are applying the stimuli. When conducting a sensory examination, note sensory loss on one side of the body compared with the other. When appropriate, check for levels of sensory functions at the clavicle, nipple line, navel, and groin (key dermatomes).

If the spinal cord is damaged at the level of C3, all the muscles of respiration are paralyzed, and no spontaneous respirations occur. You must provide total respiratory support in this situation.

Injuries at or above C5 result in loss of both the intercostal and the abdominal muscles of breathing, resulting in diaphragmatic breathing only. The diaphragm continues to function because the nerves have already exited from the spinal cord above the level of injury. The loss of the intercostal and abdominal muscles may result in smaller tidal volumes. The patient must compensate for the decreased tidal volume by increasing the respiratory rate. You may note abdominal movement only. Supplemental oxygen is required, and assistance with positive-pressure ventilation may be necessary. When the intercostal and abdominal muscles are paralyzed, the patient is unable to cough effectively and has more difficulty clearing secretions, blood, and vomitus. Suction must be available to keep the oropharynx clear.

Table 24-1 summarizes the level of spinal cord injury in relation to the patient's respiratory status and treatment.

Pulse and Blood Pressure. When assessing blood pressure and pulse, you should remember that spinal injury can alter the findings. When the spinal cord is severed at or above the upper thoracic level, the patient may become hypotensive from vasodilation. The sympathetic nerves control the tone of the blood vessels. With loss of sympathetic tone, which can result from thoracic spinal cord injury, the blood vessels dilate and the blood pressure falls (hypotension). Many patients with this type of shock *(neurogenic)* have systolic blood pressure levels in the range of 70 to 80 mm Hg. Their pulse rate appears normal in the range of 60 to 80 beats/min. They cannot compensate by increasing their heart rate because this is also a function of the sympathetic nervous system. Furthermore, because the

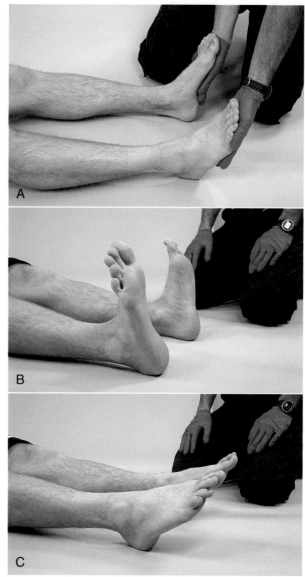

Figure 24-13 **A,** With your hands placed on the soles of the feet, ask the patient to apply downward pressure. **B,** Have the patient flex the ankles. **C,** Have the patient flex and extend the feet. When checking for motor function, note the differences in motor strength and the ability to move one extremity or the other (lateralizing signs).

Table 24-1	Level of Cervical Spinal Cord Injury in Relation to Respiratory Status and Treatment	
Level of Injury	**Respiratory Status**	**Treatment**
Above C3	Complete paralysis of all muscles of respiration	Positive-pressure ventilations, oxygen
Below C5	Paralysis of intercostal and abdominal muscles, causing decreased tidal volume and ineffective cough	Supplemental oxygen May require positive-pressure ventilation Suction of airway

vessels are dilated, the skin may be warm and perhaps flushed, in marked contrast to the cool, pale, and clammy skin of the patient with hypovolemic shock, who has a normal sympathetic nervous system.

Trauma sufficient to cause cord damage may also have caused other injuries. Because signs of hypovolemic shock may be masked by the simultaneous presence of neurogenic shock, look carefully for signs of injuries known to be associated with significant blood loss. Remember that patients with spinal cord injury also have sensory loss and may not complain of pain or tenderness.

You must have a high index of suspicion for internal bleeding when evaluating a patient with suspected spinal injury caused by trauma. Spinal injury patients may not feel pain or have signs of shock, such as rapid pulse or clammy skin from loss of sympathetic functions.

Priapism. Another sign of spinal cord injury is **priapism** (sustained penile erection). This condition is also explained by loss of sympathetic influence. The parasympathetic nerves causing dilation of the penile vessels are unopposed by the sympathetic nerves that constrict these vessels. Bladder and bowel functions also may be altered.

Unresponsive Patient. Because unresponsive patients cannot inform you of pain or tenderness or cooperate with sensorimotor examination, there is more reliance on mechanism of injury and history from bystanders. With an unresponsive patient, you should perform the initial (primary) assessment and rapid trauma assessment and look for injury and other related signs. It is critical to expose these patients and perform a thorough physical examination to identify possibly hidden injuries.

> ### REAL*World*
>
> As an EMT, you must remember that medical conditions may cause traumatic events. When you find a patient unconscious and unresponsive after a traumatic event, assess and manage the ABCs. Manage injuries as they are discovered, then consider a possible medical problem, such as a seizure, hypoglycemia, or stroke.

Ongoing Assessment (Reassessment)

The sensorimotor examination, mental status assessment, and vital signs should be repeated periodically. You should record your findings on the prehospital care report and pay particular attention to any changes in the level of motor or sensory function.

> #### LEARNING OBJECTIVES
> • Describe the airway emergency medical care techniques for the patient with a suspected spinal injury.
> • Describe how to stabilize the cervical spine.
> • Establish the relationship between airway management and the patient with head and spinal injuries.

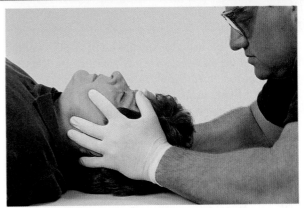

Figure 24-14 Manual inline stabilization.

Management

Airway

Patients with altered mental status or any evidence of neurologic dysfunction should be given high-concentration oxygen. Lack of an adequate airway and secretions that may obstruct the airway are major concerns. If any doubt exists about the adequacy of ventilations, you should assist with positive-pressure ventilation.

You should have suction ready because the airway may need to be cleared while the patient's head is still immobilized. If the patient vomits while immobilized on a spine board, be ready to move the patient and board as a unit onto one side (if necessary) to suction and clear vomitus and prevent aspiration.

Stabilization of Cervical Spine

After ensuring an open airway, you should ensure stabilization of the cervical spine. **Manual inline stabilization** consists of holding a patient's head in a neutral position in line with the rest of the body (**Figure 24-14**). Manual inline stabilization should be maintained throughout the assessment and management of a patient until the patient has been fully immobilized.

As with all suspected fractures, the patient with possible spinal injuries should be immobilized before being moved. The technique depends on how the patient is found—lying, sitting, or standing. These skills are demonstrated later in this chapter. The algorithm shown in **Figure 24-15** represents one method by which multiple assessment findings are used to determine the need for spinal immobilization (see also Chapter 7).

Injuries to the Head

Understanding the basis for evaluation and treatment of patients with brain and skull injuries is assisted by knowledge of the anatomy and physiology of the CNS. Disruption of the brain's blood supply can result from traumatic or medical conditions. In addition, the brain can be injured from a direct blow, loss of vital nutrients, or drugs. Considering the difference between structural and metabolic injuries assists you in understanding evaluation and management.

Structural Injuries

Injuries to the brain that cause disruption of specific sections of brain tissue or nerves result in loss of specific functions. Damage can occur to one area while other parts of the nervous system may still function. Injuries that involve specific areas are said to be structural injuries. These injuries may be traumatic or nontraumatic.

For example, a penetrating wound to the head may disrupt the tracts of nerves on the left side of the brain only and leave the right side of the brain functionally intact. Because the nerves cross to the other side of the body, the patient with a wound to the left brain may not have use of the right side of the body, but the left side of the body may still function.

Some medical conditions also can be classified as "structural," as in patients with disrupted blood supply in one artery supplying a particular area of the brain (e.g., stroke). Such patients can have weakness and loss of sensation on one side of the body.

Metabolic Injuries

When the energy processes necessary for cell function are compromised, the patient has a metabolic injury. The best example is the lack of oxygen after a cardiac arrest. All the brain's cells are affected. The patient loses consciousness, does not respond to stimuli such as pain, has no ability to move, and loses control of vital functions such as breathing. The cells on both sides of the body are affected equally.

How can you tell whether a patient has a structural or a metabolic problem? One clue to structural injury is asymmetrical findings. You will note a difference when comparing one side of the body to the other, as if certain wires had been cut on an electrical diagram. Contrast this with metabolic injuries, which will affect all CNS tissues equally. Both sides of the brain are equally affected. Such an injury affects the metabolism of all cells. Examples include hypoxia from any cause, low blood glucose levels, shock, and poisoning. For example, you would not expect the victim of cyanide poisoning to be able to move one side of the body better than the other; both sides of the brain have been poisoned.

Secondary Complications

After direct injury to the brain, complications can lead to further damage to brain tissue. These secondary complications include hypoxia, hypotension, hypoglycemia, infections, and increased _intracranial pressure_ (ICP). They can follow the primary event and further compromise the ability of the injured nerve tissue to heal or regain function. These secondary processes may exacerbate the original injury, resulting in more extensive damage or death.

These complications can result from a loss of the brain's ability to control vital organ systems after an injury, such as loss of breathing control after a blow to the head. They may also arise from other injuries, such as internal bleeding and chest trauma, which can lead to hypotension or hypoxia. Swelling or bleeding within the skull is another example of secondary brain injury. Because the brain is contained in a nonexpandable space, swelling or bleeding within the skull results in increased pressure on the brain (increased ICP).

Hypoxia

An unconscious patient with head trauma may have an obstructed airway caused by relaxation of the jaw and blockage by the tongue, causing hypoxia. A patient with multiple trauma may have both head injury and injury to the respiratory system or chest wall, such as flail chest. The resulting hypoxia from the flail chest or the obstructed airway is a further insult to the already damaged brain tissue.

Pulse oximetry can be used to determine a patient's oxygenation. Normal saturation is approximately 95% to 100%. The Brain Trauma Foundation recommends treatment to keep oxygen saturation greater than 90% to prevent secondary head injury from hypoxia.

Hypotension

A patient with head trauma and severe hemorrhage from a ruptured spleen may have both hypotension and direct brain damage. The hypotension aggravates the brain injury by decreasing brain perfusion with oxygenated blood. Patients with isolated closed head injuries would not be expected to present with hypotension because the amount of blood lost in the skull of an adult patient is usually insufficient to cause hypovolemic shock. When signs of hypovolemic shock are present (hypotension; rapid pulse; cool, pale, clammy skin), you should look elsewhere (outside the head) for signs of internal bleeding. Remember, spinal injury can also lead to hypotension caused by widespread vasodilation.

Blood pressure varies with age. The Brain Trauma Foundation recommends that hypotension be treated to prevent secondary head injury from hypoperfusion. **Table 24-2** reviews the target blood pressure of pediatric age groups.

Stabilization of blood pressure may require control of bleeding and administration of intravenous (IV) fluid; you should consider an advanced life support (ALS) intercept or rapid transport to the hospital as appropriate.

Hypoglycemia

Consider a diabetic patient working on his roof through the afternoon. He missed a meal, became faint, and fell from the roof, sustaining a head injury. If damage to brain tissue occurs from the fall, the chance of healing is further compromised by the lack of a vital brain nutrient, glucose. Because hypoglycemia may precede a traumatic brain injury, you should assess glucose level in patients, especially if a medical problem, such as fainting, occurred before the trauma or if patients are known to have diabetes.

Increased Intracranial Pressure

A patient may have sustained a head injury with a loss of consciousness, recovered, and then later experienced deterioration in mental status. Such a patient may have injured an artery or vein that resulted in bleeding within the skull. Because the space within the skull is confined, any additional content (as from bleeding) increases the pressure within the cranium. This increase in ICP is the cause of additional brain injury and occurs after the patient apparently recovered from the initial event (see Epidural Hematoma).

Infection

A patient with an open skull fracture may recover from the brain injury only to incur an infection of the brain. As much as possible, use sterile techniques to cover wounds. The importance of recognizing and managing secondary brain injury cannot be overemphasized. Little can be done for recovery of brain tissue that was destroyed as a result of direct trauma (e.g., gunshot wound). However, other areas of brain tissue, although damaged, may heal if there is no further injury. Neurosurgical centers have found that the increased ability to save patients with severe head injuries results from careful attention to and treatment of these secondary processes.

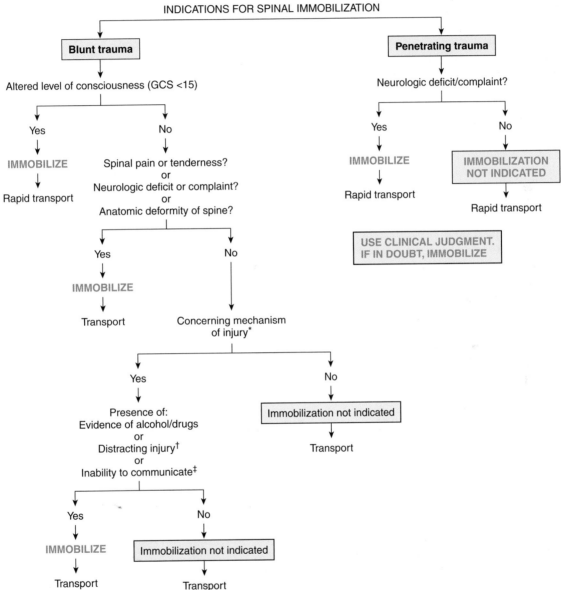

Figure 24-15 Algorithm showing one method by which multiple assessment findings are used to determine the need for spinal immobilization. *Mechanism of injury: (1) Any mechanism that produced a violent impact to the head, neck, torso, or pelvis (e.g., assault, entrapment in structural collapse). (2) Incidents producing sudden acceleration, deceleration, or lateral bending forces to the neck or torso (e.g., moderate- to high-speed motor vehicle accident, pedestrian struck, involved in explosion). (3) Any fall, especially in elderly persons. (4) Ejection or fall from a motorized or human-powered transportation device (e.g., scooters, skateboards, bicycles, motor vehicles). (5) Victim of shallow-water diving incident. †Distracting injury: Any injury that may have the potential to impair the patient's ability to appreciate other injuries. Examples of distracting injuries include (1) long-bone fracture; (2) visceral injury requiring surgical consultation; (3) large laceration, degloving injury, or crush injury; (4) large burns; or (5) any other injury producing acute functional impairment. ‡Inability to communicate: Any patient who, for reasons not specified above, cannot clearly communicate so as to participate actively in the assessment. Such patients include speech-impaired or hearing-impaired patients, those who only speak a foreign language, and small children.

Head Injury and Associated Cervical Spine Injury

Although only a small percentage of patients with a head injury have fractures of the cervical spine, these patients area at risk of paralysis and death if the cervical spine fracture is not handled properly. You should suspect that all patients with a head injury might also have an injury to the cervical spine.

Scalp Wounds

Many head injuries result in scalp lacerations. Associated skull fractures and injury to brain tissue may or may not be present (**Figure 24-16**). The scalp has numerous small blood vessels, and significant bleeding can occur from scalp lacerations. As with other wounds, bleeding from the scalp is best controlled with direct pressure. The pressure should be applied gently and just sufficient to control the bleeding; it should be distributed over a wide area with a wide dressing and bandage, especially if you suspect an underlying skull fracture. Because of the rich supply of blood vessels in the scalp, hematomas often occur, which on palpation are difficult to distinguish from depressed skull fractures. By applying direct pressure over a broad area, you are less likely to displace loose bone fragments downward into the brain.

A person can bleed to death from scalp lacerations. Often, when patients are found to be hypotensive, active bleeding from scalp wounds may have ceased. Look at the amount of obvious bleeding on the ground or floor. The patient may not bleed

Table 24-2	Targeted Blood Pressure to Age 15 Years*
Age (years)	**Systolic Blood Pressure (mm Hg)**
<1	65
1-5	70-75
5-12	75-80
12-15	80-90

Data from Ghajar J: Traumatic brain injury, *Lancet* 356(9233):923-929, 2000.
*Interventions to maintain blood pressure above the targeted systolic blood pressure levels are recommended to maintain perfusion of the brain.

again from the wound until the blood volume is replaced and the hypotension corrected.

Skull Fractures

Although a significant force is required to fracture the skull, a skull fracture in itself does not mean brain damage has occurred. A patient with a skull fracture may have remarkably few or no other signs of injury. On the other hand, patients without skull fractures may have lethal head injuries.

However, skull fractures in certain areas tend to cause more severe damage. One region is the temporal area, where a major artery, the middle meningeal artery, travels along a groove on the inside surface of the temporal bone. If the sharp bony fragments of the fracture lacerate this artery, significant bleeding can occur inside the skull (**Figure 24-17**).

As with other injuries, skull injuries may be open or closed. In an open injury the skin over the fracture site is not intact, allowing communication between the outside environment and the brain or its coverings (meninges). This results in an increased risk of infection. In a closed injury the skin above the fracture site is still intact.

Types of Skull Injuries

Injuries to the skull can vary from simple lines or cracks to depression of skull fragments into the brain (**Figure 24-18**).

When great forces strike the skull, especially if they are applied over a small surface area (as with a hammer blow), the bone fragments may be depressed downward toward the brain. The depressed skull fracture may be confused with a hematoma because both will have a soft center that is easily depressed on palpation.

With open wounds the depressed fracture may be obvious. A penetrating wound through the scalp may cause a depressed skull fracture. Bullets can drive skull fragments forward and into the brain. You should not attempt to remove penetrating objects that are lodged within the skull.

Injuries to the base or floor of the skull are often recognized by the characteristic sign of clear CSF leaking from the nose or ear, because these structures are connected to bones from the

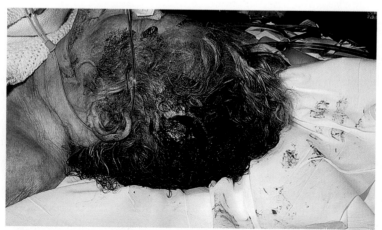

Figure 24-16 Deep laceration of scalp by fall on street after the patient was struck by a vehicle. This patient sustained a subdural hematoma underneath the area of the external laceration.

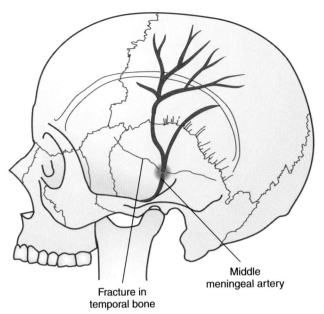

Figure 24-17 Temporal bone fractures can tear the middle meningeal artery, resulting in bleeding within the epidural space.

Fracture in temporal bone

Middle meningeal artery

base of the skull. Sometimes the CSF that leaks from the nose or ear is mixed with blood.

You should place a loose, sterile dressing over any leaking CSF or blood from the nose or ear. Do not attempt to obstruct or block the flow. The main purpose of the dressing is to minimize further contamination by outside debris or bacteria moving up through the fracture site into the brain.

Other signs of basilar skull fracture include black-and-blue areas or ecchymosis around the eyes ("raccoon eyes," **Figure 24-19**) or behind the ear (Battle's sign). These, however, may occur later, even hours after the injury.

Case in Point

Two EMTs respond to a 43-year-old man who was repairing a roof and fell 30 feet, landing on his back. Bystanders advise them that the man was unresponsive for 5 minutes and regained conscious 2 minutes before their arrival. There is a large hematoma over the right side of his head. The patient is alert and oriented with a Glasgow Coma Scale (GCS) score of 15. He is breathing at 24 breaths/min with no cyanosis. Blood pressure is 120/80 mm Hg, and the pulse is 90 beats/min, regular, and of normal quality. During transport the patient becomes unresponsive with GCS score of 8 (unequal pupils) and 8 breaths/min. The EMTs institute positive-pressure ventilation.

Traumatic Brain Injuries

Concussion

Understanding some of the common conditions that can follow a head injury helps an EMT recognize the significance of assessment findings.

A **concussion** is defined as a transient loss of consciousness or neurologic function from a blow to the brain. The blow sends shock waves that temporarily disrupt brain function.

Many degrees of brain injury exist. The least severe and most common brain injury is a momentary loss of function immediately after impact, in which case the patient may not even be sure that consciousness was lost. The patient might have a short period of confusion but will have full recall of events up to or after the point of impact.

Also common are brief periods of amnesia (memory loss). The patient cannot recall events just before impact or in the period immediately after the blow. The brain is not able to store these events in its memory.

More severe injuries cause direct damage, with bruising or contusion of the brain. Bruised brain tissue does not function properly. Specific localized findings may be present that correlate with the site of injury. Depending on the location of the bruise or contusion, a loss of motor ability on one side or perhaps an isolated visual disturbance may result.

Bleeding can occur after head injury, either within the brain tissue itself or in the spaces between the meningeal layers that cover the brain. A major complication of bleeding within the skull is increased ICP.

Increased Intracranial Pressure

As pressure within the cranium rises, certain signs and symptoms appear. The conscious patient may complain of headaches, nausea, and vomiting. Sometimes the vomiting is "projectile" (ejected from mouth forcefully).

The level of consciousness may begin to deteriorate. The patient, who was previously alert, becomes sleepy or more confused and is more difficult to arouse. Instead of responding to verbal commands, the patient may eventually respond only to painful stimuli or not at all. Children are more likely to experience drowsiness, nausea, and vomiting after even minor head injuries.

The most sensitive indicator of increasing ICP is a change (deterioration) in level of consciousness. After a head injury, the damage caused by the direct blow (concussion, contusion, or disruption of the blood supply) has been completed. Signs present immediately after the injury can be attributed to the blow itself.

EXTENDED*Transport*

During extended transport of a patient with traumatic brain injury, the EMT must monitor the patient for signs of increased intracranial pressure (ICP). The patient may initially be responsive and lucid, then become agitated and combative during transport. As the swelling continues, the patient may become unconscious and unresponsive. Nausea and vomiting may occur with increased ICP. The EMT must be prepared to suction airways and assist with ventilation. Summoning a second EMT may help if the patient becomes combative or is immobilized and requires rolling to the side to protect the airway.

Worsening of the condition might be caused by increased ICP from bleeding or swelling within the skull. This is especially the case if there is no other complication, such as hypoxia or hypotension, to explain the deterioration in status.

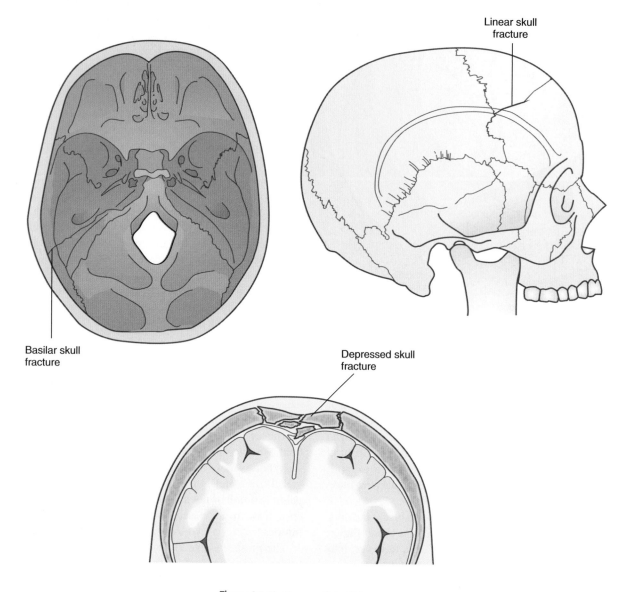

Figure 24-18 Types of skull fractures.

Eye and Motor Findings

As ICP increases, the brain may be forced down through the opening in the base of the skull (foramen magnum). Because the nerves to the eyes leave the brainstem in this area, they often are compressed between the herniating brain and bony structures; therefore eye findings may include a dilated pupil on one side. The dilated pupil may not constrict when a light shines in it. The eyelid over the dilated eye may begin to droop as well. Because nerve tracts bearing sensory and motor nerves to the entire body can also be compressed, the patient may have one-sided weakness, paralysis, sensory loss, or a combination of these findings.

As the pressure increases, the sensorimotor findings may extend to both sides. With further deterioration, the patient may assume abnormal body positions or postures. The classic postures are abnormal flexion (*decorticate posturing*), in which the arms are flexed but the legs are extended (**Figure 24-20**), and later abnormal extension (*decerebrate posturing*), in which the arms are extended and internally rotated at the shoulders, with

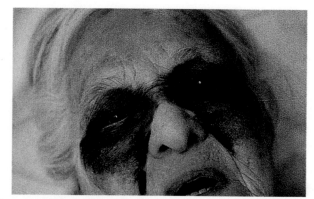

Figure 24-19 "Raccoon eyes," indicating possible basilar skull fracture.

the wrists flexed and the legs extended (**Figure 24-21**). These postures may be assumed spontaneously by the patient or in response to painful stimuli. If herniation of the brain continues, there may be no body movement, with the limbs flaccid and the muscles limp without tone. With transmission of increased ICP

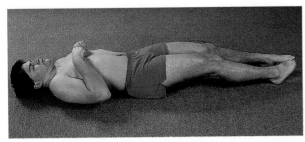

Figure 24-20 Abnormal flexion (decorticate posturing). Arms and wrists are flexed and legs and feet are extended.

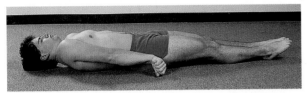

Figure 24-21 Abnormal extension (decerebrate posturing). Arms are extended and internally rotated at the shoulders with wrists flexed. Legs are extended.

to the brainstem, the centers controlling vital functions, notably breathing, also are affected.

Respirations

Abnormal respiratory patterns might occur, indicating damage to different levels of the brain **(Figure 24-22)**. You should describe the patterns during your presentation to hospital personnel.

Pulse and Blood Pressure

A late sign of increased ICP is increasing blood pressure with a slow pulse. The rising pressure within the cranium tends to collapse the blood vessels, and it is more difficult for blood to overcome this added resistance to flow. The brain makes a final effort to restore perfusion by directing a drastic increase in the blood pressure (especially the systolic) to overcome this increased ICP. Blood pressure receptors *outside* the head note this increase in blood pressure and signal for the heart to slow down. This leads to the findings of increased blood pressure and slower pulse. In addition to bleeding within the brain itself, bleeding can occur within the coverings of the brain inside the skull, exerting pressure on the brain.

Epidural Hematoma

Laceration of the arteries traveling along the inner surface of the cranium can lead to hematomas in the space outside the dura **(Figure 24-23)**. Because the bleeding is arterial, the blood accumulates quickly and can lead to rapid deterioration of the patient's mental status. Thus, early recognition of signs of increased ICP is important because the bleeding must be stopped and the clot surgically evacuated to prevent further deterioration in status and death.

Epidural hematomas typically present with a short period of unconsciousness after blunt trauma to the head, followed by a

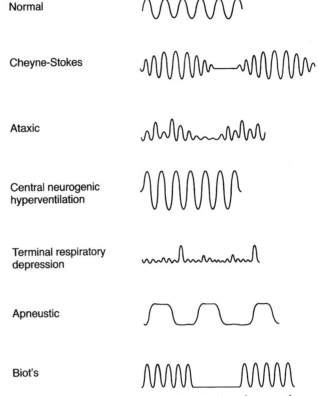

Figure 24-22 Patterns of abnormal respiration that may be present after brain injury.

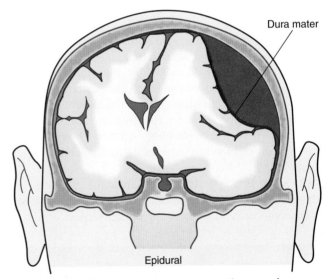

Figure 24-23 Epidural hematomas occur in the space between the dura and the skull and result from arterial bleeding.

lucid interval during which the patient regains consciousness. Some patients do not have an initial loss of consciousness immediately after impact. Shortly thereafter, however, the patient shows a decrease or alteration in the level of consciousness and has a dilated pupil on the side of the blow and weakness and sensory impairment on the opposite side of the body. Within a short time the patient has abnormal respiratory patterns,

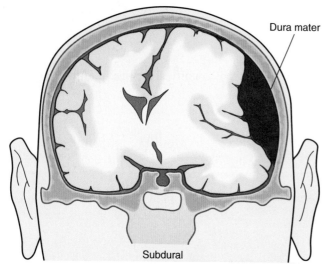

Figure 24-24 Subdural hematomas occur in the space between the dura and the arachnoid and result from venous bleeding.

abnormal posturing, possibly high blood pressure and a slow pulse, and then death occurs if the condition is left untreated. An important point to remember is that the blow itself, although severe enough to cause temporary loss of consciousness, is not the cause of subsequent deterioration. Rather, the bleeding caused by the blow results in the increased ICP (a secondary complication), which causes the subsequent deterioration.

Subdural Hematoma

Underneath the dura lies a rich venous network. When veins in this area are ruptured after trauma, bleeding is confined to the space between the dura and the arachnoid membrane, resulting in a subdural hematoma. Although bleeding from veins is under lower pressure than arterial bleeding, if a large vein or many smaller veins are ruptured, blood can accumulate rapidly. If smaller veins bleed, it takes a longer for the same amount of blood to accumulate in the subdural space (**Figure 24-24**).

Because of the speed with which hematomas in the cranium cause death, you should provide early transport of a patient with a serious head injury to an appropriate facility.

REALWorld

Subdural hematomas may take several days to present. Geriatric patients are at increased risk of subdural hematoma because they are prone to falls, and the size of their brain shrinks with age. An elderly patient may fall and then may be found unconscious hours or even days later. As an EMT, you must take a thorough history and must be complete in your assessment to determine if a traumatic event occurred.

Hospital personnel rely on an accurate and knowledgeable record of the mechanism of injury, the initial signs and symptoms, and subsequent evaluations of the patient's status en route to the hospital. As an EMT, you are responsible for a complete report.

LEARNING OBJECTIVE
• Relate mechanism of injury to potential injuries of the head.

Mechanism of Injury

More than half of all head injuries in the United States are the result of motor vehicle crashes. Other common sources of injuries include falls, home and sports accidents, and penetrating wounds from knives and guns.

Blunt Trauma

Either static or dynamic forces may cause a head injury. Most blunt head injuries are a combination of both mechanisms.

An example of a *static* injury would be a vehicle falling off a jack onto the head of a mechanic lying on the ground underneath. The force of the injury is applied in only one direction. The head and brain do not move about after the impact but are crushed between the vehicle and the ground.

Dynamic forces causing head injury are those that follow the initial blow. They are caused by movement of the brain within the skull, which has been set in motion by the impact. Dynamic forces can be applied even without a direct blow to the skull. The most common example may be in a motor vehicle crash in which the driver is wearing a seat belt. The deceleration forces after the collision cause the head and its contents to be subjected to rotational or shearing forces.

Because of the dynamic components of head injury, its effects may occur on the side of the brain opposite the site of the blow. The brain continues to move within the skull after the initial impact and can strike the opposite side of the skull. This *coup*, or blow, is opposite to (*contra*) the site of impact and is therefore known as a *contrecoup* injury.

The effects of the static and dynamic forces are usually additive. In fact, if rotation of the skull can be prevented, it takes a much greater blow to result in the same amount of brain damage.

Penetrating Trauma

Most penetrating injuries are the result of gunshot and knife wounds (**Figure 24-25**). In addition to destroying brain tissue in the path of the missile or penetrating object, associated bleeding and later swelling can extend the injury zone to brain tissue surrounding the path of penetration. Bullets cause shock waves that widen the area of damage in proportion to the speed and weight of the bullet.

Assessment

Scene Size-up

The mechanism of injury should be determined as completely as possible. In motor vehicle crashes an estimation of the speed of impact, point of impact, position of the patient in the vehicle, and whether the patient was wearing a seat belt are all important factors.

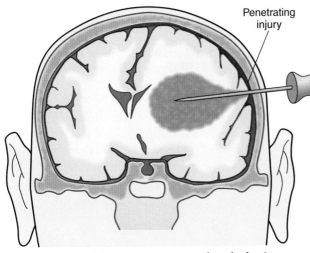

Figure 24-25 Penetrating wound to the brain.

Table 24-3	Glasgow Coma Scale Score		
Parameter	Type of Response	Point Value Assigned to Response	Comments
Eye opening	Spontaneous	4	
	To voice	3	
	To pain	2	
	None	1	
Verbal response	Oriented	5	Record patient's best verbal response.
	Confused	4	
	Inappropriate words	3	*Arouse patient with voice or painful stimulus.*
	Incomprehensible sounds	2	
	None	1	
Motor response	Obeys command	6	Record patient's best motor response.
	Localizes pain	5	
	Withdraw (pain)	4	*Response to command or painful stimulus.*
	Flexion (pain)	3	
	Extension (pain)	2	
	None	1	
Total score		3-15	

Initial (Primary) Assessment

Assessment of airway, breathing, and circulation (ABCs) is the first concern. You should approach all injured patients with the assumption that a cervical spine injury exists. Ideally, the cervical spine is stabilized manually as the initial assessment proceeds.

The airway maneuver of choice is the modified jaw thrust. You may need to insert an oropharyngeal or nasopharyngeal airway for an unconscious patient.

Suction must be available to aid in keeping the airway clear. The patient with a head injury is likely to vomit. Associated injuries to the face may cause bleeding or swelling, which can also compromise the airway.

Because terms such as "lethargic," "stuporous," and "semi-comatose" can have different meanings to various observers, you should avoid use of these terms. You should instead use the AVPU (*alert,* responds to *verbal* stimulus, responds to *painful* stimulus, *unresponsive*) method to describe findings during the check for responsiveness.

Glasgow Coma Scale

One method of objective assessment of mental status used by emergency medical service (EMS) and hospital personnel is the **Glasgow Coma Scale (GCS).** This method assesses the three parameters of eye opening, verbal response, and motor ability **(Table 24-3).**

Although the GCS was initially designed for patients with head trauma, it is also useful for evaluating and describing the neurologic status of all unresponsive patients. It enables health personnel at all levels to "speak the same language."

The GCS is intended for patients with an altered mental status. Patients who can be evaluated by the GCS range from individuals who are well oriented and able to obey commands to patients who are deeply comatose and unable to respond to any stimuli. Accordingly, stimuli are applied sequentially, starting with verbal questions and commands and followed by administration of painful stimulus if there is still no response.

A score is then assigned according to set criteria within the three general parameters. Four eye responses, five verbal responses, and six motor responses are possible. The best score is 15; the most unresponsive patient receives a score of 3. A score of 1 is the lowest score for each component of the GCS.

To apply a pain stimulus, you should apply pressure to the nail bed. Another painful stimulus used by many emergency department (ED) and prehospital personnel is to pinch the skin over the patient's forearm, shoulder, or armpit. The pain stimulus should be applied to both sides of the body because there may be a sensory deficit on one side.

Eye Opening. If the patient's eyes are open on your arrival or open spontaneously without being stimulated, the patient receives a score of 4. If the eyes open on the verbal command, "Open your eyes," the score is 3. If the eyes open after painful stimuli, the score is 2. If the eyes do not open in response to pain, the score is 1.

Verbal Response. The alert and oriented patient receives the highest score of 5. A patient who is confused but able to respond in a conversational manner receives a 4. A patient who cannot maintain a conversation and gives inappropriate responses to questions posed by the examiner receives a score of 3. This patient may respond in a disorganized manner with exclamatory or profane language. However, the key in distinguishing the confused from the inappropriate response is whether the *attention* of the patient can be maintained. The confused patient will converse with the examiner, and the patient's attention can be maintained. The inappropriately responding patient will drift off and will not answer the examiner's questions without repeated verbal stimulation. This patient has a more depressed mental status than the confused patient.

The patient who responds with incomprehensible sounds and moaning and no recognizable words receives a score of 2. The patient who does not respond verbally at all receives a score of 1.

Motor Response. The GCS score of 6 is given to a patient who appropriately responds to verbal motor commands (e.g., "Move your arms"). The assumption is that the patient has no fractures or other wounds of the extremities that will affect motor function relating to the command. The GCS is concerned with brain function, not the status of any other components necessary for movement.

A patient with a spinal injury that leaves the legs paralyzed would receive a GCS score of 6 if able to move an arm in response to a verbal command. This is evidence that the brain is intact. The inability of the patient to move the legs is a result of damage to a lower structure, in this case the spinal cord.

Painful Stimuli. The other possible motor response scores are elicited after application of painful stimuli. If a patient can localize the pain, a GCS score of 5 is given. Localizing pain is an attempt by the patient to reach for or to remove the source of a painful stimulus. For example, if the left shoulder is pinched as a painful stimulus, a patient might reach a hand up toward the examiner's fingers.

If the patient does not reach up for the examiner's hand but rather pulls away from the pain stimulus, the patient is said to "withdraw." A withdrawal response is given a score of 4.

Some patients respond with flexion of one or both arms in response to pain. This is called a *decorticate* response and indicates that the higher brain centers are damaged. This flexion of the arms is accompanied by extension of the legs in most cases. The flexion response receives a GCS score of 3.

With deeper coma or more extensive brain damage, a patient may respond to pain with the extension of both the arms and the legs. Extension of the arms is quite characteristic. The shoulders rotate internally, and the wrists flex. This response is also known as a *decerebrate* response. It indicates that the entire upper brain is functionally separate from the brainstem and the rest of the nervous system. The extension response receives a GCS score of 2. The lowest score of 1 is given if no response is observed from verbal or painful stimuli.

A patient is graded according to the best response that would give the highest score. The response does not have to be bilateral. That is, if the patient could not move one side but responded on the other side with a flexion response, the motor score would receive a grade of 3 for the flexion that was observed. You should remember to apply a pain stimulus on each side.

Scoring Approach. You should always describe the patient and record your findings according to the subcomponents of the GCS score. Your records may have space for the score as follows:

GCS: Verbal (1-5) _____, Motor (1-6) _____, Eyes (1-4) _____
___; Total score _____

Case in Point

A 30-year-old man has been shot in the head but has no other evident injuries. There is a wound over the right temporal bone and no visible exit wound. The patient was injured 10 minutes before EMT arrival. He is found to be breathing spontaneously, with deep ventilations at 26 breaths/min with no cyanosis. Blood pressure is 120/80 mm Hg, and the pulse is 60 beats/min, regular, and of normal quality. The patient is unresponsive without painful stimuli. The GCS evaluation shows eyes opening to pain, incomprehensible sounds, and flexion as the motor response. For this patient, E (2), V (2), and M (3) = GCS score of 7.

Table 24-4 Infant Glasgow Coma Scale Scoring

Eye Opening (E)= Points Assigned	Verbal Response (V)= Points Assigned	Motor Response (M)= Points Assigned
Spontaneous = 4	Coos, babbles = 5	Obeys = 6
Reaction to speech = 3	Irritable cry = 4	Localizes = 5
Reaction to pain = 2	Cries to pain = 3	Withdraws = 4
No response = 1	Moans, grunts = 2	Flexor response = 3
	No response = 1	Extensor response = 2
		No response = 1
Total score = E + V + M		

From the description in the Case in Point box, other healthcare providers can evaluate the patient's mental status. Some EMS systems use the total score for trauma *triage* (sorting of patients according to priority). Note that metabolic causes of coma may result in a low score. A patient who is "dead drunk" may have no response to verbal or painful stimuli and may receive a total score of 3.

The following systematic approach to collecting the GCS is recommended by the Brain Trauma Foundation.

Start with a check of eyes and verbal response with a series of questions, as follows:
1. "Can you tell me what happened?"
2. "Can you open your eyes?"
3. "Can you tell me the month and year?"
4. "Can you show me two fingers?"

If the patient does not respond to verbal commands, provide painful stimuli by using nail bed pressure, and observe the best response. For example, a patient who has open eyes, communicates the correct month and year, and is able to show you two fingers would receive a score of 15 (4 for eyes, 5 for voice, and 6 for motor). A patient who opened his or her eyes when prompted by the second question and is able to show you two fingers but did not know the month or year would receive a score of 13 (3 for eyes, 4 for voice, 6 for motor).

Infant Glasgow Coma Scale. The GCS technique described is used for children and adults. However, because of limited communications skills, infants require a special approach to evaluation. The Brain Trauma Foundation recommends the use of a modified GCS (**Table 24-4**). Questions appropriate for the infant's communication level are also recommended, as follows:
- To elicit eye opening, encourage the infant to look at a parent, caregiver, or toy. Stranger anxiety is common in infants older than 6 months.
- To determine verbal response and orientation, ask a question that requires an awareness and acknowledgment of something known, such as a parent.
- To determine motor response, use a simple command, preferably one that is not threatening, such as squeezing a parent's finger instead of an EMT's finger.

Special Situations. If a patient cannot be assessed for all three GCS components, you should still communicate the components of the score that can be assessed.

Box 24-2 Signs and Symptoms Associated with Brain and Skull Injury

Altered or decreasing mental status (best indicator)
Confusion, disorientation, or repetitive questioning
Deteriorating mental status if conscious
Unresponsiveness
Irregular breathing pattern
Consideration of mechanism of injury
Deformity of windshield
Deformity of helmet
Contusions, lacerations, hematomas to the scalp
Deformity to the skull
Blood or fluid (CSF) leakage from the ears or nose
Bruising (discoloration) around the eyes and behind the ears (mastoid process)
Neurologic disability
Nausea and vomiting
Unequal pupil size with altered mental status
Seizure activity

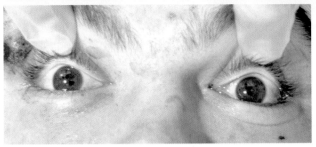

Figure 24-26 Pupils in a patient with traumatic brain injury and signs of herniation. Pupils are asymmetrical and nonreactive to light.

For the patient with an endotracheal tube in the airway who cannot speak, the score would be noted as follows:

Motor, flexion; eye, no response; verbal, not applicable (patient intubated)

For the patient with massive injuries about the eyes, the score would be noted as follows:

Verbal, incomprehensible sounds; motor, withdraws; eyes, not tested because of swelling

Focused (Secondary) Assessment

During the focused (secondary) assessment (patient history, physical examination) of the head-injured patient, you should remain alert for signs and symptoms associated with brain and skull injury (**Box 24-2**).

Head and Scalp. The scalp should be examined for signs of fractures, such as wounds, swelling, crepitus, and other deformities and signs of injury (DCAP/BTLS). You should gently palpate any swellings because depressed skull fractures may be present. Use direct pressure to control any bleeding. You should look carefully for features such as "raccoon eyes" and Battle's sign and for drainage from the ears and nose.

Pupils. Pupils should be evaluated for their size, responsiveness to light, and equality or symmetry. Always check the pupils because they give an indication of brainstem function. They are easily and readily evaluated and have good reliability.

Size. The size of the pupils is described as midposition, constricted, or dilated. They can be expressed more specifically in terms of their diameter in millimeters.

Equal Size. The pupils are generally equal to one another in size. If the pupils are not the same size, they are said to be "unequal." The finding of unequal pupils may mean that part of the brain has been injured. However, you should be aware that approximately 5% of the population has slightly unequal pupils.

Reaction to Light. Much information can be gained by shining a penlight or flashlight into the pupils. Pupils normally constrict when light is shined into the eye; this response is described as being "reactive to light."

The Brain Trauma Foundation defines significant changes in pupil findings as follows:

• Size: pupil size greater or equal to 4 mm in adults.
• Equal size: asymmetrical pupils differ by more than 1 mm.
• Reaction to light: a fixed pupil shows a change of less than 1 mm in reaction to bright light. Note findings of both right and left pupils (**Figure 24-26**).

When evaluating pupils, it is also important to understand other factors that may lead to abnormal pupillary findings. These conditions include the following:

• Hypoxemia
• Hypothermia
• Trauma to the eye and bones around the eye
• Drug use
• Hypotension
• Toxic exposure

If any of these conditions is present, note them on the prehospital record and initiate treatment. This includes treatment of hypoxia with ventilation and supplemental oxygen and body warming. Some conditions may require advanced life support, such as IV fluid therapy and antidotes for drug overdose. In these patients, you should consider the need for an ALS intercept (when transport will be delayed) or rapid transport to an appropriate hospital.

Motor and Sensory Examination. The neurologic examination for motor and sensory function in the field should be brief. The examination is performed to grossly determine the following:

1. Whether motor ability and sensation are intact.
2. Whether they are equal on both sides of the body.

You should touch the conscious patient on each side, first on the hands and then on the feet, and ask whether your touch can be felt. By touching the hand and the foot, you are testing the most distal portions of the extremities and are reasonably sure that sensation proximal is also intact.

You should then ask the patient to move both hands and then the feet. The motor examination should also begin with the hands and feet because, as with the sensation test, the most distal nerves will be tested, and the patient may have other injuries that would make movement of the rest of the extremities painful or inadvisable.

You can assess the sensation of patients with altered mental status by applying a painful stimulus to the hands and feet (e.g., pinch). Carefully observe the patient to see whether any motor and sensory responses are symmetrical (equal on both sides).

Vital Signs. Vital signs may vary as a result of head and spinal trauma. For example, while assessing the respiratory rate and depth, you should observe carefully for any abnormal respiratory patterns.

The brain controls regulation of temperature. With some brain injuries the patient is unable to maintain body temperature and feels cold or hot to the touch. The general aim is to help the patient maintain body temperature.

An increase in blood pressure with a slowing pulse should raise suspicion of increased ICP. An increase in blood pressure, decrease in pulse rate, and alteration in breathing pattern is known as Cushing's reflex. This is usually a late sign and found in patients with severe head injuries.

SAMPLE History. The following are pertinent questions:
- When did the injury occur?
- Was there immediate loss of consciousness?
- Was the injury a direct blow?
- Was there a documented period of respiratory arrest or cyanosis at the scene?
- Did the presence of blood at the scene suggest severe blood loss?
- Is the patient at risk for hypovolemic shock from a scalp laceration?
- Are there any known diseases that may have contributed to the injury?

Ongoing Assessment (Reassessment)

Critical information is gained from repeating the neurologic examination and the vital signs. Whether a patient's status improves, deteriorates, or stays the same in the prehospital phase of treatment is important information for both ED personnel and the neurosurgeon. Examinations should be repeated every 5 to 10 minutes and recorded. These examinations should include the mental status, vital signs, eye findings, and sensory and motor function.

Management

Protect yourself with body substance isolation procedures before patient contact. As with all patients, priority treatment of patients with head injuries is directed toward ensuring an open airway, adequate ventilations, and effective circulation.

Airway

The airway maneuver of choice for the patient with a head injury is the modified jaw thrust. Any blood or secretions in the oropharynx should be suctioned and the presence or absence of a gag reflex evaluated. For patients without a gag reflex, insert an oropharyngeal or nasopharyngeal airway. You should manually stabilize the cervical spine and have suction equipment readily available.

Ventilations

If the patient's ventilations are inadequate, you should assist the patient with a bag-mask or other ventilation device while maintaining cervical immobilization. Good ventilations for patients with a head injury are important to ensure an adequate supply of oxygen and prevent a buildup of carbon dioxide (CO_2), which can increase blood volume and pressure on the brain.

When CO_2 level in the blood increases (as occurs with hypoventilation), the cerebral vessels also dilate. When CO_2 level in the blood is low, the cerebral blood vessels constrict, allowing less blood to flow to the brain. The CO_2 content of the blood is low during hyperventilation.

This principle can be used in treating patients with increased ICP. By hyperventilating a patient's lungs, you can reduce CO_2 content of the blood and thereby reduce blood flow to the head. Because ICP is the sum of the skull's contents (brain, CSF, blood), reducing the amount of blood entering the head reduces the pressure within the skull.

However, hyperventilation has some risks to the patient. For example, hyperventilation of a patient *without* severe traumatic brain injury (herniation) may result in hypoxia to the brain from profound vasoconstriction. The Brain Trauma Foundation has developed specific criteria for initiating hyperventilation in the field that strongly suggest the probability of severe traumatic brain injury and herniation. These include an unconscious and unresponsive patient with the following signs:
- Significant dilation of pupil (≥ 4 mm)
- Asymmetrical pupils (differ >1 mm)
- Unresponsiveness to painful stimuli

In some EMS systems, hyperventilation is incorporated into prehospital treatment protocols. Hyperventilation may be helpful for patients with signs of severe head injury and increased ICP, such as coma, asymmetrical or unreactive pupils, and extensor posturing, or progressive deterioration in the GCS score (decrease in GCS score >2 points in patients with initial GCS score <9). The Brain Trauma Foundation recommends the following rates of hyperventilation as an option for treatment for patients with signs of herniation:

Infants: 30 breaths/min
Children: 25 breaths/min
Adults: 20 breaths/min

All patients with severe head injuries, and especially those requiring positive-pressure ventilation, should receive high-concentration supplemental oxygen.

Circulation

Treatment of shock is a high priority. For head injury wounds, you should take care when applying direct pressure to avoid compounding depressed skull fractures. The algorithm from the Brain Trauma Foundation is one method by which these assessments are used to guide treatment of patients with traumatic brain injury (**Figure 24-27**).

LEARNING OBJECTIVES
- Discuss indications for using a cervical collar.
- Describe a method for sizing a cervical collar.
- Describe how to log-roll a patient with a suspected spinal injury.
- Describe how to secure a patient to a long spine board.
- List situations when a short spine board should be used.
- Describe how to immobilize a patient with a short spine board.
- Explain the rationale for immobilizing the entire spine when a cervical spine injury is suspected.
- Explain the rationale for using immobilization methods other than the straps on the cots.
- Explain the rationale for using a short spine immobilization device when moving a patient from the sitting to the supine position.

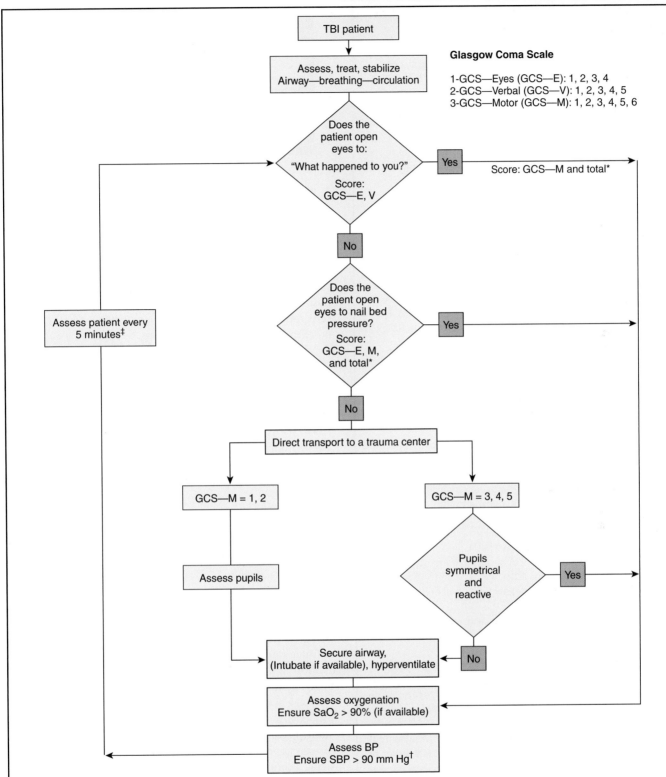

Glasgow Coma Scale

1-GCS—Eyes (GCS—E): 1, 2, 3, 4
2-GCS—Verbal (GCS—V): 1, 2, 3, 4, 5
3-GCS—Motor (GCS—M): 1, 2, 3, 4, 5, 6

Figure 24-27 Algorithm for prehospital assessment and treatment of patients with traumatic brain injury *(TBI)*.
*Patients with a total GCS score of 3 to 13 should be transported to an appropriate trauma center.
†For age less than 16 years, refer to systolic blood pressure thresholds by age (see Table 24-2).
‡Neurologic assessment may change and therefore lead to changes in ongoing assessment (reassessment).

Continued

Figure 24-27– cont'd

Algorithm Explanation

The emergency medical service (EMS) task force used a consensus method to develop an algorithm based on the scientific evidence obtained in *Guidelines for Prehospital Management of Traumatic Brain Injury*. The algorithm can be used as a framework to assess, treat, and transport the patient with TBI. Individual and regional circumstances may require prehospital healthcare providers (e.g., EMTs) to modify the algorithm because it may not be appropriate for all patients and locations. The following points provide more details for summaries of the steps in the graphic algorithm.

- The EMT's first priority in assessing, stabilizing, and treating a TBI patient is to follow basic resuscitation protocols that prioritize airway, breathing, and circulation (ABCs) assessment and treatment.
- After stabilization of ABCs, the EMT assesses the patient by first asking, "What happened to you?"
- If the patient opens the eyes, the EMT then asks the questions in the verbal and motor sections of the Glasgow Coma Scale (GCS) to determine the total score. Patients with a GCS score of 9 to 13 (moderate TBI) and patients with a GCS score of 3 to 8 (severe TBI) should be transported to a trauma center.
- If the patient does not open the eyes, the EMT applies blunt pressure to the nail bed or pinches the anterior axillary skin to elicit eye opening.
- If the patient opens the eyes with nail bed pressure or axillary pinch, the EMT assesses the verbal and motor sections of the GCS to determine the total score.
- Patients who are unresponsive with a GCS score of 3 to 8 should be transported to a trauma center with the following TBI capabilities:
  1. 24-hour computed tomography scanning capability
  2. 24-hour available operating room and prompt neurosurgical care
  3. The ability to monitor intracranial pressure and treat intracranial hypertension as delineated in the guidelines
- Patients with a GCS score of 14 to 15 can be transported to a nontrauma center hospital, which has the basic emergency department capabilities for immediate resuscitation of critically injured patients.
- If the patient does not open the eyes with nail bed pressure or axillary pinch, the patient should be transported directly to a trauma center as described above.
- For unresponsive patients who respond to nail bed pressure with extensor posturing or who are flaccid, the EMT should secure the airway (intubate, if available) and hyperventilate (20 breaths/min in an adult, 30 breaths/min in a child, and 35 breaths/min in an infant).
- For unresponsive patients who respond to nail bed pressure or axillary pinch with abnormal flexion or a higher GCS motor response, but have asymmetrical and/or dilated and fixed pupil(s), the EMT should hyperventilate at the rates described above.
- All TBI patients should have their oxygenation assessed at least every 5 minutes and their oxygen saturation maintained above 90%. Systolic blood pressure should also be measured and maintained greater than 90 mm Hg in adults and for ages 12 to 16 years, 80 mm Hg for ages 5 to 12 years, 75 mm Hg for ages 1 to 5 years, and 65 mm Hg for infants younger than 1 year.
- Because the patient's neurologic status may change, the EMT should fully assess the patient every 5 minutes and treat or modify treatment as appropriate.

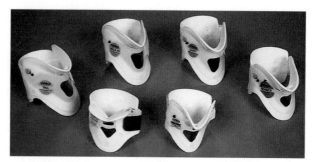

Figure 24-28 Various sizes of cervical collars.

Immobilization

All patients with head injuries must be evaluated for spinal injuries and treated accordingly. The conscious patient with an isolated head injury or nontraumatic brain injury with no suspicion of neck injury may be transported in the semisitting position. This position decreases the gravitational effect on cerebral blood flow and allows the patient to clear the airway more easily if vomiting should occur.

When definitive spinal immobilization is necessary, such as when a **long spine board** is required, the supine position is the position of choice. It is essential that the patient be secured adequately to the device to allow for rotation in the event of vomiting. Again, suction should be readily available.

For patients with nontraumatic or isolated brain injury (e.g., stroke), the left lateral recumbent (recovery) position may be used during transport. This position allows for easier drainage of secretions from the mouth and nose.

Cervical Collars

Cervical collars play an important role in immobilizing the spine. They limit flexion and extension and, to some extent, lateral movement of the neck. Several varieties of cervical collars are available, ranging from soft foam-filled to rigid plastic types. The foam-filled devices are not suitable for spinal immobilization because they allow more cervical motion.

Although cervical collars can contribute to immobilization, they are not completely immobilizing the spine. Cervical collars are an adjunct to more definitive immobilization devices, such as short and long spine boards with attachment straps for the torso and head.

When you are applying a cervical collar, the first concern is proper sizing of the device. Sizes range from infant through tall adult (**Figure 24-28**). A variety of adjustable collars also allow for easy application to a variety of patients. A simple method for sizing a cervical collar is to place the device against the anterior aspect of the neck and note the relation of the chin groove to the base of the chin. The specific manufacturers may recommend other techniques. You should become familiar with the types of cervical collars used in your area.

Spine Boards

Spine boards are essential for lifting and moving patients with suspected spinal injuries. Several varieties of long spine boards are used (**Figure 24-29**), but all provide essentially the same function: rigid support for the spinal column to prevent further injury.

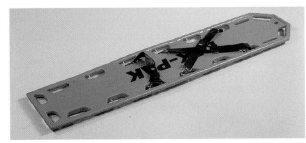

Figure 24-29   Long spine board.

The long spine board is used as the primary device for removing patients who are lying in the supine or lateral recumbent positions. It is also used to facilitate rapid extrication of motor vehicle crash patients. **Skill 24-1** shows the technique of log-rolling a patient onto a long spine board.

Kendrick Extrication Device

The **Kendrick extrication device (KED)** represents one variety of the short spine board. Its semirigid form permits easy and speedy application and provides effective immobilization of the spine when secured properly (**Skill 24-2**). This device and others like it are used to immobilize patients who are found in the sitting position.

LEARNING OBJECTIVES
- Explain the rationale for using rapid extrication approaches only when they will make the difference between life and death.
- Describe the indications for rapid extrication.
- List steps in performing rapid extrication.

Rapid Extrication

Patients who must be removed quickly from a vehicle can be evacuated directly onto the long spine board by using the **rapid extrication** procedure. This particular technique is also recommended through the Prehospital Trauma Life Support program and requires a minimum of three providers. The rapid extrication technique should be used for a patient with critical, life-threatening injuries who is found in the sitting position of a vehicle. (See Chapter 5 for the rapid extrication technique.)

Spinal Immobilization of a Standing Patient

The spine is immobilized in the "rapid takedown procedure" when a patient with a suspected spinal injury is found upright at the scene. If the mechanism of injury is sufficient to cause spinal injury, this procedure can be used to secure the patient to a spine board (**Skill 24-3**).

LEARNING OBJECTIVES
- Identify different types of helmets.
- Describe the unique characteristics of sports helmets.
- Explain the preferred methods to remove a helmet.
- Describe how the patient's head is stabilized to remove the helmet.

- Differentiate how the head is stabilized with and without a helmet.
- State the circumstances when a helmet should be left on the patient.
- Discuss the circumstances when a helmet should be removed.

Helmet Removal

Management of patients involved in a motorcycle crash or those with sports injuries is often hampered by the presence of a helmet. You must be familiar with the special assessment needs of these patients and the indications and contraindications for helmet removal. Once a decision has been made to remove a helmet, the proper procedure must be followed to avoid movement of the cervical spine during this task.

Your first concerns when faced with a helmeted patient are assessment and management of airway and ventilation. Some helmets may make airway management difficult, if not impossible. In these cases the helmet (or its face mask) must be rapidly and systematically removed to facilitate the management of the patient. A helmet may also prevent proper spinal immobilization. Large helmets may place the neck in the flexed position, and inline immobilization of the cervical spine may be difficult to achieve.

The decision to remove a helmet is often determined by the type of helmet. Sports helmets typically open anteriorly and permit easier access to the airway. Coaches and trainers may have a special backboard that allows an injured player's helmet to remain in place. You should remove the helmet (if necessary) and shoulder pads together while maintaining alignment of the spine.

Motorcycle helmets vary in design; some cover only the superior portion of the head and are simple to remove or work around during airway management and immobilization. Conversely, helmets with full face guards make airway management difficult. These helmets must almost always be removed when airway and ventilation management is required (**Table 24-5**).

The removal of a helmet requires a minimum of two providers and should be done systematically to avoid unnecessary movement of the patient. If the patient is wearing eyeglasses, they should be removed before the helmet is removed. **Skill 24-4** lists the steps for helmet removal. Keep in mind that some variation in technique may be needed depending on the type of helmet.

Immobilization of Infants and Children

Infants and children require the same attention to spinal immobilization as adult patients. Cervical collars, long and short spine boards, rapid extrication procedures, and helmet removal techniques are all appropriate approaches to spinal immobilization. It is important to pad spine boards from the shoulders to the heels of infants and small children to account for the larger head in proportion to the body (**Figure 24-30**). If the cervical collar does not properly fit the infant or child, a rolled towel and tape can be used to immobilize the neck. An improper immobilization device is likely to do more harm than good in managing the injured infant or child. Infants and small children found in car seats may be transported in these seats if assessment, treatment, and immobilization can be accomplished in the position found.

Table 24-5	Indications and Contraindications for Helmet Removal		
Consideration	**Do Not Remove Helmet**		**Remove Helmet**
Helmet fit	Good fit with little or no movement of patient's head within helmet.		Improperly fitted helmet that allows excessive movement within helmet.
Airway and breathing	No impending airway or breathing problems. No interference with the EMT's ability to assess airway and breathing.		Restriction of adequate management of airway and breathing. Inability to assess or reassess airway and/or reassess breathing or cardiac arrest.
Spinal immobilization	Ability to perform proper spinal immobilization with helmet in place or possible injury on removal of helmet. Patient has both helmet and shoulder pads. If helmet must be removed (for airway or breathing), shoulder pads should also be removed while maintaining alignment of spine.		Inability to perform proper spinal immobilization because of presence of helmet.

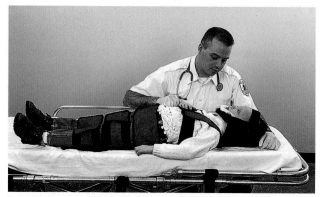

Figure 24-30 Child fully immobilized on a long spine board. The spine boards may require additional padding from the shoulders to the heels of small children to maintain neutral alignment of the spine.

Scenario Follow-up

This case illustrates some classic signs of both head and spinal injury. A sudden loss and transient loss of consciousness suggests a concussion, indicating the brain sustained a significant mechanism of injury. The patient awoke every quickly with no evidence of an immediate life-threatening problem. However, complications may follow; for example, bleeding within the brain would be evident if the patient became unresponsive again and developed other neurologic signs, such as pupillary changes, one-sided paralysis, or sensory loss.

This patient also sustained a significant cervical spine injury because there are sensorimotor deficits below the level of the clavicle. Other signs indicate a loss of sympathetic tone. When the spinal column is damaged in the cervical region, sympathetic nervous system function can be lost because these nerves arise from the thoracic and lumbar spine. Priapism is also a sign of compromised sympathetic tone. Finally, the patient appears to be breathing with only his diaphragm. Intercostal muscles in the chest arise from the thoracic vertebrae, which are not receiving impulses because of the injury in the cervical spine. Care for this patient includes positive-pressure ventilation, careful spinal immobilization, and treatment of spinal shock.

Summary

Central nervous system (CNS) problems are among the most common emergencies you will encounter. Both traumatic and medical problems arising from the CNS can result in paralysis or death. You must therefore be prepared to recognize the problem quickly and provide immediate and lifesaving prehospital care and rapid transport to an appropriate medical facility. All unconscious trauma patients, patients with a significant mechanism of injury, and patients exhibiting direct signs of spinal trauma should receive spinal immobilization. Establish spinal immobilization as a first step in your initial assessment, and continue this until arrival at the hospital.

Serious head injuries may be caused by blunt or penetrating mechanisms of injury. Management of airway and ventilation is critical to the survival of these patients. Carefully document alterations in mental status and other neurologic signs for all patients with suspected head or spinal injury. Rapid transport to surgical intervention is a critical step in the management of these patients.

Skills

Placing a Patient in Supine Position on a Long Spine Board Using the Log Roll

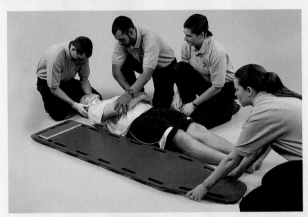

1. Apply a cervical collar, and place the patient's arms by his or her side or across the chest. One EMT maintains manual cervical stabilization throughout the procedure.

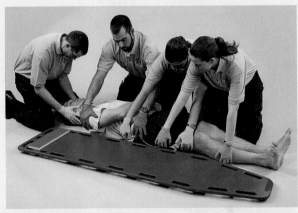

2. Three EMTs are positioned at the patient's side at the level of the chest, hips, and lower extremities while the long spine board is positioned on the other side of the patient. Check the patient's arm on the side of the EMTs for injury before log-rolling the patient. Align the lower extremities.

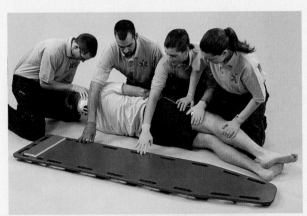

3. On command from the EMT at the head, all EMTs should rotate the patient toward themselves, keeping the body in alignment. The EMTs then reach across with one hand and pull the board toward the patient.

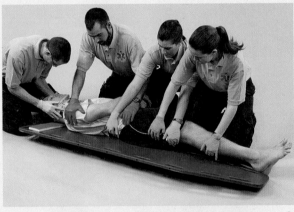

4. On command from the EMT at the head, the EMTs gently roll the patient onto the board, then roll the board to the ground.

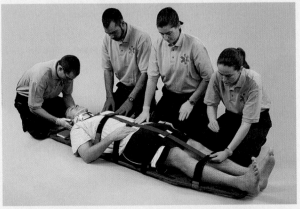

5. Strap the patient's torso and extremities securely to the board.

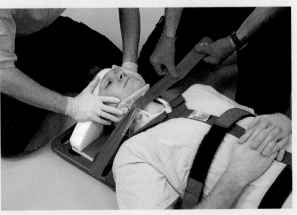

6. Immobilize the head with a head immobilizer or tape.

Skill | 24-2   *Applying the Kendrick Extrication Device*

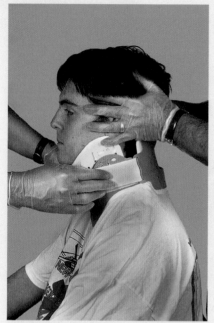

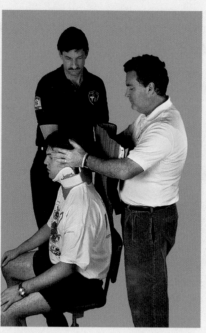

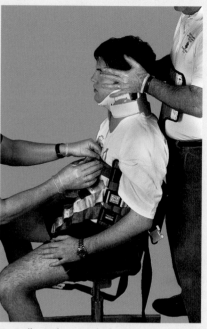

1. One EMT maintains cervical spine stabilization from behind the patient. Apply a rigid cervical collar.

2. Position the Kendrick extrication device behind the patient.

3. Pull up the Kendrick extrication device securely into the axillary region.

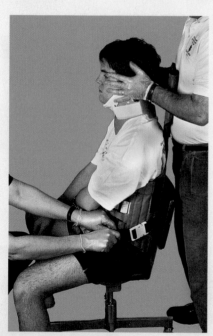

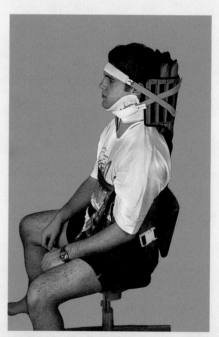

4. Attach the chest and abdominal straps securely without hindering breathing. Attach the groin straps last. Take care not to pinch the patient.

5. Secure the head by using the Velcro fasteners. Padding may be necessary.

Skill | 24-3 **Immobilizing the Spine of a Standing Patient**

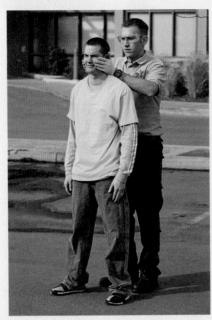

1. Position an EMT taller than the patient behind the patient, and have this EMT manually stabilize the patient's head and neck. This EMT's hands will not leave the patient's head and neck until the entire procedure is complete and the head is taped down to the board.

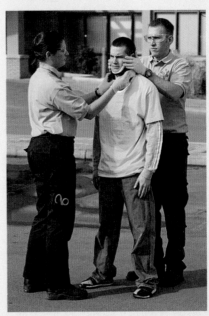

2. A second EMT applies a cervical collar to the patient.

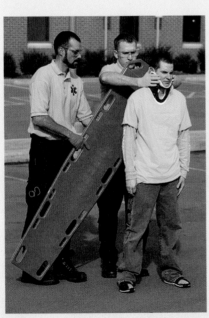

3. The second EMT carefully positions the long board behind the patient, working around the EMT who is applying manual stabilization. It is often useful to stand directly behind the patient with elbows spread to facilitate the placement of the backboard by a second EMT.

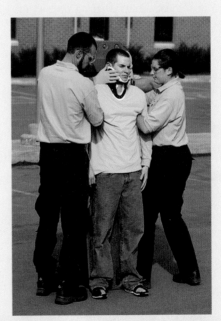

4. The second EMT ensures that the long board is centered behind the patient. The second and third EMTs, standing on either side of and facing the patient, reach under the patient's arm on their respective sides with the hand that is closest to the board and grab the backboard at a hole near the patient's armpit or higher. This will keep the patient from sliding off the board while being laid down.

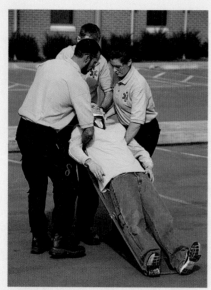

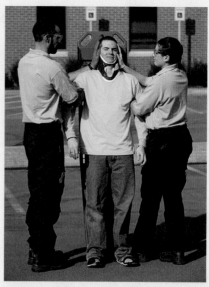

5. Once the board is tilted back, the patient will be suspended temporarily by the armpits. To keep the patient's arms secure, the EMTs grasp the backboard at the elbow level with their other hand and hold the arm next to the patient's body.

Slowly lay the board down, tilting it backward so that the head end begins to be lowered. It is important first to let the patient know what you will be doing so as not to make the patient even more anxious.

The EMT who is stabilizing the patient's head and neck walks backward and squats down, keeping up with the speed at which the board is being lowered.

6. The same technique is performed with two EMTs.

Skill |24-4   *Removing a Patient's Helmet*

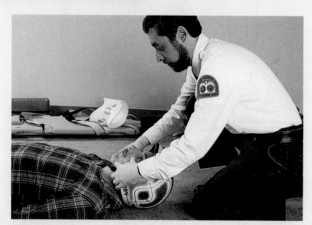

1. Remove the patient's eyeglasses and face shield before removing the helmet. One EMT stabilizes the helmet by placing the hands on each side of the helmet, with the fingers on the patient's mandible to prevent movement.

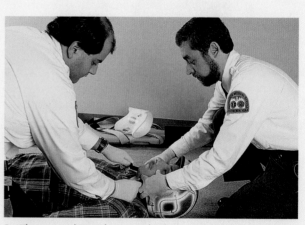

2. The second EMT loosens the helmet strap.

Skill | 24-4   *Removing a Patient's Helmet—cont'd*

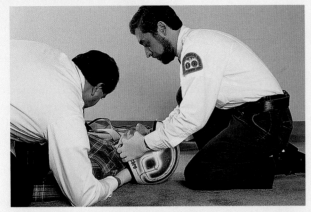

3. The second EMT places one hand on the mandible at the angle of the jaw and the other hand posteriorly at the occipital region.

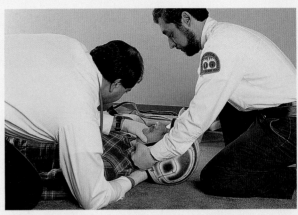

4. The EMT holding the helmet pulls the sides of the helmet apart and gently slips the helmet halfway off the patient's head, then stops.

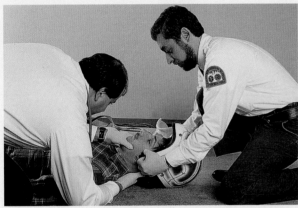

5. The EMT maintaining stabilization of the neck repositions, sliding the posterior hand superiorly to secure the head from falling back after complete helmet removal.

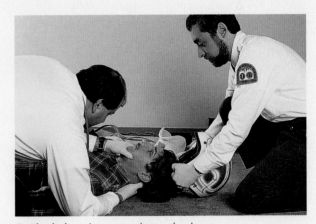

6. The helmet is removed completely.

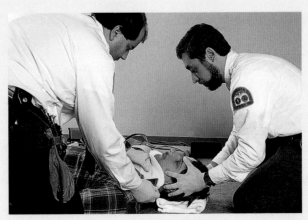

7. The EMT who removed the helmet assumes inline stabilization of the cervical spine, and the occiput is padded as needed.

The Bottom Line

Learning Checklist

✓ The nervous system includes the central nervous system (CNS; brain and spinal cord) and peripheral nervous system (PNS; motor and sensory nerves).

✓ The cerebrum is divided into areas by function: frontal lobe (motor and intellectual functions), parietal lobe (sensation), temporal lobe (hearing and smell), and occipital lobe (vision).

✓ The autonomic nervous system is concerned with involuntary activities such as control of heart rate, blood pressure, respiration, and digestion and consists of parasympathetic and sympathetic divisions.

✓ The three membranous coverings around the brain are the meninges (dura mater, arachnoid, pia mater). Cerebrospinal fluid (CSF) is contained in the space formed by the arachnoid and pia mater.

✓ The brain is protected by the bones of the skull (frontal, parietal, temporal, occipital) and the face (nasal, maxilla, mandible). The spinal cord is protected by the spinal vertebrae (7 cervical, 12 thoracic, 5 lumbar, 5 sacral, 4 coccygeal).

✓ Spinal injuries can occur from compression forces, flexion injuries, extension injuries, and penetrating injuries, including stab wounds and missile injuries.

✓ Suspect and treat spinal injuries in all unconscious trauma patients and patients with a significant mechanism of injury such as a motor vehicle crash, fall, or penetrating injury to the head or face.

✓ Signs and symptoms of spinal cord injury include tenderness in the area; pain associated with or without movement; soft tissue injuries of the head, spine, and shoulder; numbness, weakness, or tingling in the extremities; loss of sensation or paralysis below the level of injury or extremities; and incontinence.

✓ Injuries to the brain may be structural (injuries or disruptions to a specific area of the brain) or metabolic (hypoxia, hypoglycemia, or infection). Structural injuries cause one-sided or lateralizing signs.

✓ Metabolic injuries affect all portions of the brain equally and result in global physical findings.

✓ Secondary complications that occur after brain injury include hypoxia, hypotension, hypoglycemia, increased intracranial pressure (ICP), and infection.

✓ Skull fractures may include simple lines or breaks in the bone or may be depressed downward toward the brain. They may also involve the base of the skull as evidenced by "raccoon eyes" (ecchymosis around both eyes) or Battle's sign (ecchymosis behind the ear).

✓ A concussion is a sudden and temporary loss of consciousness or neurologic function from a blow to the brain.

✓ Signs of increased ICP include headaches, nausea, and vomiting (projectile); specific respiratory patterns; rising blood pressure and slowing of the pulse; dilating pupils; and changes in the Glasgow Coma Scale (GCS).

✓ The GCS is a standardized method for documenting neurologic function that consists of measurements of eye opening (score of 1 to 4), verbal response (score of 1 to 5), and motor response (score of 1 to 6).

✓ Measurement of motor and sensory function of an extremity can help identify structural causes of brain injury by the presentation of one-sided or lateralizing signs.

✓ Care for the suspected spinal injury patient should include maintaining inline immobilization, using the modified jaw thrust to open the airway, and immobilizing with a cervical collar and spinal immobilization device.

✓ Patients in a motor vehicle crash with a significant mechanism of injury or other evidence of spinal injury should be immobilized with the appropriate device (e.g., Kendrick extrication device) before removal unless the patient is unstable.

✓ A critical patient from a motor vehicle crash should be removed by the rapid extrication procedure.

Key Terms

Brainstem Lower part of the brain responsible for a variety of vital functions and regulatory activities, including respiratory and circulatory functions.

Cerebellum An outpocketing of the brain located posterior to the brainstem; primarily concerned with coordination of movement and balance.

Cerebrum Largest and most superior portion of the brain responsible for intellectual activity, motor control, sensory perception, visual stimuli, smell, hearing, and other body functions.

Cervical collar Rigid collars that provide partial immobilization and prevent some movement of the cervical spine.

Compression force Force that occurs when one spinal vertebra is driven into another; may be transmitted from above (the head) or from below.

Concussion Transient loss of consciousness or neurologic function as a result of trauma to the brain.

Cushing's reflex Reflex due to cerebral ischemia that causes an increase in blood pressure, decrease in pulse rate, and changes in breathing patterns.

Flexion force Force that involves fixed and mobile vertebrae that are bent to the point of fracture.

Glasgow Coma Scale (GCS) Brain function assessment tool that evaluates verbal, motor, and eye-opening responses and has high intraobserver reliability.

Kendrick extrication device (KED) Semirigid, short device used to immobilize and extricate victims of vehicle crashes who are found in the sitting position.

Long spine board Flat wooden, plastic, or metal device used to maintain spinal immobilization or to transport a patient.

Manual inline stabilization Holding a patient's head in a neutral position that is in line with the rest of the body.

Priapism Sustained penile erection; a sign of spinal cord injury.

Rapid extrication Specialized rescue removal technique used to extricate a critical patient quickly from a vehicle crash with minimal flexion, extension, or rotation of the spinal column.

Review Questions

1. The nervous system is structurally divided into two main divisions: the central nervous system and the _____ nervous system.
   a. peripheral
   b. autonomic
   c. medial
   d. voluntary

2. What aspect of the central nervous system is the initiator of the reflex arc?
   a. Sensory nerves
   b. Peripheral nerves
   c. Motor nerves
   d. Spinal cord

3. You respond to a patient with a slow pulse in association with a head injury. What part of the ventral nervous system mediates this finding?
   a. Autonomic
   b. Reflex
   c. Central
   d. Voluntary

4. The earliest sign of inadequate oxygenation of the brain is:
   a. Alteration in mental status
   b. Weakness
   c. Tingling
   d. Tachycardia

5. You respond to a head injured patient with CSF leaking from the ear. What approach should used to manage this finding?
   a. Attaching an occlusive dressing.
   b. Attaching a loose dressing over the ear.
   c. Providing irrigation.
   d. Placing the patient on the affected side.

6. You respond to a 43-year-old woman who has a significant head injury and severe pain in her neck and back. What airway maneuver is most appropriate when treating this patient?
   a. Head-tilt/chin-lift
   b. Head-tilt/neck-lift

   c. Jaw thrust without head tilt (modified)
   d. Triple airway maneuver

7. When immobilizing a spinal injury patient, you should *not* return the neck to the neutral position if:
   a. The neck is flexed.
   b. Resistance is encountered.
   c. The neck is extended.
   d. Contusions are noted on the neck.

Questions 8-10. Match the situation in column B to the approach to initial immobilization in column A.

Column A	Column B
8. Short spine board	**a.** Critically injured driver of vehicle
9. Long spine board	**b.** Pedestrian struck by vehicle
10. Rapid extrication	**c.** Non–critically injured driver of vehicle

11. You respond to a 23-year-old male with an altered mental status, cyanosis, and evidence of respiratory distress. What oxygen delivery system is most appropriate when treating this patient?
    a. Nasal cannula
    b. Partial rebreather mask
    c. Simple face mask
    d. Nonrebreather mask or bag-mask

12. You arrive at the scene of a single-vehicle motorcycle crash. The female rider was thrown and is in a supine position approximately 15 feet from the vehicle. The helmet is in place but has a noticeable crack in the exterior. The findings are as follows:

Stimulus	Response
"Can you tell me what happened?"	No response
"Can you open your eyes?"	No eye opening to command
	Incomprehensible sounds
"Can you tell me the month and the year?"	No response
"Can you show me two fingers?"	Eyes open; straightens limb and rotates shoulder inward
Nail bed pressure	

What is the GCS? Eyes _____ Verbal _____ Motor _____ Total GCS _____

13. You arrive at the scene of an accident to find a male patient in his mid-20s who has fallen off a garage roof. The findings are as follows:

Stimulus	Response
"Can you tell me what happened?"	No response
"Can you open your eyes?"	Opens eyes
"Can you tell me the month and the year?"	Wrong month, correct year
"Can you show me two fingers?"	Raises two fingers
Nail bed pressure (not indicated)	–

What is the GCS? Eyes _____ Verbal _____ Motor _____ Total GCS _____

14. You are at your station when a woman arrives with a 12-month-old female infant. The child had apparently fallen down the stairs when the mother was in the other room. The child initially cried but now "isn't acting right." There is a hematoma on the base of the child's head. The findings are as follows:

Stimulus	Response
"What happened to you?"	Refuses to look at you, starts crying
"Can you look at your Mom?"	Opens eyes to look at mother, continues to cry
"Who's holding you?"	Continues irritable cry
"Can you squeeze Mom's finger?"	Grasps mother's finger
Nail bed pressure (not indicated)	—

What is the GCS? Eyes _____ Verbal _____ Motor _____ Total GCS _____

For Further Review

In the Student Workbook

- Multiple-choice questions
- Matching questions
- Fill-in-the-blank questions
- True-false questions
- Case scenario questions
- Skill check questions

On Evolve

- Anatomy challenge
- Weblinks
- Lecture Notes
- Exercises

Learning Objectives

Cognitive Objectives

- State the components of the nervous system.
- List the functions of the central nervous system.
- Define the structure of the skeletal system as it relates to the nervous system.
- Relate mechanism of injury to potential injuries of the head and spine.
- Describe the implications of not properly caring for patients with potential spinal injuries.
- State the signs and symptoms of a potential spinal injury.
- Describe the method of determining if a responsive patient may have a spinal injury.
- Describe the airway emergency medical care techniques for the patient with a suspected spinal injury.
- Describe how to stabilize the cervical spine.
- Discuss indications for using a cervical collar.
- Establish the relationship between airway management and the patient with head and spine injuries.
- Describe a method for sizing a cervical collar.
- Describe how to log-roll a patient with a suspected spinal injury.
- Describe how to secure a patient to a long spine board.
- List situations when a short spine board should be used.
- State the circumstances when a helmet should be left on the patient.
- Describe how to immobilize a patient with a short spine board.
- Describe the indications for rapid extrication.
- List steps in performing rapid extrication.
- Discuss the circumstances when a helmet should be removed.
- Identify different types of helmets.
- Describe the unique characteristics of sports helmets.
- Explain the preferred methods to remove a helmet.
- Discuss alternative methods to remove a helmet.
- Describe how the patient's head is stabilized to remove the helmet.
- Differentiate how the head is stabilized with and without a helmet.

Affective Objectives

- Explain the rationale for immobilizing the entire spine when a cervical spine injury is suspected.
- Explain the rationale for using immobilization methods other than the straps on the cots.
- Explain the rationale for using a short spine immobilization device when moving a patient from the sitting to the supine position.
- Explain the rationale for using rapid extrication approaches only when they will make the difference between life and death.
- Defend the reasons for leaving a helmet in place for transport of a patient.
- Defend the reasons for removal of a helmet before transport of a patient.

Psychomotor Objectives

- Demonstrate opening the airway in a patient with suspected spinal cord injury.
- Demonstrate evaluating a responsive patient with a suspected spinal cord injury.
- Demonstrate stabilizing the cervical spine.
- Demonstrate the four-person log roll for a patient with a suspected spinal cord injury.
- Demonstrate how to log-roll a patient with a suspected spinal cord injury with two people.
- Demonstrate securing a patient to a long spine board.
- Demonstrate using the short-board immobilization technique.
- Demonstrate the procedure for rapid extrication.
- Demonstrate the preferred methods for stabilizing a helmet.
- Demonstrate helmet removal techniques.
- Demonstrate alternative methods for stabilizing a helmet.
- Demonstrate completing a prehospital care report for patients with head and spinal injuries.

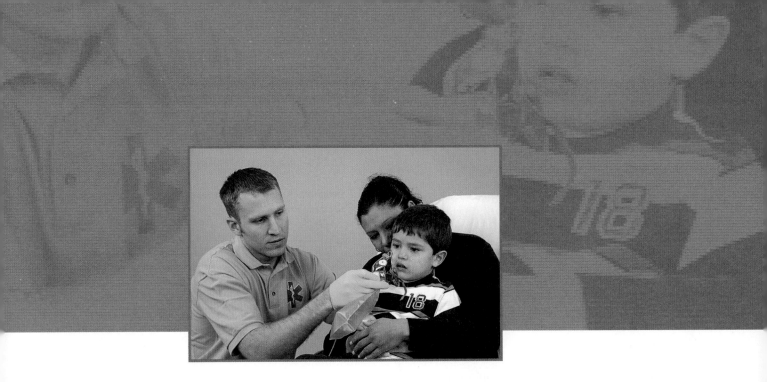

25 Infants and Children

CHAPTER OUTLINE

Epidemiology
Differences between Children and Adults
Assessment
Management
Common Pediatric Conditions
Child Abuse
Infants and Children with Special Needs
Emotional Stress
Skills

Scenario

You respond to a call for a 3-year-old boy in respiratory distress. The child is crying, alert, and agitated. You allow him to remain on his mother's lap while you conduct a torso-to-head survey. On focused physical examination, you note nasal flaring, intercostal retractions, cyanotic nail beds, and wheezing in both lungs. His vital signs are pulse 140 beats/min and regular, blood pressure 110/90 mm Hg, and respirations 28 breaths/min and labored. The mother advises you that the child has a history of asthma. The child will not tolerate oxygen by mask, so you ask the mother to administer blow-by oxygen to the child.

The call to help a child presents several challenges to the emergency medical technician (EMT). The pediatric emergency is usually emotionally charged for all concerned: the child, the parents, the bystanders, and the EMT. As an EMT, you must remember the key differences among adult, child, and infant patients and, depending on the child's age, use different approaches to obtain historical and physical information, interpret assessment findings, and provide treatment.

Children are not small adults. As an EMT you must develop the knowledge and skills to recognize the developmental, anatomic, and physiologic differences between children and adults. The range of emergencies and the response to illness in the child vary from those in the adult patient.

> **LEARNING OBJECTIVES**
> - Explain the rationale for having knowledge and skills appropriate for dealing with the infant and child patient.
> - State the usual cause of cardiac arrest in infants and children versus adults.

Epidemiology

The causes of most deaths in children are different from the causes of death in adults. After the first year of life, preventable injuries and respiratory conditions account for the majority of deaths. Deaths in children each year result from injuries caused by motor vehicles, falls, poisoning and assaults, and drowning.

Causes of respiratory arrest in children include asthma, trauma, drug ingestion, drowning, smoke inhalation, sudden infant death syndrome (SIDS), infection (e.g., sepsis, meningitis, croup, epiglottitis), and foreign body aspiration.

Unlike adults, cardiac arrest in children is rarely caused by heart disease. Children have strong hearts, except for the rare child with **congenital** heart disease, who had the disease or acquired heart damage at birth. Pediatric cardiopulmonary arrests usually follow a respiratory problem. Because the child's heart is strong, cardiac arrest usually implies that the heart has had a severe and prolonged period of decreased oxygen supply, or **hypoxia.** The heart becomes oxygen depleted until it has such slow and weak beats that no pulse is conducted and eventually there is no activity at all *(asystole).* **Figure 25-1** illustrates the downward spiral in an infant's condition that leads to cardiopulmonary arrest.

> **LEARNING OBJECTIVES**
> - Identify the developmental considerations for the infant, toddler, preschool child, school-age child, and adolescent.
> - Differentiate the response of the ill or injured infant or child (age specific) from that of an adult.
> - Attend to the feelings of the family when dealing with an ill or injured infant or child.
> - Understand the provider's emotional response to caring for infants or children.

Differences between Children and Adults

When treating a child, you should realize that you have two concerns: the child and the parent. Your primary attention is focused on the child, but you must consider the parents as well. Parents may feel anxious, fearful, and impatient as they seek help and medical attention for their child. Lacking a medical background and with considerable emotional investment in the patient, they may overreact because they may anticipate the worst possible condition or result from the emergency situation. In the face of their own panic, they may not act rationally or in the child's best interest. It is important to mobilize the parents' energies into constructive activities to gather the necessary history and to calm the child. To elicit their cooperation and support, you must gain their confidence. You can accomplish this by acting in a calm and professional manner.

Understanding and facing your own emotional reactions to a sick child are also important. We are all capable of minimizing or overestimating the seriousness of an emergency situation. Our own reactions can be influenced by the behavior and atmosphere encountered at the scene. We all tend to see children as innocent and vulnerable.

Once you understand your own and others' reactions to the sick or injured child, you can influence rather than participate in the emotional turmoil. Sick or injured children cannot always fully understand what is happening to them. Pain and fear often cause them to be uncooperative and more difficult to evaluate. Parents are often the best source of the history and can help calm the child and even participate in care by helping keep the child in a position of comfort or holding the oxygen delivery device. With a calm, objective approach, coupled with an understanding of pediatric prehospital care, you can have a positive impact on the situation.

> **REAL***World*
>
> Parents of special needs children are your best historians. They usually are fully aware of their child's condition and can inform the EMT about what needs to be done, how it needs to be done, and to what hospital the child should be transported. These parents are knowledgeable about disease processes the average EMT may see only once or twice in an entire career. Listen to them.

Developmental Differences

Children pass through developmental stages from newborn, to infant, to toddler, to preschool child, to school-age child, to adolescent. Your approach, evaluation, and treatment must consider the patient's developmental stage.

In general, you should keep the child and parent together whenever possible. Separation causes anxiety, especially when several people are hurt. An emergency places the child in a frightening environment; you are a stranger, and the last thing a child may want is to be separated from the parents. You should remain calm and remember that calming the parents is also important because children pick up signals from their parents.

Honesty is required in every situation. For example, you should not say, "This won't hurt," when it will. Once you lose a child's trust, you lose whatever cooperation you may have gained. The following sections discuss specific developmental considerations for different age groups.

Newborn to Infant

Up to 1 year of age, an infant has minimal language capability but responds to facial expressions and tone of voice. Infants are used to interacting with their parents and generally have minimal "stranger anxiety." Beginning at about 8 months, however, some infants may demonstrate anxiety when approached by strangers. When caring for infants you should obtain the history from the parents and examine the infant within sight of the parents or even while the baby is in their arms.

You should try to provide a warm environment, both emotionally and physically, for an infant. For example, warm your hands and stethoscope (rub them together) before placing them on the infant.

Infants, particularly ill infants, may cry when touched by a stranger. You should try to gather information, such as respiratory rate and quality of breathing, before you touch the baby. The baby may feel more secure and may be less likely to cry if held in one of the parent's arms. Listen to the lungs first, then perform the physical examination in a *trunk-to-head* manner. This approach is used because examination around the face is most threatening to the infant. In fact, infants, toddlers, and preschool children may perceive oxygen delivery by mask as threatening or "suffocating"; other techniques for therapy, such as blow-by oxygen, may be necessary.

Toddler

The toddler stage is 11 months to 3 years, including the "terrible twos." No matter how charming you are, a child in this age range may refuse to cooperate with the examination and treatment. Developmentally, they see themselves as individuals and are assertive, yet they fear pain and separation from their parents. You cannot really explain things to a toddler, but you can talk in a soothing tone, examine the child on the parent's lap, and approach the child at eye level. Often, you can distract the child with a colorful toy or puppet and quickly listen to the lungs before the child reacts. As with an infant, you should examine the toddler from trunk to head, leaving the more threatening head examination for last.

If possible, do not undress the toddler all at once. Toddlers do not like to be touched or have their clothing removed; therefore you should remove the clothing only if necessary for examination and then replace it if possible. You should not let the child see scissors or instruments unnecessarily because toddlers fear pain and are afraid of needles. You can, however, let the child play with your stethoscope and blood pressure cuffs.

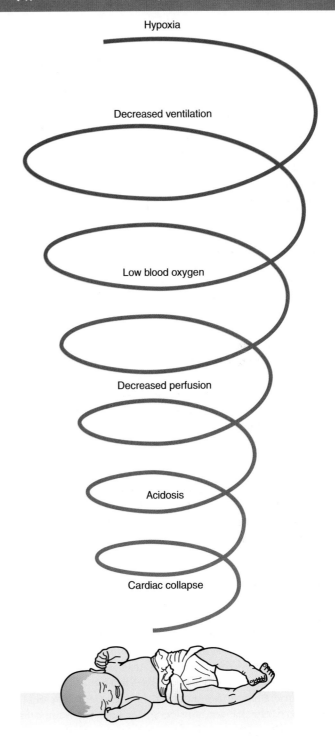

Figure 25-1 The pediatric patient rarely has a cardiac arrest as a primary event. Cardiac arrest usually follows a respiratory problem and a sustained period of poor oxygenation (hypoxia).

REAL*World*

Be careful how you talk to toddlers and preschoolers. You might tell adult patients that you are going to "take their blood pressure," but young children might become upset with this statement. They may not know what a "blood pressure" is, but they certainly do not want you to "take" anything from them. Consider using words such as "measure" and "count" when assessing pulses and blood pressure.

Preschool Child

Preschool children are between the ages of 3 and 6 years. These children are in a period of intensive learning and have varied levels of ability to express their thoughts and feelings. As with the toddler, preschool children do not like being touched, are apprehensive about separation from parents, fear pain, dislike having clothing removed, may feel "suffocated" by a face mask, and may believe they are responsible for their illness or injury. In addition, they may be afraid of blood and permanent injury and may have feelings of modesty.

Preschool children are curious and communicative. They live in a world of intense play fantasy with imaginary friends and often merge fantasy with reality. This means they possess "magical thinking" and believe what they hear. Although these children may have a strong fear of pain and separation, especially under the circumstances of an emergency, if they are not in pain and you take a few moments to play with them, they can be very cooperative. You should be friendly and talk to the parents first. This way the child is more likely to perceive you as a friend. A child may think the injury or illness is punishment for being "bad." If this is the case, you should assure the child that he or she is good and that illness or injury is not the child's fault.

You should approach the preschool child at eye level in a nonthreatening manner, perhaps offering a toy or giving simple explanations. Again, you should try not to show sharp objects; if the child sees a pair of scissors, for example, you should explain their purpose to relieve any anxiety. Children in this age group are interested in your stethoscope and blood pressure cuff. If you have to perform a procedure, wait until the last minute to explain it, and then do it immediately. You should be honest with the child. If a procedure might be painful, tell the child that it may "hurt a bit" but that it is necessary to help the child. Do not overexplain or give the child too much time to fantasize about what you are going to do.

School-Age Child

Children between the ages of 6 and 12 years are fighting between a desire to be treated as a child and a desire to be an adult. They also have many personal fears and a strong fear of disfigurement and permanent injury. They may have feelings of modesty and fear pain and blood. You should talk to the school-age child first to demonstrate that you consider his or her opinion important, and you should explain what you are doing during the examination and treatment.

Adolescent

What is true for the school-age child is also true for the adolescent (12 to 18 years of age). Adolescents, having undergone the changes of puberty, want to see themselves as adults. Under the stress of injury or sickness, however, they may feel helpless and childlike. You should respect their "space," answer their questions, respect their shyness, and allow them to retain as much control as possible. When talking to an adolescent, you should not be confrontational. It may be best to treat the adolescent as an adult, and you should respect that this patient may desire to be assessed privately, away from the parents or guardians.

LEARNING OBJECTIVE
• Describe differences in anatomy and physiology of the infant, child, and adult patient.

Anatomy and Physiology

In general, the pediatric patient has a better ability to compensate physiologically in the early phases of severe illness and injury because the main compensatory mechanisms, the cardiovascular system and respiratory system, are young and healthy. When the child's compensatory mechanisms fail, however, the condition can deteriorate rapidly, and time is crucial in reaching definitive care. Therefore, as an EMT, you must recognize early signs of stress and rapidly treat and transport the pediatric patient. Understanding the differences in the anatomy and physiology of pediatric patients will help you in this regard.

Airway

The airways of infants and children differ in some important ways from those of adults. Infants and small children have smaller airways at all levels, including the nasopharynx, oropharynx, larynx, trachea, bronchi, and bronchioles. The tongue of an infant or child is large in relation to the airway and has a greater potential for obstruction. The glottis (opening of the larynx) is in a more anterior and superior position compared with the adult airway and is protected by a relatively large, U-shaped epiglottis. The **cricoid cartilage,** or ring at the base of the larynx, is the narrowest part of the child's upper airway **(Figure 25-2)**. The vocal cords are the narrowest part of the adult's airway. The infant and child's airway is also softer and more pliable than that of an adult.

The anatomic differences at various ages become meaningful during airway management. For example, the position for opening the airway varies with age. For infants younger than 1 year old, you should place the head in the "sniffing," or *neutral,* position to avoid bending or kinking the softer trachea. You may place a folded towel beneath the shoulders to help keep the head aligned in the neutral position. For toddlers and small children (1 to 8 years), you should extend, but not hyperextend, the neck slightly. The relatively large tongue in the child

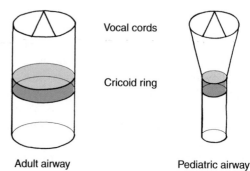

Comparison of airway anatomy

Vocal cords

Cricoid ring

Adult airway   Pediatric airway

Figure 25-2 The narrowest part of the child's airway is the cricoid ring (cricoid cartilage). The adult's airway is narrowed at the vocal cords.

Table 25-1	Normal Respiratory Rates
Group	**Range (Breaths/Min)**
Adult	12-20
Child	15-30
Infant	25-50

Table 25-2	Normal Pulse Rates	
Age	**Range (Beats/Min)**	**Average (Beats/Min)**
Newborn	85-205	140
Infant	100-190	130
Child (2-10 yr)	60-140	80
Child (>10 yr)	60-100	75
Adult	60-80	72

makes maneuvers to lift the tongue off the airway especially important. When inserting an oropharyngeal airway, you should use a tongue blade to displace the tongue because rotating the airway in the usual manner may inadvertently damage the soft tissues of the palate.

Given the smaller airway of infants, small obstructions such as secretions, swelling, or mucus can result in a significant blockage of airflow. Although 1 to 2 mm of airway edema in an adult is inconsequential, it can become a significant obstruction to an infant. Therefore, disease processes that affect the upper airway of an infant have the potential for significantly compromising the airway.

Infants prefer to breathe through the nose and are considered obligate nose breathers. Blockage of the nasal passages from mucus or swelling can significantly narrow the airway and increase a baby's work of breathing. Infants often have upper respiratory infections such as the common cold. If the infant also has a disease of the lower airway, this blockage in the nasopharynx may be sufficient to cause decompensation. Suctioning the baby's nasal passages can significantly improve the clinical picture. Humidification of the oxygen that the child breathes can also help by loosening any encrusted mucus or secretions.

Breathing

The respiratory rate in children is much faster than in the adult, and it gradually decreases with age. You should be familiar with the range of variations to evaluate the patient's respiratory status properly (**Table 25-1**).

As with adults, the rate of breathing alone is not the measure of adequate ventilation. Depth of breathing or tidal volume must also be considered. Evaluate depth by observing for chest rise and listening and feeling for the movement of air.

Infants have compliant chest walls. When the infant works harder at breathing and uses the accessory muscles of respiration, supraclavicular, substernal, and intercostal retractions may be noted along the chest wall. Retractions and nasal flaring, as well as "seesaw" or alternate abdominal and chest movement, which are signs of increased work of breathing, are often obvious on inspection. Infants and children can have a vigorous respiratory and cardiovascular response to compensate for illness.

When they need to work to breathe, infants and children develop respiratory muscle fatigue more rapidly than adults. When this occurs, there may be a sudden deterioration in their condition. For example, a child with asthma may have increased work of breathing and may be unable to sleep. Eventually the child will become exhausted. You should be watchful for the child who has been working hard to breathe who becomes tired and wants to sleep or lie down. In addition, anxiety and anxious behavior may be signs of hypoxia, which appears before the patient becomes cyanotic. EMTs must remember that the child may tire to the point that respiratory efforts are inadequate and assistance by positive-pressure ventilation is necessary.

Simple interventions, such as administering humidified oxygen and keeping the infant or child warm, may keep a child from deteriorating. By adding oxygen, you may decrease the need to work so hard at breathing. Humidifying the oxygen when possible can be helpful because dried secretions might obstruct airflow and increase airway resistance.

When positive-pressure ventilation is necessary, you should take care not to overventilate because the respiratory volumes of infants and children also vary with age. During positive-pressure ventilation, closely observe the rise of the chest to determine the end point of ventilation. Infants and small children are also more subject to gastric distention because of their small lung capacity and the tendency for excessive volumes and pressure of air to "overflow" into the esophagus.

Circulation

Pulse Rate and Blood Pressure. The average pulse rate of a child decreases with age. For example, an infant's average pulse rate is 130 beats/min, with a range of 100 to 190 beats/min. The average values decrease toward adult values with age (**Table 25-2**).

Blood pressure, on the other hand, increases with age. The following formula is used to approximate the lower limit for systolic blood pressure (SBP) in children older than 2 years:

$$SBP\,(mm\,Hg) = 70 + (2 \times Age\,in\,years)$$

You should always use the cuff size appropriate for an infant or child to prevent false readings. As a general rule, the width of the cuff should cover approximately two thirds of the length of the upper arm, and the bladder should cover approximately 75% of the arm's circumference. If the cuff is too small, readings will be falsely high; if it is too large, readings will be falsely low.

With the greater range and variability in normal vital signs, it is sometimes more difficult to interpret the significance of changes in blood pressure in the child. The American College of Surgeons (ACS) considers an SBP of less than 70 mm Hg with tachycardia and cool skin an indicator of shock in children. The Broselow tape is a tool used by many prehospital providers to reference normal vital signs. The tape measures the child's size and correlates it with vital signs, cardiopulmonary resuscitation (CPR) techniques, airway adjunct sizes, and other information. It is also advisable for prehospital providers to carry a table of vital signs, which is available in a variety of pocket guides or laminated cards.

Table 25-3	Signs of Dehydration
Stage	**Signs**
Early	Rapid pulse
	Less urine output
	Dry mucosal membranes
Intermediate	Lack of tears
	Sunken fontanel
	Sunken eyes
Late	Skin tenting
	Delayed capillary refilling time
	No urine output
	Hyperventilation
	Altered mental status
	Irritability
	Lethargy
	Thready pulse
	Hypotension (very late sign)

LEARNING OBJECTIVE
- Identify the signs and symptoms of shock (hypoperfusion) in the infant and child patient.

Bleeding and Shock. Hypovolemic shock is the most common type of shock in childhood. Acute dehydration and bleeding are the two causes of hypovolemia most often encountered by EMTs.

Hypovolemia from dehydration (not enough water) is likely in any sick child with increased metabolic needs and a decreased intake of fluid. Vomiting and diarrhea can also add to fluid loss. The smaller the child, the more vulnerable the child is to dehydration.

Signs of dehydration are progressive (**Table 25-3**). The infant or small child initially has a rapid pulse, less urine output, and dry mucosal membranes. This condition then progresses to a lack of tears, sunken fontanels (infant), and sunken eyes. Late signs of dehydration include "skin tenting" (pinched skin looks like a tent), delayed capillary refilling time, hyperventilation, and altered mental status (including irritability and lethargy).

With acute blood or fluid loss, as occurs with hemorrhage, the pediatric patient exhibits the same signs of shock as an adult. Remember that the total blood volume of children is significantly less than that of adults. The average blood volume in pediatric patients is 80 mL/kg body weight. This means that an average 10-kg 1-year-old infant would have a total blood volume of 800 mL. What might be an insignificant 200-mL blood loss in an adult is 25% of the 10-kg baby's blood volume.

With healthy compensatory mechanisms, children can maintain their blood pressure until nearly 40% of their blood volume is lost. A fall in blood pressure in the child is an even later finding than in adults. By the time children become hypotensive, they are in the late stages of shock.

Children and infants are also susceptible to other, less common causes of shock. Vasodilation is seen with sepsis (overwhelming infection), anaphylaxis, and spinal cord shock, as well as in response to certain drugs. After a trauma, the pediatric patient can go into shock from tension pneumothorax and cardiac tamponade, which obstruct flow of venous blood returning to the heart. Rarely does a child experience cardiogenic shock (shock from primary heart problems). Possible causes of cardiogenic shock in a child include previous congenital heart disease, an acute infection of the myocardium, or severe contusion to the heart.

Case in Point

You arrive on scene to evaluate a 6-year-old child who has taken her grandfather's blood pressure medication, named Catapres (clonidine). You find the child lying on the ground, unconscious and unresponsive. Her pulse rate is slow and blood pressure is low. Her mother tells you the child only took one pill. Even though it was only one pill, the child is in shock because of the medication's dramatic pediatric effects.

Many pills are known as "one-pill killers" when ingested by children. Tablet ingestion by children should always be taken seriously.

Metabolic Considerations

Keeping the child warm is a simple and valuable measure that should not be underestimated. Infants and children have a higher baseline metabolic rate than adults. Their "engine" runs at higher speeds. For their size, they need more fuel, which in humans is oxygen and glucose. To accomplish this, children have a faster normal respiratory rate to capture the oxygen and a faster normal heart rate to deliver it to the tissues. They also consume more calories per unit of weight than do adults, as any bleary-eyed new parent can attest to after nighttime feedings.

Part of the reason infants have a higher basal metabolic rate is that they are busy growing. Another explanation is that they need to expend more energy to remain warm. Infants have proportionately larger heads and a greater skin surface area relative to body weight than do adults. This means that they lose heat and moisture through the skin more easily. Their higher respiratory rate also adds to the amount of heat and water lost through the lungs.

The intake of food and water usually decreases in the sick or injured child. Because the metabolic rate is higher and because there are smaller reserves of glucose, children quickly use up their energy supplies. Fever further increases the metabolic rate and complicates this situation.

An additional problem is that infants younger than 6 months cannot shiver in response to cold and therefore cannot generate heat through muscular contraction. By keeping the child warm and well oxygenated, you help the infant conserve energy reserves.

Neurologic Differences

Because the very young pediatric patient's head is large in relation to the body, this patient is more likely to sustain head injury. An infant can lose enough blood within the cranium to cause shock. This is in contrast to adult and child patients, in whom blood loss with closed head injury alone is not sufficient to cause hypovolemic shock. Both infants and children are also more prone to episodes of *apnea* (absence of breathing) with head trauma.

Table 25-4	Differences in Anatomy and Physiology in Infants and Children and Related Actions

Difference	Problem	Action
Smaller airway overall and large tongue in relation to airway Infants are obligatory nose breathers	Respiratory distress can develop in infants and small children when the nose or other airway structures become clogged with mucus and secretions	Use humidified oxygen to loosen secretions and clear nasal passage Suction nasal passage
	Tongue can easily block airway if child unconscious	Use proper airway maneuvers and/or airway adjuncts
Soft trachea	May kink if neck is hyperextended	Maintain head and neck in neutral sniffing position during airway opening
Cricoid ring is narrowest point of the airway	Site of narrowing with "croup" (infection)	Use humidified oxygen to loosen secretions Cricoid ring serves as functional "cuff" around endotracheal intubation tube in children younger than age 8 years
Delicate soft and hard palate	May tear and bleed during oropharyngeal airway insertion	Use tongue blade and not the rotational technique during airway insertion
Larger head	Loses heat more quickly	Cover head and keep infant or child warm during care
Fontanel	Unlike the adult, the infant can bleed a large volume of blood into cranial cavity and may become hypovolemic	Look for signs of hypovolemic shock in association with head injuries

Summary

Table 25-4 summarizes the key anatomic and physiologic differences in infants and children.

> **LEARNING OBJECTIVE**
> - Describe the methods of determining end-organ perfusion in the infant and child patient.

Assessment

Variations in the specific treatment approaches primarily relate to developmental and physiologic issues. For example, the head-to-toe survey becomes the toe-to-head or trunk-to-head survey in infants and small children. Airway maneuvers used during assessment also change according to age, as do the evaluation and interpretation of vital signs.

This section addresses the special considerations associated with the evaluation of infants and children who have acute medical problems and provides helpful tips on what to look for and how to look. As with all patients, you should assess and manage any life-threatening injuries first and then gather additional information while transporting the child and parents to the hospital.

Initial (Primary) Assessment

As part of the initial (primary) assessment, evaluate the level of responsiveness, respiratory status, and skin color as you approach the patient. Pediatricians have described their ability to conduct this initial evaluation "from the doorway" as they approach a child. Their initial question, "Is this child significantly ill?" is followed by the question, "Am I dealing with a respiratory problem?" Answers may be apparent by general observation and initial handling of the child. Look for activity and playfulness, skin color, respiratory effort, and temperature. Listen to the quality of speech or crying.

A common scenario that you may encounter is a screaming and combative 3-year-old child running around and being uncooperative. In addition, the parents are hysterical and upset. Standing in the doorway, you assess the following:

- The child's airway is patent and functional because the child is pink and screaming.
- The circulatory function is adequate because the child is upright and moving around.
- The child does not have meningitis, appendicitis, or other severe infectious process, or the child would be lying very still or showing evidence of distress.
- This child does not have an immediate life-threatening problem.

By being calm and observant, you can gather useful information before actually approaching the child. You can reassure yourself and the parents that you have time for evaluation, intervention, and transportation.

On the initial observation, note the general level of activity and assess for mechanism of injury, including the child's surroundings. Is the child limp, anxious or agitated, or drowsy? Or does the child appear to have normal energy? When observing infants, you should look for eye contact with the parents and whether or not the infant follows a toy with the eyes. With a small child, observe whether the child is aware of and interacting with the environment. Is the child playful, moving around, and exhibiting age-appropriate behavior?

The infant or small child has no reason to be interested in your examination and should be appropriately upset. Be wary of a child who is "too good" or quiet during your examination.

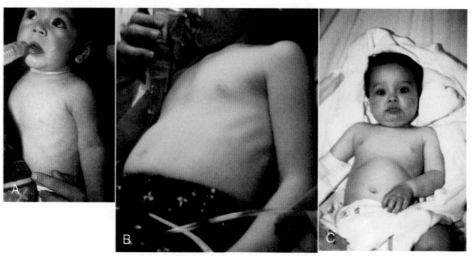

Figure 25-3 Key signs of respiratory distress. **A** and **B,** Nasal flaring and retractions. **C,** Exaggerated abdominal movement. All these key signs are indicators of significant respiratory distress in infants and children.

Your initial impression should also include a quick observation of the child's weight and nutritional status:

- Does the child appear too thin or wasted? Is there evidence of adequate nutritional and fluid intake?
- Does the child feel warm?
- Is there a history of fever?

Regardless of the underlying disease, children can quickly become dehydrated. Signs of dehydration can include poor skin *turgor* (expected resiliency of skin), sunken eyes, and dry mucous membranes. Look for evidence of a sunken fontanel in the infant.

You should look at the child's skin color and note any pallor, mottling, flushing, or cyanosis. *Cyanosis* is of immediate concern, especially if there is central cyanosis noted at the lips. Note that cyanosis of the hands and feet can occur "normally" in infants younger than 2 months when the infant is cold. Before you approach the child, ask the parents to remove or lift the child's shirt. Look for mottling of the trunk in the infant. *Mottling* is a large, blotchy pattern of mixed pale and reddish to reddish blue areas evident on the skin, which may be evidence of inadequate perfusion. A cold environment can also result in mottling in the normal infant, especially in the extremities.

Evaluation of the quality and quantity of breathing can likewise be done from across the room. Keeping the normal values for the age group in mind, you should take note of the respiratory rate and check for symmetrical chest expansion.

Notice whether the child is breathing easily or working hard to breathe, as demonstrated by the use of neck and other accessory muscles of breathing; **retractions** above the clavicles, between the ribs, and below the sternum; and increased abdominal movement (**Figure 25-3**). Look at the position the child assumes if there is respiratory distress. Children with respiratory distress may prefer to remain sitting. With obstruction of the upper airway, they may be found leaning forward, with the neck extended slightly and the chin forward (sniffing position) and the mouth open and tongue slightly protruding. How hard a child is working to breathe is as important as the rate of breathing. Look for nasal flaring (seen predominantly in infants), which is a sign of respiratory distress. Notice whether there is nasal congestion.

Listen for obvious stridor, grunting, wheezing, or cough. **Stridor** is a noisy crowing sound made on inspiration and suggests upper airway obstruction. Stridor with retractions is a concern. *Grunting* is a rhythmic sound heard at the end of exhalation. This is a sure sign of significant respiratory compromise and is rarely noted past 3 years of age. Loud wheezing and coughing may be heard without a stethoscope.

Key Respiratory Findings

Retractions. Retractions are often visible in children because of the flexibility of the chest wall. Retractions are the inward depression of muscular areas and their attached ribs, which are drawn inward and reflect an increased work at breathing caused by obstruction to airflow. Retractions may be seen in different muscular areas. In croup, for example, nasal flaring and supraclavicular retractions may be seen with moderate distress, and intercostal and substernal retractions are evident as the distress becomes more severe. Head bobbing is a form of retraction of the neck muscles seen in infants that is caused by extension of the neck during inhalation with relaxation during exhalation.

Stridor. Stridor is the high-pitched noise usually heard on inspiration caused by obstruction to airflow in the upper airway. Severe airway obstruction may result in stridor on inspiration and expiration. Stridor is audible without a stethoscope.

Wheezing. Wheezing is the high-pitched "musical" sound caused by the narrowing of the lower airways, obstructing airflow. This narrowing can be caused by swelling in the airway or narrowing of the small bronchioles. Wheezing may be heard only during exhalation, and the exhalation time may be prolonged to allow time for air to exit from the narrowed airways. Wheezing is created by turbulence generated from increased expiratory pressures forcing air through narrow airways. There are many causes of wheezing in children, including asthma, bronchiolitis, and pneumonia.

Cyanosis. As with adults, central cyanosis is a sign of low oxygen saturation of the hemoglobin in the blood. Cyanosis is not an early sign of hypoxia, and other indications, such as altered mental status, may appear before cyanosis is present. Because cyanosis appears when a certain concentration of the hemoglobin in the blood is unsaturated with oxygen, it may be late or absent in children with hemorrhage or anemia, when the total hemoglobin amount is low.

Pediatric Assessment Triangle

Table 25-5 summarizes the signs of respiratory distress and failure in children.

You should periodically repeat your assessment during transport to reevaluate the patient's condition and help determine the effectiveness of treatment.

The American Academy of Pediatrics (AAP) states that the evaluation of (1) general appearance, (2) work of breathing, and (3) signs of circulation to the skin, known as the *pediatric assessment triangle,* is an important tool to form your general impression. The pediatric assessment triangle uses this "ABC" approach (*a*ppearance, *b*reathing, *c*irculation) to evaluate the child "from the doorway" and begin to assess the child's neurologic, respiratory, and circulatory status.

Focused (Secondary) Assessment

Patient History

Obtaining a history in the child follows the same format as in the adult. After hearing the chief complaint, obtain the SAMPLE history (see Chapter 7). For the infant, inquire about any problems during pregnancy or birth. Was the baby premature or kept in the hospital for additional time? The younger the child, the more you must rely on the parents for the history. When speaking with children, you should remember to use terms appropriate for their age and vocabulary.

Physical Examination

In general, assess breath sounds first and then circulation, and perform the detailed physical examination with a trunk-to-head approach. The following considerations are helpful for obtaining vital information:

Table 25-5	Signs of Respiratory Distress

Early Signs	Increasing Distress/ Respiratory Failure	Prerespiratory Arrest
Tachypnea	Severe retractions or grunting, or both	Cyanosis or grayish hue to skin
Tachycardia	Increased tachycardia and tachypnea	Bradycardia (an ominous sign)
Mottling of skin	Altered mental state	Shallow breathing or apnea
Nasal flaring	Poor peripheral perfusion	Unconsciousness
Retractions	Cyanosis	Weak distal pulses
Stridor, wheezing, grunting	Decreased muscle tone	Limp muscle tone

- When approaching the small child or infant, you should initially listen to the lungs because you do not know how long the child will remain quiet. When listening to the lungs (with a warm stethoscope), listen for the presence or absence of air movement, and note any abnormal breath sounds, especially wheezing and stridor. Keep in mind that normal respiratory and heart rates are faster in children.
- If the child is old enough to understand, ask the child to blow at your pen as if it were a birthday candle. If able, the child will take a deep breath before blowing.
- Often the child is crying, and you may be unable to assess lung sounds adequately. However, you already know that a strong cry is a good sign because a sick child is too busy working to breathe to put up a fight.
- You should assess circulation by taking a brachial pulse in infants. Assess other peripheral pulses in children as in adults, noting the rate, quality, and regularity.
- Evaluate capillary refilling time in small children, noting delay if the return to normal color takes longer than 2 seconds.
- You should check the blood pressure in children older than 3 years, being careful to use the appropriate-size cuff.
- You should note skin temperature, moisture, and color in all patients.

Other Considerations

An infant's skull bones are not fully fused until well into the second year of life. The anterior fontanel (soft spot), between the frontal and parietal bones, is the largest space between these bony plates. The average size of the fontanel is 3 × 3 cm at birth, which slowly decreases with age. The level of the fontanel relative to the skull is significant. In the normal, sitting infant, the soft spot should be level with the bones of the skull or only slightly depressed. In the dehydrated infant, the fontanel is depressed even when the baby is lying down. Conversely, a bulging fontanel may reflect increased intracranial pressure. The most common concern with a bulging fontanel is meningitis; however, other causes, such as hematomas and bleeding within the skull, are possible. The strain of crying can also cause the fontanel to bulge.

A stiff neck is an important physical finding and may indicate infection in the brain or its coverings (meningitis). The irritable infant or small child may be difficult to assess. Try to have the child follow a toy or keys by turning the head so that the child must flex the neck. Be aware that infants and small children can have meningitis without either a stiff neck or a bulging fontanel; they may simply be listless. The only presenting sign of a severely sick infant may be the parent's opinion that the child is "just not acting right." Infants who were born prematurely are even more susceptible to serious infections in the first 2 months of life.

In a child with respiratory distress, especially stridor, you must specifically avoid examining the oropharynx. The only exception would be in the case of direct visualization of a foreign body.

Rashes are common in children. They are associated with allergic reactions and common viruses, such as measles, rubella (German measles), varicella (chickenpox), and a variety of nonspecific viral illnesses (**Figures 25-4** and **25-5**). Rashes are also seen with bacterial illness. Making a specific diagnosis in children with rashes is often difficult, even for hospital personnel.

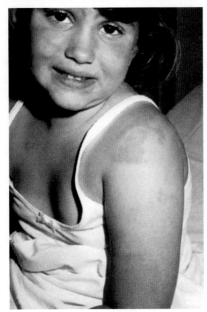

Figure 25-4 A child with hives, or urticaria, from an allergic reaction.

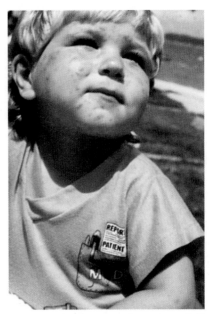

Figure 25-5 Rashes on children may be a sign of allergy or infection. This child has chickenpox.

Because the child's condition might be contagious, inform the hospital before arrival so that appropriate isolation preparations can be made. To complete the physical examination, follow the same focused (secondary) assessment guidelines used for adults, remembering that in the very young child, you should perform a complete head-to-toe survey in reverse order.

> **LEARNING OBJECTIVE**
> • Summarize emergency medical care strategies for respiratory distress and respiratory failure.

Management

Opening the Airway

As with adults, the head-tilt/chin-lift is the preferred method for opening the airway of an infant and child. However, the degree of neck extension is modified according to the age of the patient. You should not hyperextend the neck in infants age 1 year or younger. Instead, you should maintain the head and neck in a neutral or slightly extended ("sniffing") position with padding (e.g., towel, folded sheet) under the torso if necessary (**Figure 25-6**). In children up to 8 years old, slight extension of the neck may be useful, with care taken not to hyperextend the neck to avoid any kinking of the airway. The ultimate test of effectiveness for all techniques is adequate chest rise and evidence of breathing.

Figure 25-7 demonstrates the jaw thrust without head tilt for the infant and child. As with the adult, this procedure is used for patients thought to have spinal injury.

Suctioning

A rigid catheter is preferred for suctioning the child's oropharynx of blood, vomitus, and small particulate matter. You should insert the rigid catheter only as far as you can see. The suction

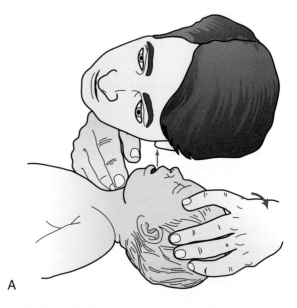

A

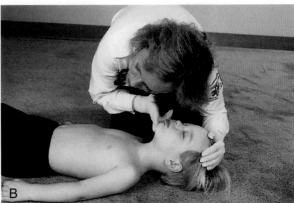

B

Figure 25-6 Using the head-tilt/chin-lift. **A,** For the infant, keep the head in the neutral position. **B,** For the child, extend the neck back slightly.

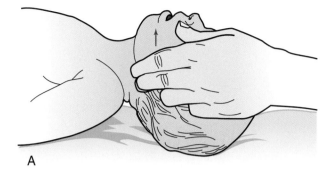

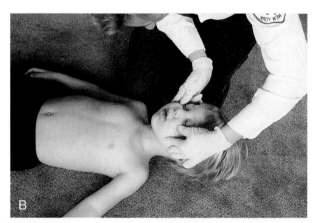

Figure 25-7 With suspected cervical spine injury in the pediatric patient, use the jaw thrust without head tilt. Place the fingers under the angle of the jaw and lift the lower jaw upward. **A,** Infant. **B,** Child.

pressure generally should be at least 300 mm Hg of vacuum. (In newborns, this pressure should not exceed 100 mm Hg of vacuum.)

A soft catheter or bulb suction can be used for suctioning the nasal passages in infants and newborns needing low to medium suction. If appropriate, you should hyperventilate the patient with oxygen before and after suctioning. Maintain short periods of suction; the 15 seconds or less in adults should be even shorter in infants and children. If the mouth is filled with secretions or emesis that cannot be removed easily by suctioning, you should log-roll the patient and help clear the oropharynx.

Airway Adjuncts

Oral airways are used for patients who do not have a gag reflex. Size the airway by measuring it from the corner of the patient's lips to the bottom of the earlobe or angle of the jaw. When introducing the airway, use a tongue blade placed at the base of the tongue to press the tongue downward and insert the oropharyngeal airway directly, without rotation.

Nasal airways might be used in patients who are responsive but who need assistance in keeping the tongue from obstructing the airway. Consider the size of the nostril, and measure from the tip of the nose to the patient's ear to help select the appropriately sized airway. Lubricate the airway with a water-soluble lubricant, and insert it posteriorly with the bevel toward the base of the nostril or toward the septum. If the airway cannot be inserted in one nostril, try the other.

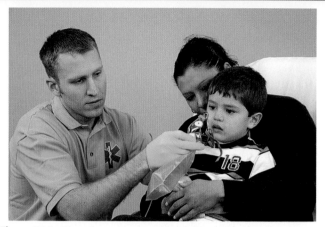

Figure 25-8 Blow-by oxygen can be delivered by mask, oxygen tubing, or nebulizer tubing, or can be improvised by placing oxygen tubing through the bottom of a paper cup.

Oxygen Therapy and Positive-Pressure Ventilation

Oxygen therapy in infants and children is generally delivered by either a nonrebreather mask or blow-by oxygen administration techniques. Because infants and small children may refuse or fight placement of a face mask, you might hold oxygen tubing (which may be inserted into a paper cup) or the mask about 2 inches from the face. The child may permit the parent to hold the tube or mask closer to the nose or mouth than the EMT would be allowed (**Figure 25-8**).

If the need for positive-pressure ventilation is established, provide two initial breaths and perform rescue breathing. You should give one breath every 3 seconds (20 breaths/min) for the infant and child up to age 8 years and one breath every 5 seconds for the older child (12 breaths/min) with volumes in proportion to the size of the patient. Breaths should be gentle and given smoothly over 1 to 1½ seconds to avoid overinflation, gastric distention, and pressure-related injury (e.g., pneumothorax). A bag-mask device can be used to administer positive-pressure ventilation; however, care should be taken when the device has a pop-off valve (pressure-release valve) because the airway resistance may exceed the pop-off valve setting, causing air leakage at the valve (**Figure 25-9**).

The pop-off valve is designed to avoid barotrauma (pressure injury to the lungs). When there is high airway resistance (e.g., resuscitation, asthma), however, the pop-off valve may release before adequate volumes of air can be delivered to cause a chest rise. Pop-off valves can be closed shut with a finger or tape or, in some cases, by twisting. Oxygen-powered breathing devices are not recommended for pediatric patients because high airway pressures may develop, causing tension pneumothorax or gastric distention.

Gentle pressure may be applied on the cricoid cartilage (Sellick maneuver) to help prevent gastric distention during positive-pressure breathing if the number of personnel available permits this action (**Figure 25-10**). Use finger pressure over the cricoid cartilage (ring directly beneath thyroid cartilage, or Adam's apple) and press down gently. Gentle pressure is enough to help close off the esophagus and airflow into the stomach. You should avoid excessive pressure, especially in infants, to prevent collapse of the trachea itself.

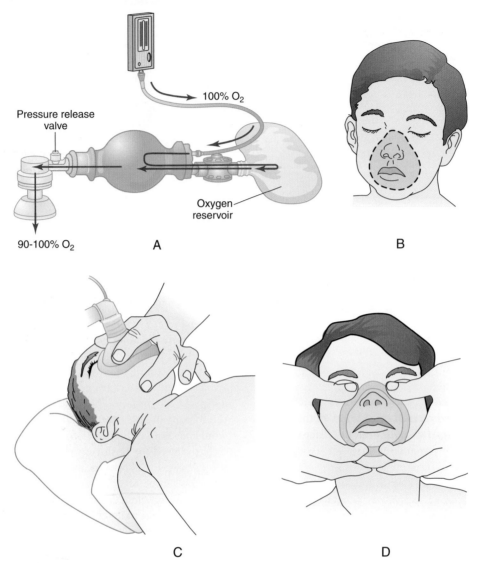

A

B

C

D

Figure 25-9 Pediatric bag-mask technique. **A,** Pediatric bag-mask with oxygen reservoir (note pressure-relief valve). **B,** Position of face mask. **C,** One-handed technique of ventilation. **D,** Two-handed technique for sealing mask. *Modified from Chameides L, Hazinski MF, eds: Textbook of pediatric advanced life support, Dallas, 1994, American Heart Association.*

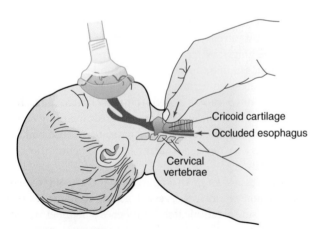

Figure 25-10 The Sellick maneuver is used with positive-pressure ventilation to avoid air flowing into the esophagus, thus preventing gastric distention. *Modified from Chameides L, Hazinski MF, eds: Textbook of pediatric advanced life support, Dallas, 1994, American Heart Association.*

The size of the mask used depends on the size of the patient. The mask should cover the nose without pressing on the eyeballs, and its lower end should rest on the chin just below the lower lip. Again, when you are determining the volume to be delivered, chest rise is the best indicator of effectiveness. When enough personnel are available, use the two-person bag-mask technique, with one person ensuring a good seal of the mask while the other squeezes the bag during each artificial breath.

Table 25-6 summarizes the key differences among adults, infants, and children in relation to airway management and ventilation.

LEARNING OBJECTIVES
- Indicate various causes of pediatric respiratory emergencies.
- List the steps in the management of choking in the infant and child.

Table 25-6	Airway Management and Ventilation Differences		
Skill	**Adult**	**Child**	**Infant**
Airway opening	Head-tilt/chin-lift with head extended	Head-tilt/chin-lift with slight extension of head by using anterior displacement of cervical spine with a blanket under occiput	Head-tilt/chin-lift with head in neutral position
Oropharyngeal airway insertion	Rotational insertion or insertion with a tongue blade	Insertion with only a tongue blade to avoid injury to soft tissues	Insertion with only a tongue blade to avoid injury to soft tissues
Rate of positive-pressure ventilation	12 breaths/min	20 breaths/min	20 breaths/min
Timing of a single rescue breath	1-2 seconds to administer a breath (with supplemental oxygen)	1-1.5 seconds to administer a breath	1-1.5 seconds to administer a breath

Common Pediatric Conditions

Your primary concern as a provider of prehospital care is to decide quickly whether emergency intervention is necessary. Therefore, learning about some of the more common childhood conditions is valuable and will help you gain confidence in evaluating and dealing with children.

Respiratory Disorders

A failing or failed respiratory system is the single most important cause of death in the pediatric age group. Control of the airway, ventilation, and oxygenation is the most important element of pediatric resuscitation. Except for the child with congenital or acquired heart disease, children normally have strong hearts. This explains the common pediatric saying, "Control or treat the respiratory system, and the heart will follow."

Upper Airway

The major upper airway diseases requiring emergency attention are croup, epiglottitis, and choking. All these conditions carry the risk of causing severe obstruction. A distinction must be made between the infectious causes (croup and epiglottitis) and the presence of a foreign body, because the management will differ. The obstructed airway maneuvers used to remove a foreign body are of no value for croup and epiglottitis. In addition, stimulation of the pharynx and epiglottis must be avoided if a patient has epiglottitis because it may cause severe spasm and closing of the airway.

Croup. Infection accounts for the majority of cases of stridor in childhood. Within this group, croup is common. **Croup** is a viral infection affecting the larynx, trachea, and bronchi. It causes airway narrowing, especially at the level of the cricoid ring, and produces stridor (**Figure 25-11**). The classic course begins with an upper respiratory infection or cold. The child with croup may exhibit the following signs and symptoms:

• Hoarseness
• Low-grade fever
• Cough that sounds like a barking seal
• Varying degrees of inspiratory stridor
• Retractions with inspiratory effort

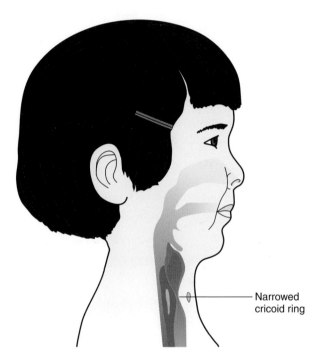

Figure 25-11 Croup can cause significant narrowing of the airway as a result of inflammation and mucus, especially at the level of the cricoid ring.

Croup is often worse at night or on awakening. It is most common from age 6 months to 3 years. Keys to effective management include humidification, hydration, and oxygenation.

Croup may appear to be "cured" by humidification or by the cool night air. In fact, many patients are asymptomatic by the time they reach the hospital or the physician's office. However, severe cases of croup can result in severe airway obstruction.

Epiglottitis. Acute **epiglottitis** is an infectious swelling of the epiglottis (caused by a bacterial infection) that has a rapid onset of approximately 10 to 12 hours (**Figure 25-12**). Epiglottitis usually affects children age 2 to 7 years but can also occur in older children and adults.

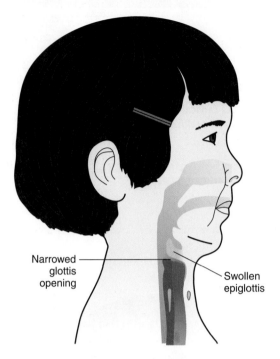

Figure 25-12 An inflamed and swollen epiglottis (epiglottitis) can obstruct the opening to the larynx. Avoid any manipulation of the posterior pharynx or any attempt to "see" the epiglottis because complete obstruction from spasm can occur.

The major signs and symptoms of epiglottitis include the following:
- High fever
- Sore throat
- Dysphagia (difficulty swallowing)
- Occasional inspiratory stridor
- Drooling

The child with epiglottitis is frequently sitting upright and leaning forward, with the weight distributed on the hands, the mouth open, the tongue protruding, and the chin thrust forward (tripod position). This maximizes the airway diameter and improves ventilation. Other key signs include restlessness, a flushed face, and signs of dehydration.

Epiglottitis is a potentially life-threatening emergency. An additional concern is that stimulation of the pharynx, as with examination with a tongue blade, can cause reflex spasm of the epiglottis, resulting in total airway obstruction. Classically, the child has a mild upper airway infection and then suddenly becomes ill.

The behavior of the child with epiglottitis is the key to management. The patient sits relatively still, holding the head in a particular position (which is keeping what little airway there is open). The approach to management follows:
1. Use gentle, calm handling, staying away from the child's airway.
2. Let the child stay in the parent's arms, even during transport, to decrease the chance of oxygen consumption that may result from anxiety.
3. Offer humidified oxygen, but if the child is alert and resists, do not persist.

Table 25-7	Signs of Croup, Epiglottitis, and Foreign Body Obstructions	
Croup	**Epiglottitis**	**Foreign Body Obstructions**
6 mo-3 yr	2-7 yr	Any age (especially 3 mo-5 yr)
Slow onset	Sudden onset (hours)	Sudden onset (history of choking)
Low-grade fever	High fever	No fever
Sick, not toxic	Toxic	Not toxic
Cough (barking seal)	Muffled or quiet	Coughing initially
Hoarse	Dysphagia	Difficulty talking
Usually not drooling	Drooling	May drool
Agitated, moving	Quiet, classic tripod position	Either quiet or agitated

4. In these circumstances, you or the parent may try to hold the mask near the child's airway.
5. If cyanosis and lethargy are evident, attempt positive-pressure ventilation. Studies have shown that ventilations with a bag-msk can be effective in patients with epiglottitis.

Choking. The child or infant with foreign body aspiration is usually a previously healthy child with a history of choking on something who now exhibits signs of upper airway obstruction (e.g., stridor, rapid breathing, difficulty moving air). For the purpose of treatment, an "infant" is defined as a patient younger than 1 year and a child as a patient age 1 year and older. These age parameters relate to an average size at these ages; a small 13-month-old child may be treated as an infant, and a large 11-month-old infant may be treated as a child.

It is important to determine whether the choking episode is mild or severe and to assess the level of consciousness, air exchange, and ability to speak or cry. You should take a brief history from the parent or caregiver regarding recent upper respiratory infections, fever, and barking cough or a history of choking after eating or playing with objects in the mouth, to help clarify the cause of obstruction.

You should treat all suspected infectious causes of obstruction as epiglottitis; that is, do not manipulate or attempt to examine the airway. Review the summary of croup, epiglottitis, and foreign body obstruction in **Table 25-7** to clarify the major differences.

The Alert Child. If the child is alert, even with severe stridor and a rapid respiratory rate, keep your management to a minimum. You should keep the child and parents calm and allow the child to remain in the parent's arms in the position of comfort that the child chooses. You should also supply humidified oxygen to the child when available without agitating the child and transport quickly.

This treatment is appropriate regardless of whether you suspect croup, epiglottitis, or a choking episode. Even if you suspect choking, do not intervene if the child is alert and moving air.

Severe Airway Obstruction (Unconscious Patient). If the infant or child is unconscious, you will usually recognize an airway obstruction during your attempts at artificial positive-pressure ventilation. During your assessment, you may note absent breathing and may attempt to ventilate. With a severe obstruction, your ventilation efforts will not result in chest rise.

You should first reopen the airway and reattempt ventilation. Because the tongue is the most common cause of airway obstruction in the unconscious patient, use the head-tilt/chin-lift procedure (modified jaw thrust if trauma is suspected), and administer positive-pressure ventilation.

If your second attempt at ventilation is not successful, treat the infant or child for a severe airway obstruction. If you suspect that the infant or child has an infectious cause of airway obstruction, continue to attempt "forced" positive-pressure ventilation, and transport rapidly to the hospital. A child with this type of obstruction often requires surgical opening of the airway (cricothyroidotomy or tracheotomy).

If you suspect that the child has a foreign body obstruction of the airway, follow the guidelines outlined in **Skills 25-1** and **25-2.**

Mild or Severe Airway Obstruction (Conscious Patient). If the infant or child is conscious but cannot speak or cry, or if the child is showing evidence of poor air exchange, including a weak ineffective cough, stridor, increased respiratory difficulty, and possibly cyanosis, you should treat the patient for a severe airway obstruction.

Other Upper Airway Conditions. Children often have upper respiratory infections. Most are the common cold or sore throat with swelling of the pharynx and tonsils. From the EMT's perspective, the following three points deserve mention:

1. Secretions in the nasal passage can narrow the pediatric airway.
2. The upper respiratory condition may precede more severe problems, such as croup and epiglottitis, or even severe tonsillitis.
3. A call for help when the child "has a cold" should prompt a search for complicating factors, such as dehydration, exhaustion, or the early, but not yet evident, onset of more severe complications.

Lower Airway

The primary diseases affecting the lower airways in pediatric patients are bronchiolitis, asthma, pneumonia, other infectious processes, and foreign bodies that are small enough to pass through the trachea and lodge in the smaller lower airways. Although it is possible to differentiate among these conditions in the field, management is the same. The patient with difficulty breathing without upper respiratory problems is treated with the following measures:

• Reducing stress and exertion.
• Administering humidified oxygen.
• Transporting to a hospital.

Bronchiolitis. Bronchiolitis is a viral illness affecting infants (usually 2 to 6 months of age but up to 2 years) and causing swelling (edema) and mucus production in the lower and smaller airways. Bronchiolitis follows an upper respiratory tract infection and often occurs in the winter. The narrowing of the airways results in turbulence and impaired airflow. Wheezing, rhonchi, and rales can be heard.

Asthma. Asthma is a common and recurrent condition that affects children and adults. Asthma causes bronchospasm with mucus and edema production, resulting in the narrowing and obstruction of lower airways. This causes an increased resistance to airflow, primarily during expiration. Wheezing (usually bilateral) is heard, and expiration is prolonged.

Patients can die of asthma when the obstruction is so severe that no effective air exchange takes place or when they become exhausted. When this occurs, no wheezing may occur, and the patient may be unable to speak. With severe bronchospasm, increased resistance is also encountered during positive-pressure ventilation.

Asthma can be triggered by different conditions in different patients. Some triggering events are infections of the respiratory tract, allergies, and the withdrawal of some medications, such as steroids. Patients with asthma often have treatment at home in the form of nebulizers, which release a mist of bronchodilator drugs, such as albuterol.

Again, you should be wary of a child with an altered mental status or who becomes lethargic and wants to lie down.

If an asthmatic patient requires positive-pressure ventilation, high resistance to flow should be anticipated. Maintain an effective seal, and use proper technique when ventilating the asthmatic patient. Note that in some cases, ventilation cannot be adequately accomplished without drugs to relax the airway constriction. In these cases, rapid transport may be lifesaving.

Pneumonia. As with adults, children can have both viral and bacterial infections of the lower airways and alveoli. Pneumonia often follows a simple upper respiratory tract infection, which may be viral or bacterial. The patient usually has a complaint or history of fever and cough. Dehydration as well as signs of a recent upper respiratory infection may be present. Children often have difficulty describing the symptoms of pneumonia. Pneumonia may cause abdominal pain because irritation of the diaphragm may be interpreted by the child as abdominal in nature. Also, signs of pneumonia, such as rales, may become apparent a day or more after the onset of fever and cough. When present, rales may be heard with or without wheezing and on one or both sides. Pleuritic pain may be noted.

The keys to management of pediatric pneumonia are appropriate attention to the signs of respiratory distress and application of humidified oxygen and ventilatory support as needed.

Foreign Bodies. Foreign bodies, such as peanuts, food, plastic, metal, and teeth, can be inhaled past the upper airway and lodge in the lower airways. In these situations a cough is usually noted. The cough is initially nagging and nonproductive. Wheezing may be heard on one side, reflecting the bronchospasm initiated by the presence of the foreign body in the airway. The problem may not be diagnosed for a time after the foreign body is inhaled. In these cases the child may have a fever and increased mucus production as part of a generalized inflammatory response. Anatomically, the foreign body is more likely to lodge on the right side because the right main stem bronchus offers the more direct pathway at the division of the trachea. Treatment in the field is directed at respiratory support (see Skills 25-1 and 25-2).

In all pediatric patients with lower airway disease, treatment is based on administration of humidified oxygen, reduction of exertion and emotional stress, and transport in the upright position (or position of comfort). Pay careful attention to signs of respiratory failure and the need for positive-pressure breathing.

LEARNING OBJECTIVE
• Differentiate between respiratory distress and respiratory failure.

Respiratory Failure and Respiratory Arrest

If you encounter a child with respiratory failure or respiratory arrest, immediate intervention is necessary. Essential lifesaving steps are performed as you look for the underlying cause. Key signs of respiratory failure include the following:
• Cyanosis or mottling
• Fast or slow respiratory rate relative to the patient's age
• Little or no air movement
• Labored breathing and retractions

You should look for evidence of inadequate oxygenation, such as altered mental status, extreme weakness or sleepiness, and possibly dilated pupils, and assess the heart rate and pulse strength. Hypoxia initially results in a rapid pulse as the heart tries to compensate, but later leads to a slow pulse as the heart muscle becomes hypoxic. The child who does not resist positive-pressure ventilation most likely needs it. Children who resist your intervention are demonstrating a degree of oxygenation through their responsiveness and skeletal muscle exertion. Remember, however, that hypoxic patients can become combative and make interventions difficult. When in doubt, ventilate and look for signs of responsiveness. If breathing is inadequate, time your ventilations with the child's efforts to breathe to augment the child's own respiratory efforts.

Children who are fully responsive but have respiratory distress should receive high-concentration oxygen. The rapid addition of oxygen at the highest concentration available can provide a small but crucial margin of safety and can increase the likelihood of continued adequate oxygenation of the brain and heart.

Children with signs of respiratory distress who are alert should be allowed to remain with their parents and should be approached gently. "Gently" does not imply slowly, but avoid increasing the child's anxiety, which may increase the work of breathing and critical oxygen consumption.

Box 25-1 summarizes the management of respiratory distress and respiratory failure.

Drowning

More than 5000 children drown each year in the United States. Drowning occurs more often in warmer areas. Children age 18 months to 3 years make up the most vulnerable population. In addition to drowning by falling into swimming pools, the inquisitive, fearless toddler also may drown in a bathtub, laundry pail, well, or rain barrel. Adolescents are also statistically overrepresented in this number because of a combination of factors, including decreased supervision, increased risk-taking behavior, and alcohol and drug use.

Children fare much better after a drowning incident than do adults. This is especially true with a cold-water submersion. There are numerous case reports in the literature of infants and children who survived prolonged ice-water submersion. A few of these children had no signs of life when they were pulled out of the water but recovered fully. Overall, survival in the water is better when the water is warmer; however, if submersion is prolonged, freezing cold water may contribute to cell preservation and survival.

The pathophysiology of drowning is the same for children as for adults. However, it is important to note that infants and children have an exaggerated *mammalian diving reflex* that shunts blood to the body core and slows down metabolism in response to sudden immersion in icy water.

All children found immersed in water should be immediately transported while CPR is performed. When the child is found in shallow water, you should consider the possibility of cervical spine injury and the need for inline immobilization of the spine. A long spine board should be used during the removal of such patients. When conditions permit, you should start rescue breathing in the water and add high-concentration oxygen at the first possible opportunity. You should also maintain the patient's body temperature.

Sudden Infant Death Syndrome (SIDS)

The leading cause of death from 1 month to 1 year of age is SIDS. Each year approximately 2500 infants die of SIDS in the United States; the incidence is 2 per 1000 live births. Most children die while asleep and are found by their parents. This explains why most ambulance calls for SIDS patients occur in the early morning. Many of the children are in perfect health or might have had a minor respiratory infection before death.

Sudden infant death syndrome is not an event associated with newborns because it occurs beyond the first 2 weeks of life. Most cases occur before 6 months of age, with a peak at 10 to 14 weeks of life. The incidence is higher in late fall and winter (**Box 25-2**). SIDS can occur in any family, but the following are significant risk factors:
• Low socioeconomic group
• Adolescent mother
• Infant sleeping on stomach
• Drug use during pregnancy (e.g., mother taking methadone poses a 25-fold increased risk)
• Prematurity, especially if the baby had respiratory complications and received ventilator assistance
• Low birth weight
• Poor prenatal care
• Mother who smoked during pregnancy

Sudden infant death syndrome does not appear to have a single cause. Various theories relate to the immaturity of the infant's neurologic system, poor control of the respiratory system, and airway compromise resulting in prolonged apnea. The "Back to Sleep" campaign to have infants sleep on their backs

---

Box 25-1 Sample Protocol for Pediatric Respiratory Distress and Respiratory Failure

1. Provide oxygen to all children with respiratory emergencies.
2. Assist ventilation for severe respiratory distress with:
   • Altered mental status
   • Cyanosis with oxygen
   • Poor muscle tone
   • Ineffective respiratory efforts
3. Provide oxygen and positive-pressure ventilation (bag-mask or mouth-to-mask) for respiratory arrest.

Box 25-2 Sudden Infant Death Syndrome (SIDS) Statistics

- 2246 deaths per year (8% of total deaths of infants younger than 1 year)
- Third leading cause of death in infants younger than 1 year
- Appearance of SIDS babies includes the following signs:
  Lividity (mottling in dependent areas)
  Cooling and rigor mortis (within 3 hours)
  Frothy drainage from mouth and nose
  Small marks (e.g., diaper rash) that look more severe
  Well-developed appearance

Data from US Department of Health and Human Services, Centers for Disease Control and Prevention: *Final data on infant health,* Hyattsville, Md, 2004, National Center for Health Statistics.

---

has reduced the death rate. Whatever the contributing abnormalities, the result is cessation of respiration during sleep.

Role of the EMT

The scene of a SIDS death or near-death is emotionally charged. There are two circumstances you may encounter. In the first the parents have found the infant in respiratory and cardiac arrest after some period of time. In the second situation the parents have observed a period of apnea (cessation of breathing) in the infant that was transient, and now the baby appears fine.

If the infant is not breathing, perform CPR and transport. If the infant is breathing, observe the baby for key signs associated with a postresuscitation or a sleep apnea event. The child may have been resuscitated by a bystander or the parents by the time you arrive. The following observations obtained by your examination or the history given by the parents indicate that the child has had a significant event:

- Presence of cyanosis, either before your arrival or currently
- Evidence of shallow respirations
- Evidence of respiratory or cardiac arrest

You should assess the child for the continued need for CPR and continue to assess the infant en route to the hospital while administering humidified oxygen and keeping the infant warm. Additional observations that may prove useful to the physician to help judge the significance of the breathless period and events surrounding the illness include the following:

- Infant is unresponsive or dazed.
- Infant's breathing is labored or irregular.
- Infant's color is pale, blue, flushed, or mottled.
- Infant is limp, hypertonic (muscle spasm), or exhibiting jerking movements.
- Blood or vomitus is present on the bed sheet.

Unless the baby has clear signs of death (e.g., rigor mortis) and the parents are clearly aware of this, you should initiate resuscitation and transport and avoid any delay at the scene. In the following months, the parents will relive this tragic event repeatedly. They will feel better knowing everything possible was done for their child.

Parents may experience denial, grief, and sometimes guilt. It is not unusual for victims of SIDS to have mottling in the dependent areas of the body, which may be confused as bruises associated with child abuse. Never be judgmental in these

circumstances. If you suspect child abuse, you should report it to the physician at the emergency department. Do not question the parents in a suspicious manner. Your professional and tactful behavior in this situation is important in helping the parents cope with the loss of their child.

Fever

Fever is common in children. In fact, a minor illness associated with a fever is the most common complaint that pediatricians encounter. Common misconceptions are that the fever itself is dangerous and that the higher the fever, the greater the risk of a seizure. About 5% of children have a simple febrile seizure during childhood. However, the increased temperature does not trigger the seizure; rather, it is caused by the *rapid rise* in temperature. Therefore the actual degree of the fever is not overly significant.

Children can have a high fever with a simple viral illness, or a fever can accompany a serious infection. In the absence of serious infection, children can tolerate high fevers well. However, any febrile child should be transported. The fever itself is not worrisome, but the cause of the fever is a concern.

A common practice to cool a febrile child is covering the child with a cloth soaked with tepid water. Alcohol or cold water should not be used because this causes shivering and vasoconstriction in the extremities. Such treatment puts the child at risk of an actual increase of core temperature resulting from peripheral vasoconstriction or, in contrast, hypothermia that may occur during transport.

Hypothermia may also occur with the use of tepid-water soaks. The towels or sheets can cool quickly from the effects of the environment and become cold soaks. Given the high risk of hypothermia at the scene or en route, you should carefully weigh the use of this option. When transporting, remember that even a febrile child is at risk for hypothermia. The prehospital evaluation of temperature is carried out by simple tactile assessment. Actual measurement of temperature with a thermometer is not necessary and would only increase the time on the scene and act to disturb the infant or child.

LEARNING OBJECTIVES
- List the common causes of seizures in the infant and child patient.
- Describe the management of seizures in the infant and child patient.

Seizures

A seizure in a child is a common and usually controllable medical emergency. However, the sight of a seizing child is frightening to parents and results in an emotional response that may interfere with optimal management. The seizure itself usually is not life threatening unless it occurs while a child is swimming, climbing, or engaging in other activities. As long as the airway is maintained, a child can tolerate a grand mal seizure in excess of 20 minutes without permanent damage.

The most common seizure you are likely to encounter with pediatric patients is a simple febrile seizure. Approximately 3% to 4% of children between age 6 months and 6 years with a febrile illness will have a febrile seizure. The seizure is often the first sign of an illness. A simple febrile seizure is brief, lasting less than 5 minutes, and is associated with fever and a *tonic-clonic* (contraction and relaxation of skeletal muscles) generalized convulsion. The child is most likely to be in the *postictal phase* (lethargic, confused state after tonic-clonic movements) of the seizure when you arrive on the scene, but the mental status is likely to improve during transport to the hospital.

A febrile seizure is considered complex if (1) it is greater than 15 minutes in duration, (2) it is localized to a part of the body, or (3) there are multiple episodes within 24 hours. Five percent of children with febrile seizures will present in *status epilepticus,* a persistent generalized seizure lasting more than 20 minutes or a series of recurrent seizures without the return of consciousness.

When you are called for a seizing child, the brief febrile seizure is usually over by the time you arrive. It is important to transport every child who has had a seizure because there may be a serious underlying cause. Ten percent of children with meningitis have seizures, and in children younger than 18 months, a meningeal sign (e.g., stiff neck) may not be present. In addition to fever, causes of seizures in children include the following:
- Infections: encephalitis, meningitis, roseola, shigellosis
- Metabolic disorders: hypoglycemia, hypoxia, fever, hyponatremia, hypocalcemia
- Toxic substances: lead, aminophylline, lidocaine, cocaine, nicotine, phenothiazine, drug withdrawal (especially from prescribed anticonvulsants)
- Structural problems: trauma, bleeding, mass lesion, scar in the brain
- Idiopathic: no known cause

The mortality rate associated with status epilepticus is 8% to 15%. You should consider any patient who is actively seizing when you arrive as being in status epilepticus.

Complications

The complications associated with seizures are caused by their effect on many organ systems. Respiratory problems encountered include decreased respiratory drive, airway obstruction by the tongue, risk of aspiration during the unconscious period, and ineffective respiratory muscles during seizure activity. All these factors can contribute to low oxygenation and retention of carbon dioxide. Metabolic problems include rise of body temperature from persistent muscular activity, depletion of glycogen stores and blood glucose, and cell damage. The central nervous system (CNS) can be affected from prolonged electrical activity of the brain as well as from respiratory and metabolic complications.

Box 25-3 summarizes the management of children with seizures.

Box 25-3   Sample Protocol for the Pediatric Seizure Patient

1. Ensure a patent (open) airway
2. Position the patient on his or her side if no cervical spine injury is suspected
3. Have suction ready
4. Provide oxygen and ventilation (if necessary)
5. Transport

Trauma

Trauma is the leading cause of death in children age 1 to 14 years and is the second most common cause of death in infants. Many more children sustain debilitating injuries from trauma, and a significant number of these deaths are preventable.

Prevention

The use of infant and child car seats, seat belts, and bicycle helmets significantly reduces morbidity and mortality. Educating the public on pedestrian and bicycle safety, the dangers of drunk driving, and child awareness is also important. Other environmental issues of importance are window guards (especially in urban areas), water safety, smoke detectors, fire prevention, and supervision of children at home. The use of childproof caps on medication containers has significantly decreased mortality from toxic ingestion in toddlers. Simple measures, such as adjusting the temperature of household water heaters to safe levels, can prevent serious scalding injuries. EMTs should play an active role in community health education and prevention to reduce death and injury rates.

Mechanism of Injury

Children are less protected than adults when subjected to blunt trauma. A child's bones are more resilient, and forces are more easily transmitted to internal organs. Because of the resilience of the child's skeleton, clues to internal damage may be less obvious than in an adult. In addition, because of the child's small size, more vital organs are located within a small space, and transmitted force can affect many organs before the force dissipates. This is important because it increases the risk of multisystem injury and therefore mortality risk. As a result of the young and vital cardiopulmonary system, the child responds dynamically with initial compensatory mechanisms that can mask signs of blood loss. Serial examinations of the vital signs are necessary before they can be considered stable in the traumatized child.

For a variety of reasons, the youngest individual in a vehicle is statistically the most vulnerable to injury and death during an accident. As the vehicle decelerates, the child or infant who is unrestrained or held in a parent's arms literally becomes a missile that smashes into dashboards and windshields, sustaining head and neck injuries. Ordinary car seats are not built to restrain a child, although some special car seats can do this effectively. Children who are restrained with lap belts only (without shoulder straps) may sustain abdominal or lower spine injuries. Infants and small children in car seats and younger children who do not fit properly in three-point restraints should be placed in the rear seat to avoid injury from airbags.

LEARNING OBJECTIVES
- Differentiate among the injury patterns in adults, infants, and children.
- Discuss the field management of the infant and child trauma patient.

Children are also often victims of pedestrian trauma. Because of their size, children are more likely to sustain direct injury to the vital organs (head, abdomen, and extremities) from the bumper of a vehicle. Most of these injuries occur in urban areas, where children often play in the streets. Children may also sustain serious injuries when they fall from a height or dive into shallow water. Spinal injury should be suspected in all falls and diving injuries.

Children are often reckless on bicycles, underestimate their chance of injuries, and may not wear helmets. They are frequently struck by motorists while playing near traffic. Common injuries from bicycle spills are abrasions, fractures, and head and spinal injuries. Children can strike the abdomen on the bicycle handle when they fly forward over the handlebar. Such injuries can damage internal organs such as the liver or spleen.

Injuries to Specific Body Regions

Head Trauma. Head trauma is a leading cause of death in children. With early attention, a greater number of children can be saved. Prevention of secondary brain damage is just as important as in the adult. Hypoxia and hypotension must be prevented and treated aggressively when encountered. The single most important maneuver to ensure an open airway is the modified jaw thrust maneuver. As with adults, any suspicion of internal bleeding requires rapid hospital intervention. Early diagnosis is important to prevent or treat brain injury. Nausea and vomiting are common signs and symptoms. Ongoing assessment (reassessment) must be performed to detect progression or deterioration. You should use the AVPU mnemonic (*a*lert, *v*erbal, *p*ainful, *u*nresponsive) and other neurologic scales employed by your system to determine responsiveness. Pupillary and motor reactions are important findings that can be elicited rapidly and repeatedly.

Infants have relatively large heads with small necks and weak cervical musculature. The head easily snaps forward on the frail neck musculature, which can result in devastating injury. As with adults, children with evidence of a head injury or violent force to the neck should be immobilized. In general, the best immobilization is accomplished with the combined use of a high-cut rigid or firm cervical collar and a rigid backboard. Infants and small children are prone to high cervical spine injuries (above C5), which can result in total loss of respiratory effort.

Chest Trauma. The child's compliant chest wall allows damaging levels of trauma to be transmitted to intrathoracic structures without causing rib fractures. For example, there can be an underlying heart or lung contusion without obvious external evidence. With healthy, pliable blood vessels, tearing of the aorta is rare in childhood. However, the compliance of structures within the chest and the decreased ability to expand lung volume make other conditions worse. The child, as with the adult, can lose a sufficient amount of blood in the thorax to bleed to death.

Rupture of the diaphragm occurs in children from severe motor vehicle injuries and falls, with the high abdominal pressure bursting the diaphragm and thrusting abdominal organs into the chest cavity, most often on the left side. Collapse of the lung from penetrating injuries or air from a rupture in the trachea, bronchus, or esophagus can result in respiratory compromise.

Box 25-4	Sample Protocol for Major Pediatric Trauma

1. Ensure airway patency with the modified jaw thrust and cervical spine precautions
2. Suction as needed with a large-bore suction catheter
3. Provide oxygen and assist with positive-pressure ventilations as needed
4. Provide spinal immobilization
5. Transport

A child may be at risk for respiratory compromise from pulmonary contusions or bruises to the lungs. Pulmonary contusions may cause slight edema or extravasation of blood and fluid into the alveoli. Symptoms of respiratory distress may not be severe initially, but they can progress over a short time and result in an inability to oxygenate the patient. Therefore, careful continued evaluation of the child en route to the hospital, looking for a change in respiratory status, is warranted.

Abdominal Trauma. Children have thin abdominal walls that provide little protection, and the organs that are subject to hemorrhage from trauma are relatively large. Force is easily transmitted across the abdomen and can affect multiple organs because they are packed closely together. Distention of the abdomen may be noted with severe hemorrhage. Because the hemorrhage from an abdominal organ can be rapid and the child's condition can suddenly deteriorate after a period of compensation, you should transport the child with suspected abdominal trauma to the hospital as soon as possible, monitoring vital signs and treating shock en route.

The most common internal injury in childhood is rupture of the spleen. A less common but more fatal injury in children is rupture of the liver. Injury to other hollow structures is also possible.

Musculoskeletal Trauma. The pliable bones of children break in different places than adult bones, and sometimes they bend rather than break. However, the basic approach to injuries to a child's musculoskeletal system is the same as that for an adult's. One difference is that traction may further injure the pediatric growth plate. Accordingly, traction sometimes is not used for fractures of the femur. Check local protocols for further clarification.

Box 25-4 reviews the overall management of the pediatric trauma patient.

LEARNING OBJECTIVES
- Summarize the indicators of possible child abuse and neglect.
- Describe the medical-legal responsibilities in suspected child abuse.

Child Abuse

Child abuse is a major problem in pediatric morbidity and mortality; only SIDS and trauma are responsible for more pediatric deaths. More than 100,000 children a year sustain permanent disability from abuse. This epidemic seems to be increasing, with more cases reported each year, whether from the problem worsening or from an increased awareness by

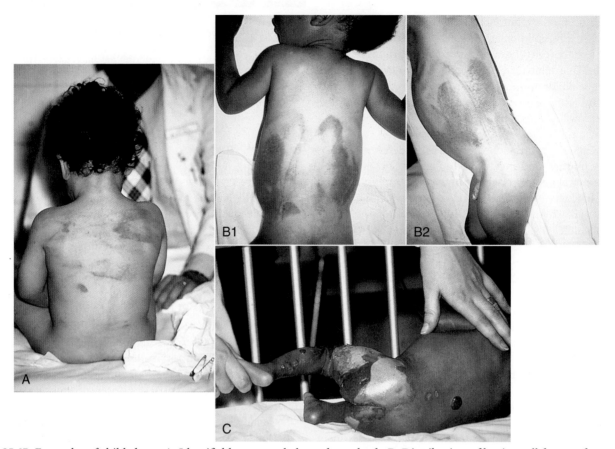

Figure 25-13 Examples of child abuse. **A,** Identifiable pattern: belt marks on back. **B,** Distribution of bruises: all four surfaces of the midbody are involved, but there are no bruises on the arms or legs. **C,** Nonaccidental immersion scald: involvement of virtually the entire posterior surface of the legs indicates that the legs were held under the water, because even an infant this young would flex the knees to avoid the hot water.

health professionals and society, resulting in increased reporting. Importantly, most children who die or are disabled from child abuse have a previous history of a suspicious injury or suspected child neglect.

The majority of abused children are younger than 3 years of age. In general, the younger the child, the higher is the risk for abuse. Unfortunately, the most vulnerable are also most frequently the victims. Abused children and their siblings are often subjected to recurrent abuse. In addition, many cases of child abuse are probably underestimated or not reported. This is certainly an area in which prehospital personnel can play an important role. Only with early recognition can the morbidity and mortality of this preventable injury be reduced.

Categories of child abuse are as follows:
- Physical abuse
- Sexual abuse
- Emotional mistreatment and neglect

Physical Abuse

Physical abuse accounts for 80% of the reported cases of child abuse. Physical abuse includes intentional trauma to the soft tissues, skeleton, CNS, viscera, teeth, and sensory organs, as well as intentional poisoning. The "four Bs" of active physical abuse are *b*attered, *b*ruised, *b*roken, and *b*urned.

Most often you will see soft tissue injuries. Bruises can be inflicted on all parts of the head and neck area and the trunk, including the flanks, buttocks, and extremities. With normal activity, children usually bruise themselves over bony prominences such as the forearm and the anterior portion of the leg. Therefore, bruising over meaty areas is suspicious. Any injury with a pattern, such as marks left by belts, teeth, or electrical cords, is suspicious, as are multiple bruises in various stages of healing (**Figure 25-13**).

Unusual patterns of burns should also trigger the suspicion of abuse. Sharp demarcations are rarely seen in burns. Note burns that have a shape or pattern. Any burn of the genitalia, or any injury to that area, should be noted.

Intentional injury to the CNS carries a particularly poor prognosis. CNS injuries account for only 15% of reported cases of child abuse but are the leading cause of death and permanent morbidity after intentional injury. An infant can sustain significant acute subdural hematomas merely from being shaken vigorously, without any external signs of injury. These babies may present with vomiting, agitation, seizures, and coma, or with only nonspecific findings such as poor feeding. Any fracture in an infant is suspicious, as are multiple fractures, especially when in various stages of healing.

Sexual Abuse

More difficult to diagnose and accept is the sexual abuse of children. This is a chronic problem, with the abuser usually being someone known and close to the child. Sexual abuse crosses all socioeconomic lines. Physical findings are often scant, but suspicion is raised by signs of external genital trauma or a child having difficulty walking. Frequently, children are reluctant to admit anything because of fear, guilt, and an unwillingness to break up the family. You should take seriously a child's statement that someone is "bothering" him or her. Children cannot usually make up details about sexual advances.

Neglect

Children can also be subjected to more subtle forms of abuse. All children are entitled to adequate food, clothing, shelter, education, medical care, dental care, emotional nurturing, and appropriate supervision. Failure to provide these basics to a child is abusive and is considered neglect. These children are at risk for various self-inflicted injuries, such as the unsupervised small child who sets the apartment on fire while playing with matches. These children are at as high a risk of growing up with severe emotional and developmental problems as children being physically abused. The following are signs and symptoms of neglect:

- Lack of adult supervision
- Malnourished appearance
- Unsafe living environment
- Untreated chronic illness (e.g., asthmatic patient with no medication)

Assessment

The information you gather surrounding the occurrence of an injury is extremely important, but it would be unwise to undertake an investigation yourself. Careful observation without accusation or confrontation allows you to transport the child to a hospital with the least amount of delay. This is in the child's best interest, and once at the hospital, you can relay your suspicions and observations.

As you obtain the child's history, the following should alert you to possible abuse:
- Repeated calls at the same address
- Parents' story not consistent with the injury (e.g., 9-month-old with obvious deformity of lower extremity whose parents claim child fell off couch)
- Changes in the history, depending on who is giving it
- Witnesses giving contradictory histories
- Parent reluctant to give a history
- A delay in obtaining medical attention
- Timing of the injury not consistent with clinical findings (e.g., "My child fell down two steps," but bruises are at various stages of healing and are scattered over child's body [**Table 25-8**])
- Parents' response not appropriate to the severity of the injury
- Child exhibiting inappropriate agitation with you or the family

Table 25-8	Appearance of Bruises in Various States of Healing
Age of Bruise	**Appearance**
1-3 days	Red/blue
3-7 days	Purple
>7 days	Yellow/brown
>3 weeks	Brown to clearing

- Obvious alcohol or drug use by the parents
- Child fearful of discussing how the injury occurred
- Conflicting stories
- Fresh burns

Pay particular attention to the environment, the sanitary state of the home, and any evidence of a struggle. You should determine the time of the incident, presence of witnesses, any history of recent illness, and the condition of the child's clothing (e.g., presence of blood or dried secretions).

The abused child may respond in various ways. The child may be overly friendly or withdrawn or may have inappropriate responses, such as to pain. Be concerned about the child who is "too good."

You should be aware of your emotional response, and be extra cautious not to ask questions in an accusatory tone. You should try not to be judgmental. It may be helpful to realize that abusive parents usually want help and may themselves be victims of complex psychosocial situations. Often, abused children grow up to be abusive parents. Bring objective information to the hospital.

Reporting laws do not vary from state to state, and you are legally mandated to report child abuse. Additionally, as an EMT you are morally and professionally responsible to communicate your suspicions if you suspect child abuse. All the laws are written so that one can report suspicions and be protected from litigation for false accusations. By careful, objective documentation of your findings at the scene and documentation of all subsequent conversations with healthcare providers regarding your findings, you are helping to alleviate the problem of child abuse. Remember, report what you see and hear, not what you think.

REAL*World*

The EMT should note how parents respond to their injured or ill child. Parents with a psychiatric illness known as *Munchausen's syndrome by proxy* like the attention they receive from family and friends when their child is sick or injured. To gain that attention, they may intentionally harm their child. This condition should be suspected when a child is treated repeatedly for illnesses or injuries that make no sense. The parents will not be concerned about the treatment provided. As with other types of abuse, report your suspicions to the receiving physician and legal authorities, as required by local law.

Infants and Children with Special Needs

The technologically dependent and medically fragile child poses special challenges to the EMT. With technological and medical advances, children survive substantial illness and injury. In many situations, they depend on technology and medical devices to breathe, eat, receive medications, or relieve pressure on the brain. These children are often cared for at home, many with minimal nursing support. The families are very important in the care of these children and provide most of their needs. It is not unusual for these medically fragile children to have relapses for which they need to seek hospital attention. As an EMT, you may be called to assist in transport under these circumstances. Children with special needs include those with substantial lung disease, heart disease, and neurologic disease.

Infants may have significant lung disease, especially those who were born prematurely and have received ventilator assistance in a hospital. Ventilator-dependent children require the placement of a special airway tube in the trachea (**Figure 25-14**). Some children require this on a long-term basis, and it is their primary breathing tube.

Infants and children may have diseases that are chronic or that have altered their normal function from birth. The baseline status can be considerably different from that of a normal child. Take this into account when you evaluate a patient with special needs. Remember that parents are taught how to care for their child's special needs at home. They know their child's baseline status and are the best source of information. In many situations, a 20% variance from their baseline respiratory rate or oxygenation levels is a cause to seek medical attention. Also, remember the differences in infants and children when estimating the need for oxygen supplementation. Although a 1- or 2-L/min flow to an adult represents 22% to 24% oxygen delivery, to an infant with little dead space and smaller total minute ventilation, this can represent a very high level of oxygen dependency. Some children are receiving less than 1-L/min flow but completely depend on this amount of oxygen. Children with heart disease may have chronic cyanosis. Again, the parents are the best source to ascertain whether their status represents a change in baseline or function.

Children with substantial or chronic neurologic disease can be susceptible to seizures that are difficult to control. Recurrent seizures that are more frequent than the child's usual baseline might be an indication for the parents to call emergency medical services (EMS) for help. Patients with neurologic problems also can be difficult to assess because some may not have normal consciousness or normal mental status as their baseline. Again, talk to the parents to obtain an indication of the change in status.

Some children may not be able to eat on their own and may have special feeding tubes. Others may be oxygen dependent or ventilator dependent and may have tracheostomy tubes and home ventilators. Patients who require continuous intravenous (IV) therapy may have central IV lines placed near the heart for long-term use. Other patients who have obstruction of cerebrospinal fluid (CSF) tracts in the brain have special shunts placed to allow CSF to drain into the central vascular space or the abdomen.

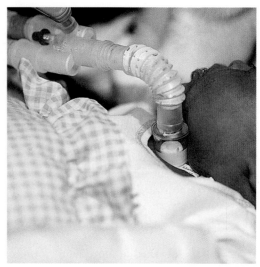

Figure 25-14 This infant depends on a ventilator and has a tracheostomy tube.

Tracheostomy Tubes

A tracheostomy is a surgical opening of the airway through which an artificial tube can be passed and remain in place to allow airflow. These tubes are inserted in children because of chronic dependence on a ventilator or perhaps obstruction in the upper airways because of congenital problems.

There are various types and sizes of tracheostomy tubes. Some have cuffs; some do not. Some have an internal cannula, whereas others are one piece (for very small infants). You need to be prepared to assist the parents in changing a tracheostomy tube. Remember, parents are taught how to care for and change a tracheostomy tube if the child receives care at home. Parents have extra tubes, tubes that are one size smaller, and equipment to suction secretions and provide artificial ventilation.

The most common complication is dislodgement of the tracheostomy tube. If parents or caregivers cannot replace the tube, they are taught to try one size smaller. If it cannot be replaced, observe the child to see if he or she is ventilating adequately through the *stoma* (opening in trachea). In general, less manipulation in the field is better if the patient can tolerate it. Give the patient supplemental oxygen, and transport as soon as possible. If there are signs of inadequate ventilation, options include the following:

- Attempting to replace the tracheostomy tube as local protocol allows.
- Covering the stoma with a small mask and ventilating with a bag-mask device.
- Ventilating with a bag-mask through the child's mouth and nose with a finger closing the stoma hole.

Tracheostomy tubes can become clogged with mucus and foreign bodies. If obstruction is apparent, suction the outer opening of the tube. Some systems allow EMTs to suction down the tube to clear the obstruction (**Figure 25-15**). Use a flexible suction catheter that is appropriate for the size of the tracheostomy tube, generally half the diameter. The parents should have the correctly sized catheter available. Remember, if you move the child to the ambulance and suction with the equipment,

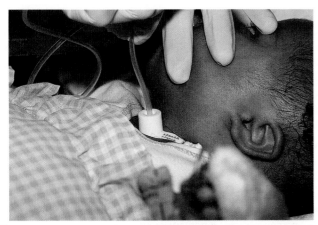

Figure 25-15 Suction of a tracheostomy tube may be required to clear an obstruction. Use an appropriately sized flexible suction catheter (generally half the diameter of the tube) and a suction pressure less than 100 mm Hg.

the setting should not exceed 100 mm Hg of pressure. Put 1 to 3 mL of saline solution down the tracheostomy tube to facilitate removal of tenacious mucus or other obstructions with a 3-mL to 5-mL syringe. If this does not work, do not spend a long time trying to remove the obstruction; instead, change the tube. This skill is usually reserved for advanced life support (ALS) providers.

REAL*World*

Even if your system does not allow you to change tubes, you may be asked assist a paramedic or flight nurse.

Changing the tube depends on the type of tube. If it has an inner cannula, it is removed and replaced. If the patient is a smaller infant with a one-cannula tube, the entire tube is removed and a new tube inserted. A child on a ventilator at home with a tracheostomy tube may have a cuff that is blown up. Deflate the cuff before removing this tube. Again, the parents or caregivers are knowledgeable on the type of equipment and their child. In general, you assist *them*.

As with adults, you may be able to ventilate an older child by covering the stoma with a smaller mask and a bag-mask device. This is difficult in infants, however, because they have such small necks. If there is no upper airway obstruction in these patients, it might be better to occlude the stoma with a gloved hand and ventilate by covering the nose and mouth with a bag-mask.

Once a tracheostomy tube is replaced, secure it in place with the ties that are provided. Bleeding may occur because of trauma to the airway, which may occur with suction. This is generally not a major problem, although it might alarm the parents and initiate a call for help. The main priority is to ensure that there is adequate air movement; if not, use suction.

Ventilator-dependent children may have tubes with cuffs, and these cuffs can occasionally leak air. This is usually noted by the pilot balloon on the outside; if this occurs, it may be necessary to change the tube. In some cases, air leaks because children grow too large for the size of the cuff previously inserted. Leaks

can occur between the outer cannula of the tracheostomy tube and the growing trachea. Because of this, the child may not receive the volumes needed from the ventilator and may show signs of poor oxygenation. In these situations the next-size tracheostomy tube is needed, which might be inserted in the hospital rather than at home. Signs of infection may occasionally be seen around the tracheostomy site.

As noted previously, the major goal in emergency medical care is to maintain an open airway and suction obstructions with minimal pressure. You should transport the child in a position that is most comfortable for breathing, usually a 45-degree elevation or in a sitting position.

Home Ventilators

Many types of ventilators are available for home use, and the parents should know how to use their particular machine. Both portable ventilators and battery packs are usually available in case of electrical failure or mechanical problems. This would be the device of choice to use during ambulance transport. Allow the parents to go with you so that they can maintain control of the ventilator en route. If the ventilation fails totally, you may have to assist with positive-pressure ventilations and supplemental oxygen.

Central Lines

Intravenous lines are placed to provide continuous IV therapy, medication administration, or nutrition. These lines can be placed in the subclavian region (under the clavicle) in the chest or in a central vein in the neck. Complications of IV lines include cracking, infection, clotting, and bleeding. Prehospital management of these types of emergencies is limited. If bleeding occurs, apply pressure to the site of bleeding, and transport the child with the IV line in place.

Gastrostomy Tubes

For some children who cannot eat by mouth, a tube is placed directly into the stomach for feeding. Some are placed through the nose and others directly through the abdominal wall into the stomach. In these cases, a balloon is usually inflated inside the stomach to keep the tube in place, and it is secured to the skin on the outside with tape. A gastrostomy tube (G-tube) comes in different shapes (**Figure 25-16**). Some devices, called G-tube "buttons," are flat with the abdominal wall and have an insertion port so that feedings can take place. Complications of gastrostomy tubes can include obstruction, leakage, and dislodgement.

Overfeeding through the G-tube can cause expansion of the stomach against the diaphragm and compromise respiratory efforts or ventilatory volumes. Advise the parents to vent the G-tube (an action they are familiar with) to relieve excess pressure in the stomach. As an EMT, you should focus on respiratory support and transport the patient. Have suction available. Infants and children may exhibit other signs if they have problems with feeding through their G-tubes, such as the following:

- Dehydration
- Lethargy
- Hypoglycemia if diabetes is present

Transport the child in a sitting position or lying on the right side with the head elevated.

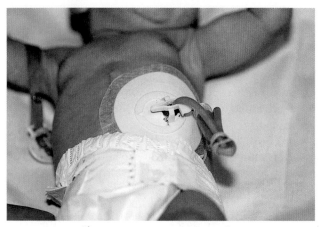

Figure 25-16 Gastrostomy tube.

Shunts

A *shunt* is a device running from the brain to the abdomen or central vasculature to drain excess CSF from the brain. You can often palpate the "reservoir" on the side of the skull and trace the shunt tubing down the neck. EMTs provide no intervention with shunts. However, you should be aware that these children sometimes have changes in their mental status, and the parents may be concerned about whether the shunt is working properly. You should focus on managing the airway, being ready to provide positive-pressure ventilation, if necessary, and transporting the patient. You should continuously watch for a change in mental status and seizures.

Case in Point

A father was changing his young child's diaper and noticed a plastic tube protruding from the child's anus. The father called 9-1-1. The child had a cerebral shunt placed several months ago. The tube was identified as the end of the shunt. The shunt had migrated into the gastrointestinal tract and eventually was excreted. Treatment consists simply of supportive care.

LEARNING OBJECTIVE
• Recognize the need for EMT debriefing after a difficult infant or child transport.

Emotional Stress

Caring for severely ill or injured children can be stressful for EMTs. The EMT can become emotionally involved when children suffer or die. EMTs may identify young patients with their own children.

It is important to realize that some anxiety may be caused by a lack of experience in treating children or a fear of failure. Remember, the basic principles you have learned about adults are used to treat children as well, although adjusted for the developmental, anatomic, and physiologic differences. Learn the differences, familiarize yourself with pediatric equipment, and take every opportunity to examine children.

You should recognize the value of discussing your feelings by using a debriefing format after a difficult infant or child transport.

Scenario Follow-up

In managing pediatric emergencies, you must understand common conditions affecting children and know developmental differences by age. In this case, for example, you allow the child to be held by his mother to decrease anxiety, which could increase oxygen consumption. This 3-year-old child had asthma, a condition common to children. The child also benefited from staying close to his mother because young children may feel threatened by strangers and may feel suffocated by an oxygen mask. By anticipating these issues, you significantly improve care. As an EMT, you also perform a trunk-to-head survey, avoiding the most threatening parts of the examination (around the head) to gain the boy's cooperation. The use of blow-by oxygen also contributes to the child's comfort.

Summary

In the management of pediatric emergencies, the EMT must deal with an emotionally charged environment. The feelings of the patient, the parents, and the EMT must all be acknowledged. A professional and caring attitude that instills calm and confidence is required to enlist the support of the parents and the trust of the child. The EMT should approach children with respect and consideration for their developmental age.

Infants and children are not small adults. The anatomic and physiologic differences are of the utmost importance in both assessment and treatment. Children depend on others for basic needs. Although their hearts are strong and can compensate for severe insults, their small size leaves them vulnerable to sudden decompensation. A careful search for early signs of shock is critical to prevent collapse.

Control of the airway is fundamental. Remember the pediatric adage: control the airway and the heart will follow. Keep anatomic differences in mind to apply correct airway and ventilation therapy. A child's small airway is easily obstructed. Humidification, suction, and administration of supplemental oxygen can make a significant difference. A youngster's store of glucose is easily depleted, and maintenance of body temperature is important to conserve the child's energy stores.

Skills

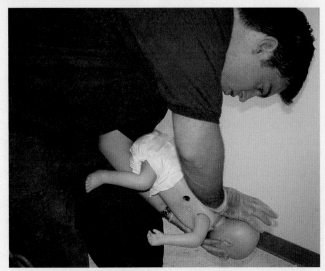

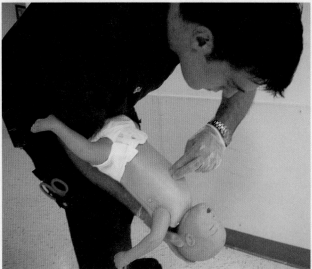

| **Skill | 25-1** | **Managing Foreign Body Airway Obstruction (Conscious or Unconscious Infant)** |

1. Confirm severe or complete airway obstruction (signs of serious breathing difficulty, ineffective cough, no strong cry). Give up to 5 forceful back blows.

2. Open the infant's airway using head-tilt/chin-lift, and look for a foreign object. Remove it if you see the object (do not perform a blind finger sweep). Give up to 5 forceful chest compressions.
3. If unable to ventilate, look in the airway again for a foreign object. Remove it if you see the object (do not perform a blind finger sweep). If infant becomes unconscious, perform CPR.

Skill | 25-2   **Managing Foreign Body Airway Obstruction (Conscious or Unconscious Child)**

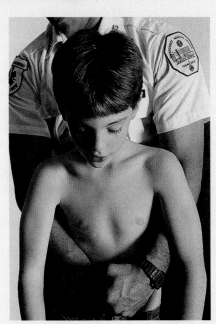

1. Ask, "Are you choking?" Give abdominal thrusts.
2. Repeat thrusts until effective or child becomes unresponsive.
3. Attempt to ventilate.
4. When you open the airway, look for a foreign object. Remove it if you see the object (do not perform a blind finger sweep).

The Bottom Line

Learning Checklist

✓ Children rarely die from sudden cardiac death. They die as a result of down-spiraling conditions that progress from hypoxia to decreased ventilation, low blood oxygen, decreased perfusion, acidosis, and cardiac collapse.

✓ Several developmental differences in children affect evaluation and treatment.

✓ Newborns and infants have minimal language ability but respond to voice and tone. They may demonstrate anxiety with strangers. They should remain in the arms of parents whenever possible and be examined in a trunk-to-head manner, taking the lung sounds first.

✓ Toddlers do not like to be touched by strangers, may refuse to cooperate, and should remain with their parents whenever possible. Distract the child with a stuffed animal or puppet. Do not undress the child all at once, and replace clothing as soon as possible.

✓ Preschool children are in a period of intensive learning and have varied communications skills. They should also remain with parents and may have an intense fear of pain. Approach the child at eye level in a nonthreatening manner with a toy or other device. Do not lie or overexplain.

✓ School-age children, ages 6 to 12 years, have a strong fear of disfigurement and permanent injury. They may have feelings of modesty and a fear of pain and blood. Explain what you are doing during the examination and treatment.

✓ When talking to adolescents, do not be confrontational; respect their personal "space," answer their questions, respect their shyness, and allow them to retain as much control as possible.

✓ Children and infants have a smaller airway at all levels. The narrowest point of the infant's airway is the cricoid cartilage.

✓ Positioning of the airway varies with infants and children. For infants, place the head in the sniffing, or neutral, position. For children, tilt the head slightly to open the airway.

✓ Respiratory rate varies with age: 12 to 20 beats/min for adults, 15 to 30 beats/min for children, and 25 to 50 beats/min for infants.

✓ Average pulse rates vary with age: 72 beats/min for adults, 75 beats/min for children 10 years or older, 80 beats/min for children age 2 to 10 years, 130 beats/min for infants, and 140 beats/min for newborns.

✓ The formula for predicting normal systolic blood pressure for children older than 2 years is 70 + (2 × age in years).

✓ Signs of dehydration are progressive: early (rapid pulse, less urine output, dry mucosal membranes), intermediate (lack of tears, sunken fontanels, sunken eyes), and late (skin tenting, delayed capillary refill, no urine output, hyperventilation, altered mental status, thready pulse, hypotension).

✓ Foreign body airway obstruction in infants is treated with back blows and chest thrusts.

✓ Foreign body airway obstruction in children is treated with abdominal thrusts.

✓ Early signs of respiratory distress include tachypnea, tachycardia, mottling of skin, nasal flaring, retractions, stridor, wheezing, and grunting.

✓ Signs of increasing respiratory distress or respiratory failure include severe retractions, grunting, increased tachypnea and tachycardia, altered mental state, poor peripheral perfusion, cyanosis, and decreased muscle tone.

✓ Signs of imminent respiratory arrest include cyanosis or grayish hue to the skin, bradycardia, shallow breathing or apnea, unconsciousness, weak distal pulses, and limp muscle tone.

✓ Signs of croup, a viral infection affecting the larynx, trachea, and bronchi, include hoarseness, stridor, barking cough, fever, and retractions.

✓ Treatment of croup includes humidification, hydration, and oxygenation.

✓ Signs of epiglottitis, a bacterial infection that causes swelling of the epiglottis, include sore throat, difficulty swallowing, stridor, high fever, and drooling.

✓ Treatment of epiglottitis includes avoiding unnecessary stimulation of the pharynx and administering humidified oxygen and positive-pressure ventilation if signs of respiratory failure or arrest occur.

✓ Diseases of the lower airway in children include bronchiolitis, asthma, and foreign body obstruction.

✓ Key signs of respiratory failure and the possible need for positive-pressure ventilation include cyanosis or mottling, fast or slow respiratory rate relative to age, little or no air movement, and labored breathing or retractions.

✓ Sudden infant death syndrome (SIDS) is the sudden death of an infant between age 1 month and 1 year. Approximately 2500 infants die from SIDS each year in the United States.

✓ Appearance of SIDS babies includes mottling in dependent areas, cooling and rigor mortis, frothy drainage from mouth or nose, and small marks on the body (e.g., diaper rash) that look more severe in an otherwise well-developed appearance.

✓ Risk factors for SIDS include prone sleeping position, winter months, low socioeconomic living conditions, adolescent mother, prematurity, smoking during pregnancy, and no prenatal care.

✓ Unless there are clear signs of death (i.e., rigor mortis), perform CPR and transport the baby with suspected SIDS.

✓ The febrile child may be cooled with tepid water soaks, but take care not to induce hypothermia.

✓ Seizures in children may be caused by high fever, idiopathic epilepsy (no known cause), metabolic disorders, toxic substances, structural problems (e.g., head injuries), and infections.

✓ The management of seizures includes maintaining a patent airway, administering oxygen, preventing injury, having suction ready, and if possible, placing the patient on his or her side to prevent aspiration.

✓ Trauma is the leading cause of death in children older than 1 year.

✓ Management of infants and children with major trauma includes ensuring a patent airway with the jaw thrust maneuver, providing oxygen and assisting with artificial ventilation as needed, and providing spinal immobilization.

✓ Child abuse includes physical abuse, sexual abuse, emotional mistreatment, and neglect.

✓ Injuries and bruises associated with child abuse may be found in all parts of the body in various states of healing, with sharp demarcations and patterns such as belt, bite, and electrical cord marks.

✓ Children may depend on technology and medical devices to breathe, eat, receive medications, or relieve pressure on the brain. Many of these children are cared for at home.

✓ Tracheostomy tubes are required in children because of chronic dependence on a ventilator or upper airway obstruction caused by congenital problems. The most common complication an EMT will see is dislodgement of the tube. If signs of inadequate ventilation are present, try to replace the tube as local protocol allows, cover the stoma with a small mask and ventilate with a bag-mask device, or ventilate with bag-mask through child's mouth and nose with a finger over the stoma hole. Transport the child in a comfortable breathing position: 45-degree angle or sitting.

✓ If transporting a child on a ventilator, allow parent to maintain control of ventilator during ambulance transport. If ventilation fails, you may have to assist with positive-pressure ventilation and supplemental oxygen.

✓ IV lines provide continuous IV therapy, medication, or nutrition. Complications include cracking, infection, and clotting and bleeding. Prehospital care is limited. If bleeding occurs, apply pressure and transport child with IV in place.

✓ Gastronomy tubes are placed directly into the stomach for feeding. Complications include obstruction, leakage, and dislodgement. You should focus on respiratory support and transport. Have child in sitting position or lying on the right side with head elevated during transport. Have suction available.

✓ Shunts drain excess CSF from the brain. EMTs provide no interventions, but must be aware of changes in mental status, seizures, and airway management.

Key Terms

Congenital Present at birth.

Cricoid cartilage Band of cartilage below the thyroid cartilage, forming a circle just above the trachea; also called *cricoid ring.*

Croup Viral infection affecting the larynx, trachea, and bronchi.

Epiglottitis Bacterial infection causing swelling of the epiglottis.

Hypoxia Prolonged period of decreased oxygen supply.

Retractions Inward depression of muscular areas and their attached ribs, which are drawn inward and reflect increased effort to breath.

Stridor High-pitched noise, audible without a stethoscope, usually heard on inspiration and caused by an obstructed airway.

Sudden infant death syndrome (SIDS) Unexplained death of an infant younger than 1 year old.

Review Questions

1. You are about to examine a 2-year-old child. She appears to be alert and in mild respiratory distress. Given the child's age, which of the following strategies might be helpful?
   a. Allow the child to be held by the mother.
   b. Carefully perform a head-to-toe survey.
   c. Tape the mask to the child's face.
   d. Remain standing above the child.

2. You are treating a 13-year-old girl who fell off a moped and sustained injuries to her torso and legs. The mother is present. You are about to perform a focused (secondary) assessment to evaluate the extent of the injuries. Given this child's age, how should you proceed?
   a. Bring her to a private location with her mother to perform the examination.
   b. Use modern slang language that identifies with the patient.
   c. Respect the privacy of the patient.
   d. Only talk to the mother because the child is a minor.

3. An infant has aspirated a small object, resulting in severe airway obstruction. What is the narrowest point in the *upper airway* where the object would likely become lodged?
   a. Pharynx
   b. Larynx
   c. Cricoid ring
   d. Tracheal ring

4. Which of the following respiratory diseases is more common in children than in adults?
   a. Croup
   b. Asthma
   c. Pneumonia
   d. A collapsed lung

5. What is the choking maneuver used in infants but not in children or adults?
   a. Heimlich maneuver
   b. Abdominal thrust
   c. Back blow
   d. Finger sweep

6. Which of the following children would require positive-pressure ventilation?
   a. A 1-year-old with nasal flaring who is crying loudly
   b. An alert and agitated 13-year-old with wheezing
   c. An unresponsive 2-year-old with a respiratory rate of 6 breaths/min
   d. An alert 6-month-old with intercostal retractions

7. Which of the following signs of perfusion is more reliable in young children than in adults?
   a. Blood pressure
   b. Capillary refilling time
   c. Skin color
   d. Skin temperature

8. What is the primary problem leading to cardiac arrest in children?
   a. Heart disease
   b. Respiratory failure
   c. Cancer
   d. Seizures

9. Which of the following is the most common cause of seizures in children?
   a. Hypoglycemia
   b. Trauma
   c. Hypoxia
   d. Fever

10. Because of developmental differences in children, which of the following statements about injury is true?
    a. Because of the child's smaller size, it is harder to damage organs.
    b. Because the child's chest is so compliant, internal injuries can occur without signs of rib fracture.
    c. Children are less likely to sustain head injuries because their skulls are softer.
    d. Because a child's bones are growing, they are more likely to fracture.

11. You respond to an injured child and suspect that the injuries may be caused by child abuse. Which of the following signs should you look for to support your concerns?
    a. Bruises over the knees and elbows
    b. An isolated cut on the chin
    c. Conflicting stories from younger siblings
    d. Injury pattern not consistent with the mechanism described

For Further Review

In the Student Workbook

- Multiple-choice questions
- Matching questions
- Short-answer questions
- True-false questions
- Case scenario questions

On Evolve

- Anatomy challenge
- Weblinks
- Lecture notes
- Exercises

Learning Objectives

Cognitive Objectives

- State the usual cause of cardiac arrest in infants and children versus adults.

- Identify the developmental considerations for the infant, toddler, preschool child, school-age child, and adolescent.
- Differentiate the response of the ill or injured infant or child (age specific) from that of an adult.
- Describe differences in anatomy and physiology of the infant, child, and adult patient.
- Identify the signs and symptoms of shock (hypoperfusion) in the infant and child patient.
- Describe the methods of determining end-organ perfusion in the infant and child patient.
- Summarize emergency medical care strategies for respiratory distress and respiratory failure.
- Indicate various causes of pediatric respiratory emergencies.
- List the steps in the management of foreign body airway obstruction in the infant and child.
- Differentiate between respiratory distress and respiratory failure.
- List the common causes of seizures in the infant and child patient.
- Describe the management of seizures in the infant and child patient.
- Differentiate among the injury patterns in adults, infants, and children.
- Discuss the field management of the infant and child trauma patient.
- Summarize the indicators of possible child abuse and neglect.
- Describe the medical-legal responsibilities in suspected child abuse.
- Recognize the need for EMT debriefing after a difficult infant or child transport.

Affective Objectives

- Explain the rationale for having knowledge and skills appropriate for dealing with the infant and child patient.
- Attend to the feelings of the family when dealing with an ill or injured infant or child.
- Understand the provider's emotional response to caring for infants or children.

Psychomotor Objectives

- Demonstrate the techniques of foreign body airway obstruction removal in the infant.
- Demonstrate the techniques of foreign body airway obstruction removal in the child.
- Demonstrate the assessment of the infant and child.
- Demonstrate bag-mask artificial ventilations for the infant.
- Demonstrate bag-mask artificial ventilations for the child.
- Demonstrate oxygen delivery for the infant and child.

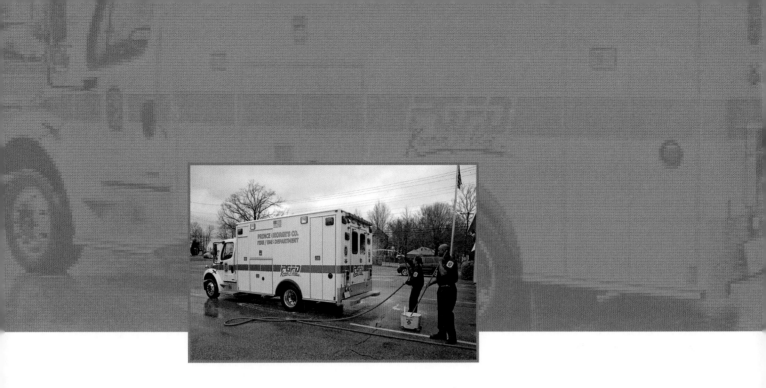

26 Ambulance Operations

CHAPTER OUTLINE

Phases of an Ambulance Call
Aeromedical Considerations

Scenario

Immediately after inspecting the ambulance and equipment, you and your partner receive a call from dispatch for a patient "in cardiac arrest." The dispatcher provides the location of the patient and the cross streets and advises you that bystanders are being given phone-directed instructions in performing cardiopulmonary resuscitation (CPR). You and your partner quickly discuss route selection, turn on the emergency lights, and carefully respond to the scene. En route to the call, you discuss your respective roles in the management of the patient.

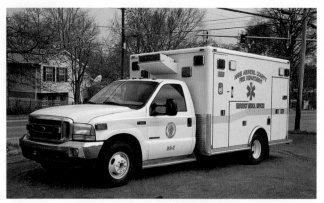

Figure 26-1 Type I ambulance.

LEARNING OBJECTIVES
- Discuss the medical and nonmedical equipment needed to respond to a call.
- List the phases of an ambulance call.
- Explain the rationale for having the unit prepared to respond.

Phases of an Ambulance Call

The phases of an ambulance call include the following:
- Preparation for a call
- Dispatch
- En route to the call
- Arrival at the scene
- Transfer of patient to the ambulance
- En route to the receiving facility
- At the receiving facility
- Back in service and after the call

Preparation for a Call

Before the first call on a shift, an emergency medical services (EMS) provider must check the vehicle and equipment with appropriate checklists to ensure readiness for communication, transport, and patient assessment and care.

Equipment

As technology advances and improves the field of EMS, the emergency medical technician (EMT) becomes more and more reliant on the use of equipment to evaluate and treat the patient. Thirty years ago, ambulance equipment was minimal and simplistic. Ambulance personnel had few options for immobilizing, oxygenating, or ventilating an acutely ill or injured patient. In current EMS systems, a wide range of equipment is more specific to a given patient's needs and therefore requires careful consideration by the prehospital provider. For example, a well-equipped ambulance may carry several types of spinal immobilization devices. The EMT must assess the situation first and then select the most appropriate option.

Complex variations within each device are another complicating factor facing EMTs today. In the past, a traction splint consisted of the simple combination of a metal frame combined with bandages. Currently, several variations of traction devices are available that use pulley systems, tension meters, and Velcro

attachments. Innovations do not necessarily make the device more complicated. Most of these splints are easier to apply than their metal and bandage "ancestors," but they represent yet another area in which training is necessary for the provider. Because most EMT courses do not have the time to orient students to all the variations of a given device, you should review the equipment stocked on your own ambulance to ensure familiarity before the first call.

The type of equipment stocked on a particular ambulance varies from region to region and system to system. Factors such as cost, types of calls, local environment, level of training, and exposure to state-of-the-art equipment are likely to account for these differences.

Ambulances

Three basic types of ambulances are used within EMS systems. Each has advantages and disadvantages, and they are often selected on the basis of regional needs or the budgetary limitations of a given provider. These vehicles differ in size, weight, turning radius, storage capacity, and interior working space.

Type I Ambulance. The **type I ambulance** consists of a box-shaped passenger compartment mounted on a truck-style chassis (**Figure 26-1**). This type of ambulance tends to be more spacious and more powerful than its counterparts. The modular unit allows for some degree of cost efficiency because it can be transferred onto a new chassis as the need arises. This type of ambulance generally has a rougher ride, and the cab is separated from the passenger compartment. This prevents the driver from going to a partner's aid if the need for assistance arises while en route to the hospital.

Type II Ambulance. The **type II ambulance** is a van-style vehicle with a raised roof and an extended rear compartment (**Figure 26-2**). Unlike the type I ambulance, the cab and patient compartments are usually joined to allow access by the driver. The van also tends to have a smoother ride. However, the space in the patient compartment is smaller, and generally less storage capacity is available. The turning radius of a van is better than that of the modular-type vehicles. This allows for greater mobility and easier parking. The enhanced maneuverability of the van-style ambulance is of great value in urban areas with congested traffic and narrow streets.

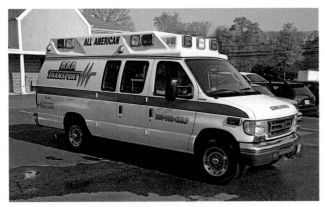

Figure 26-2 Type II ambulance.

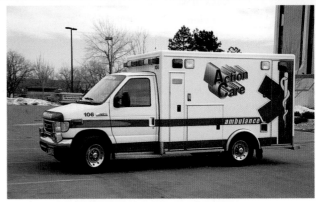

Figure 26-3 Type III ambulance.

Type III Ambulance. The **type III ambulance** is a modular box, as found in the type I ambulance, but it is mounted on a van chassis (**Figure 26-3**). As in a type II ambulance, access to the patient compartment is usually available from the cab. The combination of added storage space and better gas mileage than the truck style makes this a popular model in many EMS systems.

The equipment carried in the ambulance may vary according to regional requirements and resources, but certain equipment is recommended as standard by regulatory agencies, such as state departments of health, local EMS administrations, and national agencies (**Table 26-1**).

The personnel for a basic life support ambulance should consist of at least one EMT in the patient compartment and, for certain types of patients, two EMTs to allow for the management of the patient in the event of a cardiac arrest or other serious complication. All personnel should be prepared to respond quickly at the moment of dispatch. Some systems require that EMTs be available at quarters, and others have providers roving in the response area. In volunteer systems, providers often respond from home directly to the scene or to the ambulance station.

> **LEARNING OBJECTIVE**
> • Summarize the importance of preparing the unit for the next response.

Daily Inspection. The finest equipment available is of no value to the EMT or the patient if it is not serviceable, not stocked, or presents an infectious threat. Care of the ambulance and equipment starts at the beginning of your working tour, continues after each individual call, and ends with your tour of duty. Embarrassment is the least of your worries if you are transporting an ill or injured patient and your ambulance runs out of gas. A life may be lost if you have two cardiac calls in a row and fail to replace essential resuscitation equipment between calls. The timing of emergency calls is unpredictable, and the best way to safeguard against a poorly prepared unit is to check the equipment and vehicle at definite, regularly specified intervals (**Figure 26-4**).

The vehicle should be systematically checked at the beginning of each tour to be sure that it is fueled and in safe, serviceable condition. The easiest way to be certain that all areas of your vehicle are inspected regularly is to use a checklist that covers all the areas discussed next.

Engine Check. Fuel and oil levels should be checked and replaced as needed. The battery should be checked for appropriate fluid level, connections, and signs of corrosion. The cooling system should also be checked for fluid levels and hoses for leaks. You should also check power steering and transmission fluid levels. All belts should be checked for wear and replaced as needed.

Outside Inspection. A complete inspection of the ambulance body should be conducted to establish the condition before the first ambulance run. Record any dents not previously noticed on your check sheet. You should inspect tires for tread wear, defects, and air pressure. An outer inspection of all light systems should also be done at this time. Inspect doors, windows, and outside compartments to ensure that they are operational. The outside of the ambulance should be washed and waxed at regular intervals to prolong the life of the vehicle and convey a sense of professionalism to the public.

Cab Inspection. Test the brakes by noting the level to which the brake pedal can be depressed. Inspect turning and stopping signals, all emergency lights, sirens, and the horn. Start the ambulance and check all gauges and indicator or warning lights. Windshield wipers, ventilation, and cooling and heating systems should be evaluated. The driver should adjust the mirrors and seat position if necessary. You should check mirrors, doors, and storage compartments to ensure that they are secure and operational. The steering wheel should move freely and soundlessly. Check communication equipment by contacting dispatch and requesting confirmation.

Patient Compartment. A systematic check of the patient compartment and cabinets must be conducted to find any missing, dirty, or damaged equipment and to ensure that the compartment itself is clean. The floor and all environmental surfaces should be cleaned at the beginning of each tour and after each call when needed. Local protocols determine specific guidelines for thorough disinfection of the ambulance in special situations, such as after transportation of an infectious patient. Wipe the stretcher with a disinfectant solution after each patient and add

| Table 26-1 | Ambulance Equipment Checklist |

Item	Description	Quantity	Item	Description	Quantity
Burn sheet	Sterile	2	Masks for bag-mask device	Sizes: premature, infant, child, adult	4 (1 of each)
Cold pack	Chemical	4	Bedpan	Regular	1
Surgical clothing	Goggle, gown, mask, hat, eyewear	4 each		Fracture	1
Bandages, gauze	2 sizes	10 each	Emesis basin	Small, large	2 each
Bandages, triangular		10	Blood pressure cuff, stethoscope		1 each
HEPA respirator		4	Urinal	Plastic	1
Obstetrics kit	Disposable	1	Sharps container	Mounted forward-end squad bench	1
Obstetrics pad	Sterile	6			
Swaddler	Infant, commercially prepared	1	Spine board	Adult, pediatric	1 each
Incontinence pads	Disposable	4	Traction splint	Adult, pediatric	1 each
Dressings and tape	Multitrauma, 4 × 4–inch, occlusive	4 each	Rigid splints	4′ × 3″, 3′ × 3″, 15″ × 3″	2 each
			Head immobilizer	Adult, pediatric	1
Tissue	Facial	1 box	Padded board splint	Sizes: small, medium, large	6 (2 of each)
Restraint	Vest, extremity	1 pair			
Scissors, bandage		1 pair	Scoop stretcher	With 3 sets of straps	1
Multiple-casualty incident kit	New York State issue, sealed	1	Strap	6-foot	5
			Cervical spine immobilization collars	Sizes: tall, regular, short, no-neck, pediatric, baby no-neck	12 (2 of each)
Kendrick extrication device		1			
Oxygen tank	Full "E" cylinder	2	Immobilizer	Pediatric	1
	Regulator on tank	1	Flashlight	Large	1
	Onboard oxygen tank	1	Jumper cable	Heavy duty	1
Linen	Towel, sheet, blanket, pillowcase	4 each	PASG	Adult with pump	1
			Flare, road	Emergency, 30 minute	12
	Pillow	2	Screwdriver	Large, straight blade	1
Oral and nasopharyngeal airways	Adult, pediatric	4 each	Transport folder	Passenger side	6
			Portable suction	Various	1
Nasal cannulae	Adult, pediatric	4 each	Suction tubing, suction catheters: 5 to 18 French and rigid		1 each
Nonbreather masks	Adult, pediatric	4 each			
Bag-mask device	Adult with ETco₂ detector	1			
	Pediatric with ETco₂ detector	1	Sheet on pad, blanket, chart		1 each
	Neonatal	1	Stair chair	Folding	1

HEPA, High-efficiency particulate air; ETco₂, End-tidal carbon dioxide; PASG, pneumatic antishock garment.
Data from University Hospital and Medical Center at Stony Brook, Stony Brook, New York.

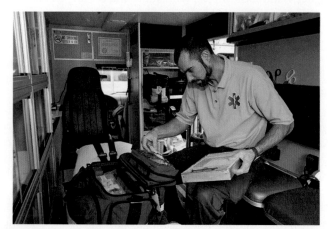

Figure 26-4 Checking equipment is an essential preresponse activity for the EMT.

clean linen. This includes blankets that have been used on a call. Dispose of all waste materials in the appropriate receptacles.

Ventilation, Airway, and Oxygen Equipment. Bag-mask devices, oxygen-powered resuscitators, other positive-pressure ventilation equipment, and suction devices should be tested to ensure that they are operational. They should be disinfected or replaced after each use according to local protocols. You should check both onboard and portable oxygen tanks to ensure a sufficient supply. You should also check the number of oxygen administration and airway devices and replace them as needed.

Bandage and Sterile Supplies. Check bandages, dressings, burn packs, obstetric kits, and other sterile supplies to ensure sterility and sufficient quantity. Store all sterile supplies in a dust-free, dry location. These supplies should be replaced if they

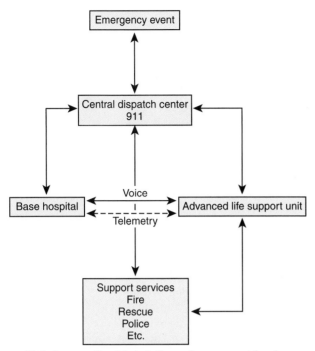

Figure 26-5 A centralized 9-1-1 dispatch system with telemetry communications to medical direction facilities. *From Stapleton E, Best J: Developing a hospital based ambulance service. In Pascarelli E, editor: Hospital based ambulatory care, Norwalk, Conn, 1983, Appleton-Century-Crofts.*

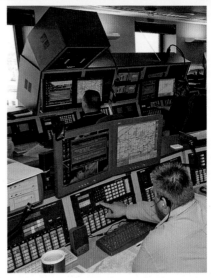

Figure 26-6 Modern communications center.

become wet because sterility can no longer be guaranteed. You should check expiration dates periodically, and pull and discard outdated items. Newly acquired supplies should be placed under existing supplies to minimize waste.

Stretchers and Immobilization Equipment. Long spine boards, short spine boards, and stretchers should be stored neatly and should be operational. You should examine straps to ensure that they are in sufficient quantity for each device. Also check traction, rigid, and other types of splinting devices. You should clean immobilization equipment after each use.

Safety and Extrication Equipment. Traffic cones, flares, and other safety devices should be checked. You should carefully inspect protective clothing, and if the ambulance carries a self-contained breathing apparatus, it should be checked to ensure it is functional. Some ambulances carry extrication equipment. If you are responsible for its use, it should be tested at regular intervals.

Other Equipment. Diagnostic and specialized equipment, such as stethoscopes, sphygmomanometers, and pneumatic anti-shock garments, should be checked to ensure that they are present and in working order.

Dispatch

Dispatch models range from dispatch directly from the ambulance quarters to a highly sophisticated, 24-hour **central access dispatch** system that coordinates various EMS units within a given area, to an **enhanced 9-1-1** computerized dispatch system that automatically identifies a caller's location. **Figure 26-5**

illustrates a communications model that links the dispatch center to emergency services and hospitals. Many systems also maintain communication from a medical control center to advanced life support (ALS) units in the field. These systems often integrate biotelemetric communications to allow for electrocardiogram (ECG) transmission for advanced EMS providers. A modern dispatch center uses personnel trained in **emergency medical dispatch (EMD),** a formal program that educates dispatchers in telephone triage and telephone-directed instructions designed to guide laypeople in the essentials of first-aid and emergency care **(Figure 26-6).**

Typical information collected at the dispatch center may include the following:
- Nature of the call
- Name, location, and call-back number for the caller
- Location of the patient
- Number of patients
- Severity of injury
- Special problems (e.g., dangers, hazards)

For a more complete discussion of communications systems, see Chapter 8.

LEARNING OBJECTIVES
- Describe the general provisions of state laws relating to the operation of the ambulance and privileges in the following categories: speed, warning lights, sirens, right of way, parking, and turning.
- List contributing factors to unsafe driving conditions.
- Describe the considerations that should be given to request for escorts, following an escort vehicle, and intersections.
- Discuss "due regard for safety of all others" while operating an emergency vehicle.
- State what information is essential to respond to a call.
- Discuss various situations that may affect response to a call.
- Identify what is essential for completion of a call.

En Route to the Call

Case in Point

In 1976, a fire department ambulance responded to the scene of a cardiac arrest with two EMTs aboard. An off-duty firefighter who lived two blocks away from the scene of the call also responded and initiated CPR with the ambulance crew. The firefighter continued resuscitation efforts while en route to the hospital, and the patient's family followed behind. The ambulance was traveling at a speed in excess of 70 mph on local streets, and the patient's family was unable to keep up with it.

At 4:30 AM, the ambulance failed to make a sharp curve, mounted the curb, and struck a tree, killing five people on impact: two firefighters, two EMTs, and the patient. On impact, the top of the ambulance was ripped completely off, scattering bodies and equipment across the lawn.

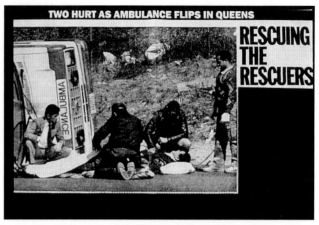

Figure 26-7 Newspaper headline on ambulance accident. _From Ambulance accident prevention student workbook, Albany, New York State Department of Health._

This single incident prompted the establishment of the Emergency Vehicle Operation Course (EVOC), sponsored by the U.S. Department of Transportation (DOT). Until this time, no standardized curriculum had been developed to train EMTs in the operation of emergency vehicles. Although more than 100 hours are dedicated to the teaching of acute emergency medicine during the EMT program and many years of experience can be accumulated, this is all wasted if the EMT never arrives at the scene or fails to deliver the patient to the hospital (**Figure 26-7**).

Ambulances are subject to special vehicle and traffic laws, and their operators are charged with the responsibility of preserving human life. Although the philosophies and procedures described in this text are a good basic introduction, it is necessary to practice these techniques in a properly supervised EVOC program to gain a full understanding of them. Actual hands-on experience reinforces these ideas, allows the EMT to practice emergency maneuvers in a controlled environment, and gives the EMT a better appreciation of the size and weight of the vehicle. Laws for emergency vehicle operation can vary from state to state and city to city. EMTs must be familiar with the laws governing the area where they work.

Driving an Emergency Vehicle

Arch of Driver Safety. Driving can be thought of as an "arch" that is constructed of many components, including physical and mental abilities, knowledge of traffic laws, and driver attitude. This concept is called the **arch of driver safety.**

The driver of an emergency vehicle must possess many attributes to perform his or her duties effectively. Physical fitness is essential to the driving task, but even though driving is considered to be primarily a physical activity, 90% of it depends on the driver's attention and concentration. Therefore, mental fitness is an integral component of the arch.

Good judgment is required to select the best alternatives in crisis situations. In this area the experienced operator, having acquired the proper skills, can anticipate and avoid hazards.

Some drivers develop good driving habits, such as using proper turning techniques, using the brake in questionable situations, and using safety restraint devices consistently. Others develop poor habits, including left-foot braking and "palming" the wheel during a turn. Motor vehicle crashes are often avoided because good driving habits have prevailed over poor habits.

Knowledge of how a particular ambulance handles and familiarity with applicable traffic laws are critical. Although certain "privileges" are granted to emergency vehicle operators to expedite the delivery of emergency care, EMTs can be held liable for abuse of any of these exemptions.

The keystone of the arch is _attitude._ The ambulance operator who assumes that the ambulance always has the right of way may cause a serious incident. The EMT's paramount concern should be the safe operation of the ambulance, without which the EMT cannot perform the job.

Although textbooks can contribute to an individual's bank of knowledge and EMTs can quickly develop skills to perform lifesaving tasks, attitudes cannot be altered as readily. EMTs should carefully assess their driving attitude before each shift and examine any personal and job-related stresses before accepting the responsibility of operating an ambulance. EMTs also have the responsibility to monitor the driving behaviors of their partners and report unsafe vehicle operation.

Control Tasks. Control of a vehicle can be divided into directional control and speed control.

**Directional Control.** Directional control depends on many factors, including the mechanical condition of the vehicle, road conditions, and the physical condition of the driver. One of the simplest but most important factors is the driver's hand position. Emergency vehicle operators should drive with two hands on the wheel whenever possible. Secondary tasks, such as radio and siren operation, should be delegated whenever possible to a second EMT so that the operator can focus full attention on the driving task. The recommended hand positions are at the 9-o'clock and 3-o'clock positions, which allow the optimal position for evasive maneuvers (**Figure 26-8**). The driver should turn the steering wheel with the hand-over-hand technique, which has proved to be a safe method (**Figure 26-9**). In another steering wheel technique, called "shuffling," the hands slide from one position to the next as the driver turns the steering wheel. With this technique, the hands never leave the wheel.

Emergency vehicle operators should not vary their driving habits when they enter their own vehicles because these

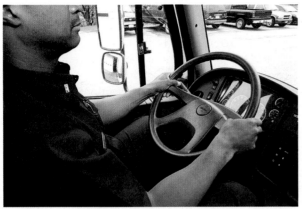

Figure 26-8 The 9-o'clock and 3-o'clock positions ensure maximum control and maneuverability.

	Table 26-2 Stopping Distances of a Light-Axle Truck		
Speed (mph)	Driver Reaction Distance (feet)	Vehicle Braking Distance (feet)	Total Stopping Distance (feet)
10	11	7	18
15	17	7	34
20	22	30	52
25	28	46	74
30	33	67	100
35	39	92	126
40	44	125	169
45	50	165	215
50	55	225	280
55	61	275	336
60	66	360	426

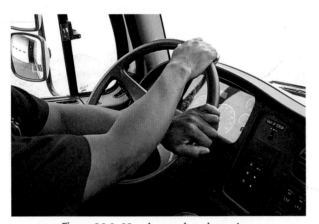

Figure 26-9 Hand-over-hand turning.

procedures are applicable to all motor vehicles and are reinforced by constant practice. You should remember that you cannot drive an ambulance like a car. The ambulance is a light truck that weighs approximately 10,000 pounds, and it cannot stop as fast as a car (**Table 26-2**).

Speed Control. Speed control depends on many of the same factors as directional control, and a loss of control in either case can be serious. Again, modern ambulances weigh up to four times more than the standard passenger vehicle and therefore have different handling characteristics. EMTs quickly learn that ambulances have substantially longer stopping distances than their own vehicles, and the additional weight, combined with improper braking technique, can cause an uncontrollable skid and loss of control. A survey of fully equipped type III ambulances found that the average vehicle weighs 10,450 pounds without the patient or crew inside. Many EMS services routine overload their ambulances. When the gross vehicle weight is exceeded, the handling and braking of the vehicle are affected.

Seat Belts. One of the simplest devices that can help maintain control of any vehicle is an ordinary seat belt. There are no valid excuses for not wearing a seat belt. Not only does a seat belt keep vehicle operators inside the vehicle in the event of a collision, but it also keeps them in position behind the controls of the vehicle. Most vehicles involved in motor vehicle crashes

actually have two collisions: the initial impact and a second crash if the driver is unable to control the vehicle after the initial impact. The second impact is frequently more severe than the first because contact is often made with a fixed object, such as a parked vehicle or a utility pole.

The theory that an occupant can be "thrown clear" of the crash has a very low probability. In most circumstances, individuals who are ejected from a moving vehicle, even at low rates of speed, sustain serious injuries. Being thrown from a vehicle increases the chance of death by a multiple of 25. Such individuals are frequently struck by other vehicles and are occasionally even run over by their own vehicle.

Questions are routinely voiced about seat belts: "What happens if I'm in a head-on collision and both my arms are broken and the car is on fire? How can I get out if my seat belt is on?"

In all probability, if the collision was severe enough to break both arms while you were wearing your seat belt, you would have been even more seriously injured or killed had the seat belt not been fastened. Statistically, 1 in 200 people involved in collisions while correctly wearing seat belts is injured by the restraints. However, these injuries are much less severe than those sustained by unrestrained occupants. In addition, less than 0.5% of motor vehicle crashes involve fires.

A person might comment, "If I see a collision about to happen, I can brace myself against the dashboard." A passenger bracing against the dashboard can be compared to a sprinter running at full speed: 15 miles per hour (mph). If the sprinter were to run into a wall at that speed with the arms extended, he or she would sustain serious injury. If the running speed were accelerated to 30 mph, the physical insult would be four times as great.

All vehicle occupants, including patients and those escorting patients in the ambulance, should wear seat belts. EMTs can be held responsible for any injuries to unrestrained passengers who are in the ambulance while a patient is being transported to the hospital. The seat belt should be worn snugly across the pelvic girdle, not across the lower abdomen, which is highly susceptible to blunt trauma in deceleration incidents (**Figure 26-10**).

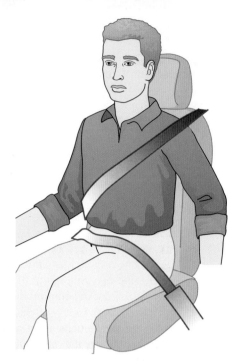

Figure 26-10 Proper position of seat belts.

Small children should be restrained in approved child seats because unrestrained children are frequently ejected from vehicles during a collision. Motor vehicle crashes are a leading cause of death in young children.

If you are still not convinced that safety belts save lives, ask any EMT how often he or she has unbuckled a dead person.

Motor Vehicle Laws. The wording of vehicle and traffic laws regarding emergency vehicle operation differs slightly from state to state, but the content is generally consistent. Emergency vehicle operators should become familiar with the specific regulations in their community regarding emergency vehicles before operating an ambulance.

Ambulances are considered emergency vehicles only while they are engaged in emergency activities. A *true emergency* is defined as any situation involving a high probability of death or serious injury to an individual or group of individuals or a significant loss of property, when the action of an emergency service may reduce the severity of the situation. Such a definition does not include returning from service to an emergency.

Specific Exemptions. The driver of an authorized emergency vehicle, when involved in an emergency operation, may exercise the following privileges:

1. The driver may proceed past a steady red signal, a flashing red signal, or a stop sign, but only after slowing down as necessary for safe operation. Some states require ambulances come to a complete stop.
2. The driver may exceed the maximum speed limit as long as he or she does not endanger life or property. Many states regulate the allowable speed above the posted limit, typically no more that 10 mph over the limit.
3. The driver may disregard regulations governing the direction of movement or turning in specified directions.

4. These exemptions apply only when the authorized emergency vehicle uses an audible warning device and displays appropriate red warning lamps.
5. Specific exemptions do not relieve the driver from the duty to drive with **due regard** for the safety of all persons. The exemptions do not protect the driver from the consequences of reckless disregard for the safety of others.

Although certain privileges are granted to an emergency vehicle operator, the driver is responsible for the outcome if an incident occurs while exercising any one of these privileges.

Drivers of emergency vehicles are actually held to a higher standard than the average driver. For example, an ambulance with lights and siren on, en route to a cardiac call, drives up a narrow one-way street against the flow of traffic. A car pulling out of a parking space strikes the ambulance head-on, causing considerable damage to both vehicles. Despite that the ambulance operator used all warning devices, because the ambulance driver was proceeding against traffic on a one-way street, he or she is responsible for the incident.

What does "due regard" in the above privilege mean, and how does it affect the driver of an ambulance? Due regard is based on the particular circumstances. In judging due regard, you should use the following criterion: Was there enough notice of approach to allow other motorists and pedestrians to clear a path and protect themselves? If you do not give notice of the ambulance's approach until a collision is inevitable, you have probably not satisfied the principle of due regard for the safety of others.

In determining whether an ambulance was exercising due regard in the use of signaling equipment, for example, the courts consider at least the following points:
- Was it reasonably necessary to use the signaling equipment under all the circumstances?
- Was the signaling equipment actually used?
- Was the signal given audible and/or visible to the motorists and pedestrians?
- Would a reasonably careful person performing similar duties under the same circumstances act in the same manner?

Ambulance personnel should respond to all calls in the same manner, keeping in mind that the general public is usually unaware of the fine points of medicine. A typical "seizure" call may in fact be the result of a serious head trauma, and the "sick" call may be cardiac arrest. Only after you have arrived on the scene and assessed the patient can you determine the severity of the call. How you return to the hospital can be adjusted according to the known condition of the patient. Rapid transportation of serious multitrauma and cardiac patients is frequently contraindicated because a high-speed ambulance ride could worsen their condition or hinder treatment. You should balance speed of transport by the need to perform procedures en route (e.g., maintain an airway, positive-pressure ventilation, CPR).

Emergency Lights. Most state traffic laws mandate the use of emergency lights and a siren when an operator is exercising emergency vehicle privileges. However, these warning devices are simply that: warning devices. They do not automatically grant right of way; they can only *request* it. Once again, use of lights and a siren does not relieve the emergency vehicle operator of liability in the event of an accident.

Emergency warning lights have been shown to be almost in-effective during periods of low light, such as at dawn and at dusk. A complete spectrum of warning lamps would be required to deal with all light and weather conditions. Each state mandates different colors for various types of emergency vehicles; red and white warning lamps are the most common. Rear-facing red lamps easily blend in with a field of tail and brake lights, reducing their effectiveness. Some people are color blind to red and are not warned by the lights. Therefore, amber and blue rear-facing warning lamps are preferred. The most effective warning lamps are mounted at the eye level of other drivers. These are the vehicle headlights. White lights contain all the colors of the light spectrum, making them most noticeable in all conditions.

As a note of caution, four-way hazard lights should not be used while operating a moving vehicle. They negate the turn signals and the brake lights and therefore create a hazard to other motorists, who cannot anticipate the actions of the ambulance. Flashing lights on the rear of an ambulance should flash simultaneously rather than one at a time. This helps the oncoming driver recognize the size of the ambulance, interpret the signal, and react properly.

Emergency Siren. The emergency vehicle siren is emitted in a cone of sound transmitted ahead of the vehicle. Its effectiveness can be reduced by a number of factors, such as reverberation, absorption, reflection, background noise, and a phenomenon called "vehicle insertion," in which the ambulance actually projects itself into its own siren cone the faster it goes, thereby limiting its advance warning. At approximately 60 mph (88 feet/second), the siren barely precedes the speeding ambulance, so vehicles ahead of it cannot respond to its warning. Studies have shown the distance for getting the attention of a motorist traveling at 60 mph is within 5 feet of the ambulance's bumper.

People respond to a warning sound in a four-step process. First, we detect the signal with our personal sensory system. We all are bombarded with so much auditory stimulation that we tend to filter out the noise and recognize only signals that we are listening for or that are unusual and well above the background threshold level.

Next, we notice the signal because it attracts our attention. Unfortunately, ambient street noise, stereo systems, and air conditioning and heating fans can all cause high sound levels within the vehicle. The combination of all this noise can easily mask even the most intense exterior sounds, such as those of a siren.

Third, we interpret the sound by attaching a purposeful meaning to it. Overuse or abuse of the use of the siren may have desensitized the public; many people frequently do not even turn their heads when they hear a siren. Couple this fact with frequent sounding of vehicle theft alarms, and it becomes evident that people often do not connect the sound of a siren with an emergency.

Last, we react, which is the desired response. Drivers who do not interpret the siren until the last minute often respond unpredictably. When a person is frightened by the siren, this "fight or flight" situation produces a snap reaction that does not always include ample time for logical decision making.

Sometimes even the best emergency warning device proves to be inadequate for the task of warning drivers in time for them to take evasive action. A DOT study found that only 26% of the occupants of a closed vehicle with the windows rolled up could tell the direction from which a siren sound was coming.

The siren physically affects ambulance operators and their abilities as drivers. A normally safe driver can feel the effects of the siren as soon as it is switched on. The siren's wail causes an immediate release of epinephrine into the driver's system. As a consequence, the pulse quickens, the vision narrows, the palms become sweaty, and the muscles tense. The driver's right foot presses down on the accelerator, and the ambulance picks up speed without any conscious effort by the driver. Because the vision is narrowed, the driver is not as aware of cross traffic, pedestrians, or other distractions and may even unconsciously ignore traffic signals in the quest to reach the scene as quickly as possible.

Being aware of this phenomenon is not enough. The ambulance operator must make a conscious effort to overcome the effects of the epinephrine by letting up on the accelerator as soon as the siren is switched on. In addition, the driver must make an effort to check peripheral vision by changing the focus of vision regularly and increasing general awareness of the environment. The driver should alternate checking ahead with checking the scene from right and left, the gauges, and the grip on the steering wheel.

The siren noise level can also be dangerous to the EMT. The National Institute for Occupational Safety and Health (NIOSH) conducted an investigation of siren noises in ambulances in 1984. The staff evaluated the effect of siren speaker location on noise levels, monitoring sound levels in the following four locations:

1. Driver compartment/driver position
2. Patient compartment/patient position
3. 10 feet from the siren speakers
4. 100 feet from the siren speakers

Exposure to high levels of noise may cause temporary or permanent hearing loss. The extent of damage depends on the intensity of the noise and the duration of the exposure. Evidence indicates that protracted noise exposure above 90 decibels (dB) causes hearing loss in a portion of the exposed population. NIOSH recommends a lower limit standard of 85 dB. **Table 26-3** lists the recommended noise limits according to exposure time.

Table 26-3	Standard Permissible Noise Exposure
Exposures (hours/day)	**Noise Level (decibels)***
8	90
6	92
4	95
3	97
2	100
1-1½	102
1	105
½	110
¼	115

*NIOSH recommends 5 dB less per level.
From U.S. Department of Transportation: *Emergency vehicle operators student manual,* Washington, DC, 1978, Department of Transportation.

The study found that when siren speakers were located on the roof above the driver, the siren noise within the ambulance had an average intensity of 109 dB in the driver's position (**Figure 26-11**) and an average of 91 dB in the patient's position. Siren noise immediately in front of the ambulance created a hazard at 122 dB, exceeding the NIOSH ceiling level of 115 dB. Siren noise 100 feet downrange from the ambulance increased from 99 to 105 dB when siren speakers were located on the roof instead of on the grill. The study recommended minimizing noise exposure by locating siren speakers in the grill area and keeping the windows in the cab closed. Under these conditions, the noise decibel range is much healthier for the ambulance crew and patients.

The same factors affect the patient being transported. A surge of epinephrine caused by a frantic ambulance ride to the hospital has several potential effects on a cardiac patient. The increased heart rate would cause a compensatory increase in myocardial oxygen demand. With already reduced oxygen levels resulting from the ischemia, more heart muscle might infarct en route. This would affect the patient in the same way as jogging to the hospital.

Escort Vehicles

Generally, the use of **escort** vehicles is not a good idea and should be avoided whenever possible. Some drivers observing an emergency vehicle crossing an intersection may falsely believe that it is the sole emergency vehicle, and this may lead them to proceed through the intersection, only to collide with the second vehicle. The only circumstance in which an escort vehicle may be practical is when the ambulance driver is not familiar with the route to the receiving hospital. Extra caution must be taken at all intersections.

Principles of Effective Operation

Route Planning. Once the EMT is dispatched, the first step should be to plan the route to the call. The shortest route is not necessarily the quickest one. A number of factors influence response route planning, depending on the environment in which the EMT works. These include traffic congestion during peak hours, construction delays, nonsequential traffic lights, and weather conditions. An area map must be carried in the ambulance so that the EMT can plan routes in unfamiliar areas and select alternate routes when detours are dictated by conditions. Effective preselection of the route allows the EMT to devote full attention to the driving task. During response, assign personnel to specific duties so that care on the scene can be provided in a rapid and efficient manner.

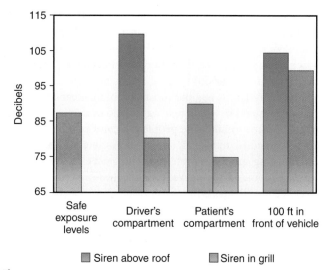

Figure 26-11 Siren decibels by location. _Modified from_ Ambulance accident prevention student workbook, _Albany, New York State Department of Health._

Natural Laws. In addition to local and state laws, other laws affect emergency vehicle operation. These are referred to as "natural laws," and they affect the two major control tasks of the emergency vehicle operator: speed control and directional control.

Gravity. Gravity is most evident when you are operating a high-top van ambulance. These vehicles have been modified by their manufacturers to include a heavy fiberglass roof that drastically changes the handling characteristics of the vehicle by raising its _center of gravity._ In contrast, consider a sports car with a much lower center of gravity (half the weight of the vehicle above and half the weight below this point). The sports car can turn a sharp corner at 50 mph. If the ambulance attempted to take the same sharp turn at the same speed, it would flip on its side because its higher center of gravity would pull it over.

During normal operation, the weight of the vehicle is distributed relatively evenly over all the wheels; during sudden braking, however, the weight of the vehicle suddenly shifts forward onto the front wheels, which makes steering more difficult and adds strain on the steering and front braking systems. With little weight on the rear wheels during this maneuver, the rear brakes are considerably less effective in stopping the vehicle and may lock up when increased pedal pressure is applied to stop the ambulance. New antilock braking systems may help considerably, but some ambulances have yet to be equipped with this system.

Centrifugal Force. Centrifugal force can be demonstrated by swinging a weight attached to a string over your head. If you let go of the string, the rock flies off in a straight line, not an arc. The force that pulls on a rock is the same as that exerted on a vehicle in a turn. Centrifugal force tends to pull a vehicle out of a curve and on a straight line to the arc. This force increases with the following factors:
- Weight of the vehicle
- Sharpness of the curve
- Speed of the vehicle
- Flatness of the "bank" (tilt of the road)

REAL_World_

In large cities and small towns, roadways and highways are often under construction. When a construction project begins, drivers often must use different routes to their destinations. This is true for EMTs driving ambulances as well. At the start of their shift, EMTs should check with their dispatch center or the police department to learn of road construction and detours. This can help keep response times short.

Modern road design compensates for centrifugal force by banking the curves in proportion to the sharpness of the curve and by adding preformed concrete barriers that redirect vehicles back onto the road before centrifugal force carries them into the opposite lanes or off the road.

Friction. Friction is required to control both the speed and the direction of a vehicle. It is important to distinguish between two types of friction: rolling friction and stopping friction.

- *Rolling friction.* Contact with the road is essential for steering the vehicle. Furthermore, the front wheels must be rolling to maintain directional control. If rolling friction is lost, such as when a patch of ice is hit, directional control is lost and *inertia* (the property of matter by which it remains at rest or in uniform motion in the same straight line unless acted on by some external force) and centrifugal force direct the movement of the vehicle. When a driver is "peeling rubber" (accelerating quickly from a stop), rolling friction is lost, and forward momentum is actually reduced.
- *Stopping friction.* Contact between the brake pads and the brake drums (or discs) slows the vehicle. At the road surface, the tires require friction with the pavement to both stop and steer the vehicle. The shortest stopping distance is achieved when the brakes do not "lock up." Locked brakes cause the tires to skid. This sudden increase in friction is converted to heat, which melts the tire rubber. Molten rubber forms beads between the tire and the pavement that actually reduce friction, thereby increasing the stopping distance.

Each tire has only 20 square inches of contact with the road, about the same as the surface area of your hand. There are a number of factors that can negatively affect friction even further: adverse weather conditions, poor road surface, and items on the road surface such as oil, gravel, and wet leaves. Poor tire condition further reduces the operator's ability to maintain control of the vehicle. The tread and air pressure of the tires are critical to vehicle performance and handling, especially for emergency vehicles, which are exposed to higher speeds and rougher handling compared with passenger vehicles.

Operation. One of the major advantages of ambulances is that the driver is positioned high and has a view of the road above other vehicles and well ahead of his or her position in traffic. You can use this advantage to avoid collisions. First, define the safest path well ahead of the ambulance. Certain lanes may be bunched tightly together and therefore may necessitate sudden stops and lane changes. Second, keep safe distances from the vehicle ahead, allowing time to scan the entire traffic situation, and keep your eyes moving, regularly checking the rear-view and side-view mirrors, the gauges, and your grip on the steering wheel.

Make sure other drivers see you. This is especially important at intersections. By having eye contact with other drivers, you ensure that they are aware of you. Make sure that they acknowledge you before you proceed into an intersection.

Leave yourself an "out." This is probably the most important concept in collision avoidance. When using the techniques just outlined, you must expect the unexpected and leave yourself an emergency exit route in case of a sudden change in the traffic situation ahead. Do not wait for a crisis to occur before you plan

---

Box 26-1	Guidelines for Safe Driving

1. Drive with your headlights on all the time. This is helpful in alerting other drivers to see you and stay away.
2. Keep a 4-second following distance whenever driving an ambulance. Remember the stopping distance is much greater than that of a car, which uses the 2-second rule.
3. Make gradual changes in acceleration.
4. Look far ahead so you can recognize the hazards, understand the defense maneuvers you may have to make, and act correctly in time.
5. Apply the brakes smoothly.
6. When stopping in traffic, always be able to see the rear tire of the vehicle in front of you.
7. Maintain adequate cushions of space to the side and rear.
8. Make gradual lane changes.
9. Always use proper signaling for turns and exits.
10. Exercise proper eye movement and use of mirrors.
11. Exercise sensible speed control, reducing speed in the following situations:
    - Decreased visibility or obstructed view
    - Reduced road grip
    - Sharp changes in direction
12. Always be prepared to brake when approaching all intersections and potential hazards.

---

a potential exit. Whenever possible, leave a space to one side of the vehicle in case the space in front suddenly disappears.

Box 26-1 provides guidelines for safe driving.

Distance. All vehicle operators are responsible for maintaining a clear following distance behind the vehicle in front of them. If you fail to do so and collide with the rear of the vehicle in front of you, you are held completely responsible, regardless of road, vehicle, or weather conditions. If a vehicle cuts in front of the ambulance and stops, the experienced emergency vehicle operator should have a preplanned escape route. In addition, the driver should keep a safe following distance by using the "4-second rule." A 4-second distance is maintained by observing the vehicle in front of you passing a stationary object (e.g., light pole, overpass, even a shadow). If your vehicle passes the same object in 4 seconds or more, you are traveling at a safe distance. If you count less than 4 seconds, you must reduce your speed until that 4-second distance is obtained. This system works at all speeds and in all types of vehicles on a dry road surface. It must be modified in rainy, snowy, or icy conditions. In rainy weather, double the time to 8 seconds. On icy or snowy roads, triple the time to 12 seconds. **Figure 26-12** illustrates braking distances and reaction time.

Speed. Speed is the greatest contributing factor to motor vehicle crashes. Fewer than 1% of people involved in crashes at speeds of 70 mph survive. On a 2-mile ambulance run, the difference in arrival time between averaging 30 mph and 60 mph is only 2 minutes. Traveling at 60 mph through most streets, except major interstate highways, is unsafe and imprudent. Operating an ambulance at excessive speeds constitutes irresponsible, dangerous driving. The risks far outweigh the potential benefits. Conditions that should decrease your speed include

Ambulance minimum stopping distance 100 feet

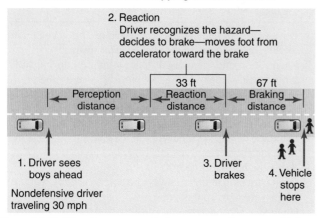

Figure 26-12 The distance needed to react and stop a vehicle when a nondefensive driver is faced with a hazard. *Modified from* Ambulance accident prevention student workbook, *Albany, New York State Department of Health.*

adverse weather conditions, a poor road surface, high-density urban traffic areas, and school zones.

Intersections. Studies have shown that 70% of emergency vehicle crashes occur at intersections, where high-speed vehicles come together at right angles, controlled only by traffic signs or signals. Many EMTs believe that lights and a siren legally grant them the right of way. In fact, these warning devices are simply accessories to warn other motorists of your approach. Each driver establishes right of way on an individual basis as he or she reacts to the approaching emergency vehicle. Intersection crashes most often occur when emergency vehicle operators assume that they have the right of way or when they misjudge the speed of their own or other vehicles. Being aware of this statistic is not enough. You must always stop at each intersection when approaching a red light or stop sign and must ensure it is safe to proceed before driving on. Realize that other motorists may try to beat changing traffic signals and that pedestrians frequently try to race across an intersection before the arrival of your vehicle.

Even green lights are unsafe for emergency vehicles. Approaching cars frequently turn left in front of the ambulance, and most motorists take full advantage of right-on-red laws. Impatient drivers may run red lights altogether. Pedestrians are also potential victims. They often seem to be "color blind," crossing regardless of the traffic signals.

What about other emergency vehicles? Depending on the type of call, other agencies (police, fire, rescue, and specialized units) may be responding to your (or a different) call from other directions. Be attentive; listen for other sirens from different directions. In many situations, responding units can talk to each other over the radio to announce their location.

If you are involved in a crash with an emergency vehicle, you may be held personally liable for damages incurred as a result of your actions. Liability may be limited to civil penalties (financial reimbursement for damages) or may involve criminal charges (e.g., manslaughter, driving while impaired).

Case in Point

During the trial of an ambulance driver in Binghamton, NY, the judge told the defendant, "Everybody keeps calling this a tragic accident; it was tragic, but I don't think it was an accident at all. Somebody propelled a 10,000-pound ambulance through an intersection at a high rate of speed against a light; that's not an accident." The defendant was convicted of a misdemeanor assault for running a red light and severely injuring an 18-year-old woman. The woman had a broken neck and was in a coma for 5 weeks, and the driver of the ambulance was sentenced to 4½ months in jail and 3 years' probation.

Backing. A certain percentage of ambulance crashes occur when the driver is backing up. Fixed objects, such as parked vehicles and emergency room canopies, are usually hit. Because these objects do not respond to back-up alarms, you must check behind the ambulance before backing up. Whenever possible, if you are backing and turning, turn from the driver's side and stay close to the driver's side of the vehicle because you can always see better and have better control of this side of the vehicle. If a police officer, firefighter, or second EMT is available, this person may assist as a spotter in this maneuver (**Figure 26-13**).

The following list summarizes some common elements of crashes that were derived from a 4-year study by a major urban EMS system:

- 70% occurred in daylight
- 70% occurred in an intersection
- 56% occurred on a clear day
- 63% occurred on dry roads
- 53% occurred at traffic signal devices

Parking at the Scene. Be certain to park the ambulance appropriately at the scene. If toxic gases, liquids, or other hazards are suspected, you should park 100 feet uphill and upwind. In general, you should park in front of or beyond the wreckage to ensure safe passage of the patient from the scene to the vehicle. Turn the front wheels toward the curb in case the ambulance is struck from behind, and be sure to set the parking brake. Engage the appropriate warning lights; however, turn headlights off when the ambulance is parked unless there is a need to illuminate the scene. Headlights can blind oncoming drivers. You should park in a location that allows for an easy exit from the scene.

Arrival at the Scene

At every phase of the call (response, arrival at scene, departure from scene, arrival at hospital, departure from hospital, and availability), it is important to notify dispatch to ensure the appropriate coordination of resources and documentation of the call. On arrival at the scene, your first concern is safety. You should take precautions, including body substance isolation precautions, and conduct your scene size-up. Park the ambulance appropriately as previously described, and quickly determine whether hazards are present that would preclude access to the scene or require immediate evacuation of the patient.

You should first determine the mechanism of injury. If it is a mass casualty incident, determine the number of patients and call for additional help. Begin patient triage by rapidly tagging or applying identifying tape to patients according to priority status. Be sure to use spinal immobilization as needed.

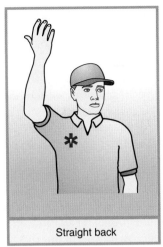
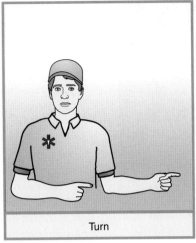
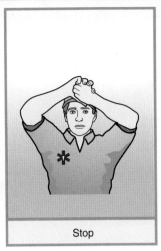

| Straight back | Turn | Stop |

Figure 26-13 Proper hand signals for directing a vehicle. *Modified from* Ambulance accident prevention student workbook, *Albany, New York State Department of Health.*

In every call, it is important to be organized and provide rapid and efficient assessment and treatment while keeping early transport in mind. EMS providers are always at risk of spending too much time at the scene. Remember, early access to definitive care is an essential part of prehospital care.

Transfer of Patient to the Ambulance

The patient should be rapidly prepared for transfer to the ambulance. Critical interventions should be completed, dressings and splints checked, and the patient covered according to the environmental conditions. Securely attach patients to the transfer device. Choose the device according to the needed patient position, immobilization, and the type of terrain. Chapter 5 describes the specifics of lifting and carrying patients.

En Route to the Receiving Facility

Once the patient is properly secured in the ambulance, you should notify the dispatcher of your response to the receiving hospital or trauma center. Ongoing assessment, including vital signs, is performed at appropriate intervals during transport. When appropriate, notify the receiving hospital as soon as possible so that the staff has adequate time to prepare for your arrival. Take care to deal with the emotional concerns of the patient, and reassure the patient during your treatment. When transporting patients who have a less serious injury, you may complete the prehospital care report en route to the hospital.

At the Receiving Facility

Again, notify the dispatcher on arrival at the hospital. The proper transfer of the patient to the emergency department staff should include a complete but concise patient history. It is important to consider information obtained at the scene that otherwise may not be known (e.g., seizures, mechanism of injury). Complete the prehospital care report and leave a copy for the patient's record (see Chapter 9).

Back in Service and After the Call

Once the transfer of your patient to hospital staff has been accomplished, you need to prepare for the next call. Clean and disinfect the ambulance and equipment as needed, restock supplies, and refuel the unit. File reports, and notify the dispatcher as soon as your unit is available.

Aeromedical Considerations

Helicopters have been used extensively for medical evacuation since the Korean War. Modern helicopters often are equipped with ALS capabilities and highly trained crews (**Figure 26-14**). The primary benefit of helicopter transport is the ability to decrease time from injury (or illness) to arrival at the hospital and definitive care. Helicopters have the distinct advantage of being able to travel at greater speeds and in a relatively straight line from the scene to the receiving hospital. Often the EMS providers are encouraged to make the decision for helicopter transport. This decision may be made based on your own judgment or in conjunction with medical direction or the EMS communications center. If you intend to call for helicopter transport, you should decide early in the care of the patient to ensure a timely arrival.

Decision to Call

The decision to call for aeromedical services is often the most critical step associated with the use of a helicopter. EMS providers must weigh several factors when initiating the call for help, including the proximity to the hospital, nature of the terrain, location of the patient, estimated extrication time, and clinical status of the patient. Your decision should ultimately be based on local protocols that are likely to address when, why, and how to call for a medical helicopter.

Again, the most common reason for selecting helicopter transport is the reduction of time from incident to arrival at the hospital. This is particularly important for rural and suburban EMS systems, where travel time from the scene to the hospital may exceed the "golden hour" (defined as 1 hour from the time of injury to arrival at definitive care). As a rule, if a helicopter transport does not decrease the arrival time to the hospital by at least 10 minutes, ground transportation may be the best strategy.

When calculating time, many issues should be considered. How long will ground transport take? What will be the expected

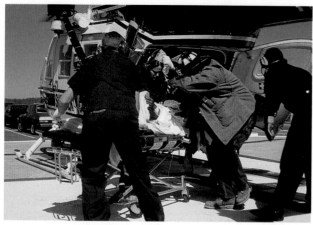

Figure 26-14 Helicopters can provide rapid transport to the hospital for critical patients.

time of arrival of the helicopter? How long will it take to extricate the patient? Can the helicopter land at the site of the incident, or will the patient have to be transported to another location for transfer to the helicopter? Will weather conditions allow for helicopter response and transport?

The estimate of helicopter arrival can be provided by the flight crew and includes engine warm-up time (if the helicopter is not in flight) and travel time to the scene. The pilot can also provide an estimate of flight time from the scene to the hospital.

The location of the patient may also establish the need to use a helicopter for evacuation and transport. For example, patients in remote locations that are not accessible by ground transport, such as islands, deep woods, and mountains, may be good candidates for aeromedical evacuation. Helicopters may also provide resources that are not otherwise available on the scene. For example, a trapped victim of a car crash may require ALS measures.

Locating and Preparing the Landing Zone

A landing zone should be selected and prepared before arrival of the helicopter. EMS systems with helicopter capability usually have specific protocols about landing area requirements and coordination with ground units and helicopters. These should be strictly followed because of the potential for danger. Many helicopters have their own crews who pick up and attend to patients from the scene.

General considerations for selecting a landing zone include the following:

1. The zone should ideally be an area larger than 100 × 100 feet to allow for a clear approach and departure route for the helicopter.
2. The area should be on relatively flat ground. Ideally, the slope of the ground should be no greater than 10 degrees because the rotor may come in contact with the ground on a more acute angle.
3. The zone should be clear of debris, such as trash, rocks, and large quantities of sand, which can become small missiles when exposed to the force of "rotor wash" or can blur the pilot's vision.

4. No major vertical structures, such as telephone poles, towers, high grasses, and tall trees, should be close to the landing zone. The approach to the landing zone should also be free of obstacles such as power and telephone wires that may be invisible to the pilot or crew from the air.
5. The area should be as close as possible to the scene to avoid the need for ambulance transport.

When possible, a designated individual with the greatest experience in helicopter operations should be assigned the task of selecting and managing the landing zone. This person can communicate with the helicopter crew and provide essential information during initial contact and on arrival at the scene. This information includes wind direction, major landmarks in proximity of the landing zone, the basic description of the terrain and surrounding area, suggested direction of approach, the status of the patient, and any other important data. The landing zone should be relatively close to the patient. However, if the area is not suitable for helicopter landing, the closest appropriate area can be selected, and the patient can be transported by ambulance. Moving the patient to another area is better than selecting an area that may be hazardous to flight operations. When possible, this type of decision is best made in conjunction with the flight crew, who are familiar with the benefits and limitations of a particular landing zone.

To prepare the landing zone for arrival, carefully secure loose gear and remove all unnecessary gear from the area. Vehicles should be positioned at least 30 feet from the landing zone, and bystanders should be positioned at least 100 feet away. Flash cameras should not be used, and flashlights should never be pointed in the direction of the helicopter because the light may temporarily blind the flight crew. Smoking should be strictly prohibited in the vicinity of the landing zone. Rescuers should wear eye protection to prevent eye injuries from flying debris. The landing zone can be marked with objects that are visible based on light conditions. Objects that may be affected by rotor wash should not be used. At night, colored lights can mark the corners of the landing zone. Ideally, white lights should not be used because they impair the crew's vision. Lights should not face the front-approach end of the landing zone because they will be projected into the pilot's eyes.

As the helicopter approaches, the pilot can be directed to the scene by radio. When directing a pilot to the scene, you can use the clock method for communicating location, keeping in mind that the pilot is facing 12 o'clock. When appropriate, you should communicate key landmarks and potential obstacles such as fences and telephone poles. Hand signals can be used to help guide the helicopter into the landing zone (**Figure 26-15**).

Safety around the Helicopter

Direct interface with helicopters can be very dangerous, particularly when providers are not acquainted with basic safety procedures. Helicopter rotor wash can spray bystanders with debris, resulting in serious soft tissue injuries. Bystanders also run the risk of being struck by a rotor, particularly the tail rotor because it is close to the ground. A rotating tail rotor can be almost invisible.

The first and most important consideration around a helicopter is *not to approach from the rear* (**Figure 26-16**). You should always approach from the front of the helicopter in clear view of the crew. After the helicopter has landed, you should make eye contact with the flight crew and wait for their signal before approaching the helicopter. If the helicopter is on a slope, never approach from the uphill side, where the main rotor is closer to the ground. Once again, never approach near the tail rotor. Often, flight crews are placed at the rear of the ship to prevent this type of injury, particularly with a rear-loading helicopter.

When approaching the helicopter, you should assume a crouching position to further minimize the possibility of injury because rotors can dip lower in response to the wind. If advanced life support is provided, you should not carry intravenous lines or other equipment above your head while in proximity of the helicopter. Stretchers should be carried waist high.

Usually the flight crew will come to your location and evaluate the patient before loading him or her into the helicopter.

Some factors may prevent transport of the patient in the helicopter. For example, patients who are thrashing about because of seizures or altered mental status may represent a serious danger to the crew. This is especially true for a small helicopter, where the patient's feet are close to the pilot. You should prepare a concise history for the aeromedical crew as you would for arrival at the hospital. If possible, provide a copy of the prehospital care report.

Hospitals, public agencies, and other entities that operate medical helicopters often conduct "hands-on" safety classes for emergency personnel. This training provides the opportunity to learn and practice techniques for safely approaching and loading a patient into the helicopter during "cold loads" (engine off, rotors not moving) and "hot loads" (engine on, rotors in motion). Participation in this training is strongly encouraged for EMTs working in a system where they may use aeromedical transport services.

Scenario Follow-up

On arrival at the scene, you notify the dispatcher and carry the appropriate equipment to the patient's side, including an airway kit, automated external defibrillator (AED), and cardiac board. After determining that the scene is safe, you perform a rapid assessment on the patient, who is apneic and pulseless. You apply the AED, which analyzes the patient's heart rhythm and confirms that "shock is advised." You call "clear" and defibrillate the patient. You perform 2 minutes of CPR, and the patient begins to move and breathe spontaneously.

You monitor the patient's airway and provide appropriate oxygen therapy as your partner prepares the patient for transport. During transport, your partner contacts both dispatch and the receiving hospital and provides information concerning the patient's status and estimated time of arrival to the emergency department.

On arrival at the hospital, your partner notifies the dispatcher, and both you and your partner transfer the patient into the emergency department. You provide a concise history to the physician and nurse and give them a copy of the prehospital care report. You and your partner then clean and disinfect the ambulance and equipment. You then inform the dispatcher of your availability to respond to another call.

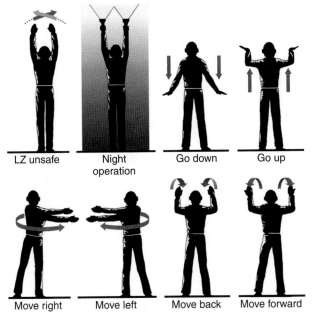

Figure 26-15 Landing zone hand signals. *From Sanders M:* Mosby's paramedic textbook, *ed 3, St Louis, 2006, Mosby-Elsevier.*

LZ unsafe   Night operation   Go down   Go up

Move right   Move left   Move back   Move forward

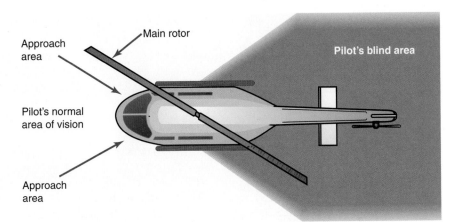

Figure 26-16 Be aware of how you should approach a helicopter. *Redrawn from* Emergency services operation manual, *New York City.*

Summary

The EMT relies on various types of equipment to respond, communicate, provide safety, perform patient assessment, and administer patient care. During the preparation (prerun) phase of a call, the EMT must check essential equipment to ensure that it is available and operational. This involves daily inspection and replacement and cleaning as needed.

Operating an emergency vehicle involves assuming several risks not normally incurred while driving a passenger car or truck. This may involve exceeding posted speed limits, traveling the wrong way down one-way streets, or passing red lights. You should minimize these risks as much as possible, thereby reducing the possibility of having a collision. When emergency vehicle exemptions are used, you must show due regard for safety at all times. The Case in Point described in this chapter shows how an ambulance operator who failed to show due regard for safety and his reckless operation were major contributors to the deaths of five people.

A professional attitude behind the wheel should be maintained at all times. Even in the busiest EMS systems, the EMT spends more time driving than performing patient care. Do not let the actions of other drivers affect your abilities as an emergency vehicle operator or as an EMT. The results can be disastrous.

In the dispatch phase, an EMT must use communication equipment to ascertain the dispatch data. En route to the call, the EMT must rely on the vehicle to provide a safe and reliable ride. This requires careful inspection and maintenance on a daily basis. At the scene, use protective clothing and other equipment to ensure the safety of EMTs and patients.

Finally, during transport to the hospital, at the hospital, and en route to the station, use equipment to provide continued assessment, treatment, and effective communication. After each call (during the postrun phase), replace needed supplies and ensure that the unit is ready for the next call.

The Bottom Line

Learning Checklist

✓ Phases of an ambulance call include preparation for a call, dispatch, en route to the call, arrival at the scene, transfer of the patient to the ambulance, en route to the receiving facility, at the receiving facility, and back in service and after the run.

✓ Before the first call, the EMT must check the vehicle and equipment with the appropriate checklist to ensure readiness for communication, transport, and patient assessment and care.

✓ Three basic types of ambulances are currently used in EMS systems: type I (truck chassis and modular box passenger compartment), type II (modified van), and type III (van chassis and modular box passenger compartment).

✓ Safe emergency vehicle operation can be thought of as an "arch" that is constructed of many components, including physical and mental abilities, knowledge of traffic laws, and driver attitude.

✓ One of the simplest devices that can help maintain control of any vehicle is the seat belt. There are no valid excuses for not wearing a seat belt.

✓ Most state traffic laws mandate the use of emergency lights and a siren when an operator is exercising emergency vehicle "privileges."

✓ Sirens may cause a fight-or-flight response for the operator of the emergency vehicle, the patient being transported, and the drivers of other vehicles. The emergency vehicle operator must make a conscious effort to overcome the effects of the siren on his or her mental attitude and related behavior.

✓ The only circumstance in which an escort vehicle may be practical is when the ambulance driver is not familiar with the route to the receiving facility. Extra caution must be taken at all intersections.

✓ A number of factors influence response route planning, including traffic congestion during peak hours, construction delays, nonsequential traffic lights, and weather conditions.

✓ The 4-second rule (counting seconds while passing a fixed object) helps establish a safe distance between the emergency vehicle and the vehicle directly in front.

✓ The most common location for emergency vehicle accidents is at intersections. You should come to a complete stop when approaching an intersection with a red light or stop sign before proceeding.

✓ If toxic gases, liquids, or other hazards are expected or observed at an emergency scene, park 100 feet uphill and upwind.

✓ When appropriate, notify the receiving facility so that the staff can prepare for your arrival.

✓ The proper transfer of the patient to the emergency department staff should include a complete but concise patient history.

Key Terms

Arch of driver safety Components that ensure safe operation of an emergency vehicle, including the driver's physical and mental abilities, knowledge of traffic laws, and attitude.

Central access dispatch Form of dispatch that coordinates numerous EMS units in a given region.

Due regard Attention that must be given to the safety of the public while driving an emergency vehicle.

Emergency medical dispatch (EMD) Nationally recognized method for training dispatchers in the systematic questioning of people calling 9-1-1 and, when necessary, providing telephone-directed instructions.

Enhanced 9-1-1 Computerized dispatch system that automatically identifies a caller's location when the 9-1-1 system is accessed and allows for computer documentation of special information about patients based on their telephone number.

Escort Use of police vehicles to direct the movements of an ambulance from the scene of an emergency to the receiving facility.

Type I ambulance Ambulance designed with a modular box patient compartment mounted on a truck-style chassis.

Type II ambulance Van-style ambulance.

Type III ambulance Ambulance designed with a modular box patient compartment mounted on a van-style chassis.

Review Questions

1. Exemptions of traffic regulations provided by law for persons driving emergency vehicles are best described as:
   a. Necessary evils
   b. Privileges
   c. Protection from crashes
   d. Legal protections

2. A passenger in the back seat is in an accident while wearing a lap belt and sustains severe injuries to the abdominal cavity and lower spine. Which "correct" lap belt position would have reduced the risk of these injuries?
   a. Umbilicus
   b. Thigh
   c. Pelvic girdle
   d. Upper thigh

3. The chances of being severely injured by a seat belt are approximately 1 in _____ crashes.
   a. 5
   b. 10
   c. 50
   d. 200

4. Your partner is driving recklessly through an intersection. He says he is allowed by law to drive this way because he is using the ambulance's lights and sirens. As an EMT, how would you characterize the use of emergency lights and sirens in this situation to your partner?
   a. Necessary to relieve the operator of liability in case of a crash
   b. Most effective in low-light situations, such as at dawn or dusk
   c. Do not relieve the operator of liability in the event of a crash
   d. Most effective at high speeds

5. Four-way hazard lights:
   a. Should not be used in a moving vehicle.
   b. Should be turned off when the vehicle is parked.
   c. Are necessary in a moving ambulance.
   d. Are most effective in low-light situations.

6. You are traveling at 60 mph while using the ambulance's lights and siren. This is hazardous because the sound emitted from an ambulance siren:
   a. Moves more quickly through the air.
   b. Barely precedes the ambulance.
   c. Is louder on the sides of the vehicle.
   d. Will not be heard inside the ambulance.

7. An escort vehicle should be used only when:
   a. The ambulance is traveling at high speeds.
   b. The operator is unfamiliar with the route.
   c. Police are available.
   d. There is more than one ambulance.

8. Most emergency vehicle crashes occur:
   a. On highways
   b. At the scene of an emergency
   c. En route to an emergency
   d. At intersections

Questions 9-11. Match the descriptions in column B to the ambulance type in column A.

Column A
 9. Type I
10. Type II
11. Type III

Column B
a. Van-type ambulance
b. Modular patient compartment with van chassis
c. Modular patient compartment with truck chassis

12. If sterile supplies, such as bandages and dressings, become wet, they should be:
    a. Dried in an autoclave
    b. Air-dried
    c. Discarded
    d. Dried under ultraviolet light

For Further Review

In the Student Workbook

- Multiple-choice questions
- Matching questions
- Fill-in-the-blank questions
- Case scenario questions

On Evolve

- Chapter challenge
- Weblinks
- Lecture notes
- Exercises

Learning Objectives

Cognitive Objectives

- Discuss the medical and nonmedical equipment needed to respond to a call.
- List the phases of an ambulance call.
- Summarize the importance of preparing the unit for the next response.
- Describe the general provisions of state laws relating to the operation of the ambulance and privileges in the following categories: speed, warning lights, sirens, right of way, parking, and turning.
- List contributing factors to unsafe driving conditions.
- Describe the considerations that should be given to request for escorts, following an escort vehicle, and intersections.
- Discuss "due regard for safety of all others" while operating an emergency vehicle.
- State what information is essential to respond to a call.
- Discuss various situations that may affect response to a call.
- Identify what is essential for completion of a call.

Affective Objectives

- Explain the rationale for having the unit prepared to respond.

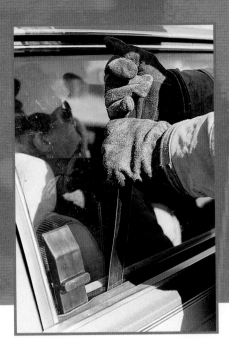

27 Gaining Access

CHAPTER OUTLINE

Response and Approach to the Scene

Gaining Access at the Scene

Scenario

Two emergency medical technicians (EMTs) respond to a motor vehicle crash. As they approach the scene, they review several variables. Is the scene safe? Are there hazards? Will assistance be needed? How many patients will there be? Are any of the patients trapped?

On their arrival at the scene, the EMTs find that the police have controlled traffic and that two vehicles are involved. One patient is pinned by the steering wheel in the first vehicle, and two patients are in the second vehicle. The arm of the driver of the second vehicle is trapped in the space between the seat and doorpost, and his feet are caught beneath the pedals. The head of the passenger in the second vehicle has struck the windshield.

The EMTs immediately call for rescue personnel to assist in gaining access and performing extrication and to begin triage and care of the patients.

Rescue and **extrication** is a specialized field in prehospital care. As an Emergency Medical Technician (EMT), however, you must be able to work closely with rescue teams to ensure safe access and removal of entrapped patients (**Figure 27-1**). Special situations in which patients may need rescue include motor vehicle crashes, heights (high-angle rescue), caves or tunnels (confined-space rescue), water (water rescue), and collapsed buildings. As an EMT, your primary role in these situations is to ensure the safety of you and your patient and to provide emergency medical care before, during, and after rescue operations. If you also have rescue responsibilities, you will participate in a related educational program to prepare for this role. Numerous programs are offered, including automobile extrication, high-angle rescue, low-angle rescue, water rescue, confined-space rescue, and other specialized areas.

LEARNING OBJECTIVES

- Describe the purpose of extrication.
- Discuss the role of the EMT in extrication.
- Identify what equipment for personal safety is required for the EMT.
- Define the fundamental components of extrication.
- State the steps to take to protect the patient during extrication.

Response and Approach to the Scene

The decisions you make while approaching a scene determine the effectiveness of the patient's rescue. As an EMT, you have the capability of making a rescue safe and efficient or creating a secondary disaster. For example, after the crash of a jet plane on Long Island, rescuers responded on a single road to the scene. The early-arriving rescuers left their vehicles in the middle of the road, blocking access and escape from the scene. Additional emergency vehicles made the same error. Eventually, the single access road was completely blocked, resulting in delays in removing patients from the crash.

When approaching the scene, stop (ideally 100 feet away, uphill, and upwind), look, and listen. Observe what is happening

(**Figure 27-2**). How many vehicles are involved? How many patients are present? What resources do you need? Are the resources with you or available to you in a timely manner?

When assessing a scene, perform a risk-benefit analysis. Determine whether a rescue attempt will pose an undue risk of injury to you or other rescuers. If the risk is greater than the benefit, take actions to reduce the risk. For example, if a vehicle is fully enveloped in flames on your arrival, you would not initially place your hands in the vehicle in an attempt to rescue the occupants; instead, you would attempt to extinguish the fire. Being capable of making risk-benefit analyses makes you an effective member of the rescue team.

When approaching the vehicle, you should perform a windshield survey (**Figure 27-3**). Are the patients moving? Are they conscious? Are they attempting to exit the vehicle?

During your approach to the vehicle, make a quick check for downed electrical wires in the immediate vicinity. If wires are down, do not touch anything, retreat to a position of safety, protect all bystanders by establishing a hazard zone, and advise the occupants of the vehicle not to attempt to exit. Contact

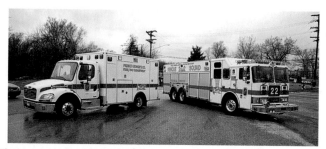

Figure 27-1 The EMS and rescue team must work cooperatively to achieve the best possible patient outcomes. The key to success is cooperation.

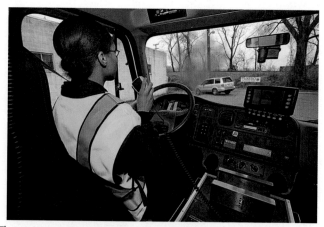

Figure 27-2 When approaching the scene, survey the area completely for hazards and indications of activity. Look for hazardous material (HAZMAT) placards, spillage, and fire. Check for patients who may have been ejected from the vehicle. Initially, survey the scene from a distance for your safety and for the safety of the patients. Decide which initial resources you need, and call for them.

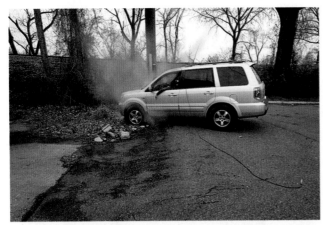

Figure 27-3 Look at the vehicle. Is this a high-velocity crash? Is there impact on the passenger area? Are the patients trapped? Some EMS systems take pictures of the vehicle so that the physician at the hospital can visualize the damage. Would that be useful here?

the appropriate support service (local utility) and ask that the power be shut off and the wires moved.

Evaluate the stability of the vehicle and determine whether it can be entered safely. Will the vehicle turn over? Is it on its side? Is it on its wheels? Is it secure? Does the vehicle rock? Could the movement of the vehicle or a rescue attempt injure the patient, because the vehicle still has the capability of moving? If this is the case, block the frame of the vehicle to prevent any movement and ensure stabilization. A vehicle resting on its side presents a significant hazard and should be stabilized before you gain access. Any crash vehicle, even if it is on its wheels, should be stabilized. It may be necessary only to chock (place a wedge under) the wheels to prevent forward motion. An unstable vehicle puts both rescuers and patients at high risk for injury.

Knowing your personal limitations relative to the rescue scene is important. The place to try new rescue equipment and technique is the garage, in a structured training program, not in the field, where the lives of the patients and rescuers may be at risk.

Case in Point

You and your partner respond to the report of a female patient with shortness of breath. On your arrival at the patient's home, you find a morbidly obese woman in a small back bedroom. She is complaining of shortness of breath and weakness. There is a small hallway to negotiate. The patient is too heavy for two persons to carry her safely. How will you transport the patient to the ambulance? The same principles discussed in this chapter for vehicle and high-angle rescues can be applied to such situations. Consider calling for additional personnel and equipment to assist. In some situations, walls have been altered or cut to allow for the removal of large patients.

Scene Size-up and Scene Safety

A basic principle of rescue operations is that the scene must be assessed for potential danger to rescuers, the public, and the patient. Performing a scene size-up, including scene safety, is

---

Box 27-1 Twelve "Never" Guidelines of Scene Safety

1. Never enter a potentially hazardous rescue scene without the appropriate personal protective equipment.
2. Never operate on an active roadway until traffic flow has been controlled.
3. Never enter an unstable vehicle until it has been appropriately stabilized.
4. Never enter a fire scene unless directed by fire rescue personnel.
5. Never enter a confined space unless directed by confined-space or cave rescue personnel.
6. Never attempt a deep-water rescue or surface-water rescue without the support of water rescue personnel.
7. Never enter a scene where toxic gases or spills are suspected until cleared by fire or rescue personnel.
8. Never enter a structural collapse unless directed by rescue personnel.
9. Never enter a scene where violence has occurred before the arrival of police.
10. Never attempt a rescue from a height without the support of rescuers trained in high-angle rescue.
11. Never approach an electrical hazard unless cleared by the appropriate rescue or utility personnel.
12. Never proceed with any potentially hazardous rescue scene unless you are fully informed that the scene is safe.

---

the most critical step of every call (see Chapter 7). Many well-intentioned providers have died entering unsafe environments without careful assessment of the hazards. It is important to recognize that not all patients who are in need of rescue can be rescued. Certain situations present such significant hazards to both rescuers and the public that an effort to attempt a rescue may be both futile and costly in terms of lives. The need for a risk-benefit analysis is essential. The rescuer who runs into a burning building without assessing the safety of the scene and becomes injured or loses his or her life becomes an additional, unnecessary patient.

Remembering and adhering to the 12 "nevers" of scene safety can almost always prevent injury to yourself and your partner **(Box 27-1)**.

Traffic Control

Traffic is among the most dangerous of all the on-scene hazards an EMT will face at a vehicle crash scene. Most recognized standards advise the arriving crews to park their heavy trucks at an angle to the traffic to "fend off" oncoming vehicles. This parking angle is not the only safety consideration you must take when working around moving traffic. Highly reflective traffic vests worn by all rescuers provide added visibility for passing motorists.

Reflective traffic cones can be used to establish a safety zone around the perimeter of the crash. Road flares work well at night; however, they must be used far from any flammable vapors or liquids. You should place the cones in a position well ahead of the incident to give approaching drivers sufficient warning distance to react. The safety zone should include the patient loading area around your ambulance. This is the only traffic control measure you should take. Law enforcement personnel or people

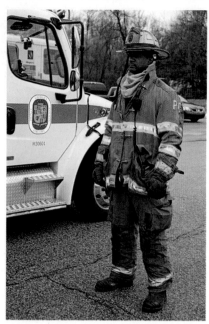

Figure 27-4 EMTs wear proper personal protective equipment (PPE) to perform a rescue. Note the reflective stripes, which make the EMT visible on the scene of an emergency.

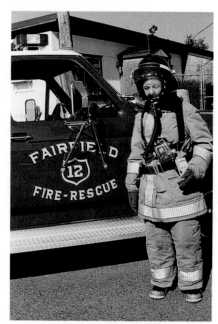

Figure 27-5 An EMT wearing PPE with self-contained breathing apparatus (SCBA). Note the yellow personal distress device on the belt. If the EMT is motionless for a set period, this device will activate. Also, if in trouble, the EMT can activate the device manually and alert others involved in the operation. The helmet is tipped back to show the face piece; in a normal operation, the helmet would be square on the head.

specially trained in controlling or diverting high-speed traffic will best accomplish total scene protection.

Personal Protection

Your personal protective equipment (PPE) represents the single most important factor in reducing the potential for injury. A complete protective "envelope" or turnout gear consists of headgear, eye protection, respiratory protection (if required), gloves, boots, and coat (**Figure 27-4**).

In dealing with a rescue situation, remember that patient care always precedes the rescue effort unless a life-safety hazard exists. A *life-safety hazard* is any situation in which the rescuers are risking serious injury or death as the result of entering the rescue area. A life-safety hazard is encountered, for example, every time an EMT stops to assist an injured motorist on a dark, unmarked roadway. Remember, your value to the patient is lost if you are injured or killed.

Unfortunately, PPE is bulky, hot, and generally not conducive to providing effective and timely treatment. Your uniform should also provide some degree of protection. In general, your uniform should be flame resistant and flame retardant and should be reflective to identify you to drivers in low-light environments.

Remember, the areas of the body you are trying to protect are the head, eyes, hands, torso, legs, and feet. The primary hazards that you face are from traffic, fire, debris, cuts, and toxic contamination. Your PPE should provide sufficient protection against these threats. Your level of involvement in a particular rescue process also determines the type of PPE that you require. (See also Chapter 7.)

Respiratory Protection

Before entering a smoke condition or any situation in which toxic gases may be present, you must put on the appropriate equipment. The use of self-contained breathing apparatus

(SCBA) should be restricted to individuals who have specific hands-on training with this equipment. If you believe that you require such training, the local fire service can probably provide it (**Figure 27-5**).

You should be able to recognize possible toxic environments and recognize the need for SCBA use. Particle masks may be necessary when sawing through glass or plastic, to prevent rescuers from inhaling glass or plastic dust.

Patient and Bystander Safety

In the various methods of gaining access, every attempt should be made to ensure the safety of the patient. Shards of glass, metal edges, and fire are examples of hazards that may occur during the rescue process. You should cover the patient with a rescue blanket or take other protective measures to decrease the possibility of injury to the patient.

It is also important to explain the nature of the extrication process to the patient. The loud sounds and activities surrounding the extrication process are likely to result in anxiety and increased secretion of epinephrine, which increases the patient's oxygen consumption and could worsen his or her condition. Psychologic first aid is important in the management of the patient during a rescue.

Stabilizing the Vehicle

The goal of stabilization is to prevent any unwanted or dangerous movement of the vehicle body on its springs. Another goal is to ensure that the structural integrity of the vehicle will not be compromised by the rescue effort, including (but not limited to) rolling, tipping, falling, or rocking. Stabilization is

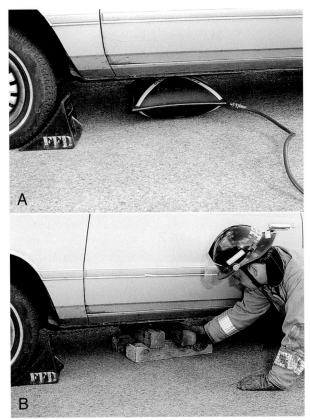

Figure 27-6 **A,** The airbag and the wheel chock stabilize the vehicle in two directions, forward and backward and up and down. **B,** The cribbing also provides vehicle stabilization.

accomplished by taking the weight of the vehicle and spreading it over as large an area as possible. Make as many points of the vehicle as possible come in contact with the ground.

Many methods are available to stabilize a vehicle with your hands. The attempt by personnel to lift or stabilize a vehicle is both unsafe and foolhardy. Although several muscular people can certainly lift a vehicle, what happens when one of them injures his or her back in the middle of the operation?

The use of **cribbing** material is the safe method of stabilizing a vehicle. Use hardwood, such as oak, and carry several different sizes. Build a base of large pieces, integrating smaller pieces toward the top. **Figure 27-6** illustrates the basic technique for vehicle stabilization with wood cribbing and chocks.

LEARNING OBJECTIVES
- Evaluate various methods of gaining access to the patient.
- Distinguish between simple and complex access.

Gaining Access at the Scene

Efforts to **gain access** to the patient should be made in the most expedient manner possible. The route by which you reach the patient is not necessarily the route by which the patient is removed. Your objective at this point is to gain entry into the vehicle and provide lifesaving care and stabilization before removal.

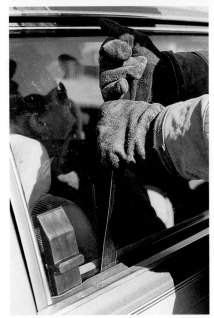

Figure 27-7 Slim Jim in operation with a wedge. The Slim Jim produced commercially is the best type to use. Much practice is required; instruction manuals are available.

There are two ways to gain access to a vehicle. **Simple access** is defined as access in which tools are not required. **Complex access** occurs when tools and other specialized equipment are necessary for access.

Once you are inside the vehicle, your assessment of the patient's condition may change, and the priorities of the rescue may be altered accordingly. When you gain access, take your rescue blanket with you and cover the patient. This aids in treating the patient for shock by maintaining body temperature, and it provides some measure of protection during the rescue.

The rescue operation should always be kept as simple as possible. For example, if the door is locked and the patient is conscious, you can ask the person to unlock the door. This action may be all that is needed to gain access. Also, check all the doors, including hatchbacks, before breaking glass.

The **Slim Jim** is a device that has been used by vehicle-repossession agents and is very effective for gaining access to locked cars, causing little or no damage to the vehicle (**Figure 27-7**). The drawback to this technique is its basic unreliability when used by individuals who have had minimal experience with the device. Unless you use the device on a regular basis, your potential for success is limited. Also, electronic locking systems in newer cars may not be able to be released using the Slim Jim.

Entering through a Window

If the door of a vehicle is locked and the patient is unconscious, the quickest way to gain access is to select the window farthest from the patient and break the glass with the *spring-loaded window punch.* Because the patient may be in need of immediate lifesaving management, breaking glass is a reasonable and necessary response. You may perform an initial patient assessment through the window before you are able to enter the vehicle with your whole body.

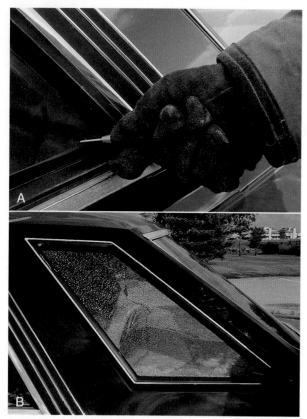

Figure 27-8 A, The spring-loaded center punch is an excellent tool for breaking window glass in a nonobstructive way. This technique is used only on a fully framed and closed window and depends on complete circumferential pressure to achieve the desired result. **B,** A vehicle side window after the spring-loaded punch has been used. Note that the center punch does not operate on the windshield because it is laminated glass. This device is effective only on side windows because they are made of tempered glass. The breaking quality of the tempered glass is what makes the device work.

Spring-loaded window punches are ideal tools to be used for gaining access and result in the least amount of glass entering the vehicle. If possible, practice this technique and become familiar with it before you encounter a real situation **(Figure 27-8).**

Other methods of breaking glass include the use of hammers, axes, and screwdrivers. All these methods have drawbacks over the spring-loaded punch. One method of reducing the amount of glass entering the vehicle is to stick contact paper over the window to be broken before breaking the glass; much of the glass will stick to the paper. One drawback to this method is that contact paper does not stick well on wet windows and therefore may not always produce the expected result.

Doors

Just as doors are a good place through which to enter a vehicle, they are also an excellent place through which to remove patients rapidly. However, the door opening may have to be widened. Often it is possible to widen a door opening by simply "walking" the door back. Before beginning, you should ensure that the vehicle is stabilized, the wheels are chocked, and the brake is set. One or two EMTs then press their body weight against the door and slowly push the door open beyond its normal operating range.

Freeing the Driver

Freeing the driver is one of the most common extrication challenges you will encounter. The steering wheel presents problems during extrication, but removal of the driver may require only a few inches of space. Moving the seat back without unduly jarring the driver is the simplest method. Seats move either manually or electrically, and either method is acceptable if done slowly.

Always disconnect the vehicle's battery during extrication. Modern vehicles usually have at least one or more undeployed airbags that are ready to fire. Disconnecting the battery is the safest way to prevent injury or death to rescuers and patients during extrication (see following section).

Supplemental Restraints (Airbags)

Virtually every vehicle built since the early 1990s has one or more supplemental restraint systems, commonly known as airbags. An **airbag** is a woven bladder that fills with an inert gas to cushion the occupant from hitting hard objects. Once it deploys and protects, the airbag rapidly deflates.

Several types of airbags are available. Front airbags include the driver's bag, which deploys from the center of the steering wheel, and the much larger passenger side bag, which deploys from the dash. Vehicles may also contain one or more styles of side-impact airbags that can fire from the back of the front seat, the roof rail area, or the door itself. Because airbags are set to fire in zones, chances are you will encounter both deployed and undeployed airbags in most vehicle crashes.

Deployed airbags pose less hazard to your efforts, but some airbags have dual-stage deployment, meaning they might refire after initially deploying. EMTs have been injured by postcrash airbag deployment during extrication activities, and you must take actions to prevent this. Observe the "5-10-20 rule" when working around undeployed airbags. Keep the area clear from the airbag's path by keeping back 5 inches from a side bag, 10 inches from the driver's airbag, and 20 inches from the passenger's airbag. You will notice dust from a deployed bag in the car and possibly on your patient. Although this packing dust, usually talc or cornstarch, may be slightly caustic, it is essentially harmless.

You can save much time dealing with the airbag issue if you can safely reach the ignition key, switch it off, and remove it. However, you should not rely on this step alone. Go the extra step by disconnecting all sources of power, including anything plugged into the cigarette lighter, such as a cell phone or laptop computer. Although this will not completely protect you from a potential airbag deployment, it is one more interruption in the electrical circuit and greatly reduces the chance of accidental deployment. Follow up by disconnecting the battery. The negative side of the battery should be disconnected first.

Other supplemental protection systems that you may encounter include the automatic roll bar and the seat belt pretensioner device. Found in some convertibles, automatic rollover protection is gained by spring-loaded *roll bars* that remain in the down position during normal operation but spring up with great force when the vehicle's wheels leave the ground, locking in their fully deployed position before the vehicle can turn over. It is essential that you learn to recognize automatic roll bars and maintain a safety zone around them while caring for the patient.

Seat belt *pretensioner devices* are found in many cars and are set to quickly take up any slack in the seat belt before an airbag deploys. To avoid the possibility of a pretensioning device harming the patient during the rescue, unbuckle the seat belt from the patient as soon as it is safe to do so, remembering to observe the potential strike zones of any undeployed airbags or roll bars.

REAL*World*

Passive restraint technology is constantly changing. The knowledge and skill set involved in disconnecting a passive restraint system requires special training. EMS agencies responsible for disconnecting restraint systems receive ongoing training as automotive technology advances. The best skill for EMTs is to be aware of systems and not to place themselves in potential danger.

Essential Emergency Care

Immediately on gaining access to the patient, one EMT should assume inline cervical stabilization while another EMT conducts the initial assessment. The mechanism of injury should be used to guide you in your assessment (see Chapter 7). If life-threatening conditions are identified, use the rapid extrication procedure if the patient is not trapped in the vehicle. If removal is not possible, make every attempt to stabilize the patient in the vehicle; you can manage front-seat passengers in need of airway maintenance and ventilation by lowering the back of the seat (when possible) to facilitate these procedures. As usual, the principles of management remain the same: airway, breathing, and circulation (ABCs) have priority.

Disentanglement represents the most pivotal stage of extrication as it relates to rapid patient removal from the scene. Your primary focus during the disentanglement stage is caring for the patient, not removal of the patient from the wreckage. Applying this principle to your operation provides the patient with the most efficient and stabilizing situation.

While the process of disentanglement progresses, prepare the patient for removal while maintaining cervical spine stabilization. A focused trauma examination can be conducted to identify additional injuries to the head, trunk, and extremities. Again, the mechanism of injury should provide the basis for identification of specific types of trauma. For example, a front-end collision would prompt the EMT to carefully examine the patient's anterior head, chest, and abdomen, as well as the knee, femur, and hip region.

When serious injuries are identified (e.g., flail chest), take immediate action to stabilize the condition. More minor injuries can be treated later. If time permits, open wounds should be dressed and bandaged. When possible, splint fractures before removal. However, the application of traction splints and long board splints to the lower extremities is usually not possible in the confines of an automobile.

The patient should be attached to a torso immobilization device such as the Kendrick extrication device (KED) and removed from the vehicle onto a long spine board. Once again, if life-threatening injuries exist and removal is possible, follow the rapid extrication procedure.

Once the patient is effectively immobilized, removal from the vehicle can proceed. Exercise care in selecting the exit route. Again, the optimal route follows the path of least resistance. For example, the rear window is a poor choice for removal of the driver or a front-seat passenger. However, the condition and location of wreckage often dictate the options available to the rescuer. Once again, the door adjacent to the occupant is the best choice.

A second consideration is personnel. Attempting removal of an adult patient with two EMTs should be avoided. Three or more prehospital providers are usually needed to perform an extrication procedure. Personnel should be recruited on the basis of their experience in handling patients and their individual physical strength. Strong rescuers should be assigned positions that require the greatest effort during movement.

Removal of the patient from the vehicle should proceed carefully, without abrupt or jerky movements that could result in loss of inline stabilization of the cervical spine. Review the path and steps of removal with the rescuers before removing the patient. Initiate each step with a verbal cue from the team leader. The patient should be protected during removal. This is particularly important when the windshield or window exit is used. On lifting the patient, rescuers should support the patient as one unit. As a rule, lift the patient, not the device. In most cases, a wheeled cot stretcher can be positioned adjacent to the exit route to facilitate transfer to the long spine board. (See Chapters 5 and 24.)

Scenario Follow-up

Every motor vehicle crash will include elements of scene and patient safety, gaining access, and extrication. This case illustrates effective analysis while approaching the scene and the appropriate use of resources. Rarely should EMTs play a primary role in the extrication process. The EMT role focuses on patient assessment, care of the patient, immobilization, and safe removal of the patient from the vehicle.

Summary

The successful extrication of injured patients from a motor vehicle crash is a challenge that you are likely to encounter. Your effectiveness depends on your ability to remain calm and to organize the available resources. Safety to yourself, bystanders, and the patient is your first priority. In most cases, rescue personnel concentrate on gaining access and disentanglement. Your role is to assess, treat, immobilize, and safely remove and transport the injured patient.

Time to definitive care should be a prime consideration. When you are called on to effect a rescue, you should be prepared to do so with a minimal amount of equipment. Selection of the safest, fastest, and often the simplest method of gaining access and disentanglement should be the guiding principle of the rescue operation.

Many extrication techniques can be used. Rescue is a skill requiring many hours of training. As an EMT, you should understand some of the rescue options available and the guiding principles. Give the highest priority to the patient and a rapid extrication. This chapter presents several options in extrication, but study of this chapter alone does not qualify you to perform the rescue techniques outlined. You also need time, experience, and training to achieve this goal.

The Bottom Line

Learning Checklist

✓ Specialized rescue personnel are usually responsible for gaining access to the patient. The EMT's role is primarily related to safety and patient assessment and care.

✓ On arrival at a scene that may require specialized rescue personnel, the EMT should communicate as a first step to ensure a timely response.

✓ The use of personal protective equipment is a critical aspect of safety at the scene of a rescue situation and includes headgear, eye wear, gloves, and other clothing or equipment appropriate for the situation.

✓ The use of self-contained breathing apparatus is critical at scenes where toxic gases might be present and should be used only by trained individuals.

✓ When approaching a suspected hazardous materials incident, the EMT should park 100 feet uphill and upwind.

✓ Simple access to a patient trapped in a vehicle does not require tools. Complex access requires the use of tools and specialized equipment.

✓ The EMT should begin the scene assessment with a "window assessment," looking at the scene as the approach for hazards

✓ Potentially unstable vehicles should be stabilized with cribbing before the EMT enters to care for an injured patient

✓ The EMT needs to remain aware of the location of airbags and take the necessary steps to disarm airbags to avoid additional injury to the patient or themselves.

✓ After assuring their own safety, the priority of the EMT on the scene is the medical assessment, care, and transport of the patient.

Key Terms

Airbag Woven bladder that fills with an inert gas to cushion the occupant from hitting hard objects.

Cribbing Materials or devices, including wood and airbags, used to support a large amount of weight during rescue operations.

Complex access Gaining access to the patient with tools or specialized equipment.

Disentanglement Part of the extrication process in which the rescuers remove materials that are trapping a patient.

Extrication Process by which entrapped patients are rescued from vehicles, tunnels, or other structures or devices.

Gain access Part of the extrication process in which the rescuers gain entry to trapped patients.

Simple access Gaining access to the patient without the use of any tools or specialized equipment.

Slim Jim Device for gaining access to locked cars.

Review Questions

1. The EMT's primary role at the scene of a motor vehicle crash is:
   a. Gaining access
   b. Extrication
   c. Disentanglement
   d. Emergency care

2. The term used to describe an extrication that can be accomplished through the use of skills, such as opening locks, is called:
   a. Disentanglement
   b. Simple access
   c. Strategic access
   d. Rapid extrication

3. Because of the possibility of spilled gasoline at a motor vehicle crash, the least appropriate method of securing the scene is through the use of:
   a. Reflectors
   b. Flares
   c. Road cones
   d. Battery-operated lights

4. Blocks of wood used to stabilize vehicles are commonly called:
   a. Stacking blocks
   b. Cribbing
   c. Stabilizers
   d. Construction blocks

5. When attempting to gain access through a window, the EMT should protect the patient by:
   a. Moving the patient away from the window.
   b. Tilting the vehicle away from the patient.
   c. Covering the patient with a rescue blanket.
   d. Shattering the window from the inside out.

6. On gaining access to the interior of the vehicle, you find a patient who is short of breath, pale, cool, sweaty, and hypotensive, with a respiratory rate of 22 breaths/min. Your immediate reaction is to:
   a. Apply oxygen and a short spine board device.
   b. Rapidly extricate the patient.
   c. Apply the pneumatic antishock garment before extrication.
   d. Begin positive-pressure ventilation.

7. The fastest and best way to create a larger door opening is to:
  a. Remove the hinges and door.
  b. Remove the inner door lining.
  c. Cut through the roof.
  d. Overbend the door outward.

For Further Review

In the Student Workbook

- Multiple-choice questions
- Case scenario questions

On Evolve

- Weblinks
- Lecture notes
- Exercises

Learning Objectives

Cognitive Objectives

- Describe the purpose of extrication.
- Discuss the role of the EMT-Basic in extrication.
- Identify what equipment for personal safety is required for the EMT-Basic.
- Define the fundamental components of extrication.
- State the steps to take to protect the patient during extrication.
- Evaluate various methods of gaining access to the patient.
- Distinguish between simple and complex access.

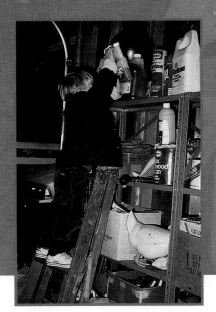

28 Disasters and Hazardous Materials

CHAPTER OUTLINE

Hazardous Materials
Disasters
Incident Management System
Roles and Responsibilities of the EMT

Scenario

On a summer afternoon, you and your partner are the first responders to the scene of a freight train derailment and bus crash at an at-grade crossing. Multiple vehicles have been stopped at the crossing and are involved in the incident. On arriving at the scene, you observe a derailed train with HAZMAT placards on the railcars, a tour bus that has rolled down a small embankment on the side of the road, and a large number of noninjured observers. Law enforcement officers are on site. They inform you the tour bus had 30 passengers of all ages on a trip to a nearby lake.

- What is your overall plan of action?
- What precautions would you take?
- How would you activate your disaster plan?
- What resources are needed?
- What roles would you and your partner assume as first responders on the scene?
- What steps can you take to prevent further injury, reduce the number of deaths, and transport the patients in a timely manner?

As an emergency medical technician (EMT), you will respond to special situations when you cannot handle the job alone. You will have patients who have been exposed to hazardous materials. At other times the number of patients will be greater than your resources. You may find yourself called to assist at a disaster where there is widespread disruption over a large area, with or without casualties.

Your role as an EMT is to provide emergency medical care after the scene is safe. You will be expected to know how to interact with others in a coordinated response. At times you may be first on the scene, so you need to know if additional help is needed and what to do until help arrives. To this end, you should learn how to recognize whether a hazardous situation exists and how to take actions to prevent further injury and contamination.

At **multiple-casualty incidents (MCIs),** in which the personnel or equipment needs exceed those readily available from responding units, your role may include performing **triage** (the sorting of patients into high, secondary, and low priorities), making sure each patient has an initial assessment, and assigning them by their priority status to responding personnel. Because there are often multiple agencies that must work together at an MCI or a disaster site, you need to know the command structure within your region.

REAL*World*

Multiple-casualty incidents (MCIs) will have different effects in different systems. In a large metropolitan system, dozens of ambulances may be available to respond. Mutual aid agreements, in which neighboring systems provide backup response, allow many ambulances on a scene in minutes. Also, large cities may have several hospitals available to receive patients. During incidents such as the Columbine shootings in Colorado, a line of ambulances waited in the staging area to receive patients. In contrast, in a small community with one volunteer ambulance and a small hospital, a motor vehicle crash with four patients could overwhelm the system.

Fortunately, the **incident management system** is widely used to control, direct, and coordinate all responding agencies at MCIs and hazardous situations. You may be asked to respond to a particular emergency medical system (EMS) sector at an MCI and report to the EMS sector officer so you can perform your task as part of a coordinated response.

LEARNING OBJECTIVES

- Explain the EMT role during a call involving hazardous materials.
- Describe what the EMT should do if there is reason to believe there is a hazard at the scene.
- Describe the actions that an EMT should take to ensure bystander safety.
- State the role the EMT should perform until appropriately trained personnel arrive at the scene of a HAZMAT situation.
- Break down the steps to approaching a hazardous situation.
- Discuss the various environmental hazards that affect EMS.
- Explain the methods for preventing contamination of self, equipment, and facilities.

Hazardous Materials

A **hazardous material** is any substance (solid, liquid, or gas) capable of causing harm to people, property, or the environment; they are found everywhere in our society. Few of us go through a day without using hazardous materials or something produced from them (**Figure 28-1**).

Exposures can range from fumes after mixing bleach and ammonia in a cleaning bucket to chemical plant spills. Mass poisonings from hazardous materials, such as the gas leak from the chemical plant in Bhopal, India, in 1984, capture worldwide

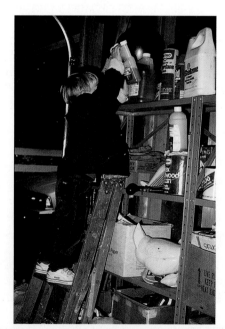

Figure 28-1 Hazardous materials are very common throughout the community and the home.

Box 28-1	Nine Classes of Hazardous Materials

Class 1: Explosives
Class 2: Gases
Class 3: Flammable/combustible liquids
Class 4: Flammable solids
Class 5: Oxidizing substances
Class 6: Poisonous and infectious substances
Class 7: Radioactive substances
Class 8: Corrosive materials
Class 9: Miscellaneous hazardous materials

attention. No community is immune. Hazardous materials (HAZMAT, hazmat) incidents and the potential for chemical emergencies are waiting to happen in virtually every industrial, commercial, agricultural, and residential area. For example, in the state of Washington, 2360 individuals had acute exposure to hazardous materials over a 4-year period in the 1990s, and 75% of these patients were transported to a healthcare facility. Because many hazardous materials have health risks, you have to be prepared to respond.

Hazardous materials can contaminate or physically remain on or in a person, animal, the environment, or equipment, thereby creating a continuing risk of injury or a risk of exposure to others. **Decontamination** is the physical or chemical process of reducing, removing, and preventing the spread of contaminants from persons at a hazmat incident. A contaminated person or item exposed at the incident site may cause secondary contamination of others who are far removed from the event. Specially trained members of a HAZMAT response team may be dispatched under an emergency response plan to handle and control actual or potential leaks or spills of hazardous materials that may require close approach to the material.

The EMT's primary duties at a hazmat incident are to provide medical care and to maintain safety, preventing unnecessary contamination of themselves and others. To perform this role, you must have some basic knowledge about the types of hazardous incidents, how to identify a hazardous agent, and how to promote safety for yourself, the patient, and others. In addition, you must know how to integrate the EMS response smoothly with other agencies within the incident command structure.

General Knowledge

Hazardous materials may be flammable, toxic, infectious, corrosive, radioactive, oxidizing, or reactive or may have a combination of these properties (**Box 28-1**). The potential for harm varies with the agent, and specific knowledge of the hazard at hand and its properties is important to guide medical treatment.

You may encounter a hazmat situation in various scenarios. You may be dispatched to an industrial incident where the on-site HAZMAT team has decontaminated the victim and given you detailed information of the medical hazards of the exposure. You may encounter a patient who spilled insecticide on his clothing hours before and does not relate his shortness of breath and increased secretions to contamination with an organophosphate, the active ingredient in many insecticides. You may be on a scene where some victims are fleeing from an exposure but have been contaminated and may spread the contaminant to you and to others.

In recognition of the potential risks in our everyday world, federal legislation has directed planning to have safer responses to hazmat incidents. The scope is comprehensive; it includes special training and equipment, creation of a written response plan, and implementation of the incident command system during the hazmat response. Federal legislation provides implementation of training programs for five levels of response through the Occupational Safety and Health Administration (OSHA) Hazardous Waste Operations and Emergency Response standard. This law, as well as related Environmental Protection Agency (EPA) regulations to cover government personnel, requires training for all personnel who would be expected to respond to a hazmat incident. The types of training are tailored to the expected role that an individual would play at the incident and are named according to specific tasks, as follows:

- *First responder/awareness.* Awareness training is appropriate for first responders likely to witness or discover a hazmat incident and then initiate an emergency response. This training includes identification of hazardous materials, their risks, and potential outcomes after exposure. The ability to recognize the presence of hazardous materials, available guidebooks and resources, and how to secure additional resources and promote safety are covered.
- *First responder/operations.* Operations training is aimed at individuals who would respond to a hazmat situation but are trained to try to contain the release from a safe distance, keep it from spreading, and prevent further exposure. In addition to awareness-level knowledge, the operations-trained provider would also learn about protective equipment; how to perform basic control, containment, and confinement operations; and how to implement basic decontamination procedures.
- *Hazardous materials technician.* The technician level is directed at appropriate individuals who would attempt to stop the release of the hazardous substance.
- *Hazardous materials specialist.* The specialist receives even more training and specific or direct knowledge of substances that might be released.
- *On-site incident commander.* The commander-level personnel receive training with broad knowledge of hazardous materials and emergency response plans.

Role of the EMT

Most EMS agencies operate at the awareness or operations level. This level of response is strictly defensive, and the EMT would not take any aggressive action at the point of the release of the hazardous substance. Instead, the EMT is concerned with patient care. Depending on his or her training, the EMT may or may not care for contaminated victims. The National Fire Protection Association (NFPA) has standards for competencies of EMS personnel that draw such a distinction. According to the NFPA 473 standard, an EMT caring for patients who have been decontaminated should be trained to responder level I; an EMT with some decontamination responsibility is trained to responder level II.

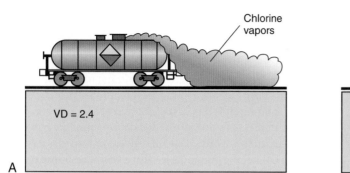
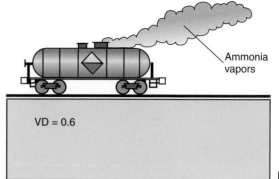

Figure 28-2 Vapor density *(VD)* will influence whether a released gas will settle near the ground (**A**) or disperse into the atmosphere (**B**).

Special training in hazmat response is required for the EMT to operate at any hazardous materials level, and EMTs should not operate outside their level of training. Consult your local protocols for the requirements of EMS responders in your area.

Safety

Safety is your first and ongoing concern at a hazmat incident. When approaching a hazmat incident, you should attempt to position your ambulance and your crew upwind and uphill from the incident. Upwind positioning is important so that wind currents do not move vapors toward you; the uphill position is preferable so that liquid spills do not flow down to you. You should ascertain information about the incident from a safe distance. Remember, as an EMT you generally will not respond with *chemical protective clothing* (CPC) or adequate respiratory protection to safeguard yourself from the toxic effects of a chemical.

Binoculars are helpful when approaching the scene, to allow the crew to look for reliable clues from a safe distance. Keep unnecessary people away from the hazmat area. Section off the area (using rope, tape, or other barriers to control and restrict passage), restrict further access, and evacuate the area. The specific actions you take will depend on your disaster plan, the specifics of the incident, and what other responders are available at the scene.

Properties of Hazardous Materials

You should understand the various ways in which hazardous materials can enter and harm the body. These include inhalation, absorption, ingestion, and injection, alone or in combination. You will need to know the substance at hand to know what risk is faced. For example, gases are problematic because they can disperse over a large area. Liquids can be absorbed through the skin but may also give off vapors that can be inhaled and absorbed.

Knowing the physical properties of a chemical will help you understand how a substance may spread. For example, *vapor density* is the weight of a volume of gas compared with an equal volume of air. If the ratio is less than 1, it is lighter than air and will rise. If the vapor density is greater than 1, it is heavier than air and will settle in low areas, presenting a greater risk of exposure for people on the ground (**Figure 28-2**). The *vapor pressure* of liquid is a measure of its volatility or rate of evaporation. The higher the vapor pressure, the greater is the inhalation hazard. Nerve gas poisons such as sarin, which was used in a Tokyo

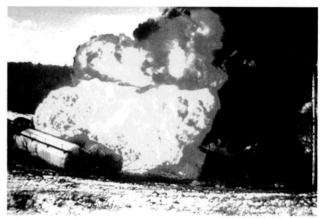

Figure 28-3 Large, boiling-liquid expanding-vapor explosions (BLEVEs) are one reason to evaluate potentially hazardous scenes from a distance. *From US Department of Transportation: North American emergency response guidebook, 2004.*

subway terrorist attack in March 1995, are spread as liquids that evaporate (similar to evaporation of water) and expose victims to the fumes.

Liquefied gases kept under pressure are also a potential hazard because the product may rapidly boil and expand if the container is suddenly punctured or breached. If flammable, a large fireball may result. This is known as a *boiling-liquid expanding-vapor explosion* (BLEVE) (**Figure 28-3**). Even if nonflammable, the container may rupture, resulting in a large vapor release, and the container or projectiles may travel great distances.

These examples help show the relevance of taking basic safety actions, following advice of experts in hazardous materials, and taking additional courses on hazmat procedures for emergency personnel.

Control Zones

A basic concept used at hazmat incidents is the establishment of control zones (**Figure 28-4**). **Control zones** are geographic areas at a hazmat incident designated on the basis of safety and the degree of hazard.

The **hot zone** is the area in which contamination occurs. It should only be entered by those with the training and *personal protective equipment* (PPE) to deal safely with the substance at

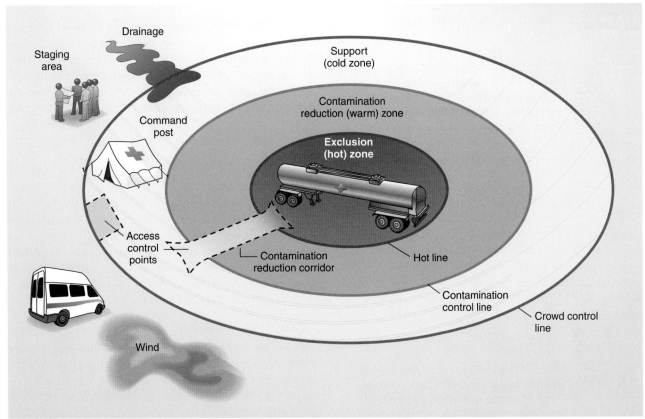

Figure 28-4 Establishing control zones is an essential safety procedure. The hot zone is where the hazardous material was spilled, and only suitably protected and trained responders should enter. The warm zone is the transition zone where decontamination occurs and access is controlled between the hot and cold zones. Suitable training and protection are necessary to enter the warm zone. The cold zone, or clean zone, is where patients are brought for EMS assessment before transport from the scene. The cold zone is also the site for staging supplies and command.

hand. Those entering the hot zone must be decontaminated when leaving. The principal patient management technique in the hot zone is patient removal.

The **warm zone** immediately surrounds the hot zone and is the place where decontamination occurs. The warm zone has control points for access corridors in and out of the hot zone and the cold zone. Restricting access assists in reducing spread of contamination. Only properly trained and protected EMS personnel should enter the hot and warm zones, and medical care should be limited to lifesaving care and triage.

Once decontaminated, patients can be brought to the **cold zone,** or *clean zone,* where EMS personnel can further assess the patient, ensure that adequate decontamination is performed before transport, and perform patient care functions as required. The cold zone is also where staging of supplies and the command center are established and rehabilitation takes place.

Anyone not essential to the incident and patient care should be kept outside these control zones. Crowd control is important because these situations may attract curious onlookers. Police may be needed to secure public safety.

Personal Protective Equipment

At a hazmat incident, PPE shields or isolates a person from the chemical, physical, and thermal hazards that may be encountered. PPE includes both protective clothing and respiratory

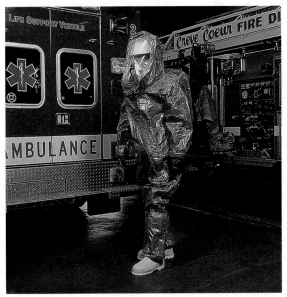

Figure 28-5 Class A personal protective equipment.

protection to safeguard the respiratory system, skin, eyes, face, hands, feet, head, body, and sense of hearing (**Figure 28-5**).

Those who enter a potentially contaminated area should have special training and specialized protective clothing and breathing apparatus. PPE, including fluid-resistant gowns and shoe covers,

Table 28-1	Chemical Protective Clothing (CPC) Classification

Protection Level	Description
A	Provides for the highest level of respiratory protection and the highest level of skin protection. This suit is fully encapsulated and protects against gases. SCBA or supplied air with an escape air bottle is required.
B	Provides for the highest level of respiratory protection but a lesser level of skin protection. SCBA is required. Level B suits come in various types, both encapsulated and nonencapsulated, and do not protect against gases.
C	Provides for a lesser level of respiratory protection and an even lesser degree of skin protection. SCBA is not required. Respirators designed to filter specific particles out of the ambient air are required. Specialty skin protection, such as acid aprons and heavy-duty gloves, is used for skin protection.
D	Offers no chemical protection and is found in the form of generalized work clothes (e.g., steel-toe work boots and hard hat). *Note:* Structural firefighting gear offers no chemical protection.

SCBA, Self-contained breathing apparatus.

is suitable for activities in the cold zone. However, for entrance to contaminated areas or to perform decontamination duties, special hazardous materials protective clothing *specifically compatible with the hazard* is required. For example, CPC is identified by its ability to protect its occupant from the dangers of contact with chemicals or chemical vapors (**Table 28-1**).

No one suit is good for all chemical emergencies, and no single level of protection is best for all situations. The chemical and its physical properties and health effects must be identified before entering a hazardous area. CPC compatibility charts must be consulted when a hazmat zone is being organized. Other protective clothing exists for high temperatures and structural firefighting.

Access to victims may have to wait until proper chemical identification and hazard analysis can be made. Do not enter the area unless you are fully protected and properly trained. You may face one of the most difficult decisions of your life: despite training and expectations, you may not be in a position to help patients until the scene is safe. Learn your limitations, and operate within them. The contaminated patient, no matter how seriously ill or injured, may have to be left alone until the appropriate personnel and equipment arrive. Avoid contact with the chemical involved. Patients may be removed to a safe area if this can be accomplished without the potential for contamination of the EMS crew.

Remember, you are of no help to your patients if you become incapacitated after exposure to the toxic effects of a chemical. Let those who are properly trained remove victims to a safe area.

Decontamination

Once a hazard is identified, simple decontamination procedures that follow local protocol can be used to reduce the risk of contamination to EMS, hospital personnel, and others. Gross decontamination during the initial phase of decontamination may significantly remove surface contaminants by *mechanical removal, clothing removal, and rinsing.* The following types of decontamination are generally used in the prehospital setting:
- Dilution
- Absorption
- Chemical washes
- Disposal and isolation

All these decontamination methods are covered in special hazardous materials training offered by OSHA and the NFPA. Although ideally the EMT does not engage in decontamination, situations occur in which a patient with substantial contamination will leave the scene, and you must conduct gross contamination, with care not to become contaminated yourself.

Hazard Identification

What if you are the first arriving unit and the first to suspect a hazmat incident? How will you identify the agent? What clues should you look for, and what resources can you use?

At your first suspicion of an incident, your early actions should include evacuating bystanders and denying further access to individuals not part of the response by sectioning off the area. Depending on available personnel at the scene, you may do this or designate the task to others. These safety measures are necessary as you seek to gain more information from your scene size-up about what exactly is at hand. Rather than moving immediately to a patient's side, you may be gathering information at a distance to avoid unnecessary exposure and contamination.

Try to approach upwind and uphill if possible; rapidly assess the situation and search for signs and clues. The following clues are useful in identifying a hazmat incident and the substance involved:
- Preplanning or simply being aware of the type of location or occupancy you are responding to will give you a sense of the potential for a chemical incident. Local emergency response plans are usually made after compiling the high-risk sites within the region.
- If you notice multiple patients at the scene with the same symptoms, such as coughing, difficulty breathing, seizures, or unconsciousness, there is a high likelihood that they were exposed to a hazardous material.
- Container shapes unique to certain types of chemicals, as specified by the U.S. Department of Transportation (DOT), often provide clues regarding the contents of a truck or trailer. Look at the size and shape of a container from as far away as possible with binoculars.
- Diamond-shaped signs (**placards**) affixed to the outside of the transport vessel are useful in helping determine the actual commodity or the classification of a hazardous material (**Figure 28-6**). Placards use colors, symbols, and numbers to identify the chemicals involved and are required to be placed on the outside of a hazardous materials carrier, such

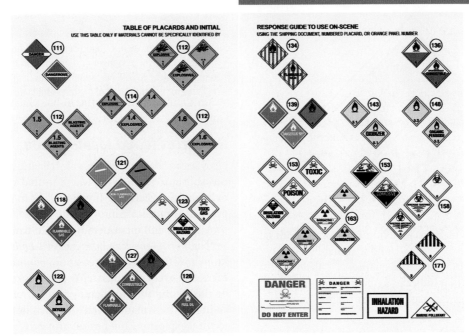

Figure 28-6 Hazardous materials (HAZMAT) warning placards. *From US Department of Transportation:* North American emergency response guidebook, *2004.*

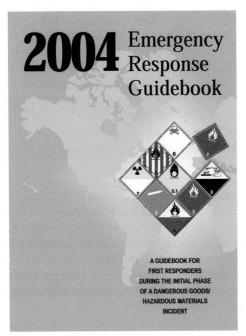

Figure 28-7 Emergency response guidebook. *From US Department of Transportation:* North American emergency response guidebook, *2004.*

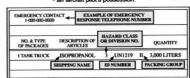

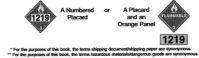

Figure 28-8 Bill of lading (shipping papers) with explanation of elements. *From US Department of Transportation:* North American emergency response guidebook, *2004.*

as a railroad car or truck. *Labels,* smaller versions of the placard, can be found on each individual package. There may be a four-digit identification (ID) number used to identify the product. Become familiar with federal and state requirements for labeling and placards as well as the use and application of the *North American Emergency Response Guidebook* as a resource for initial identification and response **(Figure 28-7).**

• Shipping papers, sometimes called *bills of lading,* are used for highway transport and can provide valuable information

about the cargo **(Figure 28-8).** Chemicals can be determined by the shipping name, classification, and ID number. Shipping papers can be found in the cab and are the responsibility of the driver. *Waybills* provide similar information for hazardous cargo transported by rail and are the responsibility of the conductor. Use extreme caution when obtaining the shipping papers as a means of identification; approaching the truck may place you close to a potentially dangerous situation.

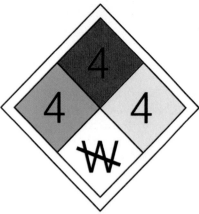

Figure 28-9 NFPA 704 placards have numbers corresponding to health (blue), reactivity (yellow), and flammability (red) risk as well as a white miscellaneous quadrant. A 4 is the most severe rating; for health, it indicates a material that on very short exposure could cause death or major residual injury.

The NFPA 704 System has developed a marking method that uses a diamond-shaped sign with four color-coded quadrants. It is often placed on tanks or on buildings where materials are used or stored. Three color-coded quadrants are used to rank fire, health, and reactivity hazards of the product on a 0 (no hazard) to 4 (severe hazard) scale, leaving one quadrant for miscellaneous information (**Figure 28-9**).

Finally, your senses aid in detecting the presence of hazardous materials. You may see a vapor cloud or leaking container; you may smell a strong odor; or you may feel irritation to your eyes, nose, or mouth. Although this may be the first clue, you must understand that sensory detection is a warning sign that there is the significant potential for danger and you are already exposed. Heed the warning signs and retreat until proper identification can be made. Remember that certain chemicals have no sensory warning properties at all. Other chemicals have warning properties that are not produced until unsafe levels have been reached. Do not rely on your senses as your primary means of detection.

Dispatch information can be helpful as you respond to an emergency. You should always use extreme caution as you approach a hazardous materials scene. Clues as previously stated will guide your approach. Remember, conditions can change without notice. Take care to stay as far away as possible until all information can be obtained. If you cannot obtain necessary information or if you do not fully understand the information you have gathered, consider the worst-case scenario and proceed accordingly.

Environmental Hazards

Whenever possible, make every effort to protect the environment from chemical hazards and secondary contamination. If there is no risk, prevent runoff by building a dike or digging a trench to minimize contamination of soil and water. Equipment that has been contaminated must either be decontaminated or disposed of as hazardous waste. Expert advice from HAZMAT team members will be useful to ensure that items are properly cleaned or disposed of.

Case in Point

On a major highway in Connecticut, a diesel tanker crossed the median and struck several passenger cars. In addition to providing medical care to multiple victims, EMS personnel dug a ditch in the grassy median of the highway to prevent runoff of the diesel fuel into a nearby river.

Resources to Aid Identification

No one can recall all the possible scenarios and details of hazardous substances. Knowing where to find reliable references and expert advice is crucial. If you are first to recognize a hazardous event, communicate information gained from placards or shipping papers and other details gleaned from the scene size-up.

The *North American Emergency Response Guidebook,* formerly known as the *DOT Emergency Response Guidebook,* should be carried in every ambulance. You can use the name of a product or the ID number to identify the substance and plan a quick response. Information available includes the hazard potential for fire, explosion, and health; protective clothing needs; evacuation concerns; basic first-aid information; and protective distances to be maintained.

Local HAZMAT response teams are specially trained and equipped to handle many types of chemical emergencies and are a valuable resource. They should be consulted in every hazardous materials incident.

Another resource available 24 hours a day, 7 days a week, is CHEMTREC. This organization is supported by the Chemical Manufacturer's Association and can be contacted by telephone toll free at 800-262-8200. Anyone can contact CHEMTREC at any time. You should be ready to provide the following information:

1. Name of the chemical (preferably trade name and shipper/manufacturer)
2. Nature of the problem or exposure
3. Current status

You may be asked to relay the nature and extent of injuries to people, the nature and extent of damage to the environment, and the prevailing weather. CHEMTREC responds with first-aid procedures; fire, spill, or leak-containment procedures; physical properties; inherent hazards; and appropriate levels of personal protective equipment to aid you in the decision-making process.

The *material safety data sheet* (MSDS) is also of great value. The MSDS is available for any chemical at a particular work site and provides essential information such as first-aid and decontamination procedures, primary routes of exposure, symptoms of overexposure, underlying medical conditions that may be aggravated by exposure to the chemical, and appropriate levels of PPE necessary for rescuers. Whenever possible, bring the MSDS with you to the hospital during transport. Reference books, computerized databases, and online consultations, such as poison control centers, are other available resources.

As mentioned, the OSHA standards were enacted to protect all emergency rescuers from the dangers of exposure to toxic substances. Other performance recommendations and guidelines, such as NFPA standards 471 (Recommended Practice for Responding to Hazardous Materials Incidents), 472 (Standard for Professional Competence of Responders to Hazardous Materials Emergencies), and 473 (Standard for Competencies for EMS Personnel Responding to Hazardous Material Incidents), essentially mirror the OSHA standard and provide compliance steps for your protection. Your employer or organization has responsibility to implement these safety provisions, including planning, training, and use of protective equipment. Consult your local emergency preparedness organization for more information.

Medical Care

The needed medical care at the scene will be dictated by the specific chemical. Examples of chemicals that require special consideration include corrosives such as acids and alkali, pulmonary irritants such as ammonia and chlorine, pesticides such as organophosphates, chemical asphyxiants such as cyanide and carbon monoxide, and hydrocarbon solvents.

In addition to general first aid that might be recommended for various types of exposure, there are situations when a patient may need an antidote to survive. Two such contaminants are cyanide and organophosphates, which can cause rapid death after severe exposure. At worksites where these chemicals are used, the antidote may be readily available. You may not be trained to administer these antidotes yourself, but an advanced life support (ALS) responder may be ordered under medical direction to give such treatment, and you should be aware that antidotes may be available at the incident site.

Case in Point

On a farm used as a pumpkin patch, careless and uneven insecticide dispersal results in the subsequent poisoning of several students on a class trip. The EMT recognizes that multiple victims at an open-air farm environment suggests a hazmat incident. ALS personnel should be requested and antidotes administered.

You may also find yourself called to the scene to monitor the health status of the other responders. Members of a HAZMAT response team are required to have EMS on scene to provide medical monitoring before, during, and at the end of a hazardous materials response. Not only are team members at risk for medical complications of possible chemical and thermal exposure, but their PPE may contribute to both heat exhaustion and dehydration from increased perspiration. You should monitor their vital signs and state of hydration as well as their medical and psychological state. Therefore, EMS providers may also become secondary responders, providing routine medical monitoring and decontamination of HAZMAT personnel. Often this occurs in the warm zone of an incident, and EMTs filling this responsibility need appropriate hazardous materials training (e.g., meeting competency at EMS responder level II by the NFPA Standard 473).

Transfer of Care to the Hospital

Patients ideally are decontaminated at the scene before transport to the hospital. In some situations, however, the medical needs of the patient must be weighed against the risk of secondary contamination. Consultation with both hazmat experts and medical direction will guide these decisions. It is important to give the receiving hospital advance notice and coordinate patient transfer with the staff to allow them time to prepare and to minimize any chance of secondary contamination on site. The hospital may have a special entrance or separate room for contaminated patients. Information important to the facility includes the type and nature of incident, the chemical involved and its physical state, and the number of potential patients, in addition to standard patient information.

Termination of the Incident

After treatment is completed and the patient has been transferred to hospital personnel, you should check yourself for possible secondary contamination and evaluate your own exposure risk. Exposure to certain substances may produce delayed and acute effects. It is important to gather product information and document the route, extent, and duration of your exposure as well as any actions taken to limit your exposure and prevent contamination. Your safety officer and medical director can assess your follow-up needs. Make sure you and your equipment are decontaminated before you use it for another patient, following instructions from the hazmat experts on whether any special cleaning is needed.

A critique of the hazardous materials incident is a good opportunity to review the local emergency response plan and identify the need for any changes or additional training.

REAL World

"Better safe than sorry." If there is any concern that a toxic substance may be involved, appropriate scene control and containment must be established. Several incidents have occurred where a hazmat scene has been established, only to discover later that the substance was benign (rust, baking powder). After such an event, it may seem much time and money were spent for nothing, but when potential hazards are ignored, people are injured.

Disasters

A **disaster** is a sudden event producing great material damage, loss, and distress. It usually encompasses a large geographic area, such as after a flood, hurricane, or mine explosion. A major disaster requires a multiagency response to minimize death and disability, protect health and property, and initiate recovery.

From the EMT's perspective, a disaster is any situation that overwhelms the resources available. For example, an ambulance capable of transporting two patients may arrive at a scene where there are five critically injured people. You may encounter situations in which there are more needs than the initial responding personnel and equipment can meet, a situation defining a *multiple-casualty incident* (MCI). Although far below the scale of a disaster, the procedures and thought processes used to respond to these overwhelming situations are similar.

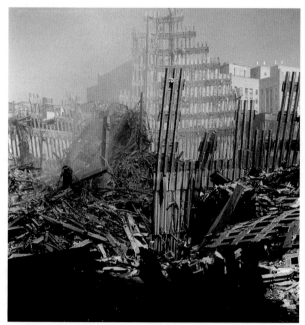

Figure 28-10 The World Trade Center attack on September 11, 2001, represents two elements of a closed disaster. People were initially trapped on the floors above the fire and then trapped when the buildings collapsed.

Case in Point

In a rural town with two ambulances, an explosion at a "meth lab" in a residential house results in six victims, two of whom are severely burned, two who have minor orthopedic injuries, and two who have minor burns and skin lacerations. The nearest burn center is 2 hours away. A medical helicopter must be called to transport the severely burned patients, and additional mutual aid is required to handle all the transports to the local emergency department (ED). Because the demands of the incident clearly outstrip the resources of this rural EMS agency, the incident can be considered a disaster from the perspective of the involved agency. A comparable incident in a large city would not be considered a disaster given the larger number of available resources.

Closed versus Open Incidents

A disaster scene can be classified as closed or open. An *open incident* allows easy access to victims from different directions. An open situation may be spread over a large area, placing additional demands on the rescuers to search a large territory. For example, a group of injured people in a field constitutes an open situation.

A *closed incident* has physical or geographic boundaries that prevent speedy access to or evacuation of patients. Examples include victims who are pinned in a bus, a high-rise fire in which victims are trapped on the top floor, a construction incident or building collapse with victims trapped beneath debris (**Figure 28-10**), or an airplane crash in a wooded area where there are no accessible roads (**Figure 28-11**).

To gain access to a closed incident, specialized resources are required. These resources may include helicopters, search and rescue teams, self-contained breathing apparatus (SCBA), and specialized extrication equipment.

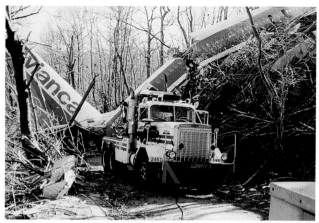

Figure 28-11 The Avianca plane crash of January 1990 evolved into a closed incident when the single-access road became clogged with onlookers, cars, and rescue vehicles.

Active versus Contained Incidents

An *active situation* exists when the forces that contributed to or were associated with the disaster are still active, evolving, and ongoing. An ongoing threat is posed to the rescuers, the public, and the victims. A *contained situation* exists when the forces responsible for the disaster are exhausted or contained; the likelihood of further injury is therefore low.

An ongoing fire is an active situation. Once the fire is extinguished or under control, it is considered contained.

Mutual Aid

Mutual aid is a prearranged response system that is established with neighboring communities to ensure a large-scale response of emergency personnel and vehicles, including police, firefighters, and ambulances, during a catastrophic incident. Even when a disaster has occurred, the regular needs of the community must still be met. Often the outside units cover the normal response load of the area during a disaster.

LEARNING OBJECTIVES
- Summarize the components of basic triage.
- Define the role of the EMT in a disaster operation.
- Describe basic concepts of incident management.
- Review the local MCI plan.

Incident Management System

An *incident management system* is an organized system of roles, responsibilities, and standard operating procedures used to manage emergency operations. An incident management system is established for the smooth operations at a disaster when multiple resources or agencies are needed. It may also be used during MCIs.

The EMS command function represents one component of the overall command structure in a community disaster plan. The response to a disaster requires an organized approach, with a central authority (or command) responsible for overall

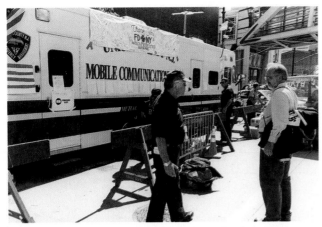

Figure 28-12 EMS command and communications center plays an important role in the management of a disaster. An EMS communications trailer from a neighboring EMS service was donated to serve New York City EMS on site for command and communications functions at the World Trade Center after the original command post was destroyed in the attack.

disaster emergency operations. EMS command is necessary and provides an essential function that is critical to success (**Figure 28-12**). The first arriving EMT may assume the responsibility of EMS command and other non–patient care functions in the initial stages of a disaster.

Subdivisions of the EMS command are called *sectors*. Sectors are named for their function, such as extrication, treatment, or transportation, to facilitate the roles and responsibilities of each function in the EMS component of care.

Triage means to sort patients in order of priority of need and proper place of treatment. Disasters call for a change in the EMT's approach to triage and priority of care. For example, on a usual EMS call for which adequate resources for all patients are available, a cardiac arrest patient would receive immediate attention. In a disaster, however, where the number of patients exceeds the resources to care for them, a patient in cardiac arrest who would consume many resources yet have little chance of survival would have the lowest priority. A cardinal rule in disaster triage is to protect and save the most people possible.

A plane crash, bus crash, or act of terrorism can overwhelm the personnel and resources of an EMS system. A structure must be in place to anticipate and respond to these events. Most regions maintain an incident management system that uses the local, state, and national resources to respond to a large-scale disaster or MCI.

An incident management system consists of a structure designed to control, direct, and coordinate all the resources available in a given region, including the following:
- Defined roles for personnel.
- Methods for communicating and managing information in an orderly manner.
- A management structure that facilitates timely and appropriate decision making.

In a large-scale disaster, a wide variety of tasks must be accomplished rapidly and effectively, as follows:
- The event must be evaluated and resources activated to deal with the specific needs of the incident.
- Patients must be systematically located and triaged.
- Provisions for extrication and other special resources must be available.
- Staging areas must be established for arriving units and supplies that will not expose these units to contamination or other risk and also will avoid blocking access roads and obstructing traffic flow.
- Patients must be treated promptly, in order of priority.
- Supplies must be available for treatment and documentation.
- Patients must be appropriately distributed to area hospitals.
- Communications must be in place that allow comprehensive coordination of resources.

All these resources must be coordinated by one central management team to ensure a systematic and efficient approach.

In an incident management system, roles and organizational sectors are developed by the incident manager or commander. Each sector is assigned personnel as they arrive, and officers are designated to oversee operations at the MCI. **Table 28-2** lists

Table 28-2	Sectors Defined by Incident Management System
Sector	**Roles and Responsibilities**
Command	A mobile center near the site of the multiple-casualty incident (MCI) where the overall command of the MCI is coordinated; this area may also contain the field communications equipment.
Extrication	Coordination of personnel and resources during an extrication process.
Triage	Initial triage usually occurs at the patient's side; the patient is then relocated to the secondary triage/treatment sector for a more definitive triage disposition.
Treatment	Organized sector where major field treatments are administered; priority treatments may be started at the side of the patient before transport to the treatment sector.
Transportation	Responsibility for overall activities related to moving patients, supplies, vehicles, equipment, and other resources associated with the event.
Staging	Area where ambulances stage for receiving patients and assignments of destination hospitals.
Supply	Area where supplies are stockpiled for the various operational needs of the MCI.
Rehabilitation	Area where care is rendered to rescuers and physical and psychological assessment and support are offered. This area is especially important for prolonged disaster operations. EMS may be called to a disaster scene where the major job is to provide medical care to the rescue team.

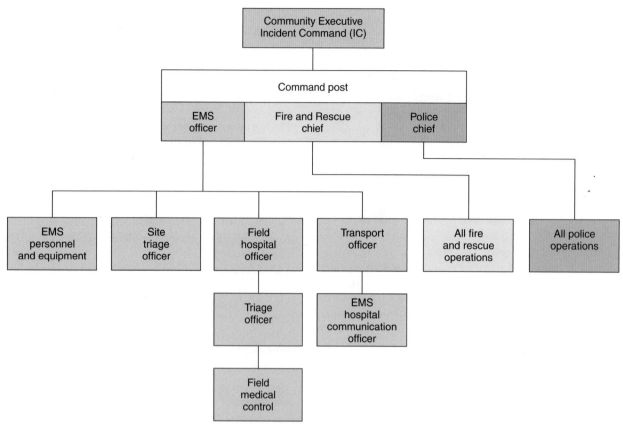

Figure 28-13 Multiple-casualty incident (MCI) community agency organization. The full scope of police or fire operational plans is not displayed in this diagram. In some cases an agency has dual responsibilities (e.g., fire and EMS or police and EMS), but for the purposes of this model the functions of EMS are emphasized separately.

examples of various sectors that are developed in an MCI to facilitate these roles and responsibilities.

When arriving at the scene of an MCI or disaster, you will be assigned a particular role and report to the sector officer associated with that role. When your assigned task is completed, you should report this fact to the sector officer and await your next assignment. Proper communication is an essential ingredient to the overall control and coordination of an event.

The three essential EMS components of disaster management are as follows:

- Command
- Triage
- Transportation

These three components constitute the basic nucleus around which all other activities are organized. Each component should have an individual assigned to it, functions necessary within each component identified (e.g., first-stage triage, second-stage triage), and individuals assigned to each function or task.

Command

Command signifies the person ultimately in charge of the disaster response, such as the fire or police chief, the EMS chief, the mayor, or the county executive. Who ultimately assumes command depends on the type of incident and the political structure within that region. For example, if there is a riot, police may be the primary command, with other public agencies assisting. At the scene of a fire, the fire chief heads overall operations, with other

agencies assisting. If a situation occurs in which the focus is primarily patient treatment, the EMS chief may assume command.

At any disaster, multiple agencies are likely to respond and should make up the command structure. The medical personnel report to the EMS command officer or his or her representative. The EMS command officer is responsible for coordinating the emergency medical response with other agencies involved in the disaster. This individual is ultimately responsible for emergency medical operations (including the care rendered) and supervises the triage and transport areas.

Figure 28-13 illustrates a plan for organization of a disaster response as well as the various areas of responsibility and the chain of command. Local plans may have different tables of organization. **Figure 28-14** specifically indicates some EMS responsibilities on the scene of a disaster.

Roles and Interagency Relationships

Effective disaster management requires cooperation among a large number of agencies and personnel. An understanding of the basic roles and responsibilities of all involved helps avoid duplication of efforts and conflicts at the disaster scene. These roles differ from community to community, but there are some universal components within most systems.

Police. The primary function of police is to protect and serve. In a disaster, police roles include scene security, traffic control, investigation, identification of the dead, and notification of families (**Figure 28-15**).

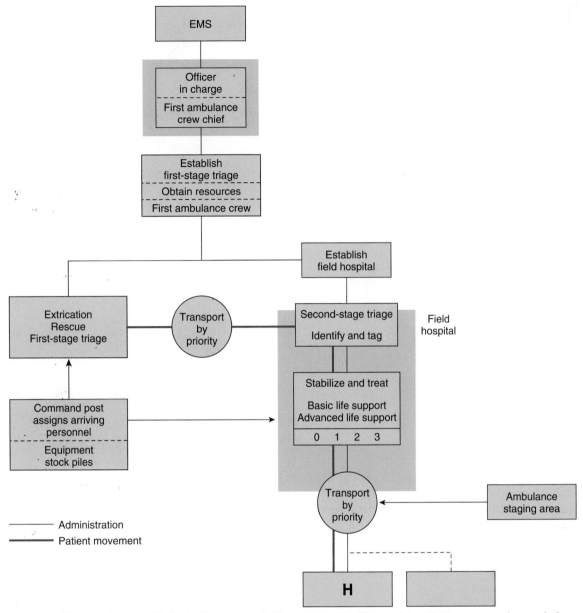

Figure 28-14 Field triage flow model, including responsibility assumed by first-arriving EMS crews until more help arrives.

Fire. The primary function of the fire service is the protection of life and property. In a disaster, fire service roles include rescue and extrication, fire suppression, hazard elimination, and scene safety (**Figure 28-16**).

Other Agencies. Other agencies included in disaster plans are public works, the Red Cross, the Salvation Army, social agencies, hospitals, and the military. These organizations operate within the sphere of their expertise, providing services as needed in coordination with the command post. Each of these agencies has its own command structure.

Communications

Communications represents one of the most essential elements of disaster management. Many disasters have had poor outcomes as a result of inadequate communications.

Within an overall plan, EMS communications should be separated from other disaster communications. Local disaster plans should identify specific communication channels for various participating agencies. The coordination of EMS communications is a function unto itself (**Figure 28-17**).

One individual must be identified as the coordinator of communications. This individual may be the dispatcher or someone at the scene. EMS command assumes this function or delegates it. All communications must go through this designated individual to avoid duplication, promote centralized record keeping, and maximize resource allocation.

Radio frequency allocation is an option available to some EMS systems. A primary rule of effective communication is to maintain radio silence unless information is requested of you or communication is necessary in the course of carrying out your assigned responsibility.

Communications may also include conveying necessary information to the public and media. Initially, this is a command post function that may be delegated by the command officer.

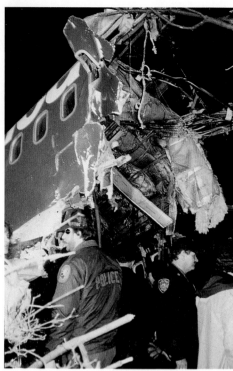

Figure 28-15 Police duties include traffic and perimeter control, identifying the dead, securing the disaster area, setting up a temporary morgue, investigating the incident, and securing valuables.

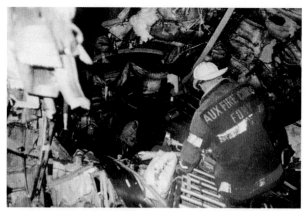

Figure 28-16 Fire roles can include extrication and heavy rescue.

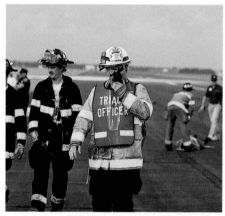

Figure 28-17 Separate radio frequencies may be used during a disaster that allow for communication of all personnel to the command center.

Documentation

Record keeping is an essential component of disaster management. It is used to maintain information about individual patients, key events, and the progress of the incident. Specific records that need to be kept at the disaster site include the following:

1. A major event log
2. The number of patients
3. Conditions and triage categories
4. Vehicles on the scene
5. Personnel on the scene
6. Hospital availability
7. The number of individuals transported
8. Hospital disposition and mode of transport

Figure 28-18 shows a patient destination log. Information should also be logged regarding any patients treated and released from the scene.

Safety

The EMS command should oversee scene safety as it relates to EMS personnel and patients. Scene safety is the responsibility of all rescuers involved in operations. Safety concerns are prioritized in the following order:

1. Rescuer
2. Public
3. Victim

A primary concern is not to add to the number of victims. Sometimes, difficult decisions must be made not to commit personnel to insurmountable or potentially life-threatening situations.

Some injuries may be prevented through the use of protective clothing, fire suppression, lighting, crowd control, and traffic control.

Resource Recruitment and Allocation

As the disaster response evolves, EMS command relays the need for additional resources (including specialized equipment or personnel) through the dispatch center. In addition, the transport officer is notified by command of the impending arrival of personnel, equipment, and vehicles.

Traffic Control

In coordination with the police department, traffic routes should be established to ensure rapid access to and from the site.

The responding units arriving first at the scene may be able to identify routes in and out for subsequent responders. This information should be transmitted to the dispatch center and to the first-responding police units. Traffic control is critical from the start.

Disaster Triage

There are three stages of triage. During the first stage, no treatment is rendered. Victims are tagged with colored surveyor's tape or tags by category of injury and likelihood of survival **(Figure 28-19)**.

MCI Patient Triage and Destination Log

Incident: _____ Completed by: _____ Date: _____

Triage tag #	Category I,D,M,X	Age	Sex	Chief complaint	Unit #	Destination	Time enroute

Figure 28-18 MCI patient destination log.

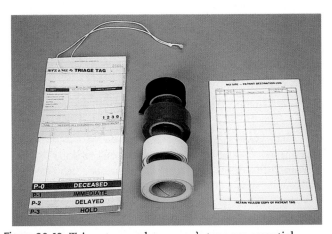

Figure 28-19 Triage tags and surveyor's tape are essential disaster supplies.

The second stage of triage begins after patients have been removed to a safe area where more thorough assessment and medical care can be given. During the second stage, patients may be recategorized by priority. This stage is a collection point for all patients to ensure appropriate priority and transport. These functions are directed by a triage officer (**Box 28-2**). Depending on the time patients remain at the scene, there will be ongoing assessment (reassessment) of patients, and, if necessary, patients may again be recategorized by priority.

In certain circumstances, a third stage of triage, the field hospital, may be created on site. This stage is initiated if long delays occur in securing hospital care (e.g., because of isolation, weather conditions, earthquakes, floods) and in communities that mobilize field hospitals as part of their disaster plan.

Advanced life support occurs during the second and third stages of triage. In some situations, multiple secondary triage sites are necessary, such as in a large building or venue with multiple points of exit. In such circumstances, designating additional triage officers will be necessary.

Box 28-2 Disaster Triage Personnel

Triage Sector Officer
Appointed by EMS command officer.
Located: triage areas.
Radio ID: triage.
- Establishes first-stage triage procedures (as dictated by incident type).
- Establishes second-stage triage procedures (before treatment or transport).
- Appoints triage support personnel as needed.
- Coordinates EMS activities, including equipment and personnel needs within the triage (rescue/extrication) sector.
- Coordinates actions with fire officers.
- Coordinates patient movement through second-stage triage to treatment or transportation sector.

Triage Support Personnel
Appointed by triage sector officer.
Located: established triage areas.
Radio ID: none assigned.
- Perform first-stage triage procedures, if established.
- Perform second-stage triage procedures, including prioritizing and tagging each patient.

In disasters, priorities are set so that the greatest number of patients survive.

Color-Coding System

A universal system of color coding is used to categorize patients at disasters, as follows:
- Red
- Yellow
- Green
- Black

Priority	Handling	Color	Description	Patient Diagnosis
Table 28-3	Triage Protocol			
P-1	Immediate	Red	Life- or limb-threatening situations requiring immediate care	Airway or respiratory difficulties, severe burns, cardiac problems, uncontrollable or severe hemorrhage, open chest or abdominal wounds, severe head injury, severe medical problems, shock
P-2	Delayed	Yellow	Patients requiring care but whose condition will not worsen with prompt (vs. immediate) treatment	Burns, multiple or major fractures, spinal cord injuries, uncomplicated head injuries
P-3	Hold	Green	Patients with minor injuries and those of an ambulatory nature	Minor fractures and wounds; minor burns of less than 10% body surface area and no respiratory involvement; psychologic problems
P-0	Deceased	Black	Patients with absence of vital signs	Casualties who have expired or those with injuries incompatible with survival

Highest Priority–Red. Red is used for critical patients with life-threatening conditions who have a chance to survive with early stabilization and transport. These patients require hospital care within 1 hour. Some systems use an emergent subclassification to identify critical patients in need of immediate physician or hospital intervention. Red-coded patients are patients in critical condition who have a good chance of recovery after immediate definitive care. They may have conditions such as readily controllable bleeding, compound fractures, or mechanical respiratory problems.

Second Priority–Yellow. Yellow is used for patients with potentially life-threatening injuries who must be treated within the next few hours. These patients do not have systemic signs of shock, but their injuries, such as multiple or major fractures, may cause death if the patients do not receive care.

In some systems, patients without life-threatening injuries are coded yellow if they are unable to walk. This color assignment is used to help estimate stretcher and transportation requirements. These patients would be transferred after the yellow-coded patients with potentially life-threatening injuries.

Lowest Priority–Green. Green-coded patients have no life-threatening injuries and generally are ambulatory. In some systems, disaster patients are asked whether they can walk as a means of rapidly assessing the number of victims who are ambulatory. Also, if there are large numbers of patients and an ongoing disaster exists with continued hazards in the hot zone, having ambulatory patients leave the danger zone by their own power allows the rescuers to assist victims who need physical removal from the scene. The ambulatory patients should be directed to the secondary triage area for further and closer triage. If the situation warrants, they may be asked to assist with removal of other patients.

In severe disasters, such as train crashes, injuries can range from minimal to fatal. However, because all passengers encountered the same force, constant reevaluation is necessary to ensure that internal injuries are not overlooked, even when patients are ambulatory. Being ambulatory does not mean that the patient has no serious injury. In some systems, no green tag is assigned until a patient has had the benefit of a detailed triage evaluation, regardless of ability to walk.

Last Priority–Black. The patient found without signs of life or with obvious mortal injuries is given a black code and is moved to the side or removed after higher-priority patients are evacuated. In some circumstances, such as a plane crash, these patients may have to be moved to gain access to other individuals. In certain situations, if leaving the dead does not impede access to other victims, investigative personnel may prefer that the dead be left in place for accident investigation purposes.

Case in Point

A terrorist explosion at a train station results in multiple victims, who are triaged with color-coded tags. Those who can walk away from the scene and have no obvious life-threatening injuries are tagged green. Those who are missing a limb and are unresponsive, or who have been decapitated, are given black tags. Those who have closed fractures of the lower extremity but no signs of shock are given yellow tags. Patients with signs of shock but who have controllable bleeding, compound fractures, or mechanical respiratory problems are given red tags.

Table 28-3 provides an example of triage priorities. Some systems use a quick method to assess the major organ systems (respiratory, circulatory, and neurologic) to help separate mortally injured patients into black and red categories.

START System

The *simple triage and rapid treatment* (START) technique is used for quick primary triage and checks the patient's ability to walk, breathing, pulse, and mental status to separate mass casualties quickly into the four categories, as follows:

1. *Walking.* Patients who can walk are the "walking wounded" and categorized as *delayed.* They are directed to remain in their location or to walk to a treatment or transportation sector.
2. *Breathing.* If breathing is absent, patients are classified as *dead/dying.* A rate of less than 10 or more than 30 breaths/min puts them in *critical* status.
3. *Pulse/perfusion.* If no pulse is present, the *dead/dying* category is used. If there is no radial pulse but a carotid pulse, patients are *critical.* If both radial and carotid pulses are present, proceed to step 4.

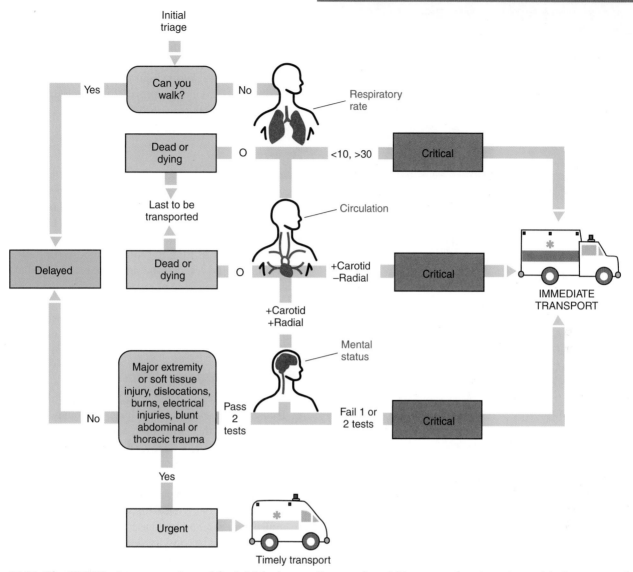

Figure 28-20 The START triage system is used for initial triage at disasters. It quickly separates patients into *critical, urgent,* and *delayed* categories. Tests to assess mental status may include a motor task (e.g., lift left arm) and mental tasks (e.g., name, date, year). *Courtesy Hoag Memorial Hospital Presbyterian and Newport Beach Fire Department.*

4. *Mental status.* Ask the patient to perform two simple tasks: a motor task such as lifting the left arm and a mental task such as stating name, date, and year. If patients can do both tasks, they are *delayed.* If they fail a test, they are *critical.*

No treatment is rendered when classifying patients except for repositioning the airway and controlling severe bleeding. However, neither action should delay the triage of other patients. Have one of the ambulatory patients assist with these treatments if no one else is available (**Figure 28-20**).

Sequence of Triage

Initial triage takes place at the site of the incident. Patients are then moved to a separate area for stabilization and reevaluation. The secondary triage area should be the central collection point for all victims removed from the debris. Proximity to the transport area is essential. This area should be hazard free and, when possible, protected from the weather.

At the secondary triage stage, patients are reevaluated with the intent of stabilizing critical injuries and beginning treatment.

After secondary triage, patients should be sorted and grouped together by triage priority. Signs or flags can be posted to identify separate areas (**Figure 28-21**). The secondary triage area is the site where arriving medical personnel and medical supplies are gathered and more advanced treatment is initiated. Triage tags may be filled out at this time, and identifying information can be elicited. **Figure 28-22** describes how to use a triage tag.

Information about the number and classes of victims is relayed to the triage officer, and a decision is made as to whether a field hospital should be established. This decision depends on the following factors:

- The number of ambulances in relation to the number of victims
- Weather conditions
- Availability of space
- The potential for advanced treatment on site

By second-stage triage, all patients with potential spinal injuries should be immobilized on a rigid stretcher and have a cervical collar placed. This may be done during the initial triage, but

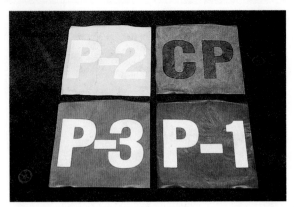

Figure 28-21 Signs can be placed at the key operation areas of the disaster site to regulate the flow of patients and identify the disaster coordinators. These four signs are used to locate patients by priority after secondary triage *(P-1, P-2, P-3)* and to define the area used for the command post *(CP)*.

conditions can make this impossible. Oxygen is administered, major fractures are splinted, and shock treatment is begun as needed. Local protocols and plans dictate the level of care to be given at the scene of a disaster.

Special Considerations

Special considerations during triage must be given to children, rescuers, and panicky or hysterical patients. Children should be kept with their parents when possible. Rescuers, when injured on site, must be removed from the scene immediately so as not to divert attention from the general rescue effort. Panic typically ensues when a victim fears death, perceives limited means of escape, and has no information about what happened. You can reduce panic by providing information, giving stable and calm direction, and initiating care. Hysterical patients who cannot be calmed should be separated from other patients and removed from the scene. However, careful medical evaluation of *all* patients is indicated to ensure they are not hypoxic or otherwise medically impaired.

Transportation

The primary function of the transport officer is ambulance staging and dispatch. In communications with the EMS command or triage officer, decisions are made to deploy personnel and vehicles and ensure smooth traffic flow. The transport officer stockpiles additional supplies and personnel arriving on the scene. *Drivers should remain with their vehicles in the event that traffic routes or staging areas are changed.* The ambulance without a driver constitutes a potential obstruction at a disaster site. If the driver leaves, vehicle keys should be given to the transport officer.

When an ambulance leaves the site with patients, the transport officer notifies the receiving hospital. To keep the airwaves clear, only the basic patient condition is relayed. Ambulance drivers transporting patients should be advised not to communicate with hospitals unless requested to do so by the communications coordinator. A transport log is maintained to track which patients were sent to particular hospitals.

Hospital Selection

Hospital selection is performed according to local protocol. In some cases the closest hospitals become overloaded or are incapable of handling critically injured trauma or burn patients. In these situations it may be necessary to transfer patients to other facilities to distribute patients by medical need and hospital capability.

Convergence

Convergence is the rapid gathering of onlookers, rescuers, and press at the scene of a disaster. It is a common problem at disasters and must be anticipated. Incoming and outgoing traffic routes must remain clear. Traffic control keeps back bystanders and onlookers and, at times, rescue personnel, who are asked to wait for instructions from the command post. Ambulances and other units should respond to staging areas to prevent a convergence of rescue vehicles in one place. An ambulance blocked by a fire truck or other rescue vehicle is of no use at the scene. The importance of maintaining traffic flow cannot be overemphasized.

The transport officer works with police to maintain traffic control.

Disaster Management Procedures

Disaster management includes the following procedures:

1. *Planning* is essential to coordinate the many resources and personnel on the scene. EMS agencies need to think about potential disasters in their local regions. Are there any industrial sites with hazmat materials (or potential terrorist targets)? How many schools are in the area? Are there home improvement stores with multiple hazardous chemicals? Are there train lines, or navigable rivers with boat traffic? What resources are available to respond to a local disaster or MCI? All potential hazards should be considered when planning your EMS agency's disaster plan. Without appropriate anticipation, success of any particular disaster management plan will be limited.

2. Depending on the type of disaster, *warning and evacuation* may or may not occur. Warning and evacuation are best exemplified by smoke/fire alarms and hurricane/tornado warning systems. Situations do occur where no warning is possible, such as in an explosion, transportation accident, or building collapse.

3. The *event* is the actual disaster that occurs—a school bus sliding off the road with 35 children on board, a plane crashing in a rural community, or an earthquake striking a major city.

   The events that take place before the arrival of emergency personnel are beyond the rescuer's control. For example, survivors from an airplane crash at night may be lost in the woods and scattered over a large area. The victims capable of walking may run from the scene. There may be unfavorable traffic conditions because of the convergence of curious onlookers and neighbors, preventing a speedy response. The latter is such a common event that traffic and crowd control are essential elements in any disaster plan. You must anticipate and assume that these conditions will exist.

4. After notification, the *organized, dispatched response* of emergency personnel and services to the scene begins. This response may last from hours to days.

How to Use the NYS-EMS Triage Tag

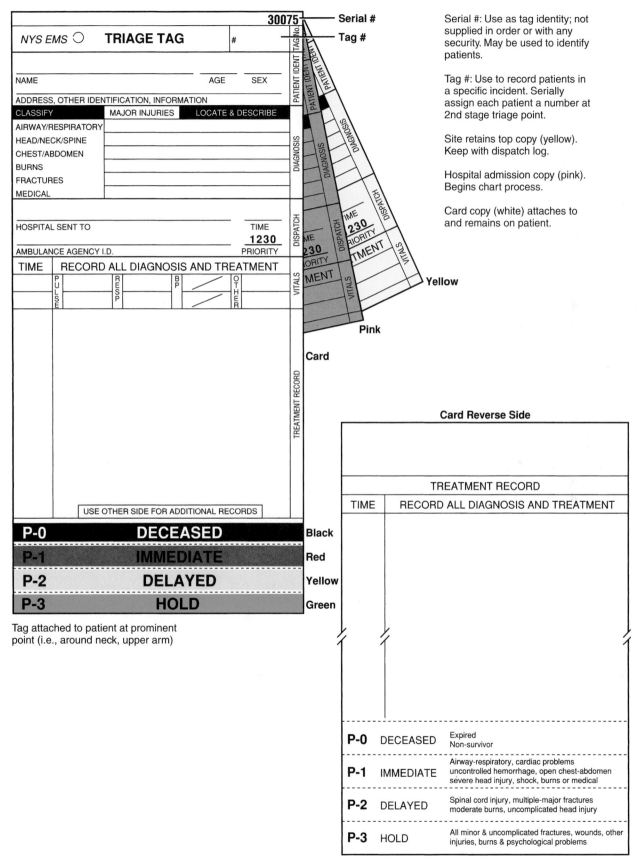

Serial #: Use as tag identity; not supplied in order or with any security. May be used to identify patients.

Tag #: Use to record patients in a specific incident. Serially assign each patient a number at 2nd stage triage point.

Site retains top copy (yellow). Keep with dispatch log.

Hospital admission copy (pink). Begins chart process.

Card copy (white) attaches to and remains on patient.

Yellow

Pink

Card

Tag attached to patient at prominent point (i.e., around neck, upper arm)

P-0	DECEASED	Black
P-1	IMMEDIATE	Red
P-2	DELAYED	Yellow
P-3	HOLD	Green

Card Reverse Side

| | TREATMENT RECORD | |
| TIME | RECORD ALL DIAGNOSIS AND TREATMENT | |

P-0	DECEASED	Expired Non-survivor
P-1	IMMEDIATE	Airway-respiratory, cardiac problems uncontrolled hemorrhage, open chest-abdomen severe head injury, shock, burns or medical
P-2	DELAYED	Spinal cord injury, multiple-major fractures moderate burns, uncomplicated head injury
P-3	HOLD	All minor & uncomplicated fractures, wounds, other injuries, burns & psychological problems

Figure 28-22 Typical triage tag (front and back) and explanation of how to complete the triage tag.

5. **Recovery** is the process of demobilizing response vehicles, apparatus, and personnel for the purpose of returning to normal operations in the community.

6. **Restoration** involves the rebuilding of the community in a physical and emotional sense. This includes critical incident stress debriefing (for victims as well as rescuers), reconstruction, and the restoration of services (e.g., water, electricity) to the area.

Roles and Responsibilities of the EMT

It is important for EMTs to have an overall sense of their regional disaster plan so that they can assume the functions required at different points in time. If EMTs arrive on the scene first, they must assume many functions beyond that of normal patient care. These functions may play a greater role in the survival of patients than direct medical care and may include triage, transport, interhospital transfer, helicopter operations, extrication, and communications. **Box 28-3** lists supplies and equipment included in an EMS disaster management field kit.

Depending on when the first EMTs arrive at the disaster scene, you should be prepared to assume any or all of the following functions: command, triage, and transport. The following discussion assumes that two EMTs are the first responders at a disaster site. If there are more than two people, some functions can be delegated.

Scene Assessment

On arrival at the disaster scene, perform a quick survey from your vehicle to obtain basic information about the type of equipment and resources needed. In a disaster, this is critical for rapid mobilization of additional resources.

1. Establish the type of incident (fire, airplane crash, building collapse) and then determine whether further injuries may occur.
   • Is there fire or the presence of hazardous materials?
   • Is your vehicle positioned safely relative to traffic, smoke, gasoline from spills, and other factors?
   • Is this incident open or closed, active or contained?
2. Determine the specific location of the incident, and identify the best access routes.
3. One EMT should leave the vehicle and walk to the scene. This EMT estimates the patient numbers and injury types and determines whether the incident is open or closed, active or contained.
4. The second EMT stays with the ambulance, identifying possible staging areas and traffic routes into the site. It may be necessary early to move the ambulance to expedite traffic control. Contact should be made with the communications center to inform the staff of the incident and to relay preliminary information.
5. As soon as the first EMT returns, both EMTs should try to ascertain the following information:
   • Approximate number of patients
   • Specific location of the incident
   • Whether the incident is open or closed (access restricted)
   • Whether the incident is active (continuing) or contained

---

Box 28-3	Emergency Medical Services (EMS) Multiple-Casualty Incident (MCI) Field Management Kit and Disaster Supplies

• Field manuals
• Command officer identification vests
• Command post and area identification signs
• Plastic ribbon for triage and area marking
• Armbands for ancillary personnel
• Pencils (no. 2) and grease pencil

Other items may be useful resources for your agency's response plan. The following items should also be considered.

Equipment and Supplies
Equipment
• All equipment must be boldly marked, identifying the agency of ownership.
• All cots/stretchers should be boldly marked to identify the agency and specific vehicle to which they are assigned.

Agency Disaster Supplies
Additional medical patient handling and administrative supplies need to be stored and made available, including:

• Ten wooden spine boards (6 feet × 16 inches)
• Bandages, dressings
• Splints
• Oxygen and resuscitation equipment
• Pencils, clipboards, and felt-tip pens or indelible markers
• Flashlights and lanterns
• Blankets
• Ground cover/tarps (conveniently colored red, yellow, and green)
• Tape
• Advanced life support (ALS) equipment
• Plastic resealable bags
• Masking tape or duct tape
• Pylons
• Stapler
• Morgue bag
• Boundary marking tape
• Rope or perimeter

Replenishment of Supplies
• At scene
• After incident
• Special supplies (ALS)

Although the kit provided is intended for one-time use, the intentional use of individual components in training can enhance MCI preparation and education. Use of triage tags on specific days, with patient types, or during all MCIs (e.g., several patients in motor vehicle crash) will familiarize ambulance personnel and hospitals with them. Staging, patient prioritizing, and patient handling are good drills for educating all agency members. Management and incident command concepts should be applied at many incidents and events occurring almost daily.

- The need for special resources (e.g., lights, cranes, boats)
- Number of additional ambulances required
- Any other relevant information
- Potential dangers to public safety and personnel

6. Once these questions are addressed, immediately relay this information to the communications center.

Communications

The two EMTs again separate and initiate the three primary functions of disaster management. Assuming the scene is safe, one EMT approaches the disaster and initiates first triage. The second EMT remains with the ambulance and assumes command and transport functions. A major event log should be initiated. Similarly, establish a transportation log with a record of all patients removed from the scene. Develop a resource list that specifies personnel already available on the scene, requested resources yet to arrive, and hospital availability. The EMT in the command function must contact the supervising police officer and fire chief to establish a centralized command post. The ambulance, with its lights, radio, and shelter, serves as a good temporary command post.

After the community disaster plan is activated, notify the local hospitals about the potential for incoming patients. Implement mutual aid plans, initiating a response to the disaster and backup coverage for the community.

In coordination with the police department, an incoming and outgoing traffic pattern is established. A site for ambulance staging is selected, and the next personnel to arrive at the scene are recruited to direct vehicles to this staging area and control their release for transport. Drivers should remain with their assigned vehicles.

In coordination with the fire department, a scene safety plan should be developed to minimize injuries to rescuers. This may involve placement of lights and ladders, fire suppression, and initiation of safe extrication and rescue maneuvers.

The second EMT's primary function is the coordination of communications and the flow of information back to the dispatch center to ensure a proper response. Until relieved, this person represents the EMS command officer on the scene.

The first EMT must communicate with the second EMT regarding resource requirements. When available, use identifying vests and helmets (**Figure 28-23**).

As other units arrive on the scene, they are directed to the ambulance staging area to await instructions. EMTs carrying supplies from these vehicles respond to the scene, and drivers remain with their vehicles. Until relieved, the second EMT is identified as the transport officer, whose function is to control traffic flow, gather supplies, stage additional vehicles, and communicate ambulance availability to the command post. The keys to any vehicles left unattended should be collected at the time of arrival by the staging or transport officer.

Psychologic Aspects

A disaster presents a situation of extreme duress for all participants—victims, families, rescuers, and the community.

Emergency medical technicians face an enormous challenge in a disaster situation. Not only are they administering psychologic first aid to the victims, but they are also affected by the enormity of the situation. It is important to acknowledge your own emotional response as you participate in a rescue. To function effectively, you must keep your own emotions in check.

Empathy with the victims is normal. However, the EMT must be wary not to *identify* with the victims. The victims need the professional skills of the rescuers to maximize their chances of survival. Victims look to rescuers for signs (spoken and unspoken) of reassurance. Because panic is easy to spread in a disaster situation, you should offer positive, encouraging, but honest feedback whenever possible.

After disasters, it is standard practice for rescuers to participate in debriefing exercises (**Figure 28-24**). These exercises serve many purposes, such as venting of emotions and sharing reactions to the experience. Professional counselors may be available, and rescuers should avail themselves of their services. Rescuers should feel free to share their emotions with fellow EMTs. Failure to acknowledge this type of stress can result in an inability to perform in the future.

Another valuable benefit that arises from debriefing is the opportunity to learn from the disaster experience. This knowledge can be used in future disaster planning and shared with other systems.

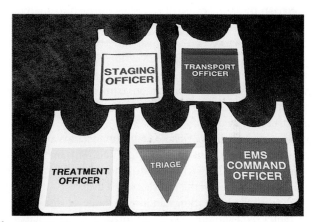

Figure 28-23 Vests that identify the key players at the disaster site help decrease the amount of confusion.

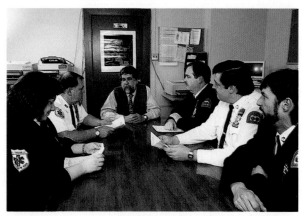

Figure 28-24 Critical incident stress debriefing is an essential process that allows rescuers, victims, and family members to express feelings and experiences associated with the event.

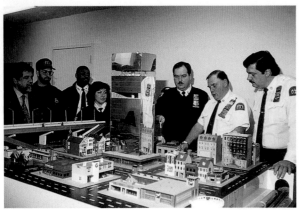

Figure 28-25 Tabletop exercises are an ideal way to practice the management of an MCI while maintaining the "big picture" of the event.

Disaster Drills

Disaster drills represent a method of training EMTs in the steps outlined in the local disaster plan. The five types of drills are as follows:

1. *Orientation.* The disaster plan is presented.
2. *Discussion.* This is a discussion of hypothetical situations in relation to the plan. Feedback is encouraged to analyze the overall approach.
3. *Tabletop exercise.* The participants try to solve a problem in a roundtable forum (**Figure 28-25).**
4. *Emergency coordination simulation.* This type of exercise requires the use of communications equipment and the physical movement of personnel and vehicles. No role-playing victims are used.
5. *Full-scale field simulation.* Role-playing victims are used for realism and are transported to hospitals. This may be a surprise exercise. It is recommended, however, that all participants be notified of the fact that it is a drill.

Each EMS organization handles the issue of disaster drills differently. You should seek out opportunities to participate in this valuable experience.

Case in Point

In concert with the local hospital, multiple EMS agencies conduct a full-scale field simulation. Months of planning result in senior citizens from the local day center agreeing to serve as patients in a simulated bus accident. Fake injuries (e.g., orthopedic fractures, lacerations, bleeding sites), called **moulage,** are placed on the victims (**Figure 28-26).** The ability of the EMS agencies to control the scene appropriately and triage victims is tested in the field, as well as their ability to communicate with each other at the scene and with the local hospital.

Transport to the local ED commences, where the hospital's disaster plan and ability to receive multiple injured patients is tested. ED physicians and nurses participate, as well as trauma and orthopedic surgeons. Hospital administrators fill their roles as defined in the hospital disaster plan.

A debriefing session takes place at the end of the drill with all participants. Strengths and weaknesses of each aspect of the actual drill process are reviewed, as well as the plans for each organization. Future training is then based on weaknesses in the drill.

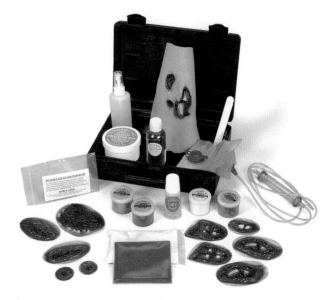

Figure 28-26 Basic moulage kit. *Courtesy Simulaids (Simulaids.com).*

Scenario Follow-up

You and your partner have ascertained that a train carrying hazardous materials has derailed and crashed into a tour bus that is now down an embankment. Police have instituted crowd control, and you determine that the scene is now closed. You and your partner survey the scene and determine that the bus and your ambulance are upwind from any potential hazard material release, rendering the scene safer. You proceed to the bus scene and determine that at least 10 passengers have significant injuries. Your partner stays at the ambulance, giving a preliminary report to your dispatch center, and requests additional EMS personnel as well as help from the local fire agency. The fire agency will control the hazardous materials as well as provide help in extricating victims from the bus.

In such situations, once the exact number of victims is known, a specific number of ambulances can be requested and the local hospital informed of the number of potential patients. In addition, a medical command post or special operations vehicle should be dispatched if available. EMS supervisors should be requested to come to the scene and given medical command of the incident so that you are free to treat victims. The on-scene supervisor, in concert with fire and police agencies, can then request special resources as needed.

Triage commences with a color-coded tag system. Victims who can walk away from the scene are given green tags. The dead are given black tags. All others are given red or yellow tags depending on their injuries; red-tagged individuals are given priority transport to the hospital, with yellow-tagged individuals given next priority. The incident commander coordinates transport of the patients to local hospitals and specialized trauma and burn centers, using multiple ambulances. An event and transportation log is maintained so that accurate information can be relayed to appropriate agencies and the public through the designated public information officer.

Once all victims are triaged and transported, additional EMS crews stay on scene and provide any needed recovery services for other emergency workers, such as HAZMAT crews and fire or police personnel.

Summary

You must be prepared to respond to a hazardous materials incident or disaster in the event one occurs in your community. Each EMT must be knowledgeable about the disaster plan and HAZMAT protocols in the community and familiar with all the elements of successful management. The first EMT at the scene of an incident often sets the tone for the future outcome of the operation.

The incident command structure is used to maintain a smooth and orderly operation when multiple agencies or multiple responding units are needed. The EMS command will designate sectors that assume the roles and responsibilities of functions such as triage, transportation, and supplies. Triage at a hazmat or disaster incident attempts to save the greatest number of victims with the resources at hand.

At a hazmat incident your primary concerns are safety and medical care. You may be first on the scene and should know how to recognize a potential hazardous materials situation, how to identify the substance involved, and how to set up a safety zone to protect yourself, bystanders, and patients. Avoid entering the hot zone (contaminated zone) or the warm zone (where decontamination occurs) unless you have the appropriate training and personal protective equipment. Take note of the health risks from the substances involved and any special treatment indicated.

Planning ahead for hazmat incidents and disasters is essential. All communities have local emergency response plans. You should be acquainted with your role by reviewing that plan—before you are needed to respond. The plan will also dictate the extent of responsibility to be assumed by EMS. You can thereby obtain the necessary training and equipment to perform your role safely and professionally.

The Bottom Line

Learning Checklist

✓ Key steps to take when approaching the scene of a potential hazardous materials (hazmat) incident include:
  ✓ Ensuring the safety of you and your crew, patients, and the public.
  ✓ Approaching the scene from a safe distance and vantage point.
  ✓ Isolating the area to prevent further contamination of the public and responders.
  ✓ Identifying the substance.
  ✓ Communicating with experts on hazardous materials.
  ✓ Removing patients to a safe zone.

✓ Your major duties as an EMT at a hazmat incident are to recognize that a hazardous situation exists, prevent further illness and injury, and provide patient treatment.

✓ To ensure bystander safety at the scene of a hazmat incident, you should establish a safety zone and notify other agencies of the need for containment and control of access roads.

✓ Until people who are trained to safely enter a hazard zone arrive, you should isolate the area, park upwind and uphill at a safe distance, keep unnecessary people away, avoid contact with the material, and only remove patients if there is no risk to yourself.

✓ Environmental hazards that affect EMS include weather, smoke and fire, natural disasters (e.g., hurricanes, floods), and contamination with hazardous materials.

✓ You can prevent contamination of yourself, your equipment, and receiving hospitals by recognizing that a hazmat situation exists and by avoiding contact with the materials, wearing personal protective equipment, decontaminating before transport whenever possible, and alerting the receiving hospital before arrival of the nature of incident.

✓ A multiple-casualty incident (MCI) is declared when the needs of patients at a scene exceed the resources of the responding EMTs.

✓ The incident management system or incident command system is designed to assist with control, direction, and coordination of emergency response resources at the scene of an MCI. It facilitates interactions with multiple agencies and provides an orderly means of communication and information for decision making and operations.

✓ The EMS sectors at an MCI can include extrication, treatment, transportation, staging, supply, triage, and mobile command.

✓ Triage at an MCI sorts victims according to three levels of priority, from highest to lowest.
  ✓ High-priority victims include those with major but potentially reversible conditions, such as airway and breathing difficulty, severe bleeding, altered mental status, shock, severe burns, and major medical problems.

✓ Secondary-priority injuries include burns without airway problems, major or multiple bone or joint injuries, and back injuries with or without spinal cord damage.

✓ Lowest-priority victims include those with minor injuries as well as those without vital signs or with mortal injuries. The latter are often categorized as a separate and lowest priority, without vital signs or with injuries incompatible with survival.

✓ Your role as an EMT at the scene of a disaster is to provide medical care and medical triage.

✓ If you are first to arrive at an MCI, you will need rapidly to estimate the nature of the incident and number of patients, evaluate scene safety, communicate the incident to dispatch to recruit needed resources, and establish a safe zone to keep unnecessary people out of the area.

✓ If you are asked to respond to a disaster incident, report to the EMS sector officer where you are assigned for specific duties, and then report back to the officer when your task is finished.

✓ After determining that the scene is safe, EMS triage begins, and the most knowledgeable EMS provider should assume the role of triage officer, performing initial assessment on all patients first and assigning available personnel and equipment to high-priority patients.

Key Terms

Cold zone The clean zone at a hazardous materials incident where EMS personnel can further assess the patient, ensure that adequate decontamination is performed before transport, and perform patient care functions as required.

Control zones Geographic areas at a hazardous materials incident that are designated based on safety and the degree of hazard.

Convergence Rapid gathering of onlookers, rescuers, and press at the scene of a disaster.

Decontamination Physical or chemical process of reducing, removing, and preventing the spread of contaminants from persons at a hazardous materials incident.

Disaster A sudden event producing great material damage, loss, and distress.

Hazardous material Any substance (solid, liquid, or gas) capable of creating harm to people, property, and the environment.

Hot zone Area at a hazardous materials incident where contamination occurs.

Incident management system Disaster response system in which resources are coordinated by one central management team to ensure a systematic and efficient approach.

Moulage Fake injuries applied to "patients" in disaster simulations.

Multiple-casualty incident (MCI) Situation in which the need is more than the initial responding personnel and equipment can meet.

Mutual aid Prearranged response system with neighboring communities to ensure a large-scale response of emergency personnel and vehicles, including police, firefighters, and ambulances, during a catastrophic incident.

Placards Specialized signage used to identify various hazardous materials.

Recovery Process of demobilizing response vehicles, apparatus, and personnel so they can return to normal operations in the community.

Restoration The rebuilding of the community, both physically and emotionally; includes critical incident stress debriefing, reconstruction, and restoration of services to the area.

Triage Sorting of casualties in a disaster to determine the priority of need and proper place of treatment.

Warm zone Area at a hazardous materials incident immediately surrounding the hot zone and where decontamination occurs.

Review Questions

1. The primary responsibility of an EMT at a hazardous materials incident is:
   a. Containment and establishment of control zones
   b. Decontamination and restoration
   c. Emergency medical care and safety
   d. Triage and removal

2. You smell a strange odor when approaching a transportation incident. You should first:
   a. Relocate upwind and assess the scene from a distance.
   b. Apply your SCBA gear and approach the scene to perform an assessment.
   c. Move away from the scene until you cannot smell the substance, and then perform an assessment.
   d. Contact CHEMTREC immediately to have an expert come to the scene.

3. When you are reacting to a documented hazmat incident, it is important to establish a place where ambulances and supplies can respond. This is called a:
   a. Command center
   b. Staging area
   c. Communications area
   d. Triage area

4. The bill of lading is most often found:
   a. In the cab of the vehicle or with the driver
   b. Posted on the back end of the vehicle
   c. Within the trailer
   d. Posted on the windshield

5. A predetermined response system with neighboring communities that ensures a large-scale response of emergency vehicles during a disaster best describes a:
   a. Transfer agreement
   b. Mutual aid agreement
   c. Disaster plan
   d. MCI

6. The sorting of casualties to determine the priority of need and proper place of treatment best defines:
   a. Categorization
   b. Stacking
   c. Triage
   d. Designation

Questions 7-10. Match the condition in column B to the appropriate color triage tag in column A.

Column A	Column B
7. Red: critical	**a.** An unconscious patient with a head injury
8. Yellow: urgent	
9. Green: delayed	**b.** Traumatic cardiac arrest
10. Black: dead or dying	**c.** Pelvic fracture
	d. Fractured humerus

11. At the site of a disaster, drivers of emergency vehicles should:
    a. Participate in early triage and treatment.
    b. Park as close to the accident as possible.
    c. Remain with their vehicles.
    d. Report to the triage officer.

12. At a disaster scene, the person whose function is to control traffic flow, gather supplies, stage additional vehicles, and communicate ambulance availability to the command post is the:
    a. Supply officer
    b. Transport officer
    c. Communications officer
    d. Triage officer

13. The process by which participants are allowed to express their feelings about the incident and thereby relieve stress associated with the situation is called the:
    a. Catharsis
    b. Debriefing
    c. Critique
    d. Field exercise

For Further Review

In the Student Workbook

- Multiple-choice questions
- Matching questions
- True-false questions
- Case scenario questions
- Crossword puzzle

On Evolve

- Weblinks
- Lecture notes
- Exercises

Learning Objectives

Cognitive Objectives

- Explain the EMT's role during a call involving hazardous materials.
- Describe what the EMT should do if there is reason to believe that there is a hazard at the scene.
- Describe the actions that an EMT should take to ensure bystander safety.
- State the role the EMT should perform until appropriately trained personnel arrive at the scene of a hazmat situation.
- Break down the steps to approaching a hazardous situation.

- Discuss the various environmental hazards that affect EMS.
- Explain the methods for preventing contamination of self, equipment, and facilities.
- Describe the criteria for a multiple-casualty incident (MCI).
- Evaluate the role of the EMT in the MCI.
- Summarize the components of basic triage.
- Define the role of the EMT in a disaster operation.
- Describe basic concepts of incident management.
- Review the local MCI plan.

Psychomotor Objective

- Given a scenario of an MCI, perform triage.

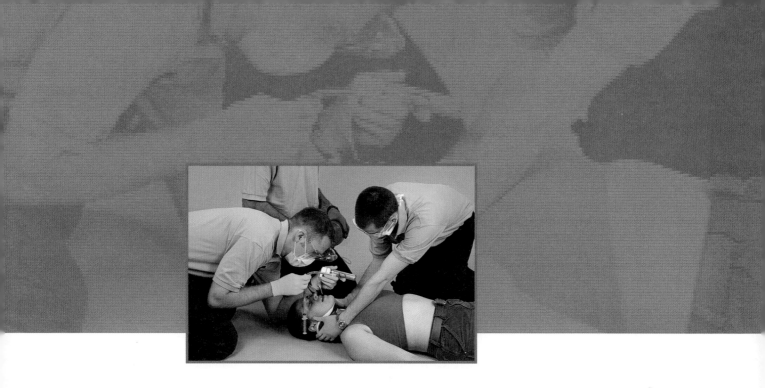

29 Advanced Airway Management

CHAPTER OUTLINE

Cricoid Pressure (Sellick Maneuver)

Endotracheal Intubation

Alternative Airway Devices

Suctioning

Advanced Airway Management in Infants and Children

Skills

Scenario

You respond to the home of a 52-year-old man who collapsed suddenly. You find him without signs of circulation. Your partner begins cardiopulmonary resuscitation (CPR), pushing hard and pushing fast using the bag-mask device to give 2 ventilations after each 30 compressions. You attach the automated external defibrillator (AED) and administer one shock. After the shock and a second 2 minutes of CPR, reassessment of the patient reveals he has regained signs of circulation and has a pulse rate of 80 beats/min. However, the patient is still not breathing. Your partner continues to ventilate with the bag-mask as you prepare the patient for transport.

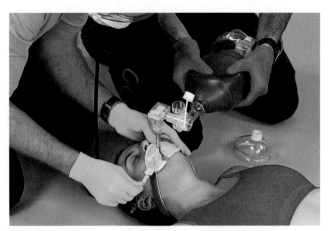

Figure 29-1 Endotracheal intubation provides the most secure airway and the most effective method for positive-pressure ventilation.

Among the most essential skills an emergency medical technician (EMT) brings to the patient are management of the airway, positive-pressure ventilation with mask devices, and oxygenation. These basic skills are all that many patients need. Manual opening of the airway may lift the tongue and establish a patent (open) airway. Insertion of an oropharyngeal airway may help keep the tongue away from the posterior pharynx. If a patient needs positive-pressure ventilation, mouth-to-mask or bag-mask ventilation techniques can be lifesaving.

For patients who are unresponsive and who require continuous positive-pressure ventilation, or when mask devices fail to provide adequate ventilation, more definitive airway management techniques may be needed, such as **endotracheal intubation (Figure 29-1),** or alternative advanced techniques using the dual-lumen esophageal-tracheal intubation device (Combitube), pharyngotracheal lumen airway, or laryngeal mask airway (or newer King LT-D supraglottic airway). These latter techniques involve the insertion of a device either directly into the trachea, into the esophagus with ventilation ports at the level of the larynx, or placed just above the larynx.

Most emergency medical services (EMS) systems do not allow the EMT to use advanced airway skills. This decision rests with individual state rules, the system medical director, and leadership within a given EMS system. Many factors guide whether to use a particular intervention, including the time and difficulty in training providers, the ability to maintain adequate skill proficiency based on frequency of use, and the cost to the local EMS system. Advanced airway devices require a level of skill proficiency greater than that needed to perform mouth-to-mask or bag-mask resuscitation. This is particularly true for tracheal intubation, which is a fairly complex psychomotor skill.

Advanced and alternative airway devices are only as good as the skill level of the provider who is using them. Inappropriate use of these devices can be fatal to the patient in need of positive-pressure ventilation. The provider must be well trained and well practiced to be good at a particular skill.

If you are working in an EMS system that has chosen to allow EMTs to use advanced airway devices, you have a responsibility to achieve and maintain the appropriate skill level. The goal of skill acquisition and retention can only be achieved by preparation, practice, reinforcement, and continued evaluation of your individual competency. This is usually measured by the EMS system medical director but ultimately is your responsibility.

Competency can be maintained by several strategies, most importantly frequent use of the skill. This often poses the most difficulty because the frequency of encounters with patients in respiratory or cardiac arrest tends to be low in many EMS systems. When actual use is low, providers depend on mannequin practice, continuing education, and in some systems, practice in the operating room (OR) under the supervision of a physician or nurse. Unfortunately, when many EMTs are using advanced or alternative airway skills in a particular EMS system, time in the OR may not be possible because of the number of providers in need of continuing education. In these situations, medical directors may rely on mannequin practice or close field observation by mentors to verify competency.

> ### Case in Point
>
> While caring for a patient in respiratory arrest, EMTs decide to place an advanced airway adjunct. Their protocols allow for placement of a laryngeal mask airway (LMA) for patients in respiratory and cardiac arrest. It has been several months since the EMTs have used the LMA. During insertion, the LMA is not placed correctly and attempts at ventilation are not effective.

Advanced and alternative airway skills do not stand alone as patient management tools. Rather, they are integrated with basic airway management techniques such as manually opening the airway, suctioning, and mechanically opening the airway with airway adjuncts (see Chapter 6). Basic life support (BLS) airway maneuvers should occur before advanced life support (ALS) maneuvers (BLS to ALS).

> ### LEARNING OBJECTIVE
> • Describe how to perform the Sellick maneuver (cricoid pressure).

Cricoid Pressure (Sellick Maneuver)

Cricoid pressure (Sellick maneuver) was developed for use during intubation of patients in the OR to prevent passive regurgitation of food related to medication and paralysis. The technique

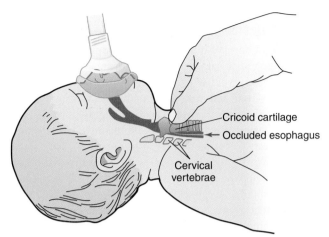

Figure 29-2 The cricoid cartilage is located just below the thyroid cartilage (Adam's apple) and is the only complete (360-degree) tracheal ring made of cartilage. When pressure is applied on the anterior surface, the posterior surface compresses the esophagus and prevents air from entering the stomach during positive-pressure ventilation.

is also useful in an unresponsive patient without a cough or gag reflex to help prevent regurgitation and aspiration during endotracheal intubation in the prehospital setting; it can be used while a patient is being ventilated with a bag-mask device.

In brief, pressure is applied to the *cricoid cartilage,* which is a complete circle of rigid cartilage (**Figure 29-2**). Pressure on the cricoid cartilage in turn presses the esophagus against the spine. This closes the esophagus and helps prevent gastric inflation and regurgitation. The cricoid cartilage is inferior to the cricothyroid membrane (discussed in Chapters 4 and 6). To find it, locate the thyroid cartilage (Adam's apple), then slide your finger to the depression just below; this is the cricothyroid membrane. The prominence below the cricothyroid membrane is the cricoid cartilage.

Ideally, a third EMT who is not providing positive-pressure ventilation or cardiac compressions should find the cricoid cartilage and compress gently with the thumb and index finger with firm pressure just lateral of midline on both sides of the

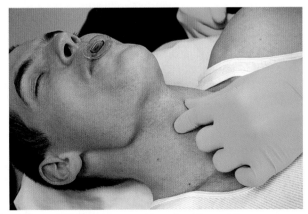

Figure 29-3 Sellick maneuver is used with positive-pressure ventilation to avoid air flowing into the esophagus, thus preventing gastric distention.

ring (**Figure 29-3**). This procedure should be maintained during positive-pressure ventilation until the patient is intubated.

During the application of cricoid pressure, you should perform the following measures:

- Verify correct anatomy to avoid damage to other structures.
- Avoid excess pressure in infants and children because the soft, pliable trachea may collapse and cause tracheal obstruction during the procedure.
- Use this technique only when sufficient personnel are available to apply it.

> **LEARNING OBJECTIVES**
> - Describe the indications for advanced airway management.
> - List complications associated with advanced airway management.
> - Explain the rationale for securing the endotracheal tube.
> - State the consequence of and the need to recognize unintentional esophageal intubation.

Endotracheal Intubation

The most effective form of airway management is endotracheal intubation. A properly placed **endotracheal (ET) tube** rests in the trachea and seals against the internal wall with a cuff that is inflated. In small children and infants a cuff is not used; instead, the tube is wedged tightly into the ring formed by the cricoid cartilage. This is sometimes referred to as the "physiologic cuff" because of the seal that is created. In either case, the seal around the ET tube helps to prevent aspiration of liquids and other materials into the lungs and allows direct ventilation of the lower airways. An ET tube can be passed through the nose into the trachea (**nasotracheal intubation**) or through the mouth (**orotracheal intubation**).

Nasotracheal intubation is considered a "blind" placement technique. In other words, the ET tube is placed into the trachea through the nose without the EMT being able to see where the tube is going. Because of this, the procedure carries a higher risk of complications and patient injury. Orotracheal intubation is used more often than nasotracheal intubation and is the focus of this section.

Purpose

Orotracheal intubation is the most effective way of controlling a patient's airway. In general, EMTs perform orotracheal intubation for patients in respiratory or cardiac arrest. Orotracheal intubation provides complete control of the airway and minimizes the risk of aspiration. Orotracheal intubation also permits better oxygen delivery, more effective ventilation, and deeper suctioning than other methods (e.g., nasotracheal).

Indications for orotracheal intubation include situations in which prolonged positive-pressure ventilation is required and cannot be effectively achieved by other methods. It is indicated for apneic patients and unresponsive patients who cannot protect their airway, as evidenced by absence of a cough or gag reflex.

The advantages of orotracheal intubation include the following:

- Prevents gastric distention.
- Minimizes aspiration risk.
- Allows access to the lower airway for suctioning.

Complications

Several complications can occur when performing tracheal intubation.

Esophageal Intubation

The most dangerous complication of orotracheal intubation is unrecognized intubation of the esophagus. The tube may pass into the esophagus rather than the trachea. It is therefore important to confirm proper tube placement after every attempt at intubation and periodically thereafter. Also, the tube may become displaced during movement and transport.

Continuous monitoring of tube placement is an important part of the technique. A tracheal tube that is inserted or dislodged into the esophagus will lead to inadequate ventilation, severe hypoxia, and gastric inflation if not corrected within minutes. In studies of pediatric and adult intubation, rates of incorrect placement or dislodgement of tracheal tubes by EMS providers ranged from 8% to 25%. These are significant rates of failure and error that are likely to harm patients in need of continued airway management and positive-pressure ventilation.

Inadequate Ventilation and Oxygenation

Prolonged attempts at intubation without intervening periods of positive-pressure ventilation can lead to inadequate ventilation and oxygenation, resulting in **hypoxia** (inadequate oxygenation) and **hypoxemia** (deficient oxygen concentration in arterial blood). As a rule, intubation attempts should take no longer than 30 seconds without intervening periods of ventilation with a mask device.

Soft Tissue Trauma

Soft tissue trauma to the lips, teeth, tongue, gums, and airway structures can occur if the laryngoscope is used forcefully. It can also occur when the top teeth are used for leverage to view the vocal cords. The laryngoscope must be carefully inserted in the mouth and used gently to *lift* the jaw and epiglottis, without tilting the blade back over the teeth.

Right Main Stem Bronchus Intubation

If the tube is inserted too far, it tends to enter the right main stem bronchus because of its relatively straight angle off the trachea and slightly larger size. This results in ventilation of only one lung. After intubation, check breath sounds on both sides. As a general rule, you should stop insertion of the tube when the proximal end of the cuffed ET tube just passes the vocal cords or use reference marks on the ET tube to assist in estimating tube location.

Vomiting

The laryngoscope can induce a gag reflex in patients who seem otherwise unresponsive, resulting in vomiting and possible aspiration of stomach contents into the lungs. Always have suction ready in case vomiting occurs.

Bradycardia and Dysrhythmias

At times, patients react to the stimulus of intubation with a slowing of the heart rate because of stimulation of the autonomic nervous system. Check the heart rate periodically.

Tube Dislodgement

Extubation (removal of tube from trachea) during patient movement is a potential hazard in every patient. When a patient is moved, the EMT who is performing ventilation may be in an awkward position and may not be able to anticipate sudden movements and thus inadvertently dislodge the tube. The best prevention against this is properly securing the tube after intubation and effective coordination of team members during patient movement. You should always reassess and confirm the tube position after moving the patient. If there is any sign of possible extubation, you should never blindly attempt to reposition or reinsert the tube. If there is any doubt about tube placement, the ET tube should be removed and the patient ventilated with a bag-mask device and oral adjunct. Continuous monitoring using waveform capnography is the standard to confirm proper tube placement.

LEARNING OBJECTIVES
- List the equipment required for orotracheal intubation.
- Describe the proper use of the curved blade for orotracheal intubation.
- Describe the proper use of the straight blade for orotracheal intubation.
- Describe the methods of choosing the appropriate-size endotracheal tube in an adult patient.
- State the reasons for and proper use of the stylet in orotracheal intubation.
- Explain the rationale for the use of a stylet.

Equipment

Personal Protective Equipment

The performance of airway and ventilation procedures may expose you to the risk of contact with blood or other body fluids. As you provide positive-pressure ventilation, fluids may be sprayed from the patient's face onto your hands or into your eyes. You should routinely use gloves when performing airway procedures, as well as mask and protective eyewear if splashing of blood or body fluids is likely.

Laryngoscope

The **laryngoscope** consists of a handle and blades that are attached by a locking bar at the end of the handle. When in use, a laryngoscope blade is hooked around the locking bar and extended to a 90-degree angle. This activates a light on the edge of the blade used to illuminate the airway to view the opening of the glottis. The handle contains batteries that power the light source and a locking bar that secures the blade. Always have a spare set of batteries available (**Figure 29-4**).

Two types of blades are used: straight and curved. The blade is used to sweep the bulk of the tongue to the side and lift the remainder of the tongue and jaw upward. This action also lifts the epiglottis and allows direct visualization of the vocal cords and glottic opening. The use of one type of blade over another is determined by factors such as provider preference, age of the patient, and anatomy of the patient.

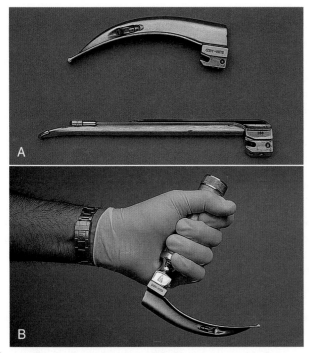

Figure 29-4 **A,** Curved and straight laryngoscope blades. **B,** Check the blades by inserting the notch into the handle. Lift the blade to form a 90-degree angle. The light should be "bright, white, and tight."

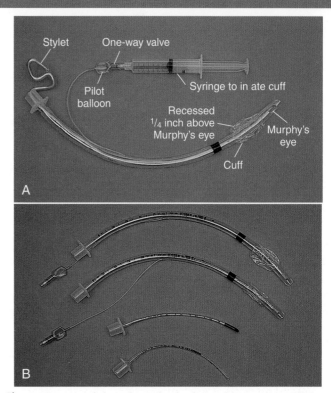

Figure 29-5 **A,** Adult endotracheal tube and its parts. **B,** Various sizes of endotracheal tubes, both cuffed and uncuffed.

The *straight blades* (Miller blades) are narrow, with a curved central channel, available in sizes numbered 0 to 4. The straight blade directly lifts the epiglottis upward to allow visualization of the vocal cords. It is recommended when intubating children and infants. The straight blade may have a lumen or channel running along the inferior edge of the blade. Providers often try to insert the ET tube through this channel, blocking visualization of the vocal cords or glottic opening. This should be avoided. Rather, the tube should be inserted in the right side of the mouth to maintain visualization of the glottic opening until the point of insertion.

The *curved blade* (MacIntosh blade) also comes in sizes numbered 0 to 4. It is inserted into the vallecula, the space anterior and superior to the epiglottis, thereby indirectly elevating the epiglottis away from the larynx and allowing visualization of the vocal cords and glottic opening.

The laryngoscope is assembled by inserting the notch on the blade onto the locking bar or the laryngoscope handle. The blade is then lifted up until it locks into place and the light comes on. You should always check to ensure that the light is "bright, white, and tight." If there is a problem with the light source, check the batteries or change the light bulb. Spare bulbs are available in sizes suitable for the various blades and should be kept in a convenient place.

Endotracheal Tubes

Endotracheal tubes come in a variety sizes and have universal features that are important to the procedure. ET tubes vary in size from 2.5 to 10.0 mm in internal diameter. The average-sized adult woman requires a 7.0-mm tube. The adult man requires a slightly larger tube, ranging from 8.0 to 8.5 mm. During the intubation procedure, it is helpful to have a tube one size larger and a tube one size smaller available (**Figure 29-5**).

A standard ET tube has several components. A 15-mm adapter is standard and allows attachment of the bag-mask or other ventilation or oxygenation devices. Larger tubes have a cuff that is filled with air to seal the space between the tube and the tracheal wall so that air does not escape up the sides during ventilation. An inflated cuff also helps prevent aspiration of vomitus or secretions into the lungs. The cuff is inflated through a one-way valve through the proximal end of the tube and has a pilot balloon outside the mouth that can be checked to ensure that it is inflated. The cuff should be filled with air by a syringe to check for leaks before intubation.

You should always make a mental note of the amount of air necessary to inflate the cuff so that the proper size of syringe (generally 10 mL) is ready to use after successful tube placement. Tubes used for infants and small children are uncuffed. Again, in these smaller patients, the cricoid ring serves as a functional cuff.

At the end of the ET tube is a small hole called "Murphy's eye" just above the opening. This allows airflow in the event that the end of the tube is occluded by blood, soft tissue, or secretions.

The length of the adult ET tube is 33 cm. Markings on the tube may assist in determining proper placement after insertion. In general, if the teeth are at the 19-to-23–cm marking in adults, the end of the tube is most likely properly positioned in the trachea and above the carina (point where trachea divides).

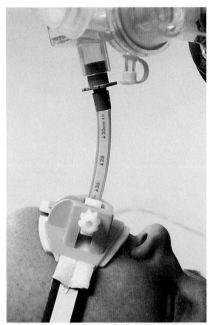

Figure 29-6 Commercial securing device.

Stylet

A **stylet** is a malleable (bendable) metal tube that is inserted into the ET tube to provide stiffness and shape to help guide the tube during intubation. You can consider lubricating the stylet before use to allow easy removal after intubation. Once inserted into the ET tube, the stylet can be shaped like a "hockey stick" to facilitate tube insertion. You should ensure that the stylet does not protrude from the distal end because it could damage the airway. The stylet should also be recessed from the tip, approximately ¼ inch above Murphy's eye.

Water-Soluble Lubricant

Use of a water-soluble lubricant can ease insertion of the ET tube into the airway. The lubricant should be placed liberally over the cuffed end of the tube.

Syringe

A 10-mL syringe is used to test the cuff for leaks before insertion. Air is then withdrawn to deflate the cuff. The syringe can remain attached and can then be used to reinflate the cuff after tube placement. After the cuff is inflated, remove the syringe and test the pilot balloon near the syringe insertion point for fullness. If the syringe remains attached after the cuff is inflated, some air may bleed back into the syringe, reducing the seal of the cuff in the trachea. If the pilot balloon collapses, select a new tube.

Securing Device

There are a number of approaches to securing the ET tube, including tape and commercial devices. You should learn and use the one advocated in your system's protocols. In general, commercial devices are more likely to secure the tube in place because tape can loosen when it becomes wet (**Figure 29-6**).

After securing the ET tube in place, you can use an oral airway as a bite block to prevent patients from occluding the tube with the teeth if they wake and bite the tube. Commercial devices usually can function as a bite block and a securing device, so additional adjuncts are unnecessary.

Suction

Suction should be readily available during the intubation procedure. A rigid, large-bore catheter should be available to evacuate secretions, blood, or vomitus from the upper airway during ET tube placement. After tube placement, attach a soft, sterile French (Fr) catheter to the suction unit for endotracheal suctioning should it become necessary.

Towels

Towels should be available to help place the head in a sniffing position or to elevate the shoulders in infants or small children. Elevating the back of the head (occiput) in adults and the shoulders in infants is often necessary to achieve visual alignment of structures between the mouth and glottic opening so that visualization of the cords is possible.

REAL*World*

The heads of pediatric patients are proportionally larger than those of adults in relation to the body. This anatomic difference must be accounted for when managing the airway of an infant or child. When placed supine, the size of the pediatric head causes forward flexion of the neck, resulting in potential airway compromise. It becomes difficult to see anatomic structures when attempting to place an orotracheal tube. When preparing to manage the airway of pediatric patients, their shoulders should be elevated with padding high enough to place the airway in neutral inline position.

Conversely, geriatric patients may develop *kyphosis*, or humpback. This change in their spine will not allow their heads to touch the ground when they are placed flat. These patients may require padding under the back of the head to provide support during an advanced airway procedure.

LEARNING OBJECTIVE
- Describe the skill of orotracheal intubation in the adult patient.

Procedure

Again, orotracheal intubation is most frequently used by advanced EMTs to secure the airway and ventilate an apneic patient in respiratory or cardiac arrest. In some systems, oral intubation may be used for any patient who is unresponsive to painful stimuli or who lacks a gag reflex to facilitate positive-pressure ventilation and prevent aspiration. The technique of orotracheal intubation is presented in **Skill 29-1**.

LEARNING OBJECTIVES
- Describe the skill of confirming endotracheal tube placement in the adult, infant, and child patient.
- Explain the rationale for confirming breath sounds.

Confirming Proper Tube Placement

After intubation, you must ensure that the ET tube has entered the trachea. Several verification procedures are available.

Primary Confirmation

Methods for primary verification of ET tube placement are as follows:

1. Direct visualization of the tube passing between the vocal cords.
2. Observation of the rise and fall of the chest with breathing.
3. Auscultation of breath sounds.

To check for breath sounds, you should begin by listening over the epigastrium. No sounds should be audible over the epigastrium. You should then listen to the left and right apexes (apices) of the lungs. Equal breath sounds on both sides of the lungs should be present (sounds are equal bilaterally).

Secondary Confirmation

Methods for secondary verification of successful endotracheal intubation include the following:

1. Carbon dioxide (CO_2) detectors
2. End-tidal CO_2 monitoring
3. Esophageal detector devices
4. Pulse oximetry (for patients who have effective circulation)

Confirmation of proper ET tube placement is critical. If sounds are present only in the epigastrium, or if confirmation of placement is in doubt, assume an esophageal intubation. An unrecognized esophageal intubation results in profound hypoxia, possible brain damage, or death. In this situation, you should deflate the cuff and remove the tube. Hyperoxygenate the patient again with a bag-mask device with 100% oxygen, and then attempt to reintubate. You should only make two attempts at intubation.

If the EMT is able to maintain the patient's airway and can ventilate the patient adequately, an advanced airway is not necessary. EMTs with the ability to place an advanced airway need to evaluate the benefit versus the risk of such placement.

Carbon Dioxide Detectors. Checking for CO_2 after placing an ET tube is helpful in confirming that the tube is properly placed in the trachea. CO_2 exists in minimal amounts in the ambient air compared with the amount present in exhaled air. CO_2 detectors are designed to monitor and identify the amount of CO_2 present in exhaled air. Some devices provide a numeric value to express the quantity of CO_2 (**Figure 29-7**). Other devices express the quantity of CO_2 with a wave on a monitor. Still other devices use a color change on paper to express the presence or absence of CO_2 in exhaled air. This is a colorimetric **end-tidal CO_2 detector,** a common device in many EMS systems. These devices can also be built into the bag-mask device.

Carbon dioxide detectors can confirm initial placement and should be used for continuous monitoring of ET tube placement. Continued monitoring of the CO_2 detector helps confirm that the tube remains in place during patient movement and transport.

Carbon dioxide detectors have limitations. For example, some patients in cardiac arrest do not produce sufficient CO_2 quantities to register on the device. In these patients there is a risk of removing a properly placed tube because of a false-negative reading (tube was in trachea, but device suggests it was in esophagus). Therefore, for patients in cardiac arrest, other measures, such as esophageal detector devices, may be used to

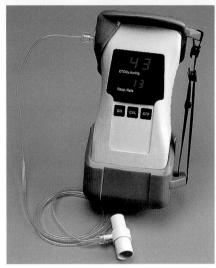

Figure 29-7 Carbon dioxide detector with digital numeric readout.

ensure proper placement in conjunction with these monitoring devices.

The EMT must remember that if any doubt exists about ET tube placement, the tube must be removed and the patient ventilated with an oral adjunct and bag-mask device.

Esophageal Detector Devices. Cardiac arrest patients may benefit from an esophageal detector device to confirm placement of the ET tube. The esophageal detector consists of a suction mechanism attached to the opening of an ET tube. Extending from the top of the device is a large syringe or bulb that generates the suction needed to confirm placement of the ET tube.

After placement of the ET tube and primary confirmation (e.g., chest rise, breath sounds), the esophageal detector device is attached to the opening of the tube. The bulb of the device is then squeezed and released, or the syringe is pulled back. If the tube is improperly placed in the esophagus, the suction of the device will cause the soft, pliable wall of the esophagus to be "sucked into" the distal end of the ET tube. This action prevents air from entering the tube or device. Thus the bulb will remain in a state of collapse, or the syringe will resist backward movement; both indicate improper placement of the ET tube. If the tube is properly placed, air will freely enter the tube and device because the trachea has a rigid lining that will not become trapped, allowing air to enter the tube and device.

If the patient has been ventilated for a prolonged period and the stomach has been inflated with air, the esophageal detector device may give a false reading.

Pulse Oximetry. A pulse oximeter is a device that monitors oxygen saturation through measurements of light transfer through capillary beds and hemoglobin. It is attached to the tip of the patient's finger over a nail bed or to an earlobe and reads the transmission of red and infrared (IR) light through the capillary bed below (**Figure 29-8**). Pulse oximeters use a *colorimetric* method of red and IR light waves to determine the percent of oxygen saturation of hemoglobin. When hemoglobin is fully saturated with oxygen, it assumes a bright-red color. Hemoglobin that is well saturated with oxygen absorbs more IR light

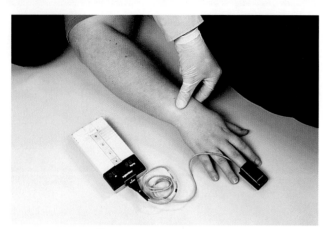

Figure 29-8 Pulse oximeter.

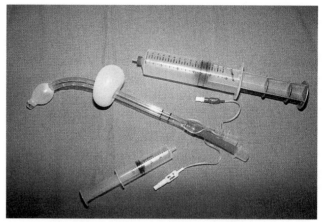

Figure 29-9 Esophageal-tracheal Combitube.

waves and fewer red light waves than unsaturated hemoglobin. On the other hand, unsaturated hemoglobin absorbs more red light waves and fewer IR light waves.

The difference in the rate of absorption of these light waves is used to generate a numeric value of the *percent of oxygen saturation*. Normal hemoglobin saturation is approximately 93% to 100%. A lower value suggests the presence of hypoxia and should be managed through adjustments in oxygen administration and positive-pressure ventilation if needed.

You should be careful when interpreting information from a pulse oximeter; several variables can affect accuracy. For example, excessive ambient light can alter the reading of a pulse oximeter. Any condition that reduces circulation to the peripheral arteries may generate a falsely low reading. These conditions include cardiac arrest, hypotension, hypothermia, and the use of drugs that cause vasoconstriction. Patients who have carbon monoxide (CO) poisoning may generate a falsely high reading because of the bright-red color of CO-saturated hemoglobin.

Because of these limitations, pulse oximetry should be considered as an *adjunct* to patient assessment, but never as the sole indicator of the effectiveness (or lack of effectiveness) of oxygen therapy.

Pulse oximeters are not useful as the only tool for confirming placement of an ET tube because data from the devices are too slow and unreliable as a source of feedback and decision making. Also, most patients intubated by EMT-Basics will be in cardiac arrest, limiting the value of pulse oximetry. In patients who have effective perfusion, however, the pulse oximeter is an important continuous-monitoring device when used with other signs of hypoxia to guide you in care of a patient.

Alternative Airway Devices

Airway devices other than those for tracheal intubation may be used to secure an airway and administer positive-pressure ventilation. These include the esophageal-tracheal Combitube (ETC), the pharyngotracheal lumen (PTL), the laryngeal mask airway (LMA), and the newer King LT-D supraglottic airway.

There is debate in the EMS community as to the appropriateness of using these alternative devices in the prehospital

setting. These devices are used more often by advanced EMTs (AEMTs, EMT-Intermediates) and as a backup for paramedics who fail to insert an ET tube successfully. Often, basic airway maneuvers and a bag-mask device are adequate to maintain a patient's airway until arrival at a hospital, where a more definitive airway can be placed.

The insertion of these devices is fairly simple because they do not require a laryngoscope and are inserted blindly into the upper airway. The ETC and PTL are used more often than the LMA (or King LT-D) in prehospital care.

Esophageal-Tracheal Combitube and Pharyngotracheal Lumen Airway

The ETC and PTL are devices that look similar to an ET tube but have two internal lumens; one communicates with the distal end of the primary tube, and the other communicates with openings in the central part of the tube. When properly inserted, the primary tube more often enters the esophagus. This places the second opening in the pharynx. After insertion, two balloons are inflated to seal off the pharynx from the esophagus and mouth. The larger balloon seals off the pharynx; the smaller balloon seals off the esophagus (**Figure 29-9**).

When a bag-mask device is attached to the appropriate port (communicating with pharyngeal openings), air is forced into the pharynx and lungs. The esophageal balloon prevents air from entering the esophagus and prevents regurgitation in the event of vomiting.

If inadvertently inserted into the trachea, the ETC or PTL device can be used the same as an ET tube, by inflating the cuff and breathing through the other external port.

Complications and Contraindications

The most significant complication with an ETC or PTL is ventilation through the wrong port after attaching the device. In one study this occurred 1.9% of the time, a significant rate of error. As with tracheal intubation, it is critical to check for primary placement (e.g., chest rise, auscultation) and secondary confirmation (e.g., end-tidal CO_2) after insertion. An esophageal detector device cannot be used to check either device. Although infrequent, the ETC or PTL may cause damage to the esophageal wall because of its invasive nature.

Because the ETC and PTL can potentially injure the esophagus, they should not be used in patients less than 5 feet tall, younger than 14 years, or with a history of caustic ingestion or known esophageal disease. These devices also should not be used in any patient who has an active gag reflex, and they should be removed if the patient becomes conscious. Ideally, patients who have an ETC or PTL inserted should be intubated with a tracheal tube as soon as possible in the hospital to avoid these potential complications.

Equipment

The equipment needed to insert an ETC or PTL includes the following:

- Personal protective equipment, including gloves, eyewear, and mask
- Stethoscope
- Suction
- End-tidal CO_2 monitoring device
- Water-soluble lubricant
- Two syringes to inflate the pharyngeal and distal cuffs
- Bag-mask device with oxygen tubing
- Oxygen
- Securing device

Procedure

Insertion of the ETC or PTL is indicated for patients in whom prolonged positive-pressure ventilation is required but cannot be effectively achieved by other methods. This is indicated for apneic patients and unresponsive patients who cannot protect the airway, as evidenced by absence of a cough or gag reflex. Either device also can be used as a backup for endotracheal intubation. The technique of inserting these devices is illustrated in **Skill 29-2**.

Case in Point

On the scene of a patient in respiratory arrest, EMTs orally intubate the patient, as confirmed by visualization of the tube passing through the cords, equal breath sounds bilaterally, and color change with CO_2 monitor. During transport, they notice gastric distention and difficulty squeezing the bag-mask. Breath sounds are absent bilaterally. The EMTs quickly remove the endotracheal tube and place an oropharyngeal airway (OPA) and begin ventilating the patient with bag-mask. The patient has a continuous flow of emesis into the posterior pharynx, which is suctioned by the EMTs. Concerned about aspiration, the EMTs place a multilumen Combitube. Both cuffs are inflated, and equal breath sounds are confirmed while ventilating through tube 1. The CO_2 monitor confirms correct placement. Transport continues without incident.

Laryngeal Mask Airway

The LMA consists of a tube (similar in appearance to ET tube) with a small, air-filled mask at the distal end. When properly inserted, the tip of the mask rests above the upper end of the esophagus and surrounds the opening of the larynx. After insertion, the mask is inflated, creating a seal around the laryngeal opening (**Figure 29-10**). A bag-mask device is then attached to the external port, and air is directed into the larynx and lungs.

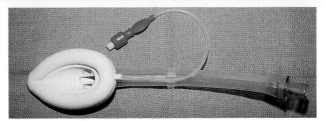

Figure 29-10 Laryngeal mask airway.

Complications and Effectiveness

The primary complication of the LMA is failure to achieve adequate placement. Studies of LMA use by EMS providers, nurses, and allied health personnel have reported success rates ranging from 64% to 100%. As with all airway devices, training and continuous reinforcement are key to maintaining the appropriate skill level.

The LMA is not as effective as other advanced or alternative airway devices in preventing gastric inflation and regurgitation. The mask seal reduces the potential for aspiration but does not provide the same degree of protection afforded by a tracheal tube or ETC. However, the LMA is better than a bag-mask in preventing regurgitation. Patients should be carefully monitored for patency of the airway, and suction should be immediately available in the event of vomiting.

Equipment

The equipment needed to insert an LMA includes the following:

- Personal protective equipment, including gloves, eyewear, and mask
- Stethoscope
- Suction
- End-tidal CO_2 monitoring device
- Water-soluble lubricant
- Syringe to inflate the mask
- Bite block or bite stick
- Bag-mask device with oxygen tubing
- Oxygen
- Securing device

Procedure

As with other advanced and alternative airway devices, the LMA is indicated for patients in whom prolonged positive-pressure ventilation is required. It is indicated for apneic patients and unresponsive patients who cannot protect the airway, as evidenced by absence of a cough or gag reflex. It is also a valuable backup for failed tracheal intubation. The technique of LMA insertion is shown in **Skill 29-3**.

King LT-D Supraglottic Airway

The King LT-D is a disposable supraglottic airway created as an alternative to tracheal intubation or mask ventilation. The King LT-D is designed for positive-pressure ventilation as well as for spontaneously breathing patients, giving it maximum versatility as an airway management tool.

The King LT-D consistently achieves a ventilatory seal of 30 cm H_2O or higher. It is easy to insert and results in minimal

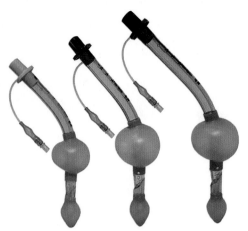

Figure 29-11 King LT-D supraglottic airway. *Courtesy King Systems, Noblesville, IN.*

airway trauma. The King LT-D comes in different sizes, is 100% latex free, and is sterile for single-patient use.

Complications and Contraindications

The King LT-D has complications similar to other blind-placement, multilumen devices. The correct-size airway must be used to avoid damage. This device should not be used on patients with esophageal varices or damage to their throat or neck. Once it is placed, the provider must ensure the airway and lungs are inflating and the patient is being ventilated. The King LT-D only has one ventilation port, so if the tube was placed incorrectly and air did not enter the lungs, the tube must be removed and the patient ventilated with an oropharyngeal airway (OPA) and bag-mask device.

Equipment

The King LT-D is a rigid tube with two distal cuffs. Both cuffs are inflated through one port. There is a side port allowing for gastrostomy tube placement. The tube is designed to slide into the trachea and provide a seal around the trachea, allowing the patient to be ventilated (**Figure 29-11**).

Procedure

- Place the patient's head in a neutral position. Ensure both cuffs on the tube are deflated.
- Slide the tube into the patient's throat until the ventilation port is at the patient's teeth.
- Inflate the cuffs.
- Attempt to ventilate the patient. The chest should not rise at this point.
- Continue to attempt to ventilate while pulling the tube gently and slowly out of the mouth. When the tube slides into place, the chest will rise with ventilation.
- Auscultate breath sounds, and then secure the tube in place.
- Document the procedure.

Again, if the chest does not rise as the tube is slowly pulled back, the tube must be removed and the patient ventilated with OPA and bag-mask.

Suctioning

Suctioning is also used for patients who are intubated with a tracheal tube. Deep suctioning is indicated when a patient has aspirated material into the lungs or copious amounts of water after a submersion incident.

Once a patient is intubated, insert the catheter through the ET tube. The size of the catheter must be small enough to fit through the tube. Because the catheter will pass through the end of the tube and down to the carina, it should be soft so as not to damage the airway. You should pay particular attention to sterile technique because you are entering deep into the body cavity. Use low to medium suction. As with other forms of suctioning, hypoxia is a common side effect; thus suction attempts should be limited to no more than 15 seconds (**Skill 29-4**).

Indications for endotracheal suctioning are obvious secretions and poor compliance (evidenced by a tight feeling when squeezing the bag) when using the bag-mask device, which may indicate an obstructed airway. Obstruction can be caused by mucus, pulmonary edema fluid, or blood, as well as aspiration of gastric contents or foreign bodies before intubation.

Complications of orotracheal suction include abnormal heart rhythms, hypoxia, coughing, mucosal damage, and bronchospasm. Proper technique minimizes the potential for these complications.

LEARNING OBJECTIVES

- Differentiate the airway anatomy in the infant, child, and adult.
- State the formula for sizing an infant or child endotracheal tube.
- Define the various alternative methods for sizing the infant and child endotracheal tube.
- Describe the skill of orotracheal intubation in the infant and child patient.
- Describe the skill of securing the endotracheal tube in the adult, infant, and child patient.
- Describe the indications, contraindications, and technique for insertion of nasogastric tubes.

Advanced Airway Management in Infants and Children

Intubation

Airway management is particularly important in infants and children because respiratory problems are a common cause of death. Because of anatomic and physiologic differences in children, modifications in equipment and techniques are often necessary (see Chapter 25).

Anatomic and Physiologic Considerations

In general, all structures are smaller and more easily obstructed in infants and children than in adults. Suctioning may be particularly important. The tongue is large and takes up more space in the mouth than it does in the adult. The epiglottis is leaf shaped and covers the glottic opening and vocal cords. It is more difficult to create a single, clear visual plane from the mouth through the pharynx to view the glottic opening for orotracheal intubation in the pediatric population than in adults. A straight blade, which provides greater displacement of the tongue, is recommended for infants and small children to enable clear visualization of the glottis.

Children have narrower and softer tracheas than do adults, and swelling can more easily obstruct their tracheas. The cricoid ring (cartilage) is the narrowest portion of the airway in infants and small children and is considered when selecting the size of endotracheal tube. Because the cartilage is less rigid and developed, a cuff is not inflated; rather, an uncuffed tube is used, with the cricoid ring serving as a functional cuff.

Equipment

The general equipment used for orotracheal intubation has been previously discussed. Remember, there are special considerations for children and infants to help determine the proper type and size of bag-mask device, laryngoscope blade, and ET tube.

The proper size of bag-mask is necessary to obtain a good seal over the mouth and nose and to provide the proper volumes of air during positive-pressure ventilation. Once again, a straight laryngoscope blade may be more helpful in infants. In general, size 1 is reserved for premature infants, infants, and small children; size 2 is used for children age 5 to 7 years; and sizes 2 and 3 are used for older children (about 8 to 10 years). Endotracheal tubes range in size from 2.5 to 10. You may use a tape or table to help you select tube size. Sizes 3 to 3.5 are used for newborns and small infants. Size 4 is used for infants up to 1 year old. For older children, you might use this formula: 16 plus the patient's age divided by 4. Other methods to estimate ET tube size include selecting a tube the size of the child's little finger or nasal opening. During intubation, it is helpful to have tubes one size smaller and one size larger than the one you think you need.

For children younger than 8 years, use an uncuffed tube. The markers on the tube can assist you in placing the tube at the proper depth in the trachea. **Table 29-1** lists approximate distances from the teeth to the midtrachea for children of various ages.

Procedure

As with adults, orotracheal intubation is the most effective means to secure the airway in pediatric patients **(Skill 29-5)**. The use of orotracheal intubation in apneic patients allows the following:

- Complete control of the airway
- Protection from aspiration
- Better delivery of oxygen
- Deeper suctioning

Confirmation of the tube placement should be performed as with adults. In infants and children, you should assess for symmetrical rise and fall of the chest as the best indicator of tube placement, because breath sounds may be misleading.

Complications

Despite the benefits of endotracheal intubation in children, significant complications can occur. In one study in an urban EMS system, endotracheal intubation did not improve survival over bag-mask ventilation when used by highly trained paramedics in the field. This was caused in part by the frequency of use of

Table 29-1	Distance from Teeth to Midtrachea as Check for Proper Endotracheal Tube Placement in Infants and Children
Age	**Distance from Teeth to Midtrachea (cm)**
6 mo-1 yr	12
2 yr	14
4-6 yr	16
6-10 yr	18
10-12 yr	20

the skill. Because cardiac arrest is relatively rare in infants and small children, however, the encounters by prehospital providers are infrequent. This study has convinced some EMS systems not to allow intubation of infants and children by prehospital providers.

You should continuously monitor the heart rate during intubation attempts because mechanical stimulation of the airway may cause a slowing of the heart rate. If a slow heart rate is noted, interrupt the intubation attempt and reventilate the patient with a bag-mask.

Table 29-2 lists specific complications of orotracheal intubation in infants and children.

Case in Point

Caring for a 6-month-old child in cardiac arrest, the EMT opens the patient's airway, places an oropharyngeal airway (OPA), and begins ventilation with a bag-mask device. The receiving emergency department is 12 miles away. The EMT considers the placement of an orotracheal tube. With the OPA, the patient has good chest rise, good skin color, minimal gastric distention, and good bag compliance. The EMT decides not to place an advanced airway because the BLS airway procedures are providing effective ventilation.

Orotracheal Suctioning

A rigid catheter should be used to suction the upper airway of infants and children. Take care not to touch the back of the airway. In general, the suction time for infants and children should be less than in the adult because this population can become significantly hypoxic with prolonged suctioning. You can perform nasal suctioning with a bulb suction or with a small-French catheter with low to medium vacuum.

Nasogastric Tube Insertion

Advanced or alternative airway adjuncts at the EMT level may include the use of a **nasogastric (NG) tube** to remove air and decompress the stomach. In unresponsive infants or children, nasogastric tubes are used when there is difficulty performing positive-pressure ventilation because of gastric inflation (distention). The distended stomach can push up against the diaphragm and cause diminished room for ventilation.

Interestingly, a major cause of gastric inflation in unresponsive children is positive-pressure ventilation with a mask device or mouth-to-mouth ventilation. Air can enter the esophagus

Table 29-2	Possible Complications of Orotracheal Intubation in Infants and Children

Complication	EMT Action*
Slow heart rate from stimulation of airway	Monitor heart rate.
Soft tissue trauma to lips, teeth, gums, airway structures	Use careful technique. Do not use undue force. Gently insert laryngoscope blade. Do not use patient's upper teeth or gums as a fulcrum. Pass tube by using direct visualization. Keep stylet recessed from tip of tube.
Hypoxia caused by prolonged intubation	Hyperoxygenate before intubation. Monitor time used to attempt intubation. If unsuccessful after 30 seconds, stop and hyperoxygenate patient.
Right main stem bronchus intubation	Observe tube passing through vocal cords. Use tube markers to determine appropriate depth. Listen to both sides of lungs for equal breath sounds. Reposition tube if one-sided breath sounds are heard.
Esophageal intubation	Observe tube passing through glottic opening. Listen for breath sounds over epigastrium and both lung fields. Look for chest rise. Look for fogging of tube. Use end-tidal CO_2 detector. Look for clinical improvement: heart rate, skin color, mental state.
Vomiting	Have suction ready.
Self-extubation	Restrain patient if intubation is essential for life support. Contact medical control to consider extubation if there are questions.
Extubation during patient movement	Reassess after every major move. Properly secure tube before movement. In difficult movement situations, detach ventilation device from tube if it cannot be securely supported during movement, so that it does not serve as fulcrum to alter tube position.

*To prevent or monitor for complication.

and fill the stomach during positive-pressure ventilation. Insertion of a tube through the nose, down the esophagus, and into the stomach allows this air to be released, relieving pressure on the diaphragm and enabling more effective ventilations to occur (**Skill 29-6**).

Complications and Contraindications

Complications of NG tube insertion include the following:
- Tracheal insertion of the tube
- Nasal trauma
- Bleeding
- Induced vomiting
- Passage into the cranium in basilar skull fractures

Contraindications to NG tube insertion include the presence of major facial, head, or spinal trauma. If the plate at the base of the skull is fractured, the NG tube might enter the cranial cavity. If used in these cases, the tube can be inserted through the mouth instead of the nose.

Equipment

The equipment required for NG tube insertion includes the following:
- Nasogastric tubes in assorted sizes (newborn/infant: 8 French [Fr]; toddler/preschooler: 10 Fr; school-age child: 12 Fr; adolescent: 14-16 Fr)

- 20-mL syringe
- Water-soluble lubricant
- Emesis basin
- Tape
- Stethoscope
- Suction unit: suction catheter
- Towels to pad the shoulders as needed

Scenario Follow-up

You attach a pulse oximeter and note that the patient has an oxygen saturation of 82%. According to protocol, you make the decision to insert a dual-lumen esophageal-tracheal Combitube. After assembling the equipment and preoxygenating the patient with the bag-mask, you insert the Combitube to the appropriate depth, inflate the pharyngeal and distal cuffs, attach the bag-mask to the appropriate lumen, ventilate, check for breath sounds, and observe chest rise. Your partner attaches a colorimetric end-tidal CO_2 detector for secondary confirmation of correct placement. You secure the device in place, and your partner continues to perform ventilation through the Combitube with the bag-mask device as you prepare to transport the patient. En route to the hospital, you continuously monitor the pulse oximeter, which reads 97%, and carbon dioxide detector, which changes color with each breath.

Summary

Advanced or alternative airway skills are available in some EMS systems for basic and advanced providers. Knowledge of the proper equipment and techniques, practicing insertion during training, and continuing medical education will allow you to provide the most secure airway for patients in great need. These techniques provide additional benefits not possible with bag-mask devices alone, including preventing gastric inflation, reducing the risk of aspiration, and allowing direct ventilation and oxygenation and suctioning of the airway.

Direct visualization of the glottis and passage of the tube through the vocal cords is the key to success. Primary confirmation by observing chest rise and auscultating breath sounds and secondary confirmation are critical to success. Careful monitoring of placement and securing the tube are important to prevent dislodging. During patient movement, be particularly vigilant and reassess tube placement after every major movement.

Skills

Skill | 29-1   *Inserting an Orotracheal Tube*

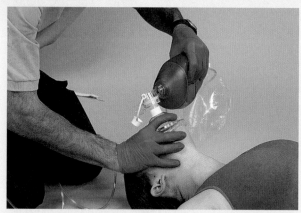

1. Take the appropriate personal precautions. Provide adequate positive-pressure ventilation by bag-mask and 100% oxygen. Hyperoxygenate the patient before any intubation attempt.

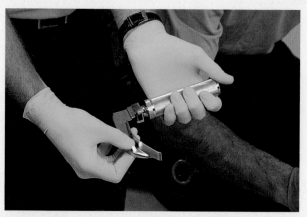

3. Assemble the blade and handle, making sure the light is "tight and bright."

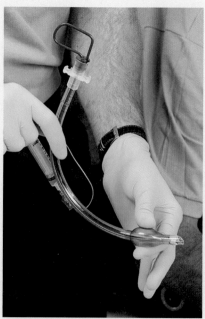

2. Assemble and test all equipment. Check the cuff for leaks by inflating it. Deflate the cuff after checking it.

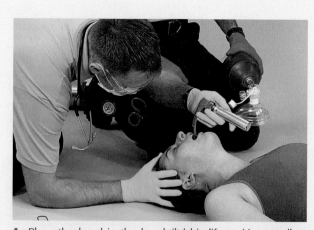

4. Place the head in the head-tilt/chin-lift position to allow for visualization. Holding the laryngoscope handle in your left hand, insert the laryngoscope blade into the right corner of the mouth. With a sweeping motion, lift the tongue up and out of the way. Lift the handle up and away from the patient in the direction it points (45-degree angle), and avoid using the teeth as a fulcrum. Insert the blade into the proper anatomic landmark based on the blade being used (straight blade lifts epiglottis; curved blade inserted into vallecula).

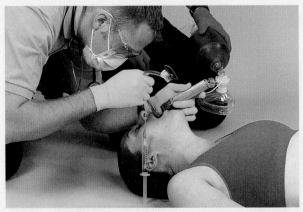

5. With the right hand, gently insert the endotracheal tube in the right side of the oral cavity and through the vocal cords. Insert the tube until the cuff just passes the vocal cords. Note markings on tube at upper teeth or gum line and record.

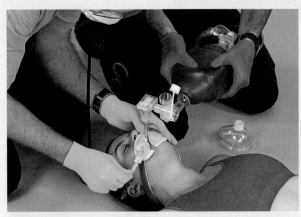

8. Confirm placement with end-tidal CO_2 monitoring, esophageal detector device, or both. Secure the tube with a commercial tube tie. Ventilate at the appropriate rate.

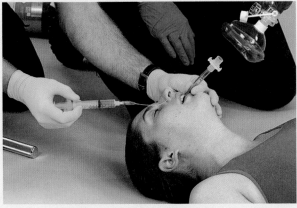

6. Remove the laryngoscope blade and extinguish the lamp. Remove the stylet if used. Inflate the cuff with 5 to 10 mL of air, and remove the syringe. Continue to hold the endotracheal tube until it is secured.

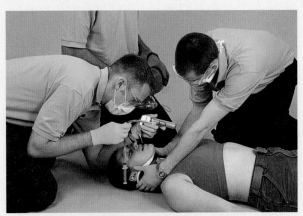

9. If trauma is suspected, use a jaw thrust maneuver, maintaining the neck in an inline position.

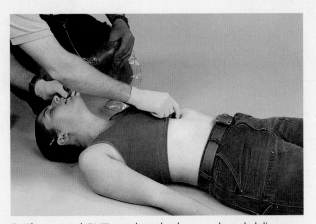

7. The second EMT attaches the bag-mask and delivers artificial ventilation while you confirm placement of the tube. Breath sounds should be equal on the right and left sides and absent in the epigastric region. If there is question about tube placement, the tube should be removed and the patient ventilated with an oropharyngeal airway and bag-mask.

Inserting an Esophageal-Tracheal Combitube

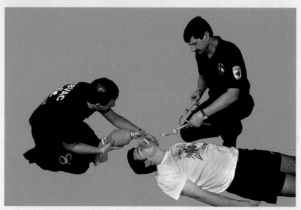

1. Take the appropriate personal precautions. Hyperoxygenate for 30 seconds at a rate of 10 to 20 breaths/min with a bag-mask device with supplemental oxygen.

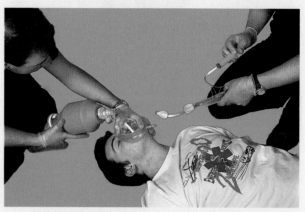

2. Check and prepare the device for insertion.

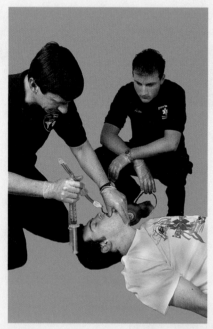

3. Place the head in the neutral position. Perform a tongue-jaw lift.

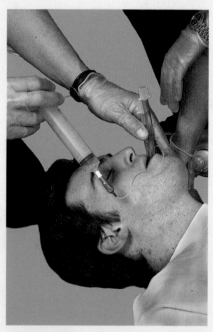

4. Insert the device midline, following the natural curvature of the pharynx. Insert until teeth are between the black rings on the tube. Inflate the pharyngeal cuff with the syringe.

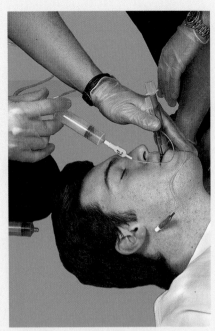

5. Inflate distal cuff using the syringe.

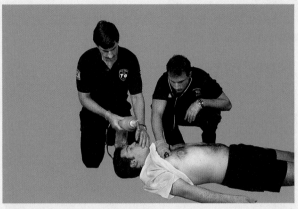

6. Attach bag-mask to appropriate port (assuming esophageal placement) and ventilate. Confirm esophageal placement by observing chest rise and auscultation over epigastrium and both lungs anterior and lateral. Continue to ventilate through the appropriate lumen.

7. No chest rise indicates tracheal placement. Ventilate through the second lumen, and confirm placement by observing chest rise and auscultation over the epigastrium and both lungs anterior and lateral. Continue to ventilate through the appropriate lumen.

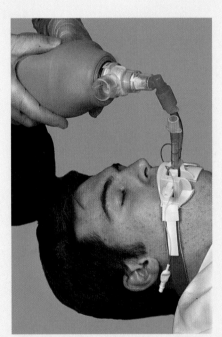

8. Obtain secondary confirmation with end-tidal CO_2 monitoring.

9. Secure device, or confirm that device remains properly secured.

Skill | 29-3   *Inserting a Laryngeal Mask Airway*

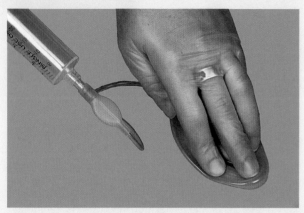

1. Take the appropriate personal precautions. Tightly deflate the cuff so that it forms a smooth "spoon shape."

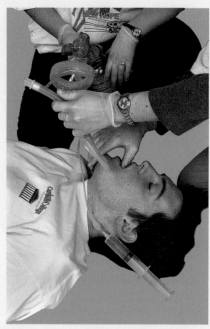

2. Lubricate the posterior surface of the mask with water-soluble lubricant. Hold the laryngeal mask airway (LMA) like a pen, with the index finger placed at the junction of the cuff and the tube.

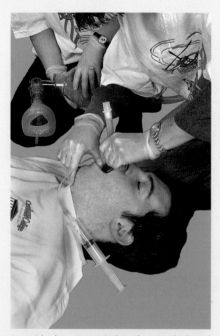

3. With the patient's head extended and the neck flexed, carefully flatten the LMA tip against the hard palate. Use the index finger to push cranially (toward the hard palate), maintaining pressure on the tube with the finger.

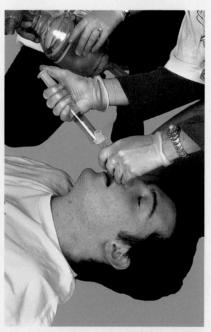

4. Advance the mask until definite resistance is felt at the base of the pharynx. Gently maintain cranial pressure with the nondominant hand while removing the index finger. Inflate the cuff with just enough air to obtain a seal. Never overinflate the cuff.

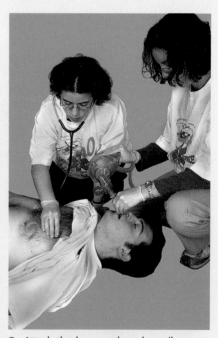

5. Attach the bag-mask and ventilate.

Skill | 29-4 *Performing Orotracheal Suctioning*

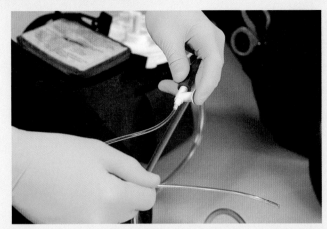

1. Check the equipment before proceeding, and use sterile technique.

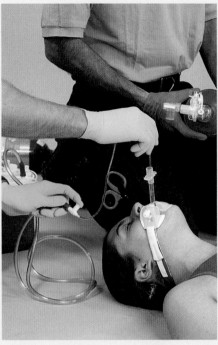

2. Insert the catheter without the suction on. Advance the catheter to the desired location (just above the carina). Apply suction, and withdraw the catheter with a twisting motion. Suctioning should not exceed 15 seconds.

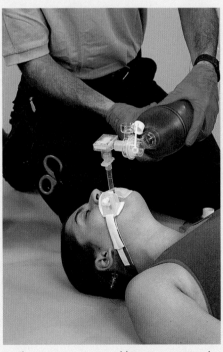

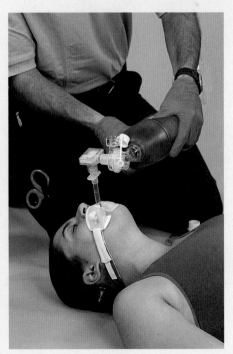

3. If necessary, stop and hyperoxygenate the patient, then repeat suctioning.

Skill | 29-5 *Intubating an Infant or Child*

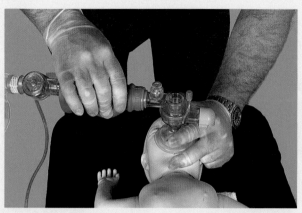

1. Take the appropriate personal precautions. Ensure adequate ventilations by bag-mask at an age-appropriate rate with 100% oxygen. Assemble and test all equipment.

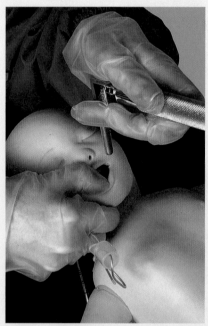

2. Align the patient's head to ensure ease of visualization. Unless trauma is suspected, tilt the head, lift the chin, and attempt to visualize the vocal cords. If you are unable to visualize the vocal cords, raise the patient's shoulder 1 inch (possibly more based on age). Again attempt visualization.

3. If trauma is suspected, intubate the patient with the head and neck in neutral position with inline stabilization.

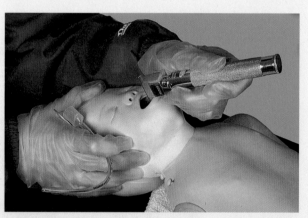

4. Use minimal force for intubation (touch is critical). Holding the laryngoscope handle in your left hand, insert the laryngoscope blade into the right corner of the patient's mouth, following the natural contour of the pharynx.

5. Once the blade is at the back of the tongue, control the tongue and lift it out of the way with a sweeping motion. Insert the blade into the proper anatomic landmark (curved blade, vallecula; straight blade, left epiglottis). Lift the handle up and away from the patient. Be careful and avoid using the patient's teeth as a fulcrum.

6. Application of the Sellick maneuver during attempts at visualization may be beneficial.

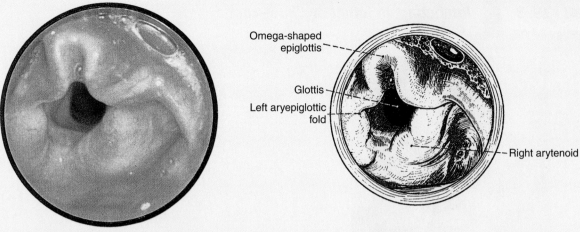

Omega-shaped epiglottis

Glottis

Left aryepiglottic fold

Right arytenoid

7. Visualize the glottic opening and vocal cords.

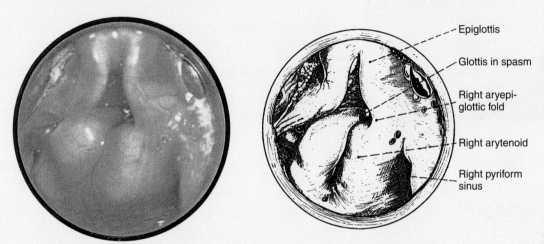

Epiglottis

Glottis in spasm

Right aryepi- glottic fold

Right arytenoid

Right pyriform sinus

8. Do not lose sight of the vocal cords.

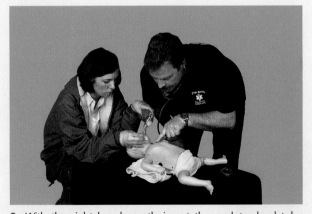

9. With the right hand, gently insert the endotracheal tube until the glottic marker, if present, is placed at the level of the vocal cords. If a cuffed tube is used, insert the tube until the cuff just passes the vocal cords. Continue to hold the endotracheal tube until it is secured. Remove the stylet if used. Remove the laryngoscope blade and extinguish the lamp. Have your partner attach the bag-mask and deliver positive-pressure ventilation. Confirm placement of the tube.

Continued

Skill | 29-5   *Intubating an Infant or Child—cont'd*

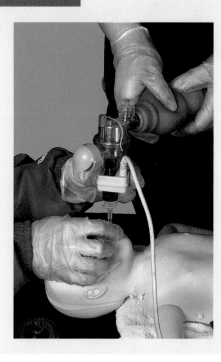

10. If breath sounds are equal bilaterally and no sounds are heard in the epigastrium, secure the endotracheal tube in place with tape or a medical director–approved commercial device. Remember to inflate the cuff if a cuffed tube was used. After securing the tube, reconfirm tube placement. Provide positive-pressure ventilation at an age-appropriate rate. You may insert an oral airway to act as a bite block.

Skill | 29-6   *Inserting a Nasogastric Tube*

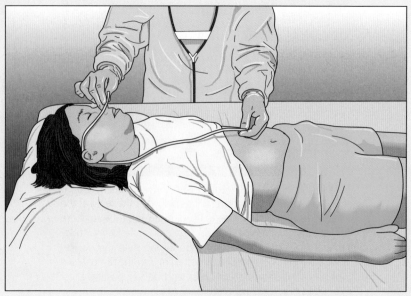

1. Prepare and assemble all equipment. Measure tube from the tip of the nose, around the ear, to below the xiphoid process.

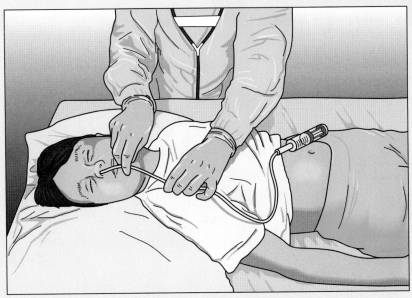

2. Lubricate the distal end of the tube. If trauma is not suspected, place the patient supine, with the head turned to the side. Pass the tube along the nasal floor.

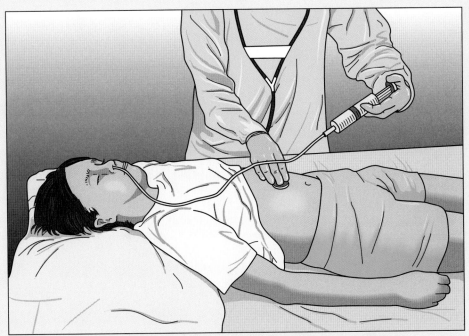

3. Check placement of the tube by aspirating stomach contents and auscultating over the epigastrium while injecting 10 to 20 mL of air into the tube.

Continued

> ## *Skill* | 29-6   *Inserting a Nasogastric Tube—cont'd*

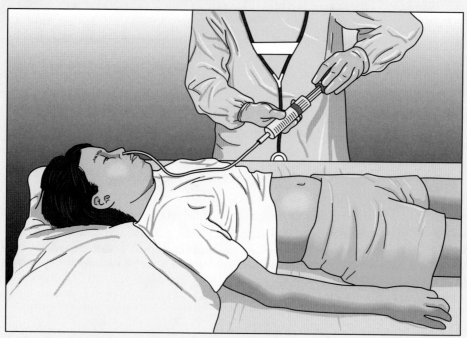

4. Aspirate stomach contents. Secure the tube in place.

The Bottom Line

Learning Checklist

✓ Cricoid pressure (Sellick maneuver) helps prevent regurgitation and aspiration in an unresponsive patient without a cough or gag reflex during intubation.

✓ Cricoid pressure is pressure applied to the cricoid cartilage, which presses the esophagus against the spine. This closes the esophagus and helps prevent gastric inflation and regurgitation.

✓ The most effective form of airway management is endotracheal intubation.

✓ An endotracheal (ET) tube can be passed through the nose (nasotracheal) or through the mouth (orotracheal).

✓ Indications for endotracheal intubation include situations in which prolonged positive-pressure ventilation is required and cannot be effectively achieved by other methods. It is indicated for apneic patients and unresponsive patients who cannot protect the airway, as evidenced by absence of a cough or gag reflex.

✓ Advantages of orotracheal intubation include preventing gastric distention, minimizing the risk of aspiration, and allowing for suctioning of the airway.

✓ Complications of intubation include esophageal intubation, inadequate ventilation and oxygenation from prolonged attempts, soft tissue trauma, right main stem bronchus intubation, vomiting, bradycardia and dysrhythmias, tube dislodgement, and self-extubation.

✓ Esophageal intubation is the most dangerous complication of endotracheal intubation because it leads to inadequate ventilation, severe hypoxia, and gastric inflation if not corrected within minutes.

✓ Intubation attempts should take no longer than 30 seconds without intervening periods of ventilation with a mask device.

✓ It is important to secure the ET tube after intubation to prevent tube dislodgement during patient movement.

✓ A straight laryngoscope blade (Miller) directly lifts the epiglottis upward to allow visualization of the vocal cords. It is often used when intubating infants and children.

✓ A curved blade (MacIntosh) is inserted into the vallecula, which indirectly elevates the epiglottis away from the larynx and allows visualization of the vocal cords and glottic opening.

✓ Endotracheal tubes vary in size from 2.5 to 10 mm in internal diameter. An adult woman generally requires a 7.0-mm tube. An adult man requires an 8.0- to 8.5-mm tube. During intubation it is important to have tubes one size larger and one size smaller available.

✓ A stylet is a malleable metal tube inserted into the ET tube to provide stiffness and shape to help guide the tube during intubation. The stylet should not protrude from the end of ET tube.

✓ The ET tube should be lubricated with water-soluble lubricant before insertion into the trachea.

✓ Confirmation of tube placement includes direct visualization of the tube passing between the vocal cords, observation of the rise and fall of the chest, auscultation of breath sounds, carbon dioxide detectors, esophageal detector devices, and pulse oximetry.

✓ Confirmation of proper tube placement is critical because unrecognized esophageal intubation results in profound hypoxia, possible brain damage, or death.

✓ Alternative airway devices include the esophageal-tracheal Combitube (ETC), pharyngotracheal lumen (PTL), laryngeal mask airway (LMA), and King LT-D supraglottic airway.

✓ The ETC and PTL are dual-lumen devices that are blindly inserted into the esophagus or trachea. Different ports are used to ventilate depending on where the tube is inserted.

✓ The most significant complication of ETC and PTL use is ventilating through the wrong port after attaching the device. An esophageal detector cannot be used to check placement with these devices.

✓ The primary complication of the LMA is failure to achieve adequate placement.

✓ Indications for endotracheal suctioning are obvious secretions and poor compliance, which may indicate an obstructed airway. Complications include abnormal heart rhythms, hypoxia, coughing, mucosal damage, and bronchospasm.

✓ Infants and children have smaller anatomic airway structures that are more easily obstructed than in adults. The tongue is larger and can impede visualization of the vocal cords with intubation. Children have narrower and softer tracheas, and swelling can more easily obstruct their tracheas. The cricoid ring is the narrowest portion of the airway in infants and children. Because the cartilage is less rigid and developed, an uncuffed endotracheal tube is used.

✓ To estimate the ET tube size for children, use this formula: 16 plus the patient's age divided by 4. Other methods include selecting a tube the size of the child's little finger or nasal opening. An uncuffed tube should be used in children 8 years and younger.

✓ In unresponsive infants or children, nasogastric (NG) tubes are used when there is difficulty performing positive-pressure ventilation because of gastric distention.

✓ Contraindications to NG tube insertion include the presence of major facial, head, or spinal trauma. Complications include tracheal insertion of the tube, nasal trauma, bleeding, vomiting, and passage into the skull.

✓ Providers must weigh the risks versus the benefits of placing an advanced airway. In many cases, basic airway procedures are adequate for prehospital airway maintenance.

Key Terms

Cricoid pressure (Sellick maneuver) Pressure around the cricoid cartilage that presses the esophagus against the spine, preventing regurgitation and aspiration.

Endotracheal intubation Process of placing an endotracheal tube in the trachea using orotracheal or nasotracheal technique.

Endotracheal (ET) tube Soft tube with an inflatable cuff that is inserted into the trachea with the aid of a laryngoscope.

End-tidal CO_2 detector Device that changes color (colorimetric) when exposed to carbon dioxide (CO_2); used to confirm placement of advanced airway device. Some CO_2 detectors give a quantitative reading; others display waveforms.

Hypoxemia Abnormal deficiency in oxygen concentration of arterial blood.

Hypoxia Inadequate oxygenation.

Laryngoscope Plastic or metal device used to visualize the vocal cords to insert an endotracheal tube.

Nasogastric (NG) tube Tube inserted into the esophagus and into the stomach to allow air to be released, relieve pressure on the diaphragm, and enable more effective ventilations to occur.

Nasotracheal intubation Intubation of the trachea through the nose.

Orotracheal intubation Intubation of the trachea through the mouth.

Stylet Malleable metal tube that is inserted into the endotracheal tube to provide stiffness and shape to help guide the tube during intubation.

Review Questions

1. Severe gastric distention and an inability to artificially ventilate an unresponsive child are indications for which of the following procedures?
   a. Inserting a nasogastric tube.
   b. Inserting a stylet.
   c. Increasing the rate and force of breathing.
   d. Placing the child in the head-down position.

2. Which of the following is an advantage of orotracheal intubation?
   a. It requires minimal practice.
   b. It is not associated with complications.
   c. It helps prevents aspiration.
   d. It is the simplest approach to airway management.

3. Which of the following endotracheal tubes is most suitable for an average adult woman?
   a. 3.5 mm
   b. 4.5 mm
   c. 5.5 mm
   d. 7.0 mm

4. When using a curved (MacIntosh) laryngoscope blade, the tip should be inserted to which of the following structures?
   a. Uvula
   b. Glottis
   c. Cricoid
   d. Vallecula

5. Which of the following is a common complication of orotracheal intubation?
   a. Esophageal intubation
   b. EMT fatigue caused by prolonged intubation attempts
   c. Trauma to the bronchioles and alveoli
   d. Left main stem bronchus intubation

6. Which of the following is not considered confirmation of correct endotracheal tube placement?
   a. Auscultation for breath sounds
   b. End-tidal CO_2 monitoring
   c. Return of spontaneous ventilations
   d. Visualization of the tube passing through the vocal cords

7. During endotracheal suctioning, when should suctioning be initiated?
   a. While inserting the catheter down the tube
   b. At the level of secretions
   c. Before inserting the catheter down the tube
   d. While withdrawing the catheter

8. A nasogastric tube is measured from the nose, around the ear, and down to what level?
   a. Stomach
   b. Nipple
   c. Xiphoid process
   d. Umbilicus

9. Which of the following presents the greatest risk for endotracheal tube dislodgement or extubation?
   a. While using a bag-mask device
   b. During endotracheal suction
   c. During major movement of the patient
   d. During nasogastric tube insertion

10. What is the most common location for an ETC or PTL when placed?
    a. Trachea
    b. Esophagus
    c. Pharynx
    d. Vallecula

For Further Review

In the Student Workbook

- Multiple-choice questions
- Matching questions
- Fill-in-the-blank questions
- Short-answer questions
- True-false questions
- Case scenario questions

On Evolve

- Weblinks
- Lecture notes
- Exercises

Learning Objectives

Cognitive Objectives

- Describe how to perform the Sellick maneuver (cricoid pressure).
- Describe the indications for advanced airway management.
- List complications associated with advanced airway management.
- State the consequence of and the need to recognize unintentional esophageal intubation.
- List the equipment required for orotracheal intubation.
- Describe the proper use of the curved blade for orotracheal intubation.
- Describe the proper use of the straight blade for orotracheal intubation.
- Describe the methods of choosing the appropriate-size endotracheal tube in an adult patient.
- State the reasons for and proper use of the stylet in orotracheal intubation.
- Describe the skill of orotracheal intubation in the infant and child patient.
- Describe the skill of confirming endotracheal tube placement in the adult, infant, and child patient.

- Identify and describe the airway anatomy in the infant, child, and adult (see Chapters 6 and 25).
- Differentiate the airway anatomy in the infant, child, and adult.
- Define the various alternative methods for sizing the infant and child endotracheal tube.
- Describe the skill of securing the endotracheal tube in the adult, infant, and child patient.
- Describe the indications, contraindications, and technique for insertion of nasogastric tubes.

Affective Objectives

- Recognize and respect the feelings of the patient and family during advanced airway procedures.
- Explain the value of performing advanced airway procedures.
- Defend the need for the EMT-Basic to perform advanced airway procedures.
- Explain the rationale for the use of a stylet.
- Explain the rationale for having a suction unit immediately available during intubation attempts.
- Explain the rationale for confirming breath sounds.
- Explain the rationale for securing the endotracheal tube.

Psychomotor Objectives

- Demonstrate how to perform the Sellick maneuver (cricoid pressure).
- Demonstrate the skill of orotracheal intubation in the adult patient.
- Demonstrate the skill of orotracheal intubation in the infant and child patient.
- Demonstrate the skill of confirming endotracheal tube placement in the adult patient.
- Demonstrate the skill of confirming endotracheal tube placement in the infant and child patient.
- Demonstrate the skill of securing the endotracheal tube in the adult patient.
- Demonstrate the skill of securing the endotracheal tube in the infant and child patient.

Reference

Rich JM, Mason AM, Bey TA, et al: The critical airway, rescue ventilation, and the Combitube. Part 2, *AANA J* 72(2), April 2004. http://www.airwayeducation.com/PDFs/AANA_ARTICLE_4-04.pdf

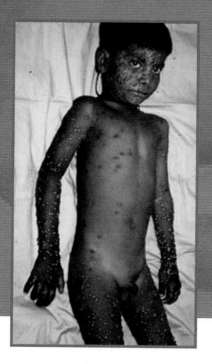

Weapons of Mass
30 Destruction and the EMT

CHAPTER OUTLINE

Scenario

You respond to a report of several casualties at a downtown bus terminal. Several emergency response units are already on scene, including police, fire, and emergency medical services (EMS). At scene size-up you note several people lying outside a bus in respiratory distress with muscular twitching. No unusual odors, fumes, or liquids have been noted.

You are directed to a staging area, upwind and several hundred feet away from the terminal, with egress for the ambulance. From there you are directed to evaluate passengers at a secondary triage unit, where EMS personnel have led ambulatory patients who are complaining of visual disturbances and shortness of breath. Many other people at the bus station are extremely anxious and asking for medical attention. You assess that most patients with visual complaints and breathing problems have small pupils and secretions. They tell you that they had just arrived on a bus from the airport, and that many people at the back of the bus had collapsed with convulsions before arriving at the station.

Many other people from the bus station also proceed to your area. Most are very anxious, without specific complaints. You direct all who can walk to retreat from the area, stay upwind, and keep onlookers away. You separate the patients with physical findings and shortness of breath from those who are anxious. You report your findings to medical command.

The previous scenario is consistent with a terrorist attack with *sarin*, a nerve agent used as an agent of war and mass destruction. Sarin is a liquid that quickly evaporates at room temperature. Within a closed space such as the bus, the vapors would accumulate and linger, exposing the passengers. This scenario is consistent with a terrorist sitting in the back of the bus and pouring liquid sarin onto the floor before exiting the bus.

The role of the emergency medical technician (EMT) in such a scenario is medical evaluation and care. Eliciting signs and symptoms of the victims with different degrees of exposure was useful in pointing to a nerve agent as the toxic agent. Stocking nerve agent antidote on the ambulance helps bring needed medication forward to the scene, where victims with great toxicity are most likely to benefit. Adjusting dosage for pediatric patients is part of the EMS care for all ages. Leaving extrication to properly prepared hazardous materials (HAZMAT) specialists prevents unnecessary casualties of emergency personnel. Police play a vital role in establishing ingress and egress for responding units, crowd control, and investigation. Indeed, the person involved in a terrorist act may indeed be one of the "victims" cared for by EMS personnel. Care for bystanders is a critical aspect of terrorist events, to prevent spread of panic and escalation of chaos at the scene and within the community.

Domestic preparedness against terrorism is part of life in the world today. Since September 11, 2001, when the World Trade Center and Pentagon were attacked by hijacked planes, the United States has been on high alert (**Figure 30-1**). The mailing of anthrax-tainted letters in the fall of 2001 left no doubt that the world had changed profoundly. In large and small communities across the country, tainted letters and look-alike hoaxes challenged emergency responders and tested response plans.

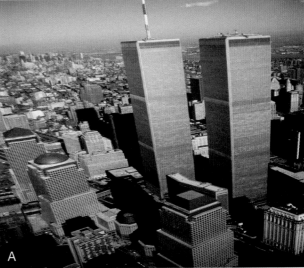

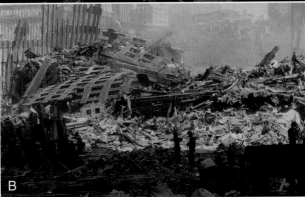

Figure 30-1 **A,** The World Trade Center was a known target since it was bombed in 1993. This picture was included in a weapons of mass destruction (WMD) awareness training course before the 2001 attack. **B,** Site of the World Trade Center disaster 6 days after the attack on September 11, 2001, when the search for victims continued.

Emergency responders across the world knew their preparations for terrorist use of chemical, biologic, or nuclear agents against the civilian population were no longer just drills. The unthinkable became openly discussed.

> **LEARNING OBJECTIVE**
> • Describe the role of an EMT at a nuclear, biologic, or chemical (NBC) event.

Terrorism Preparedness and Response

History is full of mass killings that invoke fear throughout the population. The goal of the terrorist is not just to kill or maim, but also to make the population feel unsafe, destabilize society, and spread fear and panic.

Plane hijackings, letter bombs, and building explosions are scenarios recognized as terrorist acts, but biologic and chemical terrorist acts have taken place as well. Food poisonings in Oregon in the 1980s were a terrorist plot. Terrorists have used sarin gas on at least two occasions in Japan. With reports of large-scale production of chemical and biologic agents in countries, such as the Soviet Union, Iraq, and South Africa, and terrorists' threats to use them against civilians, the potential for mass casualties has to be taken seriously. We can no longer think of these agents as acts of war, but scenarios that may be encountered on a random basis anywhere in the world.

Preparing for Terrorist Events

The United States has geared up its efforts for domestic preparedness substantially since the mid-1990s. The United States Policy on Counterterrorism, signed by President Clinton on June 21, 1995, provided the framework for the federal government response. The response offered operational support to identify and assess the threat, neutralize the toxic substance, and decontaminate victims and the environment. Cities thought to be likely targets for terrorism were given federal grants and planning assistance to bolster their emergency response plans. A Metropolitan Medical Response System was encouraged by contracts from Congress with 120 of the more populous cities in the United States. These contracts aimed to enhance local ability to respond to consequences of weapons of mass destruction terrorism. These contracts had many components, including agent detection and identification, patient decontamination, triage and medical treatment, emergency transportation of patients to local hospitals, coordination of movement of patients to more distant hospitals by the National Disaster Medical System, and plans for handling nonsurvivors. The plan seeks to enhance the capability of the local system, incorporating the local EMS system, HAZMAT personnel, law enforcement, public health agencies, and other local resources.

Preparation for all disasters must begin at home. *Emergency responders in each community will be tested first,* before help arrives. Disasters and their response may continue for days and weeks, but the actions of the first responders will greatly influence how the response evolves.

Training for Response to Terrorist Events

Terrorist incidents may involve explosive, incendiary, nuclear, biologic, or chemical agents. EMS traditionally addresses trauma and burns and multiple-casualty incidents (MCIs) and response to disasters. Training for nuclear, biologic, and chemical agents complements traditional EMS training and helps EMTs to be prepared to respond.

Courses offered by the U.S. Army, the Department of Defense (DOD), and the Department of Justice, among others, have offered first responders additional training to recognize and respond to possible *nuclear, biologic, and chemical* (NBC) terrorist threats. Materials such as the Domestic Preparedness Training Program (v8.0), available for several years now, present general awareness training as well as specific advanced courses for different responders and components of the healthcare system. (Highlights are incorporated in this chapter with permission from authors of the program.) These courses are highly recommended. The Centers for Disease Control and Prevention (CDC) website at www.cdc.gov is one of many sources to find current training modules and information about terrorist agents.

Box 30-1	Class A Biologic Agents and Four Key Classes of Chemical Agents*

Class A Biologic Agents (CDC)
Anthrax
Botulinum toxin
Plague
Smallpox
Tularemia
Viral hemorrhagic fever

Chemical Agent Categories
Nerve agents
Cyanide
Vesicants (sulfur mustard)
Pulmonary agents

*The agents listed are considered high threats and important for teaching principles of weapons of mass destruction (WMD) response to biologic and chemical incidents. Many other agents also have WMD potential.
CDC, Centers for Disease Control and Prevention.

Although not part of traditional EMT training, you must be ready to include agents of mass destruction in your analysis during a scene size-up. The goal is to recognize hazards early, take appropriate protective precautions, and respond to the medical needs of the victims in a manner that ensures your safety as well as that of bystanders and the patient.

The intent of this chapter is to raise awareness of the possibility of an NBC attack and discuss features that are similar and that differ from a hazardous materials or infectious disease incident. The role of the EMT is to recognize a possible NBC event; take actions to promote safety of self, bystanders, and the victims; and provide medical care. The EMT needs to be alert for signs and symptoms of some of the most likely agents. Awareness and recognition lead to actions, which promote safety. By briefly considering some of the chemical and biologic agents a terrorist may use, you will better understand the type of personal protection required, decontamination strategies, and first-aid and medical considerations dictated by different agents (**Box 30-1**).

LEARNING OBJECTIVES
- Describe the threat of an NBC incident by terrorists.
- Distinguish a hazardous materials incident from an NBC terrorist event.

Terrorist Weapons of Mass Destruction Events

Weapons of mass destruction (WMDs) include NBC agents. EMTs are prepared for infectious diseases as part of everyday practice. Likewise, EMTs are aware that they may respond to hazardous materials (HAZMAT, hazmat) situations as part of a medical response; in fact, many EMTs take specialized hazmat training. What additional preparation is needed to deal with WMDs? To understand the need for additional training, it is useful to understand the purpose of terrorism and the types of agents that may be used.

	Hazmat Incident	NBC Incident
Table 30-1 Hazardous Materials (Hazmat) Incident versus Nuclear, Biologic, or Chemical (NBC) Terrorism Incident		
Variable		
Deliberate attack		X
Greater agent toxicity		X
Early hazard identification	X	
Potential for mass casualties		X
Need for mass decontamination		X
Unusual risk to healthcare providers		X
Crime scene and evidence preservation	X	X
Major interaction/coordination with local, state, and federal agencies		X
EMS and hospitals quickly overwhelmed		X
Secondary device designed to kill responders		X

A distinguishing feature of terrorism is the intent to kill innocent victims, destabilize government and civil order, and wreak panic and fear throughout the population.

Features of an NBC terrorist incident that distinguish it from a hazmat incident include the following:

1. It is deliberate attack, not accidental.
2. The exact hazard is purposely hidden, and discovery requires recognition of signs and symptoms and active investigation. Contrast this to the placards and shipping papers used to identify the presence of hazardous materials.
3. The material is extremely toxic, designed to kill or cause debilitating illness or injury, and produces mass numbers of casualties, which could overwhelm the first responders and the health system.
4. There may be a need for mass decontamination.

First responders need to be especially wary of secondary devices, which are set to detonate after the first event. These secondary devices may be intended to kill those responding to the aid of the initial victims.

Terrorist events are crime scenes, and preservation of potential evidence is important to law enforcement, who will respond to the event along with multiple other local, state, and federal agencies (**Table 30-1**).

Overview of Nuclear, Biologic, and Chemical Agents

Nuclear Agents

Nuclear agents have caused fear since they were first used in World War II. In the Cold War period when Russia and the United States were in a nuclear arms race, children practiced getting under their desks at school in air-raid drills. Schools and other public buildings were designated as fallout shelters, with the familiar nuclear sign hanging on the wall. Some families even built personal fallout shelters and stocked them with water and food to sustain them for time underground if World War III were to unfold. Since then, controversy about the safety of nuclear power plants has been the topic of recurrent debates. Some power plants were forced to close because the nearby residents feared possible nuclear incidents. The nuclear accidents at Three Mile Island and Chernobyl are examples of the dangers that could occur with a nuclear leak or meltdown.

Although experts believe the threat of terrorist release of nuclear materials is less likely than the use of chemical or biologic agents, nuclear threats do exist. So-called suitcase bombs are reportedly available, and some fear they could be detonated in a crowded area. Sabotage of nuclear power plants is another fear. Dispersal of radioactive products, with or without an accompanying explosion ("dirty bomb"), is another scenario thought to be more likely. Regardless of the cause, the basic principles of radiation are useful in understanding the potential problems that a release of radiation poses to the first responders and the community. Knowing whether a victim is contaminated or irradiated makes a difference in patient handling, and the concepts of distance, time (duration of exposure), and shielding are all used to reduce risk.

Biologic Agents

Biologic agents in general do not act immediately. After a virus or bacteria is contracted by the victim, there is an incubation period (usually days) before the victim becomes symptomatic and seeks care. The public may not know a terrorist attack has taken place until some time after the actual release of the agent. Hours or days later, many victims may present to their physicians or emergency departments (EDs) with symptoms of the disease, overwhelming the health system.

Most biologic agents are not contagious, and only the victims originally exposed develop the disease. However, some agents, such as smallpox and the plague, can be spread from person to person. It has been reported that during periods of high transmission, a patient infected with smallpox can spread the disease to as many as 10 to 20 other persons. By the time a contagious disease is discovered, it may be widespread.

Biologic agents may be more difficult to discover, allowing the terrorist to escape after releasing the agent. Because they cannot see or feel the possible agent, people do not know that they have been exposed. Even the threat of a biologic attack creates fear and panic in the population. After anthrax was distributed in the U.S. mail after the September 11, 2001, terrorist attacks, hundreds of false scares caused fright among the population and extensive and expensive responses by local communities.

Chemical Agents

Chemical agents cause the most immediate havoc and destruction. From a terrorist perspective, they cause immediate disruption and stop normal activity on release. However, this means that the public is instantly aware that an attack has taken place and can begin to take defensive measures to contain the threat and treat affected persons. Nerve gases and cyanide gas can cause death in minutes after severe exposure. Blistering agents such as mustard gas cause early as well as delayed effects, which build in intensity. Other agents, such as phosgene gas, may not cause severe symptoms until hours after exposure, depending on the concentration.

LEARNING OBJECTIVE
- Recognize how an NBC weapon may be spread or disseminated.

Dissemination Devices

Dissemination devices must be matched to the properties of the NBC agent to be effective. For example, explosive devices such as munitions or rockets, with a burster charge surrounded by the agent, may be effective to break open and scatter chemical or nuclear agents, but the heat of the explosion may inactivate biologic agents, rendering them harmless.

Agents might be contained within such common elements as lightbulbs or bottles that release the agent when broken. Spraying devices are effective means to spread aerosols of chemical or biologic agents. Spraying devices include aerosol cans, garden sprayers, spraying machines on moving vehicles (as for spraying orchards), and crop-dusting airplanes.

If a moving vehicle or plane is used, a line of aerosol can contaminate a large area downwind of the release. Wind speeds between 5 and 25 miles per hour (mph) are most effective to distribute the aerosol. Alternatively, several "bomblets" or breaking devices with the agent can be distributed at different points within the target zone, saturating the area.

Other means to spread agents include *vectors,* which can include letters and packages; insects or animals; and contaminated clothing, food, or water (**Figure 30-2**).

Chemical agents are dangerous in both vapor or gas and liquid forms. Most of the biologic agents are believed to be most likely disseminated as an aerosol; however, contamination of food and water and introduction of infectious vectors (e.g., insects) are also concerns. Nuclear agents can cause damage both as particulate matter (e.g., alpha and beta particles) and as waves (gamma rays). Bursting or exploding devices may be designed with a timer and an explosive center that spreads the agent on detonation. Exploding devices have the potential to cause traumatic injuries as well as NBC agent injury.

LEARNING OBJECTIVES
- Recognize signs and symptoms of NBC agents.
- Describe the importance of surveillance in recognizing an NBC event.

Suspecting a Nuclear, Biologic, or Chemical Event

Likely Targets

Targets that arouse suspicion for an NBC event include large public gathering places such as transportation centers, sports arenas, theaters, or malls, where there are many potential victims. Because gas or aerosolized agents will dissipate into the atmosphere, closed or confined spaces such as subways or trains are potential targets because the agent would linger in toxic

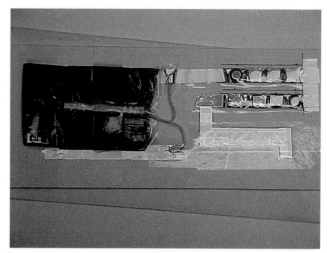

Figure 30-2 Dissemination devices can include letter bombs. *Courtesy Securesearch, Inc. In Currance, PL:* Medical response to weapons of mass destruction, *2005, St Louis, Mosby.*

concentrations. As an EMT, however, your suspicion level must remain high regardless of setting, because vectors and vehicles, food, letters, and packages have been used to spread biologic and chemical agents in rural communities and even within a single home.

Signs at an Event

Seeing multiple casualties who were previously well, all with the same complaints and at a similar time of onset, is a red flag for an intentional event. With NBC events, the first clue may be *index cases* (e.g., victims with severe effects or among the early fatalities). Because the exact agent may be unknown, looking for similar signs and symptoms among multiple victims and comparing them with possible syndromes caused by NBC agents is part of the early identification of an NBC release. Ongoing surveillance of signs and symptoms of possible NBC agents, known as *syndrome surveillance,* is now part of public health monitoring. Seeing an unexpected increase of a particular complaint or sign, such as respiratory complaints (difficulty breathing), flaccid paralysis, or bloody sputum, would result in further investigation. EMS calls and ED visits are part of the surveillance system in many communities today.

Public Health and Emergency Medical Services

The public health system and EMS are both at the front line of domestic defense against NBC events. Public health constantly monitors outbreaks of infectious disease and environmental toxins in the community. Training in infectious diseases and surveillance and epidemiology represent the process by which emerging infectious agents are identified, treated, and contained; this approach has been used for hundreds of years and in the past two decades has led to the identification of new threats such as human immunodeficiency virus (HIV) and severe acute respiratory syndrome (SARS).

The EMS system is a first responder to health events and may be called to the scene of chemical events and other disasters. In biologic terrorism, EMS may be called to the scene of an announced exposure (e.g., "this letter contains anthrax"), but EMS personnel will more likely encounter the victims after the event, when they have become symptomatic. Calls to EMS may be one of the first signs in a community that a biologic outbreak has occurred. Surveillance and reporting of EMS calls to public health authorities is a mechanism for early detection of biologic events in many communities. Individual EMTs may also contribute to surveillance and discovery of unusual trends.

Case in Point

The fact that some Tylenol (acetaminophen) capsules were poisoned with cyanide in 1982 in Chicago was discovered in part by two EMTs who overheard radio calls and alerted authorities. They were struck by the similarity of calls in which young people suddenly became ill with central nervous system and cardiac symptoms. The cause of death of a 12-year-old was initially thought to be from a stroke, highly unusual for a patient of that age. Two brothers presented to a hospital with signs of myocardial infarction. The EMTs listening to these calls noted that Tylenol was mentioned as a medication in the medical history for all these patients, and they reported this to their superiors. When authorities checked the Tylenol in these patients' homes, they discovered the capsules had been contaminated with cyanide, a poison that destroys the most oxygen-dependent organs first, the brain and the heart.

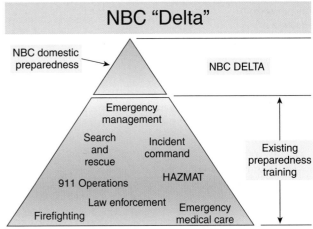

Figure 30-3 Training for WMD events builds on an EMT's existing skills and knowledge, with additional information specific to nuclear, biologic, and chemical (NBC) events referred to as NBC "delta." *Courtesy US Department of Transportation, Research and Special Programs Administration:* Emergency response guidebook, *2002.*

The NBC Delta Response

Emergency medical technicians already possess much of the needed knowledge and training to respond effectively at a WMD event. As noted, biologic agents cause infectious diseases, which EMTs, nurses, physicians, and other healthcare providers see daily and respond to with infection control practices. Hazardous materials principles are followed in response to chemical and nuclear incidents. Radiation safety principles are used daily in the healthcare setting. The incident command system is followed in disasters, MCIs, or whenever multiple agencies respond and work together at an emergency scene. All these principles are incorporated into the NBC response, and any new and specific knowledge and skills necessary to handle NBC events build on this base of information and experience and can lead to expanded scope of practice for EMTs at the time of a declared terrorist event. This additional information and training for WMDs is referred to as the NBC *delta*, or the NBC "difference" (**Figure 30-3**).

What Can EMTs Do to Become More Prepared?

To respond more effectively and safely to WMD events, EMTs must learn the NBC "delta" difference. NBC events can be so widespread that they are indeed disasters, or even acts of war, and there will be a response all the way to the federal level. In the beginning, however, as the event first unfolds, the discovery and response are local, and EMTs may be the first responders at the scene. If you are part of the emergency response in your community, you need to learn more about the NBC delta response.

Learning about specific agents likely to be used in NBC attacks is a first step in understanding potential risks. Some of the agents in each of the NBC categories are presented in this chapter along with their potential for harm; how they are spread;

signs and symptoms to aid recognition; and protection, decontamination, and first-aid measures. Dealing with the concrete rather than the theoretical concept of weapons of mass destruction will help you appreciate the principles of WMD training and response, make it more useful if an actual event unfolds, and allow you to relate it to the very real events and potential threats reported and discussed daily.

This chapter introduces you to the NBC difference and will increase your awareness. As you consider the different types of agents, relate them to the principles you have learned in previous chapters and build on that foundation. The intent is to give you working knowledge and a foundation for understanding. Know the role of EMTs within your system in an NBC response, and seek out additional training tailored to the level of your expected response, whether awareness, operations, technical, or command.

LEARNING OBJECTIVES
- Describe six biologic warfare agents, and recognize the signs and symptoms of exposure.
- Describe how to manage and care for victims of biologic agents.
- List agents that are risks for secondary transmission and actions to protect against spread with personal protective equipment and isolation measures.

Biologic Agents

Biologic agents include bacteria, viruses, and fungi (and toxins they produce) that are deliberately spread among a population to kill or immobilize large numbers of victims. Although many exist, the biologic agents that cause smallpox, plague, anthrax, botulism, tularemia, and viral hemorrhagic fevers are discussed

---

Box 30-2 Standard and Transmission-Based Precautions

Standard Precautions

- Wash hands after patient contact.
- Wear gloves when touching blood, body fluids, secretions, excretions, and contaminated items.
- Wear a mask and eye protection or a face shield during procedures likely to generate splashes or sprays of blood, body fluids, secretions, or excretions.
- Handle used patient care equipment and linen in a manner that prevents the transfer of microorganisms to people or equipment.
- Use care when handling sharps and use a mouthpiece or other ventilation device as an alternative to mouth-to-mouth resuscitation when practical.
  Standard precautions are used in the care of all patients.

Airborne Precautions

Use standard precautions, plus:

- Wear respiratory protection when entering the room.
- Limit movement and transport of the patient. Place a mask on the patient if he or she needs to be moved.
- *Notify hospital before arrival* so staff can prepare a private room that has monitored negative air pressure, a minimum of six air changes per hour, and appropriate filtration of air before it is discharged from the room.

Conventional diseases requiring airborne precautions include measles, varicella, and pulmonary tuberculosis.

Biothreat diseases requiring airborne precautions include smallpox.

Droplet Precautions

Use standard precautions, plus:

- Wear a mask when working within 3 feet of the patient.
- Limit movement and transport of the patient. Place a mask on the patient if he or she needs to be moved.
- *Notify hospital before arrival* so staff can prepare a private room or a shared room with someone with the same infection.

If not feasible, maintain at least 3 feet between patients.

Conventional diseases requiring droplet precautions include invasive *Haemophilus influenzae* and meningococcal disease, drug-resistant pneumococcal disease, diphtheria, pertussis, *Mycoplasma,* group A beta-hemolytic streptococci, influenza, mumps, rubella, and parvovirus.

Biothreat diseases requiring droplet precautions include pneumonic plague.

Contact Precautions

Use standard precautions, plus:

- Wear gloves when entering the room. Change gloves after contact with infective materials.
- Wear a gown when entering the room if contact with patient is anticipated or if the patient has diarrhea, a colostomy bag, or wound drainage not covered by a dressing.
- Limit the movement or transport of the patient from the room.
- Ensure that patient care items, bedside equipment, and frequently touched surfaces receive *appropriate disinfection or disposal (if one-time use).*
- Dedicate use of noncritical patient care equipment (e.g., stethoscopes) to a single patient or group of patients with the same pathogen. If not feasible, adequate disinfection between patients is necessary.
- *Notify hospital before arrival,* so staff can prepare a private room or shared room with someone else with the same infection.

Conventional diseases requiring contact precautions include methicillin-resistant *Staphylococcus aureus,* vancomycin-resistant enterococci, *Clostridium difficile,* respiratory syncytial virus, parainfluenza, enteroviruses, enteric infections in the incontinent host, skin infections (staphylococcal scalded-skin syndrome, herpes simplex virus, impetigo, lice, scabies), and hemorrhagic conjunctivitis.

Biothreat diseases requiring contact precautions include viral hemorrhagic fevers.

For more information, see Garner JS: Guideline for infection control practices in hospitals, *Infect Control Hosp Epidemiol* 17:53-80, 1996.

---

in this chapter. These illnesses constitute the CDC category A list, which is classified by the following features:

1. Easily disseminated or transmitted from person to person.
2. High mortality rate.
3. Ability to cause public panic and social disruption.
4. Requiring special action for public health preparedness.

Biologic agents are infectious; the agent invades the body and then multiplies and causes illness. However, not all biologic agents are *contagious* or spread from one person to another. This is a critical distinction. Although agents such as anthrax can infect large numbers of exposed individuals, they are not easily spread to a victim's family, co-workers, or healthcare workers. On the other hand, the contagious biologic agents that cause smallpox, plague, and viral hemorrhagic fever can spread through a population if proper infection control measures are not used.

Basic infection control principles are crucial to understanding how you approach patients exposed to biologic agents. Knowing how illness caused by bioterrorism is transmitted will allow you to select the appropriate personal protection precautions and decide whether airborne, droplet, or contact precautions are needed, in addition to the standard precautions that are applied to all patients (**Box 30-2**).

The EMT must follow the rules of infection control (see Chapter 2). Use of personal protection equipment during an NBC event is no different than in daily practice. Postexposure evaluation and possible treatment may be warranted. Antibiotics provide effective treatment and prophylaxis for many of bacterial agents, and more so if they are detected early. For smallpox, a vaccine is available for those exposed to an outbreak. Isolation of patients who may have contracted smallpox or plague during the contagious period of the illness will reduce the chance of transmission to others.

Biologic Agents in Warfare and Terrorism

Biologic agents have been used in warfare for more than 2000 years. The Assyrians poisoned enemy wells with rye ergot (which can cause muscle cramps and dry gangrene) in the sixth century BC. Plague victims were hurled over the city walls of Kaffa onto enemies during the Middle Ages; infected persons who fled the city may have contributed to the spread of the *Black Death*, the form of plague that was epidemic in Asia and Europe in the fourteenth century and was marked by skin hemorrhages forming large, dark patches. Smallpox was used as a biologic weapon in North America when the English gave smallpox-infested blankets to the Indians during the French and Indian War in the mid–eighteenth century. It was reported that the resulting epidemics of smallpox killed more than 50% of many affected tribes.

During World Wars I and II, many countries began biologic warfare programs, producing and stockpiling biologic agents and methods to disseminate them. The Japanese reportedly dropped plague-infected fleas over China and Manchuria in World War II. After World War II, some countries greatly increased the production of biologic agents. An international treaty, co-signed by President Nixon, was designed to stop biologic weapons production worldwide. However, some countries, notably the former Soviet Union, persisted in covertly producing, stockpiling, and experimenting with biologic agents. According to Ken Alibek, in charge of biologic weapons production for Russia until he left the Soviet Union for the United States in 1992, biologic weapons containing anthrax, smallpox, and tularemia were produced on an industrial scale, with tons of these agents manufactured in weaponized form each year. Iraq used chemical weapons against Iran in the 1980s and later the Kurds.

After the breakup of the Soviet Union, many scientists involved in biologic weapons production were no longer paid, and many were offered jobs in nations interested in biologic warfare. Both scientists and some supplies of weaponized products are missing and could have been bought by other nations or terrorist organizations. The possibility of potent biologic threats is real.

Spread of Biologic Agents

As noted, biologic weapons can be spread in different ways. In 1969 a leak of weapons-quality anthrax spores from a Soviet military microbiology facility killed at least 66 persons downwind from the facility in Sverdlovsk.

Food or water can be contaminated with a biologic agent. For example, in 1984 the Rajneeshee cult intentionally poisoned salad bars in several restaurants in The Dalles, Oregon, causing *Salmonella* food poisoning.

Aerosolized dissemination is the vehicle of most concern because it could produce the largest number of victims. Garden spray canisters can be used for point distribution of aerosols. Crop dusters and other airplanes or moving vehicles with mounted sprayers can disseminate an aerosolized agent that will move downwind over a sizable geographic area. The wind and weather conditions would have a great effect on distribution of aerosols. For example, if released outdoors, the agent would move downwind and, eventually, be dispersed and diluted by wind and atmospheric movements. Indoors, these agents would tend to stay concentrated.

Vector spread of biologic agents can include food and water as well as insects and animals. Fleas, which carry plague, feed off infected rodents and spread the disease.

Box 30-3   Epidemiologic Clues of a Biologic Warfare or Terrorist Attack

- The presence of a large epidemic with a similar disease or syndrome, especially in a discrete population.
- Many cases of unexplained diseases or deaths.
- More severe disease than is usually expected for a specific illness, or failure to respond to standard therapy.
- Unusual routes of exposure for a pathogen, such as the inhalational route for diseases that normally occur through other exposures.
- A disease that is unusual for a given geographic area or transmission season.
- A disease normally transmitted by a vector that is not present in the local area.
- Multiple simultaneous or serial epidemics of different diseases in the same population.
- A single case of disease by an uncommon agent (smallpox, some viral hemorrhagic fevers)
- A disease that is unusual for an age group.
- Higher attack rates in those exposed in certain areas, such as inside a building if released indoors, or lower rates in those inside a sealed building if released outside.
- Disease outbreaks of the same illness occurring in noncontiguous areas.
- Intelligence of a potential attack, claims by a terrorist or aggressor of a release, and discovery of munitions or tampering.

Detecting a Biologic Event

In contrast to chemical weapons, where the effects are often apparent immediately, biologic weapons may not be suspected for hours to days after release, when the exposed victim becomes ill. During this time the victims may have traveled from the site of exposure, scattered and separated, and if the illness is contagious, even spread it to others.

You must maintain a high index of suspicion to detect biologic agents. Some clues include a large number of victims with a similar illness and a high mortality rate or an illness unusual for the area or occurring out of season. A single case of an uncommon organism such as smallpox would be automatically suspect, or there could be intelligence information or a threat revealed (**Box 30-3**).

It is important to discover the cause as soon as possible because early discovery and treatment will prevent deaths and limit the spread of the illness.

Smallpox

The World Health Organization (WHO) declared smallpox eradicated in 1980. The last recorded disease outbreak was noted in 1977 (**Figure 30-4**). Immunization stopped in the United States in the early 1980s. All but two stockpiles of the virus were destroyed, one at the CDC in Atlanta, Georgia, and one in Russia. However, there is concern that there may be supplies in the hands of other nations and perhaps in the hands of terrorists. It is reported that Russia has maintained an annual stockpile of 20 tons since the 1970s and had increased their production capacity to make 80 to 100 tons a year. Now that the

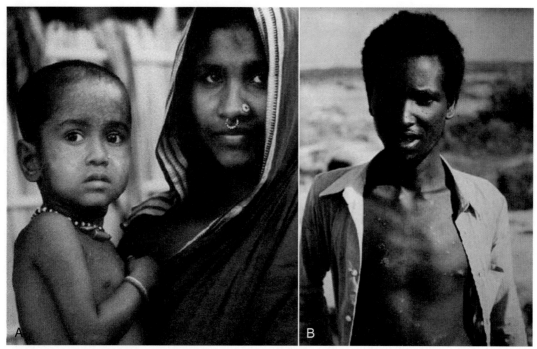

Figure 30-4 **A,** Last known case of smallpox major in Bagladesh. **B,** Last known case of smallpox minor, 1977, Somalia. *Courtesy Centers for Disease Control and Prevention Public Health Library.*

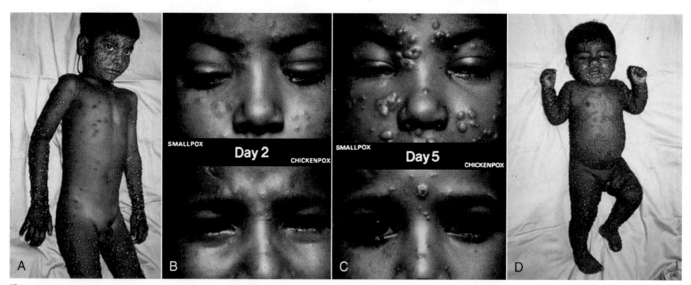

Figure 30-5 **A,** Distribution of smallpox on hands, feet, and face. **B and C,** Comparison of smallpox and chickenpox on days 2 and 5. Note the rash looks similar on day 2. **D,** Advanced smallpox. *Courtesy World Health Organization.*

world's population is no longer immunized against smallpox, the threat of an epidemic is a serious concern.

Unlike inhalational anthrax, for which spread from person to person is not a concern, smallpox is very contagious. Smallpox is spread by contact, droplet, and airborne routes. Respiratory quarantine of all secondary contacts for 17 days after exposure is needed to control the spread.

Clinical Illness. The variola virus causes smallpox. The variola major type causes the severe form of the illness. The incubation period after exposure is 12 days (range, 7-19 days), with a sudden onset of fever and chills, malaise or physically ill feeling, backache, headache, and vomiting. Two or 3 days later, a rash

appears on the face, hands, and forearms, then on the lower extremities before moving toward the trunk. The lesions initially appear round and flat, then raised, then with pus within; scabs eventually form. The lesions are all in the same stage of development at the same time. This sameness is *different* than lesions in chickenpox, for example, in which there are crops of lesions in different stages of development (flat, raised, and fluid filled) at the same time (**Figure 30-5**). In a few cases, smallpox patients have bleeding or hemorrhagic lesions.

Transmission and Personal Protection Precautions. The patient is first infectious to others about the time the rash appears and remains so until all scabs separate. Coughing and sneezing can be a source of spread to close contacts, and droplet and airborne precautions are indicated. If the patient had many skin lesions and the EMT would be in contact with the patient, contact precautions would be warranted as well. The patient should be isolated from others without the illness in negative-pressure rooms if hospitalization is required. A mask should be placed over the patient's mouth during patient movement to reduce the chance of droplet spread.

Quarantine is the isolation of patients exposed to or attacked by contagious disease until they are incapable of either developing or transmitting the disease. If there was a confirmed case of smallpox, all persons in contact with this index case would be isolated with droplet and airborne precautions for at least 17 days (outer range of incubation period). Those who contract the disease would remain in isolation until all scabs separate.

Treatment and Postexposure Considerations. A smallpox vaccine is available from the CDC, and the United States is increasing production to protect the population if an outbreak occurs. Because routine vaccination stopped in the 1980s, the younger population has no immunity at all and the immune status of those who were vaccinated so long ago is suspect. Strategic healthcare workers, including emergency responders, have been included in immunization programs on a voluntary basis.

Prehospital Considerations. As part of the healthcare team, EMTs, must remain vigilant to help detect any case of smallpox as early as possible. Airborne transmission precautions, already in place for illnesses such as tuberculosis, chickenpox, and measles, need to be followed. You should notify hospital personnel of your suspicions so that appropriate receiving and isolation arrangements can be made by the hospital staff to avoid exposure to other patients, hospital workers, and bystanders. Suspected chickenpox or measles cases are handled the same way. Many communities, as part of their bioterrorism plans, are including special arrangements for reception and treatment of suspected smallpox victims in case of an outbreak with many casualties.

If you suspect you have been exposed to smallpox, seek medical attention and as indicated, vaccine and isolation instructions, to reduce your risk of disease and prevent spread to others. Any equipment that comes in contact with a patient with known smallpox should be properly disposed of or treated with germicidal agents approved for the agent. Likewise, after transport of a known smallpox victim, an ambulance should be properly disinfected with approved agents before being put back in service for the general population.

Plague

Along with smallpox, plague is the other major bioterrorist threat capable of causing widespread person-to-person transmission with high numbers of deaths. Caused by bacteria, plague is naturally found in rodents and prairie dogs and is transmitted to humans by fleas. The flea bite transmits the bubonic form of plague, with raised and tender lymph nodes, also called *buboes* (thus the name *bubonic* plague).

The most worrisome form of plague is *pneumonic* plague, which could be spread by aerosolized distribution of the bacteria. Pneumonic plague carries an almost 100% fatality rate if untreated. Furthermore, pneumonic plague can be spread by droplets to other persons. Plague is reported to have killed one

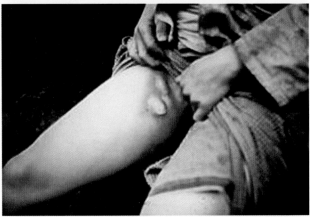

Figure 30-6 Buboes (enlarged lymph nodes) are part of bubonic plague. The bacteria are spread to humans by fleas, which generally bite the patient's lower legs. As the infection ascends, it is blocked by the lymph glands. In this illustration, the lymph nodes in the inguinal region filter infection ascending from the leg. If the lymph glands cannot contain the infection, it may enter the bloodstream and, in some cases, the lungs, with higher mortality. In a bioterrorism attack, victims may at first be overcome by inhaled toxin and directly develop pulmonic plague. As time passes, however, natural spread of plague can occur, with small animals serving as reservoirs and fleas spreading the infection to humans. *Courtesy US Department of Transportation, Research and Special Programs Administration:* Emergency response guidebook, *2002.*

quarter to one third of the population in Asia and Europe in the fourteenth century.

Although plague does occur in the United States, it is uncommon and usually in the bubonic form (**Figure 30-6**).

Clinical Illness. Pneumonic plague can result from an aerosolized exposure (as in biowarfare) or droplet exposure from a person with pneumonic plague. After an incubation period averaging 2 to 4 days, there is acute onset of fever, chills, headache, and body aches, followed by a cough with bloody sputum (*hemoptysis*)—an early suspicious sign that a patient may have this disease. Hemoptysis would be especially suspicious if seen in more than one patient with severe respiratory symptoms, especially if previously well. Without early antibiotic treatment, respiratory failure and death can ensue rapidly.

Most of EMS experience is with bubonic plague. Because fleas usually bite the lower extremities, you will find enlarged lymph nodes, the buboes, most often in the legs and groin. In most cases, spread to the blood can be found; a few patients become very ill, with a high fever, chills, and shock. In some cases, spread to the lungs occurs, and pneumonic plague results. On occasion, plague causes thrombosis of blood vessels in the extremities. This thrombosis can lead to necrosis and gangrene of the extremities, including the nose.

Transmission and Personal Protection Precautions. Coughing spreads pneumonic plague, and droplet transmission precautions must be observed in addition to the usual standard precautions. Depending on the circumstances, rodent and flea interventions may also be necessary.

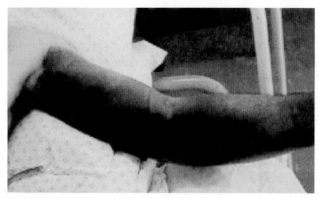

Figure 30-7 Viral hemorrhagic fever. *Courtesy US Department of Transportation, Research and Special Programs Administration:* Emergency response guidebook, 2002.

Treatment and Postexposure Considerations. Antibiotics are effective against plague, but they must be administered early. Close contacts of patients with pneumonic plague or victims exposed to aerosolized plague should be treated with antibiotics. For prophylaxis, doxycycline (100 mg twice a day) is recommended for 7 days after the last exposure.

Prehospital Considerations. The key prehospital consideration in combating pneumonic plague is a high index of suspicion. You should look for clusters of sudden and severe onset of respiratory illness in patients who are usually well, especially if they develop hemoptysis.

Droplet transmission precautions should be used in addition to standard precautions. If the disease is suspected, postexposure follow-up is essential to obtain antibiotics for prophylaxis. Soap and water is effective for decontamination, and standard disinfection procedures should be followed.

Viral Hemorrhagic Fevers

The viral hemorrhagic fevers represent a group of related illness that can cause damage to small vessels, leakage from vessels, and bleeding (**Figure 30-7**). Animals or insects often carry the viruses. Respiratory transmission by aerosol dissemination makes them a possible bioterrorism agent. Human-to-human transmission occurs by direct contact with infected blood and secretions, organs, and semen.

Many different viruses can cause viral hemorrhagic fever. The Marburg virus and the Ebola virus are two of the better known agents. The Ebola virus is of great concern because of the clusters of cases and deaths that evolved when it was described in Africa in the last three decades. As evidence of its contagious potential, 316 cases evolved from a single index case in an epidemic in Zaire in 1995. Ebola is also one of the most lethal hemorrhagic fever viruses, with 50% to 90% mortality.

Clinical Illness. Although the presentation of viral hemorrhagic fever varies, common symptoms include fever, muscle aches, and weakness. The patient may have flushing and small capillary hemorrhages on the skin; in severe cases there may be shock and bleeding from the mucous membranes. Multiple-organ involvement and failure are present in advanced stages of disease.

Late stages of viral hemorrhagic fever are marked by profuse body secretions, which are highly infectious. In hospitals in Africa with poor infection control practices (in some cases they had run out of personal protection supplies), many close contacts such as family members and healthcare workers were also infected. One hospital closed. When proper infection control practice was instituted, the epidemic stopped. *The viral hemorrhagic fevers are a good example of the need to maintain proper infection control precautions, especially body substance isolation with contact precautions.*

Transmission and Personal Protection Precautions. Because close contact with infected body fluids can transmit the disease, contact transmission precautions are necessary, including protection of the eyes and mucous membranes. Droplet transmission has been suspected in advanced stages of viral hemorrhagic fever, so respiratory precautions are also indicated.

If exposed to blood or secretions or excretions from a patient with suspected viral hemorrhagic fever, you should wash the affected skin surface with soap and water immediately. Mucous membranes should be irrigated with large amounts of water or saline solution.

Treatment. Treatment for patients with viral hemorrhagic fever is largely supportive. Vaccines are available, and antiviral agents may be helpful in some situations, but such agents would be given only after a specific agent is identified.

Prehospital Considerations. Standard precautions are the key prehospital consideration, with careful attention to prevent contact transmission. When bleeding, copious secretions, or vomiting and diarrhea are present, protective gowns, face shields, surgical masks, and eye protection should be worn by those within 3 feet of the patient. If patients have a prominent cough, vomiting, diarrhea, or hemorrhaging, a high-efficiency particulate air (HEPA) filter is recommended.

Anthrax

Anthrax is a disease caused by the bacterium *Bacillus anthracis.* This bacterium forms spores when its host dies. The spore form of the bacteria is a resistant, resting body adapted to survive unfavorable conditions in "hibernation"; it can remain dormant for many years, only to return to its active form when its conditions alter, such as when it finds a new host.

Anthrax typically occurs in animals such as cattle, sheep, goats, and horses. Spores have been found in the ground along trails used for cattle drives in the western United States. Sick animals on the drive would die, their carcass would be left to rot along the trail, and the bacteria would assume the spore form and lay dormant in the ground, only to be stirred up on a subsequent cattle drive, where it was inhaled or eaten by other cattle, who in turn became ill, died, and left more spores along the way. Even at present there are repeated outbreaks of anthrax among animals in the United States.

Humans usually contract the disease when handling contaminated animal products, such as body fluids or hides of infected animals, or from eating poorly cooked infected meat. The spore can invade the body through inhalation or a break in the skin. The disease has three forms: inhalational, cutaneous, and gastrointestinal.

The *cutaneous* form of anthrax gave the disease its name. *Antracis* means "coal" in Greek and describes the black *eschar,* or scar, that forms over the infected skin (**Figure 30-8**). Cutaneous

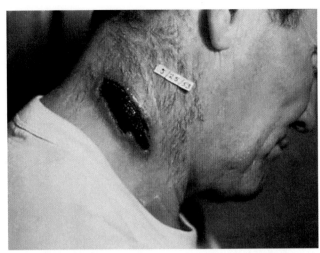

Figure 30-8 Anthrax. The name comes from the coal-colored lesion seen with cutaneous anthrax. *From Centers for Disease Control and Prevention Public Health Library. In Currance PL:* Medical response to weapons of mass destruction, *St Louis, 2005, Mosby.*

anthrax can heal spontaneously, but if it spreads to the blood, 20% of the victims can die. Fortunately, if treated with antibiotics, patients infected with the cutaneous form of anthrax can have a good outcome. *Gastrointestinal* anthrax does not occur often in humans.

Inhalational anthrax from natural sources is currently a rare event in the United States. A few persons develop this illness naturally from handling the contaminated fluids or hides of animals. Spores on animal hides are thought to be airborne and, when inhaled, can cause inhalational anthrax, also called "wool sorter's disease."

Inhalational anthrax is the most dangerous form of the disease and the primary concern in a terrorist event. Because anthrax-tainted letters were mailed in the United States after the September 11, 2001, terrorist attacks, public health, medical, and first-response personnel have learned more about its potential as a weapon. Anthrax spores can be spread by mail, aerosolized devices, and even missiles.

Clinical Illness. Inhalational anthrax is the most dangerous form and occurs when the spores are inhaled deep into the alveoli. The spore must be very small to reach this deep in the lungs. Anthrax invades the lymph nodes in the mediastinum and can cause chest pain, shortness of breath, and flulike symptoms. The few patients who contracted inhalational anthrax in the 2001 outbreak had rhinitis (runny nose) with their early symptoms. The anthrax is fast growing and makes toxins, one of which causes bloody fluid to accumulate in the lungs and around the brain. If treated early with doxycycline and other antibiotics, the chance of recovery is good. If treated late, however, the disease is often fatal.

The inhalational form of anthrax is difficult to recognize until the characteristic findings in the mediastinum (center chest cavity) are discovered on a chest radiograph, or a blood culture reveals growth of the organism. Early signs and symptoms of inhalational anthrax may appear flulike. A 2- to 6-day incubation period is followed by fever, muscle aches, cough, and fatigue. The victim may then feel better but have an abrupt onset of respiratory distress, shock, and death in 24 to 36 hours. Almost half the victims develop inflammation around the brain (meningitis).

Transmission and Personal Protection Precautions. Inhalational anthrax is not spread from person to person. Because illness develops a few days after exposure, the patient should have showered already and changed clothing, so the risk to others from casual contact is minimal. Standard precautions should be practiced. Equipment that comes in contact with body fluids should undergo standard disinfection practices.

Treatment and Postexposure Considerations. Early treatment for patients with confirmed anthrax is important for survival, especially with the inhalational form. Fortunately, common antibiotics such as doxycycline, penicillin, and ciprofloxacin have been effective in treating the illness. A vaccine is available for persons at high risk for exposure (e.g., military) or after confirmed exposure (still investigational).

Suspected exposure to anthrax spores calls for prophylactic (or preventive) treatment with an antibiotic such as ciprofloxacin, doxycycline, or amoxicillin if the substance is deemed suspicious by authorities. Ideally, laboratory testing will confirm whether the substance is anthrax. If it is proven to be anthrax and exposure is highly suspected or confirmed, prophylactic treatment may continue for up to 60 days.

If a suspicious powder is evident, the exposed individual should take off the clothing, being careful not to inhale any of the substance and preferably not to raise clothing over the head. You should offer the patient a surgical mask while clothing is removed. Some authorities recommend that garments be cut off rather than lifted over the patient's head. The clothing should be placed in a separate bag for later analysis. A shower with soap and water accomplishes decontamination of the patient who is potentially exposed. Clothing can be washed in the laundry.

Prehospital Considerations. EMS workers were often called to the scene when tainted letters were discovered to contain a powder in the months after the September 11, 2001, bombings. Exposure to a powder suspicious for anthrax does not result in sudden illness, and there is no emergency patient care needed. Although most powder incidents are hoaxes, they can cause panic and real concern. Ordinarily, you would not knowingly enter an area where a potential aerosolized powder was present. If you find yourself in such an area, you should leave and cover yourself with a mask (or if available a HEPA filter) until clear and request that any bystanders in the area leave.

Transportation of patients after suspected powder exposure who do not have symptoms is not warranted. The patient is not acutely ill; the question is whether an antibiotic should be prescribed for prophylaxis. The determination of whether prophylaxis is needed rests on whether the threat was credible and if there is evidence that anthrax spores are indeed present. This is a decision made by public health and law enforcement authorities. Public health authorities should be informed of any potentially exposed individuals and how to contact them if follow-up becomes necessary. Likewise, those potentially exposed at the scene should be given instructions and contact phone numbers if follow-up is deemed necessary or if they want further information.

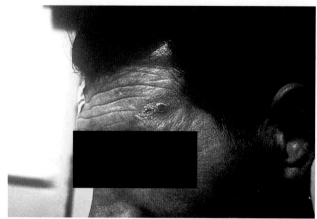

Figure 30-9 Tularemia. The illness often follows an insect bite or exposure to blood or tissue fluid from an infected animal. If it follows a bite, an ulcer may form at the site. *From Centers for Disease Control and Prevention Public Health Library. In Currance PL: Medical response to weapons of mass destruction, St Louis, 2005, Mosby.*

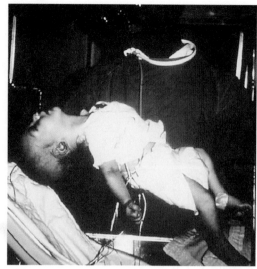

Figure 30-10 Note flaccid paralysis of this baby with botulism. *Courtesy US Department of Defense.*

Tularemia

Tularemia is usually acquired through bites of deerflies, mosquitoes, or ticks or from contact with blood or tissue fluids of infected animals. It is known to hunters as "deerfly fever" or "rabbit fever" and is caused by the bacterium *Francisella tularensis*. With an infectivity rate of 90% to 100%, most people would become ill in a bioterrorist attack. Because it can infect through the respiratory route, aerosolized delivery might be used in a bioterrorism incident.

Clinical Illness. The inhaled form of tularemia results in a sudden onset of fever and chills, aches, fatigue, headache, and loss of body fluids about 3 days after exposure. If tularemia follows a bite, an ulcer forms at the site of inoculation and the lymph glands proximal to the bite become tender and swollen. Fever and malaise follow (**Figure 30-9**).

Mortality rates for the illness vary; it is more incapacitating than lethal. Antibiotics are used for treatment. Pneumonia can be severe, and respiratory difficulty, chest pain, and cough are common complaints. Although tularemia is often thought of as more incapacitating than fatal, untreated cases of naturally acquired tularemia that involve the lungs have a 35% mortality rate.

Transmission and Personal Protection Precautions. The weaponized distribution of tularemia, by war or terrorism, would most likely be by aerosol. However, it can be contacted by vectors such as insect or tick bites or by contact with body fluids from infected animals. It is also possible to become infected by contaminated food or water. After an attack or outbreak, you should also watch for vector spread.

Treatment and Postexposure Considerations. Antibiotics are useful for treatment of tularemia, and doxycycline can be taken as prophylaxis. A vaccine is currently under investigational study.

Prehospital Considerations. Because of the high infectivity rate of tularemia, you should follow personal protection precautions, including droplet transmission precautions if there is a cough.

Botulism

Botulism causes paralysis from the head downward, resulting in hypoventilation and respiratory arrest. The paralysis is caused by a toxin produced by *Clostridium botulinum*. It is often associated with improperly canned foods. The toxin is produced by the bacterium and, once formed, blocks transmission at muscle nerve terminals.

Botulinum toxin is hazardous by the oral route, with effects manifesting within 24 hours. It has a 60% mortality rate if untreated. It is also hazardous if inhaled, and massive amounts of this agent were reportedly produced for warfare in both Russia and Iraq.

Clinical Illness. Botulism results in a classic head-downward, descending paralysis. First signs include double vision, drooping eyelids, weakness of the eye muscles, and trouble speaking and swallowing. The paralysis continues downward to involve the chest and extremities. When the diaphragm and chest muscles become involved, breathing is weak, and death from asphyxia will result without positive-pressure ventilation. The individual becomes flaccid, with no muscle tone (**Figure 30-10**).

Transmission and Personal Protection Precautions. Botulism is not transmissible from person to person. Standard personal precautions should be used.

Treatment and Postexposure Considerations. The major interventions are maintaining an airway and supporting ventilation. Antitoxin to botulism is available. Patients may require intubation and placement on a ventilator until they can resume their own respirations.

Prehospital Considerations. Because of the classic onset, EMTs may recognize botulism. Prehospital care focuses on supporting respirations.

Summary of Biologic Agents

Biologic agents will most likely be suspected once victims become symptomatic with the illness, usually days after the release. You should stay alert for signs and symptoms to recognize unusual presentations or clusters of patients with similar symptoms (**Table 30-2**).

Table 30-2 Biologic Agent Quick Reference Guide

Disease (Class)	Route of Infection*	Incubation Period/ Onset Time	Transmission to Humans	Signs and Symptoms	Decontamination or Infection Control Procedures	Prehospital Care
Smallpox (virus)	R, S, DC	10-12 days	High	Malaise, fever, rigors, vomiting, headache, backache; 2-3 days later, lesions that develop into pustular vesicles, more abundant on face and extremities, developing synchronously.	Strict quarantine with respiratory isolation for minimum of 16-17 days after exposure for all contacts. Patients are infectious until all scabs heal.	Supportive care
Pneumonic plague (bacterium)	V, R	2-3 days	High	High fever, chills, headache, hemoptysis, and toxemia, with rapid progression to dyspnea, stridor, and cyanosis; death is from respiratory failure, circulatory collapse.	Strict isolation precautions. Use of soap and water for personnel decontamination; heat, ultraviolet rays, and disinfectants for equipment.	Supportive care and respiratory and circulatory support
Viral hemorrhagic fevers (virus)	DC, V, ?R	3-21 days	Moderate	Fever, easy bleeding, petechiae, hypotension, shock, edema, malaise, myalgia, headache, vomiting, and diarrhea.	Decontamination with hypochlorite or phenolic disinfectants. Body substance isolation required.	Supportive care directed at respiratory and circulatory support
Anthrax (bacterium)	S, D, R	1-6 days	No, except for cutaneous type	Fever, malaise, fatigue, cough, and mild chest discomfort, followed by severe respiratory distress with dyspnea, diaphoresis, stridor, and cyanosis; shock and death within 24-36 hours of severe symptoms.	Universal body fluid precautions, decontamination with low-pressure soap and water wash, then 0.5% hypochlorite solution, then second soap and water wash.	Supportive care according to local protocol
Tularemia (bacterium)	V, R, D	2-10 days	No	Ulceroglandular—local ulcer and regional lymphadenopathy, fever, chills, headache, and malaise. Typhoidal or septicemic fever, headache, malaise, substernal discomfort, weight loss, nonproductive cough.	Secretion and lesion precautions, strict isolation not required, use of heat or disinfectants renders organism harmless.	Supportive care
Botulinum toxins (toxin)	D, R	24 hours to several days	No	Ptosis, weakness, dizziness, dry mouth and throat, blurred vision and diplopia, dysarthria, dysphonia, dysphagia, followed by symmetrical descending paralysis and respiratory failure.	0.5% Hypochlorite solution and/or soap and water.	Aggressive respiratory support and supportive care for other symptoms

*V, Vector; R, respiratory; D, digestive; DC, direct human-to-human contact; S, skin.

Decontamination is not a significant issue with biologic agents because most victims will usually have showered and changed clothing since exposure. The agent is not on the patient, it is *in* them.

The first rule, as always, is to protect your own health so you can be of use to others. Following the principles of infection control becomes more important than ever with biologic agents and prevents spread to self and others. Care for individual patients is no different than if they acquired the disease naturally.

A large outbreak of a biologic illness would press all health workers into service. Preplanning for biologic events is essential so that emergency responders will know what to do to maintain their own health at a time when they may be needed to provide extended periods of service.

Adhering to basic principles of infectious disease is the key to an effective response to a biologic terrorist event. Experts in the U.S. Army have summarized key points (**Box 30-4**).

LEARNING OBJECTIVES
- List four types of chemical agents that may be used in a terrorist attack.
- List two agents that cause immediate symptoms and may require antidote treatment at the scene.
- Describe the principles of decontamination for vapor exposure.
- Describe the principles of decontamination for liquid exposure.

Chemical Agents

Many chemical agents could be used by terrorists. Some are designed and manufactured only for warfare, whereas others are also used in industry. The four classes of chemicals discussed have the ability to cause large numbers of casualties and require special actions to mitigate their lethal potential. Two of these agents, *nerve agents* and *cyanide,* can kill within minutes of exposure. In high doses, victims require administration of an antidote to survive. *Mustard agents* were designed for warfare. Although some of its effects are delayed, mustard is absorbed quickly and needs to be removed from the skin immediately to avoid its consequences. The *pulmonary agents* are a class of agents that, once inhaled into the lung, begin to destroy the lung tissue, with symptoms appearing hours to days later, depending on the agent and its concentration.

Although there are many other agents, learning about these four provides an introduction to the serious threat chemical agents pose and the necessity for preplanning by EMS to address their effects and maintain safety. When responding in a medical role, the EMT will be triaging patients and evaluating the signs and symptoms to identify the possible agent, if not already known. One type of agent, the nerve agents, causes a classic presentation that is important to recognize because antidotal therapy—carried in the field—may be lifesaving if administered early.

Emergency medical technicians must also be knowledgeable about principles of contamination and decontamination of chemical agents to maintain their own safety, decrease the threat to patients, and reduce secondary contamination.

Lessons learned from previous terrorist events are instructive. For example, 10% of the 1364 first responders to the sarin poisoning in Tokyo were injured by direct or indirect exposure to the poison gas.

Nerve Agents

Nerve agents used in warfare are related to the less toxic organophosphates used as insecticides. Nerve agents act by disrupting the normal transmission of nerve impulses to muscles, organs, and glands, resulting in an excess of secretions and paralysis. *Death results from respiratory paralysis or excessive respiratory secretions.* The respiratory secretions are so great that even with positive-pressure ventilation, victims can literally drown in their own secretions. To save life, support of respiration, including positive-pressure ventilation, and antidote therapy may be needed. Nerve agents can enter the body by inhalation, ingestion, or absorption through the skin.

Dissemination

Nerve agents are in liquid form at room temperature. Depending on the agent and the temperature, the vapor (often invisible) or gaseous form results from evaporation. The *volatility,* or tendency to vaporize, will be influenced by factors such as temperature, wind currents, and the surface on which the liquid is poured. Sarin evaporates at room temperature; VX remains in liquid form and tends to persist once disseminated. Nerve agents can be dispersed by missiles, sprayers, and other devices. Liquid nerve agent can be absorbed through the skin. The vapor can be inhaled and also absorbed through the eye and the skin. However, the major threat from vapor is inhalation.

Toxicity

Nerve agents act at nerve terminals that release acetylcholine, a chemical that acts as a nerve signal. Acetylcholinesterase, an enzyme, normally limits the amount of free acetylcholine at the nerve junction. Nerve agent poisons the enzyme; acetylcholine accumulates and causes excessive stimulation of glands, organs, and muscles.

Clinical Effects

The clinical effects are directly related to an excess of acetylcholine. Most predominant is the outpouring of secretions from every organ and orifice. The eyes tear; the nose runs; secretions in the airways cause trouble breathing; and urination, vomiting, and diarrhea are present. Effects on involuntary muscles include bronchoconstriction, gastrointestinal cramps, and often constriction of the pupil, especially with vapor exposure.

Overstimulation of the skeletal muscle first appears in the patient as twitching, or fasciculations, then weakness, and, if severe, eventual paralysis. *Death results from paralysis of the respiratory muscles and the secretions in the lungs.*

Central nervous system (CNS) effects follow large exposures and include seizures, loss of consciousness, and respiratory arrest.

There are various keys to remembering these many effects. The mnemonic **SLUDGEM** is often used and stands for *s*alivation, *l*acrimation, *u*rination, *d*iarrhea, gastrointestinal cramps, *e*mesis (vomiting), *m*iosis (small pupils), and *m*uscular

Box 30-4 Ten Possible Steps for Handling Potential Bioterrorist Events

1. Maintain an index of suspicion.

In an otherwise healthy population, some associations are very suggestive, especially when seen in clusters, high numbers, or unusual presentations.

Hemoptysis (coughing blood)	Plague
Flaccid paralysis	Botulism
Bleeding purpura	Viral hemorrhagic fevers (VHFs)
Wide mediastinum (x-ray film)	Anthrax
Rash on head and extremities	Smallpox

2. Protect yourself and your patients.

Use appropriate personal protection equipment (PPE). For small-pox, triage and evaluate patient in an isolation room; wear an appropriate respirator (N-95 or higher.)

3. Adequately assess the patient.

Review and assess the patient's history. Also ask the following questions:

- Are others ill?
- Were there any unusual events?
- Was there a possible contaminated food item?
- Was there vector exposure?
- Has the patient been traveling?
- What is the patient's immunization record?
- What is the patient's occupation?

Perform a physical examination with special attention to the respiratory system, nervous system, skin condition, and hematologic and vascular status.

4. Decontaminate as appropriate.

Do not use bleach on exposed people. Soap, water, and shampoo are adequate for all biologic and most chemical agents. Chemically contaminated clothes should be removed and discarded safely. Biologically contaminated clothes can be laundered with soap, water, and perhaps bleach.

5. Establish a diagnosis.

Think clinically and epidemiologically; always send specimens for culture.

SYMPTOMS (INDIVIDUALS)	POSSIBLE DIAGNOSIS
Pulmonary	Anthrax, tularemia, plague, staph, enterotoxin B (SEB)
Neuromuscular	Botulism, Venezuelan equine encephalitis (VEE)
Bleeding/purpura	VHFs, ricin, plague (late)
Rash (various types)	VHFs, T2 mycotoxin, smallpox, plague
Flulike	Varies
Immediate symptoms (large numbers)	*Possible diagnosis*
Pulmonary	SEB, mustard, lewisite, phosgene, cyanide
Neurologic	Nerve gases, cyanide
Delayed symptoms (large numbers)	*Possible diagnosis*
Pulmonary	Biologic agents, mustard, phosgene
Neurologic	Botulism, VEE, other encephalitis

6. Render prompt treatment.

Doxycycline can be used to treat virtually everything (except viral agents or toxins) while awaiting lab results. Inhalational anthrax should be treated with two or more antibiotics, including doxycycline or ciprofloxacin plus one or more other antibiotics. Observe pediatric precautions as appropriate. Prophylaxis (antibiotics and/or vaccines) should be administered according to public health recommendations.

7. Provide good infection control.

Recommended isolation precautions (in addition to standard precautions) for biologic agents include the following:

Anthrax	Contact precautions for cutaneous anthrax
Pneumonic plague	Droplet precautions; contact precautions if draining buboes present
Smallpox	Airborne and contact precautions
Tularemia	Contact precautions if lesions present
VHFs	Contact precautions; airborne precautions, especially in late stages

8. Alert the proper authorities.

AGENCY	TELEPHONE NUMBER
FBI	_____
Municipal police/county sheriff	_____
State police	_____
County health department	_____
State health department	_____
Local emergency medical services unit	_____
Local hospitals	_____
Centers for Disease Control and Prevention Emergency Operation	770-488-7100

9. Assist in the epidemiologic investigations so as to determine who may be at risk.

Steps in an epidemiologic investigation:

- Count cases.
- Relate to the at-risk population.
- Make comparisons.
- Develop hypotheses.
- Test hypotheses.
- Make inferences.
- Conduct studies.
- Interpret and evaluate.

10. Know and spread this information.

twitching. In addition, the other classic signs are respiratory distress and altered mental status.

The route of entry dictates which symptoms appear first and the time to severe toxicity. If the agent is inhaled, the first symptoms are related to the lungs because the agent induces shortness of breath from bronchoconstriction and secretions in the airway. Then, as it is absorbed into the blood, it affects other organs. Vapor exposure also causes rhinorrhea, or excessive nasal secretions, and small pupils, a direct effect of the vapor on the eye muscle (absorbed through cornea). Inhaling vapors causes the fastest onset of symptoms, and large doses can be fatal in minutes.

Liquid on the skin will also first cause local effects, such as sweating and fasciculations of the contaminated skin and the underlying skeletal muscles. More generalized symptoms and signs follow as the poison is absorbed into the body and may include gastrointestinal (GI) distress, nausea, vomiting and diarrhea, and respiratory distress. Patients who ingest the agent, as seen in suicide attempts with organophosphate insecticides, may first present with abdominal cramps and vomiting and diarrhea, followed by respiratory distress, muscle weakness, and other generalized signs.

It is important to appreciate how nerve agent victims present after skin or vapor exposure to recognize clinical signs. Clinical signs are used to guide field treatment with the appropriate antidote.

Prehospital Considerations

The first principle with chemical agents is to eliminate continued exposure and stop absorption. In the field, this is first accomplished by removing the victim from the source and grossly decontaminating the victim.

Vapors. Decontamination of vapors is best accomplished by moving the victim to fresh air and removing outer clothing. These actions should remove up to 90% of any vapor trapped next to the victim.

For vapor exposures, victims can remove their clothing and thereby eliminate 80% to 90% of vapors trapped under or within clothing. Vapors of nerve agent, cyanide, and phosgene are not likely to be absorbed through the skin in concentrations found at a scene, but *off-gassing* of vapor trapped within outer clothing has been reported. Therefore, you should be aware of entering closed spaces where vapors can accumulate. If ambulance transport is warranted before victims receive definitive decontamination, make sure that the victim is grossly decontaminated, outer clothing is removed, ambulance airflow and ventilation are maximized, and the EMT with the patient has suitable respiratory protection. Do not enclose the patient with impermeable covering to protect the stretcher from contamination, because it may help drive any remaining poison through the skin of the victim.

Liquids. With liquid exposure, such as blotches of liquid on the skin, the most important principle is rapid removal. You should remove clothing as a first step in gross decontamination. Physically remove remaining blotches and blot the visible agent so it will not be absorbed. This includes physical removal by scraping off with a tongue blade or other flat instrument, blotting up any liquid with absorbent material (specially made or

Table 30-3	Effects of Nerve Agents	
Exposure	**Effects**	**Time of Onset**
Vapor—mild	Eyes: miosis, dim vision, headache; nose: rhinorrhea; mouth: salivation; lungs: dyspnea	Seconds to minutes after exposure
Vapor—severe	All the effects of mild exposure plus severe breathing difficulty or cessation of breathing, generalized muscular twitching, weakness or paralysis, convulsions, loss of consciousness, loss of bladder and bowel control	Seconds to minutes after exposure
Liquid—mild	Localized sweating, fasciculations, no miosis	Within 18 hours
Liquid—moderate	Gastrointestinal effects; miosis uncommon	Within 18 hours
Liquid—severe	Sudden loss of consciousness, seizures, apnea, flaccid paralysis, death	<30 minutes

readily available, such as dirt), and flushing with large amounts of water. Deactivation of the nerve agent on the skin can be accomplished with diluted bleach (0.5%) followed by flushing with water, soap and water, or use of decontamination kits developed for the military (e.g., M291, M258A1). Flush the eyes with water for 15 minutes.

Emergency medical technicians and other first responders must be careful not to become poisoned themselves. This can occur directly from vapor or liquid exposure after inadvertent entrance into a hot zone without protective equipment and from secondary contamination (see Chapter 28). The liquid on a victim's skin and the vapors trapped in clothing can cause injury to the rescuer. You should use protective clothing if encountering contaminated victims.

Advanced Aid

Advanced treatment for nerve agents includes the antidotes atropine and pralidoxime. These antidotes are packaged in autoinjector kits similar to an EpiPen and administered in a similar manner. These agents are prepackaged for field use to treat victims of nerve agents because time is crucial after severe exposure. For field use, a recommended dose schedule based on clinical presentation is used (**Table 30-3**). First responders with the appropriate training may be issued these MARK I kits, which contain fixed doses of atropine and pralidoxime for treatment of adults, or Duodote, a new version of the MARK I (**Figure 30-11**). Doses should be reduced for children. Because the MARK I kits may be lifesaving and are time dependent, they represent one of the few treatments that may be delivered in the hot zone. Only adequately protected first responders should enter the hot zone.

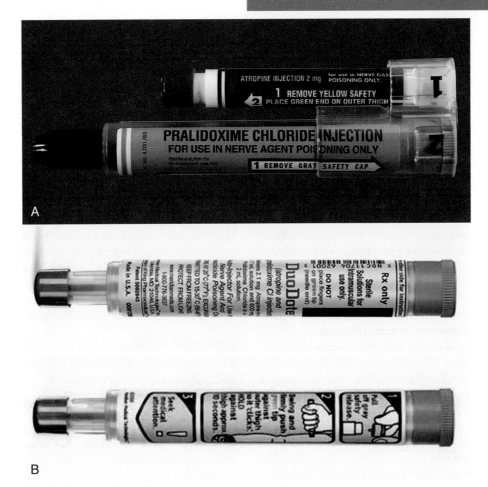

Figure 30-11 **A,** MARK I kit. **B,** Duodote (front and back). A *courtesy US Department of Transportation, Research and Special Programs Administration:* Emergency response guidebook, *2002; B courtesy Meridian Medical Technologies, Bristol, TN.*

Atropine is necessary to dry the secretions but will not improve muscle function. The pralidoxime will reverse the poisoning on the enzyme and speed overall recovery to normal function. It may be necessary to provide positive-pressure ventilation along with antidote treatment. Remember that even with positive-pressure ventilation, severely poisoned victims will still need atropine to avoid "drowning" in their own secretions. Prepackaged syringes with diazepam for treatment of seizures are also available.

Cyanide Agents

Cyanide is an effective and fast killer. In severe poisoning, antidotes are necessary to save the victim's life. Because the poison acts so quickly, these antidotes may need to be given before the victim reaches a hospital.

Several forms of cyanide exist. It is found in nature and in industry. The forms of cyanide that may be chemical agents are hydrogen cyanide and cyanogen chloride. Cyanide gas was reportedly used by the Sunni Iraqi regime against the Kurds. Cyanide gas can be formed by mixing a cyanide salt with a strong acid; these ingredients were found in Tokyo subway restrooms after the sarin release.

Cyanide is also lethal if ingested. In 1978, 913 people died when followers of a religious cult committed suicide and poisoned their children with a cyanide-laced sweet beverage at Jonestown in Guyana, South America.

Dissemination

Cyanide is very volatile. Cyanide would be in liquid form in munitions but vaporize rapidly on detonation. The major threat is from the cyanide vapor. In an open space the vapor could disperse rapidly, reducing the concentration and toxicity and ultimately the threat. In a closed space it could maintain a higher concentration and represent a continuing threat.

Toxicity

If delivered in a lethal concentration, cyanide works rapidly, causing respiratory death at the cellular level. Cyanide poisons the cell's ability to use oxygen. Cyanide attaches to the cell and renders the cell unable to use oxygen for energy. Oxygen is taken up into the blood and delivered to the cells but then returns unused in the venous blood because of the poisoning. The effects on the body are similar to being in a hypoxic environment.

Clinical Effects

Because the cells cannot burn oxygen, the most oxygen-dependent organs, the brain and the heart, are affected first. Oxygen sensors along the arteries detect a problem, and victims perceive

Table 30-4	Effects of Cyanide Vapor Exposure		
Severity	**Concentration**	**Effects**	**Time of Onset**
Moderate	Low concentration	Transient increase in rate and depth of breathing, nausea, vomiting, headache. These may progress to severe effects if exposure continues.	Time of onset of these effects depends on concentration, but often within minutes after onset of exposure.
Severe	High concentration	Transient increase in rate and depth of breathing Convulsions Cessation of respiration Cessation of heartbeat	15 seconds 30 seconds 2-4 minutes 4-8 minutes

that they are short of breath as the brain increases the rate and depth of respirations. Likewise, a transient increase in pulse and blood pressure may follow as the cardiovascular system tries to perfuse more blood to the tissues to compensate for the oxygen problem. With high concentrations, the victim quickly becomes unconscious, seizes, and stops breathing. The heart muscle itself has no fuel to continue contracting. Blood pressure and pulse rate fall and then cease. Death can occur in minutes.

What may be striking with this rapid respiratory and circulatory collapse is the initial lack of cyanosis. Rather, a patient's skin color may look good, even pinkish or red, because the hemoglobin in the venous blood returning to the heart is still loaded with the unused oxygen. As the heart and lungs fail, the victim may turn blue.

Effect of Dose. The concentration of the exposure will affect the onset and progression of symptoms. With low to moderate concentrations, a victim may experience hyperventilation, followed by apprehension and anxiety, weakness, nausea, and muscular trembling. If the victims can walk away from the vapor to fresh air, they may likely escape with no need for treatment. However, if they remain in the vapor, over time the continued cyanide exposure can be lethal. Consciousness will be lost, breathing will cease, and the heart will eventually stop.

With high concentrations of cyanide, the victim has rapid onset of hyperventilation, which can be followed within 15 to 30 seconds by seizures, then loss of respirations and cardiac activity, and death within 6 to 8 minutes.

Some refer to the lethality of cyanide exposure as an "all-or-nothing" response. If you can manage to escape the fumes, you will probably survive. If you cannot escape and are overcome, you may need an antidote to survive.

In a mass casualty situation, it is important to direct the ambulatory victims away from continued exposure while they still have the ability to escape (**Table 30-4**).

Distinguishing Cyanide from Nerve Agent Poisoning. Cyanide and nerve agents can rapidly cause loss of consciousness, convulsions, and cessation of breathing. However, it is important to distinguish the two agents because treatment differs. One clue may be the pupils. Nerve agents, especially vapors, are likely to cause small pupils. Nerve agents also cause excessive secretions and muscle twitching (fasciculations) that would not usually be seen with cyanide. These clues—small pupils, muscle twitching, and secretions—may help distinguish the two agents. In some cases you will need to look at other victims with less severe exposures, who are not in a coma, to search for findings to help recognize the agent.

Cyanogen Chloride. If the source of cyanide is cyanogen chloride, you might also notice complaints of irritation of the mucous membranes from the vapor, notably the nasal passage, airway, and eyes. The irritation may seem similar to exposure to tear gas and may give the victim a warning sign to escape. The cyanogen chloride converts to cyanide within the body and then has the same effect as hydrogen cyanide.

Prehospital Considerations

Your first priority with a cyanide outbreak is to protect yourself. You will need respiratory protection to enter the hazard area. You should remove the victim to fresh air and provide general supportive therapy, including high-concentration oxygen.

You should remove wet clothing and wash the skin with water or soap and water if there is a possibility of liquid on the skin; make sure you have proper protective clothing and are trained in its use.

Advanced Aid

One antidote for cyanide consists of two agents: nitrites and thiosulfate. The *nitrites* are generally given intravenously; however, kits to treat cyanide poisoning contain ampules of amyl nitrite, which are crushed and then inhaled by the victim. After nitrite treatment, *sodium thiosulfate* is injected in the vein, which promotes formation of thiocyanate that is then excreted in the urine.

An important note to remember is that the adult dose of nitrites cannot be given to children. An adult dose can kill a child. Nitrites act by altering some of the blood's normal hemoglobin to an altered form that does not carry oxygen but will carry cyanide. It does this only to provide a means to pull cyanide off the cells. The adult dose is calculated so that at least half of the hemoglobin remains in its normal form. If you gave an adult dose to a child, however, you could alter the child's entire hemoglobin level, and the child would be unable to carry oxygen in the blood, leading to death.

Another antidote to treat cyanide poisoning is *hydroxycobalamin*, which recently became available in the United States, after being used in France. The advantage of hydroxycobalamin is that it does not alter the hemoglobin and may have a wider margin of safety.

Great care must be given in the decision to use a cyanide antidote, and it must be under medical control. The medications in these kits are given intravenously, so they would not normally be administered by EMTs. However, they may be available as part of a WMD response plan, and EMTs should be aware of their existence and that they may be part of a field triage and treatment plan for cyanide.

Sulfur Mustard

Used extensively during World War I and more recently in the Iraq/Iran war, mustard belongs to a class of agents called *vesicants* (capable of causing blisters), or "blister agents." Mustard tends to be incapacitating rather than lethal. It can affect the skin, the eyes, and in higher concentrations, many other organs. It renders soldiers unable to continue battle and dependent on others, draining the resources of an army. In high concentrations, it can affect many organ systems, including the bone marrow and the lungs, and cause severe disability and death.

Dissemination

Sulfur mustard derives its name from the mustard-type odor, also described as similar to onion, garlic, and horseradish. It is an oily liquid with a light-yellow to brown color. Mustard is both a vapor and a liquid threat to exposed skin and mucous membranes. At room temperature, it evaporates slowly and is primarily a liquid threat. As temperatures approach 100° F (37.7° C), mustard is also a vapor hazard. Mustard freezes at temperatures below 57° F (14° C), so it is often mixed with another vesicant to lower the freezing point.

Sulfur mustard is an agent used in war. Replacing the sulfur atom with nitrogen, nitrogen mustard was developed as a vesicant. Ironically, instead of being used in war, one type of nitrogen mustard has found use in chemotherapy for cancer.

Toxicity

Sulfur mustard can cause chemical changes in other molecules within the body and has an effect similar to radiation on the body. Although the exact mechanism of sulfur mustard is unknown, it probably affects rapidly dividing cells, such as epithelium and bone marrow stem cells. The changes can lead to cell death and an inflammatory reaction.

Mustard tends to be absorbed quickly through the skin, but its clinical effects are not immediate. A victim typically notices symptoms or signs some hours after exposure.

Clinical Effects

Skin, eye, and airway findings are the most common effects from mustard. In severe cases the bone marrow is suppressed.

The first sign on the skin occurs hours after exposure. It appears red (erythema), much like a sunburn (**Figure 30-12**). Small blisters begin to form that merge together to form larger blisters. The outer skin (epidermis) separates from the dermis, with an accumulation of "blister" fluid between the layers. Danish physicians treating victims of the Iraq/Iran war noted that the skin around the blisters turned black. Some victims had large areas of dark-brown to black skin that peeled off, leaving intact skin underneath. This helps to differentiate mustard gas from a full-thickness burn. Because mustard is so reactive with the body, there is no mustard left in the blister fluid. In fact, blood, tissue, or blister fluid from mustard victims presents no chemical contamination risk to medical personnel.

At lower concentrations, victims experience irritation, soreness, and burning in the upper airway, upper pharynx, and

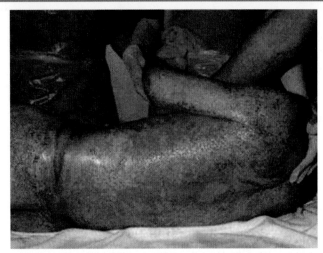

Figure 30-12 Erythema after sulfur mustard exposure. *Courtesy US Department of Transportation, Research and Special Programs Administration:* Emergency response guidebook, *2002.*

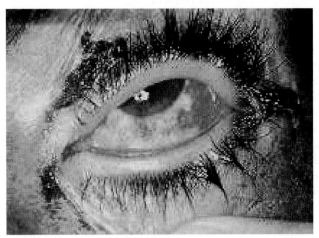

Figure 30-13 Eye injury after sulfur mustard exposure. *Courtesy US Department of Transportation, Research and Special Programs Administration:* Emergency response guidebook, *2002.*

nostrils. With higher concentrations, mustard may penetrate to the upper trachea, causing voice changes and a cough. With severe exposure, the lower airway may also be involved, with shortness of breath and a cough producing large quantities of sputum.

The eyes are sensitive to the vapors, which is clearly incapacitating to victims. Mustard is irritating to the eyes, and victims may have photophobia (avoidance of light), conjunctivitis ("pinkeye"), involuntary and spasmodic winking, lid inflammation and swelling, and brown discoloration (**Figure 30-13**). With severe exposure the cornea becomes opaque (will not transmit light), ulcers form, and it can perforate.

Because the effects of mustard are generally delayed, if signs appear early, within 2 hours, it could indicate severe exposure (**Table 30-5**).

Prehospital Considerations

Immediate decontamination is the only way to reduce damage, and it must be performed as soon as possible. Mustard can penetrate through skin surfaces in 2 minutes; therefore time

Table 30-5	Effects of Sulfur Mustard Vapor		
Organ	**Severity**	**Effects**	**Onset of First Effect**
Eye	Mild	Tearing, itchy, burning, gritty feeling	4-12 hours
	Moderate	Same as above, plus reddening, swelling of lids, moderate pain	3-6 hours
	Severe	Marked swelling of lids, possible corneal damage, severe pain	1-2 hours
Airways	Mild	Runny nose, sneezing, nosebleed, hoarseness, hacking cough	12-24 hours
	Severe	Same as above, plus severe productive cough, shortness of breath	2-4 hours
Skin	Mild to severe	Erythema (redness), blisters	2-24 hours

is of the essence. Physical removal, dry decontamination kits (M291), and flushing with water or soap and water are all priorities. Bleach solutions are also effective in deactivating mustard, but the agent will continue to be absorbed while it remains on the skin. The choice of method depends on what is immediately available.

Patient care is generally supportive. There are no specific antidotes to sulfur mustard. For example, skin care would be similar to that for a burn, with careful attention to avoid infection.

Advanced care at a medical facility is required for patients who have severe exposure with severe skin involvement, pulmonary compromise, or bone marrow suppression. Mustard patients with skin involvement do not have the increased fluid requirements seen in patients with thermal burns.

Patients with severe pulmonary signs require prioritization at triage. Most others could be triaged as "delayed." Although few patients with mustard exposure who received medical care have died in war experiences (<5%), those with severe pulmonary effects within 4 hours of exposure are at high risk, as are those who have more than 50% body surface area affected by liquid mustard.

Experimental work by a U.S. Army scientist shows promise with early use of steroids and other treatment for eye injuries. Current research shows that instilling steroid eyedrops within the first 10 minutes after mustard injury may have benefit—a time window that could lead to possible use of this treatment in the field.

Pulmonary Agents

Phosgene and chlorine were used in World War I. They are known as pulmonary agents because they can damage the alveolocapillary membrane in the lungs, resulting in pulmonary edema. *Chlorine* is more irritating than phosgene and has a more distinctive odor, giving warning to exposed victims who would

try to flee the gas. *Phosgene* smells like freshly mown grass or hay and is not as irritating; thus victims may not know they are in trouble and may not flee but rather continue to inhale the vapors.

Many other gases also belong to this class of agents. *Nitrogen oxides* are produced in fires as well as spontaneously in grain storage facilities ("silo filler's disease"). *Ammonia* is another example of an extremely irritating agent with vapors so irritating that the exposed victim would usually be impelled to escape.

Dissemination

Phosgene evaporates from its liquid form rather quickly, and the vapor represents a hazard. Phosgene is widely found in industry and at fire scenes because it is a byproduct of combustion of many common chemicals.

The concentration of the pulmonary gases and their physical properties, particularly *solubility* (reactivity with water), affect both the signs of exposure and the timing of symptoms. The more soluble the gas, the faster it reacts with the mucous membranes within the nasal passages, airway, and eyes. Ammonia is a very soluble agent and thus very reactive with water. Fumes of ammonia cause tearing and coughing almost immediately and result in a person fleeing the source and limiting exposure. Phosgene, which is much less soluble, may not react with the upper airway and eyes, giving no warning to the victim, who continues to inhale the gas, which travels deep into the alveoli. No effects from phosgene may be evident for several hours, unless the concentration is extremely high. Hours after exposure, as the phosgene reacts with the alveolocapillary membrane and fluid enters the lung, breathing becomes labored, and the victim feels shortness of breath.

Toxicity

Phosphene vapor is toxic when inhaled. The liquid form poses no threat except for the vapors it forms. Usually inhaled, the pulmonary agents can reach deep into the lungs, where they react with the delicate alveolar tissue and cause leakage of fluids across the alveolocapillary membrane, resulting in pulmonary edema.

The more soluble agents react with the eyes and upper airway, resulting in tearing, coughing, and irritation in the throat. Severe reaction can also cause narrowing of the airway.

Clinical Effects

Pulmonary agents are suspected by the signs and symptoms of lung (and upper airway) irritation and pulmonary edema. As mentioned, an odor of mown hay or freshly cut grass is described for phosgene but often not perceived or appreciated by victims.

When the lungs fill with fluid, the patient experiences shortness of breath, first noticed with exertion. Later the shortness of breath is noticeable at rest. As more fluid irritates the airways, a persistent cough develops, with frothy sputum. Oxygen exchange is impaired, and the victim becomes more and more hypoxic, as if drowning. As fluid moves into the lungs, the patient may be relatively hypovolemic (low blood volume).

With more soluble pulmonary agents, or with high concentrations of phosgene, upper airway and eye irritation may occur; in severe cases the upper airway becomes compromised.

Prehospital Considerations

The most critical treatment of patients exposed to pulmonary agents is directing victims to fresh air, away from further exposure. Patients with shortness of breath should not exert themselves unless it is to flee from the toxic vapors.

No specific antidotes for pulmonary agents exist; patient care is supportive. Supplemental oxygen and positive-pressure ventilation may be required, and in severe cases the patient may need to be intubated. Secretions may need to be cleared with suction.

Summary of Chemical Agents

Personal Protection

Do not enter chemically contaminated zones unless you are properly protected. Personal protective equipment must protect the skin and the respiratory system. Some agents require chemical protective clothing. Because the molecules of chemical agents are extremely small, special respiratory protection is needed to prevent inhalation, with filtered air or self-contained breathing apparatus. Because some of the vapors can be absorbed by the membranes around the eye, total body isolation is often required. When the chemical agent is unknown, rescuers approaching the hot zone must assume the worst and use maximal protection. EMTs should not enter without the required equipment and training.

Recognition

Early recognition of chemical agents is made by reports of clouds, odors, and onset of signs and symptoms of the victims.

Immediate casualties suggest nerve agents or cyanide. Both can cause rapid loss of consciousness, convulsions, and respiratory arrest. Cyanide causes hyperventilation initially, then circulatory and respiratory collapse, with loss of consciousness and convulsions. Pinpoint pupils, twitching muscles, excessive secretions, and respiratory distress are clues to nerve agent exposure.

Mustard and some pulmonary agents have delayed effects. Victims of these agents should be observed. With mustard, it is usually hours after exposure before the victim notices eye irritation, photophobia, blinking, redness and blistering of the skin, and cough and respiratory complaints. With pulmonary agents, hours may pass before shortness of breath is noticed, unless the concentration is very high or the agent is very reactive or soluble, in which case irritation of the eyes and nasal passage with tearing and coughing may be apparent early after exposure.

Chemical detector paper and monitoring equipment may be brought to a scene to aid detection, but it usually takes time to perform these tests.

Decontamination

Decontamination is the reduction or removal of chemical agents. The first consideration is whether exposure is a vapor or a liquid or solid.

Vapors. For vapors, remove the victim to an environment where there is clean air. Vapors from nerve agents, cyanide, and phosgene are not believed to penetrate the skin at concentrations found at the scene. Off-gassing within a closed space has been reported to cause symptoms in medical personnel. To prevent this, simply remove outer clothing so that any vapors trapped between the clothing and the victim can escape. This is judged to be 90% effective.

Liquids and Solids. Methods to remove liquids or solids include physical removal, dilution and washing, and detoxification. Chemical agents on the body must be removed immediately. For example, mustard must be removed within the first 2 minutes to prevent absorption through the skin. Nerve agents are so toxic that absorption of a small amount could be lethal.

Physical Removal. Physical removal is the fastest and most effective way to remove the largest bulk of material. A stick, a tongue blade, or a piece of cardboard can be used to scrape the substance off the outer clothing or skin. Removal of clothing is mandatory if it is contaminated with a liquid or solid.

For liquids, absorption with a powder or other dry absorbing material will help bind the chemical and slow its penetration through the skin until it can be flushed away with water. Depending on the circumstance, many different dry powders might be used, such as soap detergents, earth, or flour. The substance can then be wiped off with wet tissue paper. Flushing with large amounts of water is another option. The main point is to remove "as much as possible as early as possible." Nerve agents and mustard are both absorbed quickly through the skin.

Dilution and Washing. Another option is to wash off the agent with large amounts of water or soap and water. This may be used as the primary means of decontamination because water physically removes the agent and more slowly reacts with it. The important concept is to do what is expedient; don't wait to obtain soap or bleach if only water is available. Rather, begin to dilute and remove the agent. Only large amounts of water, normal saline, or eye solutions are recommended for the eye. Wounds that may be contaminated should be irrigated with sterile saline solution or sterile water.

Detoxification. Detoxification or deactivation of the chemical to make it harmless may be possible with common agents such as bleach (sodium hypochlorite) and soap and water. For example, you can use diluted bleach (0.5%) on the affected area, being careful to avoid the eyes, mucous membranes, and wounds, followed by a rinse with water. Soap and water can also be used.

Full-strength household bleach (5.0%) can be used, but it needs to be flushed off with water and can be irritating to some people. The diluted solution (0.5%) is made by mixing 1 part of household bleach with 9 parts of water.

The military has a dry decontamination kit that a soldier can use to remove spots of toxin on the skin by wiping it off. The M291 resin kit has carbonaceous material to absorb the agent and other materials that inactivate it; it is both reactive and absorbent.

According to U.S. Army medical experts, the half-time of VX (a liquid nerve agent) removed with bleach is 1.5 minutes; the half-times of other agents, such as mustard, are much longer. The "half-time" is the time it takes for half the agent to be rendered harmless. These time lags, during which the chemical could still be absorbed through the skin, emphasize the need first to physically remove as much agent as possible. *Once you have removed as much as possible, detoxify and wash off any chemical left on the skin.*

Medical Care at the Scene. The focus at the scene should be on critical interventions only. Decontamination must be the major priority because continued absorption of the chemical agent worsens any patient's condition. Critical interventions include airway support (as for victims of phosgene and other pulmonary agents), bleeding control, and administration of antidotes to nerve agent victims and cyanide victims. Common sense should prevail. For example, no one should bleed to death because they have a toxic exposure and are undergoing decontamination. On the other hand, you should not become involved with minor first aid while a victim absorbs a lethal dose of nerve agent from liquid on their skin.

Decontamination, Triage, and Treatment. The amount of medical care provided depends in large part on where the victim is encountered. For example, in the hot and warm zones, only rescuers with protective equipment may be present. Because the ability to evaluate will be somewhat limited, triage may use an abbreviated version of START (see Chapter 28). For example, it may be difficult to take a pulse, so more reliance is placed on observation of breathing and response to stimuli. Treatment with the MARK I kits for severe nerve agent poisoning may be lifesaving and can be administered through a victim's clothing. Only lifesaving treatment should be rendered in the contaminated zones as permitted by available personnel.

Decontamination in the warm zone may take place in separate areas for litter patients and for ambulatory victims. Serious victims who may be salvaged should receive priority. After decontamination is complete, the victim can be moved across the line into the clean zone, where the EMTs can provide further evaluation and treatment before transport. All care rendered should be documented on a triage tag. Anyone who has entered the contaminated zone needs to be decontaminated before leaving.

The concept of hot, warm, and cold zones may be unrealistic in large-scale situations. In fact, patients will self-triage and will naturally want to flee to safety, and will seek out medical care at local hospitals on their own. The threat of secondary contamination is real, and EMS agencies and nearby hospitals need to accept this as part of a possible public response so they can minimize the effects.

LEARNING OBJECTIVE
• Describe the types of radiologic hazards.

Nuclear Agents

Radiation is a form of energy transmission, as in radiation from the sun. **Nuclear radiation** refers to energy emitted from the nucleus of an unstable atom (**Box 30-5**). Nuclear radiation may be in the form of waves or particles, such as electromagnetic waves or alpha particles, beta particles, and neutrons. Nuclear

---

| **Box 30-5** | **The Atom** |

An *atom* is the smallest building block of an element. An atom consists of protons, neutrons, and electrons. Most atoms are "stable," meaning the various components stay together in a given configuration with equal numbers of protons, neutrons, and electrons. However, some elements exist in more than one form, having in common the same number of protons but different numbers of neutrons. Therefore they would have the same atomic number and similar chemical properties, but different atomic weights and possibly different physical properties. The different forms of an element are called *isotopes*. Some isotopes are "unstable" in that they have a tendency to break down spontaneously to smaller atoms *while emitting energetic rays or particles* from the nucleus in the process. Such isotopes are called *radioactive*, and the energy emitted is called *nuclear radiation* because it emanates from the nucleus.

---

radiation has the potential to alter molecules within the cell and thereby alter its function, referred to as *radiation injury*. This is sometimes referred to as *ionizing radiation* because it can convert other atoms with which it collides into charged particles (ions).

Ionizing radiation can cause instant biochemical changes in the cells. Depending on the type and dose of radiation, the effects can be immediate or delayed. High doses of radiation sustained over a short time can lead to an **acute radiation syndrome,** which can result in rapid onset of severe illness and death. Smaller doses may result in genetic effects or increased risk of cancer or cataracts, or it may affect growth, development, and life span.

Radiation Tolerance

Small amounts of radiation are not harmful. We all receive small doses of radiation each day from the sun, the earth, and other natural and artificial sources. Workers who are exposed to radioactive materials in the workplace may receive greater exposure. Limits are set on the amount of radiation to which they can safely be exposed.

Radiation cannot be perceived by our senses. We need special instruments to alert us to its presence. Workers who are exposed to radiation wear instruments to monitor the exposure encountered on the job.

Radiation Incidents

Radiation injury calls to mind threats of nuclear war and disasters such as Chernobyl and Three Mile Island. Fortunately, radiation injuries are not part of everyday emergency care. Before Chernobyl, the Federal Emergency Management Agency (FEMA) noted that in 40 years, fewer than 1000 persons in the world were known to have been involved in serious radiation incidents, with only about 450 receiving medically serious doses of radiation or contamination, and with fewer than 21 cases resulting in death. According to FEMA, "Rescuers, physicians, and nurses who were monitored while providing emergency care and treatment to victims of radiation accidents in the past received radiation exposures less than or comparable to exposures received in medical diagnostic studies."

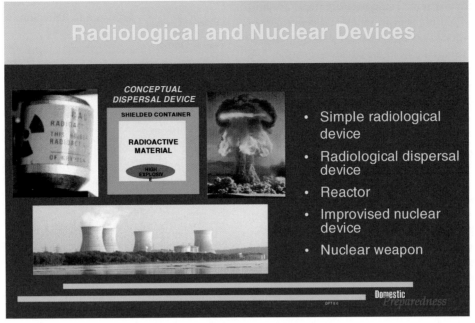

Figure 30-14 Examples of nuclear threats.

Radiation incidents usually occur in the workplace, where expert help and advice are at hand to guide the actions of emergency personnel who must care for victims who may have combined radiation and traumatic injuries. Because of the special nature of radioactive materials, special precautions are taken and plans made in advance for emergencies. Because radioactive wastes are transported along highways, an EMT might be called to the scene of a traffic incident that involves potential radiation cargo.

Threat of Radiation from Terrorism

Nuclear threats from terrorists are not judged to be as likely to occur as biologic or chemical threats, but they still must be considered. The range of threats includes detonation of a nuclear weapon, such as a "suitcase bomb"; sabotage of nuclear reactors; and dispersal of contents of radiologic agents found in medicine or industry (**Figure 30-14**).

The DOD describes five scenarios in which radioactive incidents might occur, as follows:

1. *Deliberate spread of radioactive material without explosion.* Examples cited are placing radioactive materials in a public place, exposing individuals in the area. Potent sources are found in hospitals, such as for radiation therapy. For example, thieves in Brazil stole radioactive materials (perhaps unknowingly), and 249 people were contaminated and four died.
2. *Radiologic dispersal.* An explosive disperses radiologic material over a larger area. The material may be stolen from a hospital or local industry. Both the blast from the explosion and the secondary contamination to victims and rescuers would be threats.
3. *Nuclear reactor sabotage.* The meltdown at Chernobyl resulted in 28 deaths (short term) and hundreds of severely ill patients, so the potential for a problem exists but is believed to be negligible.

4. *Improvised nuclear device.* An attempt by terrorists to build a nuclear weapon is technically very difficult but theoretically possible.
5. *Nuclear weapon.* Reportedly, suitcase-sized nuclear weapons are missing from Russia.

Regardless of the extent of actual physical injury from a nuclear incident, public reaction to news of a nuclear incident might result in widespread fear. It is important for emergency responders to prepare for nuclear incidents so that they can respond appropriately to actual events and assure the public that effects will be contained as much as possible if such an event occurs.

In addition to knowing how to summon expert help and advice, EMTs should have an understanding of the basic principles regarding radiation hazards so they can initiate lifesaving interventions and emergency care, taking precautions to prevent unnecessary radiation exposure to themselves, the public, and the victims.

> **LEARNING OBJECTIVE**
> - Describe the difference between radioactive particles (alpha, beta, neutrons) and radioactive waves.

Measuring Radioactive Activity

Units of Measurement

Ionizing radiation can result in an electronically measurable charge in the air through which it passes. This charge is measured as a *roentgen* (R). A *rad* (radiation *a*bsorbed *d*ose) is a measurement of the amount of radiation absorbed by a material or the body. A *rem* (*r*oentgen *e*quivalent *m*an) is a unit equal to the absorbed dose in rads multiplied by modifying and quality factors, allowing for some comparison of the effects of different types of radiation. All these units are also expressed as $\frac{1}{1000}$ parts, or milliroentgen (mR), millirad (mrad), and millirem (mrem).

Note that 1000 mrem = 1 rem. These measurements are how radiation is calibrated on survey instruments and personal protection badges. Radiation safety officers use such measurements to judge safety at a scene, the need for decontamination, and potential medical consequences of exposure.

Measuring Instruments

Radioactivity cannot be perceived by the senses and must be measured with instruments. Two important types are the survey instrument and the personal monitoring device. A radiation survey should be performed at the scene to guide rescue personnel. Personal dosimeters should be worn by all personnel to document the extent of their personal exposure.

Radiation safety officers or radiologic monitors should have the necessary expertise to use and interpret the results of survey and personal monitoring devices and to direct initial safety, rescue, and containment efforts. They are necessary to guide the decontamination process. EMTs should follow the advice of the radiation safety officers whenever available.

Survey Instruments

Survey instruments measure the rate of exposure and calculate it in terms of roentgens per hour or milliroentgens per hour. The Geiger-Müller counter is an example of a survey instrument. All civil defense survey meters are designed to measure gamma radiation, and some are able to detect the presence of beta radiation. Special instruments for alpha radiation detection are also available.

With survey measurements, EMTs can determine whether there is still a significant risk of irradiation at an exposure site and can predict their exposure dose over time if they enter the area. Safety officers can use this information to make risk calculations before a rescue attempt, to keep exposures within safe limits. The survey instrument can also be used to determine if a victim or rescuer has been contaminated and to monitor the decontamination process.

Dosimeters are radiation-measuring instruments used to monitor the total accumulation of radiation. Dosimeters are worn by individuals who work with radioactive particles or by rescue personnel. If the dosimeter is worn on the torso, the amount of radiation measured is estimated to be similar to the total whole-body radiation. The unit of measurement used is a roentgen or milliroentgen.

Basic types of dosimeters include film badges or photographic film, thermoluminescent devices, and pocket dosimeters, which are pocket ionization devices worn as a pencil in the breast pocket. A permanent record can be obtained from film badges and *thermoluminescent* devices, which document total exposure to beta and gamma radiation (some can measure neutron capability). The pocket dosimeter has a scale that can be read at the site to monitor total exposure at different times. Rescuers may use pocket dosimeters to ascertain whether it is safe for them to remain in the area of exposure after consultation with the radiation safety officer.

Types of Radiation

Classic types of radioactive emissions are alpha particles, beta particles, gamma rays, and neutrons. The first three are the most common because neutron-type radiation is found only

Table 30-6	Exposure to Radiation
Type of Exposure	**Amount of Exposure**
Natural background and man-made radiation	360 mrem/year
Diagnostic chest radiograph	10 mrem
Flight from Los Angeles to Paris	4.8 mrem
Barium enema	800 mrem
Smoking 1.5 packs of cigarettes per day	16,000 mrem/year
Heart catheterization	45,000 mrem
Mild acute radiation sickness	200,000 mrem
LD_{50} for irradiation	450,000 mrem

LD_{50}, Median lethal dose; *mrem* = $\frac{1}{1000}$ rem.

in high-technology installations such as nuclear reactors or linear accelerators. Again, when discussing radioactive material, it is important to remember that we are exposed to a certain amount of natural radiation every day from sources such as the atmosphere, earth, and foods. The average amount of annual exposure in the United States from these natural sources ranges from 100 to 400 mrem/year (**Table 30-6**).

Alpha Radiation

An **alpha particle** is a positively charged particle consisting of two protons and two neutrons. It is the least penetrating form of radiation and travels only a few centimeters in the air. It can be stopped by a sheet of paper, clothing, and the epidermis of the skin. It is dangerous only if ingested, inhaled, or absorbed through broken skin. Within the body, alpha radiation can affect nearby tissues. Transuranic isotopes are the most common source of alpha particles involved in nuclear incidents.

Beta Radiation

Beta particles are charged particles that have the mass of an electron. They have either a negative or a positive charge (called positrons). In air, they can travel from less than 1 foot to several feet, depending on the energy. Beta particles travel somewhat deeper than alpha particles but are stopped by the skin, where they can cause burns similar to thermal burns if left in contact with the body for a time. They can be stopped by clothing. As with alpha particles, beta particles are usually dangerous only if they cause internal contamination through ingestion, inhalation, or absorption through a break in the skin.

Because alpha and beta particles are *matter*, they can cling to the skin or clothing or contaminate a person. *Contamination* is defined as a radioactive substance dispersed in materials or places where it is undesirable. As with any other matter, these radioactive materials can be spread to other persons or things. Proper handling is required to contain the radioactive materials until they can be removed from places and people during decontamination procedures. *In practice, measures used to handle victims contaminated by radiation incidents are similar to the precautions taken with victims of communicable diseases.*

Gamma Rays

Gamma rays are high-energy electromagnetic radiation rays similar to x-rays but more energetic. They can penetrate the body and cause damage by ionizing molecules in their path. Biochemical transformation of ionized molecules is instantaneous and may lead to biologic effects manifesting later. The gamma ray does not cause contamination of the victim, and the victim is of no risk to others. The victim exposed to gamma rays is said to have been *irradiated*. Gamma rays can travel long distances and penetrate most materials with ease. Dense materials such as lead are the best shielding against gamma rays.

Neutrons

Neutrons are uncharged particles found in the nucleus of an atom. Neutron emissions occur in nuclear reactors along with other types of radioactivity. Neutrons are much more penetrating than alpha and beta particles and can cause considerable damage to underlying tissue. They can "activate" the body and materials in their path, such as rings, belt buckles, coins, and tie pins. Because they are found only in special situations, they are mentioned here only for completeness. The remaining discussion focuses primarily on alpha, beta, and gamma radiation, which are more likely to be encountered.

> **LEARNING OBJECTIVE**
> - Describe the difference between contamination and irradiation and incorporation.

Contamination versus Irradiation

The EMT must make a clear conceptual distinction between the two main types of radiation injuries: contamination and irradiation. **Contamination** is caused by radioactive particles that are physically present. **Irradiation** is caused by radioactive energy in wave or ray form and is similar to an x-ray in that it passes through but is not physically present on the body. Thus the contaminated victim can spread radioactive materials to others; the irradiated patient cannot.

Irradiation. Gamma rays, which irradiate a victim, are electromagnetic waves of energy and do not behave as particles. They pass through or penetrate the body but do not remain as radioactive materials either on or within it. The victim is "irradiated" and presents no more risk to another person than does that patient receiving radiation therapy for cancer. Any damage to the victim irradiated by gamma rays is a result of the biochemical transformations resulting from ionization of molecules during their penetration.

Contamination. Contamination may be external or internal. *External* contamination means that the presence of radioactive materials is limited to the skin and clothing. *Internal* contamination occurs when radioactive materials enter the body through swallowing, inhalation, or a break in the skin. Once within the body, radioactive materials can be incorporated as part of the body's structure.

External contamination and internal contamination demand different responses. External contamination itself is rarely a medical emergency. The primary concern with the externally contaminated patient is proper handling to prevent unnecessary spread of radioactive materials to the patient, the rescuer, and others. The presence of external contamination should not interfere with the delivery of necessary emergency care to the acutely injured patient.

Internal contamination can be treated with medical measures to eliminate, dilute, bind, or block the effects of the radioactive material before it becomes incorporated within the body. Internal contamination is no hazard to the rescuer who takes appropriate personal protection precautions.

Incorporation refers to the take-up of radioactive materials by body cells, tissues, and organs. Common sites are bone, the liver, thyroid, and kidneys. For example, radioactive iodide might be incorporated within the thyroid gland. Incorporation only happens if internal contamination occurs. Rather than being eliminated from the body, the incorporated elements are now part of it, emitting ionizing radiation to nearby cells and increasing risk of subsequent illness.

Types of Patients

Irradiation and contamination are two different results of radiation injury, and a victim may have either or both types of injuries. You might encounter four distinct types of injury after responding to the site of a possible radiation injury, as follows:

1. Irradiated with no contamination
2. External contamination
3. Internal contamination by inhalation, ingestion, or a break in the skin
4. Simple trauma

A patient may have a combination of any of these conditions.

> **LEARNING OBJECTIVE**
> - Describe acute radiation syndrome.

Acute Radiation Syndrome

High doses of radiation absorbed over a short period (minutes to hours) can cause signs and symptoms of acute radiation syndrome. This syndrome results from damage to the bone marrow, GI tract, CNS, and cardiovascular system as the dosage increases. For example, at an exposure of 50 rem, patients may have no visible effects, but a small percentage of persons who have been exposed may show a depression of white blood cells and platelets on blood testing. Physical signs and symptoms may first appear at a dose of 100 rem, with nausea and vomiting occurring in a small percentage of exposed persons. At 200 rem, most patients show signs of nausea and vomiting, with more profound depression of the bone marrow. At 400 rem, about 50% of the exposed individuals die within weeks. An exposure of 600 rem can result in almost 100% mortality if there is no medical intervention.

At doses of 1000 rem, GI complications begin to appear as nausea, vomiting, and diarrhea of immediate onset. At doses of 3000 rem, there are additional irreversible cardiovascular effects resulting in irreversible hypotension and a CNS syndrome with rapid onset of drowsiness, uncoordination, and convulsions.

Emergency Medical Care of Radiation Victims

The main focus on emergency care is treatment of associated injuries, removal from further radiation exposure, and decontamination.

Once a patient has been irradiated, little can be done at the scene. Illness usually follows hours to days later. The main focus is to limit continued exposure and treat associated injuries.

The contaminated victim requires attention to minimize the risk of internal contamination and incorporation. Through decontamination, the potential for internal contamination and secondary spread is reduced. If internal contamination has occurred, treatment to minimize the chance of incorporation should be considered as soon as possible.

> **LEARNING OBJECTIVE**
> - List factors that affect the severity of radiation exposure and how they can be used to limit exposure.

Personal Protection and Factors Affecting Severity of Exposure

The major factors used by rescuers to limit exposure are *time*, *distance*, and *shielding*. The severity of radiation exposure is affected by the strength of the radioactive source, the type of radiation, the duration of exposure, the area of the body exposed, the distance from the radioactive source, the amount of shielding between the source and the victim, and the age and condition of the patient.

Duration of Exposure. The shorter the time spent in a radiation field, the less radiation the body absorbs. For example, if the exposure rate is 100 R/hour, 15 minutes in the area may result in absorption of 25 R. Rescue workers can reduce individual exposure by sharing the time spent in the danger zone to perform a rescue.

Distance from the Source. The greater the distance from the source of radiation, the less is the radiation dose absorbed. If the source of radiation emanates from a single point, radioactivity falls inversely with the *square of the distance*. Thus, if the distance from the source is doubled, the absorbed dose decreases by a factor of 4; if tripled, it decreases by a factor of 9.

If radiation sources are scattered, this inverse square rule does not apply. However, radiation exposure is decreased significantly by increasing the distance from the material.

Shielding. Rescuers may shield themselves from the source of exposure with lead aprons or other dense materials (e.g., keeping a vehicle between themselves and the source). At times, it may be more practical to shield the source itself. Protective clothing should be worn to minimize exposure.

Penetrating radiation affects the cells through which it passes. Limitation of the exposure to an extremity, for example, may limit damage to an arm or leg and not result in the radiation syndrome. Different parts of the body can tolerate different amounts of radiation. For example, the maximal permissible occupational standards for the hands are several times the allowable limit for the gonads or the whole body. Therefore, it makes a difference which parts of the body are shielded during exposure. The routine use of shielding for parts of the body while exposing medical or dental x-ray films is an example of limiting body exposure.

Emergency Care for Radiation Injuries

Emergency medical technicians should know the scope of care expected of them in their area so they can be adequately prepared. In most events, EMTs would be called if there were a need for emergency medical attention for victims at a radiation incident site. Preplanning for radiation emergencies is done by industries that use radioactive material, all hospitals accredited by The Joint Commission (formerly Joint Commission on Accreditation of Healthcare Organizations), and responsible government agencies. These plans include the establishment of responsibility for radiologic monitoring and decontamination as well as transportation of injured victims. If EMTs are expected to participate in monitoring or rescue efforts, they should receive appropriate specialized training in each aspect of their expected performance, such as use of survey instruments, use of protective clothing, and familiarity with decontamination processes, following local protocols.

Actions for the EMT as a First Responder

Create a Safety Zone and Make Notification

If you are a first responder and discover a possible nuclear incident, your first actions should be similar to any other hazardous materials event. Establish a safety zone and prevent the public from entering the area. Stage yourself away from the incident and upwind. Notify the dispatcher so that local and regional experts can be mobilized to bring resources to guide rescue and decontamination efforts.

Use Protection Principles

Follow basic radiation protection principles; create a safety zone at least 150 feet upwind; and use protective gear to prevent unnecessary radiation exposure to self, the public, other rescuers, and victims. The basic principles used to minimize exposure to radiation include limiting the exposure to the smallest portion of the body possible and considering time, distance, and shielding, as follows:

1. Limit the time of exposure. Time in the exposure zone is minimized through use of an efficient work plan. If exposure levels are high, the patient should be removed as quickly as possible to a safe area. As in the case of fires or poisonous gases, removal of the patient to a safe environment takes priority over splinting and other aspects of emergency care. If extrication and removal are complicated, rescuers should consider sharing exposure time, which will reduce individual exposure. You should be guided by a radiation safety officer.

2. Maintain the greatest possible distance from the source. Small changes in distance can greatly reduce exposure.

3. Use suitable shielding. To protect against gamma radiation, lead shielding is required. The source itself may be shielded to prevent exposure. Other methods to place shields between the source and the victim include positioning a vehicle between them and using concrete walls or mounds of earth as shields.

4. Limit exposure to the smallest portion of the body possible. Avoid touching radioactive materials directly.

Use Protective Gear

Use protective clothing, including gloves, masks, and surgical gowns at a minimum. Shoe covers should also be used. If these are not readily available, paper bags can be secured over the shoes with tape; this offers protection if the area is not wet. A standard protocol might include the following:

1. Attach a film badge with your name to the uniform or street clothes.
2. Put large surgical trousers and pullover shirts over the uniform or street clothes. If available, tape waterproof shoe covers to the cuffs of the protective trousers.
3. Wear a surgical gown and a surgical hood and mask to offer protection to the face and head.
4. Consider wearing a second pair of surgical gloves to allow removal of the top pair should they become contaminated.
5. Attach a second dosimeter to the neck of the gown so that it can be easily read, but be careful not to place it in an area where it can be easily contaminated.

Emergency Medical Care

Medical care is the same whether the victim is contaminated or irradiated. Note that the irradiated patient poses no risk to the rescuer, whereas the contaminated patient must be approached with personal protection to avoid secondary contamination.

The first priority, as always, is to provide lifesaving emergency care. When exposures from the radioactive source are at life-threatening levels, rapidly remove the victim from the danger zone. After removal, initiate basic trauma care as necessary.

If contamination is the main hazard to the EMT, lifesaving care should be given to the victim after donning surgical gloves, gown, and mask. Avoid internal contamination from mouth-to-mouth ventilation by using other appropriate positive-pressure ventilation devices. Removing the victim's clothing generally removes 80% to 90% of the contamination. Seal it in a plastic bag, label it, and leave it in the contaminated zone for later retrieval and disposition.

Rarely is the contaminated victim a threat to the rescuers. Precautions taken during the handling of contaminated victims are aimed at preventing the spread of radioactive materials and preventing or minimizing internal contamination. The patient should be removed to a safe zone, free from threats of irradiation, where the presence and extent of contamination can be determined if a radiologic monitor is available.

Decontamination

Decontamination has three purposes: (1) prevent or minimize transfer of contaminants to an internal site, (2) reduce the amount of radiation dose from the contaminant, and (3) prevent the spread of contamination to other persons and areas. Decontamination is usually adequately accomplished with soap and water and should be conducted by individuals with appropriate training and personal protection.

Advance Hospital Notification and Plan for Orderly Transfer of Care

Hospitals have plans for caring for patients with radiation injuries. Nuclear power plants and some industries that work with nuclear materials have prior arrangements with hospitals for the care of radiation victims, which may include separate entrances and areas for care of contaminated victims. You should notify the hospital as early as possible so that staff can assemble personnel and supplies. In most situations, a decontamination room is designated and a path formed to the ambulance reception area to keep out unnecessary personnel. The floor is covered with paper or plastic coverings, as are wall switches, doorknobs, and other equipment, to limit the spread of radioactive contamination and to facilitate the cleanup. A control person is assigned to limit access into the area. You should follow this person's instructions.

The hospital staff use protective clothing and dosimeters and may provide these to ambulance personnel if needed as part of the team that implements the decontamination procedures previously noted.

The emergency physician and the radiation officer may meet the ambulance at the ED entrance. The physician assesses the patient for life-threatening injuries while the radiation safety officer determines whether the victim is contaminated. If the victim is still clothed, a decision may be made to leave it in the ambulance.

An emergency cart should be available. The ambulance stretcher is placed on the covered floor and the patient transferred to a clean stretcher and wrapped in clean blankets by hospital personnel so that a noncontaminated stretcher enters the hospital. The EMTs may be asked to remain in the ambulance until they and their equipment can be monitored and decontaminated. A buffer zone is established between contaminated and clean areas within the hospital, which is staffed with a "floating" nurse or aide.

The EMTs are monitored by the radiation safety officer. At the demarcation ("clean line") between potentially contaminated and clean areas, the EMTs should remove protective clothing in the sequence outlined, placing it in a plastic container marked "contaminated."

A complete body survey should be done of each staff member at the control line. The radiation safety officer's advice should be followed during the procedure and during decontamination of the ambulance. If an EMT was contaminated, consult a physician for postexposure follow-up.

Summary of Nuclear Agents

Understanding basic principles of radiation injuries helps the EMT to function effectively as part of a team when responding to radiation events. In addition to providing emergency care, EMTs must act to protect themselves and others from unnecessary radiation exposure and contamination. Steps involved may include identification of the substance, notification of authorities, establishment of a safety zone, and use of protective gear. Actions should be guided by radiation protection principles: time, distance, shielding, and limitation of exposure to the smallest possible body part.

The role of the radiation safety officer is crucial because special instruments and expertise are necessary to detect the presence and evaluate the significance of ionizing radiation. The survey instrument allows evaluation of the amount of exposure from an unshielded source and determines whether victims are contaminated. The dosimeter allows measurement of accumulated exposure to the patient and rescuers.

The irradiated patient presents no hazard to the EMT. The contaminated patient generally presents little threat but must be handled carefully to minimize the chance of internal contamination or secondary contamination of others. Emergency medical care should not stop because of contamination, except perhaps to don gloves and protective clothing. Decontamination may be started at the scene or in the hospital, depending on circumstances and the degree of injuries. Internal contamination is a medical emergency requiring expert advice and treatment to prevent incorporation of the radioactive material within the body.

Emergency medical care of victims at the scene follows these principles: remove the victim from the hot zone, do not delay critical emergency medical interventions unless to put on personal protective equipment, and decontaminate patients to reduce the chance of internal contamination and incorporation.

Although most radiation incidents have not resulted in any medically significant exposure to rescuers or field personnel, the EMT must be aware of the potential danger in high-technology areas, where high exposure levels may be encountered, or in terrorist events. Early onset of symptoms and signs of acute radiation syndrome mean a high dose was absorbed. Preplanning is the key to effective management of these infrequent situations. Know your role within the local protocols. Participate according to your level of training and role in your system.

Scenario Follow-up

Medical command has received reports from rescuers on the scene as well as your report. Victims on the ground who collapsed as they exited the back door of the bus have signs of increased work of breathing, muscular twitching, excessive secretions, and small pupils. Your reports of victims able to flee from the area who have visual disturbances, shortness of breath, small pupils, and tearing help confirm the suspicion of a nerve agent exposure. Medical command directs administration of nerve agent antidote (atropine and pralidoxime) to victims with severe exposure.

Rescuers with chemical protective clothing and respiratory protection board the bus and extricate the victims who have collapsed. Three victims are unconscious but have vital signs and are given oxygen and MARK I antidote injections. One victim, a child, is given a pediatric dose of the antidote. Two victims have no signs of life and are pronounced dead at the scene.

There are more victims with mild complaints than there are ambulances. Incident command directs two buses to be used for transport. Because a gas is suspected, victims are advised to remove their outer clothing, and men and women are separated on the two transporting buses. You are directed to attend the victims on one bus, bringing your MARK I antidote along as you continue to monitor the patients en route to the hospital.

People from the terminal not on the bus with the victims are separated and observed again for signs of exposure. After a period of observation, and with consultation from medical command, they are advised that they have no signs of exposure and do not require hospital evaluation. Their names and contact information are kept in a log, and they are advised to call public health authorities for any further questions or concerns.

Summary and Further Recommendations

Nuclear, biologic, and chemical (NBC) weapons are a real threat. Deployment by terrorists has occurred around the world. Military development of extremely toxic, genetically altered, and weaponized strains is well documented. Stocks of weapons are missing, and terrorist-minded states and organizations have shown interest in using them. These facts cannot be ignored. First responders must prepare as much as possible for a domestic attack.

Key and logical steps in any response include the following:
- Recognize that a terrorist event is simultaneously a mass casualty event, a hazardous materials incident, and a crime scene.
- Learn from the past. First, there may be little control over ambulatory victims; those who are able may flee the scene and overwhelm the nearby hospitals, and secondary contamination may be a major problem. Second, the medical responders who converge may not have participated in disaster training or the incident management command structure, and chaos may ensue at the scene and at area hospitals. Third, responders may rush to help without due consideration for personal protective equipment (PPE) and may become victims themselves.
- There is great psychological stress in an NBC event. It is important to provide leadership and clear direction for the lay public lest their own actions lead to further chaos.

For these and other reasons, it is essential to add NBC preparedness to existing disaster and hazmat training.

Use of an all-hazard approach is recommended in planning. Use the NBC "delta" approach, adding special preparation and drills for NBC events to the traditional disaster and hazmat drills already practiced in your region. Responders are more likely to stay organized if a familiar structure is followed.

In addition, as occurred on September 11, 2001, at the World Trade Center, real events have shown that loss of communication, command centers, and lead personnel can occur at the disaster site. When the remaining responders regroup, they are most effective when they can reestablish a structure known to all of them in advance.

In addition to standard training for hazardous materials and disasters, special needs of NBC events must be considered. These include introduction of any special equipment needed as well as including these events in yearly disaster drills. These drills are a good way to test whether the required PPE, antidotes, decontamination equipment, and plans to treat high numbers of casualties (and victims who present to hospitals) actually work, and to fix them if they do not work.

At the NBC scene, the incident management system will be established to organize and direct the response. As the most experienced medical personnel at the scene, the EMTs will assist by evaluating signs and symptoms and comparing them to known agents or classes of agents in NBC events. The evaluation may be at a distance, from reports at the scene or from bystanders, and from ambulatory victims who have fled the scene. If an NBC attack is suspected, EMTs should take protective measures and warn responding units of the potential risk.

The incident management command will decide on needed PPE; establishment of the hot, warm, and cold zones; and where triage, treatment, and transport will be conducted. EMTs will assume their role within the medical context of the incident management command structure. (See also Chapter 28.)

The EMTs need to know the appropriate use of and the limits of PPE for NBC events. Biologic PPE should be well known and reviewed. If EMTs are asked to work in a warm zone, they must know how to use and be fitted with adequate respiratory, eye, and skin PPE to protect against the responsible agent. Radiation protection is based on the principles of time, distance, and shielding. If there is threat of airborne particles, level C respiratory protection is warranted. Personal dosimeters that allow for immediate reading should be part of training and familiar to EMTs.

Familiarity with decontamination is essential for protection of self, others, and the victims. Secondary contamination and cross-contamination must be avoided through proper use of PPE; respect for hot, warm, and cold zones; and separation of contamination from equipment and the vehicle.

A chemical attack may initially be suspected after assessment of the victims. Portable devices and testing agents can detect NBC agents in the field; their value and limitations should be appreciated. Chemical devices may provide a general indication of the class of agent, but some devices will not detect low concentrations of an agent, and others may give a false-positive reading because they react with another substance.

As with disaster triage, the principles remain "to do the greatest good for the greatest number." Disaster triage often focuses on traumatic injuries. NBC events require evaluation and categorization of medical patients as well. The victims of chemical agents require special consideration. For example, nerve agent victims need to be assessed for possible emergent antidote therapy. Phosgene and mustard exposure would have unique features to consider in a triage scenario involving multiple victims.

Decontamination, triage, and treatment are dictated largely by the agent used. Useful handbooks and guidebooks to assist first responders at the scene include *Jane's Chem-Bio Handbook* and the U.S. Army's pocket-sized guidebooks for medical management of biologic and chemical casualties.

There are multiple considerations during transportation. Local hospitals may be overwhelmed by the "walking wounded." Therefore, victims who are not emergent might be directed to more distant hospitals with greater capacity. If there are multiple victims, especially ambulatory victims, alternate means of transport such as buses might be used. Ambulance transport might be reserved for more emergent victims who require care en route. At a minimum, gross decontamination should be accomplished before entrance into the relatively closed space in the vehicle, to prevent the rescuers from being subjected to

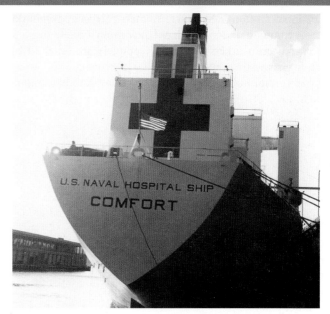

Figure 30-15 The U.S. Navy's *USS Comfort* at port on the Hudson River, prepared to accept victims of the World Trade Center attacks.

off-gassing or secondary contamination from the victim. Maintaining cleanliness of the vehicle is also important because it may be placed out of service for other transports until decontamination is accomplished.

A destination list should be maintained at the transport sector because distraught families and relatives will be searching for their loved ones soon after the incident. Without information from the transport sector, these families will be left searching directly at one hospital after another in the region, further straining resources at the facilities.

Plans may call for establishment of field treatment stations for first responders. In prolonged efforts, these may be staffed by disaster management assistance teams from outside the region. Mobile hospitals may be set up to care for survivors (**Figure 30-15**).

Plans should address evidence protection because a terrorist event is a crime scene. Dispersal equipment may be present, and a perpetrator may be one of the victims at the scene. Law enforcement personnel will be part of the response, and planning in advance for the mutual needs of all the responding agencies allows smooth interaction and understanding at a real event.

Don't wait for a disaster to see if the plan works. Work with smaller components of the plan and build on disaster and hazmat training, then incorporate NBC scenarios and conduct drills with other agencies.

This chapter is based in large part on the DOD Domestic Preparedness Program. National curricula include those from FEMA, the Department of Justice, and the military that address weapons of mass destruction preparedness. Their value cannot be overemphasized. Few people have actual experience with these agents. Many experts working on national defense against WMDs have contributed to the course content. Because federal, state, and regional agencies will all need to work together when a terrorist event occurs, it is common sense to undertake a national promulgated course so that emergency responders have a common understanding of their mutual roles.

Healthcare workers and first responders are on the front line for domestic preparedness and responses to NBC events in our communities. EMTs should receive additional training in the NBC "delta." We need to continue to prepare for NBC terrorism, and through our actions our communities are better prepared to withstand these threats. Moreover, our increased training and skills preparing for WMD events can benefit patients in our daily response to their calls for help.

The Bottom Line

Learning Checklist

✓ Terrorists have used biologic and chemical weapons of mass destruction (WMDs) in many countries, including *Salmonella* food poisoning in Oregon and nerve agent poisoning in Japan. Stockpiles of nuclear, biologic, and chemical (NBC) weapons are unaccounted for, and terrorists have threatened to use WMDs against the United States and other nations.

✓ An EMT must be aware of NBC threats to search for and recognize possible NBC scenarios during scene size-up; understand the importance of safety issues for personal, patient, and bystander safety; fulfill the medical needs to respond to various NBC agents; and participate within the regional response plans to NBC events.

✓ The EMT understands that knowledge of specific agents is necessary to recognize, triage, treat, and transport victims of WMD agents.

✓ An NBC terrorist act is distinguished from a hazardous materials incident by its intentional nature, purposely hidden hazard, extremely toxic material, need for massive decontamination, possible secondary devices, and being a crime scene.

✓ An NBC weapon can be disseminated by breaking or bursting agents, munitions, spraying devices, contamination of ventilation systems, and vectors (insects, animals, water, food).

✓ Signs of an NBC event include multiple casualties who were previously well, all with the same complaints and at a similar time of onset, as well as signs and symptoms unusual for the season, a geographic area, a particular age group, or spread by a vector unusual for a region.

✓ Surveillance of EMS and ED patients for syndromes such as respiratory complaints, GI complaints, neurologic complaints, or fever and rash, which may be caused by WMD agents, results in early investigation and early identification of an NBC release.

✓ Early signs and symptoms of biologic agents, including anthrax, smallpox, tularemia, plague, and viral hemorrhagic fever, include fever and malaise and might be mistaken for the flu. As these illnesses progress, other signs appear such as characteristic rash (smallpox), bloody sputum (plague), and bleeding tendencies (viral hemorrhagic fevers).

✓ The keys to management of patients with illness caused by biologic agents are good infection control practice; use of standard, airborne, droplet, and contact precautions; proper disposal or disinfection of equipment and the vehicle; postexposure follow-up; and notification of the hospital of the need for potential isolation of arriving patients.

✓ Biologic agents that pose a risk for secondary transmission include plague, smallpox, and viral hemorrhagic fevers.

✓ Chemical agents that might be used in a bioterrorist attack include nerve agents, cyanide, pulmonary agents, and sulfur mustard.

✓ Chemical agents that can cause immediate (seconds to minutes) symptoms, including collapse and death, include nerve agents and cyanide. Victims of severe exposure may require antidote treatment at the scene to survive.

✓ Principles of decontamination for chemical agent vapor exposure include moving away from the source of exposure to fresh air and removing outer clothing to prevent off-gassing.

✓ Principles of decontamination for chemical agent liquid exposure include (1) physical removal by scraping the agent off with a stick or other device, blotting with powder or dirt, removing clothing, and flushing with water and (2) deactivation with soap and water, bleach and water, or prepackaged kits (e.g., M291 kit for military personnel).

✓ Types of radiologic hazards include detonation of nuclear weapons, nuclear reactor sabotage, explosive dispersal of radiologic material, and nonexplosive dispersal of radiologic material.

✓ Radiation exposure can cause irradiation and contamination. Irradiation is the passage of radiation energy through the body, which can alter chemicals and cells in its path. Irradiation is no threat to the rescuer. Contamination results from radioactive particles being deposited on or in the body. These particles can be spread to the rescuer and others.

✓ Incorporation is the physical binding of a radioactive material or particle within the body's tissues or organs, where it becomes part of the organ and can continue to affect nearby tissue with its radioactive energy.

✓ The principles of prehospital treatment of radiologic casualties include self-protection, removal of victims from the source, provision of basic life support emergency care, and if necessary, decontamination of the victim.

✓ Major self-protection principles are time of exposure, distance from the source, and shielding.

✓ Concerns of contamination should not delay emergency care of radiologic victims except to don personal protective equipment to minimize cross-contamination.

✓ Radioactive particles (alpha, beta, neutrons) are matter and can contaminate or be physically present on a victim. Radioactive waves such as gamma rays pass through a victim the same as x-rays and pose no threat to a rescuer.

✓ Acute radiation syndrome results from absorption of high doses of radiation over a short time and manifests as nausea and vomiting and depression of the bone marrow; in higher doses cardiovascular and CNS effects are present.

✓ Radioactivity is detected by survey instruments that measure the amount of radiation per unit of time and personal dosimeters that record absorbed dose.

Key Terms

Acute radiation syndrome Syndrome that results from high doses of radiation absorbed over a short period that results in damage to the bone marrow, gastrointestinal tract, central nervous system, and cardiovascular system.

Alpha particles Positively charged particles consisting of two protons and two neutrons.

Beta particles Negatively or positively charged particles that have the mass of an electron.

Contamination Radiation injury caused by radioactive particles that are physically present. The contaminated patient can pass radioactive materials to others.

Dosimeter Radiation-measuring devices used to monitor the total accumulation of radiation.

Gamma rays High-energy electromagnetic radiation rays similar to x-rays but more energetic.

Incorporation Binding of radioactive materials into the body cells, tissues, and organs.

Irradiation Radioactive energy in wave or ray form passing through but not physically present on the body. The irradiated patient cannot spread radioactive materials to others.

Nuclear radiation Energy emitted from the nucleus of an unstable atom.

Quarantine The isolation of patients exposed to or having a contagious disease for a period until they are incapable of either developing or transmitting the disease.

SLUDGEM Mnemonic for salivation, lacrimation, urination, diarrhea, gastrointestinal cramps, emesis (vomiting), miosis (small pupils), and muscular twitching.

Survey instruments Instruments designed to monitor and measure radiation.

Weapons of mass destruction (WMDs) Nuclear, biologic, and chemical agents intended to do harm.

Review Questions

1. Which of the following best describes features of a terrorist incident versus a hazardous materials incident?
   a. Extremely toxic material, mass casualties, placards available for identification
   b. Secondary device intended to kill responders, hospitals overwhelmed, mass decontamination needed
   c. Law enforcement on scene, extremely toxic material, leakage accidental
   d. Potential for mass casualties, multiple agencies respond, transportation accident

2. Which of the following statements about biologic agents is *false*?
   a. Symptoms usually follow an incubation period of several hours to days.
   b. Some agents can be spread from person to person.
   c. The agent is usually not a contamination risk to rescuers.
   d. Illness after biologic agent attack is invariably fatal.

3. Passengers on a bus were exposed to a gas. Within minutes they started seizing and lost consciousness. The agents most likely to cause these symptoms include:
   a. Phosgene and cyanide
   b. Nerve agents and sulfur mustard
   c. Sulfur mustard and phosgene
   d. Nerve agents and cyanide

4. Passengers on a plane landed and went to their homes miles apart. Days later they became ill, and several days later their family members and co-workers also reported feeling ill. Of the following, which biological agents are most likely involved?
   a. Anthrax and smallpox
   b. Tularemia and viral hemorrhagic fever
   c. Plague and botulinum
   d. Plague and smallpox

5. The greatest threat after contamination with nuclear agents is:
   a. Skin burns
   b. Alpha particle syndrome
   c. Incorporation
   d. Internal contamination

6. Which of the following biologic agents and transmission-based precautions are most correct?
   a. Plague and contact precautions
   b. Smallpox and airborne precautions
   c. Botulinum toxin and airborne precautions
   d. Botulinum toxin and contact precautions

7. Three people were exposed to vapors from a nerve agent. Which of the following would be common findings?
   a. Nausea, vomiting, diarrhea, sweating
   b. Pupillary dilation, nasal congestion
   c. Tearing, nasal congestions, shortness of breath
   d. Gastrointestinal cramps, muscular twitching

8. Several people suddenly collapsed at a suspected terrorist incident. Others are running away. Which of the following would suggest the cause is nerve agent versus cyanide?
   a. Convulsions and loss of consciousness
   b. Rapid breathing and flushed skin
   c. Small pupils, excessive secretions, and muscle twitching
   d. Loss of respirations and slow pulse

9. Personal protection principles to avoid nuclear exposure include:
   a. Duration of exposure
   b. Distance from the source
   c. Shielding
   d. All the above

10. Actions of the EMT at an NBC incident are best summarized as:
   a. Medical incident command, antidote administration, and triage
   b. Recognition, safety of self and others, and provision of medical care
   c. Rescue, decontamination, and restoration
   d. Radiologic monitoring, agent detection, and treatment

For Further Review

In the Student Workbook

- Multiple-choice questions
- Matching questions
- Fill-in-the-blank questions
- Short-answer questions
- True-false questions
- Case scenario questions

On Evolve

- Weblinks
- Lecture notes
- Exercises

Learning Objectives

Cognitive Objectives

- Describe the role of an EMT at a nuclear, biologic, or chemical (NBC) event.
- Describe the threat of an NBC incident by terrorism.

- Distinguish a hazardous materials incident from an NBC terrorist event.
- Recognize how an NBC weapon may be spread or disseminated.
- Recognize signs and symptoms of likely NBC agents.
- Describe the importance of surveillance in recognizing an NBC event.
- Describe six biologic warfare agents, and recognize the signs and symptoms of exposure.
- Describe how to manage and care for victims of biologic agents.
- List agents that are a risk for secondary transmission and actions to protect against spread with personal protective equipment and isolation measures.
- List four types of chemical agents that may be used in a terrorist attack.
- List two agents that cause immediate symptoms and may require antidote treatment at the scene.
- Describe the principles of decontamination for vapor exposure.
- Describe the principles of decontamination for liquid exposure.
- Describe types of radiologic hazards.
- Describe the difference between radioactive particles (alpha, beta, neutrons) and radioactive waves.
- Describe the difference between contamination and irradiation and incorporation.
- Describe acute radiation syndrome.
- List factors that affect severity of radiation exposure and how they can be used to limit exposure.

References

Alibek K, Handelman S: *Biohazard: the chilling true story of the largest covert biological weapons program in the world—told from inside by the man who ran it*, New York, 2000, Random House.

Centers for Disease Control, www.cdc.gov.

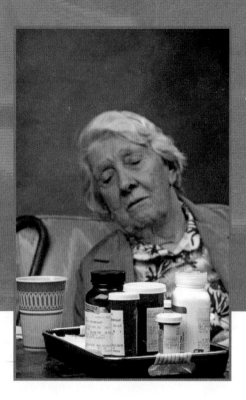

31 Geriatric Emergencies

CHAPTER OUTLINE

Physiologic Changes with Aging

Factors Complicating Patient Assessment

Common Complaints and Problems in Elderly Patients

Scenario

You are called to the home of a 79-year-old woman with altered mental status. Her son states that during dinner she complained of a queasiness and epigastric discomfort, quickly followed by her slumping down in the chair. She was eased into a recumbent position, after which she regained consciousness but remained lethargic. On your arrival the patient opens her eyes to your voice, can tell you her name, and moans occasionally, keeping her hands over her abdomen. Her pulse is 73 beats/min, blood pressure 100/66 mm Hg, and respirations 24 breaths/min. The skin is cool and dry. She has no visible trauma, but abdominal palpation reveals diffuse, moderate tenderness. Her past medical history is significant for coronary artery disease, stroke, and hypertension. Medications include aspirin, metoprolol, clopidogrel (Plavix), and fluoxetine (Prozac).

You administer oxygen by nonrebreather mask and treat the patient for shock by laying her supine, elevating her legs, and keeping her warm, with no significant change. On arrival at the hospital, the patient is quickly taken for a computed tomography (CT) scan, which reveals a ruptured abdominal aortic aneurysm. She is brought immediately to the operating room for repair.

The geriatric patient is a frequent user of the emergency medical service (EMS) system for common medical problems. As people age, they are more prone to serious medical conditions affecting every body system. Elderly patients are often difficult to evaluate, have less ability to compensate for severe illness, are prone to environmental illnesses, and are more subject to falls and serious consequences from relatively minor mechanisms of injury.

With increased life expectancy, better medical care, declining birth rate, and better living conditions, the population older than 65 years grows larger each year. The percentage of the U.S. population over 65 increased from 3% in 1900 to 12.1% in 2000. The average life expectancy in 1900 was 49 years. In 2000 it was 76.9 years. The current leading causes of death in elderly persons are heart disease, cancer, and stroke, accounting for 60% of mortality.

> **LEARNING OBJECTIVE**
> - List two physiologic changes of aging for each of these body systems: cardiovascular, respiratory, and musculoskeletal.

Physiologic Changes with Aging

As people age, a general decline occurs in the organ systems of the body.

Respiratory System

The respiratory system changes in several ways. The *vital capacity*, the total amount of air that can be moved in and out with a given breath, decreases by as much as 50%. There is decreased recoil and elasticity of lung tissue and a general loss of the muscle tissue within the walls of the lower airways. This can result in air trapping from collapsed bronchioles, an increase in the amount of air that remains in the lungs at the end of an exhalation (residual volume), and increased work of breathing.

These changes can make sudden respiratory illness a life-threatening condition because compensation for hypoxia and inadequate ventilation is less effective. For example, influenza can be a life-threatening illness to elderly persons and a reason they are encouraged to receive "flu shots." More than 90% of the deaths attributed to pneumonia and influenza occur in people older than 64 years.

Cardiovascular System

The cardiovascular system is also subject to several changes. The *stroke volume*, the amount of blood ejected from the heart with each beat, declines with age, as does the heart's pacemaker and conducting system. The maximum pulse rate decreases with age. The average maximum pulse is calculated at 220 beats/min minus an individual's age. This means that a 20-year-old has a maximum pulse rate of 200 beats/min, whereas an 80-year-old may only have a maximum pulse of 140 beats/min. When faced with internal bleeding, the elderly patient has a diminished ability to increase the heart rate and stroke volume to compensate for states of poor perfusion.

The resistance of blood vessels increases from a loss of elasticity and generalized **arteriosclerosis** (hardening of the arteries). The result is high blood pressure, or **hypertension**, a condition common in elderly persons. The ability of the cardiovascular system to respond to changes in blood pressure is slower, and they may find that sudden movement from a lying to standing position leads to symptoms of dizziness or syncope. The elderly are also more prone to blood clots, leading to heart attack, stroke, and other vascular emergencies.

Musculoskeletal System

The musculoskeletal system also degenerates with age. There is decreased total musculoskeletal weight and widening and weakening of bones. Generalized **osteoporosis** (decreased amount of bone tissue) increases the potential for fractures with relatively mild mechanisms of injury. Women are particularly prone to fractures because of osteoporosis; 75% to 80% of all hip fractures occur in women. As an emergency medical technician (EMT), you must maintain a high index of suspicion that a fracture may be present with even low falls.

> **Case in Point**
>
> Two EMTs respond to call for a "man down" on a city street. On arrival they find an 80-year-old woman complaining of pain in the hip after stepping off a curb. The patient states that she did not fall. Rather, she underestimated the distance from the top of the curb to the street and "landed hard" on her foot, causing pain in her left hip area. The EMTs splint the leg and transport the patient to the emergency department.
>
> Later, as the EMTs are cleaning their ambulance, they are called to the orthopedic suite, where a physician reviews the patient's radiograph. The physician points to an obvious fracture of the hip and congratulates the EMTs on splinting the leg despite the relatively minor mechanism of injury.

Thermoregulation

Elderly persons (and children) are also more prone to thermoregulatory problems. When exposed to environmental changes, they have a decreased ability to respond. In warm environments, they may have decreased ability to rid the body of heat through the normal mechanisms of sweating and vasodilation. In cold environments, elderly persons have a decreased ability to produce heat and maintain a normal body temperature through shivering and constriction of the vessels in the skin.

LEARNING OBJECTIVES

- List four problems affecting communication with the geriatric patient, and provide at least two ways to improve communication.
- Explain why elderly patients may be more prone to denial.
- List four factors that make physical assessment difficult in elderly patients.
- List ways to obtain information about a geriatric patient's medical history.

Factors Complicating Patient Assessment

Patient assessment of the elderly presents multiple challenges. Geriatric patients often have more than one disease at a given time, making the formation of a prehospital impression difficult. One study of elderly patients identified an average of 3.26 serious medical problems in elderly men.

Because of the number of potential problems experienced by elderly persons, chronic illnesses are often confused with symptoms of a new, acute problem. For example, it may be difficult to identify the underlying problem in a patient who presents with an altered mental status and a history of senile dementia. In these cases, clarification by family, friends, and neighbors may be extremely helpful in differentiating the chronic altered mental status from the current presenting problem.

Pain responses may also be diminished or absent in many elderly patients, causing you to underestimate the severity of a condition. For example, heart attacks without chest pain are much more common in the elderly, patients with diabetes, and women. Diminished pain response may also mask major abdominal complaints. When you evaluate elderly patients, you should be prepared to encounter more atypical presentations.

Because of changes in temperature regulatory mechanisms, elderly patients may have minimal or no fever with severe infection. This may create the appearance of a minor cold in the face of serious pneumonia, or it may mask the seriousness of any infectious disease. Again, maintain a high level of suspicion when the presenting problem seems inconsequential.

Denial of Serious Illness

Elderly persons often have a profound fear of dying and loss of independence. They dread the possibility of long-term admission to a nursing home and may see emergency hospital transport as the first step in the realization of their worst fears. As a result of these issues and other psychologic factors, elderly patients are particularly prone to denial of serious illness or injury.

Often, EMS providers respond at the home of an elderly person after a neighbor or relative has called for help, only to encounter refusal of care. In these cases, it is critical for you to maintain a high index of suspicion and to err on the side of transport to the hospital. In fact, extremes of age are a high-risk indicator when assessing refusal-of-care requests. You cannot force the patient to go to the hospital against his or her will. However, it may be helpful to enlist the aid of a friend or family member to convince the elderly patient to go to the hospital.

Some EMS systems encourage providers to contact medical direction when they encounter patients who refuse care. A physician may convince a patient to go to the hospital when prehospital personnel have been unsuccessful. Refusal of care is a serious problem if the patient needs care.

Case in Point

You and your partner respond to the home of a 72-year-old widower who fell. On arrival, he is sitting on the floor beside his bed. He normally walks with a walker and requests assistance returning to his bed. Once in bed, the patient refuses transport.

You have been called to the home numerous times for similar complaints. A home health aide treats the patient 4 hours each day. He has a complicated medical history, including end-stage renal failure and dialysis three times a week. The previous night he was transported to the hospital for injuries from a fall, but he denies any injury this morning. He has taken an unknown amount of pain medication for the injuries. His blood pressure is 120/80 mm Hg, pulse 88 beats/min, and respiratory rate 28 breaths/min; he is somewhat agitated but alert and appropriate. You accurately note that his living conditions are poor and current presentation is high risk, so you contact medical control for consultation. After reviewing the case, the physician permits the patient to refuse transport because he has no apparent acute illness or injury.

Two hours later, you are called back to the same address to find the patient in respiratory arrest. The home health aide found him prone on the floor near the bathroom. Despite resuscitative efforts, the patient expires in the emergency department.

Elderly patients may have multiple, concurrent debilitating diseases. This can result in both emotional and physical problems for the patient. The fear of long-term hospitalization or nursing home placement may cause patients to conceal an acute illness or injury. It is important to maintain a high index of suspicion and enlist expert help through medical control when caring for such a patient.

Drug-Related Factors

When taking a medication history from an elderly patient, you should exercise care in clarifying and confirming prescriptions. Elderly persons are more prone to drug reactions than younger adults or children. Confusion regarding medication is common in the elderly population. In a study of people older than 65 years, investigators found medication errors 59% of the time, with serious errors 26% of the time. The elderly patient may also confuse directions and may be taking more or less of the prescribed dose. They may also be taking multiple medications that were prescribed by multiple physicians, resulting in adverse drug interactions. Whenever possible, bring the medications to the hospital with the patient to ensure the most reliable medication history (**Figure 31-1**).

Drugs may also hamper the patient assessment process by altering normal cardiovascular function. For example, drugs classified as **beta blockers** or **calcium channel blockers,** which are taken to treat high blood pressure and heart disease, may slow the patient's heart rate. These patients normally have a slower pulse, even those with hypovolemia, who would be expected to have an increased pulse rate.

At times, medications may be the cause of the presenting problem. For example, diuretics, which promote urinary loss of

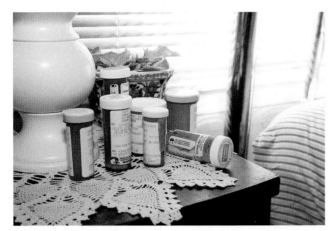

Figure 31-1 Elderly patients often take multiple medications. Confusion can lead to medication errors and drug interactions. Certain drugs can influence the physical findings during assessment. Drugs may also be a key to understanding current medical problems. Bring them to the hospital with the patient when possible.

fluids, may lead to dehydration and electrolyte imbalance. Anticoagulants may predispose to severe bleeding in an otherwise benign medical or traumatic condition. Identifying anticoagulants in the patient's medication history is critical because the treatment for heart attack, stroke, and trauma may be influenced by this information.

Considerations in Taking a Geriatric Patient's History

Obtaining a history is particularly challenging in the elderly patient because of problems with sight, hearing, and communication. You must remember to probe for significant symptoms. Often the chief complaint may seem trivial, and the patient may not volunteer information because of denial.

Visual Impairment

Impaired vision is a common and sometimes terrifying situation for the elderly patient. It can increase anxiety during movement and transport. Approximately one fifth of the population age 70 or older have visual impairment, limiting activity, increasing disability, and increasing risk of falls and other injuries. Patients with vision loss associated with aging may feel an inability to exert control over their environment and may become particularly anxious during care. They may not understand what you are doing and may be startled by seemingly simple actions. Ask if the patient uses glasses and find them. Take the time to position yourself where the patient can see you. Calmly explain your actions as you perform them so that the elderly patient can clearly appreciate what is about to happen. This is particularly important when your actions may cause pain, such as applying a splint or lifting the patient.

Hearing Impairment

Impaired hearing can also present significant challenges during the patient history. A third of older Americans are hearing impaired, and the number increases with age. According to the National Center for Health Statistics, one quarter of persons age 70 to 74 are hearing impaired, as well as more than half of those older than 85.

You should never assume that the person has difficulty hearing when you encounter elderly patients. If the patient is hearing impaired, do not shout to compensate. Shouting distorts sounds and may actually make comprehension more difficult. Instead, you should ask if the patient has a hearing aid and obtain it to help communication. Position yourself in clear view of the patient. If the patient can lip-read, speak slowly and directly to the patient. If necessary, write notes to clarify facts or retrieve information. Whenever possible, verify history with a reliable friend or relative, or seek assistance from individuals who can communicate with patients using sign language.

Elderly patients often have hearing aids, eyeglasses, or dentures. All are important in normal functioning as well as communication. Whenever possible, make sure you bring these with the patient to the hospital.

Altered Mental Status

Elderly patients may also have conditions that result in a diminished or confused mental status, such as Alzheimer's disease, senile dementia, organic brain syndrome, and stroke. Such patients are often confused and unable to recall details. Noise of radios, strange voices, and crowds of bystanders may add to the confusion. Both senility and acute organic brain syndrome may have similar signs of delirium, confusion, distractibility, restlessness, excitement, or hostility.

You should attempt to determine whether a patient's mental status represents a change from normal and, if so, how it is different. You should not assume that a confused or disoriented patient is "just senile" and fail to assess for an underlying abnormality or treatable medical cause, such as hypoglycemia. Most importantly, you should be patient and kind to these patients. A quiet, reassuring approach can assist greatly in acquiring a useful history.

> **REAL**World
>
> Change in mentation is not a normal process of aging. The geriatric patient may be slower in his or her responses or have a difficulty hearing, but altered mental status is associated with disease. The disease could be chronic such as Alzheimer's, or acute as in hypoglycemia or a stroke. The EMT should always consider other possible causes of altered mentation before assuming it is due to age.

Alcoholism

Alcoholism is more common in the elderly population than generally realized. Questions about alcohol and tobacco use are a routine and important part of any patient history. However, elderly patients may deny alcoholism. You should verify this information with the family.

Considerations in Performing the Physical Examination

Several issues are critical when performing a physical examination on an elderly patient. Elderly patients may become easily fatigued during physical assessment. During a motor examination, consider their naturally diminished physical ability, and

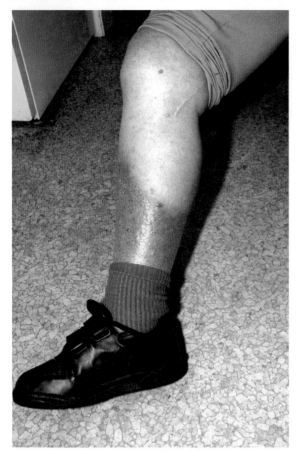

Figure 31-2 Chronic venous stasis. Swollen legs can be caused by poor venous flow in the legs. When it is chronic, discoloration of the skin occurs. Breakdown of the skin can lead to venous ulcers.

do not overexert them. Weakness may be related more to a generalized lack of fitness than a central nervous system (CNS) cause. Patients can also become fatigued when you ask them to take deep breaths during the physical examination. Proceed slowly, and be patient during this phase of assessment.

Elderly patients often wear excessive amounts of clothing that may hamper physical examination. You should not try to obtain a blood pressure reading over a sweater sleeve or listen to breath sounds through heavy clothing. Generalized arteriosclerosis may make pulse or blood pressure measurement more difficult.

The elderly patient may have rales or crackles in the lungs that are not caused by disease but by temporary collapse of alveoli that have not been used because of patient position. Often a few strong coughs or deep breaths will clear this condition.

Loss of skin elasticity may give a false appearance of dehydration. You should always look for other signs, such as rapid pulse, decreased urination, and pale conjunctiva, to confirm the presence of dehydration.

Swollen ankles and legs may be caused by varicose veins, inactivity, and position rather than by congestive heart failure. You should question the patient about the chronic nature of these signs (**Figure 31-2**).

You will increase your skills of differentiating between chronic and acute signs of illness as you gain experience as an EMT. However, you should be prepared to seek guidance from

medical direction or your partner when you are unsure of a particular physical finding, especially in the geriatric patient.

Psychosocial Issues

Once again, fear of death and loss of independence may make prehospital assessment of the elderly patient difficult. Lack of family support and sensitivity to loss of independence may make the elderly patient uncooperative.

Some general approaches may be helpful in establishing effective communication. Avoid familiarity with the patient. Greetings such as, "Hello, sweetheart," or, "We are here to help you, dear," are disrespectful. Terms such as these would rightly be perceived as condescending and insulting and are likely to engender resentment rather than cooperation. Address patients in a mature, respectful tone with their surname: "Hello, Mrs. Smith, what is the problem today?" You should avoid any tendency to treat the elderly patient like a child. A sincere, respectful, and empathetic approach will help win their confidence and cooperation.

LEARNING OBJECTIVE
• Describe common complaints and problems of geriatric patients.

Common Complaints and Problems in Elderly Patients

The following presenting problems and their related causes are common to the elderly population. Being aware of these conditions will be helpful when you respond at an elderly patient's home.

Fatigue and Weakness

Fatigue and weakness are extremely common complaints in the elderly patient. They may be caused by a serious illness or may be chronic complaints that the patient experiences daily. Your challenge is to collect an effective patient history that will help clarify the condition to the physician at the hospital. You are not responsible for making a diagnosis. However, you may need to administer treatments related to a serious illness associated with a particular complaint.

Fatigue and weakness may be a chief complaint associated with several serious cardiovascular, respiratory, and CNS problems. Cardiovascular conditions associated with these symptoms include congestive heart failure, heart attack, abnormal heart rhythms, and hypovolemic shock. It is important to search for other history details and physical examination findings that may help in your decision making.

Elderly patients with respiratory problems may also present with fatigue or weakness. Any condition that results in hypoxia may include these complaints. Chronic obstructive pulmonary disease, pneumonia, lung cancer, and numerous other severe respiratory illnesses may lead to fatigue and weakness. Again, a systematic history and physical examination will help differentiate chronic complaints from new, more serious causes.

Case in Point

Two EMTs respond to a 79-year-old woman complaining of a sudden onset of severe weakness. The patient is alert with no other serious complaints. Her vital signs are respirations 16 breaths/min and shallow, pulse 120 beats/min and thready, and blood pressure 90/70 mm Hg. Her normal blood pressure is 140/80 mm Hg. She also has pale, cool, and sweaty skin. During the focused (secondary) assessment the patient notes that she had vomited dark-red blood earlier in the day and had a bowel movement with black, tarry stools. Physical examination reveals a slightly tender abdomen in the epigastric region.

The patient initially refuses transport, but the EMTs convince her to go to the hospital. They position her supine with her legs elevated and administer high-concentration oxygen by nonrebreather mask. They maintain her body temperature by wrapping her in a warm blanket and transport her to the hospital.

When the EMTs later follow up, they found that she had severe upper gastrointestinal bleeding and hypovolemic shock.

Dizziness and Fainting

Sudden dizziness or fainting can be associated with conditions ranging from a "simple" fainting episode to stroke or even sudden cardiac death. Fainting must be taken seriously and always requires evaluation at the hospital. Conditions that present with these chief complaints include potentially fatal cardiovascular and CNS problems.

As mentioned previously, the cardiovascular system may be slow to react to changes. A patient who suddenly rises from the supine position in bed to an upright position may have a sudden onset of dizziness or fainting. This can be caused by a delayed response within the cardiovascular system in making normal adjustments with receptors that are located in the carotid arteries and aorta. The change in position generates increased oxygen demands, and the heart and blood vessels are too slow to respond. As a result, the patient's cardiovascular system fails to adequately perfuse the brain, producing dizziness or fainting.

These complaints may also be associated with stroke or a transient ischemic attack (see Chapter 12). A systematic and focused (secondary) assessment is crucial and may reveal a facial droop, weakness on one side of the body, difficulty talking, or other key signs found in the patient history and physical examination. Other serious causes of dizziness or fainting include abnormal heart rhythms (very slow or very fast rhythms), hypovolemic conditions (e.g., gastrointestinal bleeding), and aneurysms.

Falls

The potential for falls increases with age. In the United States, one of every three adults age 65 and older experiences a fall each year. Falls are the leading cause of injury death in this population, accounting for 9600 deaths in 1998. Three major reasons for this trend include decreased attentiveness, fainting, and poor posture and balance (**Figure 31-3**).

Because of decreased cerebral function, elderly persons may become briefly inattentive while walking. They may trip over objects, fall down stairs, or run into stationary objects. All these incidents may lead to serious injuries, including fractures, internal bleeding, and organ damage. As mentioned previously,

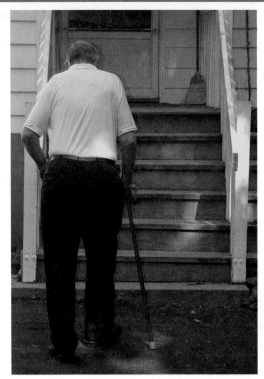

Figure 31-3 Short, uncertain steps are characteristic of gait with advancing age.

fractures are much more common among the elderly population and should be assumed when associated with any complaints of pain, contusions, or other signs or symptoms of fracture or muscular injury.

Because of alterations in CNS function, elderly persons also tend to lose their balance more easily. Poor posture is common, causing elderly patients to lose balance and fall before they can position themselves properly.

During patient assessment, you may have to establish a relationship between the fall and any existing signs or symptoms. For example, a patient may have fallen and become unconscious, or the patient may have become unconscious and then fallen. During your SAMPLE history, the events leading up to the fall will become important in establishing this association.

Headache

When called to the scene of a patient complaining of a "headache," EMTs are often prone to characterize the call as an inappropriate use of an ambulance. However, patients with many life-threatening conditions, including cerebral aneurysm, stroke, subdural hematoma, and other CNS conditions, can present with headache as the chief complaint. Serious causes of headaches are much more common in the elderly population.

Dehydration

Elderly patients are more prone to dehydration. Kidney function decreases with age. Older people are also less mobile and tend to delay fluid intake because of the effort needed to perform simple tasks.

Consider the consequences of the following scenario. An elderly man is sitting on the deck on a hot summer day. He asks his wife to bring him a glass of water. She says, "Wait until you come back in the house; if you have water now, you will have to go to the bathroom." The husband is an 80-year-old man who is taking diuretics and losing water in the hot sun through sweat. He is delaying fluid intake that will help meet his hydration needs. This type of scenario often plays out in the houses of elderly persons and can result in severe dehydration and hypovolemia.

During your assessment of an elderly patient with suspected dehydration, you should routinely ask about fluid intake, medications, and any history of renal disease. Be sure to check for signs of dehydration, including dry skin turgor and oral mucosa and sunken eyes.

Thermoregulatory Problems

Heat and cold emergencies are most common in infants and persons older than 75 years. Elderly persons may have decreased CNS function caused by arteriosclerosis, which leads to decreased thermoregulatory function. Other factors that may lead to heat and cold emergencies include the following:

- Reduced ability to regulate heat production and heat loss
- Decreased basal metabolic rate
- Decreased ability to shiver
- Effects of drugs
- Reduced ability to detect feelings of heat and cold

Hypothermia is rarely self-reported and is usually associated with patients trapped in extremely cold environments, such as those who trip and fall on ice and lie on the cold ground for a short period. However, elderly patients also may develop hypothermia in environments with moderate temperatures.

Case in Point

Emergency medical technicians respond to an 80-year-old man who has fallen at home and is discovered by his daughter, who was visiting. The patient is unresponsive and has a small laceration on his forehead; there is a large pool of dried blood on the floor near his head. The daughter states that she called him last night and he did not answer the telephone. The patient's vital signs are respirations 20 breaths/min and shallow, pulse 60 beats/min and irregular, and blood pressure 80 palp. He also has pale, cool, and dry skin. His focused (secondary) assessment reveals a very cool abdomen and rigid extremities.

The EMTs position the patient supine with his legs elevated and administer high-concentration oxygen by nonrebreather mask. They maintain his body temperature by wrapping him in a warm blanket and carefully transport him to the hospital.

At follow-up, the EMTs are told that the patient had mild hypovolemic shock and moderate hypothermia. The patient had remained on the floor for approximately 24 hours in a 70° F room. The mild hypovolemia in combination with his advanced age reduced his ability to tolerate and compensate for the exposure.

Heat-related emergencies occur in a variety of settings with the elderly population. People may be working outdoors and exerting themselves, or they may be bedridden. Elderly patients have a variety of risk factors that predispose them to *heat exhaustion* or *heat stroke*. In general, they have less ability to rid themselves of heat through normal thermoregulatory mechanisms. They also may have conditions such as Parkinson's disease that produce excess heat, or they may have febrile illnesses. Certain drugs, such as alcohol, antihistamines, and tranquilizers, also increase the likelihood of heat-related illness.

Elderly patients who are found in hot and humid environments should be evaluated for a heat-related illness. See Chapter 16 to review the key signs and symptoms of heat exhaustion and heat stroke.

Depression and Suicide

Elderly patients are a high-risk group for depression and suicide. Depression may manifest in many ways. It may mimic senility or organic brain syndrome and may inhibit the patient's cooperation. Depressed patients may be malnourished, dehydrated, overdosed with medications, and contemplating suicide.

Suicide rates increase with age and are highest in those older than 65 years. Elderly men are particularly prone to suicide. The rate of suicide in men older than 65 is at least three times that of the general population. Men account for 83% of suicides among those age 65 and older; in general; the percentage is highest for those who have lost a spouse from divorce or death. More than 10,000 persons over 60 kill themselves each year.

Common symptoms of depression include the following:

- Loss of sleep, appetite, and libido
- Loss of pleasure in normally satisfying activities
- Sadness and tearfulness
- Guilt
- Hopelessness
- Thoughts and expressions of death or suicide
- Physical symptoms

When taking a history from an elderly patient whom you suspect is depressed or suicidal, questions regarding drug ingestion or suicidal thoughts are appropriate. A history from family members or close friends may also be helpful in identifying patients at high risk.

Remember that the depressed patient may describe feelings of sadness or profound feelings of guilt. Such an individual may express *hopelessness*, a key complaint that points to a significant risk for suicide. The person may hide feelings quite effectively. Truly suicidal patients frequently seek medical attention for physical symptoms before taking their lives, but do not express their depression directly. If you see a patient whose symptoms are difficult to attribute to a medical problem, consider suicidal ideation or depression as a possible explanation.

Major risk factors for suicide associated with elderly patients include the following:

- Male gender
- Age older than 65 years
- Single, widowed, or divorced status
- Social isolation
- Unemployment
- Recent loss of significant loved one
- Alcoholism or drug abuse
- Chronic or terminal illness
- Loss of job or status

Other characteristics to note include unusual gathering of articles that can cause death, such as purchase of a gun or a large volume of pills, and verbalizing a defined lethal plan of action.

Although women attempt suicide more frequently than men, men are more often successful.

A person about to commit suicide does not always show signs of sadness or depression. In fact, severely depressed patients who decide to end their life often feel better once the decision is made because they know that their suffering is going to end. Be careful with the patient who says, "Nobody cares for me," or, "I'll never be better." Be suspicious of "accidents" that could have occurred on purpose.

Elderly patients may also have other psychiatric disorders that significantly affect their ability to care for themselves. You should observe surroundings for indications of significant hygiene problems, trash, vermin, or neglected animals. Remember, you may be the only person who is aware of these conditions. You may want to contact family members or social services if conditions warrant. Also, look for signs of dehydration, malnutrition, or other illness.

You should also look for signs of abuse. Elderly persons are a common target for abuse and neglect. As with child abuse, you should look for suspicious signs of wounds in various states of healing or marks consistent with trauma inflicted by specific objects, such as sticks, wires, ropes, and other improvised weapons (see Chapter 18).

REAL*World*

Unfortunately, many suicide attempts in elderly persons may be overlooked as "accidents." For example, an elderly man who overdosed on his pills is thought to be forgetful. Keep the possibility of a suicide attempt as part of your assessment. Direct questions such as, "Did you try to hurt yourself?" are appropriate.

Scenario Follow-up

Elderly patients often have ischemic heart disease and hypertension. These patients may take beta blockers such as metoprolol, which can blunt the tachycardia and diaphoreses often seen in hypovolemic shock. The only clue to hypovolemic shock in the elderly person may be altered mental status; even blood pressure may appear normal in the patient who is normally extremely hypertensive. Elderly patients also have a diminished physiologic response to pain, which may cause you to underestimate the severity of illness or injury. You should consider all these factors when assessing and evaluating an elderly patient.

Summary

The elderly patient is particularly prone to severe illness and injury with relatively minor mechanisms. As an EMT, you should become familiar with the common ailments associated with aging and consider the key problems associated with a particular chief complaint. An EMT should also be aware of the special considerations associated with communicating with the geriatric patient who may have impaired vision or hearing. Be aware of the reduced ability of the geriatric patient to compensate for serious illness.

The Bottom Line

Learning Checklist

✓ As people age, there is a general decline in the organ systems of the body.

✓ Respiratory system changes include decreased vital capacity, decreased recoil and elasticity of lung tissue, and a general loss of muscle tissue within the walls of the lower airway.

✓ Cardiovascular system changes include decreased stroke volume and pulse rate and a decreased ability to compensate for states of poor perfusion. The changes also include loss of elasticity and general arteriosclerosis, leading to high blood pressure. The ability of the cardiovascular system to respond to changes in blood pressure is slower, and elderly patients are more prone to blood clots.

✓ Musculoskeletal system changes include a decreased total musculoskeletal weight and widening and weakening of bones (e.g., osteoporosis).

✓ Elderly persons are more prone to thermoregulatory problems, caused by a decreased ability to respond to changes in the environment.

✓ Elderly patients may be in denial of serious injury or illness because of a profound fear of dying or loss of independence. They may also dread the possibility of long-term admission to a nursing home. It may be helpful to enlist the help of family and friends to convince an elderly person to go with you to the hospital.

✓ Medications can affect the assessment of elderly patients because of the type of medication or the number of medications.

✓ Impaired vision and hearing can affect how well an elderly patient can communicate. Elderly patients may have an altered mental status for a variety of reasons, or they may have an alcohol problem. With all elderly patients, you should be kind and patient and use a quiet, reassuring approach.

✓ Physical assessment of an elderly person may be challenging because the patient may tire easily, may wear excessive amounts of clothing, may have abnormal breath sounds that are not the result of a disease condition, and may show signs of dehydration or congestive heart failure simply because of inactivity and their age.

✓ Common complaints in the elderly patient include fatigue and weakness, dizziness and fainting, falls, headache, dehydration, and heat- and cold-related problems.

✓ Elderly persons are a high-risk group for depression and suicide.

Key Terms

Arteriosclerosis Buildup of fat on the wall of an artery, decreasing its size and elasticity.

Beta blockers Drugs that cause blood flow to increase and blood pressure to decrease; can also slow heart rate.

Calcium channel blockers Drugs that increase blood flow through vasodilation and decrease the ability of myocardial cells to respond to electrical stimulation. Patients with angina at rest or occasional rapid heart rates may be prescribed these medications.

Hypertension High blood pressure.

Osteoporosis Decrease in the amount of bone tissue occurring in older people as a result of more bone breakdown than bone formation, which leads to weaker bones.

Review Questions

1. Elderly patients may have less ability to compensate for hypovolemic shock because of their decreased ability to:
   a. Elevate their legs.
   b. Increase their pulse rate.
   c. Absorb oxygen on red blood cells.
   d. Transport carbon dioxide.

2. A disease affecting elderly persons that reduces bone strength and increases their risk of fractures with a less forceful mechanism is:
   a. Osteoporosis
   b. Osteogenesis
   c. Parkinson's disease
   d. Lou Gehrig's disease

3. Which of the following is the *least* likely cause of death in the elderly patient?
   a. Heart disease
   b. Stroke
   c. Cancer
   d. Trauma

4. Elderly patients are more prone to hypothermia because of their reduced ability to produce heat through:
   a. Shivering
   b. Sweating
   c. Vasodilation
   d. Absorption

5. Which of the following factors is a specific cause of denial in the elderly patient?

a. Poor judgment

b. Tendency not to trust healthcare providers

c. Fear of loss of independence

d. Paranoia

6. Which of the following groups has the highest mortality from suicide?

a. Elderly women

b. Elderly men

c. Young women

d. Young men

7. Which of the following factors would be *least* likely to lead to serious drug-related problems in elderly patients?

a. Prescriptions from multiple physicians

b. Confusion regarding directions of prescribed dose

c. Lack of attention when self-medicating

d. More prone to drug reactions

8. An 80-year-old man is complaining of weakness and inability to arise from his chair. During the history, he states he has been having black stools. He has history of hypertension and atrial fibrillation and is taking coumadin and a beta blocker. His pulse is 80 beats/min and his blood pressure 90/60 mm Hg. His skin is pale and cool. As you assess the patient, which of the following would best explain your findings?

a. Blood thinners such as coumadin make him susceptible to bleeding, and his age prevents him from having a compensatory heart rate.

b. His blood pressure is likely caused by an overdose of the beta blocker.

c. Blood thinners can make him prone to bleeding, and the beta blocker and his age can blunt an increase in heart rate.

d. His weakness is normal for a person of his age, and his pulse and blood pressure are consistent with signs of aging.

For Further Review

In the Student Workbook

- Multiple-choice questions
- Matching questions
- Fill-in-the-blank questions
- Short-answer questions
- True/false questions
- Case scenario questions

On Evolve

- Weblinks
- Lecture notes
- Exercises

Learning Objectives

Cognitive Objectives

- List two physiologic changes of aging for each of these body systems: cardiovascular, respiratory, and musculoskeletal.
- List four problems affecting communication with the geriatric patient, and provide at least two ways to improve communication.
- Explain why elderly patients may be more prone to denial.
- List four factors that make physical assessment difficult in elderly patients.
- List ways to obtain information about a geriatric patient's medical history.
- Describe common complaints and problems of geriatric patients.

Answers to Review Questions

Chapter 1
1. a
2. c
3. b
4. c
5. b
6. a
7. d
8. e
9. d

Chapter 2
1. c
2. a
3. a
4. a
5. a
6. b
7. b
8. a
9. c
10. c
11. b
12. d
13. c
14. a
15. b
16. a
17. d

Chapter 3
1. a
2. d
3. b
4. c
5. b
6. c
7. a
8. d
9. d
10. c
11. d
12. a

Chapter 4
1. b
2. e
3. f
4. a
5. c
6. d
7. c
8. a
9. c
10. b
11. d

12. c
13. d
14. c
15. c
16. a
17. b

Chapter 5
1. a
2. c
3. b
4. a
5. b
6. d
7. c
8. a
9. a
10. b
11. a
12. c

Chapter 6
1. b
2. b
3. d
4. c
5. b
6. a
7. b
8. c
9. c
10. c
11. d
12. a
13. a
14. b
15. d
16. a
17. b
18. d
19. a
20. c

Chapter 7
1. a
2. b, c, d, e
3. b
4. b
5. a, b, c
6. a
7. b
8. b
9. c
10. a
11. a, b, c
12. a, c, d

13. b
14. d
15. a
16. a
17. d
18. b
19. a
20. b
21. a
22. Onset, Provocation, Quality, Radiation, Severity, Time
23. c
24. b, c, d
25. a, b, c, d
26. a
27. a
28. a
29. b
30. a
31. a
32. c
33. c

Chapter 8
1. b
2. a
3. b
4. d
5. a
6. a
7. a
8. b
9. a
10. d

Chapter 9
1. b
2. a
3. b
4. b
5. c
6. a
7. b
8. b
9. a

Chapter 10
1. e
2. f
3. b
4. c
5. d
6. a
7. c
8. c

9. b
10. d
11. a
12. e
13. b
14. d
15. a
16. f

Chapter 11
1. a
2. b
3. b
4. b
5. b
6. b
7. a
8. a, c, d
9. b
10. b
11. b
12. b
13. d

Chapter 12
1. b, a, c, d
2. c
3. b
4. c
5. Oxygen, aspirin, and nitroglycerin
6. Defibrillation is the only effective treatment for ventricular fibrillation, and the chance of survival decreases with every minute that passes after collapse from ventricular fibrillation. Early defibrillation may save the patient's brain and limit organ damage. Delays decrease the chance of successful defibrillation.
7. a
8. d
9. c
10. a
11. c
12. b
13. a

Chapter 13
1. b
2. b
3. a

4. a
5. a
6. b
7. a
8. a
9. c
10. b
11. b
12. b
13. c
14. d

Chapter 14
1. c
2. c
3. b
4. d
5. d
6. c
7. c
8. c

Chapter 15
1. a
2. d
3. d
4. b
5. b
6. a
7. b
8. a
9. c
10. b

Chapter 16
1. b
2. d
3. e
4. a
5. c
6. c
7. c
8. b
9. b
10. c

Chapter 17
1. c
2. d
3. a
4. c
5. c
6. d

Chapter 18
1. c
2. b
3. a

4. c
5. d
6. a
7. b
8. d

Chapter 19
1. b
2. c
3. a
4. b
5. b
6. b
7. c
8. b
9. c
10. b

Chapter 20
1. b
2. a
3. c
4. d
5. b
6. c
7. d
8. a

Chapter 21
1. c
2. d
3. c
4. e
5. c
6. d
7. a
8. b
9. a
10. b
11. b
12. b
13. c
14. b
15. b
16. b
17. b
18. c
19. b
20. c

Chapter 22
1. a
2. d
3. b
4. d
5. b
6. b
7. a

Chapter 23
1. d
2. b
3. b
4. d
5. a
6. c
7. c
8. b
9. d
10. c

Chapter 24
1. a
2. d
3. a
4. a
5. b
6. c
7. b
8. c
9. b
10. a
11. d
12. Eyes, 2; Verbal, 2; Motor, 2; Total GCS, 6
13. Eyes, 3; Verbal, 4; Motor, 6; Total GCS, 13
14. Eyes, 3; Verbal, 4; Motor, 6; Total GCS, 13

Chapter 25
1. a
2. c
3. c
4. a
5. c
6. c
7. b
8. b
9. d
10. b
11. d

Chapter 26
1. b
2. c
3. d
4. c
5. a
6. b
7. b
8. d
9. c
10. a
11. b
12. c

Chapter 27
1. d
2. b
3. b
4. b
5. c
6. b
7. d

Chapter 28
1. c
2. a
3. b
4. a
5. b
6. c
7. a
8. c
9. d
10. b
11. c
12. b
13. b

Chapter 29
1. a
2. c
3. d
4. d
5. a
6. c
7. d
8. c
9. c
10. b

Chapter 30
1. b
2. d
3. d
4. d
5. c
6. b
7. c
8. c
9. d
10. b

Chapter 31
1. b
2. a
3. d
4. a
5. c
6. b
7. c
8. c

Glossary

The numbers in parentheses refer to the chapter in which the term is discussed.

Abandonment Discontinuation of a professional provider-patient relationship without providing the patient the time or opportunity to obtain continuation of care at the same level or higher. (3)

Abdominal aortic aneurysm Localized abnormal dilation of the descending aorta that becomes a life-threatening emergency on rupture. (12)

Abduction Movement away from the midline. (4)

Abortion Loss of a pregnancy before 20 weeks' gestation. (19)

Abrasion Scrape on the surface of the skin or mucous membrane. (7, 21)

Accessory muscles Muscles in the neck, chest, and abdomen that can increase the forces of inhalation and exhalation in patients with respiratory distress. (4, 6)

Activated charcoal Residue of the distillation of organic materials (charcoal) that has been treated to increase its absorptive properties; used often to absorb ingested drugs and poisons. (10, 15)

Acute coronary syndromes Group of diseases (e.g., myocardial infarction, angina) characterized by ischemia of heart tissue. (12)

Acute mountain sickness (AMS) General weakness, lethargy, and cognitive changes after rapid ascent to a high altitude. (16)

Acute radiation syndrome Syndrome that results from high doses of radiation absorbed over a short period, causing damage to the bone marrow, gastrointestinal tract, central nervous system, and cardiovascular system. (30)

Adduction Movement toward the midline. (4)

Adrenaline See *epinephrine*. (4)

Advance directive Specific statement or documentation made by an individual to withhold care, such as blood transfusions or CPR, if that person becomes mentally incapacitated or otherwise unable to communicate. (3)

Advanced emergency medical technician (AEMT) AEMTs provide basic and limited advanced care, including administration of certain drugs under medical oversight to critical and emergent patients who access the EMS system; also called *EMT-Intermediate* (EMT-I). (1)

Advanced life support (ALS) intercept Call for ALS to acquire resources on the scene that can be lifesaving for the patient (e.g., intubation). (7)

Aerosol Medicinal particles suspended in a gas or in air. (10)

Agonal breathing Irregular, gasping breaths that can be seen during the early onset of cardiac arrest. (6)

Air embolism Air bubble introduced into the circulatory system, such as through an open wound, that can obstruct blood flow. (21)

Airbag Woven bladder that fills with an inert gas to cushion the occupant from hitting hard objects. (27)

Alpha particles Positively charged particles consisting of two protons and two neutrons. (30)

Altered mental status Any change from normal of a patient's mental state; alterations can range from mild confusion and abnormal behavior to deep coma, a condition in which the patient is totally unresponsive to verbal or painful stimuli. (13)

Amputation The cutting away of a limb or protruding structure from a person's body. (21)

Anaphylaxis Allergic condition in which an antibody-antigen reaction results in a release of substances that can cause shock, bronchoconstriction, and airway obstruction. (14)

Angina pectoris Temporary chest pain caused by lack of blood flow to the heart to meet the oxygen needs; usually caused by exertion or stress and relieved by rest. (12)

Angioedema Condition that results from vasodilation and causes hives and swelling of the face, airway, and other tissues. (14)

Anterior Toward the front of the body. (4)

Antidote Remedy that counteracts a poison. (15)

Anxiety Fearful emotional state characterized by increased nervousness, tension, pacing, hand wringing, and trembling. (17)

Apgar score System of quickly evaluating an infant's heart rate, respiratory effort, muscle tone, reflex irritability, and color at birth. The score is determined at 1 minute and repeated at 5 minutes after birth. (19)

Arch of driver safety Components that ensure safe operation of an emergency vehicle, including the physical and mental abilities of the driver, knowledge of traffic laws, and driver attitude. (26)

Arteriosclerosis Progressive disease of the arteries that results in narrowing of the lumen caused by deposits of fat and hardening of the arterial wall. (12, 31)

Artery Muscular blood vessel that carries blood away from the heart. (4)

Asphyxiation Lack of oxygen or excess of carbon dioxide causing unconsciousness and often death. (15)

Assault Creating the fear of injury (e.g., as by lifting fist in threatening manner) or the willful attempt to harm someone (3, 18)

Asthma Acute obstructive respiratory disease with narrowing of the lower airways; often precipitated by stress, infection, or an allergic response. (6, 11)

Asystole Cardiac standstill, or an absence of any cardiac rhythm; "flatline." (12)

Auditory ossicles Malleus, incus, and stapes bones, which transmit sound waves to the inner ear. (21)

Auscultation Method of listening for sounds produced within the body; usually performed with a stethoscope. (7)

Automated external defibrillator (AED) Defibrillation that interprets the patient's electrocardiographic (ECG) rhythm and automatically initiates or advises defibrillation as needed. (12)

AVPU Mnemonic to help EMS personnel remember the level of patient responsiveness: **A**wake, patient is awake and responds without stimuli; **V**erbal, patient responds to verbal stimuli; **P**ain, patient requires some form of tactile or painful stimuli to generate a response; **U**nresponsive, patient is unresponsive to any form of stimulation. (7, 13)

Avulsion Tearing away of a body part or structure. The part is often still attached to the body by a small flap of skin. (21)

Bag-mask device Mechanical aid used to administer positive-pressure ventilation; usually consists of a bag with an oxygen inlet, a unidirectional valve, a mask, and an oxygen reservoir. (6)

Bandage Material used to secure a dressing in place and provide pressure over the dressing to aid in control of bleeding. (21)

Base station Central coordination area of a communication system that is in contact with other components of the system. (8)

Basket stretcher Type of stretcher that is useful for removing patients on rough terrain or during high-angle rescues where a patient must be either lowered from a height or lifted, as from a ditch or well. (5)

Battery The act of physically touching someone without that person's expressed consent. (3, 17)

Behavior Manner in which a person acts or performs, including physical and mental activities. (17)

Behavioral emergency Any situation in which the patient exhibits abnormal behavior that is unacceptable or intolerable to self, family, or community. (17)

Beta blockers Drugs that cause blood flow to increase and blood pressure to decrease; can also slow heart rate. (31)

Beta particles Negatively or positively charged particles that have the mass of an electron. (30)

Bilateral Occurring or appearing on two sides. (4)

Biotelemetry Transmission of biologic data by a radio or other form of communication to a distant location such as a hospital. (1, 8)

Blanket drag Rescue evacuation technique in which a blanket is used to drag the patient from the hazardous situation. (5)

Blood pressure Force exerted by the blood volume on the walls of the vessels. (7, 20)

Body mechanics Scientific use of specific methods of efficiently lifting large weights so as not to injure oneself. (5)

Body substance isolation Procedures used to protect the EMT from contact with communicable diseases, including the use of gloves, goggles, masks, and gowns. (2)

Brainstem Lower part of the brain responsible for a variety of vital functions and regulatory activities, including respiratory and circulatory functions. (24)

Braxton Hicks contractions Weak, irregular contractions of the uterus felt intermittently throughout pregnancy that strengthen the uterus in preparation for delivery. (19)

Breach of duty Negligent act or omission that has violated the standards of care expected from an EMT under the circumstances. (3)

Breech presentation A birth in which the buttocks are the presenting part. (19)

Calcium channel blockers Drugs that cause blood flow to increase through vasodilation and decrease the ability of myocardial cells to respond to electrical stimulation. Patients with angina at rest or occasional rapid heart rates may be prescribed these medications. (31)

Capillary Thin-walled blood vessel where exchange of nutrients and waste products between blood and tissue fluid through the process of diffusion occurs. (4)

Capillary refilling time Diagnostic test in which the nail bed is compressed to empty the capillaries and determine the time it takes to refill (for color to return). (7)

Cardiac arrest Cessation of a functional heartbeat. (4)

Cardiac tamponade Mechanical compression of the heart by large amounts of fluid or blood within the pericardial space. (22)

Carrier Person who shows no signs of disease yet harbors an infectious organism and may be a source of infection to others. (2)

Causal connection Clear connection between the patient's injuries and actions taken or omitted by a healthcare provider. (3)

Central Situated at, in, or near the center. (4)

Central access dispatch Form of dispatch that coordinates numerous EMS units in a given region. (26)

Cerebellum Outpocketing of the brain located posterior to the brainstem; primarily concerned with coordination of movement and balance. (24)

Cerebrovascular accident (CVA) Blockage or disruption of blood flow in an artery feeding the brain; also called *stroke.* (13)

Cerebrum Largest and most superior portion of the brain, responsible for intellectual activity, motor control, sensory perception, visual stimuli, smell, hearing, and other body functions. (24)

Cervical collar Rigid collars that provide partial immobilization and prevent some movement of the cervical spine. (24)

Chain of evidence Accountability of evidence at a crime scene, from time of possession until it is turned over to the authorities. (2, 3)

Chief complaint The reason, best stated in the patient's own words, for the medical problem that prompted the patient to seek emergency medical assistance. (7)

Cholecystitis Inflammation or low-grade, chronic infection of the gallbladder. (22)

Chronic bronchitis Disease characterized by a productive cough for at least 3 months of the year for at least 2 consecutive years; caused by inflammation of the bronchi, with repeated attacks of coughing and sputum production. (11)

Chronic obstructive pulmonary disease (COPD) Chronic respiratory condition in which air becomes trapped in the alveoli as a result of bronchospasm, mucus plugs, or collapse of the bronchioles; includes chronic bronchitis and emphysema; usually caused by smoking. Shortness of breath is the primary complaint; these patients need greater force to exhale. (6, 11)

Cincinnati Prehospital Stroke Scale Type of screening device used to rapidly identify stroke patients. (13)

Cirrhosis Scarring of the liver. (22)

Clothes drag Rescue evacuation technique that uses the patient's clothing to drag the patient along the long axis of the body from a hazardous situation. (5)

Cold zone The clean zone at a hazardous materials incident or disaster where EMS personnel can further assess the patient, ensure that adequate decontamination is performed before transport, and perform patient care functions as required. (28)

Communicable Classification of disease in which the causative agent may pass or be carried from one person to another directly or indirectly. (2)

Communicable period Time period during which a person can transmit an infectious disease to others. (2)

Communications center Part of the communication system that coordinates receiving calls, triage, dispatch, and other activities of an EMS system. (8)

Complex access Gaining access to the patient with tools or specialized equipment. (27)

Compression forces Forces that occur when one spinal vertebra is driven into another; may be transmitted from above (the head) or from below. (24)

Computerized mobile data terminals Terminals located in the ambulance that allow the EMTs to communicate with the dispatcher by computer screen; units can also be tracked. (8)

Concussion Transient loss of consciousness or neurologic function as a result of trauma to the brain. (24)

Conduction Transfer of heat to objects (including air) in direct contact with the body. (16)

Congenital Present at birth. (25)

Conjunctiva Membrane that lines the interior surface of the eyelids and covers the anterior surface of the sclera of the eye. (7)

Constrict To narrow and become smaller. (7)

Contamination Radiation injury caused by radioactive particles that are physically present. The contaminated patient can pass radioactive materials to others. (30)

Continuous quality improvement (CQI) Working toward the goal of optimal excellence in the services rendered to every patient; includes review of the prehospital care report. (9)

Contraction Cramps that occur in the lower abdomen over the pubic bone and sometimes in the lower back during labor. (19)

Contraindication Any condition that renders a particular line of treatment improper or undesirable. (10)

Control zones Geographic areas at a hazardous materials incident or disaster that are designated based on safety and the degree of hazard. (28)

Contusion Compression or blunt-force injury with no skin break in which blood vessels may leak or rupture; bruise. (7, 21)

Convection Transfer of heat through the movement of air currents. (16)

Convergence Rapid gathering of onlookers, rescuers, and the press at a scene of a disaster. (28)

Crepitus Grating or crackling sound or sensation caused by air beneath the skin or broken bone ends rubbing together; also called *crepitation.* (7, 23)

Cribbing Materials or devices, including wood or airbags, used to support a large amount of weight during rescue operations. (27)

Cricoid cartilage Band of cartilage below the thyroid cartilage, forming a circle just above the trachea; also called *cricoid ring.* (25)

Cricoid pressure (Sellick maneuver) Compression of the esophagus between the cricoid cartilage and the thoracic spine to reduce the chances of air entering the esophagus during positive-pressure ventilation and help prevent gastric distention and regurgitation. (6, 29)

Critical incident stress debriefing Psychological, emotional, and educational group process to lessen the impact of a critical incident. (2)

Critical stress incident A particularly overwhelming incident that results in emotional stress. (2)

Croup Viral infection affecting the larynx, trachea, and bronchi. (25)

Crowing See *stridor.* (7)

Crush injury Injury resulting from severe compressing force that damages and sometimes tears soft tissues and underlying structures. (21)

Cushing reflex Reflex due to cerebral ischemia that causes an increase in blood pressure, decrease in pulse rate, and changes in breathing patterns.

Cyanosis Bluish discoloration of the mucous membranes or skin caused by oxygen-depleted hemoglobin. (6, 7)

Cycle of violence Repeated phases of tension, violence, and "honeymoon" brought on by the victim's desire to be perfect and the perpetrator's anger. (18)

DCAP/BTLS Mnemonic used to remember possible physical findings identified during the head-to-toe survey: **d**eformities; **c**ontusions; **a**brasions; **p**unctures or penetrations; **b**urns; **t**enderness; **l**acerations; **s**welling. (7)

Decontamination Physical or chemical process of reducing, removing, and preventing the spread of contaminants from persons at a hazardous materials incident. (28)

Defibrillation External application of an electric shock across the heart of sufficient energy to convert ventricular fibrillation into an organized rhythm. (12)

Defibrillator Device capable of delivering electric shock therapy to reverse an otherwise lethal cardiac rhythm. (12)

Deformity Structural distortion or bend that alters the normal appearance of the body or a body part. (7)

Delirium Acute confusional state marked by an altered mental state resulting in changed behavior. (17)

Delirium tremens ("DTs") Shakes, tremors, and seizures accompanied by hyperactivity; increased respiration, pulse, and temperature; hypertension; and sometimes hallucinations associated with drug withdrawal. (15)

Dependent lividity Black-and-blue discoloration of most gravity-dependent body portions, caused by the collection of coagulated blood and seen after death. (2, 9)

Depression Condition characterized by loss of pleasure, deep sadness, feelings of hopelessness, difficulty sleeping, loss of sex drive, and feelings of guilt. (17)

Dermis Skin layer below epidermis composed of dense connective tissue that contains the nerves, blood vessels, sweat and sebaceous glands, and hair follicles. (4, 21)

Detailed physical examination Deliberate and comprehensive head-to-toe assessment to identify secondary injuries. (7)

Diabetes Disease that results from the failure of the pancreas to produce sufficient amounts of insulin. (13)

Diabetic ketoacidosis Condition resulting from a relatively prolonged insulin deficiency in which the blood glucose level rises and fatty acids are produced in the blood. (13)

Diastolic blood pressure Blood pressure measured during the relaxation phase (diastole) of the heart. The pressure at which the sounds heard through a stethoscope disappear or significantly diminish. (4)

Dilate To widen or become larger. (7)

Direct pressure First step in controlling bleeding. This pressure is applied over the site of the wound. Use a gloved hand or absorbent material, such as gauze. (20)

Disaster Sudden event producing great material damage, loss, and distress. (28)

Disentanglement Part of the extrication process in which the EMTs/rescuers remove materials that are trapping a patient. (27)

Dislocation Displacement of the bones in a joint from their normal anatomic position. (23)

Dispatcher The individual who receives the call for help and dispatches the appropriate resources through the EMS system. (8)

Distal Farther away from the trunk. (4)

Diverticulum Outpouching of the inner wall of bowel tissue into the muscular layer of the bowel. (22)

Do not resuscitate (DNR) Legal order signed by a physician that allows withholding of lifesaving measures in the event of a respiratory or cardiac arrest. (3, 9)

Domestic violence Physical, emotional, psychological, sexual or other forms of abuse perpetrated on a person in domestic relationship; the goal is usually to exert dominance or control. (18)

Dorsal Toward the back (or ventral) surface. (4)

Dorsalis pedis Artery in the foot that is palpable on the dorsal (top) surface of the foot. (7)

Dose Quantity of a substance to be administered at one time, as in a specified amount of medication. (10)

Dosimeter Radiation-measuring devices used to monitor the total accumulation of radiation. (30)

Dressing Any material that covers a wound, prevents introduction of further contamination into the wound, and aids in bleeding control. (21)

Drowning Respiratory impairment from submersion or immersion in a liquid medium which may or may not result in death. (16)

Drug Any medicinal substance. (10)

Due regard Attention that must be given to the safety of the public while driving an emergency vehicle. (26)

Duty to act Legal requirement to evaluate and treat a patient. (3)

Dyspnea Difficulty breathing. (6)

Ecchymosis Black-and-blue marks caused by bleeding beneath or within layers of the skin. (21)

Economic abuse Financial exploitation of a person by another to gain control. (18)

Electrode pads Adhesive pads that transmit electrical signs from the body through cables to detect the heart's electrical activity and in turn transfer electrical energy from the defibrillator to the body. (12)

Emancipated minor Individual who is younger than the legal adult age but who is living independently, is (or was) married, or is (or was) a parent. (3)

Emergency medical dispatch Nationally recognized method for training dispatchers in the systematic questioning of people calling 9-1-1 and, when necessary, providing phone-directed instructions. (8, 26)

Emergency medical responder (EMR) Often arriving before the ambulance, EMRs such as police and firefighters are equipped with oxygen, automated defibrillators, and airway equipment and may respond in first responder cars or police or fire vehicles. They possess knowledge and skills to provide lifesaving interventions while awaiting additional EMS response and can assist higher-level personnel on the scene. (1)

Emergency medical technician (EMT) EMTs provide basic emergency medical care and transportation for critical and emergent patients who access the EMS system. They perform interventions with basic equipment typically found on an ambulance under medical oversight, linking the patient from the scene to the emergency health care system. Also called *EMT-Basic.* (1)

Emergency move Variety of lifting and moving techniques used to remove someone rapidly from a hazardous situation. (5)

Emotional abuse Emotional injury inflicted on a person by another to demonstrate power. (18)

Emphysema Disease caused by a destruction of alveoli and the loss of elastic recoil within the lung; type of chronic obstructive pulmonary disease. (6, 11)

Endotracheal intubation Process of placing an endotracheal tube in the trachea using orotracheal or nasotracheal technique. (29)

Endotracheal (ET) tube Soft tube with an inflatable cuff that is inserted into the trachea with the aid of a laryngoscope. (29)

End-tidal CO$_2$ detector Device that changes color (colorimetric) when exposed to carbon dioxide; used to confirm placement of advanced airway device. Some CO$_2$ detectors give a quantitative reading; others display waveforms. (29)

Enhanced 9-1-1 Computerized dispatch system that automatically identifies a caller's location when the 9-1-1 system is accessed and allows for computer documentation of special information about patients based on their telephone number. (26)

Epidermis Outermost layer of skin. (4, 21)

Epiglottis Flap of cartilage that covers the larynx during swallowing to prevent food from entering the lungs. (4)

Epiglottitis Inflammation of the epiglottis usually caused by a bacterial infection; usually seen in children but also occurring in adults. Severe cases can obstruct the trachea. (6, 25)

Epinephrine Hormone secreted by the adrenal glands that increases sympathetic activity throughout the body. Effects include increased heart rate and force of contraction, increased bronchodilation and rate of breathing, increased blood flow to skeletal muscles with decreased flow to other organs (digestive and skin), and increased blood glucose; also called adrenaline. Also, a potent drug that can block the effects of histamine and slow the anaphylactic process. (4, 10, 14)

Epistaxis Nosebleed; hemorrhage from the nose. (20)

Escort Use of police vehicles to direct the movements of an ambulance from the scene of an emergency to the hospital. (26)

Evaporation Loss of heat when moisture vaporizes on the body's surface. (16)

Evisceration Spilling of the abdominal contents through a wound in the abdominal wall. (22)

Exposure Process of coming in contact with, but not necessarily being infected by, a disease-causing agent. (2)

Expressed consent Consent given by a patient for treatment to be performed; may be given verbally or through an affirming gesture such as a nod of the head. (3)

Extension Straightening of a joint. (4)

Extremity lift Rescue evacuation technique in which one EMT supports the patient's legs and a second EMT supports the torso to remove the patient from a hazardous situation. (5)

Extrication Process by which entrapped patients are rescued from vehicles, tunnels, or other structures or devices. (27)

Fascia Fibrous membrane covering that separates tissue from bone. (21)

Febrile seizure Seizure in a child that is caused by a rapidly rising body temperature. (13)

Federal Communications Commission (FCC) Government agency responsible for regulating all aspects of radio communications in the United States. (8)

Femur The thighbone, the largest bone in the body. (4)

Fetus Developing baby in the uterus (major structures outlined) from about 9 weeks after fertilization until delivery. (19)

Flail chest Condition in which two or more ribs are fractured in two or more places, resulting in a dissociation of part of the chest wall structure. (22)

Flexible stretcher (rescue stretcher) Type of stretcher that can be used to carry a patient through narrow corridors or over difficult terrain. (5)

Flexion Bending of a joint. (4)

Flexion forces Forces that involve fixed and mobile vertebrae that are bent to the point of fracture. (24)

Flow-restricted, oxygen-powered ventilation device Manually triggered positive-pressure ventilator administered by using oxygen under pressure. (6)

Focused physical examination Physical examination directed to the specific area of injury for patients who do not have a special mechanism of injury; part of focused (secondary) assessment. (7)

Focused (secondary) assessment Part of assessment devoted to identifying history and physical findings needed to treat the patient. (7)

Foot drag Rescue evacuation technique that uses the patient's feet to drag the patient along the long axis of the body from a hazardous situation. (5)

Fowler's position Posture assumed by the patient when the head of the bed is elevated. (4, 5)

Fracture Break in the continuity of bone. (23)

Frostbite Injury to the skin caused by prolonged exposure to cold; may be superficial (frostnip) or deep. The liquid content of the skin cells freezes. (16)

Frostnip Completely reversible superficial cold injury caused by intense vasoconstriction that affects only the topmost portions of the skin. (16)

Full-thickness burns Burns that involve the entire thickness of the epidermis and dermis; also called *third-degree burns.* (21)

Gain access Part of the extrication process in which EMS providers gain entry to trapped patients. (27)

Gamma rays High-energy electromagnetic radiation rays similar to x-rays but more energetic. (30)

Gasping Short breaths with a rapid inspiratory phase associated with respiratory distress and fatigue. (7)

Gel Gelatinous substance that is firm in consistency but contains much liquid. (10)

General impression First part of the initial (primary) assessment during which the EMT notes the patient's age and gender, nature of illness or mechanism of injury, and any obvious life-threatening conditions. (7)

Generic name Drug name not protected by a trademark that is usually descriptive of the chemical nature of the drug. (10)

Glasgow Coma Scale (GCS) Brain function assessment tool that evaluates verbal, motor, and eye-opening responses and has high intraobserver reliability. (13, 24)

Glucagon Substance secreted by the pancreas that can cause stored forms of glucose to be released and glucose to be made from other molecules. (13)

Glucose Sugar molecule (carbohydrate) in a form that is used by the cells for energy. (13)

Grand mal seizure Seizure that involves three phases: *tonic* (sustained contraction of all voluntary muscles), *clonic* (characterized by intermittent contractions and relaxations of skeletal muscles), and *postictal* (depressed level of consciousness and confusion). (13)

Grunting Rhythmic sound heard at the end of exhalation; key sign of respiratory distress in infants. (6, 7)

Gurgling Sound created by air moving through fluid in the airway. (7)

Hazardous material Any substance (solid, liquid, or gas) capable of creating harm to people, property, and the environment. (28)

HAZMAT, hazmat Term used for a hazardous materials incident (or special team, equipment). (2, 28)

Head-to-toe survey A rapid head-to-toe examination to identify and treat any life-threatening injuries. (7)

Healthcare proxy Legal empowerment of a third party to make decisions regarding the health care of an individual. (3)

Heart failure Condition resulting when destruction of the heart muscle reduces the heart's power of contraction. (12)

Hematoma Collection of blood beneath the skin. (21)

Hemorrhage Profuse bleeding. (20)

Hemothorax Bleeding within the pleural cavity. (22)

Hepatitis Inflammation of the liver. (22)

High-altitude cerebral edema (HACE) Cerebral edema after rapid ascent to a high altitude. (16)

High-altitude pulmonary edema (HAPE) Pulmonary edema after rapid ascent to a high altitude. (16)

High-efficiency particulate air (HEPA) respirator Specialized filtering mask designed to protect the EMT from airborne pathogens. (2)

History See Patient history.

History of the present illness Portion of the patient history that clarifies the chief complaint or presenting problem through a series of questions (e.g., OPQRST). (7)

Host Susceptible person who, if exposed to a source of infectious disease, may become ill. (2)

Hot zone Area in a hazardous materials incident or disaster where contamination occurs. (28)

Hypertension Increased or high blood pressure. (7, 31)

Hypnotic Frequently prescribed agent that induces sleep. (15)

Hypoglycemia Abnormally low blood glucose (sugar) level. (13)

Hypoperfusion Decreased blood flow through an organ, as in shock. Prolonged hypoperfusion can result in permanent cellular dysfunction and death. (4, 20)

Hypothermia Abnormal and dangerous condition in which the body temperature falls below 95° F (35° C) and the body's normal functions are impaired; usually caused by prolonged exposure to cold. (16)

Hypovolemic shock Shock resulting from low blood volume caused by excessive bleeding, burns, metabolic disorders, or other causes of loss of body fluid. (20)

Hypoxemia Abnormal deficiency in the concentration of oxygen in arterial blood. (29)

Hypoxia Prolonged period of decreased oxygen supply. (25, 29)

Immunity The body's ability to resist infection after exposure to an infectious agent. The state of being protected from (immune from) disease. (2)

Implanted cardioverter-defibrillator (ICD) Automated device implanted in a person's chest that delivers a number of low-energy shocks directly to the myocardium; also called *automated ICD (AICD).* (12)

Implied consent Type of consent in which verbal or written consent is not possible but circumstances warrant that a reasonable person would want and expect emergency treatment to be rendered. (3)

Incident management system Disaster response system in which resources are coordinated by one central management team to ensure a systematic and efficient approach. (28)

Incorporation Binding of radioactive materials into the body cells, tissues, and organs. (30)

Incubation period Time between contact with an infectious agent and occurrence of signs and symptoms of infection. (2)

Indication Condition or disease for which a drug is expected to have a beneficial effect. (10)

Infection control The practice of actions taken to block the spread of infectious agents. (2)

Inferior Toward the feet. (4)

Informed consent Consent made when the patient has been made fully aware of the risks, benefits, and consequences of the care being provided and any alternatives to that care. (3)

Initial (primary) assessment Early part of assessment devoted to identifying and treating life-threatening conditions related to airway, breathing, and circulation (ABCs) and mental status. (7)

Insulin Hormone produced by the pancreas necessary for glucose metabolism. (4, 13)

Intramuscular (IM) Within the muscular substance; route of drug administration. (10)

Irradiation Caused by radioactive energy in wave or ray form that passes through but is not physically present on the body. The irradiated patient cannot spread radioactive materials to others. (30)

Ischemia Insufficient blood supply to an area. (12)

Ischemic chest pain Characteristic pain resulting from inadequate blood supply to the myocardium. (12)

Jaundice Yellow color to the skin caused by buildup of bilirubin in the blood in liver failure. (7, 15)

Jugular venous distention Enlargement of the neck veins associated with increased venous pressure. (7)

Kendrick extrication device (KED) Semirigid, short device that is used to immobilize and extricate victims of vehicle crashes who are found in the sitting position. (24)

Laceration Tear or cut in the skin or other tissues. (7, 21)

Laryngectomy Surgical removal of part of the larynx. (6)

Laryngoscope Plastic or metal device used to visualize the vocal cords to insert an endotracheal tube. (29)

Lateral Toward the side of the body. (4)

Lateral recumbent position Position of the body when the person is lying on his or her side. (5)

Limb presentation When one of the baby's extremities is the presenting part of the birth. (19)

Locked-in position Technique in which the back is maintained in straight alignment during a lift so as not to cause strain or injury. (5)

Log roll Rotation technique used to slide an immobilization device under a patient with minimal flexion, extension, or rotation of the spinal column. (5)

Long spine board Long, flat, rigid device, usually made of plastic, used to maintain spinal immobilization or to transport a patient. (5, 24)

Los Angeles Prehospital Stroke Screen Screening device used to rapidly identify stroke patients. (13)

Malpractice Legal finding that negligence has occurred. (3)

Manual inline stabilization Holding a patient's head in a neutral position that is in line with the rest of the body. (24)

Mechanism of injury Manner in which an injury was sustained/incurred; knowing the mechanism helps in recognizing the type and extent of injury. (7)

Meconium Substance that makes up the first stool of a fetus or newborn. (19)

Medial Toward the midline of the body. (4)

Medical direction Active participation of physicians overseeing medical care in an EMS system; includes protocol development, needs assessment of the system, education, quality improvement, and outcome studies, as well as online medical direction; also called *medical control.* (1)

Medication Drug or remedy for a certain condition. (10)

Menarche Onset of menstruation occurring around age 12 to 14. (19)

Menopause Cessation of menstruation occurring around age 40 to 60. (19)

Menstruation The 28-day cycle involving release of the egg and preparation of the uterus for pregnancy; also called *menstrual cycle.* (19)

Metered-dose inhaler (MDI) Method for delivering medications through inhalation that allows for a controlled, precise dose. (10, 11)

Microorganisms Organisms not visible to the naked eye. (2)

Midaxillary Imaginary line on the body that extends from the armpit down through the lower chest wall. (4)

Midclavicular Imaginary line on the body that extends from the middle section of the clavicle down through the lower chest wall. (4)

Midline Imaginary line that divides the body into right and left halves. (4)

Minute volume Total volume of air inhaled in a minute, calculated by tidal volume multiplied by respiratory rate. (6)

Mobile two-way radios Radio contained within vehicles that allows transmission through the dispatch or medical direction system. (8)

Moulage Fake injuries applied to "patients" in disaster simulations. (28)

Multiple-casualty incident (MCI) Situation in which the need is more than the initial responding personnel and equipment can provide. (7, 28)

Mutual aid Prearranged response system that is established with neighboring communities to ensure a large-scale response of emergency personnel and vehicles, including police, firefighters, and ambulances, during a catastrophic incident. (28)

Myocardial infarction Severe and sustained oxygen deprivation of the myocardium resulting in the death of heart cells; commonly known as a "heart attack." (12)

Nasal cannula Low-flow oxygen delivery system consisting of a thin tube with prongs at the end that slip into the nares; capable of delivering 24% to 40% oxygen. (6)

Nasal flaring Characteristic flaring of the nostrils in infants and small children that suggests respiratory distress. (6, 7)

Nasogastric (NG) tube Tube inserted into the esophagus and into the stomach to allow air to be released, relieve pressure on the diaphragm, and enable more effective ventilations to occur. (29)

Nasopharyngeal airway (NPA) Soft rubber tube that extends from the nares down into the oropharynx and used to elevate the tongue away from the oropharynx. (6)

Nasotracheal intubation Intubation of the trachea through the nose. (29)

National Emergency Medical Services Information System (NEMSIS) National organization that defines what to document in prehospital care reports, setting standards with EMS experts, and ultimately to serve as data collection center to promote research. (9)

Nature of illness Type of medical complaint that a patient exhibits. (7)

Nebulizer Device for producing a fine spray or mist that includes medication to be inhaled. (11)

Neglect Failure to fulfill duties and obligations and to provide for the necessities of daily living. (18)

Negligence Deviation from the accepted standard of care that results in injury to the patient. For negligence to occur, there must be a duty to act, a breach of duty, injury to the patient, and a causal connection. (3)

Nitroglycerin Medication that works to reduce the work of the heart by decreasing peripheral vascular resistance while improving blood flow to the myocardium by dilating the coronary arteries; usually placed under the tongue for absorption. (10)

Nonrebreather mask High-flow, high-concentration oxygen (O_2) delivery device consisting of a reservoir bag (of O_2) beneath a one-way valve that prevents the patient from exhaling into the bag; used when high O_2 concentrations are needed, up to 90%. (6)

Nuclear radiation Energy emitted from the nucleus of an unstable atom. (30)

Objective finding Physical sign that can be visualized by the EMT, such as pale skin or deformed extremity. (9)

Offline medical direction Accountability by a physician for EMS providers through the use of protocols, quality improvement activities, educational endeavors, and other measures to ensure effective field care. (1)

Ombudsman An official, usually appointed by the government, who is charged with representing the interests of the public by investigating and addressing complaints reported by individual citizens. (18)

One-handed carrying technique Carrying technique used when multiple personnel are available for the carry and persons are placed strategically around the device. (5)

Ongoing assessment Reevaluation of the patient (repeat initial [primary] assessment, vital signs, focused [secondary] assessment, check of interventions); or reassessment. (7)

Online medical direction Accountability of field care by a physician though the use of radio or telephone communications. (1)

Onset When and how a patient's complaint first occurred. (7)

Open pneumothorax Pneumothorax in which the chest wall is punctured; also called a *sucking chest wound.* (22)

Opioids Narcotic agents with opiate or morphinelike affects. (15)

OPQRST Mnemonic used to remember the key questions in the history of present illness: **o**nset; **p**rovocation; **q**uality; **r**adiation; **s**everity; and **t**ime. (7)

Oral glucose Form of glucose gel that is administered orally to patients with suspected hypoglycemia. (10, 13)

Oral mucosa The lining of the mouth. (7)

Orientation A person's awareness of person, place, and time. (7)

Oropharyngeal airway (OPA) Mechanical airway device designed to elevate the tongue away from the oropharynx when the patient is unconscious. (6)

Orotracheal intubation Intubation of the trachea through the mouth. (29)

Osteoporosis Decrease in the amount of bone tissue occurring in older people as a result of more bone breakdown than bone formation, which leads to weaker bones. (31)

Overdose Result of drug being taken in excess or in combination with other agents to the point where poisoning occurs. (15)

Pacemaker Group of cells in the heart that initiates electrical impulses of the heart. Also, a mechanical device implanted to control certain dysrhythmias or provide a backup if the heart's natural pacemaker fails. (12)

Palpation Act of feeling with the hand; applying light pressure with the fingers to the surface of the body to determine the condition of the parts underneath. (7)

Pandemic flu Virulent virus for which there is little or no preexisting immunity in the population; causes illness in humans and has the potential for sustained transmission from person to person. (2)

Panic Sudden, overwhelming anxiety of such intensity that it produces terror and physiologic changes. (17)

Paradoxical motion Type of breathing in which the chest wall moves opposite to normal chest movement; also called *paradoxical breathing.* (22)

Paramedic Allied health professional whose primary focus is to provide advanced emergency medical care for critical and emergent patients. Paramedics possess complex knowledge and skills necessary to perform basic and advanced interventions with equipment found on an ambulance, under medical oversight. (1)

Paranoia Condition in which the patient feels unduly threatened by the environment and those in contact with the patient. (17)

Partial-thickness burns Burns that involve the epidermis and extend into but not through the dermis; also called *second-degree burns.* (21)

Passive immunity Immunity that is injected into a body (not produced by it), such as injection of an antibody against tetanus. (2)

Patient data Identification information provided by the patient or by family or friends; includes the patient's name, gender, age, date of birth, and address. (9)

Perfusion Fluid passing through an organ or part of the body. The surrounding and bathing of a tissue or cell with blood or the fluid part of blood. (4)

Pericardial tamponade Mechanical compression of the heart by large amounts of fluid or blood within the pericardial space; also called *cardiac tamponade.* (22)

Perineum The pelvic floor. (19)

Peripheral Away from the center of the body. (4)

Peritonitis Inflammation of the peritoneum. (22)

Personal protective equipment (PPE) Variety of safety equipment used to prevent direct contact with blood and other body fluids, including gloves, eye protection, masks, and gowns, or used to prevent contact with hazardous materials, including turnout gear, chemical-resistant clothing, and self-contained breathing apparatus. (1, 2)

Physical abuse Physical injury inflicted on a person by another to demonstrate power. (18)

Pin index safety system System of gas cylinders that allows tanks of different types of gas to accept special regulators designed specifically for that gas. (6)

Placard Specialized signage used to identify various hazardous materials. (2, 28)

Placenta Organ of pregnancy through which nutrients and waste products are exchanged between mother and fetus. *Afterbirth* refers to the expelled placenta and fetal membranes following the baby's birth. (19)

Pleuritic chest pain Pain worsened by breathing. (6)

Pneumatic (air) splint Plastic splints filled with air to provide circumferential support to an injured extremity. (23)

Pneumatic antishock garment (PASG) Air-filled pants that surround the legs and abdomen; when inflated, can be used to treat shock, immobilize fractures, and control bleeding. (20)

Pneumothorax Air within the pleural space. (22)

Poison Substance that, on ingestion, inhalation, absorption, or injection, may cause structural damage or functional disturbance. (15)

Portable stretcher Type of stretcher that can be easily carried to and from the scene of an emergency. (5)

Positive-pressure ventilation The act of forcing air into the lungs. (6)

Posterior Structures toward the rear of the body. (4)

Posterior tibial Artery passing just behind the ankle bone, where it is palpable between the medial malleolus and the Achilles tendon. (7)

Power grip Technique for holding a stretcher with your palms and fingers in complete contact with the device to ensure a safe transport. (5)

Power lift (squat lift) Effective lifting method that maximizes lifting power while avoiding injury. (5)

Prehospital care report (PCR) Standardized patient record used in the EMS system. (9)

Pressure point Common pulse location where pressure can be applied to collapse an artery and thereby reduce or stop blood flow to a wound. (20)

Priapism Abnormal sustained penile erection; a sign of spinal cord injury. (7, 24)

Prolapsed cord Slipping of the umbilical cord down past the presenting part of the fetus into the vagina. (19)

Prone Lying face downward, or on the ventral or anterior surface of the body. (4, 5)

Protocol Written procedure for a clinical treatment. (3)

Provocation Any factor that improves or worsens a patient's complaint. (7)

Proximal Closer to the trunk. (4)

Psychobehavioral disorder Any of various forms of behavior that are considered inappropriate by members of the social group to which an individual belongs. (17)

Public access defibrillation (PAD) Strategy of placing automatic external defibrillators in public places such as airports and encouraging their use by trained laypersons. (12)

Pulmonary embolism Obstruction of the pulmonary artery, often caused by a blood clot from leg veins. (12)

Pulse oximetry Measurement of hemoglobin oxygenation by a pulse oximeter; read as a percentage of oxygen saturation. (6)

Pulseless electrical activity Condition in which the heart has an organized electrical rhythm but there is no palpable pulse. (12)

Puncture Penetrating injury caused by a sharp, pointed object; to pierce or penetrate with a pointed object or instrument. (7, 21)

Pyelonephritis Severe infection of the kidney. (22)

Quality Subjective description of the complaint in the patient's own words. (7)

Quality improvement (QI) Methods of ensuring a high level of patient care. (1)

Quarantine Isolation of patients exposed to or having a contagious disease for a period until they are incapable of either developing or transmitting the disease. (30)

Radiation Transfer of heat by infrared heat rays, which are radiated by the body and other objects in the environment. If the temperature of the body is greater than the temperature of the surroundings, heat is lost from the body. In assessment of the patient's chief complaint, the spread of pain from one area of the body to another. (7, 16)

Rape Unwanted penetration of the genitalia. (18)

Rapid extrication Specialized rescue removal technique used to extricate a critical patient quickly from a vehicle crash with minimal flexion, extension, or rotation of the spinal column. (5, 24)

Reassessment. See **Ongoing assessment.**

Receiving operator The individual who receives the call for assistance. (8)

Recovery Process of demobilizing response vehicles, apparatus, and personnel so they can return to normal operations in the community. (28)

Recovery position Position of the patient lying on his or her side to help maintain a clear airway. (5)

Repeater systems Strategically based receivers and transmitters that accept signals from a portable unit or mobile radio and relay them with a more powerful transmitter. (8)

Rescue breathing Providing artificial breathing for patients who cannot breathe on their own. (6)

Respiratory arrest Cessation of breathing. (6)

Respiratory distress Condition in which there is an increased work of breathing. (6)

Respiratory failure State that exists when the respiratory system becomes so ineffective that it can no longer support life. (6, 11)

Restoration Rebuilding of the community, both physically and emotionally; includes critical incident stress debriefing, reconstruction, and restoration of services to the area. (28)

Retractions Inward depression of muscular areas and attached ribs, which are drawn inward; reflect increased effort to breathe. (6, 7, 25)

Rigid splint Splints made of rigid material such as cardboard, wood, metal, or plastic; should be well padded. (23)

Rigor mortis State of body stiffness caused by the depletion of proteins in muscles after death. (2, 9)

Route of drug administration Method through which a drug is administered to a patient, such as intramuscularly, orally, or intravenously. (10)

Run data Part of the documentation that records the location, type of call, and times related to the response. (9)

SAMPLE Mnemonic used to remember the key questions in a patient history: **s**igns and symptoms, **a**llergies, **m**edications, **p**ertinent past history, **l**ast oral intake, and **e**vents leading up to the present illness. (7)

Scene safety First step in the scene size-up phase of patient assessment; ensures safety of the providers, patients, and bystanders by effectively securing the scene. (7)

Scene size-up First phase of patient assessment that includes scene safety, appropriate use of personal protective equipment, and determination of the mechanism of injury or nature of illness. (7)

Sclera Outer layer of eye. (4, 21)

Scoop stretcher Specialized device consisting of an aluminum frame and a rectangular tube with shovel-type lateral flaps for sliding under the patient. (5)

Scope of practice Range of duties and services that may be performed by a given medical provider. (3)

Sebum Oily substance secreted by the sebaceous glands that helps moisturize the skin. (21)

Sedative Frequently prescribed agent with calming effects. (15)

Seesaw breathing Physical finding in small children and infants characterized by alternate use of the abdominal and chest wall muscles and indicating respiratory distress. (6)

Seizure Temporary alteration in behavior caused by abnormal electrical activity in the brain. (13)

Self-contained breathing apparatus (SCBA) Specialized mask and regulator used by EMS personnel in environments that may be dangerous, such as those containing smoke, carbon monoxide, or other hazardous materials. (2)

Severity Measurement of the degree of pain a patient is experiencing. (7)

Sexual abuse Unwilling or unlawful touch of genitalia, which may include rape. (18)

Sharps container Special container designed for the disposal of needles and other sharp instruments used in the care of a patient. (2)

Shock Failure of the circulatory system to adequately perfuse and oxygenate the vital organs of the body; also called *hypoperfusion.* (4, 20)

Shock position Placement of a patient supine with the legs elevated 8 to 12 inches to facilitate venous return. (5)

Short spine board Device used to immobilize and extricate patients who are found in a sitting position; evolved into *vest-type device.* (5)

Side effect A consequence other than the desired effect for which a substance is used. (10)

Sign Any objective evidence of disease or dysfunction; a clue to the patient's condition that can be observed (seen, smelled, heard, or felt) by the EMT. (7)

Simple access Gaining access to the patient without the use of any tools or specialized equipment. (27)

Slim Jim Device for gaining access to locked cars. (27)

Sling Triangle-shaped bandage used to support the weight of the arm. (23)

SLUDGEM Mnemonic for **s**alivation, **l**acrimation, **u**rination, **d**iarrhea, **g**astrointestinal cramps, **e**mesis (vomiting), **m**iosis (small pupils), and **m**uscular twitching. (30)

Snoring Harsh, low-pitched sound usually caused by the tongue blocking the airway. (7)

Source Person, insect, object, or another substance that carries or is contaminated by an infectious agent. (2)

Special situation report Report used to document unusual occurrences, such as an injury to the patient during transport. (9)

Sphygmomanometer Device for measuring blood pressure. (7)

Sprain Injuries to ligaments, usually resulting from stretching forces. (23)

Stair chair Folding chair used to carry patients who can assume the sitting position. (5)

Standard of care The body of knowledge, laws, policies, common practices, standards, protocols, and guidelines that provide the basis for care. Doing the *right thing* properly. (3)

Standard precautions Incorporate the older universal precautions and body substance isolation. Precautions used in all situations to avoid transmission from both recognized and unrecognized sources of infection. Standard precautions apply to the blood, body fluids, secretions, excretions (except sweat), nonintact skin, and mucous membranes. (2)

Status epilepticus Rapid succession of seizures without an intervening period of consciousness, or a prolonged period of continuous seizures. (13)

Stimulant Drug that causes excitability and can induce seizure with overdose; can be prescription (e.g., amphetamines) or street (e.g., PCP) drug. (15)

Stoma Permanent opening in the trachea or larynx. (6)

Strain Injury to muscles or their tendons, usually from overstretching or violent contractions. (23)

Stridor Harsh, high-pitched sound created by air flowing through a narrowed upper airway, usually heard on inspiration; also called *crowing.* (7)

Stroke Usually sudden onset of symptoms caused by blockage or disruption of blood flow in an artery feeding the brain; also called *cerebrovascular accident* (CVA). (13)

Stylet Malleable metal tube that is inserted into the endotracheal tube to provide stiffness and shape to help guide the tube during intubation. (29)

Subcutaneous emphysema Entrapment of air beneath the skin as a result of trauma to the airways, lungs, esophagus, or skin; characterized by deformity and crepitus of the skin. (7)

Subjective finding Symptom reported by the patient but cannot be seen by the EMT, such as a headache. (9)

Sublingual Under (beneath) the tongue; route of drug administration. (10)

Submersion episode Any submersion into water that requires field care and transport to a hospital for treatment or observation of the patient. (16)

Sudden infant death syndrome (SIDS) Unexplained death of an infant younger than 1 year old. (25)

Superficial burns Burns that involve the epidermis, the superficial layer of the skin; also called *first-degree burns.* (21)

Superior Toward the head. (4)

Supine Position of the body when a person is lying on his or her back. (4)

Survey instruments Instruments designed to monitor and measure radiation. (30)

Suspension Preparation of a finely divided, undissolved substance dispersed in a liquid vehicle. (10)

Swathe Folded triangular bandage or roller bandage used to bind the upper arm to the chest wall. (23)

Symptom Anything that the patient perceives as part of his or her complaint and communicates to the EMT. (7)

Systolic blood pressure Blood pressure measured during the contraction phase (systole) of the heart, noted by the first sound heard through a stethoscope when blood pressure is obtained. (4)

Tachypnea Rapid breathing. (6)

Telemedicine Bidirectional audiovisual communication between EMT at scene and medical direction. (8)

Tenderness Pain that is elicited on palpation. (7)

Tension pneumothorax Air trapped in the pleural space caused by a one-way valve effect created on the chest wall or lung wall; results in increased intrathoracic pressure, respiratory failure, and shock. (22)

Therapeutic dose Dose of a medication required to have the desired effect on a patient. (10)

Thoracic aortic dissection Tear in the wall of the aorta that causes the vessel to split (dissect), forming a false passage; proximal and distal types. (12)

Thrombus Clot that develops within a blood vessel. (12)

Tidal volume Volume of air inspired and expired during one breath. Normal tidal volume at rest for an adult is approximately 500 mL. (4)

Time Duration of the chief complaint and significant associated complaints. (7)

Tourniquet Constricting band applied over an extremity with enough pressure to stop blood flow completely beyond the site of application. (20)

Toxic Poisonous. (15)

Toxicology The study of poisons. (15)

Trachea Hollow tube with several horseshoe-shaped rings of cartilage on the anterolateral surface that support and provide structure for this portion of the airway; commonly referred to as the "windpipe." (4)

Tracheal deviation Position of the trachea to either side of the midline of the neck. (7)

Tracheostomy Surgical opening in the trachea to provide an airway. (6)

Traction splint Device consisting of a metal frame and a pulley system to apply traction to the lower extremity. (23)

Trade name Trademarked name that a manufacturer uses in marketing a given drug; also called *brand name.* (10)

Traffic delineation devices Devices used to alter traffic flow around an emergency scene. (7)

Transient ischemic attack (TIA) Temporary loss of brain function caused by diminished blood supply to part of the brain; completely resolves within 24 hours. (13)

Transmission Method by which an infectious agent travels from the source to its host. (2)

Transmission-based precautions Special precautions over and above standard precautions that are used for patients documented or suspected to be infected with highly transmissible disease. (2)

Trend Tendency toward improvement or deterioration in a patient's condition. (7)

Trendelenburg position Supine position on a surface inclined 45 degrees, with the head at the lower end and the legs at the upper end. (5)

Triage Sorting of casualties in a hazardous materials incident or disaster to determine the priority of need and proper place of treatment. (7, 28)

Triage tag Special tag with more limited but critical information on a patient's status, attached to the patient in multiple-casualty incidents. (9)

Tripod position Position characterized by a posture that is upright and leaning forward with the head and neck thrust forward; associated with respiratory distress. (7, 11)

Turnout gear Heavy clothing that is puncture resistant and gives some protection from hazardous materials and materials at extremes of temperature. (2)

Type I ambulance Ambulance designed with a modular box patient compartment mounted on a truck-style chassis. (26)

Type II ambulance Van-style ambulance. (26)

Type III ambulance Ambulance designed with a modular box patient compartment mounted on a van chassis. (26)

Umbilical cord Structure that connects the fetus to the mother, allowing the exchange of nutrients and waste products; contains three blood vessels surrounded by a clear, gelatinous substance. (19)

Universal precautions Approach to protect self in every patient contact against exposure to body substances and fluids that may carry blood-borne pathogens (e.g., HIV, hepatitis B or C virus). (2)

Urticaria Raised, red patches of skin; also called *hives.* (14)

Vaccination Inoculation with a vaccine to establish immunity to a particular disease. (2)

Vector Insects, animals, or inanimate objects that carry and transmit disease. For example, malaria is transmitted by mosquitoes. (2)

Vein Blood vessel that returns blood to the heart. (4)

Ventral Toward the abdomen or anterior. (4)

Ventricular fibrillation Chaotic quivering of the heart resulting in cardiac arrest. (12)

Ventricular tachycardia Rapid dysrhythmia (100-200 beats/min) that may or may not be capable of producing a pulse. (12)

Vertebrae Irregular bones that form the spinal column. (4)

Vital signs Measurement of the function of the vital body systems, including respirations, pulse, blood pressure, temperature, and pupils. (7)

Warm zone Area immediately surrounding the hot zone at a hazardous materials incident or disaster, where decontamination occurs. (28)

Weapons of mass destruction (WMDs) Nuclear, biologic, and chemical (NBC) agents intended to do harm. (30)

Wheeled cot stretcher Primary transport stretcher used by prehospital providers; has a wheeled base and comes in a variety of types. (5)

Wheezing High-pitched whistling sounds created by narrowed bronchioles. (6)

Index

Note: Page numbers followed by *t* indicated tables; *f,* figures; *b,* boxes.